Clinical Pharmacy and Therapeutics

EDITED BY

Roger Walker BPharm PhD MRPharmS HonMFPHM

Professor of Pharmacy Practice
Welsh School of Pharmacy, Cardiff;
Director of Pharmaceutical Public Health, Gwent, Wales, UK

Clive Edwards BPharm PhD MRPharmS

Prescribing Adviser
North Tyneside Primary Care Trust, Newcastle upon Tyne, UK

THIRD EDITION

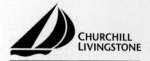
CHURCHILL
LIVINGSTONE

EDINBURGH LONDON NEW YORK OXFORD PHILADELPHIA ST LOUIS SYDNEY TORONTO 2003

CHURCHILL LIVINGSTONE
An imprint of Elsevier Limited

First edition 1994
Second edition 1999
Third edition 2003
Reprinted 2003 (twice)

ISBN 0443 071373
International edition 0443 071381

British Library Cataloguing in Publication Data
A catalogue record for this book is available from the British
Library

Library of Congress Cataloging in Publication Data
A catalog record for this book is available from the Library of
Congress

Note
Medical knowledge is constantly changing. Standard safety precautions must be followed, but as new research and clinical experience broaden our knowledge, changes in treatment and drug
therapy may become necessary or appropriate. Readers are
advised to check the most current product information provided
by the manufacturer of each drug to be administered to verify the
recommended dose, the method and duration of administration,
and contraindications. It is the responsibility of the practitioner,
relying on experience and knowledge of the patient, to determine
dosages and the best treatment for each individual patient. Neither
the Publisher nor the editors/contributor assumes any liability for
any injury and/or damage to persons or property arising from this
publication.

 ELSEVIER SCIENCE
your source for books,
journals and multimedia
in the health sciences
www.elsevierhealth.com

Typeset by IMH(Cartrif), Loanhead, Scotland
Printed in Spain

The
publisher's
policy is to use
paper manufactured
from sustainable forests

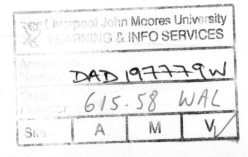

Preface

Whether in primary care or secondary care, the use of medicine is the most common intervention in health care. National strategies have emerged to promote safe, appropriate and cost effective prescribing that maximizes benefit, minimizes harm and respects patient choice. Prescribing is increasingly complex and demanding and undertaken as part of a multidisciplinary process that includes pharmacists, doctors and nurses. It is our intention that this textbook will be of value to individuals from these groups as they embark on that part of their career which specifically focuses on medicine use.

We have made every effort to update each chapter and make the content ever more relevant to practice. For the first time we have included key references in the body of the text to assist those who wish to explore the underlying evidence. In addition, and in recognition of our growing international readership, we have appointed a panel of reviewers from overseas to ensure the wider relevance of the content.

Throughout the text when using drug names we have opted to use the format Recommended International Non-proprietary Name (British approved name). With the exception of adrenaline, noradrenaline and aspirin, there will be a move to solely using rINNs and the dual naming approach of rINN (BAN) will be dropped. Given that it may be some years before full implementation, we have decided to retain the dual naming approach for this edition. We hope this helps and does not confuse.

Progress of knowledge in therapeutics is rapid, changes to dose regimens and licensed indications frequent, new medicines appear at regular intervals and guidelines for treatment of specific disorders are continually revised. Yesterday another landmark study was published. It is therefore inevitable that some sections of the book will date more quickly than others. The reader must use this text, as any other, cautiously and critically. It will then serve as a valuable learning resource, help the reader understand therapeutics and, hopefully, play a small part in achieving positive patient outcomes.

Roger Walker
Clive Edwards

Acknowledgements

We remain indebted to all the authors who have contributed to the third edition of this textbook. Their hard work, patience, tolerance and ability to meet punishing deadlines never cease to amaze. The help of many secretaries and colleagues is also acknowledged along with the wise comments from our team of international advisers. The finished product is a testament to the staff at Churchill Livingstone, who patiently edit and correct our many oversights professionally.

On a personal note we thank our close colleagues who have supported and tolerated our indulgence in editing this text. Our undergraduate and postgraduate students in clinical pharmacy at universities in Newcastle, Sunderland and Cardiff were the inspiration to produce the first edition. The feedback we continue to receive from students and practitioners, at home and abroad, sustains our commitment.

Finally, without the forbearance and understanding of our wives, Ann and Joy, there would be no book. It has been part of our lives for more than twelve years. Many domestic, social and family events have taken second place during the course of producing three editions. We are eternally grateful for their continued support.

Roger Walker
Clive Edwards

Contributors

Christopher Acomb BSc MPharm MRPharmS MCPP
Clinical Pharmacy Services Manager, United Leeds
Teaching Hospitals, Leeds; Honorary Senior Lecturer
in Pharmacy Practice, University of Bradford,
Bradford, UK
47. Anaemia

Andrew Alldred BPharm MRPharmS AdvDipClinPharm
Pharmacy Procurement Manager, formerly Clinical
Pharmacy Manager, Leeds Teaching Hospitals NHS
Trust, Leeds, UK
51. Rheumatoid arthritis and osteoarthritis
52. Gout and hyperuricaemia

Rosalyn Anderson MRPharmS BSc(Pharm) DipTher
Lead Pharmacist, Borders LHCC, Borders Primary
Care NHS Trust, Melrose, Roxburghshire, UK
56. Pressure sores and leg ulcers

Sharon D. Andrew BSc MPharm MRPharmS
Former Directorate Pharmacist, Manchester Royal Eye
Hospital, Manchester, UK
53. Glaucoma

C. Heather Ashton DM FRCP
Emeritus Professor of Clinical Psychopharmacology,
Royal Victoria Infirmary, Newcastle upon Tyne, UK
26. Insomnia and anxiety

Catrin Barker BSc MSc PGDipClinPharm
Head of Service, DIAL, National Paediatric Medicines
Information Unit, Alder Hey Children's Hospital,
Liverpool, UK
8. Paediatrics

Andrew W. Berrington MRCP MRCPath
Specialist Registrar, Department of Microbiology,
Newcastle upon Tyne Hospitals NHS Trust, Newcastle
upon Tyne, UK
33. Respiratory infections
34. Urinary tract infections

Adrian J. Bint MB ChB FRCPath
Consultant Microbiologist, Royal Victoria Hospital,
Newcastle-upon-Tyne
34. Urinary tract infections

Denise Blake BSc MSc BCOP MRPharmS
Lead Pharmacist, North London Cancer Network,
London, UK
49. Lymphomas

David Branford PhD MRPharmS
Director of Pharmacy, Derbyshire Mental Health
Services, Kingsway Hospital, Derby, UK
28. Schizophrenia

David J. Burn FRCP MD MA MBBS
Consultant and Senior Lecturer in Neurology, Regional
Neurosciences Centre, Newcastle General Hospital,
Newcastle upon Tyne, UK
30. Parkinson's disease

Brit E. Cadman BSc(Pharm) Dip Clin Pharm
Principal Pharmacist, Addenbrookes NHS Trust,
Cambridge, UK
13. Adverse effects of drugs on the liver

Judith A. Cantrill BSc MSc MPharmS
Professor of Medicines (Usage, Evaluation and Policy),
School of Pharmacy and Pharmaceutical Studies,
University of Manchester, Manchester, UK
41. Thyroid and parathyroid disorders
42. Diabetes mellitus

Mary M. Carr MD BSc FRCP
Consultant Dermatologist, University Hospital of North
Durham, Durham, UK
55. Eczema and psoriasis

John K. Clayton MB ChB FROCG
Consultant Obstetrician and Gynaecologist, Bradford
Royal Infirmary, Bradford, UK
43. Menstrual cycle disorders
44. Menopause and hormone replacement therapy

Jonathan Cooke BPharm MPharm PhD MRPharmS
Director of Research and Development and Chief
Pharmacist, South Manchester University Hospitals
NHS Trust, Manchester, UK
6. Pharmacoeconomics

Michael J. Daly BSc(Pharm) BSc MRPharmS
Acting Director of Pharmacy, Robert Jones and Agnes
Hunt Orthopaedic Hospital, Oswestry, UK
14. Liver disease

Soraya Dhillon BPharm PhD MRPharmS
Director of Taught Postgraduate Studies, Department of
Practice and Policy, The School of Pharmacy,
University of London, UK
29. Epilepsy

Stephen B. Duffull MPharm(Clin) PhD
School of Pharmacy, University of Queensland,
Brisbane, Australia
45. Drugs in pregnancy and lactation

Sarah J. Dunnett BPharm MRPharmS Dip Clin Pharm
Pharmacy Information Manager, Baxter Healthcare
Ltd, Northampton, UK
5. Parenteral nutrition

Clive Edwards BPharm PhD MRPharmS
Prescribing Adviser, North Tyneside Primary Care
Trust, Newcastle upon Tyne, UK
4. Laboratory data

Brian K. Evans PhD BPharm FRPharmS
Clinical Research Pharmacist, The Pharmaceutical
Unit, SMPU, Cardiff, UK
11. Inflammatory bowel disease

Bridget Featherstone BSc Pharm Dip Clin Pharm
Lead Pharmacist Transplantation and Surgery,
Addenbrookes NHS Trust, Cambridge, UK
13. Adverse effects of drugs on the liver

Martin Fisher MBBS BSc FRCP
Consultant Physician in HIV/GUM, Brighton and
Sussex University Hospitals NHS Trust, The Lawson
Unit, Royal Sussex County Hospital, Brighton
39. HIV infection

Ray Fitzpatrick BSc(Pharm) PhD MRPharmS
Clinical Director of Pharmacy, North Staffordshire
Hospital; Senior Lecturer, Keele University, UK
1. Practical pharmokinetics

Kevin P. Gibbs BPharm DipClinPharm MRPharmS
Clinical Pharmacy Manager, Bristol Royal Infirmary,
Bristol, UK
23. Asthma
24. Chronic obstructive pulmonary disease

Subrata Ghosh MD(Edin) FRCP FRCP(E)
Professor of Gastroenterology, Imperial College School
of Medicine, Hammersmith Hospital, London, UK
10. Peptic ulcer disease

Richard L. Gower FRCS
Clinical Director for Urological Services, Gwent
Healthcare NHS Trust, Royal Gwent Hospital,
Newport, UK
46. Benign prostatic hyperplasia

Jonathan C. Graham MBBS MRCP DTM&H
Specialist Registrar, Department of Clinical
Microbiology, Royal Victoria Infirmary, Newcastle
upon Tyne, UK
37. Surgical antibiotic prophylaxis

James W. Gray MRCP FRCPath
Consultant Microbiologist, Birmingham Children's
Hospital, Birmingham, UK
35. Gastrointestinal infections
36. Infective meningitis

Steve A. Hudson MPharm BPharm FRPharmS
Boots Professor of Pharmaceutical Care, University of
Strathclyde, Glasgow, UK
19. Congestive heart failure

Graham Jackson MA MBBS FRCP FRCPath MD
Consultant Haematologist and Honorary Senior
Lecturer, Royal Victoria Infirmary, Newcastle upon
Tyne, UK
48. Leukaemia

Dilip Kapur MBChB FRCA
Consultant in Pain Management, Pain Management
Unit, Flinders Medical Centre, Adelaide, South
Australia
31. Pain

Elizabeth A. Kay BPharm MSc MRPharmS MCPP DipMan
Chief Pharmacist, Leeds Teaching Hospitals, Leeds,
UK
51. Rheumatoid arthritis and osteoarthritis
52. Gout and hyperuricaemia

Niall P. Keaney BSc MB PhD FRCP
Consultant Physician and Head of Medical Education
and Research, City Hospitals NHS Trust, Sunderland
Royal Infirmary, Sunderland, UK
25. Drug-induced lung disease

Moira Kinnear BSc MSc ADCPT MRPharmS
Head of NHS Lothian Pharmacy Education, Research
and Development, Western General Hospital; Lecturer
in Clinical Practice, University of Strathclyde, Glasgow
10. Peptic ulcer disease

Heather Leake Date BSc MSc MRPharmS
Principal Pharmacist (HIV/Sexual health), Brighton
and Sussex University Hospital NHS Trust, The Elton
John Centre, Brighton General Hospital, Brighton, UK
39. HIV infection

Anne Lee MPhil MRPharmS
Principal Pharmacist, Area Medicines Information
Centre, Glasgow Royal Infirmary; Visiting Lecturer,
University of Strathclyde, Glasgow, UK
2. Drug interactions
3. Adverse drug reactions

Mary Maclean BSc DipPharmPrac BCOP MRPharmS
Senior Directorate Pharmacist, Cancer Services, Barts
and the London NHS Trust, London, UK
49. Lymphomas

Pamela Magee BSc MSc MRPharmS
Director of Pharmaceutical Services, University
Hospitals Coventry and Warwickshire, Coventry, UK
54. Drug-induced skin disorders

John Marriott PhD BSc MRPharmS
Senior Lecturer in Pharmacy Practice, Aston
University, Birmingham, UK
15. Acute renal failure
16. Chronic renal failure

Kay Marshall BPharm MRPharmS PhD
Senior Lecturer in Pharmacology, School of Pharmacy,
University of Bradford, Bradford, UK
43. Menstrual cycle disorders
44. Menopause and hormone replacement therapy

John McAnaw BSc MRPharmS
Research Fellow, University of Strathclyde, Glasgow,
UK
19. Congestive heart failure

Lika K. Nehaul LRCPI LRCSI MSc MFPHM
Consultant in Communicable Disease Control, Gwent
Health Authority, Pontypool, Gwent, UK
38. Tuberculosis

Anthony J. Nunn BPharm FRPharmS
Director of Pharmacy, Alder Hey Children's Hospital,
Liverpool, UK
8. Paediatrics

Stephen J. Pedler MB ChB FRCPath
Consultant Microbiologist, Department of
Microbiology, Royal Victoria Infirmary,
Newcastle upon Tyne, UK
33. Respiratory infections
37. Surgical antibiotic prophylaxis
40. Fungal infections

Peter Pratt BSc(Pharm) MPhil MRPharmS
Chief Pharmacist, Community Health, Sheffield NHS
Trust and Doncaster and South Humber NHS Trust,
Sheffield, UK
27. Affective disorders

Fiona Reid
Principal Pharmacist and Lecturer in Clinical Practice,
Royal Infirmary of Edinburgh, Lothian University
Hospitals NHS
19. Congestive heart failure

Philip A. Routledge MD FRCP FRCPE
Professor of Clinical Pharmacology, University of
Wales College of Medicine, Cardiff; Honorary
Consultant Physician, Cardiff and Vale NHS Trust,
Cardiff, UK
21. Thrombosis

Josemir W. Sander MD MRCP PhD
Professor of Neurology, Honorary Consultant
Neurologist, UCL Institute of Neurology, London, UK
29. Epilepsy

David Scott BSc PhD DipMedEd MRPharmS
Regional Clinical Training Pharmacist, Oxford
Radcliffe Hospital, Oxford, UK
18. Coronary heart disease
20. Cardiac arrhythmias

Judith Senior BPharm MRPharmS PhD
Consultant Pharmacologist, Examiner for the College
of Optometrists, University of Bradford, UK
43. Menstrual cycle disorders
44. Menopause and hormone replacement therapy

Hamasaraj G. M. Shetty BSc MBBS FRCP(London)
Consultant Physician, University Hospital of Wales,
Cardiff, UK
9. Geriatrics
21. Thrombosis

Michelle Small BPharm DipClinPharm MRPharmS
Teacher-Practitioner Pharmacist, St Mary's Hospital,
Portsmouth, UK
23. Asthma
24. Chronic obstructive pulmonary disease

Steve Smith MB ChB FRCP MD
Clinical Director of Renal Services, Birmingham
Heartlands Hospital, Birmingham, UK
15. Acute renal failure
16. Chronic renal failure

June So BSc MRPharmS
Chief Pharmacist, Christie Hospital NHS Trust,
Manchester, UK
50. Solid tumours

Gail Stark BMedSci BMBS MRCP DipRCPath
Specialist Registrar in Haematology, Royal Victoria
Infirmary, Newcastle upon Tyne, UK
48. Leukaemia

Ivan H. Stockley BPharm PhD FRPharmS
Consultant Pharmacologist, formerly Lecturer in
Pharmacology, University of Nottingham, Medical
School, Nottingham, UK
2. Drug interactions

Katherine Teahon MB BCh MD MRCP
Consultant Gastroenterologist, Nottingham City
Hospital NHS Trust, Nottingham, UK
32. Nausea and vomiting

Lucy C. Titcomb BSc MRPharmS MCPP
Directorate Pharmacist, Ophthalmology, Birmingham
and Midland Eye Centre, City Hospital NHS Trust,
Birmingham, UK
53. Glaucoma

Simon H. L. Thomas MD FRCP
Senior Lecturer in Clinical Pharmacology, Wolfson
Unit of Clinical Pharmacology, University of
Newcastle, Newcastle upon Tyne, UK
3. Adverse drug reactions
17. Hypertension

Sean Turner BPharm MSc DipClinPharm
Pharmacist in Charge, Clinical Services, King Edward
Memorial and Princess Margaret Hospitals, Perth,
Australia
8. Paediatrics

Roger Walker BPharm PhD MRPharmS HonMFPHM
Professor of Pharmacy Practice, Welsh School of
Pharmacy, Cardiff; Director of Pharmaceutical Public
Health, Gwent, UK
12. Constipation and diarrhoea
22. Dyslipidaemia

Fiona M. Ward BPharm Dip Clin Pharm MEd MRPharmS
Senor Lecturer/Practitioner, Pharmacy Department,
Arrowe Park Hospital, Wirral, UK
14. Liver disease

Martin P. Ward Platt MD FRCPCH
Consultant Paediatrician (Neonatal Medicine), Royal
Victoria Infirmary, Newcastle upon Tyne, UK
7. Neonates

Jayne Wood BSc MPhil MRPharmS MCPP
Head of Pharmaceutical Services, Pennine Acute
Hospitals NHS Trust, North Manchester General
Hospital, Manchester , UK
41. Thyroid and parathyroid disorders
42. Diabetes mellitus

Ken Woodhouse MD FRCP
Professor of Geriatric Medicine/Vice Dean of
Medicine, University of Wales College of Medicine,
Cardiff, UK
9. Geriatrics

David J. Woods BSc MPharm FHPA MRPharmS
Senior Lecturer, School of Pharmacy, University of
Otago, Dunedin, and Consultant Pharmacist,
Pharminfotech, New Zealand
45. Drugs in pregnancy and lactation

Sheila Woolfrey BSc PhD MRPharmS FCPP
Principal Pharmacist, Clinical Services, Wansbeck
General Hospital, Ashington, Northumberland, UK
31. Pain

Hilary A. Wynne MA MD FRCP
Consultant Physician and Senior Lecturer, Royal
Victoria Infirmary, Newcastle-upon-Tyne, UK
4. Laboratory data

International advisers

Saafan Al-Safi PhD
Faculty of Pharmacy, Jordan University of Science and Technology, Jordan

Yaacov Cass MSc FRParms
Regional Pharmaceutical Officer, Israel Ministry of Health, Israel

Matthew C. E. Gwee PhD MEd BPharm FIBio CBiol
Professor of Pharmacology, National University of Singapore, Singapore

Edmund Lee MB BS MMed PhD
Professor of Pharmacology, National University of Singapore, Singapore

G Parthasarathi MPharm PhD GradDipClinPharm(Australia)
Professor and Head of Department of Clinical Pharmacy, JSS Medical College Hospital, Mysore, India

A. Adij Prajitno Setiadi MSApt
Director, Centre for Medicine Information and Pharmaceutical Care, University of Swabaya, Kompleks Fakultas Farmasi, Gedung FA, Surabaya, East Jave, Indonesia

Zeinab Nabil Ahmed Said
Assistant Professor, Microbiology Department, Al-Azhar University, Cairo, Egypt

Yulia Trisna Dra Apt MPharm
Clinical Pharmacist, Department of Pharmacy, Dr Cipto Mangunkusumo Hospital, Jakarta, Indonesia

Peter T-H Wong PhD
Professor of Pharmacology, National University of Singapore, Singapore

Contents

Section 1 General

1. **Practical pharmacokinetics** 3
   R. Fitzpatrick

2. **Drug interactions** 21
   A. Lee, I. H. Stockley

3. **Adverse drug reactions** 33
   A. Lee, S. H. L. Thomas

4. **Laboratory data** 47
   H. A. Wynne, C. Edwards

5. **Parenteral nutrition** 67
   S. J. Dunnett

6. **Pharmacoeconomics** 91
   J. Cooke

Section 2 Life stages

7. **Neonates** 101
   M. P. Ward Platt

8. **Paediatrics** 111
   C. Barker, A. J. Nunn, S. Turner

9. **Geriatrics** 127
   H. G. M. Shetty, K. Woodhouse

Section 3 Therapeutics

Gastrointestinal disorders

10. **Peptic ulcer disease** 143
    S. Ghosh, M. Kinnear

11. **Inflammatory bowel disease** 163
    B. K. Evans

12. **Constipation and diarrhoea** 179
    R. Walker

Hepatic disorders

13. **Adverse effects of drugs on the liver** 193
    B. E. Cadman, B. Featherstone

14. **Liver disease** 209
    F. M. Ward, M. J. Daly

Renal disorders

15. **Acute renal failure** 229
    J. Marriott, S. Smith

16. **Chronic renal failure** 247
    J. Marriott, S. Smith

Cardiovascular disorders

17. **Hypertension** 265
    S. H. L. Thomas

18. **Coronary heart disease** 279
    D. Scott

19. **Congestive heart failure** 299
    S. A. Hudson, J. McAnaw, F. Reid

20. **Cardiac arrhythmias** 321
    D. Scott

21. **Thrombosis** 339
    P. A. Routledge, H. G. M. Shetty

22. **Dyslipidaemia** 353
    R. Walker

Respiratory disorders

23. **Asthma** 375
    K. P. Gibbs, M. Small

24. **Chronic obstructive pulmonary disease** 397
    K. P. Gibbs, M. Small

25. **Drug-induced lung disease** 413
    N. P. Keaney

Neurological and psychological disorders

26. **Insomnia and anxiety** 423
    C. H. Ashton

27. **Affective disorders** 439
    P. Pratt

28. **Schizophrenia** 455
    D. Branford

29. **Epilepsy** 465
    S. Dhillon, J. W. Sander

30. **Parkinson's disease** 483
    D. J. Burn

31. **Pain** 495
    S. Woolfrey, D. Kapur

xiii

32. Nausea and vomiting 509
K. Teahon

Infections

33. Respiratory infections 519
S. J. Pedler, A. W. Berrington

34. Urinary tract infections 533
A. J. Bint, A. W. Berrington

35. Gastrointestinal infections 543
J. W. Gray

36. Infective meningitis 555
J. W. Gray

37. Surgical antibiotic prophylaxis 569
J. C. Graham, S. J. Pedler

38. Tuberculosis 583
L. K. Nehaul

39. HIV infection 597
H. Leake Date, M. Fisher

40. Fungal infections 623
S. J. Pedler

Endocrine disorders

41. Thyroid and parathyroid disorders 639
J. A. Cantrill, J. Wood

42. Diabetes mellitus 657
J. A. Cantrill, J. Wood

Obstetric and gynaecological disorders

43. Menstrual cycle disorders 679
K. Marshall, J. Senior, J. K. Clayton

**44. Menopause and hormone replacement
therapy** 695
K. Marshall, J. Senior, J. K. Clayton

45. Drugs in pregnancy and lactation 707
S. B. Duffull, D. J. Woods

Urological disorders

46. Benign prostatic hyperplasia 717
R. L. Gower

Haematopoietic disorders

47. Anaemia 725
C. Acomb

Malignant disorders

48. Leukaemia 743
G. Jackson, G. Stark

49. Lymphomas 759
M. Maclean, D. Blake

50. Solid tumours 775
J. So

Rheumatic disorders

51. Rheumatoid arthritis and osteoarthritis 791
E. A. Kay, A. Alldred

52. Gout and hyperuricaemia 813
A. Alldred, E. A. Kay

Eye disorders

53. Glaucoma 825
L. C. Titcomb, S. D. Andrew

Skin disorders

54. Drug-induced skin disorders 843
P. Magee

55. Eczema and psoriasis 853
M. M. Carr

56. Pressure sores and leg ulcers 871
R. Anderson

Section 4 Appendices

Appendix 1 Medical abbreviations 889

Appendix 2 Glossary 897

Appendix 3 Changes to the names of certain
medical substances 901

Index 905

GENERAL

Practical pharmacokinetics

R. Fitzpatrick

KEY POINTS

- Pharmacokinetics can be applied to a range of clinical situations with or without therapeutic drug monitoring (TDM).
- TDM can improve patient outcomes but is only necessary for drugs with a low therapeutic index, where there is a good concentration response relationship, and where there is no easily measurable physiological parameter.
- Sampling before steady state is reached or before distribution is complete leads to erroneous results.
- The volume of distribution can be used to determine the loading dose.
- The elimination half-life determines the time to steady state and the dosing interval.
- Kinetic constants determine the rate of absorption and elimination.
- Clearance determines the maintenance dose.
- Creatinine clearance can be reliably estimated from population values.
- Wherever possible use actual blood level data to assist dose adjustment. However, population pharmacokinetic values can be used for digoxin, theophylline, and gentamicin.
- Once daily dosing of gentamicin is a realistic alternative to multiple dosing.
- TDM is essential in the dose titration of lithium and phenytoin, but of little value for valproate, or the newer anticonvulsants.

Clinical pharmacokinetics may be defined as the study of the time course of the absorption, distribution, metabolism and excretion of drugs and their corresponding pharmacological response. In practice, pharmacokinetics makes it possible to model what may happen to a drug after it has been administered to a patient. Clearly, this science may be applied to a wide range of clinical situations, hence the term 'clinical pharmacokinetics'.

General applications

Clinical pharmacokinetics can be applied in daily practice for drugs with a low therapeutic index, even if drug level monitoring is not required.

Time to maximal response

By knowing the half-life of a drug, the time to reach a steady state may be estimated (Fig. 1.1), and thus when maximal therapeutic response is likely to occur, irrespective of whether drug level monitoring is needed.

Need for a loading dose

The same type of information can be used to determine whether a loading dose of a drug is necessary, since drugs with longer half-lives are more likely to require loading doses for acute treatment.

Dosage alterations

Clinical pharmacokinetics can be useful in determining dosage alteration if the route of elimination is impaired through end organ failure (e.g. renal failure) or drug interaction. Using limited pharmacokinetic information such as the fraction excreted unchanged (f_e value), which can be found in most pharmacology textbooks, quantitative dosage changes can be estimated.

Choosing a formulation

An understanding of the pharmacokinetics of absorption may also be useful in evaluating the appropriateness of particular formulations of a drug in a patient.

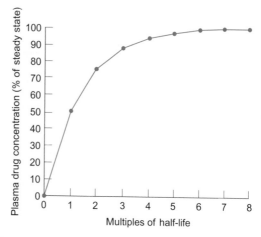

Figure 1.1   Time to steady state.

Application to therapeutic drug monitoring (TDM)

Clinical pharmacokinetics is usually associated with therapeutic drug monitoring (TDM), and its subsequent utilization. When TDM is used appropriately, it has been demonstrated that patients suffer fewer side-effects than those who were not monitored (Reid et al 1990). Although TDM is a proxy outcome measure, a study with aminoglycosides (Crist et al 1987) demonstrated shorter hospital stays for patients where TDM was used. Furthermore, a study on the use of anticonvulsants (McFadyen et al 1990) showed better epilepsy control in those patients where TDM was used.

There are various levels of sophistication for the application of pharmacokinetics to TDM. Knowledge of the distribution time and an understanding of the concept of steady state can facilitate determination of appropriate sampling times.

For most drugs that undergo first-order elimination, a linear relationship exists between dose and concentration, which can be used for dose adjustment purposes. However, if the clearance of the drug changes as the concentration changes (e.g. phenytoin), then an understanding of the drug's pharmacokinetics will assist in correct dose adjustments.

More sophisticated application of pharmacokinetics involves the use of population pharmacokinetic data to produce initial dosage guidelines, for example nomograms for digoxin and gentamicin, and to predict drug levels. Pharmacokinetics can also assist in complex dosage individualization using actual patient-specific drug level data.

Given the wide range of clinical situations in which pharmacokinetics can be applied, pharmacists must have a good understanding of the subject and how to apply it in order to maximize their contribution to patient care.

Basic concepts

Volume of distribution

The apparent volume of distribution (V_d) may be defined as the size of a compartment which will account for the total amount of drug in the body (A) if it were present in the same concentration as in plasma. This means that it is the apparent volume of fluid in the body which results in the measured concentration of drug in plasma (C) for a known amount of drug given, i.e.

$$C = \frac{A}{V_d}$$

This relationship assumes that the drug is evenly distributed throughout the body in the same concentration as in the plasma. However, this is not the case in practice, since many drugs are present in different concentrations in various parts of the body. Thus, some drugs such as digoxin have a very large apparent volume of distribution. This concept is better explained in Figure 1.2.

Apparent volume of distribution may be used to determine the plasma concentration after an intravenous loading dose:

$$C = \frac{\text{loading dose}}{V_d} \tag{1}$$

Conversely, if the desired concentration is known, the loading dose may be determined:

$$\text{loading dose} = \text{desired } C \times V_d \tag{2}$$

In the previous discussion, it has been assumed that after a given dose a drug is instantaneously distributed between the various tissues and plasma. In practice this

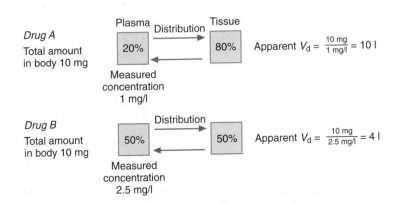

Figure 1.2 Distribution: more of drug A is distributed in the tissue compartment resulting in a higher apparent volume of distribution than drug B, where more remains in the plasma.

is seldom the case. Although a drug may be distributed into many tissues, it is reasonable for practical purposes to generalize by referring to tissue as if it were a single entity or compartment. Thus, the body may be described in pharmacokinetic terms as if it were divided into two compartments: the plasma and the tissues.

Figure 1.3 depicts the disposition of a drug immediately after administration and relates this to the plasma concentration–time graph.

Initially, the plasma concentration falls rapidly, due to distribution and elimination (α phase). However, when an equilibrium is reached between the plasma and tissue (i.e. distribution is complete) the change in plasma concentration is due to elimination from the plasma (β phase), and the plasma concentration falls at a slower rate. The drug is said to follow a two-compartment model.

However, if distribution is completed quickly (within minutes), then the α phase is not seen, and the drug is said to follow a one-compartment model.

The practical implications of a two-compartment model are that any sampling for serum concentration monitoring purposes should be carried out after distribution is complete, and intravenous bolus doses should be given slowly to avoid transient side-effects due to high peak concentrations.

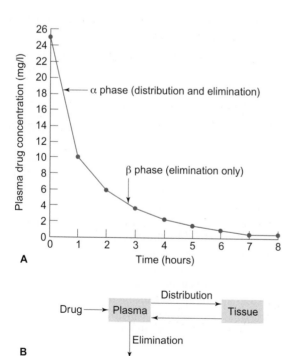

A

B

Figure 1.3 **A** Two-compartment model showing two phases in the plasma concentration-time profile. **B** representation of a two-compartment model showing distribution of drug between plasma and tissue compartments.

Elimination

Drugs may be eliminated from the body by a number of routes. The primary routes are metabolism (usually in the liver) into an inactive compound, excretion of the unchanged drug in the kidneys, or a combination of both.

The main pharmacokinetic parameter describing elimination is clearance *(CL)*. This is defined as the volume of plasma completely emptied of drug per unit time. For example, if the concentration of a drug in a patient is 1 g/l and the clearance is 1 l/h, then the rate of elimination will be 1 g/h.

Thus, a relationship exists:

$$\text{rate of elimination} = CL \times C \qquad (3)$$

Total body elimination is the sum of the metabolic rate of elimination and the renal rate of elimination. Therefore:

$$\text{total body clearance} = CL \text{ (metabolic)} + CL \text{ (renal)}$$

Thus, if the fraction eliminated by the renal route is known (f_e), then the effect of renal impairment on total body clearance can be estimated.

For most drugs, clearance is constant. Therefore, it is clear from equation (3) that as the plasma concentration changes so will the rate of elimination. However, when the rate of administration is equal to the rate of elimination, the plasma concentration is constant (C^{ss}) and the drug is said to be at a steady state. At steady state:

$$\text{rate in} = \text{rate out}$$

At the beginning of a dosage regimen the plasma concentration is low. Therefore, the rate of elimination is less than the rate of administration, and accumulation occurs until a steady state is reached (see Fig. 1.1).

$$\text{rate of administration} = \text{rate of elimination} = CL \times C^{ss} \qquad (4)$$

It is clear from equation (3) that as the plasma concentration falls (e.g. on stopping treatment or after a single dose), the rate of elimination also falls. Therefore, the plasma concentration–time graph follows a non-linear curve characteristic of this type of first-order elimination (Fig. 1.4). This is profoundly different from a constant rate of elimination irrespective of plasma concentration, which is typical of zero-order elimination.

For drugs undergoing first-order elimination, there are two other useful pharmacokinetic parameters in addition to the volume of distribution and clearance. These are the elimination rate constant and elimination half-life.

The elimination rate constant (k_e) is the fraction of the amount of drug in the body eliminated per unit time. For example, if the body contains 100 mg of a drug and 10% is eliminated per unit time, then $k_e = 0.1$. In the first unit of time, 0.1×100 mg or 10 mg is eliminated, leaving 90 mg. In the second unit of time, 0.1×90 mg or 9 mg is

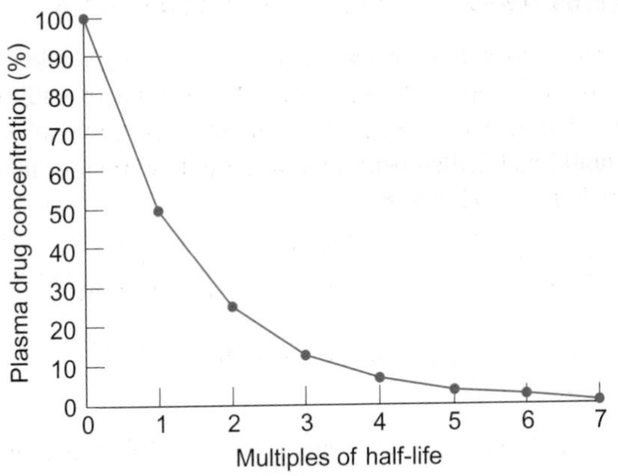

Figure 1.4 First-order elimination.

eliminated, leaving 81 mg. Elimination continues in this manner. Therefore:

$$\text{rate of elimination} = k_e \times A \tag{5}$$

Combining equations (3) and (5) gives

$$CL \times C = k_e \times A$$

and since

$$C = \frac{A}{V_d}$$

then

$$CL \times \frac{A}{V_d} = k_e \times A$$

Therefore

$$CL = k_e \times V_d \tag{6}$$

Elimination half-life ($t_{1/2}$) is the time it takes for the plasma concentration to decay by half. In five half-lives the plasma concentration will fall to approximately zero (see Fig. 1.4).

The equation which is described in Figure 1.4 is

$$C_2 = C_1 \times e^{-k_e \times t} \tag{7}$$

Where C_1 and C_2 are plasma concentrations and t is time.

If half-life is substituted for time in equation (7), C_2 must be half of C_1.

Therefore

$$0.5 \times C_1 = C_1 \times e^{-k_e \times t_{1/2}}$$

$$0.5 = e^{-k_e \times t_{1/2}}$$

$$\ln(0.5) = -k_e \times t_{1/2}$$

$$-0.693 = -k_e \times t_{1/2}$$

$$t_{1/2} = \frac{0.693}{k_e} \tag{8}$$

There are two ways of determining k_e, either by estimating the half-life and applying equation (8) or by substituting two plasma concentrations in equation (7) and applying natural logarithms:

$$\ln C_2 = \ln C_1 - (k_e \times t)$$

$$k_e \times t = \ln C_1 - \ln C_2$$

$$k_e = \frac{\ln C_1 - \ln C_2}{t}$$

In the same way as it takes approximately five half-lives for the plasma concentration to decay to zero after a single dose, it takes approximately five half-lives for a drug to accumulate to the steady state on repeated dosing or during constant infusion (see Fig. 1.1).

This graph may be described by the equation

$$C = C^{ss} [1 - e^{-k_e \times t}] \tag{9}$$

where C is the plasma concentration at time t after the start of the infusion, and C^{ss} is the steady state plasma concentration. Thus (if the appropriate pharmacokinetic parameters are known), it is possible to estimate the plasma concentration any time after a single dose or the start of a dosage regimen.

Absorption

In the preceding sections, the intravenous route has been discussed, and with this route all of the administered drug is absorbed. However, if a drug is administered by any other route it must be absorbed into the bloodstream. This process may or may not be 100% efficient.

The fraction of the administered dose which is absorbed into the bloodstream is the bioavailability (F). Thus, for oral administration, the dose or rate of administration must be multiplied by F.

In addition to bioavailability, the other useful pharmacokinetic parameter is the absorption rate constant (k_a). This term is the fraction of the dose remaining which is absorbed per unit of time. It is the converse of k_e, which describes the fraction eliminated per unit time. Thus, the absorption rate constant (k_a) is a quantitative measure of how quickly a formulation is absorbed. This is useful when comparing different formulations, particularly slow-release preparations. It is related to the absorption half-life in the same way as k_e is related to the elimination half-life. K_a may be any value < 1; the lower the K_a the slower the absorption.

Dosing regimens

From the preceding sections, it is possible to derive equations which can be applied in clinical practice.

From equation (1) we can determine the change in plasma concentration ΔC immediately after a single dose:

$$\Delta C = \frac{S \times F \times \text{dose}}{V_d} \qquad (10)$$

where F is bioavailability, and S is the salt factor, which is the fraction of active drug when the dose is administered as a salt (e.g. aminophylline is 80% theophylline, therefore $S = 0.8$).

Conversely, to determine a loading dose:

$$\text{loading dose} = \frac{\text{desired change in } C \times V_d}{S \times F} \qquad (11)$$

At the steady state it is possible to determine maintenance dose or steady state plasma concentrations from a modified equation (4):

$$\text{rate in} = \frac{S \times F \times \text{dose}}{T} = CL \times \text{average } C^{ss} \qquad (12)$$

where T is the dosing interval.

Peak and trough levels

For oral dosing and constant intravenous infusions, it is usually adequate to use the term 'average steady state plasma concentration' (average C^{ss}). However, for some intravenous bolus injections it is sometimes necessary to determine peak and trough levels (e.g. gentamicin).

At the steady state, the change in concentration due to the administration of an intravenous dose will be equal to the change in concentration due to elimination over one dose interval:

$$\Delta C = \frac{S \times F \times \text{dose}}{V_d} = C_{max} - C_{min}$$

Within one dosing interval the maximum plasma concentration (C^{ss}_{max}) will decay to the minimum plasma concentration (C^{ss}_{min}) as in any first-order process.

Substituting C^{ss}_{max} for C_1 and C^{ss}_{min} for C_2 in equation (7):

$$C^{ss}_{min} = C^{ss}_{max} \times e^{-k_e \times t}$$

where t is the dosing interval.

If this is substituted into the preceding equation:

$$\frac{S \times F \times \text{dose}}{V_d} = C^{ss}_{max} - C^{ss}_{min} \times e^{-k_e \times t}$$

Therefore:

$$C^{ss}_{max} = \frac{S \times F \times \text{dose}}{V_d\,[1 - e^{-k_e \times t}]} \qquad (13)$$

$$C^{ss}_{min} = \frac{S \times F \times \text{dose}}{V_d\,[1 - e^{-k_e \times t}]} \times e^{-k_e \times t} \qquad (14)$$

Interpretation of drug concentration data

The availability of the technology to measure the concentration of a drug in serum should not be the reason for monitoring. There are a number of criteria that should be fulfilled before therapeutic drug monitoring is undertaken. These are:

- the drug should have a low therapeutic index
- there should be a good concentration–response relationship
- there are no easily measurable physiological parameters.

In the absence of these criteria being fulfilled, the only other justification for undertaking TDM is to monitor compliance or to confirm toxicity. When interpreting TDM data a number of factors need to be considered.

Sampling times

In the preceding sections, the time to reach the steady state has been discussed. When TDM is carried out as an aid to dose adjustment, the concentration should be at the steady state. Therefore, approximately five half-lives should elapse after initiation or changing a maintenance regimen, before sampling. The only exception to this rule is when toxicity is suspected. When the steady state has been reached, it is important to sample at the correct time. It is clear from the discussion above that this should be done when distribution is complete (see Fig. 1.3).

Dosage adjustment

Under most circumstances, providing the preceding criteria are observed, adjusting the dose of a drug is relatively simple, since a linear relationship exists between the dose and concentration if a drug follows first-order elimination (Fig. 1.5A). This is the case for most drugs.

Capacity limited clearance

If a drug is eliminated by the liver, it is possible for the metabolic pathway to become saturated, since it is an enzymatic system. Initially the elimination is first order, but once saturation of the system occurs, elimination becomes zero order. This results in the characteristic dose–concentration graph of Figure 1.5B. For the majority of drugs eliminated by the liver, this effect is not seen at normal therapeutic doses and only occurs at very high supra-therapeutic levels, which is why the kinetics of some drugs in overdose is different from normal. However, one important exception is phenytoin, where saturation of the enzymatic pathway occurs at

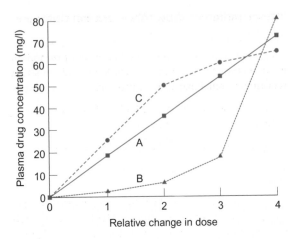

Figure 1.5 Dose-concentration relationships. **A** First-order elimination. **B** Capacity-limited clearance. **C** Increasing clearance.

therapeutic doses. This will be dealt with in the section on phenytoin.

Increasing clearance

The only other situation where first-order elimination is not seen is where clearance increases as the serum concentration increases (Fig. 1.5C). Under normal circumstances, the plasma protein binding sites available to a drug far outnumber the capacity of the drug to fill those binding sites, and the proportion of the total concentration of drug which is protein bound is constant. However, this situation is not seen in one or two instances (e.g. valproate and disopyramide). For these particular drugs, as the concentration increases the plasma protein binding sites become saturated, and the ratio of unbound drug to bound drug increases. The elimination of these drugs increases disproportionately to the total concentration, since elimination is dependent on the unbound concentration.

Therapeutic range

Wherever TDM is carried out, a therapeutic range is usually used as a guide to the optimum concentration. The limits of these ranges should not be taken as absolute. Some patients may respond to levels above or below these ranges, whereas others may experience toxic effects within the so-called therapeutic range. These ranges are only adjuncts to dose determination, which should always be done in the light of clinical response.

Clinical applications

Estimation of creatinine clearance

Since many drugs are renally excreted, and the most practical marker of renal function is creatinine clearance, it is often necessary to estimate this in order to undertake dosage adjustment in renal impairment. The usual method is to undertake a 24-hour urine collection coupled with a serum creatinine measurement. The laboratory then estimates the patient's creatinine clearance. The formula used to determine creatinine clearance is based upon the pharmacokinetic principles in equation (3).

The rate of elimination is calculated from the measurement of the total amount of creatinine contained in the 24-hour urine sample divided by 24, i.e.

$$\frac{\text{amount of creatinine}}{24} = \text{rate of excretion (mg/h)}$$

Using this rate of excretion and substituting the measured serum creatinine for C^{ss} in equation (4), the creatinine clearance can be calculated.

However, there are practical difficulties with this method. The whole process is cumbersome and there is an inevitable delay in obtaining a result. The biggest problem is the inaccuracy of the 24-hour urine collection.

An alternative approach is to estimate the rate of production of creatinine (i.e. rate in) instead of the rate of elimination (rate out). Clearly this has advantages, since it does not involve 24-hour urine collections and requires only a single measure of serum creatinine. There are data in the literature relating creatinine production to age, weight and sex, since the primary source of creatinine is the breakdown of muscle.

Therefore, equations have been produced which are rearrangements of equation (4), i.e.

$$\text{creatinine clearance} = \frac{\text{rate of production}}{C^{ss}}$$

Rate of production is replaced by a formula which estimates this from physiological parameters of age, weight and sex.

It has been shown that the equation produced by Cockcroft & Gault (1976) appears to be the most satisfactory. A modified version using SI units is shown below:

$$\text{creatinine clearance (ml/min)} = \frac{F \times [(140 - \text{age in years}) \times \text{weight (kg)}]}{\text{serum creatinine (μmol/l)}}$$

where $F = 1.04$ (females) or 1.23 (males).

Digoxin

Action and uses

Digoxin is the most widely used of the digitalis glycosides. Its primary actions on the heart are those of increasing the force of contraction and decreasing conduction through the atrioventricular node. Currently, its main role is in the treatment of atrial fibrillation by slowing down the ventricular response although it is also used in the treatment of heart failure in the presence of sinus rhythm. The primary method of monitoring its clinical effect in atrial fibrillation is by measurement of heart rate but knowledge of its pharmacokinetics can be helpful in predicting a patient's dosage requirements.

Serum concentration–response relationship

- < 0.5 micrograms/litre: no clinical effect
- 0.7 micrograms/litre: some positive inotropic and conduction blocking effects
- 0.8–2 micrograms/litre: optimum therapeutic range
- 2–2.5 micrograms/litre: increased risk of toxicity, although tolerated in some patients
- > 2.5 micrograms/litre: gastrointestinal, cardiovascular system and central nervous system toxicity.

Distribution

Digoxin is widely distributed and extensively bound in varying degrees to tissues throughout the body. This results in a high apparent volume of distribution. Digoxin volume of distribution can be estimated using the equation 7.3 l/kg (lean body weight (BWt)) which is derived from population data. However, distribution is altered in patients with renal impairment, and a more accurate estimate in these patients is given by:

$$V_d = 3.8 \times \text{lean BWt} + (3.1 \times \text{creatinine clearance (ml/min)})$$

A two-compartment model best describes digoxin disposition (see Fig. 1.3) with a distribution time of 6–8 hours. Clinical effects are seen earlier after intravenous doses, since the myocardium has a high blood perfusion and affinity for digoxin. Sampling for TDM must be done no sooner than 6 hours post-dose, otherwise an erroneous result will be obtained.

Elimination

Digoxin is eliminated primarily by renal excretion of unchanged drug (60–80%), but some hepatic metabolism occurs (20–40%). The population average value for digoxin clearance is:

$$\text{digoxin clearance (ml/min)} = 0.8 \times \text{BWt} + (\text{creatinine clearance (ml/min)})$$

However, patients with severe congestive heart failure have a reduced hepatic metabolism and a slight reduction in renal excretion of digoxin:

$$\text{digoxin clearance (ml/min)} = 0.33 \times \text{BWt} + (0.9 \times \text{creatinine clearance (ml/min)})$$

Lean body weight should be used in these equations.

Absorption

Digoxin is poorly absorbed from the gastrointestinal tract, and dissolution time affects the overall bioavailability. The two oral formulations of digoxin have different bioavailabilities:

$$F \text{ (tablets)} = 0.65$$
$$F \text{ (liquid)} = 0.8$$

Practical implications

Using population averages it is possible to predict serum concentrations from specific dosages, particularly since the time to reach the steady state is long. Population values are only averages, and individuals may vary. In addition, a number of diseases and drugs affect digoxin disposition.

As can be seen from the preceding discussion, congestive heart failure, hepatic and renal disease all decrease the elimination of digoxin. In addition, hypothyroidism increases the serum concentration (decreased metabolism and renal excretion) and increases the sensitivity of the heart to digoxin. Hyperthyroidism has the opposite effect. Hypokalaemia, hypercalcaemia, hypomagnesaemia and hypoxia all increase the sensitivity of the heart to digoxin. There are numerous drug interactions reported of varying clinical significance. The usual cause is either altered absorption or clearance.

Theophylline

Theophylline is an alkaloid related to caffeine. It has a variety of clinical effects including mild diuresis, central nervous system stimulation, cerebrovascular vasodilatation, increased cardiac output and bronchodilatation. It is the latter which is the major therapeutic effect of theophylline. Theophylline does have some serious toxic effects. However, there is a good serum concentration–response relationship.

Serum concentration–response relationship

- < 5 mg/l: no bronchodilatation[*]

---

[*] Some patients exhibit a clinical effect at these levels which has been attributed to possible anti-inflammatory effects.

- 5–10 mg/l: some bronchodilatation and possible anti-inflammatory action
- 10–20 mg/l: optimum bronchodilatation, minimum side-effects
- 20–30 mg/l: increased incidence of nausea, vomiting[*] and cardiac arrhythmias
- > 30 mg/l: cardiac arrhythmias, seizures.

Distribution

Theophylline is extensively distributed throughout the body, with an average volume of distribution based on population data of 0.48 l/kg.

Theophylline does not distribute very well into fat, and estimations should be based on lean body weight. A two-compartment model best describes theophylline disposition, with a distribution time of approximately 40 minutes.

Elimination

Elimination is a first-order process primarily by hepatic metabolism to relatively inactive metabolites.

The population average for theophylline clearance is 0.04 l/h/kg, but this is affected by a number of diseases/drugs/pollutants. Therefore, this value should be multiplied by:

- 0.5 where there is cirrhosis, or when cimetidine, erythromycin or ciprofloxacin are being taken concurrently
- 0.4 where there is congestive heart failure with hepatomegaly
- 0.8 where there is severe respiratory obstruction ($FEV_1 < 1$ l)
- 1.6 in patients who smoke (defined as more than 10 cigarettes per day), since they metabolize theophylline more quickly.

Neonates metabolize theophylline differently, with 50% being converted to caffeine. Therefore, when it is used to treat neonatal apnoea of prematurity a lower therapeutic range is used (usually 5–10 mg/l), since caffeine contributes to the therapeutic response.

Product formulation

Aminophylline (the ethylenediamine salt of theophylline) is only 80% theophylline. Therefore, the salt factor *(S)* is 0.8. Most sustained-release (SR) preparations show good bioavailability but not all SR preparations are the same. The absorption rate constant (k_a) provides a good guide to slow-release

characteristics. Generally, the lower the k_a value the better the slow-release capabilities.

Practical implications

Intravenous bolus doses of aminophylline need to be given slowly (preferably by short infusion) to avoid side-effects due to transiently high blood levels during the distribution phase. Oral doses with slow-release preparations can be estimated using population-average pharmacokinetic values and titrated proportionally according to blood levels and clinical response. In most circumstances, slow-release preparations may be assumed to provide 12 hours' cover. However, more marked peaks and troughs are seen with fast metabolizers (smokers and children). In these cases, the slow-release preparation with the lowest k_a value may be used twice daily (e.g. Theo-Dur ($k_a = 0.18$) or Uniphyllin ($k_a = 0.22$)). Alternatively, thrice-daily dosage is required if a standard ($k_a = 0.3–0.4$) slow-release product is used (e.g. Phyllocontin ($k_a = 0.37$) or Nuelin SA ($k_a = 0.33$)).

Gentamicin

Clinical use

The spectrum of activity of gentamicin is similar to other aminoglycosides but its most significant activity is against *Psuedomonas aeruginosa*. It is still regarded by many as first choice for this type of infection.

Therapeutic range

Gentamicin has a low therapeutic index, producing dose-related side-effects of nephro- and ototoxicity. The use of TDM to aid dose adjustment is essential if these toxic effects which appear to be related to peak and trough serum levels are to be avoided. It is generally accepted that the peak level (drawn 1 hour post-dose after an intravenous bolus or intramuscular injection) should not exceed 12 mg/l and the trough level (drawn immediately pre-dose) should not exceed 2 mg/l.

The above recommendations relate to multiple daily dosing of gentamicin. If once daily dosing is to be used, then different monitoring and interpretation parameters apply as described at the end of this section.

Distribution

Gentamicin is relatively polar and distributes primarily into extracellular fluid. Thus, the apparent volume of distribution is only 0.25 l/kg. Gentamicin follows a two-compartment model with distribution being complete within 1 hour.

---

[*] Nausea and vomiting can occur within the therapeutic range.

Elimination

Elimination is by renal excretion of the unchanged drug. Gentamicin clearance is approximately equal to creatinine clearance.

Practical implications

Since the therapeutic range is based on peak (1 hour post-dose to allow for distribution) and trough (pre-dose) concentrations, it is necessary to be able to predict these from any given dosage regimen.

Initial dosage. This may be based on the patient's physiological parameters. Gentamicin clearance may be determined directly from creatinine clearance. The volume of distribution may be determined from lean body weight. The elimination constant k_e may then be estimated using these parameters in equation (6). By substituting k_e and the desired peak and trough levels into equation (7), the optimum dosage interval can be determined (add on 1 hour to this value to account for sampling time). Using this value (or the nearest practical value) and the desired peak or trough value substituted into equation (13) or (14) it is possible to determine the appropriate dose.

Changing dosage. This is not as straightforward as for theophylline or digoxin, since increasing the dose will increase the peak and trough levels proportionately. If this is not desired, then use of pharmacokinetic equations is necessary. By substituting the measured peak and trough levels and the time between them into equation (7), it is possible to determine k_e (and the half-life from equation (8) if required). To estimate the patient's volume of distribution from actual blood level data, it is necessary to know the C^{ss}_{max} immediately after the dose (time zero), not the 1-hour value which is measured. To obtain this, equation (7) may be used, this time substituting the trough level for C_2 and solving for C_1. Subtracting the trough level from this C^{ss}_{max} at time zero, the volume of distribution may be determined from equation (10). Using these values for k_e and V_d, derived from actual blood level data, a new dose and dose interval can be determined as before.

Once daily dosing. There are theoretical arguments for once-daily dosing of gentamicin, since aminoglycosides display concentration-dependent bacterial killing, and a high enough concentration to mean inhibitory concentration (MIC) ratio may not be achieved with multiple dosing. Furthermore, aminoglycosides have a long post-antibiotic effect. Aminoglycosides also accumulate in the kidneys, and once daily dosing could reduce renal tissue accumulation. There have been a number of clinical trials comparing once-daily administration of aminoglycosides with conventional administration. A small number of these trials have shown less nephrotoxicity, no difference in ototoxicity, and similar efficacy with once-daily administration. Initial dosage for a once-daily regimen is 5–7 mg/kg/day for patients with a creatinine clearance of >60 ml/min. This is subsequently adjusted on the basis of blood levels. However, monitoring of once-daily dosing of gentamicin is different to multiple dosing. One approach is to take a blood sample 6–14 hours after the first dose and plot the time and result on a standard concentration-time plot (the Hartford nomogram, Nicolau et al 1995; Fig. 1.6). The position of the individual patient's point in relation to standard lines on the nomogram indicate what the most appropriate dose interval should be (either 24, 36 or 48 hours). Once-daily dosing of gentamicin has not been well studied in children, pregnant or breastfeeding women, patients with major burns, renal failure, endocarditis or cystic fibrosis. Therefore, it cannot be recommended in these groups and multiple daily dosing should be used.

Lithium

Lithium is effective in the treatment of acute mania and in the prophylaxis of manic depression. The mechanism of action is not fully understood, but it is thought that it may substitute for sodium or potassium in the central nervous system. Lithium is toxic, producing dose-dependent and dose-independent side-effects. Therefore, TDM is essential in assisting in the management of the dosage.

Dose-dependent effects

The serum concentration–response relationship derived on the basis of the 12-hour standardized lithium level (measured 12 hours after the evening dose of lithium) is shown below:

- < 0.4 mmol/l: little therapeutic effect
- 0.4–1.0 mmol/l: optimum range for prophylaxis
- 0.8–1.2 mmol/l: optimum range for acute mania
- 1.2–1.5 mmol/l: causes possible renal impairment
- 1.5–3.0 mmol/l: causes renal impairment, ataxia, weakness, drowsiness, thirst, diarrhoea
- 3.0–5.0 mmol/l: causes confusion, spasticity, dehydration, convulsions, coma, death. (Levels above 3.5 mmol/l are regarded as a medical emergency.)

Dose-independent effects

These include tremor, hypothyroidism (approximately 10% of patients on chronic therapy), nephrogenic diabetes insipidus, gastrointestinal upset, loss in bone density, weight gain (approximately 20% of patients gain more than 10 kg) and lethargy.

If result available within 24 h
- Use graph below to select dose interval. Use plasma concentration and time interval between start of infusion and sample to plot intercept (see example given on graph).
- Give next dose (7 mg/kg by infusion as above) after interval indicated by graph.
  If result falls above upper limit for Q48 h, abandon once daily regimen. Measure gentamicin concentration after another 24 h and adopt multiple daily dose regimen if result <2 mg/l
  If result falls on Q24 h sector it is not necessary to recheck gentamicin concentration within 5 days unless patient's condition suggests renal function may be compromised.

- **Graph:**   Use values of plasma concentration and time interval to find intercept
  (Example given of 6 mg/l after 10 h yields dose interval of 36 h)

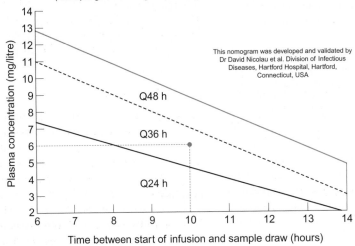

MONITORING
- Repeat U&E daily. Calculate creatinine clearance from serum creatinine to check dose interval has not changed.
- If dose interval has to be changed, check gentamicin concentration 6–14 h after start of next infusion note time of start of infusion and time of sampling and use graph to verify correct dose interval.

This protocol is based on that used at the Tayside area hospitals, Scotland

Figure 1.6   Nomogram for adjustment of once daily gentamicin dosage (Nicolau et al 1995).

Distribution

Lithium is unevenly distributed throughout the body, with a volume of distribution of approximately 0.5–1 l/kg. Lithium follows a two-compartment model (see Fig. 1.3) with a distribution time of 8 hours (hence, 12-hour sampling criterion).

Elimination

Lithium is excreted unchanged by the kidneys. Lithium clearance is approximately 20% of creatinine clearance, since there is extensive reabsorption in the renal tubules.

In addition to changes in renal function, dehydration, diuretics (particularly thiazides), angiotensin-converting enzyme inhibitors (ACE inhibitors) and non-steroidal anti-inflammatory drugs (NSAIDs) (except aspirin and sulindac) all decrease lithium clearance.

Conversely, aminophylline and sodium loading increase lithium clearance.

Notwithstanding the above factors, there is a wide inter-individual variation in clearance, and the lithium half-life in the population varies between 8 and 35 hours with an average of approximately 18 hours. Lithium clearance shows a diurnal variation, being slower at night than during the day.

Practical implications

In view of the narrow therapeutic index, lithium should not be prescribed unless facilities for monitoring serum lithium concentrations are available. Since lithium excretion is a first-order process, changes in dosage result in a proportional change in blood levels. Blood samples should be drawn 12 hours after the evening dose, since this will allow for distribution and represent the slowest excretion rate. Population pharmacokinetic data (particularly the volume of distribution) cannot be relied upon to make initial dosage predictions, although renal function may give an approximate guide to clearance. Blood level measurements are reported in SI units and therefore it is useful to know the conversion factors for the various salts.

- 100 mg of lithium carbonate is equivalent to 2.7 mmol of lithium ions
- 100 mg of lithium citrate is equivalent to 1.1 mmol of lithium ions.

Phenytoin

Phenytoin is effective in the treatment of generalized tonic–clonic and partial seizures. It is associated with dose-independent side-effects which include hirsutism, acne, coarsening of facial features, gingival hyperplasia, hypocalcaemia and folic acid deficiency. However, phenytoin has a narrow therapeutic index and has serious concentration related side-effects.

Serum concentration–response relationship

- < 5 mg/l: generally no therapeutic effect
- 5–10 mg/l: some anticonvulsant action
- 10–20 mg/l: optimum concentration for anticonvulsant effect
- 20–30 mg/l: nystagmus, blurred vision
- > 30 mg/l: ataxia, dysarthria, drowsiness, coma.

Distribution

Phenytoin follows a two-compartment model with a distribution time of 30–60 minutes. The apparent volume of distribution is 1 l/kg.

Elimination

The main route of elimination is via hepatic metabolism. However, this metabolic route can be saturated at normal therapeutic doses. This results in the characteristic non-linear dose/concentration curve seen in Figure 1.5B. Therefore, instead of the usual first-order pharmacokinetic model, a Michaelis–Menten model, used to describe enzyme activity, is more appropriate.

Using this model, the daily dosage of phenytoin can be described by

$$\frac{S \times F \times \text{dose}}{T} = \frac{V_{\max} \times C^{\text{ss}}}{K_{\text{m}} + C^{\text{ss}}} \qquad (15)$$

K_{m} is the plasma concentration at which metabolism proceeds at half the maximal rate. The population average for this is 6 mg/l, although this value varies greatly with age and race.

$V_{\max}$ is the maximum rate of metabolism of phenytoin and is more predictable at approximately 7 mg/kg/day.

Elimination half-life

Since clearance changes with blood concentration, the half-life also changes. The usual reported value is 22 hours, but this increases as concentration increases. Therefore, it is difficult to predict when the steady state will be reached; however, as a rule of thumb, 1–2 weeks should be allowed to elapse before sampling after a dosage change.

In overdose, it can be assumed that metabolism of the drug is occurring at the maximum rate of $V_{\max}$. Therefore, the decline in plasma concentration is linear (zero order) at approximately 7 mg/l/day.

Practical applications

Since the dose/concentration relationship is non-linear, changes in dose do not result in proportional changes in plasma concentration (see Fig. 1.5B). Using the Michaelis–Menten model, if the plasma concentration is known at one dosage, then $V_{\max}$ may be assumed to be the population average (7 mg/kg/day), since this is the more predictable parameter, and K_{m} calculated using equation (15). The revised values of K_{m} can then be used in equation 15 to estimate the new dosage required to produce a desired concentration. Alternatively, a nomogram may be used to assist in dose adjustments (Fig. 1.7).

Care is needed when interpreting TDM data and making dosage adjustments when phenytoin is given concurrently with other anticonvulsants, since these affect distribution and metabolism of phenytoin. Since phenytoin is approximately 90% protein bound, hypoalbuminaemia and renal failure will affect this, and care is needed when estimating doses in these clinical situations.

The oral formulations of phenytoin show good bioavailability. However, tablets and capsules contain the sodium salt ($S = 0.9$), whereas the suspension is phenytoin base ($S = 1$). Intramuscular phenytoin is slowly and unpredictably absorbed, due to crystallization in the muscle tissue, and is, therefore, not recommended. Fosphenytoin, a prodrug of phenytoin, is better absorbed from the intramuscular site. Doses should be expressed as phenytoin equivalent. Fosphenytoin sodium 1.5 mg is equivalent to phenytoin sodium 1 mg.

Carbamazepine

Carbamazepine is a drug of choice for simple and complex partial seizures, and for tonic–clonic seizures secondary to a focal discharge. There are a number of dose-independent side-effects, including various dermatological reactions and, more rarely, aplastic anaemia and the Stevens–Johnson syndrome. However, the more common side-effects are concentration related.

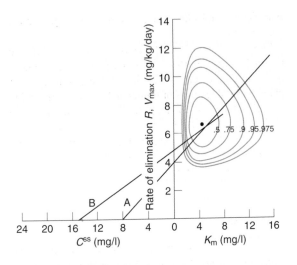

Figure 1.7 Orbit graph. The most probable values of V_{max} and K_m for a patient may be estimated using a single steady-state phenytoin concentration and a known dosing regimen. The eccentric circles or 'orbits' represent the fraction of the sample patient population whose K_m and V_{max} values are within that orbit. (1) Plot the daily dose of phenytoin (mg/kg/day) on the vertical line (rate of elimination). (2) Plot the steady-state concentration (C^{ss}) on the horizontal line. (3) Draw a straight line connecting C^{ss} and daily dose through the orbits (line A). (4) The coordinates of the mid point of the line crossing the innermost orbit through which the line passes are the most probable values for the patient's V_{max} and K_m. (5) To calculate a new maintenance dose, draw a line from the point determined in Step 4 to the new desired C^{ss} (line B). The point at which line B crosses the vertical line (rate of elimination) is the new maintenance dose (mg/kg/day). The line A represents a C^{ss} of 8 mg/l on 276 mg/day of phenytoin acid (300 mg/day of sodium phenytoin) for a 70 kg patient. Line B has been drawn assuming the new desired steady-state concentration was 15 mg/l (μg/ml). The original figure is modified so that R and V_{max} are in mg/kg/day of phenytoin acid (modified from Evans et al 1992).

Serum concentration–response relationship

- < 4 mg/l: little therapeutic benefit
- 4–12 mg/l: optimum therapeutic range for monotherapy
- > 9 mg/l: possible side-effects of nystagmus, diplopia, drowsiness and ataxia, particularly if patients are on other anticonvulsant therapy
- > 12 mg/l: side-effects common, even on monotherapy.

Distribution

Carbamazepine is distributed widely in various organs, with the highest concentration found in liver and kidneys. Carbamazepine is 70–80% protein bound and

shows a wide variation in the population-average apparent volume of distribution (0.8–1.9 l/kg). This wide variation is thought to be due to variations in absorption (since there is no parenteral form) and protein binding.

Elimination

Carbamazepine is eliminated almost exclusively by metabolism, with less than 2% being excreted unchanged in the urine. Elimination is a first-order process, but carbamazepine induces its own metabolism. Therefore, at the beginning of therapy, clearance is 0.01–0.03 l/h/kg, rising to 0.05–0.1 l/h/kg on chronic therapy. Auto-induction begins in the first few days of commencing therapy and is maximal at 2–4 weeks.

Since clearance changes with time, so does half-life, with reported values as long as 35 hours after a single dose, decreasing to 5–7 hours on regular dosing.

Absorption

Absorption after oral administration is slow, with peak concentrations being reached 2–24 hours post-dose (average 6 hours). Absorption is incomplete, with bioavailability estimated at approximately 80% (F = 0.8).

Practical implications

Use of pharmacokinetic equations is limited, due to the auto-induction effect. However, there are a number of important practical points:

- Blood samples should not be drawn before the steady state, which will not be achieved until 2–4 weeks after starting therapy or 3–4 days after subsequent dose adjustments.
- When sampling, the trough level should be measured because of the variable absorption pattern.
- Complex calculations are not helpful, but as a rule of thumb each 100 mg dose will increase the plasma concentration at the steady state by approximately 1 mg/l in adults.
- A number of other drugs (including phenytoin) when given concurrently will affect carbamazepine metabolism and subsequent blood levels.

Phenobarbital

Phenobarbital is effective in the treatment of tonic–clonic and partial seizures, and is also useful in the treatment of febrile seizures. Although there is a clear concentration–response relationship, routine serum concentration monitoring is less useful than for other drugs, since tolerance occurs.

Serum concentration–response relationship

- < 15 mg/l: little therapeutic effect
- 15–40 mg/l: optimum range
- 40–50 mg/l: sedation, confusion (elderly), although may be tolerated by some patients
- > 60 mg/l: serious toxic effect of ataxia, lethargy, stupor, coma.

The sedation which commonly manifests early on in therapy becomes less with continued therapy.

Distribution

Phenobarbital readily distributes into most body tissues and is 50% protein bound. The population-average volume of distribution is 0.7–1 l/kg.

Elimination

Phenobarbital is primarily (80%) metabolized by the liver, with approximately 20% being excreted unchanged in the urine. Elimination is a first-order process, but is relatively slow with a population-average clearance of approximately 0.004 l/h/kg. However, as with theophylline, clearance in children is increased. In the case of phenobarbital, the adult clearance value is doubled in children. Applying equations (6) and (8) to these population values gives an estimate of the half-life of the order of 5 days. This is much shorter in children and longer in the elderly.

Practical application

In view of the long half-life, single daily dosage is possible with phenobarbital. Samples for therapeutic monitoring may be drawn any time during a dose interval, since concentration fluctuation between doses is minimal. However, the patient should be at the steady state, which takes 2–4 weeks (1–2 weeks in children). The pharmacokinetics of phenobarbital may be altered by liver and (less markedly) renal disease, but are not affected by the concurrent administration of other anticonvulsants.

Primidone

Like phenobarbital, primidone is effective in the treatment of tonic–clonic and partial seizures. Much of the anticonvulsant activity of primidone is due to the metabolites phenobarbital and phenylethylmalonamide. Therefore, primidone serum concentrations are only useful to confirm transient toxicity. Toxic manifestations such as sedation, nausea and ataxia are seen at concentrations greater than 15 mg/l. The plasma concentration should be drawn approximately 3 hours post-dose, which corresponds to the peak concentration.

Phenylethylmalonamide assays are not available routinely, although this metabolite probably contributes to anticonvulsant activity. Measurement of phenobarbital levels is of limited value, since conversion of primidone to phenobarbital is variable between individuals. However, phenobarbital levels may be helpful in dosage selection, where seizures are not adequately controlled despite regular dosage, or where there is suspected toxicity.

Valproate

Sodium valproate as valproic acid in the bloodstream has a broad spectrum of anticonvulsant activity, being useful in generalized absence, generalized tonic–colonic and partial seizures.

Serum concentration–response relationship

There is no clear concentration–response relationship for valproate, although a range of 50–100 mg/l is often quoted as being optimal. Levels exceeding this range do not confer any additional therapeutic benefits. Although there is no clear relationship between serum levels and toxic effects, the rare hepatotoxicity associated with valproate appears to be related to very high levels of over 150 mg/l.

Distribution

Valproate is extensively bound to plasma protein (90–95%), and unlike other drugs, it can saturate protein-binding sites at concentrations greater than 50 mg/l, altering the free fraction of drug. Therefore, the apparent volume of distribution of valproate varies from 0.1 to 0.5 l/kg.

Elimination

Elimination of valproate is almost entirely by hepatic metabolism, with less than 5% being eliminated by the kidneys.

As a result of the saturation of protein-binding sites and the subsequent increase in the free fraction of the drug, clearance of the drug increases at higher concentrations. Therefore, there is a non-linear change in plasma concentration with dose (illustrated in Fig. 1.5C).

Practical implications

In view of the lack of a clear concentration/response relationship and the variable pharmacokinetics, there are limited indications for the measurement of valproate levels. In most cases, dosage should be based on clinical response. However, in a few cases where seizures are not controlled at high dosage, a serum level may be helpful in confirming treatment failure. If monitoring is to be undertaken, levels should be drawn at steady state (2–3 days). A trough sample will be the most useful, since wide fluctuations of blood levels may occur during a dose interval.

Lamotrigine, vigabatrin, gabapentin, tiagabine and topiramate

These newer anticonvulsants are indicated for the treatment of a range of types of epilepsy. All are used as adjunctive treatment with other anticonvulsants, with only lamotrigine indicated for monotherapy.

Serum concentration–response relationship

There is no clear relationship between serum concentration and response for these newer anticonvulsants. The situation is further complicated by the fact that these preparations are usually used as an add-on therapy with other anticonvulsants.

Practical implications

While these newer anticonvulsants have narrow therapeutic indices and inter- and intra-individual variation in pharmacokinetics, there is not enough evidence to support routine TDM, and dosage should be titrated to clinical response.

Ciclosporin

Ciclosporin is a neutral lipophilic cyclic endecapeptide extracted from the fungus *Tolypocladium inflatum gams.* It is a potent immunosuppressive agent, used principally to reduce graft rejection after kidney, heart, heart–lung, liver, pancreas and bone marrow transplants. The drug has a low therapeutic index, with a number of toxic effects including nephrotoxicity, hepatotoxicity, gastrointestinal intolerance, hypertrichosis and neurological problems. Efficacy in reducing graft rejection as well as the main toxic effect of nephro- and hepatotoxicity appear to be concentration related.

Serum concentration–response relationship

With all drugs that are monitored the therapeutic range is a window with limits, which are not absolute. It is even more difficult to define a therapeutic range for ciclosporin, since there are a number of influencing factors. First, the measured concentration varies depending on sampling matrix (i.e. whole blood, plasma or serum). Second, it depends on whether the assay is specific for ciclosporin alone or non-specific to include metabolites. A target concentration range of 200–400 micrograms/litre is generally accepted for the immediate postoperative phase following renal transplants. Levels below the lower limit of this window are associated with an increased incidence of graft rejection. Levels above the upper limit are associated with an increased incidence of nephrotoxicity and hepatotoxicity, although an upper limit of 800 micrograms/litre has also been suggested. This target range can be reduced to 100–200 micrograms/litre 3–6 months post-transplant. These target ranges are based on assays specific for the ciclosporin parent compound.

Distribution

Ciclosporin is highly lipophilic and is distributed widely throughout the body with a volume of distribution of 4–8 l/kg. There is variable distribution of ciclosporin within blood, since the whole blood concentration is approximately twice the plasma concentration. Within plasma, ciclosporin is 98% protein bound.

Elimination

Ciclosporin is eliminated primarily by hepatic metabolism, with wide inter-individual variation in clearance (0.1–2 l/h/kg). In children these values are approximately 40% higher, with a resulting increased dosage requirement on a milligram per kilogram basis. In elderly patients or patients with hepatic impairment a lower clearance rate has been observed.

Practical implications

In addition to the wide inter-patient variability in distribution and elimination pharmacokinetic parameters, absorption of standard formulations of ciclosporin is variable and incomplete ($F = 0.2$–0.5 in normal subjects). In transplant patients this variation in bioavailability is even greater, and increases during the first few months after transplant. Furthermore, a number of drugs are known to interact with ciclosporin. All these factors suggest that therapeutic drug monitoring will assist in optimum dose selection, but the use of population averages in dose prediction is of little benefit, due to wide inter-patient variation. When using TDM with ciclosporin a number of practical points need to be considered:

- The sampling matrix should be whole blood, since there is a variable distribution of ciclosporin between blood and serum.
- Samples should represent trough levels and be drawn at the steady state, which is achieved 2–3 days after initiating or changing the dosage (average half-life is 9 hours).

- Ciclosporin concentration monitoring should be undertaken every 2–3 days in the immediate postoperative phase until the patient's clinical condition is stable. Thereafter, monitoring can be undertaken every 1–2 months.
- TDM should be performed when changing brands of ciclosporin, since there are marked differences in the bioavailability of different brands.

Summary pharmacokinetic data for drugs with therapeutic serum concentrations are listed in Table 1.1.

CASE STUDIES

Case 1.1

Mr B. is a 55-year-old 65 kg man with chronic obstructive airways disease (COAD). He has been taking Nuelin SA 250 mg tablets in a dose of two tablets twice a day for many years. He has been admitted to hospital with congestive heart failure (CHF). On examination he has ankle oedema, hepatomegaly and raised jugular venous pressure (JVP).

Three days after admission Mr B. starts fitting and anticonvulsants are considered. You suggest that high theophylline levels can cause this but unfortunately (this is late Friday) there is no possibility of obtaining a level quickly.

Questions

1. If theophylline is the cause of the fitting, why has this occurred now since he has been on the medicine for some time?
2. Estimate Mr B.'s theophylline level at the time of the fitting.
3. How long after stopping Nuelin will Mr B.'s theophylline be within the therapeutic range (assume first-order elimination)?

Answers

1. Development of severe congestive heart failure reduces theophylline clearance by 50% therefore it is the same as doubling Mr B.'s current dose.
2. Using population averages, the normal clearance for a man of his weight would be 65 kg × 0.04 l/h = 2.6 l/h. However, his clearance is reduced by 50% as a result of his CHF. Therefore, CL = 1.3 l/h. Applying equation (12), assuming F=1, S=1, then his predicted C^{ss} is 32 mg/l.
3. You first need an estimate of V_d which from population data = 0.48 l/kg × 65 kg = 31.2 l. Assuming the value of clearance calculation in the previous section and applying equation (6) we find $CL = k_e × V_d$. Therefore 1.3 l/h = 31.2 l × K_e.

Table 1.1 Summary of pharmacokinetic data[a]

Drug	Therapeutic range of serum concentrations	V_d(l/kg)	CL(l/h/kg)	Half-life (h)
Digoxin	0.8–2.0 micrograms/litre 1–2.6 nmol/l	7.3	See text	36
Theophylline	10–20 mg/l 55–110 µmol/l	0.48	0.04	8
Gentamicin	Peak 5–12 mg/l, trough < 2 mg/l	0.25	1 × CL (creatinine)	2
Lithium	0.4–0.8 mmol/l	0.5–1	0.2 × CL (creatinine)	18
Phenytoin	10–20 mg/l 40–80 µmol/l	1	K_m = 6 mg/l V_{max} = 7 mg/kg/day	
Carbamazepine	4–12 mg/l 17–50 µmol/l	0.8–1.9	0.05–1	
Phenobarbital	15–40 mg/l 65–172 µmol/l	0.7–1	0.004	120
Primidone	< 15 mg/l < 69 µmol/l	0.6		
Valproate	< 100 mg/l < 693 µmol/l			
Ciclosporin	200–400 micrograms/litre			9

[a] Estimates based on the average patient. See text for variability.

Therefore $k_e = 0.042$ h^{-1}. Applying equation (8) using this k_e value gives a half-life of 16.5 h. It will take one half-life (16.5 h) for the theophylline level to fall to 16 mg/l, which is within the therapeutic range.

Case 1.2

Miss J.M. is a 50 kg woman taking phenytoin at a dose of 100 mg three times a day for the last 2 months and is seen at out-patients complaining of blurred vision and exhibiting nystagmus. Her phenytoin level is 25 mg/l.

Questions

1. Calculate V_{max} and K_m values for this patient.
2. Calculate the dose required to achieve a level of 12 mg/l.
3. Check your answer using the orbit graph.
4. How long will it take for the level to fall within the therapeutic range?

Answers

1. From population data $V_{max} = 7$ mg/day/kg $\times$ 50 kg = 350 mg/day. Substitute this into equation (15) using the measured C^{ss} of 25 mg/l and her current dose of 300 mg/day, and assuming $S = 0.9$ Solve for $K_m = 7.4$ mg/l.
2. Substitute these Km and V_{max} values into equation (15) with a desired C^{ss} of 12 mg/l and assume $S = 0.9$. This gives a dose of 240 mg day. This could be rounded up to 250 mg per day. (Note: to half the level does not mean halving the dose since phenytoin exhibits non-linear kinetics.)
3. Using the orbit graph (Fig. 1.7) the new dosage would be 250 mg/day after correcting for S.
4. At supra-therapeutic levels it can be assumed that metabolism is occurring at V_{max}. By dividing V_{max} (amount eliminated from the body per day) by V_d (volume of distribution) you can calculate rate of fall of blood level; V_d can be calculated from population data $V_d = 1$ l/kg $\times$ 50 kg = 50 l. Therefore, concentration falls at a rate of

$$\frac{350 \text{ mg/day}}{50 \text{ l}} = 7 \text{ mg/l per day}$$

Therefore, withhold dosage for 1 day to allow the levels to fall from 25 mg/l to $25 - 7 = 18$ mg/l, before starting new regimen.

Case 1.3

A 35-year-old 55 kg patient is commenced on gentamicin i.v. in a dose of 80 mg every 8 hours. Unfortunately, the hospital guidelines have not been followed and the blood levels taken 1 hour and 4 hours after the first dose are 4.5 mg/l and 2.3 mg/l, respectively. Your advice is sought on an appropriate regimen.

Questions

1. Calculate the patient's pharmacokinetic parameters of K_e, half-life and V_d.

2. Calculate a new regimen to achieve a peak level of 9 mg/l and a trough level of 1 mg/l.

Answers

1. Since you have blood level data taken after effectively a single dose, you can use this to calculate the patient's parameters. Substitute the two blood levels and the time between them (3 h) into equation (7) and solve for k_e

$$2.3 \text{ mg/l} = 4.5 \text{ mg/l} \times e^{-k_e \times 3}$$
$$\ln 2.3 = \ln 4.5 - k_e \times 3$$
$$0.83 = 1.5 - k_e \times 3$$

Therefore $K_e = 0.22$ h^{-1}.

Substitute this into equation (8) to obtain half-life = 3.15 hours. To find V_d we need to know the blood level immediately after the dose was given (you cannot use the 1 h value). Therefore, substitute either the 1 h level or the 4 h level as C_2 into equation (7) with the appropriate time (1 or 4 h) and the k_e (0.22 h^{-1}) to find C_1 which is the concentration at time 0 = 5.6 mg/l. Substitute this into equation (10) to find $V_d = 14.2$ l.
2. The first part of the regimen is the time interval. Substitute the desired peak and trough (9 and 1) into equation (7) with K_e calculated in the previous section (0.22 h^{-1}) and solve for $t = 10$ h. This is the time between the peak and trough. The peak is measured 1 h post-dose, therefore the dose interval is 11 h. The nearest practical dose interval would be 12 h.
   We now need to calculate the actual C^{ss}_{max} immediately after the dose is given. Substitute 9 mg/l (the desired 1 h post-dose level) as C_2 in equation (7) where $t = 1$ and solve for C_1.
   This will give a C^{ss}_{max} of 11.25 mg/l.
   Substitute this into equation (13) with a dose interval of 12 h and solve for dose = 148 mg. Check C^{ss}_{min} using equation (14). A practical dose would be 140 mg 12 hourly.

Case 1.4

Mr E.F., a 77-year-old 67 kg man, is admitted in uncontrolled atrial fibrillation. The doctor decides to commence him on digoxin, but is unsure of the dosage in view of his age. He seeks your views. The patient has a serum creatinine level of 140 µmol/l.

Questions

1. Calculate a suitable loading dose for this patient.
2. Calculate a suitable maintenance dose for this patient.

Answers

1. Since the patient is elderly, first calculate his creatinine clearance using the Cockroft & Gault (1976) equation, since this will be used in calculation of both volume of distribution and maintenance dose.

$$CL(\text{creatinine}) = \frac{1.23 \times [(140 - 77) \times 67]}{140}$$
$$= 37.1 \text{ ml/min}$$

Since renal function is relatively low, use $V_d = 3.8 \times$ Lean Bwt $+ (3.1 \times$ creatinine clearance).

Therefore $V_d = 254 + 115 = 369$ l (compare this V_d to that calculated from body weight only).

To calculate the appropriate loading dose substitute 369 l into equation (11) where desired concentration is 1.5 micrograms/litre using F for digoxin tablets = 0.65. Solve for dose = 850 micrograms. A practical dose of 750 micrograms will suffice. Check using equation (10) to show it will produce a level of 1.32 micrograms/litre.

2. To calculate maintenance dose substitute the estimated creatinine clearance 37.1 ml/min into the equation.

Digoxin clearance = 0.8 × Bwt + creatinine clearance which gives a value of 90.7 ml/min. Convert into l/h = 5.44 l/h. Substitute this into equation (12) and solve for dose ($F = 0.65$, $T = 24$ h, and desired C^{ss} is 1.5 micrograms/litre) which gives a dose of 299 micrograms per day. The nearest practical dose is 312.5 (1 × 250 micrograms and 1 × 62.5 microgram tablet). 250 micrograms per day would also suffice to produce a level of 1.24 micrograms/litre.

REFERENCES

Cockroft D W, Gault M H 1976 Prediction of creatinine clearance from serum creatinine. Nephron 16: 31–41

Crist K D, Nahata M C, Ety J 1987 Positive impact of a therapeutic drug monitoring program on total aminoglycoside dose and hospitalisation. Therapeutic Drug Monitoring 9: 306–310

Evans W E, Shentag J J, Jusko W J (eds) 1992 Applied pharmacokinetics, 3rd edn. Applied Therapeutics, Spokane, pp. 586–617

McFadyen M L, Miller R, Juta M et al 1990 The relevance of a first world therapeutic drug monitoring service to the treatment of epilepsy in third world conditions. South African Medical Journal 78: 587–590

Nicolau D P, Freeman C D, Belliveau P P et al 1995 Experience with a once daily aminoglycoside program administered to 2,184 adult patients. Antimicrobial Agents and Chemotherapy 39: 650–655

Reid L D, Horn J R, McKenna D A 1990 Therapeutic drug monitoring reduces toxic drug reactions: a meta-analysis. Therapeutic Drug Monitoring 12: 72–78

FURTHER READING

Begg E J, Barclay M L, Duffull S B 1995 A suggested approach to once daily aminoglycoside dosing. British Journal of Clinical Pharmacology 39: 605–609

Elwes R D C, Binnie C D 1996 Clinical pharmacokinetics of newer antiepileptic drugs. Clinical Pharmacokinetics 30(6): 403–415

Jermain D M, Crismon M L, Martin E S 1991 Population pharmacokinetics of lithium. Clinical Pharmacy 10(5): 376–381

Lemmer B, Bruguerolle B 1994 Chronopharmacokinetics: are they clinically relevant? Clinical Pharmacokinetics 26(6): 419–427

Luke D R, Halstenson C E, Opsahl J A et al 1990 Validity of creatinine clearance estimates in the assessment of renal function. Clinical Pharmacology and Therapeutics 48: 503–508

Rambeck B, Boenigk H E, Dunlop A et al 1980 Predicting phenytoin dose: a revised nomogram. Therapeutic Drug Monitoring 1: 325–354

Tserng K, King K C, Takieddine F N 1981 Theophylline metabolism in premature infants. Clinical Pharmacology and Therapeutics 29: 594–600

Winter M E 1990 Basic clinical pharmacokinetics, 2nd edn. Applied Therapeutics, Vancouver

Yukawa E 1996 Optimisation of antiepileptic drug therapy: the importance of serum drug concentration monitoring. Clinical Pharmacokinetics 31(2): 120–130

Drug interactions 2

A. Lee   I. H. Stockley

KEY POINTS

- Clinically significant drug interactions are an uncommon but none the less important cause of morbidity.
- Most clinically important drug interactions occur as a result of either decreased drug activity with diminished efficacy or increased drug activity with exaggerated or unusual effects. Drugs with a narrow therapeutic range, such as theophylline, lithium and digoxin, are often implicated.
- The most important pharmacokinetic interactions involve drugs that can induce or inhibit enzymes in the hepatic cytochrome P450 system. Pharmacists should be aware of frequently used drugs with these properties.
- Pharmacodynamic interactions are difficult to classify but their effects can often be predicted when the pharmacology of co-administered drugs is known.
- In many cases potentially interacting drugs can be given concurrently provided the possibility of interactions is kept in mind and any necessary changes to dose or therapy initiated promptly. In some situations, however, concurrent use of potentially interacting drugs should be avoided altogether.
- Clinical pharmacists should reduce the impact of adverse drug interactions on patient care by having a sound understanding of the drugs most commonly involved, the most important mechanisms and the most vulnerable patients.

Drug interactions are an increasingly important cause of adverse drug reactions (ADR) and it is vital that pharmacists have a sound understanding of the issue. This problem was recognized over 100 years ago, when it was noted that an adrenal extract, when given to a dog anaesthetized with chloroform, could cause arrhythmias. Today, with the increasing availability of complex therapeutic agents and widespread polypharmacy, the potential for drug interactions is enormous. Despite rigorous attempts to ensure that the safety profile of new medicines is as fully defined as possible at the time they are marketed, the potential for adverse interactions is not always evident. This was illustrated by the worldwide withdrawal of the calcium channel blocker mibefradil, within months of launch, following reports of serious drug interactions (Li Wan Po & Zhang 1998). More recently there has been concern about the risk of important drug interactions with bupropion (amfebutamone), used in smoking cessation (Cox et al 2001). Patients are now more likely to self-treat with herbal and other complementary preparations and awareness of their involvement in drug interactions is increasing. For example, a growing body of evidence has emerged to implicate the herbal preparation St John's wort as a cause of serious interactions due to its enzyme inducing properties.

Although the medical literature is awash with case reports of adverse drug interactions, serious problems occur infrequently. However, there are so many potential interactions that continued vigilance by pharmacists is essential. The pharmacist should be able to anticipate when a potential drug interaction might have clinically significant consequences for the patient and, in such situations, be able to advise on how to minimize the risk of harm, for example by recommending an alternative treatment in order to avoid the combination of risk, or by making a dose adjustment, or by monitoring the patient closely. To do this effectively the pharmacist needs to have a practical knowledge of the pharmacological mechanisms involved in drug interactions and an awareness both of high risk drugs and of the most vulnerable patient groups.

Definition

An interaction is said to occur when the effects of one drug are changed by the presence of another drug, food, drink or an environmental chemical agent (Stockley 1999). The net effect of the combination may be:

- synergism or additive effect of one or more drugs
- antagonism of effect of one or more drugs
- alteration of effect of one or more drugs or the production of idiosyncratic effects.

When a therapeutic combination could lead to an unexpected change or complication in the condition of the patient, this would be described as an interaction of potential clinical significance. Although recognized drug interactions are sometimes used with the aim of therapeutic benefit, in this chapter we are concerned only with drug–drug interactions which have the potential to adversely affect patient care.

Epidemiology

It is difficult to give an accurate estimate of the incidence of drug interactions, mainly because published studies have frequently used different criteria for definition, particularly in distinguishing between clinically significant and non-significant interactions. Some of the early studies uncritically compared prescribed drugs with lists of possible drug interactions without taking into account their potential clinical significance. A review of nine studies of the epidemiology of drug–drug interactions in hospital admissions found that the reported incidence ranged from 0% to 2.8% (Jankel & Fitterman 1993). However, the authors considered all studies reviewed to be flawed to some extent. In the Harvard Medical Practice study of adverse events, 20% of events in acute hospital in-patients were drug related. Of these, 8% were considered to be due to a drug interaction, suggesting that interactions are responsible for fewer than 2% of adverse events in this patient group (Leape et al 1992). Few studies have attempted to quantify the incidence of drug–drug interactions in the community. A US community pharmacy study revealed a 4.1% incidence of interactions (Rupp et al 1992), while in a Swedish study the incidence was 1.9% (Linnarsson 1993). Although the overall incidence of adverse drug interactions is probably quite low (< 1%), it is still a considerable problem in terms of the global number of patients at risk and the potential for morbidity and mortality.

Susceptible patients

Certain patients are at increased risk of drug interactions. Polypharmacy is common, and the more drugs a patient takes the greater is the likelihood of an ADR. One hospital study found an ADR rate of 7% in patients taking 6–10 drugs, increasing to 40% in those taking 16–20 drugs (Smith et al 1969). This exponential rise is partly due to drug interactions. Drug interactions are more likely to have serious consequences when they affect elderly or seriously ill patients. Patients at particular risk include those with hepatic or renal disease, those on long-term therapy for chronic disease, for example those with human immunodeficiency virus (HIV) infection, epilepsy or diabetes, those in intensive care, transplant recipients, patients undergoing complicated surgical procedures and those with more than one prescribing doctor. Critically ill and elderly patients are at increased risk not only because they take more medicines, but also because of impaired homoeostatic mechanisms that might otherwise counteract some of the unwanted effects. Interactions

may occur in some individuals but not in others. The effects of interactions involving drug metabolism may vary greatly in individual patients because of differences in the rates of drug metabolism and in susceptibility to microsomal enzyme induction. Certain drugs are frequently implicated in drug interactions and require careful attention. These are listed in Table 2.1.

Mechanisms of drug interactions

Drug interactions are conventionally discussed according to the mechanisms involved. There are some situations where drugs interact by unique mechanisms, but certain mechanisms are encountered time and time again. These mechanisms can be conveniently divided into those with a pharmacokinetic basis and those with a pharmacodynamic basis. Drug interactions often involve more than one mechanism.

Pharmacokinetic interactions

Pharmacokinetic interactions are those which can affect the processes by which drugs are absorbed, distributed, metabolized or excreted. There is marked inter-individual variability in these processes, and although these interactions may be expected, their extent cannot easily be predicted. Such interactions may result in a change in the drug concentration at the site of action with subsequent toxicity or decreased efficacy.

Table 2.1 Some drugs with high risk of interaction

Concentration dependent toxicity
Digoxin
Lithium
Aminoglycosides
Cytotoxic agents
Warfarin

Steep dose-response curve
Verapamil
Sulphonylureas
Levodopa

Patient dependent on therapeutic effect
Immunosuppressives, e.g. ciclosporin, tacrolimus
Glucocorticoids
Oral contraceptives
Antiepileptics
Antiarrhythmics

Saturable hepatic metabolism
Phenytoin
Theophylline

Absorption

Most drugs are given orally for absorption through the mucous membranes of the gastrointestinal tract. Most of the interactions which occur within the gut result in reduced rather than increased absorption. It is important to recognize that the majority result in changes in the absorption rate, although in some instances the total amount (i.e. the extent) of drug absorbed is affected. For drugs which are given chronically on a multiple dose regimen (for example the oral anticoagulants) the rate of absorption is usually unimportant provided the total amount of drug absorbed is not markedly altered. On the other hand, delayed absorption can be clinically significant where the drug affected has a short half-life, or where it is important to achieve high plasma concentrations rapidly, as may be the case with analgesics or hypnotics. Drug absorption interactions can often be avoided if an interval of 2–3 hours is allowed between the administration of the interacting drugs.

Changes in gastrointestinal pH. The absorption of a drug across mucous membranes depends on the extent to which it exists in the non-ionized, lipid-soluble form. The ionization state depends on the pH of its milieu, the pKa of the drug and formulation factors. Weakly acidic drugs, such as the salicylates, are better absorbed at low pH because the unionized form predominates. An alteration in gastric pH due to antacids, histamine H_2 antagonists or proton pump inhibitors therefore has the potential to affect the absorption of other drugs. The clinical significance of antacid-induced changes in gastric pH is not certain, particularly since relatively little drug absorption occurs in the stomach. Changes in gastric pH tend to affect the rate of absorption rather than the total bioavailability, provided that the drug is acid labile. Theoretically antacids could be expected markedly to influence the absorption of other drugs via this mechanism, but in practice there are very few clinically significant examples. Antacids, histamine H_2 antagonists and omeprazole can significantly decrease the bioavailability of ketoconazole and itraconazole, as both require gastric acidity for optimal absorption. The absorption of fluconazole, however, is not significantly altered by changes in gastric pH. The alkalinizing effects of antacids on the gastrointestinal tract are transient and the potential for interaction may be minimized by leaving an interval of 2–3 hours between the antacid and the potentially interacting drug.

Adsorption, chelation and other complexing mechanisms. Certain drugs react directly within the gastrointestinal tract to form chelates and complexes which are not absorbed. The drugs most commonly implicated in this type of interaction include tetracyclines and the quinolone antibiotics which can complex with iron, and antacids containing calcium, magnesium and aluminium. Tetracyclines can chelate with divalent or trivalent metal cations such as calcium, aluminium, bismuth and iron to form insoluble complexes, resulting in greatly reduced serum tetracycline concentrations.

Bisphosphonates such as etidronate are often co-prescribed with calcium supplements in the treatment of osteoporosis. If these are ingested concomitantly, the bioavailability of both is significantly reduced with the possibility of therapeutic failure (Fogelman et al 1986).

The absorption of some drugs may be reduced if they are given with adsorbents such as charcoal or kaolin, or anionic exchange resins such as colestyramine or colestipol. The absorption of propranolol, digoxin, warfarin, tricyclic antidepressants, ciclosporin and thyroxine is reduced by colestyramine. Acarbose, an agent used in the management of diabetes mellitus, inhibits intestinal alpha glucosidase, thereby delaying the digestion and absorption of starch and sucrose. Case reports suggest that this drug can significantly decrease plasma concentrations of digoxin. Digoxin levels increased to within the therapeutic range after acarbose was discontinued (Ben-Ami et al 1999). Patients taking both acarbose and digoxin should separate dosing by an interval of at least 6 hours. Most chelation and adsorption interactions can be circumvented by separating doses of the interacting drugs by a period of several hours.

Drug effects on the gastrointestinal flora. Bacterial flora predominate in the large bowel, and are present in much smaller numbers in the stomach and small bowel. Thus drugs which are well absorbed from the small bowel are less likely to be affected by changes in gut flora. In about 10% of individuals a substantial amount of digoxin is inactivated by gut bacteria, and the introduction of a broad-spectrum antibiotic may lead to substantially increased plasma digoxin concentrations. Antibiotics may also prevent the intestinal bacterial hydrolysis of drug conjugates secreted into bile and thus reduce reabsorption of the active parent drug. In this way, antibiotics may reduce the enterohepatic circulation of ethinylestradiol in oral contraceptives, leading to reduced circulating oestrogen levels with the potential for therapeutic failure. This is likely to be an extremely rare interaction; the enterohepatic circulation of ethinylestradiol is probably of very minor importance in most people, as judged from data from women with ileostomies.

Effects on gastrointestinal motility. Since most drugs are largely absorbed in the upper part of the small intestine, drugs which alter the rate at which the stomach empties its contents can affect absorption. Anticholinergic drugs delay gastric emptying. These drugs are commonly used in the control of movement disorders but they have been shown to reduce the bioavailability of levodopa by as much as 50% and to reduce plasma chlorpromazine concentrations significantly. Other drugs with anticholinergic effects that might influence gastrointestinal motility include tricyclic antidepressants, phenothiazines, and some antihistamines.

Opioids such as diamorphine and pethidine strongly inhibit gastric emptying and greatly reduce the absorption rate of paracetamol. Codeine, however, has no significant effect on paracetamol absorption. Morphine and diamorphine have been shown to reduce the absorption of antiarrhythmics such as mexiletine in patients with myocardial infarction. Metoclopramide increases gastric emptying and increases the absorption rate of paracetamol, an effect which is used to therapeutic advantage in the treatment of migraine. It also accelerates the absorption of propranolol, mefloquine, lithium, and ciclosporin. In general, this type of interaction is rarely clinically significant (Greiff & Rowbotham 1994).

Drug displacement (protein-binding) interactions

Once absorbed a drug is distributed to its site of action and during this process it may interact with other drugs. In practice the main mechanism behind such interactions is displacement from protein-binding sites. A drug displacement interaction is defined as a reduction in the extent of plasma protein binding of one drug caused by the presence of another drug, resulting in an increased free or unbound fraction of the displaced drug. Many drugs and their metabolites are highly bound to plasma proteins. Albumin is the main plasma protein to which acidic drugs such as warfarin are bound, while basic drugs, such as tricyclic antidepressants, lidocaine (lignocaine), disopyramide and propranolol, are generally bound to α_1-acid glycoprotein. Displacement from these proteins can be demonstrated in vitro for many drugs and in the past it was thought to be an important mechanism underlying many interactions. Current evidence suggests that, for most drugs, if displacement occurs, then the concentration of free drug will rise temporarily, but metabolism and distribution will return the free concentration to its previous level. The time this takes will depend on the half-life of the displaced drug. The biological significance of the short-term rise of free concentration is generally of minor importance but may need to be taken into account in therapeutic drug monitoring. For example, if a patient taking phenytoin is given a drug which displaces some phenytoin from its binding sites, the total (i.e. free plus bound) plasma phenytoin concentration will fall even though the free (active) concentration remains the same. There are few examples of clinically important interactions which are entirely due to protein-binding displacement. It has been postulated that a sustained change in steady state free plasma concentration could arise with the parenteral administration of some drugs which are extensively bound to plasma proteins and non-

restrictively cleared (i.e. the efficiency of the eliminating organ is high). Drugs meeting these criteria include alfentanil, fentanyl, hydralazine, lidocaine (lignocaine), midazolam and verapamil. However, no documented cases of problems in clinical practice as a result of such interactions have been found (Rolan 1994, Sansom & Evans 1995).

Drug metabolism

Most clinically important interactions involve the effect of one drug on the metabolism of another. Metabolism refers to the process by which drugs and other compounds are biochemically modified to facilitate their degradation and subsequent removal from the body. The liver is the principal site of drug metabolism although other organs, such as the gut, kidneys, lung, skin and placenta, are involved. Drug metabolism consists of phase I reactions, such as oxidation, hydrolysis and reduction, and phase II reactions, which primarily involve conjugation of the drug with substances such as glucuronic acid and sulphuric acid. Phase I metabolism generally involves the hepatic CYP450 mixed function oxidase system.

Cytochrome P450 isoenzymes. The cytochrome P450 system comprises about 40–50 isoenzymes, each derived from the expression of an individual gene. As there are many different isoforms of these enzymes a classification for nomenclature has been developed (Anon 2000, Slaughter & Edwards 1995, Horsmans 1997). Four main subfamilies of P450 isoenzymes are thought to be responsible for most (about 90%) of the metabolism of commonly used drugs in humans, CYP1, CYP2, CYP3 and CYP4. Individual isoenzymes that have been specifically identified are given a further number (e.g. CYP2D6; this is the most extensively studied isoenzyme, debrisoquine hydroxylase). Although there is overlap, each CYP isoenzyme tends to metabolize a discrete range of substrates. Of the many isoenzymes, just a few (CYP1A2, CYP2C9, CYP2C19, CYP2D6, CYP3A3, and CYP3A4) seem to be responsible for the metabolism of most commonly used drugs. The genes which encode specific CYP isoenzymes can vary between individuals and, sometimes, ethnic groups. These variations (polymorphisms) may affect metabolism of substrate drugs. For example, some people have CYP2D6 isoenzymes with decreased or absent activity and so have reduced capacity to metabolize drugs, such as nortriptyline, that are substrates for this enzyme, leading to their accumulation during therapy and an increased risk of adverse effects.

The effect of a CYP isoenzyme on a particular substrate can be altered by interaction with other drugs. Drugs may be themselves substrates for a CYP isoenzyme and/or may inhibit or induce the isoenzyme. In most instances, oxidation of a particular drug is brought about by several

CYP isoenzymes and results in the production of several metabolites. So, inhibition or induction of a single isoenzyme would have little effect on plasma levels of the drug. However, if a drug is metabolized primarily by a single CYP isoenzyme, inhibition or induction of this enzyme would have a major effect on the plasma concentrations of the drug. For example, if erythromycin (an inhibitor of CYP3A4) is taken by a patient being given carbamazepine (which is extensively metabolized by CYP3A4), this may lead to toxicity due to higher concentrations of carbamazepine. Table 2.2 gives examples of some drug substrates, inducers and inhibitors of the major CYP450 isoenzymes.

Enzyme induction. The most powerful enzyme inducers in clinical use are the antibiotic rifampicin and antiepileptic agents such as barbiturates, phenytoin and carbamazepine, the last being able to induce its own metabolism (autoinduction) (see also Table 2.2). Cigarette smoking, chronic alcohol use and the herbal preparation St John's wort can also induce drug-metabolizing enzymes. Since the process of enzyme induction requires new protein synthesis, the effect usually develops over several days or weeks after starting an enzyme inducing agent. Similarly, the effect generally persists for a similar period following drug withdrawal. Enzyme inducing drugs with short half-lives

Table 2.2   Some drug substrates, inducers, and inhibitors of the major cytochrome P450 enzymes

P-450 isoform	Substrate	Inducer	Inhibitor
CYP1A2	Amitriptyline Imipramine Theophylline *R*-warfarin	Omeprazole Cigarette smoke	Fluvoxamine Ciprofloxacin Cimetidine
CYP2A6	Halothane	Phenytoin	Tranylcypromine
CYP2C9	Diazepam Diclofenac Fluvastatin Losartan *S*-warfarin	Barbiturates Carbamazepine Dexamethasone Primidone Rifampicin St John's wort	
CYP2C19	Citalopram Omeprazole	Rifampicin	Omeprazole Tranylcypromine
CYP2D6	Amitriptyline Codeine Dihydrocodeine Flecainide Fluoxetine Haloperidol Imipramine Nortriptyline Olanzapine Propranolol Risperidone Thioridazine Venlafaxine	Quinidine	Amiodarone Cimetidine Ritonavir SSRIs (selective serotonin reuptake inhibitors)
CYP2E1	Enflurane Halothane	Alcohol (chronic) Isoniazid	Cimetidine Disulfiram
CYP3A4	Amiodarone Terfenadine Ciclosporin Corticosteroids Oral contraceptives Tacrolimus *R*-warfarin	Carbamazepine Phenytoin Barbiturates Dexamethasone Primidone Rifampicin St John's wort	Erythromycin Itraconazole Cimetidine Ketoconazole Fluconazole Ritonavir
CYP4A1	Testosterone	Clofibrate	

(e.g. rifampicin) will induce metabolism more rapidly than inducers with longer half-lives (e.g. phenytoin) because they reach steady state concentrations more rapidly. Enzyme induction usually results in a decreased pharmacological effect of the affected drug, except perhaps in the case of drugs with active metabolites. The effects of enzyme induction vary considerably between patients, and are dependent upon age, genetic factors, concurrent drug treatment and disease state. There is evidence that the enzyme-induction process is dose dependent, although some drugs may induce enzymes at any dose. Some examples of interactions due to enzyme induction are shown in Table 2.3.

Enzyme inhibition. Enzyme inhibition is an extremely common mechanism behind drug interactions. Just as some drugs can stimulate the activity of CYP450 enzymes, there are many which have the opposite effect and act as inhibitors. The rate of metabolism of drugs given concurrently can be reduced and they begin to accumulate within the body. Some enzyme inhibitors are shown in Table 2.4. Enzyme inhibition appears to be dose-related; inhibition of metabolism of the affected drug begins as soon as sufficient concentrations of the inhibitor appear in the liver, and the effects are usually maximal when the new steady state plasma concentration is achieved. Thus, for drugs with a short half-life, the effects may be seen within a few days of administration of the inhibitor. The effects are not seen until later for drugs with a long half-life. The clinical significance of this type of interaction depends on various factors, including dosage (of both drugs), alterations in pharmacokinetic properties of the affected drug, such as a half-life, and patient characteristics such as disease state. Interactions of this type are again most likely to affect drugs with a narrow therapeutic range, such as theophylline, ciclosporin, oral anticoagulants and phenytoin. For example, the initiation of treatment with an enzyme inhibitor such as ciprofloxacin or cimetidine in a patient taking chronic theophylline could result in a doubling of plasma concentrations. The ability to inhibit drug metabolism may be related to specific chemical structures. For example, a number of known enzyme inhibitors contain an imidazole ring, including cimetidine, ketoconazole, itraconazole, metronidazole and omeprazole. Some examples of interactions due to enzyme inhibition are shown in Table 2.5.

Predicting interactions involving metabolism. Predicting drug interactions is not easy because individual drugs in the same class may have different effects on an isoenzyme. For example, the quinolone antibiotics ciprofloxacin and norfloxacin inhibit CYP1A2 and have been reported to increase plasma theophylline levels, whereas lomefloxacin is a much weaker inhibitor and appears not to interact in this way. The relationship between drugs and the cytochrome P450 system is often tested early in drug development using in vitro techniques. Increasingly, the resulting information about potential drug interactions is included in manufacturers' summaries of product characteristics. However, the clinical significance of these interactions is often unknown. Pharmacists should be aware of the key sources of information on interactions and should use them to help predict and tackle clinically important interactions.

Drug transportation

P-glycoprotein (P-gp) is now known to have a role in drug interactions. A recognized cause of multiple drug resistance in malignant disease, more recent work indicates that P-gp also mediates the transcellular transport of many drugs. It acts as a drug transporter pump in the gut, kidneys and many other organs. There have been several published case reports of macrolide antibiotics increasing blood concentrations of digoxin. Initially the underlying mechanism was not understood as digoxin is renally excreted and not significantly metabolized by the liver. It is now known that digoxin is transported by, and macrolides inhibit, P-gp. If the transport pump is inhibited,

---

Table 2.3 Some examples of interactions due to enzyme induction

Drug affected	Inducing agent	Clinical outcome
Oral contraceptives	Rifampicin Rifabutin Modafinil	Therapeutic failure of contraceptive Additional contraceptive precautions required Increased oestrogen dose required
Ciclosporin	Phenytoin Carbamazepine St John's wort	Decreased ciclosporin levels with possibility of transplant rejection
Paracetamol	Alcohol (chronic)	In overdose, hepatotoxicity may occur at lower doses
Corticosteroids	Phenytoin Rifampicin	Increased metabolism with possibility of therapeutic failure

Table 2.4   Some enzyme inhibitors frequently implicated in interactions

Antibacterials	**Cardiovascular drugs**
Ciprofloxacin	Amiodarone
Erythromycin	Diltiazem
Isoniazid	Quinidine
Metronidazole	Verapamil

Antidepressants	**Gastrointestinal drugs**
Fluoxetine	Cimetidine
Fluvoxamine	Omeprazole
Nefazodone	
Paroxetine	
Sertraline	

Antifungals	**Anti-rheumatic drugs**
Fluconazole	Allopurinol
Itraconazole	Azapropazone
Ketoconazole	Phenylbutazone
Miconazole	

Antivirals	**Other**
Indinavir	Disulfiram
Ritonavir	Propoxyphene
Saquinavir	Sodium valproate

Table 2.5   Some examples of interactions due to enzyme inhibition

Drug affected	Inhibiting agent	Clinical outcome
Anticoagulants (oral)	Ciprofloxacin Clarithromycin	Anticoagulant effect increased and risk of bleeding
Azathioprine	Allopurinol	Enhancement of effect with increased toxicity
Carbamazepine	Cimetidine	Antiepileptic levels increased with risk of toxicity
Phenytoin		
Sodium valproate		
Sildenafil	Ritonavir	Enhancement of sildenafil effect with risk of hypotension

the result will be an increased concentration of the substrate drug in the body. Many, but not all, of the drugs transported by P-gp are also metabolized by CYP3A4 which can confuse the interpretation of interactions. Other common substrates for P-gp are ciclosporin, fluoroquinolones, protease inhibitors, lignocaine, quinidine and ranitidine. Common inhibitors are diltiazem, verapamil and macrolide antibiotics.

Elimination interactions

Most drugs are excreted either in the bile or in the urine. Blood entering the kidneys is delivered to the glomeruli of the tubules where molecules small enough to pass across the pores of the glomerular membrane are filtered through into the lumen of the tubules. Larger molecules, such as plasma proteins and blood cells, are retained. The blood then flows to other parts of the kidney tubules where drugs and their metabolites are removed, secreted or reabsorbed into the tubular filtrate by active and passive transport systems. Interactions can occur when drugs interfere with kidney tubule fluid pH, active transport systems, or blood flow to the kidney thereby altering the excretion of other drugs.

Changes in urinary pH.   As with drug absorption in the gut, passive reabsorption of drugs depends on the extent to which the drug exists in the non-ionized lipid-soluble form. Only the unionized form is lipid soluble and able to diffuse back through the tubule cell membrane. Thus, at alkaline pH weakly acidic drugs (pKa 3.0–7.5) largely exist as unionized lipid-insoluble molecules which are unable to diffuse into the tubule cells and will therefore be lost in the urine. The renal clearance of these drugs is increased if the urine is made more alkaline. Conversely, the clearance of weak bases (pKa 7.5–10) is higher in acid urine. Strong acids and bases are virtually completely ionized over the physiological range of urine pH and their clearance is unaffected by pH changes.

This mechanism of interaction is of very minor clinical significance since most weak acids and bases are inactivated by hepatic metabolism rather than renal excretion. Furthermore, drugs that produce large changes in urine pH are rarely used clinically. Urine alkalinization or acidification has been used as a means of increasing drug elimination in poisoning with salicylates and amphetamines respectively.

Changes in active renal tubule excretion. Drugs which use the same active transport system in the kidney tubules can compete with one another for excretion. Such competition between drugs can be used to therapeutic advantage. For example, probenecid may be given to increase the serum concentration of penicillins by delaying their renal excretion. Increased methotrexate toxicity, sometimes life-threatening, has been seen in some patients concurrently treated with salicylates and some other non-steroidal anti-inflammatory drugs (NSAIDs). The development of toxicity is more likely in patients treated with high dose methotrexate and those with impaired renal function. The mechanism of this interaction may be multifactorial, but competitive inhibition of methotrexate's renal tubular secretion is likely to be involved. If salicylates or NSAIDs are essential in patients treated with methotrexate for malignancy, the dose of methotrexate should be halved. Patients taking low doses for rheumatoid arthritis may take concurrent NSAIDs, but close monitoring for bone marrow toxicity is vital (Brouwers & de Smet 1994).

Changes in renal blood flow. Blood flow through the kidney is partially controlled by the production of renal vasodilatory prostaglandins. If the synthesis of these prostaglandins is inhibited (e.g. by indometacin), the renal excretion of lithium is reduced with a subsequent rise in serum levels. The mechanism underlying this interaction is not entirely clear, as serum lithium levels are unaffected by some potent prostaglandin synthetase inhibitors (e.g. aspirin). If a NSAID is prescribed for a patient taking lithium the serum levels should be closely monitored.

Pharmacodynamic interactions

Pharmacodynamic interactions generally involve additive, synergistic or antagonistic effects of drugs acting on the same receptors or physiological systems. These interactions are much less easy to classify than those with a pharmacokinetic basis.

Antagonistic interactions

It is to be expected that a drug with an agonist action at a particular receptor type will interact with antagonists at that receptor. For example, the bronchodilator action of a selective β_2 adrenoreceptor agonist such as salbutamol will be antagonized by β adrenoreceptor antagonists. There are numerous examples of interactions occurring at receptor sites, many of which are used to therapeutic advantage. Specific antagonists may be used to reverse the effect of another drug at receptor sites; examples include the opioid antagonist naloxone and the benzodiazepine antagonist flumazenil. Alpha-adrenergic agonists such as metaraminol and methoxamine may be used in the management of priapism arising due to excessive α-adrenergic antagonism by phentolamine and related compounds.

Additive or synergistic interactions

If two drugs with similar pharmacological effects are given together, the effects can be additive (see Table 2.6). Although not strictly drug interactions, the mechanism frequently contributes to adverse drug reactions. For example, the concurrent use of drugs with central nervous system (CNS) depressant effects, such as antidepressants, hypnotics, antiepileptics and antihistamines, may lead to excessive drowsiness, yet such combinations are frequently encountered. Combinations of drugs with arrhythmogenic potential, for example antiarrhythmics, neuroleptics, tricyclic antidepressants, and those producing electrolyte imbalance (e.g. diuretics) may lead to ventricular arrhythmias and should be avoided. Another example which has assumed greater importance of late is the risk of ventricular tachycardia and torsade de pointes associated with the concurrent use of more than one drug with the potential to prolong the QT interval on the electrocardiogram (see Chapter 3, Case 3.2).

Interactions due to changes in drug transport mechanisms

The antihypertensive effect of adrenergic neurone blocking drugs such as bethanidine and debrisoquine is prevented or reversed by indirectly acting amines and the tricyclic antidepressants, though these antihypertensives are now seldom used. Tricyclic antidepressants also prevent the re-uptake of noradrenaline (norepinephrine) into peripheral adrenergic neurones so that its pressor effects are increased.

Table 2.6   Some additive or synergistic interactions

Interacting drugs	Pharmacological effect
NSAID and warfarin	Increased risk of bleeding
ACE inhibitors and K-sparing diuretic	Increased risk of hyperkalaemia
Verapamil and β-adrenergic antagonists	Bradycardia and asystole
Neuromuscular (NM) blockers and aminoglycosides	Increased NM blockade
Alcohol and benzodiazepines	Increased sedation
Thioridazine and halofantrine	Increased risk of QT interval prolongation
Clozapine and co-trimoxazole	Increased risk of bone marrow suppression

Interactions due to disturbances in fluid and electrolyte balance

Changes in electrolyte balance may alter the effects of drugs, particularly those acting on the myocardium, neuromuscular transmission and the kidney. An important interaction is the potentiation of the effects of cardiac glycosides such as digoxin by diuretics and other drugs which decrease plasma potassium concentrations. Similarly, diuretic induced hypokalaemia increases the risks of ventricular arrhythmias associated with antiarrhythmic drugs such as sotalol, procainamide, quinidine and amiodarone. Angiotensin-converting enzyme (ACE) inhibitors have a potassium sparing effect, such that the concurrent use of potassium supplements or potassium sparing diuretics may lead to dangerous hyperkalaemia. Coadministration of tacrolimus with potassium sparing diuretics and potassium supplements can also lead to life-threatening hyperkalaemia, especially in patients with renal failure.

Lithium intoxication can be precipitated by the use of diuretics, particularly thiazides and metolazone, and ACE inhibitors. NSAIDs can also precipitate lithium toxicity, mainly due to NSAID inhibition of prostaglandin-dependent renal excretion mechanisms. NSAIDs also impair renal function and cause sodium and water retention, effects which can predispose to interactions. Many case reports describe the antagonistic effects of NSAIDs on diuretics and anti-hypertensive drugs. The combination of triamterene and indometacin appears particularly hazardous as it may result in acute renal failure. NSAIDs may also interfere with the beneficial effects of diuretics and ACE inhibitors in heart failure. It is not unusual to see patients whose heart failure has deteriorated in spite of increased doses of furosemide (frusemide) who are also concurrently taking an NSAID.

Indirect pharmacodynamic interactions

There are many indirect pharmacodynamic interactions of potential clinical significance. In insulin-dependent diabetics the normal recovery from an episode of hypoglycaemia may be impaired to some extent by propranolol. In addition, the hypoglycaemic effects of the sulphonylureas may occasionally be reduced by β-adrenoreceptor antagonists. Non-selective β-blockers block the mobilization of glucose from the liver so that recovery from hypoglycaemia is delayed. They can also block β_2 receptors in the pancreas that mediate insulin release, preventing the effects of the sulphonylureas. These interactions have been well studied and marked effects on blood glucose control appear to be unusual. Patients whose diabetes is controlled by insulin or oral hypoglycaemics can be treated with selective β-blockers, but they should be aware that the familiar warning signs of hypoglyacaemia may be masked and blood glucose should be carefully monitored.

Monoamine-oxidase inhibitors. Monoamine-oxidase inhibitors (MAOIs) reduce the breakdown of noradrenaline (norepinephrine) in the adrenergic nerve ending. This leads to the nerve ending having large stores of noradrenaline (norepinephrine) which can be released into the synaptic cleft in response to either a neuronal discharge or an indirectly acting amine. The action of directly acting amines – adrenaline (epinephrine), isoprenaline, noradrenaline (norepinephrine) – appears to be unchanged or only moderately increased in patients taking MAOIs, although in patients with underlying cardiovascular disease there may be some adverse consequences. In contrast, the concurrent use of MAOIs and indirectly acting sympathomimetic amines (e.g. amphetamines, tyramine, methylenedioxymethamfetamine (MDMA), phenylpropanolamine, pseudoephedrine) can result in a potentially fatal hypertensive crisis. Some of these compounds are contained in proprietary cough and cold remedies. Tyramine is normally present in foodstuffs (e.g. cheese and red wine) and is metabolized in the gut wall by MAO to inactive metabolites. In patients taking MAOIs, however, tyramine will be absorbed intact. If patients taking MAOIs also take these amines there may be a massive release of noradrenaline (norepinephrine) from adrenergic nerve endings with a resulting syndrome of sympathetic overactivity characterized by hypertension, headache, excitement, hyperpyrexia, and cardiac arrhythmias. Fatal intracranial haemorrhage and cardiac arrest may result. The risk of interactions continues for several weeks after the MAOI is stopped as new MAO enzyme must be synthesized. Patients taking irreversible MAOIs should not take any indirectly acting sympathomimetic amines. All patients must be strongly warned about the risks of cough and cold remedies, illicit drug use and the necessary dietary restrictions.

Serotonin syndrome. Serotonin syndrome is a rare condition which is becoming increasingly well recognized in patients receiving combinations of serotonergic drugs (Sporer 1995, Lane & Baldwin 1997). It can occur when two or more drugs affecting serotonin are given at the same time or after one serotonergic drug is stopped and another started. The syndrome is characterized by symptoms including confusion, disorientation, abnormal movements, exaggerated reflexes, fever, sweating, diarrhoea and hypotension or hypertension. Diagnosis is made when three or more of these symptoms are present and no other cause can be found. Symptoms usually develop within hours of starting the second drug but occasionally they can occur later.

Drug-induced serotonin syndrome is generally mild and resolves when the offending drugs are stopped. However, it can be severe and deaths have occurred. A large number of drugs have been implicated including tricyclic antidepressants, monoamine-oxidase inhibitors (MAOIs), selective serotonin re-uptake inhibitors (SSRIs), pethidine, lithium, and dextromethorphan (Gravlin 1997). The most severe type of reaction has occurred with the combination of selective serotonin re-uptake inhibitors and monoamine-oxidase inhibitors. Both non-selective MAOIs such as phenelzine and selective MAOIs such as moclobemide and selegiline have been implicated.

Serotonin syndrome is best prevented by not using serotonergic drugs in combination. Special care is needed when changing from an SSRI to an MAOI and vice versa. The SSRIs, particularly fluoxetine, have long half-lives and serotonin syndrome may occur if a sufficient wash-out period is not allowed before switching from one to the other. When patients are being switched between these two groups of drugs the guidance in manufacturers' summaries of product characteristics should be followed.

Conclusions

It is impossible to remember all drug interactions of potential clinical significance. Practitioners should be continually alert to the possibility of drug interactions and take appropriate steps to minimize their occurrence. In general, where the combination of potentially interacting drugs is unavoidable, the dose of any drug likely to have increased effects as a result of the interaction should be reduced (e.g. by one-third to one-half) and the patient monitored for toxic effects using clinical variables or plasma drug levels for at least 2 weeks or until these are stable. For drugs that are likely to have reduced effects as a result of the interaction, the patient similarly should be monitored for therapeutic failure for at least 2 weeks or until stable, and the dose increased if necessary. Alternatively, it may be appropriate to switch one of the treatments to one which does not interact. Patients should be advised to seek guidance about their medication if they plan to stop smoking or start a herbal remedy, as they may need close monitoring during the transition.

CASE STUDIES

Case 2.1

A 19-year-old woman is well-controlled on carbamazepine 400 mg twice daily for the treatment of epilepsy. When visiting the local community pharmacy to collect her repeat prescription she mentions that she has recently begun taking St John's wort.

Question

What is the nature of the potential drug interaction and what advice do you give?

Answer

St John's wort, a herbal remedy commonly taken for depression, induces activity of CYP1A2, CYP2C9 and CYP3A4, thereby increasing the metabolism and reducing the plasma concentrations of drugs such as warfarin, theophylline, ciclosporin, antiepileptics, oral contraceptives, protease inhibitors, non-nucleoside reverse transcriptase inhibitors and SSRIs. Most herbal remedies are unlicensed and the amount of the active ingredients unregulated, and so the extent of any effect of St John's wort on other drugs is unpredictable. Carbamazepine is a substrate of the CYP3A4 isoenzyme, so its effect may be reduced if St John's wort is taken concurrently and the patient placed at increased risk of seizures.

The UK Committee on Safety of Medicines has issued guidance on the problem of drug interactions between St John's wort and prescribed medicines. This states that a clinically important interaction with carbamazepine is likely and that the combination should not be used. It also suggests that patients already taking the combination should stop the St John's wort and the carbamazepine level should be checked.

Case 2.2

A consultant cardiologist would like to prescribe orlistat for weight reduction for a 56-year-old patient who received a heart transplant several months ago. He is taking amlodipine, fluconazole, atorvastatin, ciclosporin, prednisolone and aciclovir.

Questions

1. Are there likely to be any clinically significant drug interactions?
2. What advice do you give?

Answers

1. There is a potential interaction with ciclosporin. Orlistat inhibits fat absorption and it is possible that it reduces the bioavailability of ciclosporin, a highly lipid-soluble drug. There have been occasional reports of subtherapeutic ciclosporin blood concentrations occurring after initiation of orlistat therapy.
2. Although the effect of separating doses of ciclosporin from orlistat is not known, it would be prudent to give ciclosporin 2 hours before or several hours after the orlistat. If the combination is used, plasma levels of ciclosporin should be carefully monitored when orlistat is initiated, discontinued, or if the dose is changed.

Case 2.3

A customer in the pharmacy asks to buy some cimetidine tablets for dyspepsia. When asked about other medicines she tells you that she is also taking an oral contraceptive and that she is midway through a prescribed course of bupropion (amfebutamone) to help her stop smoking.

Question

Is the sale of over-the-counter (OTC) cimetidine appropriate in this situation?

Answer

No. Bupropion (amfebutamone) has recently been made available as a therapy for smoking cessation and its considerable potential for interaction with other medicines has since been recognized. The main concern relates to a dose-related risk of seizures and an increase of seizures occurring in the presence of factors which lower the seizure threshold.

Cimetidine is known to be a potent inhibitor of the CYP450 enzyme system and it could allow bupropion (amfebutamone)to accumulate in the body if given concurrently. Famotidine and ranitidine do not inhibit liver enzymes and either would be a better choice of H_2 antagonist in this patient.

Case 2.4

A general practitioner asks your advice about prescribing the non-steroidal anti-inflammatory drug celecoxib for osteoarthritis in a 68-year-old man who is also taking warfarin, atenolol and levothyroxine (thyroxine).

Question

Do you anticipate any problems with the addition of celecoxib?

Answer

The combination of celecoxib and warfarin is best avoided as bleeding and increased prothrombin time have been reported. Both celecoxib and warfarin are metabolized through the same cytochrome P450 pathway (CYP2C9) so it is possible that a competitive inhibition could occur, resulting in decreased elimination of either or both drugs. If treatment with celecoxib is considered essential in a patient already taking warfarin the international normalized ratio (INR) should be checked frequently at the start of treatment.

REFERENCES

Anon 2000 Why bother about cytochrome P450 enzymes? Drug and Therapeutics Bulletin 38: 93–95

Ben-Ami H, Krivoy N, Nagachandran P et al 1999 An interaction between digoxin and acarbose. Diabetes Care 22: 860–861

Brouwers J R B, de Smet P A G. 1994 Pharmacodynamic – pharmacokinetic drug interactions with non-steroidal anti-inflammatory drugs. Clinical Pharmacokinetics 27: 462–485

Cox A, Anton C, Ferner R 2001 Take care with Zyban. Pharmaceutical Journal 266: 721

Fogelman I, Smith L, Mazess R et al 1986 Absorption of oral diphosphonate in normal subjects. Clinical Endocrinology 24: 57–62

Gravlin M A 1997 Serotonin syndrome: what causes it, how to recognise it and ways to avoid it. Hospital Pharmacy 32 (4): 570–575

Greiff J M C, Rowbotham D 1994 Pharmacokinetic drug interactions with gastrointestinal motility modifying agents. Clinical Pharmacokinetics 27: 447–461

Horsmans Y 1997 Major cytochrome P450 families: implications in health and liver diseases. Acta Gastro-Enterologica Belgica 60: 2–10

Jankel C A, Fitterman L K 1993 Epidemiology of drug–drug interactions as a cause of hospital admissions. Drug Safety 9 (1): 55–59

Lane R, Baldwin D 1997 Selective serotonin reuptake inhibitor-induced serotonin syndrome: a review. Journal of Clinical Psychopharmacology 17 (3): 208–221

Leape L L, Brennan T A, Laird N et al 1992 The nature of adverse events in hospitalised patients: results of the Harvard Medical Practice Study II. New England Journal of Medicine 324: 377–384

Li Wan Po A, Zhang W Y 1998 What lessons can be learnt from withdrawal of mibefradil from the market? Lancet 351: 1829–1830

Linnarsson R 1993 Drug interactions in primary health care: a retrospective database study and its implications for the design of a computerised decision support system. Scandinavian Journal of Primary Health Care 11: 181–186

Rolan P E 1994 Plasma protein binding interactions – why are they still regarded as clinically important? British Journal of Clinical Pharmacology 37: 125–128

Rupp M T, De Young M, Schondelmeyer S W 1992 Prescribing problems and pharmacist interventions in community practice. Medical Care 30: 926–940

Sansom L N, Evans A M 1995 What is the true clinical significance of plasma protein binding displacement interactions? Drug Safety 12 (4): 227–233

Slaughter R L, Edwards D J 1995 Recent advances: the cytochrome P450 enzymes. Annals of Pharmacotherapy 29: 619–624

Smith J W, Seidl L G, Cluff L E 1969 Studies on the epidemiology of adverse drug reactions. V. Clinical factors influencing susceptibility. Annals of Internal Medicine 65: 629

Sporer K A 1995 The serotonin syndrome. Drug Safety 13 (2): 94–104

Stockley I H 1999 Drug interactions: a source book of adverse interactions, their mechanisms, clinical importance and management, 5th ed. Pharmaceutical Press, London

FURTHER READING

Stockley I H 1999 Drug interactions: a source book of adverse interactions, their mechanisms, clinical importance and management, 5th edn. Pharmaceutical Press, London

Pirmohamed M, Orme M L'E 1998 Drug interactions of clinical importance. In: Davies D M, Ferner R E, and de Glanville H, eds Davies's Textbook of Adverse Drug Reactions, 5th edn. Chapman and Hall Medical, London, ch 33

Fugh-Berman A 2000 Herb–drug interactions. Lancet 355: 134–138

Li Wan Po A 1999 Interactions with over the counter medicines. Prescribers' Journal 39 (4): 249–254

Anon. 2000 Why bother about cytochrome P450 enzymes? Drug and Therapeutics Bulletin 38: 93–95

Adverse drug reactions 3

A. Lee   S. H. L. Thomas

KEY POINTS

- Adverse drug reactions (ADRs) are an important cause of morbidity and mortality. They are responsible for a considerable number of hospital admissions and significantly increase health care costs.
- The World Health Organization defines an adverse drug reaction as any response to a drug which is noxious and unintended and which occurs at doses normally used in man for prophylaxis, diagnosis or therapy.
- Adverse drug reactions can be classified as either type A or type B. Type A (augmented) reactions are normal pharmacological effects which are undesirable. They are usually dose-dependent and fairly predictable. They are an important cause of morbidity, but death is unusual.
- Type B (bizarre) reactions are effects unrelated to the known pharmacology of a drug. These reactions are rare, unpredictable and generally unrelated to dose. Reactions are often severe or fatal.
- Important predisposing factors to adverse drug reactions include extremes of age, polypharmacy, intercurrent disease and genetic factors. Mechanisms of reactions may be pharmaceutical, pharmacokinetic or pharmacodynamic.
- Early recognition of potential adverse drug reactions is critical. Type B reactions are unlikely to be detected during clinical trials. Post-marking surveillance, including spontaneous reporting of suspected adverse drug reactions, is essential for monitoring drug safety.
- The pharmacist should always ensure that medicines are used safely, and should endeavour to minimize the impact of adverse drug reactions on pharmaceutical care. The pharmacist also has an important role in pharmacovigilance procedures.

An adverse drug reaction (ADR) is any undesirable effect of a drug beyond its anticipated therapeutic effects occurring during clinical use (Pirmohamed et al 1998). It has been recognized since the earliest times that drug therapy can be a significant cause of morbidity and mortality. About 400 BC Hippocrates warned of the dangers of drugs, recommending that they should never be prescribed unless the patient had been thoroughly examined. In 1785, when William Withering described the benefits of digitalis, he also described the vomiting, alteration of vision, bradycardia, convulsions and death it could cause. In the 20th century great therapeutic advances were accompanied by a growing awareness of the problem of adverse reactions to medicines among both health care professionals and consumers. In particular, the thalidomide tragedy in the late 1950s and early 1960s was the seminal event leading to the development of modern drug regulation. Thalidomide, prescribed as a 'safe' hypnotic to many thousands of pregnant women, caused a severe form of limb abnormality known as phocomelia in many of the babies born to these women.

Drug-induced disease is rarely specific and almost invariably mimics naturally occurring disease. Few adverse drug reactions are associated with diagnostic clinical or laboratory findings which demarcate them from the features of a spontaneous disease. Moreover, many of the subjective effects frequently attributed to drugs (such as headache, nausea and dizziness) occur commonly in healthy individuals taking no medication and in patients taking a placebo. Pharmacists have a key role in minimizing the occurrence of adverse drug reactions. This requires some knowledge of the adverse effects of drugs, including their frequency and severity, the most common predisposing factors, and the relationship to dosage and duration of treatment. There is a huge literature on adverse drug reactions, including several comprehensive textbooks, and this chapter is no more than an introduction to the subject. It concentrates on the epidemiology, mechanisms and classification of adverse drug reactions, important predisposing factors, and how adverse reactions are identified and evaluated.

Epidemiology

Many studies have attempted to determine the incidence of adverse drug reactions in a variety of settings. The estimates of incidence vary widely and this reflects differences in the methods used to detect suspected reactions and differences in the definition of an ADR. Nevertheless, several important studies in the 1960s helped establish the epidemiological basis of drug-induced disease. One of these was the Boston Collaborative Drug Surveillance Program (BCDSP), which made a great impact in the field; data were collected on over 50 000 consecutive patients admitted to medical wards over a 10-year period (Borda et al 1968). This allowed much original research on the association between short-term drug exposure and acute ADRs to be carried out. In an interim analysis of 19 000 patients monitored there were approximately 171 000 drug exposures and an adverse reaction rate of 30% (Jick 1974). However, many ADRs were minor and the author concluded that drugs were 'remarkably non-toxic'. Detailed analysis of the data provided much information on patient characteristics predisposing to ADRs and allowed some established adverse effects of drugs, such as excessive drowsiness or 'hangover' with flurazepam, to be quantified.

The Harvard Medical Practice study showed that in 1984, 3.7% of 30 195 patients admitted to acute non-psychiatric hospitals experienced adverse reactions during their stay (Brennan et al 1991). Further data from this group suggested a 6% incidence of adverse drug events and a 5% incidence of potential adverse drug events among 4031 medical and surgical admissions over a 6-month period (Bates et al 1995). Of all events observed, 1% were fatal, 12% life-threatening, 30% serious and 57% significant. Of observed adverse drug events, 28% were considered preventable, with a greater proportion of the life-threatening and serious reactions in that category. The drug classes most frequently implicated in those reactions were analgesics, antibiotics, sedatives, cytotoxics, cardiovascular drugs, anticoagulants, antipsychotics, antidiabetics and electrolytes. A recently published study of adverse events in hospital in-patients in Colorado and Utah in 1992 found a similar frequency and type of adverse events to those observed in the Harvard study (Thomas & Brennan 2000). A review of data on nearly 15 000 patients discharged from 28 hospitals in the two states identified adverse events (not necessarily drug related) associated with 2.9% of hospitalizations in each state. Adverse drug reactions were the second most common type of adverse event, accounting for 19.3% of those identified. A quarter (24.9%) of the ADRs were associated with antibiotics, 17.4% with cardiovascular agents, 8.9% with analgesics and 8.6% with anticoagulants. More than a third of the ADRs were considered avoidable and nearly 1 in 10 caused irreversible harm. UK data from a study carried out in Oxford suggested that 7% of over 20 000 medical in-patients experienced an ADR during their stay in hospital (Smith et al 1996).

Adverse reactions to drugs are responsible for a significant number of hospital admissions, with reported rates ranging from 0.3% to as high as 11% (Beard 1992, Lazarou et al 1998). Overall, the incidence of ADR-induced admissions, as estimated from large early studies, is of the order of 3% of medical admissions. For ADRs occurring in the community, the reported

incidence ranges from 2.6% to 41% of patients, but this is a much more difficult area to study and there are fewer well-designed studies (Martys 1979, Mulroy 1973). Despite the problems with definition and incidence studies, ADRs undoubtedly increase hospital admission rates, increase morbidity and mortality, and have a significant impact on health care costs. Two recent US studies showed that the length of hospital stay was significantly greater in patients who experienced an ADR while in hospital (Classen et al 1997, Bates et al 1997). Both studies estimated substantial cost implications: the Classen study estimated that the occurrence of an ADR increased the cost of patient care by $2262 per patient and Bates et al estimated the cost of preventable ADRs in a 700-bed hospital to be $2.8 million per annum.

Definition and classification

An adverse drug reaction has been defined by the World Health Organization as 'any response to a drug which is noxious, unintended and occurs at doses used in man for prophylaxis, diagnosis or therapy'. There are several ways of classifying adverse reactions, but the simplest is to separate them into types A and B as proposed by Rawlins and Thompson in 1977 (Table 3.1). Type A reactions are the result of an exaggerated, but otherwise normal, pharmacological action of a drug given in the usual therapeutic doses. Examples include bradycardia with a β adrenoreceptor blocker, haemorrhage with anticoagulants or hypoglycaemia with a sulphonylurea. Type A reactions are predictable from a drug's known pharmacology. They are usually dose-dependent and their incidence and morbidity are generally high. Their mortality, however, is usually (but not invariably) low. Some type A adverse reactions have a long latency. Examples include teratogenicity, chloroquine retinopathy, and delayed effects such as the vaginal clear-cell adenocarcinoma which may occur in the daughters of women who received diethylstilbestrol during pregnancy.

In contrast, type B reactions are aberrant effects that are not to be expected on the basis of a drug's pharmacology. Examples include malignant hyperthermia of anaesthesia, acute porphyria and many immunological reactions. Type B reactions are generally unrelated to dosage and, although comparatively rare, they often cause serious illness and death. These reactions are often not observed during conventional pharmacological and toxicological screening programmes and consequently they account for many drug withdrawals from the market.

It has been suggested that the type A and B classification be extended by adding types C (chronic, long-term effects), D (delayed effects), E (end of use or

Table 3.1 Comparison between type A and type B adverse drug reactions (Rawlins & Thompson 1977, Rawlins & Thomas 1998)

	Type A augmented response	Type B (bizarre response)
Pharmacologically predictable	Yes	No
Dose-dependent	Yes	No
Incidence	High	Low
Morbidity	High	Low
Mortality	Low	High
Management	Dosage adjustment often appropriate	Stop

withdrawal effects) and F (failure of therapy) (Edwards & Aronson 2000). In our view these additional classes do not assist in understanding either the mechanisms of ADRs or their management.

Predisposing factors

Factors predisposing to ADRs may relate either to the properties of the drug or to the characteristics of the patient.

Multiple drug therapy

The incidence of adverse drug reactions and interactions has been shown to increase sharply with the number of drugs taken. This suggests that the effects of multiple drug use are not simply additive. There is likely to be a synergistic effect, but the concept of confounding by multiple disease states must be borne in mind.

Age

The very old and the very young are more susceptible to adverse drug reactions. The elderly often have multiple and chronic disease and are major consumers of medicines. They are particularly vulnerable to the adverse effects of drugs because of the physiological changes that accompany ageing. Most studies have shown a positive correlation between age and the number of adverse drug reactions but this is a complex issue (Castleden & Pickles 1988, Lawson 1998, Thomas & Brennan 2000). It is difficult to determine whether age alone renders these patients more susceptible to ADRs or whether this simply reflects increased drug exposure, multiple disease states and age-related pharmacokinetic changes. Drug metabolism is impaired in the elderly. In

fit elderly people, changes in the rates of drug metabolism are mainly due to the age-related decrease in liver blood flow and liver mass. Consequently there is greater systemic exposure to drugs which normally undergo substantial biotransformation in the liver during absorption. In the frail elderly there appears to be, in addition, a reduction in the intrinsic hepatic drug-metabolizing activity, which increases their vulnerability to type A reactions (Kinirons & Crome 1997). There is also evidence that age-related pharmacodynamic changes make the elderly more sensitive to the effects of some drugs. Adverse reactions in elderly patients often present in a vague, non-specific fashion. Mental confusion, constipation, hypotension and falls may be the presenting features of illness but may also suggest ADRs. Drugs which commonly cause problems in elderly patients include hypnotics, diuretics, non-steroidal anti-inflammatory drugs, antihypertensives, psychotropics and digoxin.

All children, and particularly neonates, differ from adults in the way they handle and respond to drugs. Some drugs are particularly likely to cause problems in neonates but are generally well tolerated in older children, for example morphine. Others are associated with an increased risk of problems in children of any age, for example sodium valproate. Hazardous drugs for neonates include chloramphenicol, morphine and antiarrhythmics. Specific examples of concern in children are Reye's syndrome with aspirin and hepatotoxicity with sodium valproate (Choonara et al 1996).

Gender

Women may be generally at greater risk of ADRs than men; increased drug exposure does not seem to account for this difference. Women are reputed to be more susceptible to blood dyscrasias with phenylbutazone and chloramphenicol, to histaminoid reactions to neuromuscular blocking drugs, to reactions involving the gastrointestinal tract and to drug-induced prolongation of the QT interval on the electrocardiogram (Lawson 1998).

Intercurrent disease

Patients with impaired renal or hepatic function are at substantially increased risk of developing ADRs to drugs eliminated by these organs. There are, however, specific disease states which may predispose to adverse drug reactions, such as human immunodeficiency virus (HIV)-positive patients who suffer an increased incidence of the adverse effects of co-trimoxazole. Immune deficiency is a complex clinical area with multiple drug exposures, multiple illness events and consequent difficulty in interpreting drug toxicity data.

Race and genetic polymorphism

Inherited factors that affect the pharmacokinetics of numerous drugs are of great importance in determining an individual's risk of ADR. The discipline of pharmacogenetics deals with those variations in drug response that are under hereditary control. Genetic variations in genes for drug metabolizing enzymes, drug receptors and drug transporters have been associated with individual variability in the efficacy and toxicity of drugs (Meyer 2000). These genetic polymorphisms of drug metabolism produce the phenotypes of 'poor metabolizers' or 'rapid metabolizers' of numerous drugs. Polymorphisms in the cytochrome P450 enzymes in the liver can have a profound effect on drug efficacy. In poor metabolizers the genes encoding specific cytochrome P450 enzymes often contain inactivating mutations, which result in a complete lack of active enzyme and a severely compromised ability to metabolize drugs.

All pharmacogenetic variations studied to date occur at different frequencies among sub-populations of different ethnic or racial origins. This ethnic diversity implies that ethnic origin has to be considered in pharmacogenetic studies and in pharmacotherapy.

Mechanisms of type A adverse drug reactions

The individual response to drugs shows great variation. This is manifest either as different doses being required to produce the same pharmacological effect, or as different responses to a defined dose. Such inter-individual variation is the basis of type A adverse reactions. Dose-related adverse reactions may occur because of variations in the pharmaceutical, pharmacokinetic or pharmacodynamic properties of a drug, and are often due to the underlying disease state or pharmacogenetic characteristics of the patient (Rawlins & Thomas 1998). In some cases a combination of these causes may be responsible.

Pharmaceutical causes

Adverse reactions can occur due to pharmaceutical aspects of a dosage from either because of alterations in the quantity of drug present, or in its release characteristics. As a result of stringent requirements laid down by regulatory authorities, such reactions are now rare in developed countries. In 1983 a rate-controlled preparation of indometacin (Osmosin) was withdrawn following the receipt of a significant number of reports of gastrointestinal bleeding and haemorrhage. This was probably due to the irritant effects of a very high concentration of the active ingredient on a localized area of intestinal mucosa.

Pharmacokinetic causes

Quantitative alterations in the absorption, distribution, metabolism and elimination of drugs may lead to alterations in the concentration of a drug at its site of action with corresponding changes in its pharmacological effects. Such alterations may produce either an exaggerated response or therapeutic failure as a consequence of abnormally low drug concentrations.

Absorption

Differences in both the rate and extent of drug absorption may cause adverse effects. Factors which can influence the extent of absorption of a drug include dosage, pharmaceutical factors, gastrointestinal tract motility, the absorptive capacity of the gastrointestinal mucosa, and first-pass metabolism in the liver and gut wall before it reaches the systemic circulation. The rate of absorption of orally administered drugs is largely determined by the rate of gastric emptying, which is influenced by factors including the nature of the gastric contents, disease and concomitant drugs. The majority of adverse reactions resulting from changes in drug absorption are reduced therapeutic efficacy or therapeutic failure.

Distribution

The distribution of drugs to various tissues and organs is dependent on factors including regional blood flow, plasma protein and tissue binding. Changes in how a drug is distributed may, theoretically, predispose to adverse effects, although the clinical importance of such mechanisms is unclear.

Elimination

Most drugs are excreted in the urine or bile or metabolized by the liver to yield metabolites which are then excreted by the kidneys. Changes in drug elimination rates are probably the most important cause of type A adverse drug reactions. Reduced elimination leads to drug accumulation, with potential toxicity due to increased plasma and tissue levels. Conversely, enhanced elimination leads to reduced plasma and tissue drug levels, resulting in therapeutic failure.

Renal excretion

Impaired glomerular filtration leads to reduced elimination of drugs which undergo renal excretion. Individuals with reduced glomerular filtration (such as patients with intrinsic renal disease, the elderly and neonates) are liable to develop type A adverse reactions to 'normal' therapeutic doses of drugs which are mainly excreted by the kidney. Some of the most potentially toxic drugs in this respect are digoxin, ACE inhibitors, aminoglycoside antibiotics, some class I antiarrhythmic agents (disopyramide, flecainide), and many cytotoxic agents. The occurrence of these ADRs may be minimized by adjusting the dosage given to individual patients on the basis of their renal function.

Drug metabolism

Lipid-soluble agents are frequently metabolized to water-soluble compunds which then undergo excretion by the kidney. Metabolism occurs predominantly in the liver, although the kidney, lungs, skin and gut also have some metabolizing capacity. In man, drug metabolism can be divided into two phases. Phase I (oxidation, reduction or hydrolysis) exposes functionally reactive groups or adds them to the molecule. Phase II (sulphation, glucuronidation, acetylation or methylation) involves conjugation of the drug at a reactive site produced during phase I. Drugs that already have reactive groups undergo phase II reactions only. Others are sufficiently water-soluble after phase I metabolism to be eliminated by renal excretion.

Inter-individual differences or alterations in the rate at which drugs are metabolized result in appropriate variations in elimination rates. Reduced rates of metabolism may lead to drug accumulation and an increased risk of type A adverse drug reactions, while enhanced rates of metabolism may result in therapeutic failure. There is wide inter-individual variation in some routes of metabolism, even among normal individuals, because of genetic and environmental influences. This particularly applies to oxidation, hydrolysis and acetylation. Competition for glucuronidation may occur when two drugs metabolized by this pathway are given concurrently.

Microsomal oxidation

Drug oxidation occurs mainly in the smooth endoplasmic reticulum of the liver by the cytochrome P450 enzyme system. It is mediated by a group of enzymes known as the cytochrome P450 superfamily. Four main subfamilies of P450 isoenzymes are thought to be responsible for most (about 90%) of the metabolism of commonly used drugs in humans, CYP1, CYP2, CYP3 and CYP4. Individual isoenzymes that have been specifically identified are given a further number (e.g. CYP2D6, which is the most extensively studied isoenzyme, debrisoquine hydroxylase). Although there is overlap, each CYP isoenzyme tends to metabolize a discrete range of substrates. Of the many isoenzymes, just a few (CYP1A2, CYP2C9, CYP2C19, CYP2D6, CYP3A3 and CYP3A4) seem to be responsible for the metabolism of most commonly used drugs. The genes which encode specific CYP isoenzymes can vary between individuals and, sometimes, ethnic groups.

Inter-individual variability in debrisoquine metabolism is well-recognized. Poor metabolizers tend to have reduced first-pass metabolism, increased plasma levels, and exaggerated pharmacological response to this drug, resulting in postural hypotension. By contrast, rapid metabolizers may require considerably higher doses for a standard effect. The antidepressants nortriptyline and desipramine are metabolized by similar mechanisms to those of debrisoquine and as a result the steady state plasma levels reached with these drugs are dependent on the individual's phenotype. The enzyme showing polymorphism in this situation is debrisoquine hydroxylase or CYP2D6. This enzyme is inactive in about 6% of white people. In the UK several million people are thus at risk of compromised metabolism or ADRs when prescribed drugs that are CYP2D6 substrates. Many such drugs are used in the treatment of psychiatric, neurological and cardiovascular diseases. Clinical problems can also arise from the co-administration of drugs that inhibit or compete for CYP2D6. A drug may interact with and inhibit CYP2D6 to the extent that it is no longer functionally active, resulting in a patient responding like a poor metabolizer even though he or she has an extensive metabolizer genotype. Thus quinidine, a powerful CYP2D6 inhibitor, may exaggerate the effects of other drugs that are prescribed concomitantly or may prevent the metabolic activation of drugs such as codeine by CYP2D6. Genotyping the CYP2D6 enzyme to assist individual dose selection for psychiatric drugs is currently the most widely accepted application of pharmacogenetic testing.

The potential effects of enzyme induction and inhibition on other drugs are discussed in the chapter on drug interactions (see Chapter 2).

Hydrolysis

Suxamethonium apnoea is the best-known example of an alteration in drug response due to individual variation in drug hydrolysis. The neuromuscular blocking effects of suxamethonium are usually short lived, as the drug is rapidly inactivated in plasma by hydrolysis. The hydrolysis is catalysed by plasma pseudocholinesterase which exists in several different genetically determined forms. Individuals homozygous for the atypical gene (about 1 in 2500 of the UK population) may develop prolonged neuromuscular blockade. Suxamethonium apnoea may also be somewhat prolonged in individuals who are heterozygous for the gene (i.e. who possess both the usual and the atypical gene). The frequency of the atypical genes shows marked racial variation. Phenotypic studies of patients who develop prolonged neuromuscular blockade after suxamethonium do not always reveal recognizable genetic abnormalities. In some instances these type A reactions are secondary to liver or renal disease, both of which can influence the activity of plasma cholinesterase.

Acetylation

A number of drugs are metabolized by acetylation including dapsone, isoniazid, hydralazine, phenelzine, procainamide and many sulphonamides. Acetylation is under genetic control and shows a polymorphism such that individuals may be phenotyped as either 'slow' or 'rapid' acetylators. The variability is due to differences in the activity of the liver enzyme N-acetyltransferase. In the UK about half the population are rapid acetylators, but there are considerable racial differences. The incidence of rapid acetylation is highest among the Japanese and among Canadian Inuit.

Slow acetylators are at increased risk of developing type A adverse reactions. Thus, isoniazid-induced peripheral neuropathy, the haematological adverse effects of dapsone, and the adverse effects of sulfapyridine are more likely to occur in these individuals. Slow acetylators of hydralazine and procainamide are also at greater risk than fast acetylators of developing systemic lupus erythematosus.

Glucuronidation

Several drugs commonly used in clinical practice (e.g. morphine, paracetamol, and ethinylestradiol) are eliminated at least partly by glucuronide conjugates. There is evidence that, like the CYP450 enzyme system, glucuronyltransferases exist in multiple forms with many drugs acting as substrates for more than one isoenzyme. Glucuronyltransferases are also inducible and the administration of an inducing drug can lead to loss of efficacy of combined oral contraceptives.

Pharmacodynamic causes

Many, if not most, type A ADRs have a pharmacokinetic basis. Some, however, are due to enhanced sensitivity of target organs or tissues. Moreover, in some individuals, ADRs may result from a combination of the two mechanisms. The reasons why tissues from different individuals should respond differently to drugs are still largely unknown, but evidence is accumulating to show that target organ sensitivity is influenced by the drug receptors themselves, by physiological homoeostatic mechanisms and by disease (Rawlins & Thomas 1998).

Mechanisms of type B adverse drug reactions

Type B reactions are inexplicable in terms of the normal pharmacology of the drug. The cause may be pharmaceutical or pharmacokinetic, or may lie in target organ response (pharmacodynamic).

Pharmaceutical causes

Pharmaceutical apects of the medicine itself may be the cause of type B adverse reactions. Such reactions can occur due to the presence of degradation products of the active constituents, the effects of the non-drug components of the formulation, such as excipients and other compounds (i.e. colourings, preservatives and antioxidants), or the actions of synthetic by-products of the active constituents. In most cases the administration of a decomposed drug will result in therapeutic failure, but in some cases the decomposition product may be toxic and potentially lethal (e.g. earlier formulations of tetracycline). Adverse reactions have resulted from the incorporation of clearly toxic substances such as diethylene glycol (which caused 105 deaths in the USA in 1937 when it was used as a solvent in sulphanilamide elixir); the use of certain excipients in susceptible patient groups, such as asthmatics or neonates; and the alteration of an excipient mixture resulting in changes in the bioavailability of drugs such as digoxin and phenytoin. A number of adverse reactions caused by pharmaceutical excipients are recognized.

Nowadays, with stringent manufacturers' controls and monitoring by regulatory authorities, it is extremely unusual for pharmaceutical preparations to be adulterated with synthetic by-products. A relatively recent example is the potentially fatal syndrome of eosinophilia and myalgia associated with L-tryptophan, which was probably due to a contaminant, although genetic factors may have been involved.

Pharmacokinetic causes

There are no documented type B adverse reactions that can be attributed to abnormalities of absorption or distribution. However, there is, emerging evidence that to suggest that the bioactivation of drugs to yield reactive species is responsible for a significant proportion of type B adverse effects (Knowles et al 2000). Binding of such reactive metabolites may result in either direct or immune-mediated toxicity (Pirmohamed et al 1994). Examples of type B reactions postulated to occur as a result of bioactivation to reactive metabolites include tacrine (hepatotoxicity), clozapine (agranulocytosis), halothane (hepatotoxicity) and carbamazepine (hypersensitivity reactions). The reasons why only some individuals develop such type B reactions remains unclear. Suspectible people may have overactive or underactive specific bioinactivation pathways, or immunological characteristics that render them more responsive to haptogens or immunogens.

Pharmacodynamic causes

Individual patients vary widely in their responses to drugs. Even after allowance has been made for the patient's age, gender, bodyweight, disease state and concurrent drug regimens there is still variation between individuals. Qualitative differences in the target organ response to drugs may be considered as genetic, immunological, neoplastic or teratogenic.

Genetic causes for abnormal response

Many type B adverse reactions have been labelled as idiosyncratic reactions that were assumed to be due to some qualitative abnormality in the patient. Until recently, drug 'idiosyncrasies' have tended to form a 'dustbin'category for ADRs that could not be classified under any other heading. This situation is now changing slowly as their underlying mechanisms are better understood and it is becoming apparent that many have a genetic basis (Table 3.2 gives some examples).

Erythrocyte glucose-6-phosphate dehydrogenase (G6PD) deficiency

A well known example of qualitative difference in the response to drugs is G6PD deficiency, which affects between 100 and 400 million people worldwide. G6PD is an enzyme required for the stability of red blood cells. Individuals with a sex-linked inherited deficiency in this enzyme have weakened red cell membranes and are predisposed to haemolysis due to oxidant drugs such as primaquine, sulphonamides and sulphones, and nitrofurantoin. There are many variants of G6PD and not all are associated with drug-induced haemolysis. The frequency of the enzyme deficiency also varies widely between and within various populations. The African type G6PD (A⁻) is characterized by mild enzyme deficiency with a mean activity of 8–20% of normal. The Mediterranean type, on the other hand, is characterized

Table 3.2 Examples of genetically determined adverse reactions

Condition	Drug	Effects
Erythrocyte enzyme deficiencies • Glucose-6-phosphate dehydrogenase • Methaemoglobin reductase	Oxidant drugs (see Table 3.3) Oxidant drugs (see Table 3.3)	Haemolytic anaemia Methaemoglobinaemia
Haemoglobin variants • Haemoglobin H, Zurich, Torino • Haemoglobin Zurich	Oxidant drugs (see Table 3.3) Sulphonamides	Haemolytic anaemia Haemolytic anaemia
Porphyria (hepatic)	Barbiturates, sulphonamides, griseofulvin	Precipitates attack of porphyria
Malignant hyperthermia	General anaesthetics (halothane) Muscle relaxants	Hyperthermia with prolonged muscle rigidity, acidosis
Genetic predisposition to raised intraocular pressure	Topical corticosteroids	Increased intraocular pressure
Familial dysautonomia (Riley–Day syndrome)	General anaesthetics Parasympathomimetics	Exaggerated reponse

by severe enzyme deficiency (0–4% enzyme activity). Consequently, a potentially haemolytic drug is likely to produce only mild haemolysis in patients with the African type, but it may have severe and potentially fatal effects in patients with the Mediterranean type. Many drugs have been associated with haemolysis in G6PD deficiency, but the severity of the reaction varies between drugs and also depends on the type of enzyme deficiency. Haemolytic episodes can be provoked by drugs or illness in G6PD-deficient individuals and some drugs have been wrongly implicated as a cause of haemolysis. The number of currently available medicines with proven haemolytic potential in G6PD-deficient individuals is relatively small; primaquine is probably the best-known example. Drugs that should be avoided in G6PD deficiency are shown in Table 3.3.

Hereditary methaemoglobinaemias

An inherited deficiency of methaemoglobin reductase in erythrocytes renders affected individuals susceptible to the development of methaemoglobinaemia and cyanosis in response to oxidant drugs. Drugs that are oxidizing agents, nitrites, and all of the drugs listed in Table 3.3 may have this effect.

Porphyrias

The porphyrias are a heterogeneous group of inherited disorders of haem biosynthesis. The disorders are transmitted as autosomal dominants, with the exception of the rare congenital porphyria, which is recessive. The effects of drugs are of most importance in patients with acute porphyrias, in whom certain commonly prescribed agents may precipitate life-threatening attacks. Other trigger factors include alcohol and endogenous and exogenous steroid hormones. In the acute porphyrias, patients develop abdominal and neuropsychiatric disturbances, and they excrete in their urine excessive amounts of the porphyrin precursors 5-aminolaevulinic acid (ALA) and porphobilinogen. A number of drugs may induce excess porphyrin synthesis. However, it is extremely difficult to predict whether or not a drug will cause problems in patients with porphyria and the only factors shown to be clearly linked with porphyrinogenicity are lipid solubility and membrane fluidization (i.e. the ability to disrupt the phospholipid bilayer of the cell membrane). A number of commonly used drugs induce ALA synthetase in the liver, but there is wide variation between porphyric patients in their sensitivity to drugs which may trigger attacks. Thus, whereas a single dose of a drug may be sufficient to trigger an acute attack in one patient, another may require a number of relatively large doses of the same drug to produce any clinically significant effect. Lists of drugs which are known to be unsafe and drugs which are thought to be safe for use in acute porphyria are available in the British National Formulary.

Malignant hyperthermia

Malignant hyperthermia is a rare but potentially fatal condition in which there is a rapid rise in body temperature (at least 2°C per hour) occurring without obvious cause after administration of anaesthetics or muscle relaxants. The condition usually follows the administration of an inhalational general anaesthetic, often halothane, in combination with suxamethonium. In addition to the temperature rise, the syndrome is characterized by stiffness of skeletal muscles, hyperventilation, acidosis, hyperkalaemia and signs of increased activity of the sympathetic nervous system. It is likely that the condition is triggered by an abnormal release of intracellular ionized calcium, which may be due to an inherited defect of cellular membranes. The condition is associated with a mortality rate of up to 40%.

Glucocorticoid glaucoma

In genetically predisposed individuals, glucocorticoids can cause a rise in intraocular pressure leading to blindness. Development of increased intraocular pressure appears to be correlated with dosage, and may persist for several months after stopping steroid treatment. It is important to remember that this complication may arise in patients treated with glucocorticoid eye drops.

Cholestatic jaundice induced by oral contraceptives

Oral contraceptives are known to cause jaundice in some women, especially during the first month of medication; this recovers rapidly on discontinuation of treatment. Available evidence suggests that a genetic component is important for the development of the reaction. The underlying mechanism for this reaction is unclear, but it

Table 3.3 Drugs to be avoided in G6PD deficiency
Dapsone
Niridazole
Methylthioninium chloride (Methylene blue)
Primaquine
Quinolones (including ciprofloxacin, nalidixic acid, norfloxacin and ofloxacin)
Sulphonamides (including co-trimoxazole)

is likely that oestrogen-induced changes in the composition of the hepatocyte membrane are involved.

Immunological reasons for abnormal response

Some drugs (e.g. peptides of foreign origin such as streptokinase) are immunogenic and may cause immunological reactions in their own right (Assem 1998). Drug allergy is the most frequently encountered type of immunological adverse reaction. True allergic reactions are immunologically mediated effects. The features of these reactions are:

- there is no relation to the usual pharmacological effects of the drug
- there is often a delay between the first exposure to the drug and the occurrence of the subsequent adverse reaction
- very small doses of the drug may elicit the reaction once allergy is established
- the reaction disappears on withdrawal of the drug
- the illness is often recognizable as a form of immunological reaction.

Allergic reactions vary from rash, serum sickness and angio-oedema to life-threatening bronchospasm and hypotension associated with anaphylaxis. Many factors influence the development of allergic reactions. Patients with a history of atopic or allergic disorders are at greatest risk. Table 3.4 lists some examples of adverse reactions with an immunological basis.

Delayed adverse effects of drugs

A number of adverse effects may only become apparent after long-term treatment, for example the relatively harmless melanin deposits in the lens and cornea that are seen after years of phenothiazine treatment and which should be distinguished from pigmentary retinopathy, a dose-related adverse effect occurring within several months of initiation of treatment. Other examples include the development of vaginal carcinoma in the daughters of women given diethylstilbestrol during pregnancy for the treatment of threatened abortion, and immunosuppressives and chemotherapeutic agents which can induce malignancies that may not be apparent until years after treatment has been given.

Adverse effects associated with drug withdrawal

Some drugs cause symptoms when treatment is stopped abruptly, for example the benzodiazepine withdrawal syndrome, rebound hypertension following discontinuation of antihypertensives such as clonidine and the acute adrenal insufficiency that may be precipitated by the abrupt withdrawal of corticosteroids. These are all type A reactions.

Detection and monitoring of adverse drug reactions

By the time a drug receives a marketing authorization it will usually have been given to an average of 1500 people, and it is likely that clinical trials will have detected only the most common adverse drug reactions. It follows that type B reactions, particularly those with an incidence of 1 in 500 or less, are unlikely to have been identified before the drug appears on the market. It is only after much wider use that rare reactions or those which occur predominantly in certain subgroups within populations, such as the elderly, are detected. It is therefore essential to monitor safety once a drug has been marketed. Some methods used commonly in post-marketing surveillance are described below.

Case reports

The publication of single case reports, or case series, of adverse drug reactions in the medical literature is an important means of detecting new and serious reactions, particularly type B reactions. In the past, case reports

---

Table 3.4 Immunological mechanisms of adverse drug reactions (according to the Coombs and Gell classification, 1968)

Immunological reaction	Immunological mechanism	Clinical manifestation	Drugs
Type I	IgE mediated	Anaphylaxis	Penicillin
Type II	Humoral cytotoxic	Haemolysis	Methyldopa
Type III	Humoral immune complex (IgM, IgG) mediated	Serum sickness Acute glomerulonephritis Systemic lupus erythematosus	Streptokinase Hydralazine
Type IV	Cell-mediated injury	Morbilliform skin eruptions	Amoxicillin

have been vital in alerting the professions to several serious adverse reactions, for example the oculomucocutaneous syndrome associated with practolol and halothane-induced hepatitis. In recent years, published single case reports have become less important with the emergence of formalized spontaneous reporting systems.

Cohort studies

Cohort studies are prospective studies which study the fate of a large group of patients taking a particular drug. The best studies compare adverse event rates in groups of patients taking the drug of intent with a comparative group. Cohort studies include ad hoc investigations set up to investigate specific problems (e.g. the Royal College of General Practitioners' oral contraceptive study), studies sponsored by pharmaceutical companies, prescription event monitoring (PEM), and a variety of record linkage schemes.

Case–control studies

Case–control studies compare drug usage in a group of patients with a particular disease with use among a matched control group who are similar in potentially confounding factors, but who do not have the disease. The prevalence of drug taking is then compared between the groups and a significant excess of drug takers in the disease group may be evidence of an association with the drug. This is a useful retrospective method which can provide valuable information on the incidence of type B reactions and the association between drugs and disease. Examples of associations which have been established by case–control studies are Reye's syndrome and aspirin, and the relationship between maternal diethylstilbestrol ingestion and vaginal adenocarcinoma in female offspring. The case–control method is an effective means for confirming whether or not a drug causes a given reaction once a suspicion has been raised. It is not capable of detecting previously unsuspected adverse reactions.

Spontaneous reporting schemes

The thalidomide tragedy led to the institution, in many countries, of national schemes for the voluntary collection of adverse drug reaction reports. In the UK the Committee on Safety of Medicines (CSM) adverse reactions reporting scheme ('yellow card' scheme) has been operating for more than 30 years. The scheme has received over 300 000 reports of suspected adverse reactions. Doctors and pharmacists are asked to report all suspected serious adverse reactions, and all suspected reactions to newer products (marked with an inverted black triangle symbol in product information and in the British National Formulary). Spontaneous reporting schemes cannot provide estimates of risk because the true number of cases is invariably underestimated, and the denominator (i.e. the total number of patients treated with the drug in question) is not known. However, the CSM's spontaneous reporting scheme has been shown to provide valuable early warnings or signals of possible adverse drug reactions and to enable the study of associated factors. The main advantages of the scheme are:

- it is easily available for all doctors and pharmacists to report
- it covers all therapeutic agents, including vaccines and herbal medicines
- it is capable of detecting both rare and common reactions
- it is relatively inexpensive to operate.

The main disadvantage of the scheme is the level of under-reporting of reactions; it is likely that fewer than 10% of serious reactions are notified. The scheme operates on the basis that reports should be made despite uncertainty about a causal relationship, irrespective of whether or not the reaction is well recognized, and regardless of other drugs having been given concurrently.

Identification of adverse drug reactions

The establishment of a causal relationship between a specific drug and a clinical event is a fundamental problem in adverse reaction assessment. First, adverse drug reactions frequently mimic other diseases and, second, many of the symptoms attributed to them occur commonly in healthy individuals taking no medication. Thus clinicians may fail to recognize the features of an adverse drug reaction because they do not fit into a clearly defined pattern.

When a suspected adverse reaction has occurred, it may be helpful to try to assess whether it is definitely, probably or possibly due to the drug. This process, known as causality assessment, is fraught with difficulties, although some decision on the likelihood that a drug caused a particular reaction is usually taken, perhaps subconsciously in some cases. Various systematic approaches, or algorithms, have been developed in an attempt to rationalize causality assessment of adverse reactions, but these are of limited value.

Factors taken into account when assessing the likelihood of an adverse drug reaction

Where an adverse drug reaction is suspected, a full history – in particular details of other drugs taken by the patient, including over-the-counter and herbal medicines – is important (Gruchalia 2000). The patient should be asked about the nature and timing of the symptom or event, and whether such effects have occurred in the past. The temporal relationship of a suspected adverse drug reaction is important. It is relatively easy to recognize an adverse reaction that occurs soon after drug administration and an event predating prescription is clearly unlikely to be drug related. However, once more than a few weeks have elapsed the association between the drug and the event is more difficult. This is well illustrated by the practolol syndrome. There are very few cases where it is certain that a given drug caused a particular reaction in a specific patient, even though the drug is known to cause the reaction in some recipients. Unlike other conditions in medicine, adverse drug reactions rarely produce characteristic physical signs and laboratory investigations. It is reassuring to find that an adverse reaction resolves once a drug is stopped, but this may take time. Occasionally the adverse reaction is irreversible, as in tardive dyskinesia which may actually deteriorate when the offending drug is withdrawn. Rechallenge sometimes occurs inadvertently but is only rarely justified clinically to confirm a diagnosis. Positive rechallenge is often taken as proof of a causal relationship, but this may not always be the case, particularly where the suspected reaction is subjective in nature.

Patients and adverse drug reactions

There is some evidence that patients themselves are capable of correctly distinguishing probable adverse drug reactions from other types of adverse clinical event (Mitchell et al 1994, Egberts et al 1996). An increasing proportion of patients and their carers wish to be involved in decisions about medication. In an investigation of the attitudes of patients with ankylosing spondylitis, 47% reported serious adverse drug reactions associated with their medication. They regarded insufficient information and inadequate monitoring by the doctor as important causes of adverse drug reactions (O'Brien et al 1990). A recent US study of 2500 hospital out-patients attempted to determine whether patients believed the physician should use discretion in the amount of information given to them on potential adverse drug reactions. It found that most individuals wanted to be told of all possible adverse effects and did not favour physician discretion (Ziegler et al 2001). It seems reasonable to expect that providing education for patients about their drug therapy could assist in preventing or minimizing ADRs. Such intervention needs to be carefully constructed and balanced, with

risks and benefits being kept in perspective. This type of educational initiative is costly but it could turn out to be money well spent in the long term by reducing ADRs and associated morbidity.

The pharmacist's role

Ensuring that medicines are used safely is fundamental to the pharmacist's role. Pharmacists' involvement in patient care should result in prevention of some, and early detection of other ADRs. Recent studies have demonstrated that pharmacist involvement with patients averted a large number of potential adverse reactions (Lesar at al 1997, Leape et al 1999). Based on knowledge of relevant patient and medication factors, pharmacists can ensure that prescribing is as safe as reasonably possible. Medication counselling should include alerting the patient to potential adverse effects. The pharmacist also has a significant role in the education of other health care professionals about the prevention, detection and reporting of ADRs.

Regulatory authorities in many countries accept reports of adverse reactions from pharmacists; in the USA, pharmacists initiate most reports submitted to the Food and Drug Administration (FDA) via the Medwatch system. In the UK, the involvement of hospital pharmacists has been shown to increase the number of yellow cards submitted to the CSM with no discernible difference in the quality of reports submitted from hospital doctors and hospital pharmacists (Lee et al 1997). Similarly, yellow card reports from community pharmacists have been shown to be comparable to those received from GPs (Davis & Coulson 1999). All pharmacists in the UK are now able to contribute to yellow card reporting. Community pharmacists are well placed to assist in monitoring for problems with over-the-counter medicines, complementary therapies and new medicines.

Conclusion

Adverse drug reactions are an inevitable risk associated with the use of modern medicines. However, careful attention to dosage, taking into account factors such as age and renal function, will minimize the risk of type A reactions in many patients. Genetic status should be taken into account in the few cases where this is appropriate, and it is now possible to genotype individuals, using recombinant DNA methods, for some of the known polymorphisms.

CASE STUDIES

Case 3.1

A 45-year-old black man presented at the accident and emergency department with extreme swelling of his lips and surrounding face. His current medication comprised ramipril 5 mg daily, bendroflumethiazide (bendrofluazide) 2.5 mg daily and reboxetine 4 mg twice daily. He had been taking ramipril and bendroflumethiazide (bendrofluazide) for about 6 months and reboxetine for the last 2 months.

Questions

1. What drug-induced complication do these symptoms suggest?
2. How should it be managed?

Answers

1. Angioedema is the term used to describe soft tissue swelling of the eyes, lips and hands; it is a severe form of urticaria. In severe cases the mouth and larynx can be involved. Angioedema is a recognized problem with all angiotensin-converting enzyme (ACE) inhibitors. The estimated incidence is 0.1–0.5% in Caucasians but may be higher in other racial groups.

   In most cases the reaction occurs in the first week of treatment, often within hours of the initial dose. However, in some cases it has developed after prolonged therapy of up to several years. The mechanism of ACE inhibitor-induced angioedema is thought to involve bradykinin, but angiotensin-II receptor antagonists, which do not affect this substance, can also induce angioedema.

2. Treatment of ACE inhibitor-induced angioedema is governed by the severity of the reaction. ACE inhibitors should be withdrawn immediately in any patient presenting with angioedema. In mild cases, with no airway obstruction, withdrawal of the ACE inhibitor may be sufficient. More serious cases may require stabilization of the airway and administration of i.v. corticosteroids, subcutaneous adrenaline (epinephrine) and antihistamines. Affected patients should not receive further treatment with ACE inhibitors. An alternative drug from a different class (not an angiotensin II antagonist) should be substituted. Angioedema has been described in association with angiotensin II antagonists in patients who have previously experienced this problem with an ACE inhibitor. Angiotensin II antagonists should therefore be used with extreme caution in such patients.

Case 3.2

A 58-year-old woman was admitted to hospital for investigation after several episodes of syncope. On admission she was taking tibolone 2.5 mg daily, indapamide 2.5 mg daily, sumatriptan and co-codamol, as necessary, for migraine and mizolastine 10 mg daily for hayfever. The ECG showed a prolonged QT interval (the corrected QT interval, QTc, measured 550 ms). All electrolyte concentrations were normal.

Questions

1. Could any of the current medication have contributed to the patient's problem?
2. How should QT interval prolongation be managed?

Answers

1. A number of drugs have the potential to prolong the QT interval on the electrocardiogram (ECG). The QT interval is an indirect measure of the duration of the ventricular action potential and ventricular repolarization. Prolongation of ventricular repolarization can cause arrhythmias, the most characteristic of which is torsade de pointes (twisting of the points), a specific form of ventricular tachycardia. The name describes the characteristic 'twisting' of the QRS complexes around the electrical axis on the ECG, which can appear as an intermittent series of rapid spikes lasting a few seconds during which the heart fails to pump effectively. This is usually a self-limiting arrhythmia that may cause dizziness or syncope, but it can lead to ventricular fibrillation which can cause sudden death. The cause of malfunction may be genetic (congenital long QT syndrome (LQTS)) or related to metabolic disturbance or drug therapy (acquired LQTS). Drugs are thought to prolong repolarization either by blocking potassium channels and thus delaying potassium outflow, or by enhancing inward sodium or calcium currents. QT prolongation is usually assumed to be present when the QT interval corrected for changes in the heart rate (QTc) is greater than 450 ms (men) or 470 ms (women), although arrhythmias are most often associated with values of 550 ms or more.

   The antihistamine mizolastine has a weak potential to prolong the QT interval in a few individuals. The degree of prolongation is described as modest and cardiac arrhythmias have not been reported. This patient is also taking the diuretic indapamide; diuretic use, independent of electrolyte concentrations, is a known risk factor for torsade de pointes.

2. If a patient is suspected to have drug-induced prolongation of the QT interval, the drug(s) implicated should be stopped immediately. In this case, the patient's syncopal episodes may have been related to an arrhythmia. Some patients with torsade de pointes may be asymptomatic, while others experience dizziness, light-headedness, syncope, collapse, irregular heart beat and palpitations. The arrhythmia should be controlled by accelerating the heart rate, either by atrial pacing or by an isoprenaline infusion. Electrolyte abnormalities should be corrected and magnesium sulphate infusion may effectively terminate the arrhythmia, even in the presence of normal magnesium levels. Antiarrhythmic drugs may worsen the problem and should be avoided. Torsade de pointes that degenerates to ventricular fibrillation requires DC shock for termination.

Case 3.3

A 25-year-old woman presents with a prescription for fexofenadine 120 mg daily for an itchy rash. Patient medication records show that she has been taking carbamazepine 200 mg three times daily for the past 3 months.

Question

What action should be taken?

Answer

Carbamazepine causes skin eruptions in about 3% of patients. Eruptions include erythematous, morbilliform, urticarial or purpuric rashes. Toxic epidermal necrolysis and exfoliative dermatitis are well recognized. The time to onset for these reactions after the initiation of carbamazepine is variable, but is generally 6 months or less.

In this case, it may be that the prescriber has overlooked carbamazepine as a possible cause of the rash. The woman should be questioned about the nature of the rash, whether she has a history of skin disease or allergic reactions, and about other potential trigger factors. The prescriber should be contacted to discuss whether the rash may be drug related. If so, carbamazepine should be stopped.

Case 3.4

A consultant psychiatrist asks your advice about a 49-year-old woman who is taking olanzapine 10 mg daily for schizophrenia. The patient has type 2 diabetes which is managed by diet only. Within 6 weeks of starting olanzapine, the patient noted a deterioration in her blood glucose control. Her fasting blood glucose levels before treatment was started were generally in the range 6–9 mmol/l but have now increased to around 12 mmol/l. The patient has gained 2.5 kg in weight since olanzapine was started.

Questions

1. Is olanzapine likely to have worsened diabetic control in this patient?
2. If so, which alternative antipsychotics may be used?

Answers

1. All atypical antipsychotics are associated with weight gain. Olanzapine has been reported to cause or exacerbate diabetes in several published case reports. The exact cause of glucose dysregulation with olanzapine is unclear, but weight gain does not seem to be the sole aetiology.

   It has been postulated that serotonin ($5-HT_{1A}$) antagonism may decrease the responsiveness of the pancreatic beta cells. This would result in inappropriately low insulin secretion and hyperglycaemia. Further examination of the incidence and aetiology of this problem is needed.
2. Olanzapine is not contraindicated in patients with diabetes, but should be used with careful monitoring of blood glucose control. In this case, where the patient's diabetic control has worsened during therapy, it would be reasonable to discontinue olanzapine and switch to another antipsychotic. Risperidone or quetiapine are alternative atypical antipsychotics not associated with problems in diabetic patients.

REFERENCES

Assem E-S K 1998 Drug allergy and tests for its detection. In: Davis D M, Ferner R E, de Glanville H (eds) Davies's textbook of adverse drug reactions, 5th edn. Chapman and Hall Medical, London, ch 27, pp 790–815

Bates D W, Cullen D J, Laird N et al 1995 Incidence of adverse drug events and potential adverse drug events: implications for prevention. Journal of the American Medical Association 274 (1): 29–34

Bates D W, Spell N, Cullen D J et al 1997 The costs of adverse drug events in hospitalized patients. Journal of the American Medical Association 277: 307–311

Beard K 1992 Adverse reactions as a cause of hospital admission in the aged. Drugs and Aging 2 (4): 356–367

Borda I T, Slone D, Jick H 1968 Boston Collaborative Drug Surveillance Program. Assessment of adverse reactions within a drug surveillance program. Journal of the American Medical Association 205: 645–647

Brennan T A, Leape L L, Laird N et al 1991 The nature of adverse events in hospitalized patients: the results of the Harvard medical practice study II. New England Journal of Medicine 324: 377–384

Castleden C M and Pickles H 1988 Suspected adverse drug reactions in elderly patients reported to the Committee on Safety of Medicines. British Journal of Clinical Pharmacology 26: 347–353

Choonara I, Gill A, Nunn A 1996 Drug toxicity and surveillance in children. British Journal of Clinical Pharmacology 42: 407–410

Classen D C, Pestotnik S L, Evans R S et al 1997 Adverse drug events in hospitalized patients: excess length of stay, extra costs, and attributable mortality. Journal of the American Medical Association 277: 301–306

Coombs R R A, Gell P G H 1968 Classification of allergic reactions responsible for clinical hypersensitivity and disease. In: Gell P G H, Coombs R R A (eds) Clinical aspects of immunology, 2nd edn. Blackwell, Oxford, p. 575

Davies D M, Ferner R E, de Glanville H (eds) 1998 Davies's textbook of adverse drug reactions, 5th edn. Chapman and Hall Medical, London

Davis S, Coulson R 1999 Community pharmacist reporting of suspected ADRs: the first year of the yellow card demonstration scheme. Pharmaceutical Journal 263: 786–788

Edwards I R, Aronson J K 2000 Adverse drug reactions: definitions, diagnosis, and management. Lancet 356: 1255–1259

Egberts T C, Smulders M, de Koning F H, Mayboom R H, Leufkens H G 1996 Can adverse drug reactions be identified earlier? A comparison of reports by patients and professionals. British Medical Journal 313: 530–531

Gruchalia R S 2000 Clinical assessment of drug-induced disease. Lancet 356: 1505–1510

Jick H 1974 Drugs – remarkably non-toxic. New England Journal of Medicine 291: 824

Kinirons M T, Crome P 1997 Clinical pharmacokinetic considerations in the elderly: an update. Clinical Pharmacokinetics 33: 302

Knowles S R, Uetrecht J, Shear N H 2000 Idiosyncratic drug reactions: the reactive metabolite syndromes. Lancet 356: 1587–1591

Lawson D H 1998 Epidemiology. In: Davies D M, Ferner R F, de Glanville H (eds) Davies's textbook of adverse drug reactions, 5th edn. Chapman and Hall Medical, London, ch 2, pp 40–64

Lazarou J, Pomeranz B H, Corey P N 1998 Incidence of adverse drug reactions in hospitalised patients: a meta-analysis of prospective studies. Journal of the American Medical Association 279: 1200–1205

Leape L L, Cullen D J, Clapp M D et al 1999 Pharmacist participation on physician rounds and adverse drug events in the intensive care unit. Journal of the American Medical Association 282: 267–270

Lee A, Bateman D N, Edwards C, Smith J M, Rawlins M D 1997 Reporting of adverse drug reactions by hospital pharmacists: pilot scheme. British Medical Journal 315: 519

Lesar T S, Briceland L, Stein D S et al 1997 Factors related to errors in medication prescribing. Journal of the American Medical Association 277: 312–317

Martys C R 1979 Adverse reactions to drugs in general practice. British Medical Journal ii: 1194–1197

Meyer U A 2000 Pharmacogenetics and adverse drug reactions. Lancet 356: 1667–1671

Mitchell A S, Henry D A, Hennrikus D et al 1994 Adverse drug reactions: can consumers provide early warning? Pharmacoepidemiol Drug Safety 3: 257–264

Mulroy R 1973 Iatrogenic disease in general practice: its incidence and effects. British Medical Journal ii: 407–410

O'Brien B J, Ellswood J, Calin A 1990 Perception of prescription drug risks: a survey of patients with ankylosing spondylitis. Journal of Rheumatology 17: 503–507

Pirmohamed M, Breckenridge A M, Kitteringham N R et al 1998 Adverse drug reactions. British Medical Journal 316: 1295–1298

Pirmohamed M, Kitteringham N R, Park B K 1994 The role of active metabolites in drug toxicity. Drug Safety 11 (2): 114–144

Rawlins M D, Thomas S H L 1998 In: Davies D M, Ferner R E, de Glanville H (eds) Mechanisms of adverse drug reactions. Davies's textbook of adverse drug reactions, 5th edn. Chapman and Hall Medical, London, ch 5, pp 40–64

Rawlins M D, Thompson J W 1977 Pathogenesis of adverse drug reactions. In: Davies D M (ed) Textbook of adverse drug reactions. Oxford University Press, Oxford

Smith C C, Bennett P M, Pearce H M et al 1996 Adverse drug reactions in a hospital general medical unit meriting notification to the Committee on Safety of Medicines. British Journal of Clinical Pharmacology 42: 423–429

Thomas E J, Brennan T A 2000 Incidence and types of preventable adverse events in elderly patients: population based review of medical records. British Medical Journal 320: 741–744

Ziegler D K, Mosier M C, Buenaver M et al 2001 How much information about adverse effects of medication do patients want from physicians? Archives of Internal Medicine 161 (5): 706–713

FURTHER READING

Davies's textbook of adverse drug reactions, 5th edn. Davies D M, Ferner R E, de Glanville H (eds) 1998 Chapman and Hall Medical, London

Edwards I R, Aronson J K 2000 Adverse drug reactions: definitions, diagnosis, and management. Lancet 356: 1255–1259

Pirmohamed M, Kitteringham N R, Park B K 1994 The role of active metabolites in drug toxicity. Drug Safety 11 (2): 114–144

Pirmohamed M, Breckenridge A M, Kitteringham N R et al 1998 Adverse drug reactions. British Medical Journal 316: 1295–1298

Knowles S R, Uetrecht J, Shear N H 2000 Idiosyncratic drug reactions: the reactive metabolite syndromes. Lancet 356: 1587–1591

Gruchalla R S 2000 Clinical assessment of drug-induced disease. Lancet 356: 1505–1510

Meyer U A 2000 Pharmacogenetics and adverse drug reactions. Lancet 356: 1667–1671

Laboratory data 4

H. A. Wynne   C. Edwards

This chapter will consider the common biochemical and haematological tests that are of clinical and diagnostic importance. For convenience, each individual test will be dealt with under a separate heading and a brief review of the physiology and pathophysiology will be given where appropriate to explain the basis of biochemical and haematological disorders.

It is usual for a reference range to be quoted for each individual test (Table 4.1). This range is based on data obtained from a sample of the general population which is assumed to be disease-free. Many test values have a normal distribution and the reference values are taken as the mean ± 2 standard deviations (SD). This includes 95% of the population. The 'normal' range must always be used with caution since it takes little account of an individual's age, sex, weight, height, muscle mass or disease state, many of which variables can influence the value obtained. Although reference ranges are valuable guides, they must not be used as sole indicators of health and disease. A series of values rather than a simple test value may be required in order to ensure clinical relevance and to eliminate erroneous values caused, for example, by spoiled specimens or by interference from diagnostic or therapeutic procedures. Furthermore, a disturbance of one parameter often cannot be considered in isolation without looking at the pattern of other tests within the group.

Further specific information on the clinical and therapeutic relevance of each test may be obtained by referral to the relevant chapter in this book.

Table 4.1   Biochemical data: typical normal adult reference values measured in serum (or plasma)

Laboratory test	Reference range
Urea and electrolytes	
Sodium	135–145 mmol/l
Potassium	3.5–5.0 mmol/l
Calcium (total)	2.15–2.46 mmol/l
Calcium (ionized)	1.19–1.37 mmol/l
Phosphate	0.80–1.44 mmol/l
Creatinine	50–110 µmol/l
Urea	3.0–8.0 mmol/l
Glucose	
Fasting	3.3–6.0 mmol/l
Non-fasting	< 11.0 mmol/l
Glycated haemoglobin	< 5.5%
Liver function tests	
Albumin	38–50 g/l
Bilirubin (total)	< 19 µmol/l
Bilirubin (conjugated)	< 4 µmol/l
Enzymes	
Alanine transaminase	< 60 U/l
Aspartate transaminase	< 35 U/l
Alkaline phosphatase	35–130 U/l
γ-glutamyl transpeptidase	< 70 U/l
Cardiac markers	
Cardiac troponin (cTnT)	< 0.1 microgram/l
Creatine kinase	< 175 U/l
Lactate dehydrogenase	< 430 U/l
Other tests	
Osmolality	282–295 mmol/kg
Uric acid	0.15–0.47 mmol/l

Biochemical data

The homeostasis of various elements, water and acid–base balance are closely linked, both physiologically and clinically. Standard biochemical screening includes several measurements which provide a picture of fluid and electrolyte balance and renal function. These are commonly referred to colloquially as 'U and Es' (urea and electrolytes) and the major tests are described below.

Sodium and water balance

Sodium and water metabolism are closely interrelated both physiologically and clinically, and play a major role in determining the osmolality of serum.

Water constitutes approximately 60% of body weight in men and 55% in women (women have a greater proportion of fat tissue which contains little water). Approximately two-thirds of body water is found in the intracellular fluid (ICF) and one-third in the extracellular fluid (ECF). Of the ECF 75% is found within interstitial fluid and 25% within serum (Fig. 4.1).

In general, water permeates freely between the ICF and the ECF. Cell walls function as semipermeable membranes, with water movement from one compartment to the other being controlled by osmotic pressure: water moves into the compartment with the higher osmotic concentration. The osmotic content of the two compartments is generally the same, i.e. they are isotonic. However, the kidneys are an exception to this rule.

The osmolality of the ECF is largely determined by sodium and its associated anions, chloride and bicarbonate. Glucose and urea have a lesser but nevertheless important role in determining ECF osmolality. Protein (especially albumin) makes only a small (0.5%) contribution to the osmolality of the ECF but is a major factor in determining water distribution between the two compartments. The contribution of proteins to the osmotic pressure of serum is known as the colloid osmotic pressure, or oncotic pressure.

The major contributor to the osmolality of the ICF is potassium.

The amount of water taken in and lost by the body depends on intake, diet, activity and the environment. Over time the intake of water is normally equal to that lost (Table 4.2). The minimum daily intake necessary to maintain this balance is approximately 1100 ml. Of this, 500 ml is required for normal excretion of waste products in urine, while the remaining volume is lost via the skin in sweat, via the lungs in expired air, and in faeces.

Water depletion

Water depletion will occur if intake is inadequate or loss excessive. Excessive loss of water through the kidneys is unusual except in diabetes insipidus or following the overenthusiastic use of diuretics.

Patients with fever will lose water through the skin and ventilated patients will lose it through the lungs. Diarrhoea causes water depletion. Water loss is usually compensated for if the thirst mechanism is intact or can be responded to, but this may not occur in patients who are unconscious, have swallowing difficulties or are disabled. Severe water depletion may induce cerebral dehydration, causing confusion, fits and coma, and circulatory failure can occur.

The underlying cause for the water depletion should be identified and treated. Replacement water should be given orally where possible, or by nasogastric tube, intravenously or subcutaneously if necessary. About two-thirds of the deficit should be corrected within 24 hours and the remainder during the following 24 hours.

Water excess

Water excess is usually associated with an impairment of water excretion such as that caused by renal failure or the

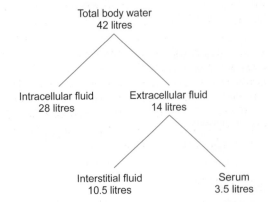

Total body water
42 litres

Intracellular fluid
28 litres

Extracellular fluid
14 litres

Interstitial fluid
10.5 litres

Serum
3.5 litres

Figure 4.1 Approximate distribution of water in a 70 kg man.

Table 4.2 Typical daily water balance for a healthy 70 kg adult				
	Input (ml)		Output (ml)	
Oral fluids	1400	Urine	1500
Food	700	Lung	400
Metabolic oxidation	400	Skin	400
		Faeces	200
Total	2500		2500

syndrome of inappropriate secretion of antidiuretic hormone (SIADH). This syndrome has several causes including chest infections and some tumours. Excess intake is rarely a cause of water excess since the healthy adult kidney can excrete water at a rate of up to 2 ml/min. Patients affected usually present with signs consistent with cerebral overhydration, although if it is of gradual onset, over several days, they may be asymptomatic. Hyponatraemia is usually present.

Water and ECF osmolality

If the body water content changes independently of the amount of solute, osmolality will be altered (the normal range is 282–295 mmol/kg of water). A loss of water from the ECF will increase its osmolality and result in the movement of water from the ICF to ECF. This increase in ECF osmolality will stimulate the hypothalamic thirst centres to promote a desire to drink while also stimulating the release of vasopressin or antidiuretic hormone (ADH). ADH increases the permeability of the renal collecting ducts to water and promotes water reabsorption with consequent concentration of urine.

If the osmolality of the ECF falls, there is no desire to drink and no secretion of ADH. Consequently a dilute urine is produced which helps restore ECF osmolality to normal.

The secretion of ADH is also stimulated by angiotensin II, arterial and venous baroreceptors, volume receptors, stress (including pain), exercise and drugs such as morphine, nicotine, tolbutamide, carbamazepine and vincristine. If blood volume decreases by more than 10% the hypovolaemia stimulates ADH release and overrides control based on osmolality.

Sodium distribution

The body of an average 70 kg man contains approximately 3000 mmol of sodium. Most of this sodium is freely exchangeable and is extracellular. The normal serum range is 135–145 mmol/l. In contrast, the ICF concentration of sodium is only about 10 mmol/l.

Each day approximately 1000 mmol of sodium is secreted into the gut and 25 000 mmol filtered by the kidney. The bulk of this is recovered by reabsorption from the gut and renal tubules. It should be clear therefore that partial failure of homeostatic control can potentially have major consequences.

Sodium and ECF volume

The ECF volume is dependent upon total body sodium since sodium is almost entirely restricted to the ECF, and water intake and loss are regulated to maintain a constant concentration of sodium in the ECF compartment.

Sodium balance is maintained by renal excretion. Normally, 70% of filtered sodium is actively reabsorbed in the proximal tubule, with further reabsorption in the loop of Henle. Less than 5% of the filtered sodium load reaches the distal tubule where aldosterone can stimulate further sodium reabsorption.

Other factors such as natriuretic peptide hormone can also affect sodium reabsorption. This hormone is secreted by the cardiac atria in response to atrial stretch following a rise in atrial pressure associated with, say, volume expansion. It is natriuretic (increases sodium excretion in urine) and, among other actions, reduces aldosterone concentration.

Sodium depletion

Inadequate oral intake of sodium is rarely the cause of sodium depletion although inappropriate parenteral treatment may occasionally be implicated. Sodium depletion commonly occurs with water depletion, resulting in dehydration or volume depletion. The normal response of the body to the hypovolaemia includes an increase in aldosterone secretion (which stimulates renal sodium reabsorption) and an increase in ADH secretion if ECF volume depletion is severe.

The serum sodium level can give an indication of depletion, but it must be borne in mind that the serum sodium may be:

- increased – e.g. where there is sodium and water loss but with predominant water loss, as occurs in excessive sweating
- normal – e.g. where there is isotonic sodium and water loss, as occurs from burns or a haemorrhage
- decreased – e.g. sodium loss with water retention as would occur if an isotonic sodium depletion were treated with a hypotonic sodium solution.

Sodium excess

Sodium excess can be due to either increased intake or decreased excretion. Excessive intake is not a common cause although iatrogenic hypernatraemia can be associated with excessive intravenous saline infusion.

Sodium excess is usually due to impaired excretion. It may also be caused by a primary mineralocorticoid excess (for example Cushing's syndrome or Conn's syndrome), but is often due to a secondary hyperaldosteronism associated with, for example, congestive cardiac failure, nephrotic syndrome, hepatic cirrhosis with ascites, or renal artery stenosis. Sodium and water retention causes oedema.

Hypernatraemia

The signs and symptoms of hypernatraemia include muscle weakness and confusion.

Drug-induced hypernatraemia is often the result of a nephrogenic diabetes insipidus-like syndrome whereby the renal tubules are unresponsive to ADH. The affected patient presents with polyuria, polydipsia or dehydration. Lithium and phenytoin are the most commonly implicated drugs.

- The diabetes insipidus-like syndrome with lithium has been reported after only 2 weeks of therapy. The syndrome is usually reversible on discontinuation. While affected, however, many patients are unresponsive to exogenous ADH.
- Demeclocycline can also cause diabetes insipidus and has been used in the management of patients with the syndrome of inappropriate ADH secretion (SIADH).
- Phenytoin generally has a less pronounced effect on urinary volume than lithium or demeclocycline, and does not cause nephrogenic diabetes insipidus. It inhibits ADH secretion at the level of the central nervous system.

Hypernatraemia can be caused by a number of other drugs (Table 4.3) and by a variety of mechanisms; for example, hypernatraemia secondary to sodium retention is known to occur with corticosteroids while the administration of sodium-containing drugs parenterally in high doses also has the potential to cause hypernatraemia.

Table 4.3   Examples of drugs known to cause hypernatraemia

Adrenocorticotrophic hormone
Anabolic steroids
Androgens
Carbenoxolone
Clonidine
Corticosteroids
Diazoxide
Lactulose
Methyldopa
Oestrogens
Oral contraceptives
Phenylbutazone
Sodium bicarbonate

Hyponatraemia

A fall in the serum sodium level can be the result of sodium loss, water retention in excess of sodium, or a combination of both factors. A number of drugs have also been implicated as causing hyponatraemia (Table 4.4).

The inappropriate secretion of ADH is the mechanism underlying many drug-induced hyponatraemias. In this syndrome the drug may augment the action of endogenous ADH (e.g. chlorpropamide), increase the release of ADH (e.g. carbamazepine), or have a direct ADH-like action on the kidney (e.g. oxytocin). Hyponatraemia can also be induced by mechanisms different from those described above. Lithium may cause renal damage and a failure to conserve sodium. Likewise the natriuretic action of diuretics can predispose to hyponatraemia.

Table 4.4   Examples of drugs known to cause hyponatraemia

Aminoglutethimide
Amitriptyline and other tricyclic antidepressants
Amphotericin
Captopril and other angiotensin-converting enzyme (ACE) inhibitors
Carbamazepine
Chlorpropamide
Cisplatin
Clofibrate
Cyclophosphamide
Diuretics
Heparin
Lithium
Miconazole
Non-steroidal anti-inflammatory drugs (NSAIDs)
Opiates
Oxcarbazepine
Tolbutamide
Vasopressin
Vincristine

Potassium

The total amount of potassium in the body, like sodium, is 3000 mmol. About 10% of the body potassium is bound in red blood cells, bone and brain tissue and is not exchangeable. The remaining 90% of total body potassium is free and exchangeable with the vast majority having an intracellular location. Only 2% of the exchangeable total body potassium is in the ECF, the compartment from which the serum concentration is sampled and measured. Consequently, the measurement of serum potassium is not an accurate index of total body potassium, but together with the clinical status of a patient it permits a sound practical assessment of potassium homeostasis.

The serum potassium concentration is controlled mainly by the kidney with the gastrointestinal tract normally having a minor role. The potassium filtered in the kidney is almost completely reabsorbed in the proximal tubule. Potassium secretion is largely a passive process in response to the need to maintain membrane potential neutrality associated with active reabsorption of sodium in the distal convoluted tubule and collecting duct. The extent of potassium secretion is determined by a number of factors, including:

- the amount of sodium available for exchange in the distal convoluted tubule and collecting duct
- the availability of hydrogen and potassium ions for exchange in the distal convoluted tubule or collecting duct
- the ability of the distal convoluted tubule or collecting duct to secrete hydrogen ions
- the concentration of aldosterone
- tubular fluid flow rate.

As described above, both potassium and hydrogen can neutralize the membrane potential generated by active sodium reabsorption and consequently there is a close relationship between potassium and hydrogen ion homeostasis. In acidosis, hydrogen ions are normally secreted in preference to potassium – i.e. hyperkalaemia is often associated with acidosis (except in renal tubular acidosis). In alkalosis fewer hydrogen ions will be present and potassium is excreted – i.e. hypokalaemia is often associated with alkalosis.

The normal daily dietary intake of potassium is of the order of 60–200 mmol, which is more than adequate to replace that lost from the body. It is unusual for a deficiency of normal intake to account for hypokalaemia. A transcellular movement of potassium into cells, loss from the gut or excretion in the urine are the main causes of hypokalaemia.

Hypokalaemia

Transcellular movement into cells. The shift of potassium from the serum compartment of the ECF into cells accounts for the hypokalaemia reported following intravenous or, less frequently, nebulized administration of β-adrenoceptor agonists such as salbutamol. Parenteral insulin also causes a shift of potassium into cells, and is used for this purpose in the acute management of patients with hyperkalaemia.

Loss from the gastrointestinal tract. Although potassium is secreted in gastric juice, much of this, together with potassium ingested in the diet, is reabsorbed in the small intestine. Stools do contain some potassium, but in a patient with chronic diarrhoea or a fistula considerable amounts of potassium may be lost and precipitate hypokalaemia. Likewise, the abuse of laxatives increases gastrointestinal potassium loss and may precipitate hypokalaemia. Analogous to the situation with diarrhoea, the potassium secreted in gastric juice may be lost following persistent vomiting and can also contribute to hypokalaemia.

Loss from the kidneys. Mineralocorticoid excess, whether it be due to primary or secondary hyperaldosteronism or Cushing's syndrome, can increase urinary potassium loss and cause hypokalaemia. Likewise, increased excretion of potassium can result from renal tubular damage. Nephrotoxic antibiotics such as gentamicin have been implicated in this.

Many drugs which can induce hypokalaemia do so by affecting the regulatory role of aldosterone upon potassium–sodium exchange in the distal tubule and collecting duct. Administered corticosteroids mimic aldosterone and can therefore increase potassium loss.

Perhaps the most commonly used groups of drugs that can cause hypokalaemia are thiazide and loop diuretics. Both groups of drugs increase the amount of sodium delivered and available for reabsorption at the distal convoluted tubule and collecting duct. Consequently, this will increase the amount of potassium excreted from the kidneys. Some of the drugs known to cause hypokalaemia are shown in Table 4.5.

Clinical features. The patient with moderate hypokalaemia may be asymptomatic, but the symptoms of more severe hypokalaemia include muscle weakness, hypotonia, paralytic ileus, depression and confusion. Arrhythmias may occur. Typical changes on the electrocardiogram (ECG) are of ST depression, T wave depression/inversion and prolonged P–R interval. Insulin secretion in response to a rising blood glucose concentration requires potassium and this mechanism may be impaired in hypokalaemia. Rarely there may be impaired renal concentrating ability with polyuria and polydipsia.

Hypokalaemia is managed by giving either oral potassium or intravenous potassium, depending on its severity.

Hyperkalaemia

Hyperkalaemia may arise from excessive intake, decreased elimination or shift of potassium from cells to

Table 4.5 Examples of drugs known to cause hypokalaemia
Amphotericin
Aspirin
Corticosteroids
Diuretics
Gentamicin
Glucose
Insulin
Laxatives
Benzylpenicillin (penicillin G) (sodium salt)
Piperacillin + tazobactam
Salicylates
Sodium bicarbonate
Sodium chloride
Terbutaline
Ticarcillin + clavulanate

Table 4.6 Examples of drugs known to cause hyperkalaemia
Angiotensin-converting enzyme (ACE) inhibitors
Antineoplastic agents (e.g. cyclophosphamide, vincristine)
Non-steroidal anti-inflammatory drugs (NSAIDs)
β-adrenoceptor blocking agents
Ciclosporin
Digoxin (in acute overdose)
Diuretics, potassium sparing (amiloride, triamterene, spironolactone)
Heparin
Isoniazid
Lithium
Penicillins (e.g. potassium salt)
Potassium supplements
Succinylcholine chloride
Tetracycline

the ECF. It is rare for excessive oral intake to be the sole cause of hyperkalaemia. The inappropriate use of parenteral infusions containing potassium is probably the most common iatrogenic cause of excessive intake. Hyperkalaemia is a common problem in patients with renal failure due to their inability to excrete a potassium load.

The combined use of potassium-sparing diuretics such as amiloride, triamterene or spironolactone with an angiotensin-converting enzyme (ACE) inhibitor, which will lower aldosterone, is a recognized cause of hyperkalaemia, particularly in the elderly. Mineralocorticoid deficiency states such as Addison's disease where there is a deficiency of aldosterone also decrease renal potassium loss and contribute to hyperkalaemia.

The majority of body potassium is intracellular. Severe tissue damage, catabolic states or impairment of the energy-dependent sodium pump, caused by hypoxia or diabetic ketoacidosis, may result in apparent hyperkalaemia due to potassium moving out of and sodium moving into cells. Table 4.6 gives examples of some drugs known to cause hyperkalaemia.

Haemolysis during sampling or a delay in separating cells from plasma will result in potassium escaping from red blood cells into plasma and causing an artefactual hyperkalaemia.

Clinical features. Hyperkalaemia can be asymptomatic but fatal. An elevated potassium level has many effects on the heart, notably the resting membrane potential is lowered and the action potential shortened. Characteristic changes of the ECG precede ventricular fibrillation and cardiac arrest.

In emergency management of a patient with hyperkalaemia (>6.5 mmol/l ± ECG changes), intravenous calcium gluconate (or chloride) at a dose of 10 ml of 10% solution is given intravenously over 5 minutes. This does not reduce the potassium concentration but antagonizes the effect of hyperkalaemia on cardiac tissue. Immediately thereafter, glucose 50 g with 20 units soluble insulin, for example, by intravenous infusion, will lower serum potassium levels within 30 minutes by increasing the shift of potassium into cells.

If acidosis is present, bicarbonate administration may be considered.

The long-term management of hyperkalaemia may involve the use of oral or rectal polystyrene cation-exchange resins which remove potassium from the body.

Chronic hyperkalaemia in renal failure is managed by a low potassium diet.

Calcium

The body of an average man contains about 1 kg of calcium and 99% of this is bound to bone. Calcium is present in serum bound mainly to the albumin component of protein (46%), complexed with citrate and phosphate (7%), and as free ions (47%). Only the free ions of calcium are physiologically active. Calcium metabolism is regulated by parathyroid hormone (PTH) which is inhibited by increased serum concentrations of calcium ions. PTH is secreted in response to low calcium concentrations and increases serum calcium by actions on osteoclasts, kidney and gut.

The serum calcium level is often determined by measuring total calcium, i.e. that which is free and bound, but the measurement of free or ionized calcium offers advantages in some situations.

In alkalosis, hydrogen ions dissociate from albumin, and calcium binding to albumin increases, together with an increase in complex formation. If the concentration of ionized calcium falls sufficiently, clinical symptoms of hypocalcaemia may occur despite the total serum calcium concentration being unchanged. The reverse effect (i.e. increased ionized calcium), occurs in acidosis.

Changes in serum albumin also affect the total serum calcium concentration independently of the ionized concentration. A variety of equations are available to estimate the calcium concentration. A commonly used formula is shown in Figure 4.2. Caution must be taken when using such a formula in the presence of disturbed blood hydrogen ion concentrations.

Hypercalcaemia

Hypercalcaemia may be caused by a variety of disorders, the most common being hyperparathyroidism and malignancy. Hypercalcaemia of malignancy is seen in multiple myeloma and carcinomas which metastasize in bone. It is also seen in squamous carcinoma of the bronchus, as a result of a peptide with PTH-like activity,

produced by the tumour. Hypercalcaemia also occurs in thyrotoxicosis, vitamin A and D intoxication, renal transplantation and acromegaly.

Thiazide diuretics, lithium, tamoxifen and calcium supplements used in the management of osteoporosis are examples of some of the drugs which can cause hypercalcaemia.

An artefactual increase in total plasma calcium may sometimes be seen as a result of a tourniquet being applied during venous sampling. The resulting venous stasis may cause redistribution of fluid from the vein into the extravascular space, and the temporary haemoconcentration will affect albumin levels.

Management of hypercalcaemia involves correction of any dehydration with normal saline followed by furosemide (frusemide) which inhibits tubular reabsorption of calcium. Bisphosphonates are used to inhibit bone turnover.

Hypocalcaemia

Hypocalcaemia can be caused by a variety of disorders including hypoalbuminaemia, hypoparathyroidism, pancreatitis and those that cause vitamin D deficiency, e.g. malabsorption, reduced exposure to sunlight, liver disease and renal disease. In alkalaemia (for instance as may occur when a patient is hyperventilating) there is an increase in protein binding of calcium, which can result in a fall in plasma levels of ionized calcium, manifesting itself as paraesthesiae or tetany.

Drugs that have been implicated as causing hypocalcaemia include phenytoin, phenobarbital, aminoglycosides, phosphate enemas, calcitonin, mithramycin and furosemide (frusemide).

Phosphate

About 80% of body phosphate is in bone, 15% in intracellular fluid and only 0.1% in extracellular fluid. Its major function is in energy metabolism. Plasma levels are regulated by absorption from the diet, which is partly under the control of vitamin D, and PTH which controls its excretion by the kidney.

Hypophosphataemia

Excessive use of antacids may result in binding of dietary phosphate in the gut. Phosphate moves into cells as a result of increased glycolysis such as occurs in alkalosis and insulin treatment during diabetic ketoacidosis promotes cellular uptake of the anion. Hypophosphataemia is also seen in renal failure, parenterally fed patients and chronic alcohol abuse.

Clinical features. Severe hypophosphataemia can cause muscle weakness and wasting and some skeletal wasting.

For albumin < 40 g/l:

Corrected calcium = [Ca] + 0.02 × (40 − [alb]) mmol/l

For albumin > 45 g/l:

Corrected calcium = [Ca] − 0.02 ([alb] − 45) mmol/l

Figure 4.2 Formula for correction of total plasma calcium concentration for changes in albumin concentration: albumin concentration = [alb] (albumin units = g/l); calcium concentration = [Ca] (total calcium units = mmol/l).

Hyperphosphataemia

Hyperphosphataemia occurs in chronic renal failure and hypoparathyroidism.

Creatinine

Serum creatinine concentration is largely determined by its rate of production, rate of renal excretion and volume of distribution. It is frequently used to evaluate renal function.

Creatinine is produced at a fairly constant rate from creatine and creatine phosphate in muscle. Daily production is a function of muscle mass and declines with age from 24 mg/kg/day in a healthy 25-year-old to 9 mg/kg/day in a 95-year-old. Creatinine undergoes complete glomerular filtration with little reabsorption by the renal tubules. Its clearance is therefore usually a good indicator of the glomerular filtration rate (GFR). As a general rule, and only at the steady state, if the serum creatinine doubles this equates to a 50% reduction in the GFR and consequently renal function. The serum creatinine level can be transiently elevated following meat ingestion (but less so than urea) or strenuous exercise. Individuals with a high muscle bulk produce more creatinine and therefore have a higher serum creatinine level compared to an otherwise identical but less muscular individual.

The value for creatinine clearance is higher than the true GFR due to the active tubular secretion of creatinine. In a patient with a normal GFR this is of little significance. However, in an individual in whom the GFR is low (< 10 ml/min) the tubular secretion may make a significant contribution to creatinine elimination and overestimate the GFR. In this type of patient, the breakdown of creatinine in the gut can also become a significant source of elimination.

Urea

The catabolism of dietary and endogenous amino acids in the body produces large amounts of ammonia. Ammonia is toxic and its concentration is kept very low by conversion in the liver to urea. Urea is eliminated in urine and represents the major route of nitrogen excretion. The urea is filtered from the blood at the renal glomerulus and undergoes significant tubular reabsorption. This tubular reabsorption is pronounced at low rates of urine flow. Moreover, urea levels vary widely with diet, rate of protein metabolism, liver production and the GFR. A high protein intake from the diet or following haemorrhage in the gut, and consequent absorption of the protein from the blood, may produce elevated serum urea levels (up to 10 mmol/l). Urea concentrations of more than 10 mmol/l are usually due to renal disease or decreased renal blood flow following shock or dehydration. As with serum creatinine levels, serum urea levels do not begin to increase until the GFR has fallen by 50% or more.

Production is decreased in situations where there is a low protein intake and in some patients with liver disease. Thus non-renal as well as renal influences should be considered when evaluating changes in serum urea concentrations.

Bicarbonate and acid–base

Bicarbonate acts as part of the carbonic acid–bicarbonate buffer system which is important to maintain acid–base balance in the blood. Bicarbonate concentrations in the plasma change when there is a metabolic acid–base disorder and bicarbonate levels, together with plasma P_{CO_2} concentrations, can help to differentiate the cause of an alkalosis or acidosis.

For example, in metabolic acidosis such as occurs in renal failure, diabetic ketoacidosis or salicylate poisoning bicarbonate levels fall. In metabolic alkalosis the plasma bicarbonate concentration is high. This can occur, for instance, when there is a loss of hydrogen ions from the stomach, as in severe vomiting, or loss through the kidneys, as in mineralocorticoid excess or severe potassium depletion. In the latter situation an increase in sodium reabsorption in the kidney results in bicarbonate retention and a loss of hydrogen ions.

Glucose

The serum glucose concentration is largely determined by the balance of glucose moving into, and leaving, the extracellular compartment. In a healthy adult, this movement is capable of maintaining serum levels below 10 mmol/l, regardless of the intake of meals of varying carbohydrate content.

The renal tubules have the capacity to reabsorb glucose from the glomerular filtrate, and little unchanged glucose is normally lost from the body. Glucose in the urine (glycosuria) is normally only present when the concentration in serum exceeds 10 mmol/l, the renal threshold for total reabsorption.

Normal ranges for serum glucose concentrations are often quoted as non-fasting (< 11.1 mmol/l) or fasting (3.3–6.0 mmol/l) concentration ranges. Fasting blood glucose levels between 6.1 and 7.0 mmol/l indicate impaired glucose tolerance and levels above 7.0 mmol/l are consistent with a diagnosis of diabetes. Other signs and symptoms if present, notably those attributable to an osmotic diuresis, will suggest clinically the diagnosis of diabetes mellitus.

Glycated haemoglobin

Glucose binds to a part of the haemoglobin molecule to form a small glycated fraction. Normally about 5% of haemoglobin is glycated, but this amount is dependent on the average blood glucose concentration over the lifespan of the red cells (about 120 days). The major component of the glycated fraction is referred to as HbA_{1C}.

Measurement of HbA_{1C} is well established as an indicator of chronic glycaemic control in patients with diabetes. Several methods exist for its determination, and until standardization is achieved, clinicians should be aware that the ranges indicating good or poor glycaemic control can vary markedly between different assays and laboratories.

Uric acid

Uric acid is the end product of purine metabolism. The purines, which are used for nucleic acid synthesis, are produced by the breakdown of nucleic acid from ingested meat or synthesized within the body.

Monosodium urate is the form in which uric acid usually exists at the normal pH of body fluids. The term urate is used to represent any salt of uric acid.

Two main factors contribute to elevated serum uric acid levels: an increased rate of formation and reduced excretion. Uric acid is poorly soluble and an elevation in serum concentration can readily result in deposition, as monosodium urate, in tissues or joints. Deposition usually precipitates an acute attack of gouty arthritis. The aim of treatment is to reduce the concentration of uric acid and prevent further attacks of gout. Low serum uric acid levels appear to be of no clinical significance.

Liver function tests

Routine liver function tests (LFTs) give information mainly about the activity or concentrations of enzymes and compounds in serum rather than quantifying specific hepatic functions. Results are useful in confirming or excluding a diagnosis of clinically suspected liver disease, and monitoring its course.

Serum albumin levels and prothrombin time indicate hepatic protein synthesis; bilirubin is a marker of overall liver function.

Transaminase levels indicate hepatocellular injury and death, while alkaline phosphatase levels estimate the amount of impedance of bile flow.

Albumin

Albumin is quantitatively the most important protein synthesized in the liver, with 10–15 g per day being produced in a healthy man. About 60% is located in the interstitial compartment of the ECF, the remainder in the smaller, but relatively impermeable, serum compartment where it is present at a higher concentration. The concentration in the serum is important in maintaining its volume since it accounts for approximately 80% of serum colloid osmotic pressure. A significant reduction in serum albumin concentration often results in oedema.

Albumin has an important role in binding, among others, calcium, bilirubin and many drugs. A reduction in serum albumin will increase free levels of agents which are normally bound and adverse effects can result if the 'free' entity is not rapidly cleared from the body.

The serum concentration of albumin depends on its rate of synthesis, volume of distribution and rate of catabolism. Synthesis falls in parallel with increasing severity of liver disease or in malnutrition states where there is an inadequate supply of amino acids to maintain albumin production or in response to inflammatory mediators such as interleukin. A low serum albumin concentration will occur when the volume of distribution of albumin increases, as happens for example in cirrhosis with ascites, in fluid retention states such as pregnancy, or where a shift of albumin from serum to interstitial fluid causes dilutional hypoalbuminaemia after parenteral infusion of excess protein-free fluid. The movement of albumin from serum into interstitial fluid is often associated with increased capillary permeability in postoperative patients or those with septicaemia. A shift of protein is known to occur physiologically when moving from the lying to the upright position. This can account for an increase in the serum albumin level of up to 10 g/l and can contribute to the variation in serum concentration of highly bound drugs which are therapeutically monitored.

Other causes of hypoalbuminaemia include catabolic states associated with a variety of illnesses and increased loss of albumin, either in urine from damaged kidneys, as occurs in the nephrotic syndrome, or via the skin following burns or a skin disorder such as psoriasis, or from the intestinal wall in a protein-losing enteropathy.

Albumin's serum half-life of approximately 20 days precludes its use as an indicator of acute change in liver function but levels are of prognostic value in chronic disease.

An increase in serum albumin is rare and can be iatrogenic (for example inappropriate infusion of albumin) or the result of dehydration or shock.

Bilirubin

At the end of their life, red blood cells are broken down by the reticuloendothelial system, mainly in the spleen. The haemoglobin molecules, which are subsequently liberated, are split into globin and haem. The globin enters the general protein pool, the iron in haem is reutilized, and the remaining tetrapyrrole ring of haem is degraded to bilirubin. Unconjugated bilirubin, which is water insoluble and fat soluble, is transported to the liver tightly bound to albumin; there it is actively taken up by hepatocytes, conjugated with glucuronic acid and excreted into bile. The conjugated bilirubin is water soluble and secreted into the gut where it is broken down by bacteria into urobilinogen, a colourless compound, which is subsequently oxidized in the colon to urobilin, a brown pigment excreted in faeces. Some of the urobilinogen is absorbed and most is subsequently re-excreted in bile (enterohepatic circulation). A small amount is absorbed into the systemic circulation and excreted in urine, where it too may be oxidized to urobilin.

The liver produces 300 mg of bilirubin each day. However, because the mature liver can metabolize and excrete up to 3 g daily, serum bilirubin concentrations are not a sensitive test of liver function. As a screening test they rarely do other than confirm the presence or absence of jaundice. In chronic liver disease, however, changes in bilirubin concentrations over time do convey prognostic information.

An elevation of serum bilirubin concentration above 50 µmol/l (i.e. approximately 2.5 times the normal upper limit) will reveal itself as jaundice, seen best in the skin and sclerae. Elevated bilirubin levels can be caused by increased production of bilirubin (e.g. haemolysis, ineffective erythropoiesis), impaired transport into hepatocytes (e.g. interference with bilirubin uptake by drugs such as rifampicin or hepatitis), decreased excretion (e.g. with drugs such as rifampicin and methyltestosterone, intrahepatic obstruction due to cirrhosis, tumours, etc.) or a combination of these factors.

The bilirubin in serum is normally unconjugated, bound to protein, not filtered by the glomeruli and does not normally appear in the urine. Bilirubin in the urine (bilirubinuria) is usually the result of an increase in serum concentration of conjugated bilirubin and indicates an underlying pathological disorder.

Enzymes

The enzymes measured in routine liver function tests are listed in Table 4.1. Enzyme concentrations in the serum of healthy individuals are normally low. When cells are damaged, increased amounts of enzymes are detected as the intracellular contents are released into the blood.

It is important to remember that the assay of 'serum enzymes' is a measurement of catalytic activity and not actual enzyme concentration and that activity can vary depending on assay conditions. Consequently the reference range may vary widely between laboratories.

While the measurement of enzymes may be very specific, the enzymes themselves may not be specific to a particular tissue or cell. Many enzymes arise in more than one tissue and an increase in the serum activity of one enzyme can represent damage to any one of the tissues which contain the enzymes. In practice, this problem may be clarified because some tissues contain two or more enzymes in different proportions which are released on damage. For example, alanine and aspartate transaminase both occur in cardiac muscle and liver cells, but their site of origin can often be differentiated, because there is more alanine transaminase in the liver than in the heart. In those situations where it is not possible to look at the relative ratio of enzymes, it is sometimes possible to differentiate the same enzyme from different tissues. Such enzymes have the same catalytic activity but differ in some other measurable property, and are referred to as isoenzymes.

The measured activity of an enzyme will be dependent upon the time it is sampled relative to its time of release from the cell. If a sample is drawn too early after a particular insult to a tissue there may be no detectable increase in enzyme activity. If it is drawn too late, the enzyme may have been cleared from the blood.

Alkaline phosphatase

Alkaline phosphatases are found in the canalicular plasma membrane of hepatocytes, in bone where they reflect bone building or osteoblastic activity, and in the intestinal wall and placenta. Each site of origin produces a specific isoenzyme of alkaline phosphatase, which can be electrophoretically separated if concentrations are sufficiently high.

Disorders of the liver which can elevate alkaline phosphatase include intra- or extrahepatic cholestasis, space-occupying lesions (e.g. tumour, abscess) and hepatitis.

Physiological increases in serum alkaline phosphatase activity also occur in pregnancy due to release of the placental isoenzyme and during periods of growth in children and adolescents when the bone isoenzyme is released.

Pathological increases in serum alkaline phosphatase of bone origin may arise in disorders such as osteomalacia and rickets, Paget's disease of bone, bone tumours, renal bone disease, osteomyelitis and healing fractures. Alkaline phosphatase is also raised as part of the acute phase response, for example intestinal alkaline phosphatase may be raised in active inflammatory bowel disease.

Transaminases

The two transaminases of diagnostic use are aspartate transaminase (AST; also known as aspartate aminotransferase) and alanine transaminase (ALT; also known as alanine aminotransferase). These enzymes are found in many body tissues, with the highest concentration being in hepatocytes and muscle cells.

Serum AST levels are increased in a variety of disorders including liver disease, crush injuries, severe tissue hypoxia, myocardial infarction, surgery, trauma, muscle disease and pancreatitis. ALT is elevated to a similar extent in the disorders listed which involve the liver, though to a lesser extent, if at all, in the other disorders. In the context of liver disease, increased transaminase activity indicates deranged integrity of hepatocyte plasma membranes and/or hepatocyte necrosis. They may be raised in all forms of viral and non-viral, acute and chronic liver disease, most markedly in acute viral, drug induced (e.g. paracetamol poisoning), alcohol related and ischaemic liver damage.

γ-Glutamyl transpeptidase

γ-Glutamyl transpeptidase (gamma GT; also known as γ-glutamyl transferase) is present in high concentrations in the liver, kidney and pancreas, where it is found within the endoplasmic reticulum of cells. It is a sensitive indicator of hepatobiliary disease but does not differentiate a cholestatic disorder from hepatocellular disease. It can also be elevated in alcoholic liver disease, hepatitis, cirrhosis, pancreatitis and congestive cardiac failure.

Serum levels of γ-glutamyl transpeptidase activity can be raised by enzyme induction by certain drugs such as phenytoin, phenobarbital and rifampicin.

Serum γ-glutamyl transpeptidase activity is usually raised in an individual with alcoholic liver disease. However, it can also be raised in heavy drinkers of alcohol who do not have liver damage, due to enzyme induction. Its activity can remain elevated for up to 4 weeks after stopping alcohol intake.

Cardiac markers

Troponins

Cardiac troponin I (cTnI) and cardiac troponin T (cTnT) are component proteins of the contractile apparatus in cardiac muscle cells. The cardiac specific isoforms are released into plasma as a result of myocardial damage, when raised levels can be detected. They are the preferred marker for the detection of myocardial damage, and they contribute significantly to stratification of individuals with acute coronary syndromes, either alone or in combination with admission ECG or a predischarge exercise stress test. The decision whether to monitor cTnT or cTnI in a given laboratory is a balance between cost, availability of automated instrumentation and assay performance.

Creatine kinase

Creatine kinase (CK) is an enzyme which is present in relatively high concentrations in heart muscle, skeletal muscle and brain in addition to being present in smooth muscle and other tissues. Levels are markedly increased following shock and circulatory failure, myocardial infarction and muscular dystrophies. Less marked increases have been reported following muscle injury, surgery, physical exercise, muscle cramp, an epileptic fit, intramuscular injection and hypothyroidism.

Creatine kinase has two protein subunits, M and B, which combine to form three isoenzymes, BB, MM and MB. BB is found in high concentrations in the brain, thyroid and some smooth muscle tissue. Little of this enzyme is present in the serum, even following damage to the brain. The enzyme found in serum of normal subjects is the MM isoenzyme which originates from skeletal muscle.

Cardiac tissue contains more of the MB isoenzyme than skeletal muscle. Following a myocardial infarction there is a characteristic increase in serum creatine kinase activity. Although measurement of activity of the MB isoenzyme was used in the past to detect myocardial damage when there was a possibility of a contribution of creatinine kinase from another source, such as after exercise, trauma or an intramuscular injection, troponin measurement is now superseding these assays.

Lactate dehydrogenase

Lactate dehydrogenase has five isoenzymes (LD1 to LD5). Total lactate dehydrogenase activity is rarely measured because of the lack of tissue specificity. Levels of activity are elevated following damage to the liver, skeletal muscle and kidneys and in both megaloblastic and haemolytic anaemias. In lymphoma, a high LD activity indicates a poor prognosis. Elevation of LD1 and LD2 occurs after myocardial infarction, renal infarction or megaloblastic anaemia; LD2 and LD3 are elevated in acute leukaemia; LD3 is often elevated in some malignancies, and LD5 is elevated after damage to liver or skeletal muscle.

Tumour markers

While only a few markers contribute to the diagnosis of cancer, serial measurements can be useful in assessing the presence of residual disease and response to treatment. A detailed discussion of each marker (they include prostatic-specific antigen, human chorionic gonadotrophin, α-fetoprotein, carcinoembryonic antigen, cancer antigen (CA) 125, and CA 15-3) is beyond the scope of this chapter.

Prostatic specific antigen (PSA) is a serine protease produced by normal and malignant prostatic epithelium and secreted into seminal fluid. Only minor amounts leak into the circulation from the normal prostate, but the release is increased in prostatic disease. It is involved not only in screening for early detection of prostatic cancer, but also in the detection of recurrence, disease progression and response to therapies. In order to improve the specificity of PSA testing, a number of refinements to measurement including free to total PSA ratio, PSA density, and age-specific reference ranges have been proposed.

Immunoglobulins

Immunoglobulins are antibodies which are produced by B lymphocytes. They are detected on electrophoresis as bands in three regions: α, β and γ, most occurring in the γ region. Hypergammaglobulinaemia may result from stimulation of B cells and produces an increased staining of bands in the γ region on electrophoresis. This occurs in infections, chronic liver disease and autoimmune disease.

In some diseases such as chronic lymphatic leukaemia, lymphoma and multiple myeloma, a discrete, densely staining band (paraprotein) can be seen in the γ region. In multiple myeloma, abnormal fragments of immunoglobulins are produced (Bence-Jones protein) which clear the glomerulus and are found in the urine.

Haematology data

The haematology profile is an important part of the investigation of many patients and not just those with primary haematological disease.

Typical measurements reported in a haematology screen, with their normal values, are shown in Table 4.7, while a list of the common descriptive terms used in haematology are presented in Table 4.8.

Red blood cell count (RBC)

Red blood cells are produced in the bone marrow by the process of erythropoiesis. One of the major stimulants of this process is erythropoietin, produced mainly in the kidney. Immature erythroblasts develop into mature erythrocytes which are then released into the circulation:

erythroblasts
↓
normoblasts
(nucleated)
↓
reticulocytes
(non-nucleated)
↓
erythrocytes

Normally only reticulocytes and non-nucleated mature erythrocytes are seen in the peripheral blood.

The lifespan of a mature red cell is usually about 120 days. If this is shortened, as for instance in haemolysis, the circulating mass of red cells is reduced and with it the supply of oxygen to tissues is decreased. In these circumstances, red cell production is enhanced, in healthy bone marrow by an increased output of erythropoietin. Under normal circumstances red cells are destroyed by lodging in the spleen due to decreasing flexibility of the cells. They are removed by the reticuloendothelial system.

Table 4.7 Haematology data: typical normal adult reference values

Haemoglobin	13.5–17.0 g/dl (men)
	11.5–16.5 g/dl (women)
Red blood cell count (RBC)	$4.5–5.9 \times 10^{12}$/l (men)
	$3.8–5.2 \times 10^{12}$/l (women)
Reticulocyte count	$50–100 \times 10^9$/l
Packed cell volume (PCV)	0.40–0.52 (men)
	0.37–0.47 (women)
Mean cell volume (MCV)	80–96 fl
Mean cell haemoglobin (MCH)	27–32 pg
Mean cell haemoglobin concentration (MCHC)	315–345 g/l
White cell count (WBC)	$3.5–11.0 \times 10^9$/l
Differential white cell count:	
Neutrophils (30–75%)	$1.5–7.5 \times 10^9$/l
Lymphocytes (5–15%)	$1.0–4.0 \times 10^9$/l
Monocytes (2–10%)	$0.2–0.8 \times 10^9$/l
Basophils (< 1%)	$< 0.1 \times 10^9$/l
Eosinophils (1–6%)	$0.04–0.4 \times 10^9$/l
Platelets	$150–400 \times 10^9$/l
Erythrocyte sedimentation rate (ESR)	< 10 mm/h
Serum iron	13–32 μmol/l
Transferrin	1.2–2.0 μmol/l
Ferritin	21–300 microgram/l
	15–150 microgram/l (women)
Total iron binding capacity (TIBC)	47–70 μmol/l
Serum B_{12}	160–760 ng/l
Red cell folate	160–640 microgram/l

A high RBC (erythrocytosis or polycythaemia) indicates increased production by the bone marrow and may occur as a physiological response to hypoxia, as in chronic airways disease, or as a malignant condition of red cells such as in polycythaemia rubra vera.

Reticulocytes

Reticulocytes are the earliest non-nucleated red cells. They owe their name to the fine net-like appearance of their cytoplasm which can be seen, after appropriate staining, under the microscope and contains fine threads of ribonucleic acid (RNA) in a reticular network. Reticulocytes normally represent between 0.5% and 1.0% of the total RBC and do not feature significantly in a normal blood profile. However, increased production

(reticulocytosis) can be detected in times of rapid red cell regeneration as occurs in response to haemorrhage or haemolysis. At such times the reticulocyte count may reach 40% of the RBC. The reticulocyte count may be useful in assessing the response of the marrow to iron, folate or vitamin B_{12} therapy. The count peaks about 7–10 days after starting the therapy and then subsides.

Mean cell volume (MCV)

The mean cell volume (MCV) is the average volume of a single red cell. It is measured in femtolitres (10^{-15} l). Terms such as 'microcytic' and 'macrocytic' are descriptive of a low and high MCV, respectively. They are useful in the process of identification of various types of anaemias such as those caused by iron deficiency (microcytic) or vitamin B_{12} or folic acid deficiency (megaloblastic or macrocytic).

Packed cell volume (PCV) (haematocrit)

The packed cell volume (PCV) or haematocrit is the ratio of the volume occupied by red cells to the total volume of blood. It can be measured by centrifugation of a capillary tube of blood and then expressing the volume of red cells packed in the bottom as a percentage of the total volume. It is reported as a fraction of unity or as a percentage (e.g. 0.45 or 45%). The PCV is calculated nowadays as the product of the MCV and RBC. The PCV often reflects the RBC and will therefore be decreased in any sort of anaemia, in haemorrhage or in haemolysis. It will be raised in polycythaemia. It may, however, be altered irrespective of the RBC, when the size of the red cell is abnormal, as in macrocytosis and microcytosis.

Mean cell haemoglobin (MCH)

The mean cell haemoglobin (MCH) is the average weight of haemoglobin contained in a red cell. It is measured in picograms (10^{-12} g) and is calculated from the relationship:

$$MCH = \frac{haemoglobin}{RBC}$$

The MCH is dependent on the size of the red cells as well as the concentration of haemoglobin in the cells. Thus it is usually low in iron deficiency anaemia when there is microcytosis and there is less haemoglobin in each cell, but it may be raised in macrocytic anaemia.

Mean cell haemoglobin concentration (MCHC)

The mean cell haemoglobin concentration (MCHC) is a measure of the average concentration of haemoglobin in 100 ml of red cells. It is usually expressed as grams per

Table 4.8 Descriptive terms in common use in haematology

Anisocytosis	Abnormal variation in cell size (usually refers to RBCs), e.g. red cells in iron deficiency anaemia
Agranulocytosis	Lack of granulocytes (principally neutrophils)
Aplastic	Depression of synthesis of all cell types in bone marrow (as in aplastic anaemia)
Basophilia	Increased number of basophils
Hypochromic	Mean cell haemoglobin concentration (MCHC) low, red cells appear pale microscopically
Leucocytosis	Increased white cell count
Leucopenia	Reduced white cell count
Macrocytic	Large cells
Microcytic	Small cells
Neutropenia	Reduced neutrophil count
Neutrophilia	Increased neutrophil count
Normochromic	MCHC normal; red cells appear normally pigmented
Pancytopenia	Decreased number of all cell types: it is synonymous with aplastic anaemia
Poikilocytosis	Abnormal variation in cell shape, e.g. some red cells appear pear shaped in macrocytic anaemias
Thrombocytopenia	Lack of platelets

litre but may be reported as a percentage. The MCHC will be reported as low in conditions of reduced haemoglobin synthesis such as in iron deficiency anaemia. In contrast, in macrocytic anaemias the MCHC may be normal or only slightly reduced because the large red cells may contain more haemoglobin, thus giving a concentration approximating that of normal cells. The MCHC can be raised in severe prolonged dehydration. If the MCHC is low, the descriptive term 'hypochromic' may be used (for example a hypochromic anaemia) whereas the term 'normochromic' describes a normal MCHC.

Haemoglobin

The haemoglobin concentration in men is normally greater than that in women, reflecting in part the higher RBC in men. Lower concentrations in women are due, at least in part, to menstrual loss.

Haemoglobin is most commonly measured to detect anaemia. In some relatively rare genetic diseases, the haemoglobinopathies, alterations in the structure of the haemoglobin molecule can be detected by electrophoresis. Abnormal haemoglobins which can be detected in this manner include HbS (sickle haemoglobin in sickle cell disease) and HbA_2 found in β-thalassaemia carriers.

Platelets (thrombocytes)

Platelets are formed in the bone marrow. A marked reduction in platelet number (thrombocytopenia) may reflect either a depressed synthesis in the marrow or destruction of formed platelets.

Platelets are normally present in the circulation for 8–12 days. This is useful information when evaluating a possible drug-induced thrombocytopenia, since recovery should be fairly swift when the offending agent is withdrawn.

A small fall in the platelet count may be seen in pregnancy and following viral infections. Severe thrombocytopenia may result in spontaneous bleeding. A reduced platelet count is also found in disseminated intravascular coagulation, which manifests clinically as severe haemorrhages, particularly in the skin and results in rapid consumption of clotting factors and platelets.

An increased platelet count (thrombocytosis) occurs in malignancy, in inflammatory disease, and in response to blood loss.

White blood cell count (WBC)

White cells (leucocytes) are of two types of cell – the granulocytes and the agranular cells. They are made up of various types of cells (Fig. 4.3) with different functions and it is logical to consider them separately. A haematology profile often reports a total white cell count and a differential count, the latter separating the composition of white cells into the various types.

Neutrophils

Neutrophils or polymorphonucleocytes (PMNs) are the most abundant type of white cell. They have a phagocytic function, with many enzymes contained in the lysosomal granules. They are formed in the bone marrow from the stem cells which form myoblasts and these develop through a number of stages into the neutrophil with a multiple-segmented nucleus. Neutrophils constitute approximately 40–70% of circulating white cells in normal healthy blood. Their lifespan is 10–20 days. The neutrophil count increases in the presence of infection, tissue damage (e.g. infarction) and inflammation (e.g. rheumatoid arthritis, acute gout). Neutropenia – also described as agranulocytosis in its severest forms – is associated with malignancy and drug toxicity, but may also occur in viral infections such as influenza, infectious mononucleosis and hepatitis.

Basophils

Basophils normally constitute a small proportion of the white cell count. Their function is poorly understood but basophilia occurs in various malignant and premalignant disorders such as leukaemia and myelofibrosis.

Eosinophils

Eosinophils normally constitute less than 6% of white cells. Their function appears to be concerned with inactivation of mediators released from mast cells, and eosinophilia is therefore apparent in many allergic

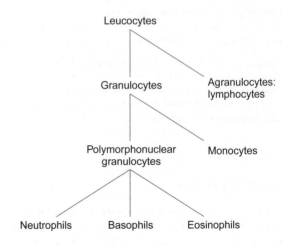

Figure 4.3   Types of white cells

conditions such as asthma, hay fever and drug sensitivity reactions as well as some malignant diseases.

Lymphocytes

Lymphocytes are the second most abundant white cells in the circulating blood, but the majority of them are found in the spleen and other lymphatic tissue. They are formed in the bone marrow. An increase in lymphocyte numbers occurs particularly in viral infections such as rubella, mumps, infectious hepatitis and infectious mononucleosis.

Monocytes

Monocytes are macrophages. Their numbers increase in some infections such as typhoid, subacute bacterial endocarditis, infectious mononucleosis and tuberculosis.

Other blood tests

Erythrocyte sedimentation rate (ESR)

The erythrocyte sedimentation rate (ESR) is a measure of the settling rate of red cells in a sample of anticoagulated blood, over a period of 1 hour, in a cylindrical tube.

In youth the normal value is less than 10 mmol/h, but normal values rise with age. The Westergren method, performed under standardized conditions, is commonly used in haematology laboratories. The ESR is strongly correlated with the ability of red cells to aggregate into orderly stacks or rouleaux. In disease, the most common cause of a high ESR is an increased protein level in the blood, such as the increase in acute phase proteins seen in inflammatory disease. Proteins are thought to affect the repellent surface charges on red cells and cause them to aggregate into rouleaux and hence the sedimentation rate increases. Although some conditions may cause a low ESR, the test is principally used to monitor inflammatory disease. The ESR may be raised in the active phase of rheumatoid arthritis, inflammatory bowel disease, malignant disease and infection. The ESR is non-specific and therefore of little diagnostic value, but serial tests are helpful in following the progress of disease, and its response to treatment.

C-reactive protein

Although C-reactive protein is measured by the hospital clinical biochemistry rather than the haematology laboratory, it is described here, since it is an acute phase reactant which is used for a similar purpose to the ESR.

C-reactive protein is secreted by the liver in response to a variety of inflammatory cytokines. It recognizes altered self and foreign molecules, as a result of which it activates complement and generates pro-inflammatory cytokines and activation of the adaptive immune system. Raised levels are a non-specific indicator of inflammation, trauma and infection and serial measurements can be used to monitor response to treatment and resolution of the condition.

Monitoring anticoagulant therapy

Blood clotting in the body is mediated through a cascade of coagulation factors which can be split into an extrinsic and an intrinsic element. The extrinsic and intrinsic pathways can be evaluated in the laboratory by the prothrombin time (PT) and the activated partial thromboplastin time (APTT), respectively.

Extrinsic pathway. Factor III (tissue thromboplastin), which is normally extrinsic to the circulation, is released from damaged tissue into the blood and forms a complex with factor VII. The latter becomes activated (factor VIIa) and in turn activates factor X to Xa in the presence of calcium ions.

$$VII + Ca^{2+} + III \text{ (tissue factor)} \rightarrow VIIa \rightarrow X \rightarrow Xa$$

Intrinsic pathway. The intrinsic system depends on substances normally present in blood for its activation. The intrinsic mechanism is initiated when factor XII is adsorbed in vivo onto subendothelial collagen which is exposed in a damaged blood vessel or, in vitro, adsorbed onto a surface such as glass or kaolin. Surface adsorption activates factor XII by exposing an active enzyme site. Factor XIIa then activates XI and so on:

$$XII \rightarrow XIIa \rightarrow XI \rightarrow XIa \rightarrow IX \rightarrow IXa \rightarrow X \rightarrow Xa$$
$$\uparrow$$
Factor VII as co-factor

Common pathway. The extrinsic and intrinsic pathways converge at the level of factor X, from which there is a common pathway whereby thrombin (factor IIa) and fibrin (factor I) are eventually formed, leading to formation of a fibrin clot.

One-stage prothrombin time (PT)

The prothrombin time (PT) is a test used to measure the clotting time of plasma in the presence of tissue extract (thromboplastin, factor III) and indicates the overall efficiency of the extrinsic system. It is used to monitor warfarin therapy (warfarin inhibits the formation of factors II, VII, IX and X). The test involves adding extrinsic thromboplastin to citrated plasma and adding calcium to clot the mixture. The time to form the fibrin clot is recorded. Control blood has a PT of 12–15 seconds.

International normalized ratio (INR)

The results of the test are commonly expressed as a ratio of the PT time of the patient compared with that of the normal control. This is known as the international normalized ratio (INR).

$$INR = \left[\frac{\text{patient's PT}}{\text{control PT}} \right]^{ISI}$$

The ISI is the international sensitivity index, which is allocated to commercial preparations of thromboplastin to standardize them.

The target value varies according to the indication for the anticoagulant. For example, patients with atrial fibrillation usually have a target INR of 2.5, whereas for those with recurrent deep vein thrombosis and pulmonary embolism, the target is higher at 3.5.

The most common use of the PT and INR is to monitor oral anticoagulant therapy, but it can also be used to assess liver function.

Activated partial thromboplastin time (APTT)

The activated partial thromboplastin time (APTT) is used to assess the intrinsic pathway and is the most common method for monitoring unfractionated heparin therapy.

A thromboplastic reagent is added to an activator such as activated silicone or kaolin. If the activator is kaolin, the test may be referred to as the PTTK (partial thromboplastin time kaolin) or the KCCT (kaolin–cephalin clotting time). Cephalin is a brain extract supplying the thromboplastin.

The mixture of thromboplastin and activator is mixed with citrated plasma to which calcium is added, and the time for the mixture to clot is recorded. The desirable APTT for optimal heparin therapy is between 1.5 and 2.5 times the normal control.

Low molecular weight heparins are effective and safe for the prevention and treatment of venous thromboembolism; because they provide more predictable anticoagulant activity than unfractionated heparin it is usually not necessary to monitor the activated partial thromboplastin time during treatment. Laboratory monitoring using an anti-factor Xa assay may be of value in certain clinical settings, including patients with renal insufficiency, and use of fractionated heparin for prolonged periods in pregnancy or in newborns and children.

D-dimers

D-dimers are degradation products of cross-linked fibrins, formed when plasmin degrades fibrin clots. Several methods for their analysis are available. There is no standard unit of measurement. Levels of D-dimers in the blood are raised in conditions associated with coagulation and are used to detect venous thromboembolism, although they are influenced by the presence of co-morbid conditions such as cancer, surgery and infectious diseases. Rapid tests have been developed, feasible for use in emergency conditions. D-dimers are not specific to venous thromboembolism and there is no consensus as to a critical cut-off value for screening for deep vein thrombosis (DVT), but a cut off level of about 0.3–0.5 mg/l is often used. Diagnosis of DVT should include a clinical probability assessment as well as D-dimer measurements, backed up with the availability of ultrasound or radiology.

Coombs's test

Coombs's reagent is a mixture of anti-human immunoglobulin antibody and anticomplement antibody. When added to washed red blood cells, it will detect antibody or complement on the cell surface and cause agglutination of the red cells. The test is positive (i.e. agglutination occurs) in cases of autoimmune anaemia.

Iron, transferrin and iron binding

Iron circulating in the serum is bound to transferrin. It leaves the serum pool and enters the bone marrow where it becomes incorporated into haemoglobin in developing red cells. Serum iron levels are extremely labile and fluctuate throughout the day and therefore provide little useful information about iron status.

Transferrin, a simple polypeptide chain with two iron binding sites, is the plasma iron binding protein. Measurement of total iron binding capacity (TIBC), from which the percentage of transferrin saturation with iron may be calculated, gives more information. Saturation of 16% or lower is usually taken to indicate an iron deficiency, as is a raised TIBC of greater than 70 μmol/l.

Ferritin is an iron store protein found in cell cytosol. Serum ferritin measurement is the test of choice in patients suspected of having iron deficiency anaemia.

In normal individuals, the serum ferritin concentration is directly related to the available storage iron in the body. The serum ferritin level falls below the normal range in iron deficiency anaemia, and its measurement can provide a useful monitor for repletion of iron stores after iron therapy. Ferritin is an acute phase protein and levels may be normal or high in the anaemia of chronic disease, such as occurs in rheumatoid arthritis or chronic renal disease.

Iron overload causes high concentrations of serum ferritin, as can liver disease and some forms of cancer.

Free protoporphyrin concentration increases in red blood cells in iron deficiency. These can be estimated with an assay which measures the fluorescence of zinc protoporphyrin (ZPP). ZPP is increased in iron deficiency, but also in chronic disease. In general, ZPP levels provide less information about iron storage in anaemic patients than does serum ferritin.

Soluble transferrin receptors (STFR) are a sensitive index of tissue iron availability, increasing in response to functional iron deficiency. Measurement of their levels does not offer sufficient additional information to serum ferritin to warrant routine use, but it may be a useful adjunct in the evaluation of anaemic patients whose ferritin values may be increased as part of the acute phase reactions.

Vitamin B$_{12}$ and folate

In the haematology literature, B$_{12}$ refers not only to cyanocobalamin, but also to several other cobalamins with identical nutritional properties. Folic acid, which can designate a specific compound, pteroylglutamic acid, is also more commonly used as a general term for the folates. Deficiency of cobalamin can result both in anaemia, usually macrocytic, and in neurological disease, including neuropathies, dementia and psychosis. Folate deficiency produces anaemia, macrocytosis, depression, dementia and neural tube defects.

There is some controversy about the definition of the lower limit of normal for serum B$_{12}$. Liver disease tends to increase B$_{12}$ levels, and they may be inexplicably reduced in folate deficient patients. Serum folate levels tend to increase in B$_{12}$ deficiency, and alcohol can reduce levels. Red blood cell folate is a better measure of folate tissue stores.

CASE STUDIES

Case 4.1

Mrs A. is a 70-year-old lady being treated by her general practitioner. She has a history of osteoarthritis and hypertension. Her drugs (listed below) are dispensed in a medicines organizer, but she is complaining that she has too many tablets and finds it difficult to remove them from the organizer. Her medicines, which have been unchanged for several years, are: paracetamol, diclofenac, nifedipine, lisinopril, ferrous sulphate, temazepam, bezafibrate.

The GP orders clinical biochemistry tests and a full blood profile. The results of the test show the following:

Haemoglobin, MCV, RBC and folate levels are all in the normal range
Urea   12.5 mmol/l
Creatinine   185 μmol/l
All other results are normal.

Questions

1. With respect to Mrs A.'s blood results, which drugs could be considered for discontinuation?
2. How should she be monitored in the future?

Answers

1. Since she has been taking iron and folic acid for several years, it would be wise to check the original reason for starting these drugs and whether she has been monitored regularly in the past. Iron stores should be repleted within 6 months after starting oral iron therapy providing there is no pathology, and her iron tablets could be discontinued.

    The high urea and creatinine results suggest the possibility of renal problems. The renal malfunction may be caused, or aggravated, by the NSAID diclofenac. This should be considered for discontinuation. Paracetamol may be sufficient to give the required analgesia. ACE inhibitors can cause progressive renal failure in patients with renovascular disease. They are best avoided in patients with known or suspected renovascular disease, and blood pressure controlled by other drugs.
2. A full blood profile should be requested every 3 months for 1 year and annually thereafter to check that her iron stores do not become depleted again. The cause of Mrs A.'s renal failure should be investigated, as ACE inhibitors do have a valuable role in heart failure, which might be an underlying cause. Her renal function should be monitored within 3 months to check any progression of the renal dysfunction.

Case 4.2

A 50-year-old man on a hospital medical ward has a fast pulse rate and falling blood pressure. His recent drug history is bendroflumethiazide (bendrofluazide) and aspirin. He has the following blood results:

Haematology results: Hb 8.8 g/dl
RBC 4.7 × 10^{12}/l
Platelets   570 × 10^9/l

MCV, MCH and the rest of the blood profile are normal
Clinical biochemistry: Urea 11.6 mmol/l
Creatinine is normal, and sodium and potassium concentrations are normal

Questions

1. What cause of this patient's low haemoglobin should be considered and investigated?
2. What is the likely cause of his raised urea level?
3. What terms describe this type of anaemia?

Answers

1. The most likely cause of a low haemoglobin in a man with this clinical picture is haemorrhage, particularly a gastrointestinal bleed. The picture is one of blood loss, manifested by a loss of red cells and haemoglobin. The red cells are of normal size and colour.
2. A raised urea in the presence of a normal creatinine may signify dehydration or gastrointestinal bleeding. In this case,

given the blood picture, the latter is more likely. Blood in the gastrointestinal tract is a source of protein which will be absorbed into the hepatic portal system and converted to urea in the liver.

3. The blood picture is one of a normocytic, normochromic anaemia, typically seen in haemorrhage.

Case 4.3

A 75-year-old man with a history of chronic obstructive pulmonary disease (COPD) is admitted to hospital with pneumonia, which has been treated by his general practitioner with oxytetracycline. His medication includes a salbutamol inhaler, a beclometasone inhaler, amitriptyline and oral prednisolone (when required for exacerbations of COPD).

His biochemistry profile shows the following abnormalities:

Sodium   126 mmol/l
Urea   9.0 mmol/l
Creatinine levels are in the normal range

Question

What are the possible causes of the patient's abnormal sodium and urea results?

Answer

Hyponatraemia can be caused by antidepressants such as amitriptyline. However, lung infections can give rise to secretion inappropriate antidiuretic hormone (SIADH) by producing an ectopic site of antidiuretic hormone (ADH) secretion.

This would result in a low serum sodium concentration. It could be confirmed by a low serum osmolality and a high urine osmolality. In SIADH, a low urea would be expected.

The high urea in the presence of a normal creatinine may suggest dehydration, as urea is more sensitive to haemoconcentration than creatinine. It may also signify a degree of renal damage caused by the oxytetracycline. Tetracyclines are also catabolic and would tend to cause protein to be broken down and converted to urea in the liver.

Case 4.4

A 60-year-old man presents with a 2 month history of pain in his lower back. X-ray shows a lytic bone lesion in the 4th lumbar vertebra.

Biochemistry tests of urea and electrolytes, bone chemistry and full blood count reveal the following abnormalities:

Ca^{2+} 1.51 mmol/l
Urea   13.1 mmol/l
Creatinine   184 µmol/l
Haemoglobin   11.1 g/dl

Questions

1. What is the most likely diagnosis?
2. What investigations would support the diagnosis?

Answers

1. (Multiple) myeloma.
2. The diagnosis would be supported by a paraproteinaemia, low serum immunoglobulins (excluding the monoclonal component), the presence of Bence Jones protein in the urine.

Case 4.5

A patient with a history of insulin dependent diabetes, heart failure and ischaemic heart disease is admitted to hospital after vomiting. His medication includes lisinopril, furosemide (frusemide) with potassium, nifedipine and isosorbide mononitrate.

Biochemistry results show:

Potassium   5.5 mmol/l
Urea   15 mmol/l
Creatinine   150 µmol/l
Random blood glucose 23 mmol/l

Arterial blood gases:

pH   7.25
Pco_2 2.8 kPa
Actual bicarbonate 9.5 mmol/l
Po_2 12.7 kPa

Questions

1. What is the likely cause of this patient's raised serum potassium level?
2. Why are the urea and creatinine raised?
3. What do his blood gases suggest?

Answers

1. Insulin deficiency causes a reduction in absorption of potassium into the tissues.
   The patient has metabolic ketoacidosis, evidenced by his raised blood glucose and reduced pH and bicarbonate.
   Hyperkalaemia may also be caused by renal failure. The potassium supplements and lisinopril may also have contributed.
2. Renal failure is a complication of diabetes. The patient will be dehydrated because of vomiting, furosemide (frusemide) and the osmotic diuresis caused by hyperglycaemia.
3. An acid plasma pH together with a low plasma bicarbonate concentration suggests a metabolic acidosis. The low Pco_2 reflects the body's attempt to blow off CO_2 from the lungs (Kussmaul respiration) in order to restore the plasma pH to normal. This is a typical picture seen in metabolic ketoacidosis in diabetic patients, but may also occur as a result of diarrhoea (loss of bicarbonate-rich intestinal fluid) or renal failure.

FURTHER READING

Marshall W J 2000 Clinical chemistry, 4th edn. Mosby, London

Laker M F 1996 Clinical biochemistry for medical students. W B Saunders, London

Howard M R, Hamilton P J 1997 Haematology: an illustrated colour text. Harcourt Brace, Edinburgh

Parenteral nutrition 5

S. J. Dunnett

KEY POINTS

- Parenteral nutrition (PN) is indicated when the gastrointestinal tract is inaccessible, inadequate or inappropriate to meet the patient's ongoing nutritional needs.
- Combinations of oral diet, enteral feeding and PN (either peripherally or centrally) may be appropriate.
- PN regimens, tailored to the nutritional needs of the patient, should contain a balance of seven essential components: water, L-amino acids, glucose, lipid with essential fatty acids, vitamins, trace elements and electrolytes.
- Advances in PN technology often permit the required nutrients to be administered from a single container. Increasingly, standard formulations are used, including licensed presentations.
- PN must be compounded under aseptic conditions.
- PN prescriptions are guided by baseline nutritional assessment, knowledge of the patient's disease status and ongoing monitoring.
- The incidence of complications with PN is reducing; knowledge of management is improving.

Introduction

Malnutrition

Malnutrition can be described as: 'a deficiency or excess (or imbalance) of energy, protein, and other nutrients that causes measurable adverse effects on the tissue/body size, shape, composition and function and clinical outcome.'

In UK hospitals, most malnutrition appears to be a general undernutrition of all nutrients (protein, energy and micronutrients) rather than marasmus (insufficient energy provision) or kwashiorkor (insufficient protein provision). Alternatively, there may be a specific deficiency, such as thiamine in severe hepatic disease.

Multiple causes may contribute to malnutrition. They may include inadequate or unbalanced food intake, increased demand due to clinical disease status, defects in food digestion or absorption, or a compromise in nutritional metabolic pathways. Onset may be acute or insidious.

Even mild malnutrition can result in problems with normal body form and function, with adverse affects on clinical, physical and psychosocial status. For example, impaired immune response, reduced skeletal muscle strength and fatigue, reduced respiratory muscle strength, impaired thermoregulation, impaired skin barrier and wound healing may all be a consequence of mild malnutrition. In turn, these predispose the patient to a wide range of problems including infection, delayed clinical recovery, increased clinical complications, inactivity, psychological decline and reduced quality of life. Symptoms may be non-specific and so the underlying malnutrition may be left undiagnosed.

Nutrition screening

Only when the assessment of every patient's nutritional status has become routine will the full benefits of nutritional treatment be realized (Lennard-Jones 1992). A range of screening criteria and tools have been developed and refined to assess nutritional status. For example, the British Association of Parenteral and Enteral Nutrition (BAPEN) recommend utilizing the relatively simple and reproducible body mass index tool with consideration of other key factors, as in Table 5.1 (Elia 2000). This basic screening tool should not be used in isolation; significant weight fluctuations may reflect fluid disturbances, and muscle wasting may be due to immobility rather than undernutrition.

Table 5.1 Body mass index as a screening tool

$$\text{Body mass index (BMI)} = \frac{\text{weight (kg)}}{\text{height (m)}^2}$$

BMI category	Likelihood of chronic protein-energy undernutrition
< 18.5 kg/m²	Probable
18.5–20 kg/m²	Possible
> 20 kg/m²	Unlikely

67

Incidence of undernutrition

The incidence of undernutrition in hospitalized patients is not accurately known. Reports vary between 13% and 40% (Stratton & Elia 2000).

Evidence is growing that nutritional intervention can release resources in the health service, given that hospital malnutrition may be evaluated in terms of both patient outcome and total hospital costs (Tucker & Miguel 1996). Early nutrition intervention is associated with reduced average length of hospital stay and linked cost savings.

Indications for parenteral nutrition

Parenteral nutrition (PN) is the intravenous administration of a nutritionally balanced and physicochemically stable sterile combination of the six main groups of nutrients with water: amino acids, glucose, lipid emulsion including essential fatty acids, vitamins, trace elements and electrolytes. PN may fulfil the total nutritional requirements, or may be supplemental to an enteral feed or diet.

The simplest way to correct or prevent undernutrition is through conventional balanced food. However, this is not always possible. Nutritional support may then require oral supplements or enteral feeding. Assuming the gut is functioning normally, the patient will be able to digest and absorb their required nutrients. These include water, protein, carbohydrate, fat, vitamins, minerals and electrolytes. However, if the gut is not accessible or functioning adequately to meet the patient's needs, or gut rest is indicated, then PN is used. While the enteral route is first-line, this may still fail to provide sufficient nutrient intake in a number of patients (Woodcock et al 2001). Complications and limitations of enteral nutrition need to be recognized.

A decision pathway can be followed to guide initial and ongoing nutritional support. While many are published, a locally tailored and regularly updated pathway is favoured. Figure 5.1 may provide a useful starting point.

Close monitoring should ensure the patient's needs are met; a combination of nutrition routes is sometimes the best course. Where possible, PN patients should also receive enteral intake. Even minor gut stimulation has been linked with a reduction in the incidence of bacterial translocation through maintaining gut integrity and preventing overgrowth and cholestatic complications (Maroulis & Kalfarentoz 2000). Adaptation and re-establishment of enteral and oral diet is improved. PN should not be stopped abruptly but should be gradually reduced in line with the increasing enteral diet.

Nutrition teams

Multidisciplinary nutrition teams have been formed in many hospitals, notably the larger tertiary centres and teaching hospitals. They function in a variety of ways, depending on the patient populations and resources. In general, they adopt either a consultative or an authoritative role in nutrition management. Many studies

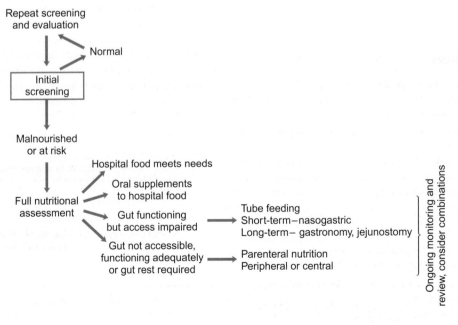

Figure 5.1   Decision pathway to guide initial and ongoing nutritional support.

have shown their positive contribution to the total nutritional care of the patient through efficient and appropriate selection and monitoring of feed and route. Recommendations to guide the initial set-up and development of such teams have been published (Howard 1999).

Components of a parenteral nutrition regimen

In addition to water, six main groups of nutrients need to be incorporated in a PN regimen (Table 5.2). The aim is to provide appropriate sources and amounts of all the equivalent building blocks in a single daily admixture.

Water volume

Water is the principal component of the body and accounts for approximately 60% and 55% of total body weight in men and women, respectively. Usually, homeostasis maintains appropriate fluid levels and electrolyte balance and thirst drives the healthy person to drink. However, some patients are not able physically to respond by drinking and so this homeostasis can readily be disrupted. There is risk of over or underhydration if the range of factors affecting fluid and electrolyte balance are not fully understood and monitored (see Chapter 4). In general, an adult patient will require 20–40 ml/kg/day fluid. However, Table 5.3 describes other factors that should be considered in tailoring input to needs.

Table 5.2 Oral and equivalent parenteral nutrition source

Oral diet	Parenteral nutrition source
Water/volume	Water/volume
Protein	L-amino acids mixture
Carbohydrate	Glucose
Fat with essential fatty acids	Lipid emulsions with essential fatty acids
Vitamins	Vitamins
Minerals	Trace elements
Electrolytes	Electrolytes

Amino acids

Twenty L-amino acids are required for protein synthesis and metabolism. A majority of these can be synthesized endogenously. Eight are called 'essential' amino acids because they cannot be synthesized (isoleucine, leucine, lysine, methionine, phenylalanine, threonine, tryptophan and valine). A further group of 'conditionally essential' amino acids, arginine, choline, glutamine, taurine and *S*-adenosyl-L-methionine, are defined as the patient's needs exceed the synthesis in clinically stressed conditions. Also, due to the immature metabolic pathways of neonates, infants and children, some other amino acids are essential in the young patient, and these include histidine, proline, cysteine, tyrosine and taurine.

Table 5.3 Factors affecting fluid requirements

Consider increasing the fluid input	Consider reducing the fluid input
• Signs/symptoms of dehydration	• Signs/symptoms of fluid overload
• Fever: increased insensible losses from lungs in hyperventilation and from skin in sweating. Allow 10–15% extra water per 10°C above normal	• High humidity: reduced rate of evaporation
• Acute anabolic state: increased water required for increased cell generation	• Blood transfusion: volume input
• High environmental temperature or low humidity: increased rate of evaporation	• Drug therapy: assess volume and electrolyte content of infused drug
• Abnormal GI loss (vomiting, ostomies, diarrhoea): consider both volume loss and electrolyte content	• Cardiac failure: may limit tolerated blood volume
• Burns or open wound(s): increased water evaporation	• Renal failure: fluid may accumulate so reduce input accordingly, or provide artificial renal support
• Blood loss: assess volume lost and whether replaced by transfusion, colloid, crystalloid	

Immature neonatal metabolism does not fully metabolize glycine, methionine, phenylalanine and threonine and so requirements are reduced.

To balance the patient's amino acid requirements and the chemical characteristics of the amino acids (solubility, stability and compatibility), a range of commercially available licensed solutions have been formulated with a range of amino acid profiles (Table 5.4). Aminoplex, Intrafusin, Synthamin and Vamin are designed for adult patients. The amino acid profiles of Primene and Vaminolact are specifically tailored to neonates, infants and children (reflecting the amino acid profile of maternal cord blood and breast milk, respectively).

L-glutamine was initially excluded from formulations due to its low solubility and relatively poor stability in the aqueous environment. However, it is recognized that there is a clinical need for this amino acid in catabolic stress, and it is now available as a free L-glutamine additive and as a dipeptide (with alanine and lysine; the peptide bond cleaves in the blood releasing free L-glutamine). Research is also considering the rationale and merits of supplementing arginine, glutathione and ornithine α-ketoglutarate.

For adults, PN solutions are generally prescribed in terms of the amount of nitrogen they provide, rounding to the nearest gram, for example 9 g, 11 g, 14 g or 18 g nitrogen regimens may be prescribed. Assuming adequate energy is supplied, most adult patients achieve nitrogen balance with 0.2 g nitrogen/kg/day.

In paediatrics, the term amino acid is preferred when formulating PN solutions. The term 'protein content' is no longer favoured as the solutions contain amino acids, not protein. The conversion factor for g of protein to g of nitrogen varies depending on the amino acid profile, with different amino acid profiles releasing a different proportion of water molecules as the peptide bonds are formed. However, some publications refer to a conversion factor of 1 g of nitrogen per 6.25 g of protein. This should be used with caution.

Amino acid solutions are hypertonic to blood and should not be administered alone into the peripheral circulation.

Energy

Many factors affect the energy requirement of individual patients. These include age, activity and illness (both severity and stage). Predictive formulae can be applied to estimate the energy requirement. Alternatively, calorimetry techniques can be used. However, no single method is ideal or suits all scenarios. It is not unusual to find that two methods result in different recommendations. The majority of adults can be appropriately maintained on 25–35 non-protein kcal/kg/day.

There is debate whether to include amino acids as a source of calories since it is simplistic to assume they are either all spared for protein synthesis or fed into the metabolic pathways (Krebs cycle) and contribute to the release of energy rich molecules. In general, we refer to 'non-protein energy' and sufficient lipid and glucose energy is supplied to spare the amino acids. As a rough guide, the non-protein energy to nitrogen ratio should be approximately 150:1, increasing towards 200:1 in hypercatabolic patients, and decreasing towards 100:1 in non-catabolic patients.

Table 5.4 Amino acid and consequential nitrogen content of licensed amino acid solutions available in the UK (alphabetical)

		Amino acid content (g/l)	Nitrogen content (g/l)
Paediatric	Primene 10%	100	15
	Vaminolact	65.3	9.3
Adult	Glamin	134 g (inc. dipeptide)	22.4 (total)
	Hyperamine 30	179	30
	Intrafusin 11	73.28	11.4
	Intrafusin 22	152.3	22.8
	Synthamin 9/9EF	55	9.1
	Synthamin 14/14EF	85	14
	Synthamin 17/17EF	100	16.5
	Vamin 9/9 Glucose	70.2	9.4
	Vamin 14/14EF	85	13.5
	Vamin 18EF	114	18.0

Dual energy

In general, energy should be sourced from a combination of lipid and glucose. This is termed 'dual energy' and is more physiological than an exclusive glucose source.

Dual energy can minimize the risk of giving too much lipid or glucose since complications increase if the metabolic capacity of either is exceeded. A higher incidence of acute adverse effects is noted with faster infusion rates and higher total daily doses, especially in patients with existing metabolic stress. It is therefore essential the administered dose complements the energy requirements and the infusion rate does not exceed the metabolic capacity.

While effectively maintaining nitrogen balance, lipid inclusion is seen to confer a number of advantages (Table 5.5).

Some patients, notably long-term home patients, do not tolerate daily lipid infusions and need to be managed on an individual basis. Depending on the enteral intake and nutritional needs, lipids are prescribed for a proportion of the days. A trial with the newer generation lipid emulsions may be appropriate.

Glucose

Glucose is the recommended source of carbohydrate (1 g anhydrous glucose provides 4 kcal). Table 5.6 indicates the energy provision and tonicity for a range of concentrations. Glucose 5% is regarded as isotonic with blood. The higher concentrations cause phlebitis if administered directly to peripheral veins and should therefore be given by a central vein or in combination with compatible solutions to reduce the tonicity.

PN formulations classically contain one or more concentrations of glucose, selected to provide both the required glucose calories and to meet total volume requirement.

The glucose infusion rate should generally be between 2 and 4 mg/kg/min. An infusion of 2 mg/kg/min (equating to approximately 200 g (800 kcal) per day for a 70 kg adult) represents the basal glucose requirement, whereas 4 mg/kg/day is regarded as the physiological optimal rate. Higher levels (up to 7 mg/kg/min) are tolerated by some patients but are not generally recommended; glucose oxidation occurs but there is an increased conversion to glycogen and fat. If excess glucose is infused and the glycogen storage capacity exceeded, the circulating glucose level rises, de novo lipogenesis occurs (production of fat from glucose) and there is an increased incidence of metabolic complications.

Lipid emulsions

Lipid emulsions are used as a source of energy and for the provision of the essential fatty acids, linoleic and α-linolenic acid. Supplying 10 kcal energy per gram of oil, they are energy rich and can be infused directly into the peripheral veins since they are relatively isotonic with blood.

Typically, patients receive up to 2.5 g lipid/kg/day. For practical compounding reasons, and assuming clinical acceptance, this tends to be rounded to 100 g or 50 g. Table 5.7 gives details of the lipid emulsions available on the UK market.

Lipid emulsions are oil-in-water formulations. Figure 5.2 shows the structure of triglycerides (three fatty acids on a glycerol backbone) and a lipid globule, stabilized at the interface by phospholipids. Ionization of the polar phosphate group of the phospholipid results in a net negative charge of the lipid globule and an

Table 5.5 Examples of the advantages of dual energy systems over glucose-only energy systems

- Minimize risk of hyperglycaemia and related complications
- Prevent and reverse fatty liver (steatosis)
- Reduce carbon dioxide production and respiratory distress
- Meet higher calorie requirements of septic and trauma patients when glucose oxidation reduced and lipid oxidation increased
- Reduce metabolic stress
- Support immune function
- Improve lean body mass and reduce water retention
- Permit peripheral administration, through reduced tonicity
- Facilitate fluid restriction, as lipid is a concentrated source of energy
- Source of essential fatty acids, preventing and correcting deficiency

Table 5.6 Energy provision and tonicity of glucose solutions

Concentration (w/v)	Energy content (kcal/l)	Approximate osmolarity (mOsmol/l)
5%	200	278
10%	400	555
20%	800	1110
50%	2000	2775
70%	2800	3885

Table 5.7   Licensed lipid emulsions available in the UK

Lipid emulsion type	Details of products with kcal per litre
Soybean oil (egg phospholipids)	• Intralipid 10% (1100 kcal), 20% (2000 kcal), 30% (3000 kcal) • Ivelip 10% (1100 kcal), 20% (2000 kcal) • Lipofundin N 10% (1022 kcal), 20% (1908 kcal)
Olive oil (80%)/soybean oil (20%) (egg phospholipids)	• ClinOleic 20% (2000 kcal)
MCT (50%)/LCT (50%) (egg phospholipids)	• Lipofundin MCT/LCT 10% (1054 kcal), 20% (1904 kcal)
Structured triglyceride (egg phospholipids)	• Structolipid 20% (1960 kcal)

MCT, medium chain triglyceride; LCT, long chain triglyceride.

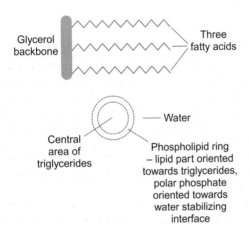

Figure 5.2   Triglyceride structure and composition of lipid emulsion globule.

electromechanically stable formulation. The lipid globule size distribution is similar to that of the naturally occurring chylomicrons (80–500 nanometers), as indicated in Figure 5.3.

The first generation lipid emulsions have been in use since the 1970s and utilize soybean oil as the source of long chain fatty acids. They have a good safety and efficacy record.

More recent research on lipid metabolic pathways and clinical outcomes has indicated that the fatty acid profile of soybean oil is not ideal. For example, it is now recognized that these lipid emulsions present excess essential fatty acids resulting in a qualitative and quantitative compromise to the metabolites that have important roles in haemodynamics, platelet function, inflammatory response and immune response. This has resulted in the development of newer lipid emulsions, including the use of medium chain triglycerides, olive oil, fish oil and structured triglycerides where the

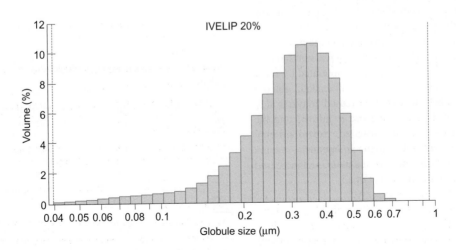

Figure 5.3   Lipid globule size distribution curve of Ivelip 20%.

glycerol backbone is esterified with a mix of medium chain and long chain fatty acids.

Both egg and soybean phospholipids include a phosphate moiety. There is debate as to whether this is bioavailable or not and some manufacturers include the phosphate content in their stability calculations while others do not.

The 20% lipid emulsions are favoured, especially in paediatrics, as they contain less phospholipid than the 10% emulsions in relation to triglyceride provision. If there is incomplete clearance of the infused phospholipids, lipoprotein X, an abnormal phospholipid-rich low density lipoprotein is generated, and a raised blood cholesterol observed. The incidence of raised lipoprotein X levels is greater with the 10% emulsions as they present proportionally more phospholipid.

Lipid clearance monitoring is particularly important in patients who are at risk of impaired clearance, including those who are hyperlipidaemic, diabetic, septic, have impaired renal or hepatic function, or are critically ill (Crook 2000).

Micronutrients

Micronutrients have a key role in intermediary metabolism, as both co-factors and co-enzymes. For example, zinc is required by over 200 enzyme systems and affects many diverse body functions including acid–base balance, immune function and nucleic acid synthesis. It is evident, therefore, that the availability of micronutrients can affect enzyme activity and total metabolism. When disease increases the metabolism of the major substrates, the requirement for micronutrients is increased. Some of the micronutrients also play an essential role in the free-radical scavenging system. These include:

- copper, zinc and manganese: in the form of superoxide dismutase, dispose of superoxide radicals
- selenium: in the form of glutathione peroxidase, removes hydroperoxyl compounds
- vitamin C: a strong reducing agent
- vitamins A, E and beta-carotene: react directly with free-radicals.

By the time a patient starts parenteral nutrition, they may have already developed a deficiency of one or more essential nutrients. By the time a specific clinical deficiency is observed, for example as depigmentation of hair in copper deficiency or skin lesions in zinc deficiency, the patient will already have tried to compensate to maintain levels, compromised intracellular enzyme activity and antioxidant systems and expressed non-specific symptoms such as fatigue and impaired immune response. A summary of factors that affect micronutrient needs is presented in Table 5.8.

Micronutrient monitoring can be costly and complex. Results require careful interpretation alongside clinical symptoms (Misra & Kirby 2000). Deficiency states are clinically significant but, with non-specific symptoms, they are often difficult to diagnose.

In general, daily administration of all micronutrients is recommended from the start of the parenteral nutrition. If a patient requires only a few days parenteral nutrition before a full enteral diet is reinstated and absorption achieved, and does not have existing deficiency or increased requirements, a few days omission may not present a clinical problem.

Additional oral or enteral supplements may be considered if there is some intestinal absorption. However, copper deficiency can increase iron absorption and zinc intake can decrease copper absorption.

The micronutrients naturally fall into two groups, the trace elements and vitamins.

Trace elements

Trace elements are generally maintained at a relatively constant tissue concentration and are present to a level of less than 1 mg/kg bodyweight. They are essential; deficiency results in structural and physiological disorders, but if identified early enough, can be resolved by readministration. Ten essential trace elements are known: iron, copper, zinc, fluorine, manganese, iodine, cobalt (or as hydroxycobolamin), selenium, molybdenum and chromium.

Various recommended baseline doses have been published but no single licensed preparation provides all

Table 5.8 Factors affecting micronutrient requirements
Baseline nutritional state on starting parenteral nutrition:
• Acute or chronic onset of illness
• Dietary history
• Duration and severity of inadequate nutritional intake
Increased loss:
• Small bowel fistulae/aspirate – rich in zinc
• Biliary fluid loss – rich in copper
• Burn fluid loss – rich in zinc, copper, selenium
Increased requirement:
• Increased metabolism – acute in anabolic phase following catabolic phase of critically ill
• Active growth
Organ function:
• Liver failure – copper and manganese clearance reduced
• Renal failure – aluminium, chromium, zinc and nickel clearance reduced

trace elements at the dose required (Table 5.9). Concern over neurotoxicity with accumulated manganese, especially in liver failure, led to a reduction in the advised daily dose and recommendations for plasma monitoring. Recognizing the benefits of zinc and selenium on the free-radical scavenging system, some specialists advise an increase in the administered dose.

Vitamins

There are two groups of vitamins, the water-soluble vitamins and the fat-soluble vitamins. Fat-soluble vitamins are stored in the body whereas excess water-soluble vitamins are renally cleared. Therefore, if there is inadequate provision, deficiency states for the water-soluble vitamins reveal themselves first.

Table 5.10 indicates the recommended (FDA 2000) daily requirements of vitamins and the formulation of commercial licensed preparation. No preparation meets the guideline requirements, therefore it is common practice for preparations to be used in combination. For example, daily Cernevit is frequently used in combination with weekly doses of Konakion MM and

Solivito N is frequently used with Vitlipid N Adult. Vitamins should be added to the daily parenteral nutrition bag.

Electrolytes

Sodium, potassium, calcium, magnesium and phosphate are included to meet patient needs. Depending upon the stability of the patient's clinical state, they are kept relatively constant or adjusted on a near daily basis, reflecting changes in blood biochemistry. Tables (e.g. British National Formulary) can be used to guide electrolyte replacement if there is excessive gastrointestinal waste or high losses through burns.

To prevent frequent minor adjustments in electrolyte prescriptions many practitioners define the minimum prescription dose change, for example, 15 mmol for potassium in an adult bag.

Some crystalloid and amino acid solutions contain electrolytes, whereas others are electrolyte-free. Table 5.11 indicates the electrolyte content of a selection of concentrated sources that may be added to PN formulations, assuming stability is confirmed.

Table 5.9   Trace element requirements and content of UK licensed products (adapted from data in Okada et al 1995)

	Units	American Medical Association 1979	Shenkin 1995	Flemming 1989	Additrace 1 ampoule	Decan 1 vial
Iron	µmol		17.5–70		20	17.9
	mg		1–4		1.12	1.000
Zinc	µmol	38–61.5	49–210	38.5–61.5	100	153
	mg	2.5–4	3–14	2.4–4	6.54	10.00
Copper	µmol	9.1–27.3	5–30	5–9.1	20	7.55
	mg	0.5–1.6	0.3–1.8	0.3–0.5	1.27	0.480
Manganese	µmol	2.7–14.5	6–36		5	3.64
	mg	0.15–0.8	0.3–2		0.275	0.200
Fluorine	µmol		49		50	76.3
	mg		0.9		0.95	1.450
Cobalt	µmol					0.025
	mg					1.470
Iodine	µmol		1		1	0.012
	mg		130		126.9	1.520
Selenium	µmol		0.4	0.5–1	0.4	0.887
	mg		0.03	0.04–0.08	0.032	0.070
Molybdenum	µmol		0.2	1–2	0.2	0.261
	mg		0.02	0.1–0.2	0.019	0.025
Chromium	µmol	0.19–0.29	1	0.19–0.38	0.2	0.289
	mg	0.01–0.015	0.05	0.01–0.02	0.01	0.015

Table 5.10 Vitamin requirements and UK licensed products (alphabetical)

	Vitamin	Recommended daily parenteral dose	Cernevit 1 vial	Konakion MM 10 mg/ml	Multibionta	Solivito N 1 vial	Vitlipid N Adult 10 ml
Fat-soluble	A (retinol)	1 mg (3330 IU)	3500 IU	–	10 000 IU as palmitate	–	3300 IU
	D	5 micrograms (200 IU)	(D3) 220 IU	–	–	–	(D2) 200 IU
	E (α-tocopherol)	10 mg (15 IU)	11.2 IU	–	5 mg as acetate	–	10 IU
	K_1	150 micrograms	–	Flexibility from 10 mg/ml presentation	–	–	150 micrograms
Water-soluble	B_1 (thiamine)	6.0 mg	3.51 mg	–	50 mg as hydrochloride	2.5 mg	–
	B_2 (riboflavin)	3.6 mg	4.14 mg	–	10 mg as sodium phosphate	3.6 mg	–
	B_6 (pyridoxine)	4.0 mg	4.53 mg	–	15 mg as hydrochloride	4.0 mg	–
	B_{12}	5 micrograms	6 micrograms	–	–	5 micrograms	–
	C	200 mg	125 mg	–	500 mg	100 mg	–
	Folic acid	600 micrograms	414 micrograms	–	–	400 micrograms	–
	Pantothenic acid	15 mg	17.25 mg	–	25 mg pantethenol	15 mg	–
	Biotin	60 micrograms	69 micrograms	–	–	60 micrograms	–
	Niacin	40 mg	46 mg	–	100 mg nicotinamide	40 mg nicotinamide	–

Administration of parenteral nutrition

Routes of administration

PN can be administered peripherally or centrally.

Peripheral route

Peripheral administration should be considered first-line for parenteral feeding. Supported by good techniques, line care and low tonicity feeds, patients can be successfully maintained with this route for many weeks. Peripheral lines are less costly than central lines, they can be inserted by less specialized staff, there is no requirement for a chest X-ray to confirm placement, and line care protocols are simpler. A mid-line should be considered as a peripheral line as it does not reach the central circulation.

Some indications and contraindications to the use of the peripheral route are summarized in Table 5.12.

Peripheral administration is sometimes complicated or delayed by phlebitis, where an insult to the endothelial vessel wall causes inflammation, redness, pain and possible extravasation. Peripheral tolerance can be influenced by a range of factors (Table 5.13).

Many consider that the tonicity of the infused solution or emulsion is a key factor defining peripheral infusion tolerance. The total number of osmotically active particles in the intracellular and extracellular fluids is essentially the same, approximately 290–310 mOsmol/l. When a lipid emulsion is included, infusions of

Table 5.11 Electrolyte and micronutrient content of additives used in parenteral nutrition compounding

	Content per ml									
	Na^+ (mmol)	K^+ (mmol)	Mg^{2+} (mmol)	Ca^{2+} (mmol)	$PO_4^{2-} HPO_4^-$ (mmol)	Cl^- (mmol)	Acetate (mmol)	Iron (micromol)	Selenium (micromol)	Zinc (micromol)
Sodium chloride 10%	1.7	–	–	–	–	1.7	–	–	–	–
Sodium chloride 23.5%	4	–	–	–	–	4	–	–	–	–
Sodium chloride 30%	5.1	–	–	–	–	5.1	–	–	–	–
Sodium acetate 40 mmol/10 ml	4	–	–	–	–	–	4	–	–	–
Sodium glycero-phosphate 21.6%	2	–	–	–	1	–	–	–	–	–
Potassium chloride 15%	–	2	–	–	–	2	–	–	–	–
Potassium acid phosphate 13.6%	–	1	–	–	1	–	–	–	–	–
Calcium chloride 1 mmol/ml	–	–	–	1	–	2	–	–	–	–
Calcium chloride 0.5 mmol/1 ml	–	–	–	0.5	–	1	–	–	–	–
Calcium chloride 13.4%	–	–	–	0.91	–	1.82	–	–	–	–
Calcium gluconate 10%	–	–	–	0.22	–	–	–	–	–	–
Magnesium sulphate 10%	–	–	0.4	–	–	–	–	–	–	–
Magnesium sulphate 50%	–	–	2	–	–	–	–	–	–	–
Addiphos	1.5	1.5	–	–	2	–	–	–	–	–
Iron chloride 100 micrograms/ml	–	–	–	–	–	–	–	1.79	–	–
Iron chloride 300 micrograms/ml	–	–	–	–	–	–	–	5.37	–	–
Sodium selenite 16 micrograms/ml	–	–	–	–	–	–	–	–	0.2	–

Table 5.12 Indications and contraindications to the use of peripheral parenteral nutrition

Indications:

- Duration of feed likely to be short term
- Supplemental feeding
- Compromised access to central circulation (e.g. local trauma, surgery or thrombosis)
- No immediate facilities or trained staff to insert central catheter
- High risk of fungal or bacterial sepsis (e.g. patients with purulent tracheostomy secretions, immune deficiency state, history of repeated sepsis)
- Contraindication to central venous catheterization

Contraindications:

- Inadequate or inaccessible peripheral veins
- High calorie/nitrogen requirements alongside fluid restrictions (admixture osmolarity too high)

Table 5.13 Factors that improve tolerance to peripheral lines

- Aseptic insertion and line care
- Selection of large vessel with good blood flow and direct path (e.g. cephalic vein)
- Fine bore catheter (22 g) for minimal trauma on insertion and disturbance of blood flow
- Fine polyurethane catheter
- Secure catheter to minimize physical trauma
- Glyceryl trinitrate patch distal to insertion site, over tip to vasodilate vein
- Regular replacement of catheter, using alternate arms (12 hourly)
- Flushing of lines not in use
- Low tonicity infusions
- Inclusion of lipid emulsion – venoprotective and isotonic with blood
- Inclusion of heparin and/or hydrocortisone where stability confirmed

approximately three times this osmolarity are generally well tolerated via the peripheral route and there are reports of success with higher levels. However, other factors should also be considered. Patient factors, such as vein fragility and blood flow may mean that some infusion episodes are better tolerated than others. One administration of a high tonicity value may indeed be more successful than another with a lower value.

The osmolarity of a PN formulation can be estimated by applying the following equation:

Osmolarity of PN formulation

$$= \frac{\Sigma \left[\text{osmolarity}_n \ (\text{mOsmol/l}) \times \text{volume}_n \ (\text{l}) \right]}{\text{Total volume (l)}}$$

where n indicates the component.

By considering the macronutrients included in the regimen, i.e. the amino acids, glucose and lipid, an estimation of the osmolarity can be made. The value will be increased by electrolyte or micronutrient additions. However, since the peripheral tolerance is affected by so many factors including tonicity, and because estimations of limits are given, the effect of these additions is relatively low unless high levels of monovalent ions are included.

Central route

The central venous route is indicated when longer-term feeding is anticipated, high tonicity formulations are required or the peripheral route is inaccessible. The rapid and turbulent blood flow in the central circulation and the constant movement of the heart ensures rapid mixing and reduces the risk of osmotically induced injury to the endothelium.

A range of single, double, triple and quadruple lumen central lines are available and one lumen must be dedicated for the nutrition. These lines require skilful insertion, usually into the jugular or subclavian vein, and confirmation of their position by X-ray. This relatively invasive and costly procedure is performed by trained medical staff. Tunnelling of the line to an appropriate exit site facilitates line care and may reduce the incidence of significant line sepsis.

PICCs

Peripherally inserted central catheters (PICCs) are typically inserted into a peripheral vein, usually the cephalic or basilic in the upper arm, with the exit tip in the superior vena cava just above the right atrium. As the name suggests, they are used for the central administration of infusions. Single and double lumen versions are available. Some also have a one-way valve to prevent backflow. Insertion is less invasive than for conventional central lines and can be undertaken by nurse practitioners.

Infusion control

Pumps

PN must always be administered under the control of an infusion pump. Acute overload of fluid, nutrition and electrolytes can have morbid consequences.

Infusion pumps should be used with an appropriate infusion or giving set which is compatible with both the infusion pump and the PN admixture. For home patients, small, simple battery powered ambulatory pumps are favoured.

Temperature

PN should be at room temperature when it is infused. It must, therefore, be removed from the refrigerator in which it is stored approximately 3 hours before connection and left to warm naturally to room temperature (for a $2^{1}/_{2}$ litre regimen). No external heat should be applied, although intermittent inversion of the bag may help.

If a cold admixture is infused, the patient may experience infusion discomfort and the acute release of gas from where it was dissolved in the admixture may cause the pump to alarm 'air-in-line'.

Compounded formulations

Historically, PN was administered from a series of separate bottles. Health care staff had to accurately and safely manage a combination of giving sets, infusion rates and total infusion times. While this system proved effective in nourishing many patients to recovery, this practice is now little used in the UK. Most patients now receive their complete nutrition from a single daily bag of a pharmaceutically stable PN formulation. The advantages of such a system far out-weigh the disadvantages, as indicated in Table 5.14.

Various terms are used to describe the PN formulation, depending on whether lipid is included. If it contains lipid, it is called a 3-in-1, ternary or all-in-one admixture. If no lipid is present, the terms 2-in-1, binary or aqueous admixture are used.

Standardized formulations

It is estimated that up to 80% of adult patient needs can be met with standard PN formulations.

Depending on the type (size and speciality) of the hospital, a range of standard formulations are maintained and supported with prescribing guidelines. These may be compounded from scratch, compounded from 'base-bags' locally or by a licensed unit, or purchased as licensed ready-to-use presentations.

The range is specifically selected to meet the needs of the patients managed by the hospital and will typically include a low tonicity regimen suitable for peripheral administration, a high calorie and high nitrogen regimen for central administration to catabolic patients and a high tonicity regimen for fluid restricted patients. Baseline electrolytes will generally be included although the flexibility for reduced levels is usually offered.

Table 5.14 Advantages and disadvantages of compounded PN formulations compared to bottle system

Advantages:

- Convenience and time saving for care staff and patient – single bag, single pump and rate, single line
- Simultaneous infusion of all nutrients – permitting optimal utilization
- Reduced infection risk – fewer connections and disconnections at ward level
- Reduced risk of error – pharmacy compounding in controlled environment with controlled procedures, single infusion managed at ward level
- Home management possible
- Storage and stock management of single item, rather than multiple nutrition sources
- Reduced scope for incompatible formulations to be compounded

Disadvantages:

- Physical and chemical stability needs to be known for both the storage and infusion time (separate bottle system offers an informed practitioner the scope to infuse incompatible parts separately, in contact for a shorter time)
- Potential time delay in compounding to unique specification
- Potential wastage of original admixture if patient's needs change
- Fridge storage required

Licensed ready-to-use products

A range of licensed ready-to-use preparations are available. For convenience, baseline electrolyte levels are included in many formulations and meet the needs of most patients; electrolyte-free options are becoming more readily available. Some are licensed in paediatrics and/or for peripheral use. Manufacturers advise on stability and shelf-life for electrolyte and micronutrient additions. The range of ready-to-use products includes:

- Triple chamber bags (OliClinomel, Compleven, Kabiven and Nutriflex Lipid ranges): chambers separately pre-filled with lipid, amino acid and glucose and terminally sterilized. Activated by applying external pressure so weak peal seals open, mixing the contents to a 3-in-1 formulation.
- Dual chamber bags (Clinimix and Nutriflex ranges): chambers separately pre-filled with amino acid and glucose and terminally sterilized. Activated to a 2-in-1 formulation. Flexibility to omit or add a compatible lipid.
- Two bottle system (Vitrimix-KV): transfer set and vacuum used to transfer lipid emulsion into the amino acid and glucose mix.

Cyclic infusions

Cyclic PN is when the daily requirements are administered over a short period. A classic example is the stable home patient who administers their feed overnight, freeing themselves from the constraints of an infusion during the day. This enables them to have more physical freedom and improves their quality of life.

Since cyclic feeding more closely simulates the human feeding pattern and is a closer match to normal hormonal and metabolic cycles, it also offers a range of metabolic and clinical advantages. Steatosis, fatty infiltration of the liver, is less common and may be corrected by employing cyclic feeding because the feed-free period facilitates lipolysis and fat mobilization. Peripheral tolerance may be improved as the endothelia recover between infusion periods.

Initially, the patient should receive the PN infusion slowly over the full 24 hours. As tolerated, the rate of infusion can be increased slowly to decrease the infusion time. This should be done over a series of days. During this period, the patient must be monitored closely for any signs of fluid, electrolyte or acid–base imbalance and hyper/hypoglycaemia. For example, on stopping the infusion, rebound hypoglycaemia may occur. The patient should also be monitored for the recognized side-effects of lipid and amino acid infusions such as nausea, vomiting, sweating and flushing which occur more frequently when infused at faster rates.

Pharmaceutical issues

Having identified the balance of nutrients required for a patient in a single day, it is necessary to formulate a physically and chemically stable sterile admixture.

PN admixtures contain over 50 chemical entities and, as such, are extremely complex. Professional advice or reference material should be used before compounding and administering PN. Manufacturers and third party experts can advise on stability issues (Allwood & Kearney 1998).

Physical stability

Physical instability takes a number of forms including precipitation of solids and cracking of the lipid emulsion.

Precipitation

Precipitation carries two key risks. First, the potential to infuse solid particles to the narrow pulmonary capillaries may result in fatal emboli. Second, the prescribed nutrients may not be infused.

Clinically dangerous precipitates may not always be visible to the naked eye, especially if lipid emulsion is present. They may also develop over time, and an apparently 'safe' admixture may develop a fatal precipitate in use.

Precipitation of solid is epitomized by the formation of calcium phosphate. This is of special concern in neonatal admixtures where the requirements to prevent hypophosphataemic rickets and severe osteopenia may exceed the safe concentrations.

It is known that calcium and phosphate can form a number of different salt forms with different solubility profiles, for example $Ca(H_2PO_4)_2$ which is highly soluble in comparision to $CaHPO_4$ and $Ca_3(PO_4)_2$. $Ca_3(PO_4)_2$ precipitation is relatively immediate, and has a white, fluffy amorphous appearance. However, $CaHPO_4.2H_2O$ precipitation is time-mediated and has a more crystalline appearance.

Factors affecting calcium phosphate precipitation are shown in Table 5.15. Practical measures can be taken to minimize the risks; these include accurate calculation of the proposed formulation, comparison against professionally defined comprehensive matrices and thorough mixing. Solubility curves and algorithms should be used with extreme caution, even if they are quoted for a specific amino acid source. This is because they do not consider all the factors and do not consistently identify risk. Assuming the sodium content can be tolerated, use of an organic phosphate salt form may be beneficial.

Trace elements have also been associated with clinically significant precipitation. These include iron phosphate and copper sulphide (hydrogen sulphide from the minor degradation of cysteine/cystine).

Lipid destabilization

The oil-in-water lipid emulsions are sensitive to destabilization by a range of factors including the presence of positively charged ions and heat. The lipid globules may come together and coalesce to form larger globules and release free oil. This could occlude the lung microvasculature and cause respiratory and circulatory compromise and lead to death.

Positively charged ions destabilize the admixture by drawing the negatively charged lipid globules together, overwhelming the electromechanical repulsion of the charged phospholipids and increasing their tendency to join or coalesce. The divalent and trivalent ions have a more significant effect. Therefore, there are tightly defined limits for the amount of Ca^{2+} and Mg^{2+} that can be added to a 3-in-1 admixture. Although the limits for the other polyvalent ions (such as zinc and selenium) are also controlled, because they are given in micromolar or nanomolar quantities they are less of a problem.

Low concentrations of amino acids and glucose also reduce the stability of the emulsion and increase the tendency for creaming.

Table 5.15 Factors affecting calcium phosphate precipitation

	Mechanism and effect
pH	Low pH supports solubility, whereas a higher pH supports precipitation Depending on the amount and buffering capacity of the amino acids, this can be affected by different concentrations and sources of glucose solution and acetate salt forms
Temperature	Higher temperatures associated with greater precipitation – increased availability of free calcium to interact and a shift to the more insoluble salt forms
Amino acids	Buffer pH changes Complex with calcium so less available to react with phosphate Both the source of amino acid and the relative content are important
Magnesium	Complex with phosphate forming soluble salts rather than less soluble calcium salts
Calcium salt form	Calcium chloride dissociates more readily than calcium gluconate, releasing it to react with the phosphate
Phosphate salt form	Monobasic salts (e.g. dipotassium phosphate) dissociate more readily than dibasic salts (e.g. potassium acid phosphate), releasing phosphate to react with the calcium Organic salts, such as sodium glycerphosphate and glucose-1-phosphate are more stable
Mixing order	Optimum stability achieved by only permitting calcium and phosphate to come together in a large volume admixture Agitate between additions to avoid pockets of concentration

The naked eye can identify large-scale destabilization, as shown in Table 5.16. However, the limitations of this method need to be recognized; clinically significant destabilization might not be visible to the naked eye. In practice, stability laboratories apply specific technical equipment and defined criteria to establish the physical stability of a formulation. These include assessing changes in lipid globule size distribution with the optical microscope and particle size counters applying defined limits of pharmaceutical acceptance. A wide safety margin is applied.

Chemical stability

Chemical stability takes many forms, notably chemical degradation of the vitamins and amino acids.

Vitamin stability

Many vitamins readily undergo chemical degradation, and vitamin stability often defines the shelf-life of the formulation.

Vitamin C (ascorbic acid), the least stable, is generally regarded as the marker for vitamin degradation. Vitamin C oxidation is accelerated by heat, oxygen and certain trace elements, including copper. Other examples include vitamin A photolysis and vitamin E photo-oxidation. Measures that minimize oxygen presence, such as minimal aeration during compounding, evacuation of air at the end of compounding and use of oxygen barrier bags, and light protection are recommended.

Amino acid stability

The amino acid profile should be maintained for the shelf-life of the formulation and manufacturers perform assays to confirm this prior to issuing stability reports.

Maillard reaction

The Maillard reaction is a complex pathway of chemical reactions that starts with a condensation of the carbonyl group of the glucose and the amino group of the amino acid. At present, relatively little is known about the clinical effects of these Maillard reaction products; however, it is prudent to minimize their presence by protecting from light and avoiding high temperatures.

Microbial stability

PN is a highly nutritious medium although hypertonicity will partially limit microbial growth potential. Growth in lipid alone is greater. Pharmaceutical developments have enabled terminal sterilization of many of the components, including the multi-chamber bag presentations. Manipulations should only be performed using validated aseptic techniques. Nurses, patients and carers must be trained to apply aseptic methods when connecting and disconnecting infusions. Many centres have documented line care and PN protocols.

Table 5.16   Lipid instability

	Description		Visual observation
Stable, normal emulsion		Lipid globules equally dispersed Suitable for administration	Normal emulsion 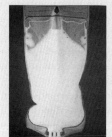
Light creaming	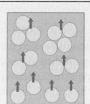	Lipid globules rising to the top of the bag. Slight layering visible. Readily redisperses on inverting the bag. Suitable for administration	Light creaming 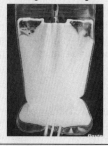
Heavy creaming, flocculation	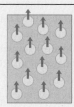	Lipid globules coming together but not joining. Rising to the top of the bag. More obvious layering visible. Readily redisperses on inverting the bag. Acceptable for administration	Heavy creaming 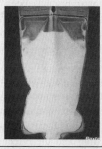
Coalescence	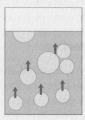	Lipid globules come together, coalesce to form larger globules and rise to the surface. Larger globules join releasing free-oil. Irreversible destabilization of the lipid emulsion. Not suitable for administration	Cracked, example 1 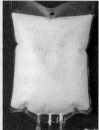 (Bag lying horizontally) Oil layer, close up 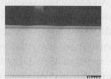 (Bag hanging vertically)

Shelf-life and temperature control

The manufacturer may be able to provide physical and chemical stability data to support a formulation for a shelf-life of up to 90 days at 2–8°C followed by 24 hours at room temperature for infusion. This assumes a strict aseptic technique is used during compounding. Units holding a manufacturing license covering aseptic compounding of PN are able to assign this full shelf-life. Unlicensed units are limited to a maximum shelf-life of 7 days.

PN must be stored and transported within the defined temperature limits. A validated cold-chain must be employed. Pharmaceutical grade fridges should be used and monitored to ensure appropriate air-cycling and temperature maintenance. The temperature during the infusion period should be known; neonatal units and incubators are classically maintained at higher temperatures, and formulations used must have been validated at these temperatures.

Drug stability

The addition of drugs to PN admixtures, or Y-site co-administration, is actively discouraged unless the compatibility has been formally confirmed. Wherever possible, the nutrition should be administered through a dedicated line. Multi-lumen catheters can be used to infuse PN separately from other infusion(s).

However, extreme competition for i.v. access may prompt consideration of drug and PN combinations. Many factors need to be considered. They include the physical and chemical stability of the PN, the physical and chemical stability of the drug, the bioavailability of the drug and the effect of stopping and starting Y-site infusions on the actual administration rates. It is not possible to reliably extrapolate data from a specific PN composition, between brands of solutions and salt forms or between brands or doses of drugs. A range of studies have been performed and published; however, these should be used with caution.

In practice, drugs should only be infused with PN when all other possibilities have been exhausted. These may include gaining further i.v. access and changing the drug(s) to clinically acceptable non-i.v. alternatives.

The relative risks of stopping and starting the PN infusion and repeatedly breaking the infusion circuit should be fully considered before sharing a line for separate infusions of PN and drug. In most cases, the risks outweigh the benefits. However, if this option is adopted, the line must be flushed before and after with an appropriate volume of solution known to be stable with both the PN and the drug. Strict aseptic technique should be adopted to minimize the risk of contaminating the line and infusions.

Filtration

All intravenous fluids pass through the delicate lung microvasculature with its capillary diameter of 8–12 μm. The presence of particulate matter has been demonstrated to cause direct embolization, direct damage to the endothelia, formation of granulomata, formation of foreign body giant cells and to have a thombogenic effect. In addition, the presence of microbial and fungal matter can cause a serious infection or inflammatory response.

Precautions taken to minimize the particulate load of the compounded regimen must include:

- use of in-lead filters (25 μm) and filter needles or straws (5 μm) during compounding to catch larger particles such as cored rubber from bottles and glass shards from ampoules
- air particle levels kept within defined limits in aseptic rooms by the use of air filters and non-shedding clothing and wipes
- use of quality raw materials with minimal particulate presence, including empty bags and leads
- confirmation of physical and chemical stability of the formulation prior to aseptic compounding applying approved mixing order (stability for the required shelf-life time and conditions).

There is ongoing debate as to whether in-line filters should be routinely used during PN infusion. Guidelines have been published that endorse their use, especially for patients requiring intensive or prolonged parenteral therapy, including home patients, the immuno-compromised, neonates and children (Bethune et al 2001). The filter should be placed as close to the patient as possible and validated for the PN to be used. For 2-in-1 formulations, 0.2 μm filters may be used. For 3-in-1 formulations, validated 1.2 μm filters may be used.

Light protection

It is widely recognized that exposure to light, notably phototherapy light and intense sunlight, may increase the degradation rate of certain constituents such as vitamins A and E. It is recommended that all regimens should be protected from light both during storage and during infusion (Allwood & Martin 2000), since:

- lipid does not totally protect against vitamin photodegradation
- Maillard reaction (see above) is influenced by light exposure
- ongoing research suggests lipid peroxidation is accelerated by a range of factors including exposure to certain wavelengths of light
- in order to minimize confusion.

Validated bag covers should always be used.

Nutritional assessment and monitoring

Initial assessment

Once screening has identified a patient is in need of nutritional intervention, a more detailed assessment is performed. This will include an evaluation of nutritional requirements, the expected course of the underlying disease, consideration of the enteral route and, where appropriate, identification of access routes for parenteral nutrition. This will be supported by a clinical assessment that will include:

- clinical history
- dietary history
- physical examination
- anthropometry including muscle function tests
- biochemical, haematological and immunological review.

Monitoring

PN monitoring has a number of objectives. It should:

- evaluate ongoing nutritional requirements, including fluid and electrolytes
- determine the effectiveness of the nutritional intervention
- facilitate early recognition of complications
- identify any deficiency, overload or toxicity to individual nutrients
- determine discrepancies between prescribed, delivered and received dose.

A monitoring protocol should be in place for each patient receiving PN. Baseline data should be recorded so deviations can be recognized and interpreted. In the early stages, while the patient is in the acute stage of their illness and the nutritional requirements are being established, the frequency of monitoring will be greatest. Some tests may be defined by the underlying disease state, rather than by the presence of PN per se. As the patient's status stabilizes, the frequency of monitoring will reduce although the range of parameters monitored is likely to increase. Examples of parameters monitored include:

- *Clinical symptoms or presentation.* May be specific (e.g. thrombophlebitis) or non-specific (e.g. confusion).
- *Weight.* Acute changes reflect fluid gain or loss and prompt review of the volume of the PN. Slow, progressive changes more likely to reflect nutritional status.
- *Nitrogen balance.* An assessment of urine urea and insensible loss and their relation to nitrogen input. Difficult to obtain accurate figures.
- *Visceral proteins.* While albumin levels may indicate malnutrition, the long half-life limits its sensitivity to detect acute changes in nutritional status. Other markers with a shorter half-life may be more useful, e.g. transferrin.
- *Haematology.* For example platelet counts and clotting studies for thrombocytopenia.
- *Blood glucose.* Hyperglycaemia is a relatively frequent complication that prompts reduction in the infused dose. Insulin is not routinely recommended. May indicate sepsis. Hypoglycaemia may be rebound to a reduction in the input.
- *Lipid tolerance.* Turbidity, cholesterol and triglyceride profiles required.
- *Electrolyte profile.* Indicates appropriate provision or other complicating clinical activity. In the first few days, low potassium, magnesium and/or phosphate with or without clinical symptoms may reflect the refeeding syndrome (see below).
- *Liver function tests.* An abnormal liver profile may be observed and it is often difficult to identify a single cause. PN and other factors such as sepsis, drug therapy, underlying disease may all interplay. In adults, PN induced abnormalities tend to be mild, reversible and self-limiting. In the early stages, fatty liver (steatosis) is seen. In longer-term patients, a cholestatic picture tends to present.
- *Anthropometry.* Assesses longer-term status.
- *Acid–base profile.* Indicative of respiratory or metabolic compromise and may require review of PN formulation.
- *Vitamin and trace element screen.* A range of single compounds or markers to consider tolerance and identify deficiencies, although of limited value as some tests are non-specific and inaccurate.

Complications

Complications of PN fall into two main categories, catheter-related and metabolic (Table 5.17). Overall the incidence of such complications has reduced because of increased knowledge and skills together with more successful management (Maroulis & Kalfarentoz 2000).

Line blockage

Line occlusion may be caused by a number of factors, including:

- fibrin sheath forming around the line, or a thrombosis blocking the tip
- internal blockage of lipid, blood clot or salt and drug precipitates
- line kinking
- particulate blockage of a protective line filter.

Management will depend on the cause of the occlusion. In general, the aim is to save the line and resume feeding with minimum risk for the patient. The use of locks and flushes with urokinase (for fibrin and thrombosis), ethanol (for lipid deposits) and dilute hydrochloric acid (for salt and drug precipitates) may be considered. In some cases, the lines may need to be replaced.

Refeeding syndrome

This metabolic complication occurs when the infused nutrition exceeds the tolerance of a previously malnourished patient. High glucose infusions result in hyperinsulinaemia and an anabolic effect with the intracellular shift of magnesium, potassium and phosphate. Acute hypophosphataemia, hypokalaemia and hypomagnesaemia may present with cardiac, haematological and neurological dysfunction; death has been reported.

Some centres selectively increase to the full nutritional regimen over 2 days to avoid this acute refeeding syndrome. Thiamine affords some protection and may be administered before the nutrition is started and over the first few days of infusion.

Table 5.17 Examples of complications during parenteral nutrition

Catheter-related:

- Thrombophlebitis (peripheral)
- Catheter-related infection – local or systemic
- Venous thrombosis
- Line occlusion (lipid, thrombus, particulate)
- Pneumothorax, catheter malposition, vessel laceration, embolism, hydrothorax, dysrhythmias, incorrect placement (central)

Metabolic:

- Hyperglycaemia or hypoglycaemia
- Electrolyte imbalance
- Lipid intolerance
- Refeeding syndrome
- Dehydration or over-hydration
- Specific nutritional deficiency or overload
- Liver disease or biliary disease
- Gastrointestinal atrophy
- Metabolic bone dysfunction (in long term)
- Thrombocytopenia
- Adverse events with PN components
- Essential fatty acid deficiency

Specific disease states

Liver

Due to the complexity of liver function, the range of potential disorders and its role in metabolism, the use of PN in liver disease is not without problems. Consensus guidelines for the use of PN in liver disease have been published (Plauth et al 1997). Nutritional intervention may be essential for recovery, although care must be exercised with amino acid input and the risk of encephalopathy, calorie input and metabolic capacity, and the reduced clearance of trace elements such as copper and manganese (Maroulis & Kalfarentoz 2000). Cyclic feeding appears useful, especially in steatosis.

Renal

Fluid and electrolyte balance demand close attention. A low volume and quality urine output may necessitate a concentrated PN formulation with a reduction in electrolyte content, particularly potassium and phosphate. In the polyuric phase or the nephrotic syndrome, a higher volume formulation may be required.

The metabolic stress of acute renal failure and the malnutrition of chronic renal failure may initially demand relatively high nutritional requirements. However, nitrogen restriction may be necessary to control uraemia in the absence of dialysis or filtration and avoid uraemia-related impaired glucose tolerance, because of peripheral insulin resistance, and lipid clearance.

Micronutrient requirements may also change in renal disease. For example, renal clearance of zinc, selenium, fluoride and chromium is reduced and there is less renal 1α-hydroxylation of vitamin D.

Lipid emulsions can usually be administered at the same time as dialysis and filtration procedures. Chronic renal failure patients are predisposed to malnutrition and an enteral diet may be supplemented with intradialytic parenteral nutrition (IDPN) during the dialysis session (Foulks 1999).

Pancreatitis

Acute pancreatitis is a metabolic stress and requires high-level nutritional support.

While enteral nutrition stimulates the pancreas, parenteral amino acids and glucose do not. There is some concern that parenteral lipids may induce or exacerbate pancreatitis. However, so long as there is no familial hyperlipidaemia and the pancreatitis is not secondary to a lipid disorder, lipid can generally be safely and beneficially administered. A test dose and gradual increase from 100 ml of lipid 20% may be considered.

Lipid clearance and the clinical state of the pancreas should be monitored.

Hyperglycaemia may occur and require exogenous insulin.

Sepsis and injury

Significant fluctuations in macronutrient metabolism are seen during sepsis and injury. An initial hyperglycaemia, reflecting a reduced utilization of glucose, is followed by a longer catabolic state with increased utilization of lipid and amino acids. The effect of the different lipid emulsions on immune function is the subject of much research.

Respiratory

While under-feeding and malnutrition can compromise respiratory effort and muscle function, over-feeding can equally compromise respiratory function due to increased carbon dioxide and lipid effects on the circulation. While chronic respiratory disease may be linked with a long-standing malnutrition, the patient with acute disease will generally be hypermetabolic.

Cardiac

Cardiac failure and multiple drug therapy may limit the volume of PN that can be infused. Concentrated formulations are used and, as a consequence of the high tonicity, administered via the central route.

Close electrolyte monitoring and adjustment is required. Cardiac drugs may affect electrolyte clearance.

Although central lines may already be in use for other drugs or cardiac monitoring, it is essential to maintain a dedicated lumen or line for the feed.

Diabetes mellitus

Diabetic patients can generally be maintained with standard dual-energy regimens.

Close glucose monitoring will guide exogenous insulin administration. This should be given as a separate infusion or, if the patient is stable, in bolus doses. Insulin should not be included within the PN formulation due to stability problems and variable adsorption to the equipment. Y-site infusion with the PN should be avoided as changes in insulin rates will be delayed and changes in feed rates will result in significant fluctuations in insulin administration.

Cancer and palliative care

Nutritional support in cancer and palliative care is guided by the potential risks and benefits of the intervention, alongside the wishes of the patient and their carers. Further research is required to evaluate the effects of PN on length and quality of life.

Standard PN may be useful during prolonged periods of gastrointestinal toxicity, as in bone marrow transplant patients. The use of PN is not thought to stimulate tumour growth (Nitenberg & Raynard 2000).

Long-term parenteral nutrition

Home care is well established in the UK with some patients successfully supported for over 20 years. Total or supplemental PN may be appropriate.

Most patients are extremely well informed about their underlying disease and their PN; many also benefit from the PINNT support group.

Paediatric parenteral nutrition

Nutritional requirements

Early nutritional intervention is required in paediatric patients due to their low reserve, especially in neonates. In addition to requirements for the maintenance of body tissue, function and repair, it is important to also support growth, especially in the infant and adolescent.

Typical guidelines for average daily requirements of fluid, energy and nitrogen are shown in Table 5.18. The dual-energy approach is favoured in paediatrics. Approximately 30% of the non-protein calories are provided as lipid using a 20% emulsion. Most centres gradually increase the lipid provision from day 1 from 1 g/kg/day to 2 g/kg/day and then 3 g/kg/day, monitoring lipid clearance through the serum triglyceride level. This ensures the essential fatty acid requirements of premature neonates are met.

Formulation and stability issues

Many centres use standard PN formulations including the specific paediatric amino acid solutions (Primene or Vaminolact). Prescriptions and formulations are tailored to reflect clinical status, biochemistry and nutritional requirements.

Micronutrients are included daily. Paediatric licensed preparations are available and are included on a ml/kg basis up to a maximum total volume (Peditrace, Solivito N and Vitlipid N Infant). Electrolytes are also monitored and included in all formulations on a mmol/kg basis. Potassium and sodium acetate salt forms are sometimes used in balance with the chloride salt forms. This is to avoid excessive chloride input contributing to acidosis. Acetate is metabolized to bicarbonate, an alkali.

Table 5.18 Typical average daily parenteral nutrition requirements

Age (years)	Fluid (ml/kg/day)	Energy (kcal/kg/day)	Nitrogen (g/kg/day)
Preterm	200–150	130–150	0.5–0.65
0–1	150–110	130–110	0.34–0.46
1–6	100–80	100–70	0.22–0.38
6–12	80–75	70–50	0.2–0.33
12–18	75–50	50–40	0.16–0.2

Due to the balance of nutritional requirements, a relatively high glucose requirement with high calcium and phosphate provision, the neonatal and paediatric prescription may be supplied by a separate 2-in-1 bag of amino acids, glucose, trace elements and electrolytes and a lipid syringe with vitamins. These are generally given concurrently, joining at a Y-site. Older children can sometimes be managed with 3-in-1 formulations. A single infusion is particularly useful in the home care environment. Some ready-to-use formulations are licensed for use in paediatrics and include Kabiven Peripheral and the OliClinomel range.

Improved stability profiles with the new lipid emulsions, and increasing stability data, may support 3-in-1 formulations that meet the nutritional requirements of younger children.

Concerns over the contamination of calcium gluconate with aluminium, and the association between aluminium contamination of neonatal PN and impaired neurological development have favoured the use of calcium chloride over gluconate (Bishop et al 1997).

Heparin

Historically, low concentrations of heparin were included in 2-in-1 formulations in an attempt to improve fat clearance through enhanced triglyceride hydrolysis,

prevent the formation of fibrin around the infusion line, reduce thrombosis and reduce thrombophlebitis during peripheral infusion. However, this is no longer recommended. It is recognized that when the 2-in-1 formulation comes into contact with the lipid phase, calcium-heparin bridges form between these lipid globules, destabilizing the formulation. Also, there is limited evidence of clinical benefit of the heparin inclusion.

Route of administration

Peripheral administration is less common in neonates and children due to the risk of thrombophlebitis. However, it is useful when low concentration, short-term PN is required and there is good peripheral access. The maximum glucose concentration for peripheral administration in paediatrics is generally regarded to be 12%. However, considering all the other factors that can affect the tonicity of a regimen and peripheral tolerance, it is clear that this is a relatively simplistic perspective. Many centres favour a limit of 10% with close clinical observation.

Central administration is via long line (peripheral long line or peripherally inserted central catheters), Broviac or Hickman catheter. There is limited experience with the Port-a-Cath devices in paediatric PN.

CASE STUDIES

Case 5.1 (Prepared with David Hoole, Aseptic Services Manager, Royal Hospital for Sick Children, Edinburgh)

Female neonate weighing 1.5 kg.
Known gastroschisis in utero with intrauterine growth retardation.
Spontaneous vaginal delivery at 35 weeks gestation.

Day	Clinical observation/event	PN changes
1	Surgical reduction of gastroschisis Negligible urine output, metabolic acidosis Ventilated with sedation, analgesia, antibiotics Receiving 0.18% NaCl/10% glucose (4 ml/h). No K^+ supplement	No PN
2	Cr 117 (μmol/l), urine output low LFTs noted and increased ALT, (possible surgical tissue release, tailed off over 4–5 days)	PN started via dedicated central long line (64 ml/kg) Low K^+, otherwise standard day 1 formula, reflecting electrolytes of previous fluids and U&Es Acetate salt form used because of acidotic state
3	PPS (plasma protein solution) started (3 ml/h) Cr reduced, urea stable, K^+ reduced from day 2	Increased to 75 ml/kg Almost standard day 2 formula; K^+ increased to 2 mmol/kg
4	Serum Na^+ raised at 146 (mmol/l) PPS	Na^+ reduced to 0.6 mmol/kg Otherwise standard day 3 formula
5	PPS stopped Extubated	Increased to 123 ml/kg, Na content increased Standard day 4 formula from this day onwards
8	EBM (expressed breast milk) started (1 ml/h) First meconium passed Weight = 1.7 kg	Volume of PN increasing in line with weight gain
10	Triglyceride and cholesterol levels normal Serum K^+ slightly raised	K^+ reduced to 1.6 mmol/kg
12	Increasing tolerance to EBM 1 ml/h	
15	Slightly raised triglyceride, upper normal of cholesterol Alkaline phosphatase increasing (still within reference range)	Phosphate content of bag increased (within stability limits)
17	Rechecked lipids; both reduced and within reference range Total protein and albumin; both at lower end of reference range throughout EBM increased to 2 ml/h. Slowly increasing tolerance to feed	
20	EBM now at 7 ml/h	PN reducing in line with increasing enteral intake
25	Erythromycin commenced (to assist gut motility) Weight = 2.1 kg	
29	PN stopped Weight = 2.2 kg Enteral supplements – iron and multivitamins	
36	Weight = 2.34 kg Discharged	

Questions

1. How is the PN route of administration chosen?
2. What were the main factors that needed to be considered in this neonate before starting PN?
3. Why were acetate salts chosen?
4. How should liver function tests be interpreted?
5. Why was the serum sodium raised on day 4?
6. How should PN be managed as enteral feeding is established?

Answers

1. PN must be administered via a dedicated intravenous line. For a regimen with a glucose concentration of > 12%, this should be a central line. The line should be inserted by a suitably trained and qualified clinician or nurse practitioner. Correct positioning should be assessed by X-ray of the radio-opaque tip. While regimens with a glucose concentration of less than 10% may be tolerated by the peripheral route, tolerance is also highly dependent on insertion technique, line care and vein patency.

   It was anticipated that this neonate would require a couple of weeks PN and the central route was first-line.

2. Poor nutritional reserves in a low birth weight premature neonate, the surgical trauma, the need to achieve relative metabolic stability with clear fluids and supportive therapies prior to commencing PN and recognizing the volume and electrolyte contribution of other concurrent therapies. Neonatal serum reference ranges, not adult values, should be applied.

3. A balance of chloride and acetate salt forms were used in the PN formulae. This neonate had metabolic acidosis and acetate salts were included to reduce the chloride input and, being metabolized to bicarbonate, as a source of alkali. However, the acid–base balance of this neonate was more dependent on the renal and respiratory status and support.

4. Daily liver function tests were reviewed. The independent rise in ALT was considered to be due to the surgical trauma and resolved within a few days. The independent rise in alkaline phosphatase probably represented an increased requirement of phosphate.

   Liver function tests are non-specific and increases could have been due to a wide range of causes including (not exclusively) sepsis, trauma, drug-induced liver complication, PN complication, e.g. induced cholestasis, and primary liver pathology.

5. In the initial stages, neonates tend to hypernatraemia due to relatively poor clearance. This should be reflected in the standard formulae used. However, this neonate also received plasma protein solution that contains 130–150 mmol/l of both sodium and chloride. At 3 ml/h, this supplied 9.4–10.8 mmol of both sodium and chloride.

6. The volume should be gradually reduced as the enteral feed is absorbed. The ratio of nutritional components is likely to remain unchanged. The PN should not be stopped abruptly; the infusion rate should be reduced over the final hours to avoid rebound hypoglycaemia.

Case 5.2 (Prepared with Fionnula King, Senior Pharmacist (Nutrition and Production), Barts and London NHS Trust)

Mr M. G. is a 46-year-old man who presented with a mesenteric artery infarct.

Day	Clinical observation/event	PN changes
1	Surgical small bowel resection and jejunostomy formation (30 cm of small bowel from DJ flexure attached to colon)	
2	ITU admission with Gram negative sepsis, isolates included *Proteus*, *E. coli* and *Klebsiella* Reviewed by multidisciplinary nutrition team Height 1.8 m, weight 85 kg, BMI 26 kg/m^2, BMR 1839 kcal	PN prescribed (considering both fluid and electrolytes from other therapies): Volume 2000 ml Nitrogen 16.5 g Carbohydrate 1200 kcal Lipid 1000 kcal
	Enteral feeding with standard whole feed throughout ICU stay (10 ml/h)	Na$^+$ 85 mmol, K$^+$ 85 mmol, Ca^{2+} 6 mmol, Mg^{2+} 6 mmol, PO$_4^{2-}$ 20 mmol Vitamins and trace elements
7	Transferred from ICU to specialist nutrition ward Drug therapy: piptazobactum, atenolol, simvastatin, loperamide, codeine phosphate	
8	Jejunostomy output: 4–6 litres per day Octreotide and omeprazole commenced	
9–11	Jejunostomy output: 2–4 litres per day	
14	Jejunostomy output: 8–10 litres per day (had increased with increasing oral intake) U&Es: Na$^+$ 134, K$^+$ 4.1, Urea 36.8, Cr 828, Mg^{2+} 0.55 Referral to dietitian. Commenced oral rehydration with modified WHO formula (the only rehydration to be taken between meals) – 20 g glucose, 2.5 g sodium bicarbonate and 3.5 g sodium chloride in a litre of water	PN volume, Na, Mg increased: Volume 4500 ml Nitrogen 16.5 g Carbohydrate 1200 kcal Lipid 1000 kcal Na$^+$ 200 mmol, K$^+$ 85 mmol, Ca^{2+} 6 mmol, Mg^{2+} 10 mmol, PO$_4^{2-}$ 20 mmol Vitamins and trace elements
17	Jejunostomy output reduced to 3 litres per day U&Es: Na$^+$ 143, K$^+$ 3.6, Urea 25.4, Cr 564, Mg^{2+} 0.95	

Day	Clinical observation/event	PN changes
19	Spiking temperature 39.5°C Peripheral and central line blood cultures taken Stat doses of gentamicin and vancomycin	
20	Gram-positive cocci prompting vancomycin 1 g twice a day for 7 days Vancomycin monitoring commenced	
21	Pre-dose vancomycin level 30.1 mg/litre and so further doses omitted until pre-levels between 5 and 10 mg/litre	
22	Identified as *Staph. aureus* prompting line removal and continuation of vancomycin for 10 days Tunnelled central line inserted and PN continued	
23	Renal function and stoma output improved onwards Urine analysis: Urea 350 micrograms/24 h Multidisciplinary team led structured and tailored training for the self-administration of the PN Patient reported feeling nauseous. Possibly related to lipid component of 3-in-1 bag Discharged home on day 43	PN volume and nitrogen reduced in line with 24 hour urea and reduced stoma output Electrolytes adjusted in line with U&Es Lipid included for 2 days per week: Volume 3500 ml Nitrogen 14 g Carbohydrate 1200 kcal Lipid 1000 kcal Na$^+$ 200 mmol, K$^+$ 80 mmol, Ca^{2+} 6 mmol, Mg^{2+} 10 mmol, PO$_4^{2-}$ 15 mmol Vitamins and trace elements Lipid-free for 5 days per week: Volume 3500 ml Nitrogen 14 g Carbohydrate 2200 kcal Na$^+$ 200 mmol, K$^+$ 80 mmol, Ca^{2+} 6 mmol, Mg^{2+} 10 mmol, PO$_4^{2-}$ 15 mmol Vitamins and trace elements

Questions

1. Why was rehydration therapy started on day 14?
2. How was the urea level used to indicate nitrogen requirement?
3. Outline the rationale for the management of line infection.
4. Why was Mr M. G. discharged with a combination of 2-in-1 and 3-in-1 regimens?

Answers

1. With such a high stoma output, Mr M. G. was at acute risk of dehydration. A balanced oral rehydration fluid was used to supply electrolytes and fluid; inclusion of > 90 mmol/litre of sodium with glucose helped facilitate fluid absorption.
2. A 24 hour urine collection can be used as an indicator of nitrogen loss, assuming all urine is collected and urea or volume output is not compromised by renal failure. However, a true nitrogen output determination requires measurement of nitrogen output from all body fluids, including urine, sweat, faeces, skin and wounds. Nitrogen balance studies can indicate the metabolic state of the patient (positive balance in net protein synthesis, negative balance in protein catabolism).

   Urinary urea constitutes approximately 80% of the urinary nitrogen. A number of predictive equations have been developed to estimate the nitrogen output from urinary urea. For example: urea (micrograms/24 h) × 0.035 = nitrogen loss (g/24 h). For Mr M. G. 350 × 0.035 = 13.25 g/24 h and so the nitrogen input was reduced from 18 g to 14 g.

3. Blood samples were taken from both the central nutrition line and a peripheral point. Subsequent comparison of the results may indicate the site of infection. Empirically, a single dose of gentamicin and vancomycin was administered to commence treatment against the most likely pathogens (Gram-negative and Gram-positive). On identification of a cocci infection, the vancomycin was continued. Sepsis and dehydration had probably contributed to renal failure and the raised vancomycin level. On identification of the *Staph. aureus* infection, the central line was removed and replaced with a new tunnelled central line.
4. Mr M. G. expressed concern that he felt nauseous when receiving the 3-in-1 regimen. In the absence of complications from a glucose-only system, the dual-energy formula was used for just 2 days per week. The patient received sufficient lipid for the provision of the essential fatty acids. Ongoing monitoring would ensure that he did not suffer complications of the glucose-only system.

REFERENCES

Allwood M C, Kearney M C J 1998 Compatibility and stability of additives in parenteral nutrition admixtures. Nutrition 14: 697–706

Allwood M C, Martin H J 2000 The photodegradation of vitamin A and E in parenteral nutrition mixtures during infusion. Clinical Nutrition 19: 339–342

American Medical Association 1979 Guidelines for essential trace element preparations for parenteral use. Journal of the American Medical Association 241: 2051

Bethune K, Allwood M, Grainger C et al 2001 Use of filters during the preparation and administration of parenteral nutrition: position paper and guidelines prepared by a British Pharmaceutical Nutrition Group Working Party. Nutrition 17: 403–408

Bishop N J, Morley R, Day J P et al 1997 Aluminium neurotoxicity in preterm infants receiving intravenous feeding solutions. New England Journal of Medicine 336: 1557–1561

Crook M A 2000 Lipid clearance and total parenteral nutrition: the importance of monitoring of plasma lipids. Nutrition 16: 774–775

Elia M 2000 Guidelines for detection and management of malnutrition. British Association of Parenteral and Enteral Nutrition, Maidenhead

Food and Drug Administration 2000 Parenteral multivitamin products. Reference DESI 2847. Federal Register 65: 21200–21201

Fleming C R 1989 Trace element metabolism in adult patients requiring total parenteral nutrition. American Journal of Clinical Nutrition 49: 573

Foulks C J 1999 An evidence-based evaluation of intradialytic parenteral nutrition. American Journal of Kidney Disease 33: 186–192

Howard P 1999 Clinical nutritional support team. Educational Supplement, 21st ESPEN Congress 1999, pp. 23–25

Lennard-Jones J E (ed) 1992 A positive approach to nutrition as treatment. King's Fund, London

Maroulis J, Kalfarentoz F 2000 Complications of parenteral nutrition at the end of the century. Clinical Nutrition 19: 295–304

Misra S, Kirby D F 2000 Micronutrient and trace element monitoring in adult nutrition support. Nutrition in Clinical Practice 15: 120–126

Nitenberg G, Raynard B 2000 Nutritional support of the cancer patient: issues and dilemmas. Critical Reviews in Oncology/Haematology 34: 137–168

Okada A, Takagi Y, Nezu K et al 1995 Trace element metabolism in parenteral and enteral nutrition. Nutrition 11 (1 Suppl.): 106–113

Plauth M, Merli M, Kondrup J et al 1997 ESPEN guidelines for nutrition in liver disease and transplantation. Clinical Nutrition 16: 43–55

Shenkin A 1995 Trace elements and inflammatory response: implications for nutritional support. Nutrition 11: 100–105

Stratton R, Elia M 2000 How much undernutrition is there in British hospitals? British Journal of Nutrition 84: 257–259

Tucker H N, Miguel S G 1996 Cost containment through nutrition intervention. Nutrition Reviews 54: 111–121

Woodcock N P, Zeigler D, Palmer M D et al 2001 Enteral vs parenteral nutrition: a pragmatic study. Nutrition 17: 1–12

FURTHER READING

British Pharmaceutical Nutrition Group. http://www.bpng.co.uk

Matarese L, Gottschlich M (eds) 1998 Contemporary nutrition support practice: a clinical guide. W B Saunders, Philadelphia

Milla P J (ed) 2000 Current perspectives on paediatric parenteral nutrition. British Association of Parenteral and Enteral Nutrition, Maidenhead

Pennington C R (ed) 1996 Current perspectives on adult parenteral nutrition. British Association of Parenteral and Enteral Nutrition, Maidenhead

Rombeau J L, Rolandelli R H (eds) 2000 Clinical nutrition – Parenteral nutrition. W B Saunders, Philadelphia

Pharmacoeconomics 6

J. Cooke

KEY POINTS

- Expenditure on medicines is increasing at a higher rate than general inflation, requiring many governments to introduce cost-effectiveness programmes.
- Pharmacoeconomics is the measurement of the costs and consequences of therapeutic decision making.
- There are a wide range of different costs associated with the economics of health care.
- In economic evaluations of health care, consequences can be expressed in monetary terms, (cost–benefit), in natural units of effectiveness (cost-effectiveness) or in terms of patient preference or utility (cost–utility).
- Decision analysis techniques provide an effective instrument for detailed analysis of cost-effectiveness studies.
- The economics of concordance and risk management are considerable.
- Guidelines for economic evaluations are becoming widespread and will be a quality assurance tool for the design and interpretation of health economic studies.

The demand for and cost of health care is increasing in all countries as the improvement and sophistication of health technologies increase. Many governments are focusing their activities on promoting the effective and economic use of resources allocated to health care.

Medicines form a small but significant proportion of total health care costs and one that has been growing consistently as new medicines are marketed. The writing of a prescription is the most common therapeutic intervention in medicine with about 1.5 million prescriptions being written by general practitioners each day and a further 0.5 million in hospitals daily in the UK. However, there is much evidence to suggest that this simple task is not conducted optimally.

In the UK, almost £7000 million was spent on medicines in 2000 and there is an annual increase in expenditure of about 12%. Each individual receives on average 9.4 medicinal items per year, at a cost of £115 per person, although this tends to be skewed towards the elderly population. Eighty-one per cent of prescribing costs are incurred in primary care and constitute up to 50% of the primary care revenue costs. Within an average general hospital, 5% of the total revenue expenditure is spent on medicines.

There are a number of reasons why prescribing costs are increasing. These include:

- demographic changes in the population that have resulted in an ageing population which is living longer and has greater pharmaceutical needs
- health screening programmes and improved diagnostic techniques that are uncovering previously non-identified diseases which subsequently require treatment
- the marketing of new medicines that offer more effective and less toxic alternatives to existing agents, and which are invariably more expensive
- the use of existing agents becoming more widespread as additional indications for their use are found
- Medicines being used in preference to invasive treatments.

In the UK, the government's recent health reforms have addressed the quality of care through promotion of clinical governance. The formation of the National Institute for Clinical Excellence (NICE) in 1998 to 'improve standards of patient care, and to reduce inequities in access to innovative treatment' has formalized this process. NICE undertakes technology appraisals of medicines and other treatments (health technologies) and addresses the clinical and cost effectiveness of therapies and compares them with alternative use of NHS funds. The increased use of evidence-based programmes not only concentrates on optimizing health outcomes but also utilize health economic evaluations. Formalized health technology assessments provide an in-depth and evidence-based approach to this process.

Definitions used in economics in health care

Pharmacoeconomics can be defined as the measurement of both the costs and consequences of therapeutic decision making. Pharmacoeconomics provides a guide for decision makers on resource allocation but does not offer a basis on which decisions should be made. Pharmacoeconomics can assist in the planning process and help assign priorities where, for example, medicines with a worse outcome may be available at a lower cost and medicines with better outcome and higher cost can be compared. Figure 6.1 summarizes the dilemmas facing decision makers when a new drug is introduced.

When economic evaluations are conducted it is important to categorize various costs. Costs can be direct to the organization: i.e. physicians' salaries, the acquisition costs of medicines, consumables associated with drug administration, staff time in preparation and administration of medicines, laboratory costs of monitoring for effectiveness and adverse drug reactions. Indirect costs include lost productivity from a disease which can manifest itself as a cost to the economy or taxation system as well as economic costs to the patient and the patient's family. All aspects of the use of medicines may be allocated costs, both direct, such as acquisition and administration costs, and indirect, such as the cost of a given patient's time off work because of illness, in terms of lost output and social security payments. The consequences of drug therapy include benefits for both the individual patient and society at large, which may be quantified in terms of health outcome and quality of life, in addition to purely economic impact.

It is worthwhile here to describe a number of definitions that further qualify costs in a health care setting. The concept of opportunity cost is at the centre of economics and identifies the value of opportunities which have been lost by utilizing resources in a particular service or health technology. This can be valued as the benefits that have been forsaken by investing the resources in the best alternative fashion. Opportunity cost recognizes that there are limited resources available for utilizing every treatment, and therefore the rationing of health care is implicit in such a system.

Average costs are the simplest way of valuing the consumption of health care resources. Quite simply they represent the total costs (i.e. all the costs incurred in the delivery of a service) of a health care system divided by the units of production. For example, a large teaching trust hospital might treat 75 000 patients a year (finished consultant episodes, FCEs) and have a total annual revenue cost of £150 million. The average cost per FCE is therefore £2000.

Fixed costs are those which are independent of the number of units of production and include heating, lighting and fixed staffing costs. Variable costs, on the other hand, are dependent on the numbers of units of productivity. The costs of the consumption of medicines is a good example of variable costs.

The inevitable increases in the medicines budget in a particular institute which is treating more patients, or treating those with a more complex pathology, have often been erroneously interpreted by financial managers as a failure effectively to manage the budget. In order to better describe the costs associated with a health care intervention, economists employ the term 'marginal costs' to describe the costs of producing an extra unit of a particular service. The term 'incremental cost' is used to define the difference between the costs of alternative interventions.

Choice of comparator

Sometimes a claim is made that a treatment is 'cost effective'. But against what? As in any good clinical trial a treatment has to be compared against a reasonable comparator. The choice of comparator is crucial to this process. A comparator that is no longer in common use or in a dose that is not optimal will result in the evaluated treatment being seen as more effective than it actually is. Sadly many evaluations of medicines fall into this trap as sponsors seldom wish to undertake 'back to back' studies against competitors. Again the reader has to be careful when interpreting economic evaluations from a setting which is dissimilar to that in local practice. A common error can be made when viewing international studies that have different health care costs and ways of treating patients and translating them directly into own practice.

Type of health economic evaluations

Cost–benefit analysis (CBA)

In cost–benefit analysis (CBA), consequences are measured in terms of the total cost associated with a programme where both costs and consequences are measured in monetary terms. While this type of analysis

	Lower cost	Same cost	Higher cost
Worse outcome	Consider	Reject	Reject
Same outcome	Consider	Optional	Reject
Better outcome	Adopt	Adopt	Consider

Figure 6.1 Dilemma matrix for decision makers dealing with the economics of a new treatment.

is preferred by economists, its employment in health care is problematical as it is frequently difficult to ascribe pecuniary values to clinical outcomes such as pain relief, avoidance of stroke or improvements in quality of life.

Methods are available for determing cost–benefit for particular groups of patients that centre around a concept known as contingent valuation (CV). Specific techniques include willingness to pay (WTP), where patients are asked to state how much they would be prepared to pay to avoid a particular event or symptom, for example pain or nausea following day care surgery. WTP can be fraught with difficulties of interpretation in countries with socialized health care systems which are invariably funded out of general taxation. Willingness to accept (WTA) is a similar concept but is based on the minimum amount an individual person or population would receive in order to be prepared to lose or reduce a service.

CBA can be usefully employed at a macro level for strategic decisions on health care programmes. For example, a countrywide immunization programme can be fully costed in terms of resource utilization consumed in running the programme. This can then be valued against the reduced mortality and morbidity that occur as a result of the programme.

CBA can be useful in examining the value of services, for example centralized intravenous additive (CIVA) services where a comparison between a pharmacy-based intravenous additive service and ward-based preparation by doctors and nurses demonstrates the value of the pharmacy service, or a clinical pharmacokinetics service where the staffing and equipment costs can be offset against the benefits of reduced morbidity and mortality. A theoretical model for the CBA of a clinical pharmacokinetics service is set out in Table 6.1.

Cost-effectiveness analysis (CEA)

Cost-effectiveness analysis (CEA) can be described as an examination of the costs of two or more programmes which have the same clinical outcome as measured in physical units, for example lives saved or reduced morbidity. Treatments with dissimilar outcomes can also be analysed by this technique. Where two or more interventions have been shown to be, or are assumed to be, similar then, if all other factors are equal (e.g. convenience, side-effects, availability, etc.), selection can be made on the basis of cost. This type of analysis is called cost minimization analysis (CMA). CMA is frequently employed in formulary decision making where often the available evidence for a new product appears to be no better than for existing products. This is invariably what happens in practice as clinical trials on new medicines are statstically powered for equivalence as a requirement for licensing submission. For example, the use of CMA in conjunction with a drug use evaluation (DUE) for the use of intravenous nitrate preparations resulted in an educational programme that saved a large teaching hospital about £25 000 a year.

An example of the use of cost-effectiveness analysis is shown in a study of the addition of recombinant human granulocyte–macrophage colony-stimulating factor (rhGM-CSF) after autologous bone marrow transplantation for lymphoid cancer. A randomized controlled double-blind trial was undertaken in 40 patients to ascertain the effect of rhGM-CSF with placebo. Outcomes measured included length of stay; economic inputs included costs of medicines, total charges, departmental charges, re-hospitalization and out-patient charges. In all outcomes, with the exception of pharmacy costs, the charges were lower with the rhGM-CSF treatment and indicated an overall saving to the organization and a better treatment outcome.

As previously described, CEA examines the costs associated with achieving a defined health outcome. While these outcomes can be the relief of symptoms such as nausea and vomiting and pain, etc., CEA frequently employs years of life gained as a measure of the success of a particular programme. This can then offer a method of incrementally comparing the costs associated with two or more interventions. For example, consider a hypothetical case of the comparison of two drug treatments for the management of malignant disease. Treatment A represents a 1 year course of treatment for a particular malignant disease. Assume that this is the current standard form of treatment and that the average total direct cost associated with this programme is £40 000 a year. This will include the costs of the medicines, antiemetics, in-patient stay, radiological and pathology costs, and so on. Treatment B is a new drug treatment for the malignancy which, as a result of comparative controlled clinical trials, has demonstrated an improvement in the average life expectancy for this group of patients from 3.5 years for treatment A to 4.5 years for treatment B. The average annual total costs for

Table 6.1 Hypothetical summary of a cost–benefit analysis for a pharmacokinetic service		
	Amount (US$)	
Item	Cost	Savings
Programme costs (equipment, supplies, personnel)	38 150	
Mortality savings (based on 18.4 years)		71 575
Morbidity savings		10 362
Total savings		81 937
Benefit–cost ratio: 2.15		

treatment B is £55 000. A comparative table can now be constructed:

Strategy	Treatment costs	Effectiveness
Treatment A	£40 000	3.5 years
Treatment B	£55 000	4.5 years

Incremental cost-effectiveness ratio:

$$= \frac{55\,000 - 40\,000}{4.5 - 3.5}$$

$$= £15\,000 \text{ per life year gained}$$

Cost–utility analysis (CUA)

An alternative measurement for the consequences of a health care intervention is the concept of utility. Utility provides a method for estimating patient preference for a particular intervention in terms of the patient's state of well-being. Utility is described by an index which ranges between 0 (representing death) and 1 (perfect health). The product of utility and life years gained provides the term 'quality-adjusted life year' (QALY).

There are a number of methods for the calculation of utilities:

- The Rosser–Kind matrix relies on preferences from population samples from certain disease groups.
- The visual analogue scale method seeks to obtain patient preferences for their perceived disease state by having patients score themselves on a line scaled between 0 and 1, as above.
- In the standard gamble method, individuals are required to choose between living the rest of their lives in their current state of health or making a gamble on an intervention which will restore them to perfect health. Failure of the gamble will result in instant death. The probabilities of the gamble are varied until there is indifference between the two events.
- The time trade-off method requires individuals to decide how many of their remaining years of life expectancy they would be prepared to exchange for complete health.

Using the previous model, supposing treatment A provides on average an increase of 3.5 years life expectancy but that this is valued at a utility of 0.9, then the health gain for this intervention is $0.9 \times 3.5 = 3.15$ QALYs. Similarly, supposing the increase in life expectancy with treatment B only had a utility of 0.8 (perhaps because it produces more nausea), then the health gain for this option becomes $0.8 \times 4.5 = 3.6$ QALYs. An incremental CEA can be undertaken as follows:

Strategy	Treatment costs	Effectiveness	Utility
Treatment A	£40 000	3.5 years	0.9
Treatment B	£55 000	4.5 years	0.8

Incremental–cost utility ratio:

$$= \frac{55\,000 - 40\,000}{(4.5 \times 0.8) - (3.5 \times 0.9)}$$

$$= £33\,000 \text{ per QALY gained}$$

The calculation of QALYs provides a method which enables decision makers to compare different health interventions and assign priorities for decisions on resource allocation. However, the use of QALY league tables is a matter of contentious debate among stakeholders of health care.

Valuation of costs and consequences over time: discounting

Discounting is an economic term based mainly on a time preference that assumes individuals prefer to forego a part of the benefits of a programme if they can have those benefits now rather than fully in an uncertain future. The value of this preference is expressed by the discount rate. There is intense debate among health economists regarding the value for this annual discount level and whether both costs and consequences should be subjected to discounting. Generally speaking, if a programme does not exceed 1 year, then discounting is felt to be unnecessary.

Decision analysis techniques

Decision analysis offers a method of pictorial representation of treatment decisions. If the results from clinical trials are available, probabilities can be placed within the arms of a decision tree and outcomes can be assessed in either monetary or quality units.

A simple decision tree might look, for example, at two options for the management of deep-vein thrombosis. Option A is the traditional method whereby a patient is admitted into hospital and receives continuous infusions of unfractionated heparin. Option B uses low-molecular-weight heparin which is administered subcutaneously on an out-patient basis or at home. The costs of the two treatments can be represented as in Table 6.2.

The quickest way to undertake decision analysis is by a computerized programme. Using published information, the probabilities of complications can be put into the decision tree, and from hypothetical or actual hospital cost data the two treatment can be assigned total direct costs.

A decision tree can then be constructed to describe the major pathways. This is depicted in Figure 6.2. By

Table 6.2 Costs associated with two treatments for deep-vein thrombosis

Option A: unfractionated heparin	Option B: low-molecular-weight heparin
Cost of drug	Cost of drug
Cost of in-patient stay (10 days)	Cost of in-patient stay (2 days)
Cost of administering drug (nurse labour)	Self-administered
Cost of monitoring	Not necessary
Cost of staff	Cost of staff
Cost of complications (e.g. bleeds, readmissions)	Cost of complications (e.g. bleeds, re-admissions)

rolling back the tree, the costs and probabilities of the model can be seen, and the tree identifies a preference for the most cost-effective option (Fig. 6.3). The model also calculates the costs of the programme at each node, and by the assignment of probabilities for each decision

arm an overall cost of the preferred option is shown to be £1038.

If there is uncertainty about the robustness of the values of the variables within the tree they can be varied within defined ranges to see if the overall direction of the tree changes. This is referred to as sensitivity analysis and is one of the most powerful tools available in an economic evaluation. Thus, if the variables are the probability of bleeding in each arm of the analysis, then overall costs can be varied either in turn (one-way analysis) or together (two- or three-way analysis).

A one-way sensitivity analysis for the model is shown in Figure 6.4. The variable cost for no bleeding with low-molecular-weight heparin is varied between £0 and £1500. The threshold value at which the tree is equivocal occurs at a cost of £1388, and is the same as the expected value for the unfractionated arm. Above this value unfractionated heparin is more cost-effective.

A decision analysis model can be used for a number of clinical situations. For example, it has been used to describe the incidence of wound infections which occurred by giving prophylactic antibiotics too early or too late in the surgical process compared to giving them on induction. A decision tree can be created for the costs associated with surgery, together with the published

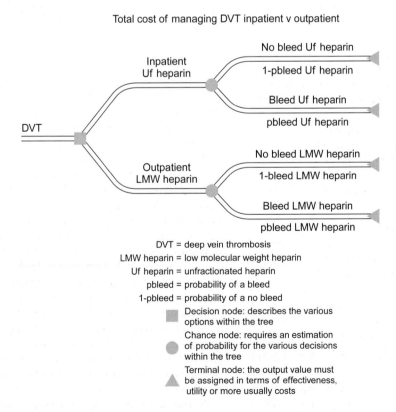

Figure 6.2 Decision analysis for management of deep-vein thrombosis.

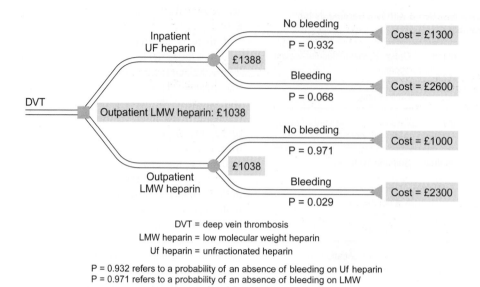

DVT = deep vein thrombosis
LMW heparin = low molecular weight heparin
Uf heparin = unfractionated heparin

P = 0.932 refers to a probability of an absence of bleeding on Uf heparin
P = 0.971 refers to a probability of an absence of bleeding on LMW

Figure 6.3   Decision analysis for management of deep-vein thrombosis: costs and probabilities.

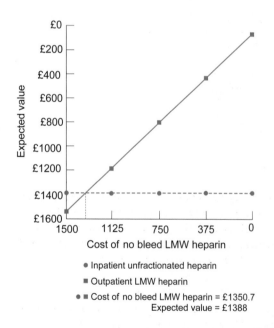

Figure 6.4   One-way sensitivity analysis on cost for no bleed for low-molecular-weight (LMW) heparin.

wound infection rates. Using this model it can be shown that there is an average £51 saving for each operation if the antibiotic is given on time. Commuted to an average hospital undertaking 10 000 surgical operations a year, this reflects a potential cost saving of £0.5 million. These decision trees are shown in Figures 6.5 and 6.6.

Guidelines for economic evaluations of medicines

A number of countries have introduced explicit guidelines for the conduct of economic evaluations of medicines. Others require economic evaluations before allowing a medicine onto an approved listing. Guidelines have been published which aim to provide researchers and peer reviewers with background guidance on how to conduct an economic evaluation and how to check its quality prior to submission for publication (Drummond & Jefferson 1996).

Unwanted drug effects: clinical risk management

The importance of avoidance of the adverse effects of medicines has become a desirable goal of therapeutic decision makers as well as those who promote quality assurance and risk management. Not only can there be significant sequelae in terms of increased morbidity associated with adverse drug effects, but also the economic consequences can be considerable. Unwanted drug effects are of two kinds: adverse drug reactions, and errors in the prescribing, dispensing and administration of medicines. For example, gentamicin is often regarded as a relatively inexpensive antibiotic. However, in the USA each case of gentamicin-induced nephrotoxicity has been reported to cost £1562 in terms of additional

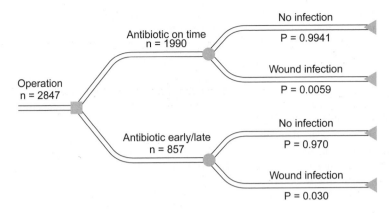

Figure 6.5   Decision tree on timing of surgical prophylaxis.

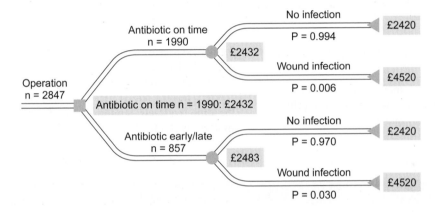

Figure 6.6   Decision tree on timing of surgical prophylaxis: costs and probabilities.

resources consumed, even without any assessment of the reduction in a patient's quality of life. The increasingly litigious nature of society has also resulted in economic valuations of perceived negligence being undertaken, for example with irreversible vestibular toxicity associated with prolonged unmonitored aminoglycoside therapy. The Department of Health (2001) in the UK has set a target for a 40% reduction in the number of serious errors in the use of prescribed medicines by 2005 through its publication *Building a Safer NHS for Patients*.

Medication adherence

The costs of poor adherence when taking prescribed medicines are considerable. In the USA it has been calculated that 11.4% of all admissions to hospital have been directly associated with some form of poor adherence at a cost of £1344 per patient. In the UK about half of all patients with chronic disease do not take their medicines as prescribed. The additional cost of extra treatment, cost production and earnings and other costs associated with this exceeds £1 billion.

Health economics viewpoint

A fundamental element of the use and interpretation of pharmacoeconomics in practice is the background against which the analysis is undertaken. Ideally this should be from a societal perspective, but frequently it is from a government, or Deparatment of Health viewpoint. Purchasers of health care may also have a different perspective to provider units, and the viewpoint of clinicians may differ from that of patients. The pharmaceutical industry will probably have still another viewpoint, focused on their particular products. All economic evaluations should be clear as to the perspective from which they have been analysed.

Conclusions

The problems of having financial budgets that are rigorously defended in any section of the health service, as occurs with the medicines budget, is to deny the application of economic decision making in the most efficient way for the country. It does not matter how good an economic evaluation is if there is not a mechanism in place to use the results. It is clear that there is an identified need for more formalized education in health economic evaluation.

Inflexibility in moving resources between the primary and secondary health care sectors is a major barrier to making the best use of cost-effectiveness studies and economic evaluations.

Glossary

Contingent valuation A method for the valuation of costs of a programme. The concept employs techniques such as willingness to pay and willingness to accept.

Discounting A technique which allows the calculation of costs (inputs) and consequences (benefits) which occur in the future. Discounting assumes that individuals prefer to forego part of the value of the benefits if they can have them now rather than in the future.

Efficiency Making the best use of available resources.

Allocative efficiency Assessing competing programmes and judging the extent to which they meet objectives.

Technical (or X) efficiency Assessing the best way of achieving a given objective.

Equity Fair distribution of resources or benefits.

Marginal analysis The process which examines the effects of small changes in the existing pattern of health care expenditure in any setting.

Sensitivity analysis A technique which repeats the comparison between inputs and consequences, varying the assumptions underlying the estimates. In so doing, sensitivity analysis tests the robustness of the conclusions by varying the items around which there is uncertainty.

Utility A term used to describe the satisfaction accrued by an individual receiving a health technology. Utility is a value on a scale between 1 (perfect health) and 0 (death). Utility is measured by the **time trade-off, standard gamble** or **Rosser–Kind matrix method.**

REFERENCES

Deparatment of Health 2001 Building a safer NHS for patients. Department of Health/Stationery Office, London
Drummond M F, Jefferson T O 1996 Guidelines for authors and peer reviewers of economic submissions to the BMJ. British Medical Journal 313: 275–283

FURTHER READING

Audit Commission 1994 A prescription for improvement: towards more rational prescribing in general practice. HMSO, London
National Prescribing Centre, MeReC Briefing 2000 An introduction to health economics. Parts 1 and 2. September 2000

LIFE STAGES

Neonates 7

M. P. Ward Platt

KEY POINTS

- The survival of very premature babies has been greatly increased through the use of antenatal dexamethasone and neonatal surfactant treatment to prevent and treat surfactant deficiency.
- The fetoplacental unit creates a unique route for drug delivery.
- Drug disposition and metabolism in the neonate is very different to that at any other time of life.
- The optimal treatment of patent ductus arteriosus and bronchopulmonary dysplasia remains challenging and controversial.

The definitions of some important terms used of babies are given in Table 7.1. The earliest in pregnancy at which newborn babies can sometimes survive is 23–24 weeks' gestation, but conventionally any baby born at less than 32 weeks is regarded as being at relatively high risk of death or disability. Just over 1% of all births take place before 32 weeks of gestation. It is the gestation at birth rather than the birth weight which is of more practical and prognostic value.

Because mothers with high-risk pregnancies will often be transferred for delivery at a hospital capable of providing neonatal intensive care, the proportion of preterm and low birth weight (LBW) – (Table 7.1) babies cared for in such units is greater than in smaller maternity units in peripheral hospitals. Depending on the population and the nature of the hospital, between 6% and 10% of all babies will be LBW, and about 2% will be very low birth weight (VLBW). In the population as a whole, between 1% and 2% of all babies will receive intensive care, and the most common reason for this among preterm babies is the respiratory distress syndrome of the newborn (RDS).

Babies of less than 32 weeks' gestation invariably need some degree of special care, and generally go home when they are feeding adequately, somewhere between 35 and 40 weeks of postmenstrual age. So although in epidemiological terms the neonatal period is the first 28 postnatal days (see Table 7.1), babies may be 'neonatal' in-patients for as long as 3 or 4 months: during this time their weight may triple and their physiology and metabolism will change dramatically.

Drug disposition

An important and unique source of drug absorption, available until birth, is the placenta. Maternal drugs pass to the fetus and back again during pregnancy, but from delivery, any drugs present in the neonatal circulation can no longer be eliminated by that route, and must be dealt with by the baby's own systems. Important examples of maternal drugs which may adversely affect the newborn baby include opiates given for pain relief during labour, β-blockers given for pregnancy-induced hypertension, or benzodiazepines for seizures. In addition, a mother may be given a drug with the intention of treating not her, but her fetus. An example of this is the use of corticosteroids to promote fetal lung maturation when preterm delivery is planned or expected.

Enteral drug absorption is erratic in any newborn baby, and unavailable in the ill baby because the stomach does not empty. Therefore most drugs are usually given intravenously to ensure maximum bioavailability. Some drugs, such as paraldehyde and diazepam (for neonatal seizures) and paracetamol (for simple analgesia), can be given rectally. The trachea is used for surfactant, and adrenaline (epinephrine) can be given this way in resuscitation. Glucose gel can be absorbed buccally in the

Table 7.1 Definitions of terms

The normal length of human pregnancy (term):	37 up to 42 completed weeks of gestation
Preterm	< 37 weeks of gestation at birth
Post-term	≥ 42 weeks onwards
The neonatal period	The first 28 postnatal days
Low birth weight (LBW)	< 2500 g
Very low birth weight (VLBW)	< 1500 g
Extremely low birth weight (ELBW)	< 1000 g

treatment of hypoglycaemia. In the very preterm baby of 28 weeks' gestation or less, the skin is extremely thin and a poor barrier to water loss; consequently it is also permeable to substances in contact with it (Rutter 1996). This is harmful to the baby if there is prolonged skin contact with alcohol (as in chlorhexidine in 70% methylated spirit), which as well as causing a severe chemical burn can result in systemic methyl alcohol poisoning. The intramuscular route is normally avoided, except for vitamin K and naloxone, because of the small muscle bulk, particularly in premature babies (see the section on principles and goals of therapy, below).

Drugs are distributed within a baby's body as a function of their lipid and aqueous solubility, as at any other time of life. The main difference in the neonate is that the size of the body water pool under renal control is related not to the baby's surface area but to body weight (Coulthard 1985); furthermore, the absolute glomerular filtration rate increases logarithmically with post-conceptional age irrespective of the length of a baby's gestation. This has implications for predicting the behaviour of water soluble drugs such as gentamicin. The amount of adipose tissue can vary substantially between different babies: any baby born more than 10 weeks early and babies of any gestation who have suffered intrauterine growth restriction may have little body fat; conversely the infant of a diabetic mother may have a particularly large fat layer. This affects retention of predominantly lipid-soluble drugs. Protein binding in the plasma is influenced by the amount of albumin available, and this in turn is related to gestation, with albumin values found 12 weeks prior to term being only two-thirds of adult concentrations (Reading et al 1990).

The metabolic fate of drugs in the newborn is not qualitatively different to that in the older child, e.g. hydroxylation, oxidation and conjugation to sulphate or glucuronide. It is the efficiency with which these processes are carried out that distinguishes the baby from the older person. In addition to the immaturity of the metabolic pathways for drug disposal, drug metabolism is also affected by the physiological hyperbilirubinaemia of the newborn. The bilirubin can compete both for enzyme-binding sites and for glucuronate, and may thus affect drug metabolism for as long as unconjugated hyperbilirubinaemia persists.

The relative immaturity of hepatic and renal function results in correspondingly slow elimination of most drugs from the neonate. This is not necessarily a disadvantage, so long as due account is taken of the slow elimination and dose intervals are modified accordingly. It may even be a useful property, as with phenobarbital, which when given as a loading dose (usually 20 mg/kg) will remain in circulation for days in useful therapeutic quantities, often avoiding the need for further doses. On the other hand, drugs such as gentamicin and vancomycin, which have a relatively narrow therapeutic index, must be given far less frequently than in children or adults and plasma drug levels must be assayed in order to avoid toxicity.

There has been little study of pharmacodynamics in the term or preterm neonate. Most clinicians work on the assumption that the kinetics of drug behaviour are so different in this group of patients that the pharmacodynamic properties must follow the same pattern. In practice the most important pharmacodynamic effect is probably that of the behaviour of opiates derived from the mother in labour. Pethidine and diamorphine are the opiates most likely to cause significant respiratory depression in the neonate. Such respiratory depression is treated with naloxone, and a special neonatal preparation (20 micrograms/ml) is available. However, after birth the opiates and their metabolites have a long plasma half-life in the baby whereas the naloxone is rapidly eliminated (Brice et al 1979). The initial dramatic effect of naloxone can give a false sense of security, as the baby may become narcosed after a few hours following transfer to the postnatal ward. To try to prevent such late-onset narcosis many paediatricians use adult naloxone (400 micrograms/ml) instead, and give it intramuscularly to ensure that it remains active over several hours.

Major clinical disorders

Respiratory distress syndrome (RDS)

Among preterm babies the most commonly encountered disorder is respiratory distress syndrome (RDS, also called hyaline membrane disease (HMD) from its appearance on lung histology). The root cause of this disease is the lack of sufficient pulmonary surfactant. The condition is rare in babies born at or near term and becomes increasingly likely the more preterm a birth takes place.

Clinically, RDS is manifested by obvious difficulty with breathing, with nasal flaring, rib recession, tachypnoea, and a requirement for oxygen therapy. A relatively big baby born around 32–34 weeks of gestation may need no more treatment than extra oxygen. The natural history is that RDS becomes worse over the first 2 days, reaches a plateau, and then gradually improves. Smaller, more premature and more severely affected babies commonly go into respiratory failure and require mechanical ventilation. The introduction of surfactant therapy (see below) has transformed the clinical course of this condition and greatly reduced its mortality.

Some babies require high inspired concentrations of oxygen (up to 100%) for days on end during this time; in such pharmacological concentrations the therapeutic index becomes an important issue. Fortunately, pulmonary oxygen toxicity is not as much a problem to the neonate as it is to the adult (though it may have a causal role in the onset of bronchopulmonary dysplasia, see below). The major concern is the damage that prolonged arterial hyperoxia can do to the retina, resulting in retinopathy of prematurity. The goal is to give enough inspired oxygen to keep the arterial partial pressure within a band of about 6–12 kPa.

Mechanical ventilation is not a comfortable experience, for adults or children, but it has taken a long time to appreciate that this may also be true for premature babies. Paralysing agents such as pancuronium are often given to ventilated neonates, but these only prevent the baby from moving, and are not sedative. Pancuronium is widely used, partly because it wears off slowly so that the baby is not suddenly destabilized. Shorter acting agents such as atracurium are often used for temporary paralysis for intubation. Whether or not the baby is paralysed, morphine is commonly given either as intermittent doses or as an infusion, to provide narcosis and analgesia to reduce the distress of neonatal intensive care.

The incidence, severity and mortality of RDS caused by surfactant deficiency may be reduced by giving corticosteroids antenatally to the mother. Antenatal steroids have been shown to reduce mortality by up to 40% among the infants of mothers so treated; unfortunately it is not possible to identify and treat all mothers whose babies could benefit. Babies of less than 32 weeks gestation gain most benefit because they are at greatest risk of death and disability from RDS. Optimum treatment is betamethasone or dexamethasone as four oral doses of 6 mg each given 12-hourly, or two doses of 12 mg intramuscularly 24 hours apart (Crowley 2001).

The introduction of exogenous surfactant, derived from the pig or calf, has revolutionized the management of RDS. Natural surfactants are currently more effective than artificial ones, but better artificial surfactants are being developed. The first dose should be given as soon as possible after birth since the earlier it is given, the greater the benefit (Yost & Soll 2001).

There are several other important ways of treating babies in respiratory failure. For some babies of at least 34 weeks of gestation and at least 2 kg birth weight, extracorporeal membrane oxygenation (ECMO), in which a baby is in effect put on partial heart–lung bypass for a few days, may be life-saving when conventional ventilation fails (ECMO Collaborative Trial Group 1996). The inhaled vasodilator nitric oxide (NO) is now widely used, and reduces the need for ECMO in some babies of 34 weeks or more, but there is little evidence of benefit for more premature babies (Barrington & Finer 2001). Partial liquid ventilation is a technique which involves the instillation of perfluorocarbons, in which oxygen is highly soluble, into the bronchial tree to abolish the water–air interface in the terminal airways.

This is a highly experimental technique at present, but may well come to prominence in the future.

Patent ductus arteriosus (PDA)

PDA can be a problem in the recovery phase of RDS, and usually shows itself as a secondary increase in respiratory distress and/or ventilatory requirement, an increasing oxygen requirement, wide pulse pressure, and often a characteristic heart murmur. Physiologically, as pressure in the pulmonary artery falls because the RDS is improving, an open duct allows blood from the aorta to flow into the pulmonary artery, which engorges the lungs and reduces their compliance, while putting strain on the heart. Echocardiography is used to confirm the clinical suspicion. About one-third of all babies with birth weights less than 1000 g will develop signs of PDA (e.g. the characteristic heart murmur), but treatment is only needed when the baby is haemodynamically compromised. When treatment is needed the options are either medical treatment with indometacin, or surgical ligation.

Indometacin is usually given intravenously in the UK, but can be given enterally although absorption is unpredictable. Serious potential side-effects are renal impairment, gastric haemorrhage and gut perforation. These unwanted features are dose related, and a low-dose, prolonged course (0.1 mg/kg daily for 6 days) has been shown to be as effective, with fewer side-effects, than the same total dose given as 0.2 mg/kg, 12 hourly for three doses (Kumar & Yu 1997). Surgery is considered when one or more courses of indometacin fails to close the PDA, or if indometacin is contraindicated for any reason.

The prophylactic use of indometacin in preterm babies is controversial. As well as reducing the incidence of PDA, as expected, a course of indometacin started as soon as possible after birth also has the desirable effect of reducing the incidence of cerebral haemorrhage (Fowlie 2001), but whether this additional property translates into better long-term neurodevelopment is not yet known.

Bronchopulmonary dysplasia (BPD)

Bronchopulmonary dysplasia (BPD) most frequently occurs in very immature babies who have undergone prolonged respiratory support. It can be defined as oxygen dependency lasting more than 28 days from birth, but this definition is not very useful in that many babies born at less than 28 weeks of gestation require oxygen for 28 days or more, but few still need it after 8 weeks. A more useful functional and epidemiological definition of established BPD is oxygen dependency at 36 weeks of postmenstrual age, in a baby born before 32 weeks. The likelihood of getting BPD depends on the degree of prematurity, the severity of RDS, infection, the occurrence of PDA, and possibly the use of lipids in parenteral nutrition solutions.

Established BPD not severe enough to need continuing mechanical ventilation is treated with oxygen, either as increased ambient oxygen delivered in the incubator or through a head box, or through nasal cannulae if the baby is in a cot. Enough oxygen must be used to maintain an oxygen saturation high enough to control pulmonary artery pressure, while avoiding chronic low-grade hyperoxia which could contribute to retinopathy of prematurity.

Although there was enthusiasm for using dexamethasone to wean babies off ventilation and perhaps to reduce the severity of BPD, there is increasing evidence that its routine use does not improve mortality and increasing concern about steroid related side-effects, including effects on brain development. A wide variety of treatment regimens have been tested in trials and there is no standard approach. Side-effects such as hypertension and glucose intolerance are common but usually reversible; but the effects on growth and development are more serious.

BPD leads to increases in both pulmonary artery pressures and lung water content. The consequent strain on the heart can lead to heart failure for which the treatment, as in any age group, is to use a diuretic. Thiazides improve pulmonary mechanics as well as treating heart failure (Brion et al 2001). Sometimes furosemide (frusemide) is used, but its side-effects are significant urinary loss of potassium and calcium, and renal calcification. An alternative is to combine a thiazide with spironolactone which causes less calcium and potassium loss. By reducing lung water content, diuretics can also improve lung compliance and reduce the work of breathing. However BPD is not routinely treated with diuretics, since many babies do well without them. Systemic hypertension is common among babies with BPD and sometimes needs to be treated with antihypertensive drugs such as nifedipine or hydralazine.

Infection

Infection is a constant hazard in any intensive care situation, but as local ecology is unique to each unit no blanket recommendations can easily be made for antibiotic policy. Important pathogens in the first 2 or 3 days after birth are group B β-haemolytic streptococci, and a variety of Gram-negative organisms, especially *Escherichia coli*. Coagulase-negative staphylococci and *Staphylococcus aureus* are more important subsequently. Superficial candida infection is common in all babies, and systemic candida infection is a risk particularly in babies receiving prolonged courses of broad-spectrum antibiotics. In general, it is wise to use narrow-spectrum agents and short courses of antibiotics whenever

possible, and to discontinue blind treatment quickly (e.g. after 48 hours) if confirmatory evidence of bacterial infection, such as blood culture, is negative. The most serious neonatal infections are listed in Table 7.2.

It is usual to start antibiotics prophylactically whenever preterm labour is unexplained, where there has been prolonged rupture of the fetal membranes prior to delivery, where the baby is very premature and when a baby is ventilated from birth; but local policies vary according to local experience. A standard combination for such early treatment is penicillin G and an aminoglycoside, to cover group B streptococci and Gram-negative pathogens; treatment can be stopped after 48 hours if cultures prove negative. Blind treatment starting when a baby is more than 48 hours old has to take account of the expected local pathogens, but will always include cover for *Staph. aureus*. The newer cephalosporins such as cefotaxime and ceftazidime have been heavily promoted for use in the blind treatment of neonatal infection on the grounds of lower toxicity than aminoglycosides, and a wide therapeutic index, so there is no need to monitor plasma concentrations. Their main disadvantage is that the breadth of their spectrum favours fungal infection and the spread of resistance, although they compare favourably with ampicillin in this regard (Tullus & Burman 1989). Also, since courses of blind treatment are often only for 48 hours, because antibiotics can often be stopped when cultures are negative, there is often no need to measure aminoglycoside levels, so much of the apparent advantage of cephalosporins is lost.

Necrotizing enterocolitis (NEC)

Necrotizing enterocolitis (NEC) is an important complication of neonatal intensive care, and can arise in any baby. However, it most commonly occurs in premature babies and those already ill for other reasons. It is especially associated with being small for gestational age, birth asphyxia, and the presence of a PDA. Since many sick babies have multiple problems it has been difficult to disentangle causal associations from spurious

Table 7.2 Serious neonatal infections and pathogens

Septicaemia	*Staphylococcus epidermidis*, group B streptococci, *Escherichia coli*
Systemic candidiasis	*Candida*
Necrotizing enterocolitis	No single causal pathogen
Osteomyelitis	*Staphylococcus aureus*
Meningitis	Group B streptococci, *Escherichia coli*

links to conditions that occur anyway in ill infants, such as the need for blood transfusion. There is general agreement that the pathophysiology is related to damage of the gut mucosa, which may occur because of hypotension or hypoxia, coupled with the presence of certain organisms in the gut; and that these organisms then invade the gut wall to give rise to the clinical condition. It almost never arises in a baby who has never been fed, but early feeding, and initiating feeding with human breast milk, appears to be protective (Lucas & Cole 1990).

A baby who becomes ill with NEC is often septicaemic and may present acutely with a major collapse, respiratory failure and shock, or more slowly with abdominal distension, intolerance of feeds with discoloured gastric aspirates and blood in the stool. A fulminant course does not always develop. The medical treatment is respiratory and circulatory support if necessary, antibiotics, and switching to intravenous feeding for a period of time, usually a week to 10 days. One of the most difficult judgements is deciding if and when to operate to remove necrotic areas of gut, or deal with a perforation.

The antibiotic strategy for NEC is to cover Gram-positive, Gram-negative and anaerobic bacteria. Metronidazole is used to cover anaerobes in the UK, but clindamycin is preferred in some other countries. As with other drugs in the neonate, metronidazole behaves very differently in adults as compared with children, having an elimination half-life of over 20 hours in term babies. The elimination half-life is up to 109 hours in preterm babies, partly due to poor hepatic hydroxylation in infants born before 35 weeks' gestation. There is probably a case to be made for monitoring plasma levels of this drug, but in practice this is seldom done.

Haemorrhagic disease of the newborn

Except in the very rare case of malabsorption, haemorrhagic disease of the newborn (better described as vitamin K-dependent bleeding) affects only breast-fed babies because they get very little vitamin K in maternal milk. Bottle fed infants get sufficient vitamin K in their formula. Even without active prevention it is a rare condition, but it may cause death or disability when it presents with an intracranial bleed.

There are several possible strategies for giving vitamin K. An intramuscular injection of phyto-menadione 1 mg (0.5ml) can be given either to every newborn baby, or selectively to babies who have certain risk factors such as instrumental delivery, preterm birth, etc. Vitamin K can be given orally, so long as an adequate number of doses is given, and this has been shown to be effective in preventing disease (Wariyar et al 2000). Intramuscular injections are an invasive and unpleasant intervention for the baby since muscle bulk is small in the newborn (and particularly the preterm), and

other structures such as the sciatic nerve can be damaged even if the intention is to give the injection into the lateral thigh. There has also been widespread publicity about a possible link between intramuscular vitamin K and childhood malignancy which has made many parents wary of assenting to its administration. Intramuscular injections can be reserved for those babies with doubtful oral absorption (e.g. all those admitted for special care), or at high risk because of enzyme inducing maternal drugs such as anticonvulsants (Hey 1999).

Apnoea

Apnoea is the absence of breathing. Babies (and adults) normally have respiratory pauses, but preterm babies in particular are prone to prolonged pauses in respiration (over 20 seconds) which can be associated with significant falls in arterial oxygenation. Apnoea usually has both central and obstructive components, is often accompanied by bradycardia, and requires treatment to prevent life-threatening episodes of arterial desaturation leading to convulsions and brain damage.

Apnoeic and bradycardic episodes can be treated in three ways: intubating and mechanically ventilating the baby; giving continuous positive airway pressure (CPAP); or giving respiratory stimulants such as one of the methylxanthines, or doxapram. The main goal of treatment is to reduce the number and severity of the episodes without having to resort to artificial ventilation. Of the methylxanthines, caffeine appears to be as effective as theophylline or aminophylline (and these two are in any case partly metabolized to caffeine). Caffeine has a much wider therapeutic index than theophylline and aminophylline and there is no need to measure plasma concentrations. Most clinicians stop giving respiratory stimulants when the baby is around 34 weeks of postmenstrual age, after which time most babies will have achieved an adequate degree of cardiorespiratory stability and no longer need even the most basic forms of monitoring device. Doxapram is occasionally given as an adjunct to both a methylxanthine and CPAP, to avoid putting the baby on a ventilator.

Seizures

Seizures may arise as part of an encephalopathy, when they are accompanied by altered consciousness, or as isolated events when the baby is neurologically normal between seizure episodes. Investigations are directed to finding an underlying cause, but in about half of all babies having fits without an encephalopathy, no underlying cause can be found.

Just as with children and adults, treatment may be needed to control an acute seizure which does not terminate quickly, or given long term to prevent the occurrence of fits. In the neonate, the first choice anticonvulsant for the acute treatment of seizures is phenobarbital because it is effective, seldom causes respiratory depression, and is active for many hours or days because of its long elimination half-life. Diazepam is sometimes used intravenously or rectally, but it upsets temperature control, causes unpredictable respiratory depression, and is very sedating compared to phenobarbital. Paraldehyde is sometimes given because it is easy to give rectally, is relatively non-sedating, and short acting. It is excreted by exhalation and the smell can make the working environment quite unpleasant for staff. Phenytoin is often used when fits remain uncontrolled after two loading doses of phenobarbital (total 40 mg/kg) but is not given long term because of its narrow therapeutic index. When seizures are intractable, options include clonazepam or an infusion of lidocaine (lignocaine). There is little experience with intravenous sodium valproate in the neonate. Longer term treatment is commonly with phenobarbital, but after the first few months carbamazepine or sodium valproate are more suitable.

Hypoxic–ischaemic encephalopathy (HIE), which usually results either from intrapartum asphyxia or from an antepartum insult such as placental abruption, is an important cause of seizures. Convulsions are a marker of a more severe insult; they usually occur within 24 hours of birth, and may last for several days, after which they spontaneously resolve. The less severely affected babies quickly return to neurological normality. No drug has been shown to improve outcome when given after the insult has occurred, and routine use of phenobarbital or any other medication is not recommended (Evans & Levene 2001).

The therapeutic dilemma lies in the degree of aggression with which convulsions should be treated, since no conventional anticonvulsant is very effective in reducing electrocerebral seizure activity, even when the clinical manifestations of seizures are abolished, and as stated before, convulsions tend naturally to cease after a few days. The question as to whether strenuous attempts to gain control of seizures have any effect on subsequent developmental outcome remains unanswered. On the other hand, seizures which compromise respiratory function need to be treated to prevent serious falls in arterial oxygen tension and possible secondary neurological damage. Also, babies with frequent or continuous seizure activity are difficult to nurse and cause great distress to their parents. Therefore in practice it is usual to try to suppress the clinical manifestation of seizure activity, and phenobarbital remains the most commonly used first-line treatment. Where a decision is taken to keep a baby on anticonvulsant medication, therapeutic drug monitoring can provide helpful information and may need to be repeated from time to time during follow-up.

Principles and goals of therapy

The ultimate aim of neonatal care at all levels is to maximize disability-free survival and identify treatable conditions which would otherwise compromise growth or development. The treatment of most newborn babies is routine and preventative, and emergency intervention is needed in only a select few; these approaches are completely different and must be considered separately. For babies born preterm, the aim is to anticipate potential problems and avoid as far as possible the complications of intensive care.

Effects of rapid growth

The growth of a premature baby, once the need for intensive care has passed, can be very rapid indeed if the child is being fed with a high-calorie formula modified for use with VLBW infants; indeed, most babies born at 27 weeks (and weighing around 1 kg) can be expected to double their birth weight by the time they are 8 weeks old. Since the dose of all medications is calculated on the basis of body weight, constant review of dose is necessary to maintain efficacy, particularly for drugs which may be given for weeks on end such as respiratory stimulants, diuretics and anticonvulsants. Conversely, all that is necessary to gradually wean a baby from a medication is to hold the dose constant so that the baby gradually 'grows out' of the drug. This practice is frequently used with diuretic medication in BPD, the need for which becomes less as the baby's somatic growth reduces the proportion of damaged lung in favour of healthy tissue.

Therapeutic drug monitoring

The assay of plasma concentrations of various drugs has a place in neonatal medicine, particularly where the therapeutic index of a drug is narrow. It is routine to assay levels of antibiotics such as aminoglycosides and vancomycin, of which the trough measurement is of most value since it is accumulation of the drug which must be avoided. More rarely it may be necessary to assay minimal inhibitory or bactericidal concentrations of antibiotics in blood or cerebrospinal fluid if serious infections are being treated, but constraints on sampling limit the frequency with which this may be undertaken. Interpretation of plasma concentrations of chloramphenicol is problematic as active metabolites are not included, and safer antibiotics such as ceftazidime and cefotaxime have replaced chloramphenicol in the treatment of Gram-negative septicaemia and meningitis.

Theophylline and aminophylline are handled unpredictably and assay of plasma theophylline concentrations is a useful guide to therapy; since a baby may be on such medication for several weeks assays need to be repeated regularly (probably weekly, for convenience). The use of caffeine, which has a much wider therapeutic index, abolishes the need for routine measurement of levels, although it may occasionally be useful to measure blood levels if a normal dose appears to be ineffective. Where phenobarbital or other anticonvulsants are given long term, intermittent measurement of plasma levels can be a useful guide to increasing the dose, as with methylxanthines. Digoxin is now rarely used in this age group but regular assay of plasma concentrations is of obvious importance. All of these drugs have a long half-life so it is most important that drug concentrations are not measured too early, or too frequently, to prevent inappropriate changes in dose being made before a steady state is reached.

Avoiding harm

Intramuscular injections are considered potentially harmful because of the small muscle bulk of babies; there are very few situations in which intramuscular injections are required. However, it is not always easy to establish venous access, and occasionally it may be necessary to use the intramuscular route instead.

For sick preterm infants ventilated for respiratory failure, handling of any kind is a destabilizing influence, so the minimal necessary intervention should be the rule. Even opening the doors of an incubator can cause the interior temperature to fall in all but the newest incubators. It is therefore good practice to minimize the frequency of drug administration and to try to coordinate the doses of different medications.

Time-scale of clinical changes

In babies, the time-scale for starting drug treatments is very short because the clinical condition of any baby can change with great rapidity. For example, surfactant should be given as soon as possible after birth to premature babies who are intubated and ventilated.

Similarly, infection can be rapidly progressive, so starting antibiotics is a priority when the index of suspicion is high, or where congenital infection is likely.

For the sick preterm infant this model applies to a wide range of interventions. It is seldom possible to wait a few hours for the availability of a drug, and this has obvious implications for the quality of support required of a pharmacy for a neonatal service.

Patient and parent care

It is all too easy to take a 'veterinary' approach to neonatal medicine, on the grounds that premature infants cannot communicate their needs and can be treated, especially while receiving intensive care, as little more than a physiological preparation. Such an approach to therapy is fundamentally flawed. Even when receiving intensive care, any infant who is not either paralysed or very heavily sedated does in fact respond with a wealth of cues and non-verbal communication in relation to current needs. Monitors therefore do not replace clinical skills, but provide supplementary information and advance warning of problems. Even the most premature babies show individual characteristics, which emphasizes that individualized care is as important in this age group as in any other.

Involvement of parents in every aspect of care is a necessary goal in neonatal clinical practice, and care within a special care baby nursery is increasingly regarded as a partnership between professionals and parents rather than the province of professionals alone. Routine administration of oral medication is thus an act in which parents may be expected to participate, and for those whose baby has to be discharged home still requiring continuous oxygen, the parent will rapidly obtain complete control, with support from the hospital and the primary health care team. The increasing number of babies who survive very premature birth but whose respiratory state requires continued support after discharge presents an increasing therapeutic challenge for the future.

CASE STUDY

Case 7.1

A. went into labour as a result of an antepartum haemorrhage at 28 weeks of gestation. There was no time to give her steroids when she arrived at the maternity unit, and her son, J., was born by vaginal delivery in good condition. However, he required intubation and ventilation at the age of 10 minutes to sustain his breathing. He was not weighed at that moment but was given intramuscular vitamin K and then taken to the special care unit. On arrival in the unit, J. was weighed (1270 g) and was placed in an incubator for warmth. He was connected to a ventilator. Surfactant was given, blood taken for culture and basic haematology, and he was prescribed antibiotics. A radiograph confirmed the diagnosis of RDS.

Question

1. Which antibiotic(s) would be appropriate initially for J.?

Over the next 2 days J. required modest ventilation and remained on antibiotics. A second dose of surfactant was given 12 hours after the first. Parenteral feeding was commenced on day 2 as per unit policy, and on day 3 very slow continuous milk feeding into his stomach was started. Blood cultures were negative at 48 hours and the antibiotics were stopped. On day 4 he was extubated into 30% oxygen.

On day 5, J. looked unwell with a rising oxygen requirement, increased work of breathing and poor peripheral perfusion. Examination revealed little else except that his liver was enlarged and a little firm, his pulses rather full and easy to feel and there was a moderate systolic heart murmur. One possibility was infection.

Question

2. Which antibiotics would be appropriate for J. on day 5?

Another possibility was a patent arterial duct leading to heart failure.

Question

3. How could his heart failure and PDA be treated?

After appropriate treatment he looked progressively better, and when the blood culture was negative after 2 days, the antibiotics were stopped. By the age of 2 weeks, J. was on full milk feeds and the duct had closed. He was in air.

However, he began to have increasingly frequent episodes of spontaneous bradycardia, sometimes following apnoeic spells in excess of 20 seconds' duration. Examination between episodes showed a healthy, stable baby. Investigations such as haematocrit, serum sodium and an infection screen were normal.

Question

4. At 2 weeks, which drug of choice could be used to treat his apnoea and bradycardia? What would be the expected duration of treatment with this drug?

Answers

1. Blind antibiotic cover is usually started until negative blood cultures are received. Penicillin and gentamicin would provide good cover for streptococci and Gram-negative organisms, which are the most likely potential pathogens at this stage. A suitable dose would be 30 mg/kg of penicillin every 12 hours and 2.5 mg/kg of gentamicin every 12 hours. Alternatively, a third-generation cephalosporin such as cefotaxime could be used for initial 'blind' treatment. If cultures were negative at 48 hours, antibiotics could be stopped provided that there were no clinical indications to continue.

2. At day 5, antibiotic treatment should take account of the likely pathogens such as *Staph. aureus* and others causing nosocomial infections. A suitable choice for the former would be vancomycin in a dose of 15 mg/kg every 12 hours. The addition of another agent with good Gram-negative activity such as ceftazidime would provide a broad spectrum of cover, including against *Pseudomonas*.

3. A low dose of intravenous indometacin (e.g. 100 micrograms/kg) would be suitable for the treatment of PDA over 6 days to reduce the incidence of adverse effects which may occur if the same total dose were to be given over 3 days. Furosemide (frusemide) (1 mg/kg as a single dose) is the drug of choice for acute heart failure.

4. Caffeine is as effective and safer than theophylline to treat the apnoea of prematurity. A metabolic pathway in the immature liver, which is virtually absent in mature livers, methylates theophylline to caffeine, and thus by administering the active metabolite the complications of giving the parent drug, theophylline, are avoided. Theophylline has a narrow therapeutic range and requires plasma level monitoring. A suitable dose of caffeine for J. would be a loading dose of 20 mg/kg with maintenance dose of 5 mg/kg/day increasing to 10 mg/kg/day, if necessary. The frequency of episodes of apnoea and bradycardia should decline immediately. The treatment is likely to continue until he is about 34 weeks of postmenstrual age, when his control of breathing should be mature enough to maintain good respiratory function.

REFERENCES

Barrington K J, Finer N N 2001 Inhaled nitric oxide for respiratory failure in preterm infants. Cochrane Review. In: The Cochrane Library, Issue 1. Update Software, Oxford

Brice J E, Moreland T A, Walker C H 1979 Effects of pethidine and its antagonists on the newborn. Archives of Disease in Childhood 54: 356–361

Brion L P, Primhak R A, Ambrosio-Perez I 2001 Diuretics acting on the distal renal tubule for preterm infants with (or developing) chronic lung disease. Cochrane Review. In: The Cochrane Library, Issue 1. Update Software, Oxford

Coulthard M G 1985 Maturation of glomerular filtration in preterm and mature babies. Early Human Development 11: 281–292

Crowley P 2001 Prophylactic corticosteroids for preterm birth. Cochrane Review. In: The Cochrane Library, Issue 1. Update Software, Oxford

ECMO Collaborative Trial Group 1996 UK collaborative randomised trial of neonatal extracorporeal membrane oxygenation. UK Collaborative ECMO Trial Group. Lancet 348: 75–82

Evans D J, Levene M I 2001 Anticonvulsants for preventing mortality and morbidity in full term newborns with perinatal asphyxia. Cochrane Review. In: The Cochrane Library, Issue 1. Update Software, Oxford

Fowlie P W 2001 Intravenous indometacin for preventing mortality and morbidity in very low birth weight infants. Cochrane Review. In: The Cochrane Library, Issue 1. Update Software, Oxford

Hey E 1999 Effect of maternal anticonvulsant treatment on neonatal blood coagulation. Archives of Disease in Childhood. Fetal and Neonatal Edition 81: F208–210

Kumar R K, Yu V Y H 1997 Prolonged low-dose indomethacin therapy for patent ductus arteriosus in very low birthweight infants. Journal of Paediatrics and Child Health 33: 38–41

Lucas A, Cole T J 1990 Breast milk and neonatal necrotising enterocolitis. Lancet 336: 1519–1523

Reading R F, Ellis R, Fleetwood A 1990 Plasma albumin and total protein in preterm babies from birth to eight weeks. Early Human Development 22: 81–87

Rutter N 1996 The immature skin. European Journal of Pediatrics 155(Suppl. 2): S18–20

Tullus K, Burman L G 1989 Ecological impact of ampicillin and cefuroxime in neonatal units. Lancet 1: 1405–1407

Wariyar U, Hilton S, Pagan J et al 2000 Six years' experience of prophylactic oral vitamin K. Archives of Disease in Childhood. Fetal and Neonatal Edition 82: F64–68

Yost C C, Soll R F 2001 Early versus delayed selective surfactant treatment for neonatal respiratory distress syndrome. Cochrane Review. In: The Cochrane Library, Issue 1. Update Software, Oxford

FURTHER READING

Halliday H L 1996 Natural versus synthetic surfactants in neonatal respiratory distress syndrome. Drugs 51: 13–20

Rennie J M, Robertson N R C 2002 A manual of neonatal intensive care. Arnold, London

Speidel B, Fleming P, Henderson J et al (eds) 1998 A neonatal vade-mecum, 3rd edn. Arnold, London

Paediatrics 8

C. Barker   A. J. Nunn   S. Turner

KEY POINTS

- Children are not small adults.
- Patient details such as age, weight and surface area need to be accurate to ensure appropriate dosing.
- Weight and surface area may change significantly in a relatively small time period.
- Pharmacokinetic changes in childhood are important and have a significant influence on drug handling and need to be considered when choosing an appropriate dosing regimen for a child.
- The availability of a product does not ensure its suitability for use in children.
- The use of an unlicensed medicine in children is not illegal although it must be ensured that the choice of drug and dose is appropriate.

Paediatrics is the branch of medicine dealing with the development, diseases and disorders of children. Infancy and childhood is a period of rapid growth and development. The various organs, body systems and enzymes that handle drugs develop at different rates hence drug dosage, formulation, response to drugs and adverse reactions vary throughout childhood. Compared with adult medicine, drug use in children is not extensively researched and the range of licensed drugs in appropriate dosage forms is limited.

For many purposes it has been common to subdivide childhood into the following periods:

- neonate: the first 30 days of life
- infant: from 1 month to 1 year
- child: from 1 year to 12 years.

For the purpose of drug dosing, children over 12 years of age are often classified as adults. This is inappropriate because many 12-year-olds have not been through puberty and have not reached adult height and weight. The International Committee on Harmonization (2000) has suggested that childhood be divided into the following age ranges for the purposes of clinical trials and licensing of medicines:

- preterm newborn infant
- term newborn infants (0–27 days)
- infants and toddlers (28 days to 23 months)
- children (2–11 years)
- adolescents (12 to 16–18 years).

These age ranges are intended to reflect biological changes. The newborn (birth to 1 month) covers the climacteric changes after birth, 1 month to 2 years the early growth spurt, 2–12 years the gradual growth phase and 12–18 years puberty and the adolescent growth spurt to final adult height. Manufacturers of medicines and regulatory authorities have not yet standardized the age groups quoted in summaries of product characteristics.

Demography

In 1992 there were 11.8 million children aged less than 16 years in the UK. This is projected to have increased by nearly 5% between 1992 and 2001 and will be verified in the population census conducted in April 2001 (results available in 2003). Children can expect to live longer than ever before. On the mortality rates expected in 1994 a baby boy would live to 74 years while a baby girl would live to 79 years.

Infant mortality has fallen dramatically since the beginning of this century. In 1901, 149 per 1000 babies died before their first birthday; by 1992 this had fallen to just seven. Despite these dramatic reductions in infant mortality, variations remain between different social classes. Mortality is also higher among babies with a low birth weight. Recent recommendations to help prevent sudden infant death syndrome (SIDS, also called cot death) which include placing the baby to sleep on its back, keeping the room temperature between 16 and 20°C, not over-wrapping the baby with clothes and avoiding exposure to cigarette smoke, have led to a marked reduction in mortality. Between 1991 and 1992 mortality from SIDS halved to 0.7 per 1000 live births; one-third the rate of 5 years earlier.

Three areas have been targeted as part of a national strategy to address the major causes of premature death and preventable illness in children. These are accidental death, smoking and teenage conception. In 1992 there were about 1 million accidents in the home in England involving children under 15 years of age but only a small proportion of these were fatal. In England, about 30 000 children are admitted annually to hospital due to the ingestion of a poison, and an additional 25 000 are treated as out-patients. The majority of these are less than 5 years of age, with the peak incidence being 18–36 months of age. Fortunately there are only approximately eight deaths annually by this cause. Most poisonings are accidental ingestions although some subjects are child abuse victims. Over the age of 10 years, poisons may be taken as a suicide attempt or as a 'cry for help'. The range of substances involved in poisonings is wide. Prescribed and over-the-counter medicines account for approximately 60% of cases. Household products and chemicals represent 35% of cases, with plants and fungi and the bites and stings of venomous animals comprising the remainder. Typical ingestants are analgesics, cough syrups, oral contraceptives, bleach, detergents, disinfectants, petroleum products, berries and leaves.

Road accidents in England remain the major cause of accidental death in childhood, accounting for half the fatal accidents in those less than 15 years of age in 1992 and 71% among 10–14 year olds. A quarter of fatal accidents among 1–4 year olds were caused by fire.

Hospital episode statistics provide details of why children are admitted to hospital in England. Injury and poisoning are major causes of hospitalization in the older age group, accounting for 1 in 6 of all diagnoses in children aged 5–14 years. Respiratory problems make up one-fifth of all diagnoses. The 10 most common admission diagnoses in a specialist children's hospital over an 18 month period are shown in Table 8.1.

Table 8.1 Top 10 admission diagnoses to a specialist children's hospital

Ranking	Diagnosis
1	Respiratory tract infections
2	Chronic diseases of tonsils and adenoids
3	Asthma
4	Abdominal and pelvic pain
5	Viral infection (unspecified site)
6	Non-suppurative otitis media
7	Inguinal hernia
8	Unspecified head injury
9	Gastroenteritis/colitis
10	Undescended testicle

Congenital malformations are one of the main causes of serious illness and death in childhood. The national monitoring system set up in 1964 following the thalidomide tragedy gives an estimate of the number of babies born with congenital anomalies in England and Wales. In 1991 this was 1% of live births. Neural tube defects (spina bifida) are one example of devastating congenital malformations that have been influenced by dietary therapy. In 1964 it was suggested that folate might be involved in these defects. In 1991 the results of a long-term study (MRC Vitamin Study Research Group 1991) showed that folate supplementation prevented 72% of neural tube defects when given to women who were at high risk of having a pregnancy with a neural tube defect. Folate supplementation is now part of the routine advice given in antenatal clinics.

Cancer in childhood is rare. In Britain about one child in 600 develops cancer during the first 15 years of life. About 30% of cases are leukaemia (mostly acute lymphocytic leukaemia) and about one-fifth are various types of brain tumour. Chemotherapy and other treatments have improved 5-year survival rates dramatically over the last 30 years from 0% to 70% for acute lymphocytic leukaemia and up to 60% for childhood cancers in general. These improvements in outcome are associated with treatment in highly specialized centres. Treatment for children with cancer in the UK is based in the 22 centres of the UK Children's Cancer Study Group (UKCCSG). The UKCCSG was established in 1977 to improve the management of children with cancer and to advance the knowledge and study of childhood malignancies. The group coordinates and implements clinical trials nationally and internationally and maintains a register of all cases of childhood cancer in the UK.

Some infectious diseases occur in epidemics and are liable to large annual fluctuations. Despite this, a decline in diseases such as measles and whooping cough has occurred due to improved immunization rates. By 1997 uptake rates for whooping cough immunization had reached 94%. Recent publicity about the measles, mumps and rubella (MMR) combined vaccine and a possible association with autism and bowel disorders, has led to a reduction in uptake of the vaccine, although between 1991 and 1998 about 90% of children had been vaccinated by their second birthday. Reports from the UK (Kaye et al 2001) do not support an association between these adverse effects and the MMR vaccine.

The normal child

Growth and development are important indicators of a child's general well-being and paediatric practitioners should be aware of the normal development milestones in childhood. In the UK development surveillance and screening of babies and children is well established through child health clinics.

Weight is one of the most widely used and obvious indicators of growth, and progress is assessed by recording weights on a percentile chart (Fig. 8.1). A weight curve for a child, which deviates from the usual pattern requires further investigation. Separate recording charts are used for boys and girls and since percentile charts are usually based on observations of the white British population, adjustments may be necessary in some groups.

Height (or length in children less than 2 years of age) is another important tool in developmental assessment. In a similar way to weight, height or length should follow a percentile line. If this is not the case, or if growth stops completely, then further investigation is required. The normal rate of growth is taken to be 5 cm or more per year and any alteration in this growth velocity should be investigated.

For infants up to 2 years of age, head circumference is also a useful parameter to monitor. In addition to the above, assessments of hearing, vision, motor development and speech are undertaken at the child health clinics. A summary of age related development is shown in Figure 8.2.

Child health clinics play a vital role in the national childhood immunization programme, which commences at 2 months of age. Immunization is a major success story for preventative medicine, preventing diseases that have the potential to cause serious damage to a child's health, or even death. An example of the impact that immunization can have on the profile of infectious diseases is demonstrated by the meningitis C immunization campaign, which began in November 1999. Among children under the age of 18 years the incidence of meningitis C has dropped by 75%.

Advice on the current immunization schedule can be found in the British National Formulary, while supplementary information is published by the Department of Health (1996).

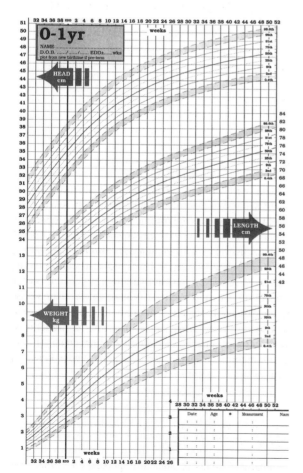

Figure 8.1 Example of a centile chart (© Child Growth Foundation).

Drug disposition

Pharmacokinetic factors

An understanding of the variability in drug disposition is essential if children are to receive rational and appropriate drug therapy. For convenience, the factors that affect drug disposition will be dealt with separately. However, when treating a patient all the factors have a dynamic relationship and none should be considered in isolation.

Absorption

Oral absorption. The absorption process of oral preparations may be influenced by factors such as gastric and intestinal transit time, gastric and intestinal pH and gastrointestinal contents. Posture, disease state and therapeutic interventions such as nasogastric aspiration or drug therapy can also affect the absorption process. It is not until the second year of life that gastric acid output increases and is comparable on a per kilogram basis to that observed in adults. In addition, gastric emptying time only approaches adult values at about 6 months of age.

The bioavailability of sulphonamides, digoxin and phenobarbital has been studied in infants and children of a wide age distribution. Despite the different physiochemical properties of the drugs, a similar bioavailability pattern was observed in each case. The rate of absorption was correlated with age, being much slower in neonates than in older infants and children. However, few other studies have specifically reported on the absorption process in older infants or children. The

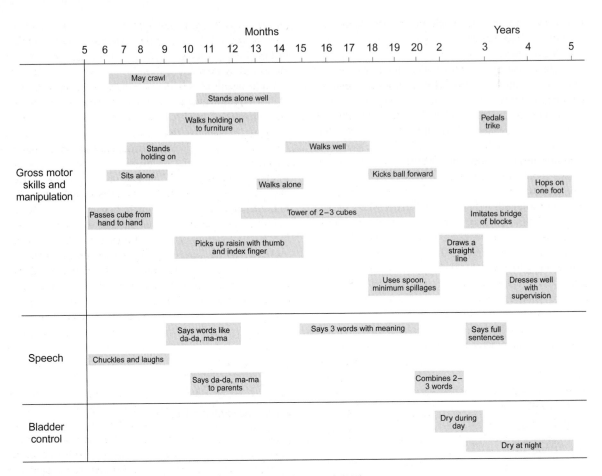

Months | Years

| 5 | 6 | 7 | 8 | 9 | 10 | 11 | 12 | 13 | 14 | 15 | 16 | 17 | 18 | 19 | 20 | 2 | 3 | 4 | 5 |

Gross motor skills and manipulation

May crawl

Stands alone well

Walks holding on to furniture

Pedals trike

Stands holding on

Walks well

Sits alone

Kicks ball forward

Hops on one foot

Walks alone

Passes cube from hand to hand

Tower of 2–3 cubes

Imitates bridge of blocks

Picks up raisin with thumb and index finger

Draws a straight line

Uses spoon, minimum spillages

Dresses well with supervision

Speech

Says words like da-da, ma-ma

Says 3 words with meaning

Says full sentences

Chuckles and laughs

Says da-da, ma-ma to parents

Combines 2–3 words

Bladder control

Dry during day

Dry at night

Figure 8.2   A summary of the various stages of development (Scott et al 1995).

available data suggest that in older infants and children orally administered drugs will be absorbed at a rate and extent similar to those in healthy adults. Changes in the absorption rate would appear to be of minor importance when compared to the age-related differences of drug distribution and excretion.

Intramuscular absorption. Absorption in infants and children after intramuscular (i.m.) injection is noticeably faster than in the neonatal period, since muscle blood flow is increased. On a practical note, intramuscular administration is very painful and should, where possible, be avoided. The route should not be used for the convenience of staff if alternative routes of administration are available.

Intraosseous absorption. This is a useful route of administration in patients in whom intravenous access cannot be obtained. It is especially useful in paediatric cardiorespiratory arrests where rapid access is required. A specially designed needle is usually inserted into the flat tibial shaft until the marrow space is reached. This route is considered equivalent to the intravenous route for rate of drug absorption, and most drugs can be given by this route.

Topical   absorption. Recent   advances   in transdermal drug delivery systems have led to an increased use of this route of administration, for example patch formulations of hyoscine hydrobromide have been found to be very useful to dry up secretions in children with excess drooling. Percutaneous absorption, which is inversely related to the thickness of the stratum corneum and directly related to skin hydration, is generally much greater in the newborn and young infant than in the adult. This can lead to adverse drug reactions. For example, the topical application of a preparation containing prilocaine and lidocaine (lignocaine) (Emla) is not recommended for use in children under 1 year of age. This is because of concerns about significant absorption of prilocaine in this younger age group, which may lead to methaemoglobinaemia. The development of needle-free subcutaneous jet injection systems appear to bring many benefits as a method of drug administration. They have been shown to give comparable levels to standard subcutaneous injections and overcome the problems of needle phobia, with less pain on administration. This system has been used with growth hormone, insulin, sedation prior to procedures and vaccination in children.

Another means of topical absorption is ophthalmically. Significant amounts of drugs may be absorbed from ophthalmic preparations through ophthalmic or nasolacrimal duct absorption, for example administration of phenylephrine eye drops can lead to hypertensive episodes in children.

Rectal absorption. The rectal route of administration is generally less favoured in the UK than in other European countries. It can be useful in patients who are vomiting, or in infants or children reluctant or unable to take oral medication. The mechanism of rectal absorption is probably similar to that of the upper part of the gastrointestinal tract, despite differences in pH, surface area and fluid content. Although some products, such as theophylline, are erratically absorbed from the rectum, the rapid onset of action of other preparations can be invaluable, for example rectal diazepam solution produces a rapid cessation of seizures in epilepsy and can be easily administered by parents in an emergency.

Buccal absorption. The buccal cavity is a potentially useful route of administration in patients who cannot tolerate medications via the oral route, for example postoperative patients or those with severe nausea. Highly lipophilic drugs can rapidly cross the buccal mucosa. Fentanyl is available in the USA as a 'lollipop' formulation (Actiq®) which is used to relax children before painful procedures; in the UK such formulations are manufactured as unlicensed 'specials'. Midazolam has also been administered via this route for the acute treatment of seizures.

There are a number of 'melt' and 'wafer' formulations available, for example piroxicam and ondansetron. These preparations have the advantage of palatability; however, they are not absorbed via the buccal muscosa but require swallowing and enteral absorption of the active constituent.

Intranasal absorption. The intranasal route is another useful route of administration. Medicines can be administered intranasally for their local action (e.g. sympathomimetics), or for their systemic effects (e.g. desmopressin in the treatment of diabetes insipidus). Midazolam has been widely used intranasally in children for the treatment of anxiety prior to procedures and also for the treatment of childhood seizures.

Significant systemic absorption of medicines given intranasally for their local effect can also occur; for example corticosteroids used in the treatment of allergic rhinitis have led to cushingoid symptoms and growth suppression.

Distribution

A number of factors that determine drug distribution within the body are subject to change with age. These include vascular perfusion, body composition, tissue-binding characteristics and the extent of plasma protein binding.

As a percentage of total body weight, the total body water and extracellular fluid volume decrease with age (Table 8.2). Thus, for water-soluble drugs such as aminoglycosides, larger doses on a milligram per kilogram of body weight basis are required in the neonate than in the older child to achieve similar plasma concentrations.

Protein binding. Despite normal blood pH, free fatty acid and bilirubin levels in infants, binding to plasma proteins is reduced as a result of low concentrations of both globulins and albumin. It has been suggested that binding values comparable with those seen in adults are reached within the third year of life for acidic drugs, whereas for basic drugs adult values are not reached until between 7 and 12 years of life. The clinical significance of this reduction in infants and older children is minimal. The influence of disease states, such as renal impairment, on plasma protein binding is more important.

Drug metabolism

At birth the majority of the enzyme systems responsible for drug metabolism are either absent or present in considerably reduced amounts compared with adult values, and evidence indicates that the various systems do not mature at the same time. This reduced capacity for metabolic degradation at birth is followed by a dramatic increase in the metabolic rate in the older infant and young child. In the 1–9 year age group in particular, metabolic clearance of drugs is shown to be greater than in adults, as exemplified by theophylline, phenytoin and carbamazepine. Thus to achieve plasma concentrations similar to those observed in adults, children in this age group may require a higher dosage than adults on milligram per kilogram basis (Table 8.3).

Metabolic pathways that play only a minor role in adults may play a more significant role in children and

Table 8.2 Extracellular fluid volume and total body water as a percentage of body weight

Age	Total body water %	Extracellular fluid %
Preterm neonate	85	50
Term neonate	75	45
3 months	75	30
1 year	60	25
Adult	60	20

Table 8.3 Theophylline dosage in children older than 1 year

Age	Dosage (mg/kg/day)
1–9 years	24
9–12 years	20
12–16 years	18
Adult	13

compensate for any deficiencies in the normal adult metabolic pathway. For example glucuronidation accounts for up to 70% of the metabolic pathway of paracetamol in adulthood; however, in the early newborn period glucuronidation is deficient, accounting for less than 20% of paracetamol metabolism. This is compensated for by a more pronounced sulphate conjugation and this leads to an apparently normal half-life in newborns. Paracetamol appears to be less toxic in children than in adults and this may be in part explained by the compensatory routes of metabolism.

Renal excretion

The anatomical and functional immaturity of the kidneys at birth limits renal excretory capacity. Below 3–6 months of age the glomerular filtration rate is lower than that of adults, but may be partially compensated by a relatively greater reduction in tubular reabsorption. Tubular function matures later than the filtration process. Generally, the complete maturation of glomerular and tubular function is reached only towards 6–8 months of age. After 8 months of age the renal excretion of drugs is comparable with that observed in older children and adults. Changes in renal clearance of gentamicin provide a good example of the maturation of renal function (Table 8.4).

Table 8.4 Renal clearance of gentamicin

	Plasma half-life
Small premature infants weighing less than 1.5 kg	11.5 h
Small premature infants weighing 1.5–2 kg	8 h
Term infants and large premature infants less than 1 week of age	5.5 h
Infants 1 week to 6 months	3–3.5 h
Infants more than 6 months to adulthood	2–3 h

Other factors

In addition to age-related changes in drug disposition, nutritional status and disease states can influence drug handling. High plasma clearance of antibiotics such as penicillins and aminoglycosides has been demonstrated in children with cystic fibrosis; increased elimination of furosemide (frusemide) has been reported in children with nephrotic syndrome, while prolonged elimination of furosemide (frusemide) has been reported in infants with congestive cardiac failure. Altered protein binding has been demonstrated in hepatic disease, nephrotic syndrome, malnutrition and cardiac failure.

Drug therapy in children

Dosage

Doses of medicines in children should be obtained from a paediatric dosage handbook and should not be extrapolated from the adult dose. There are a number of such texts available internationally. The information within them may be based on evidence from clinical studies in children or reflect the clinical experience of the contributors. In the UK, *Medicines for Children* (see further reading section), a joint publication of the Royal College of Paediatrics and Child Health and the Neonatal and Paediatric Pharmacists Group, is a national formulary which includes prescribing guidelines and drug monographs. It contains information on licensed, unlicensed and off-label use of medicines. When consulting any dosage reference resource, care should be taken to identify the dosage convention being used. Some formularies (such as *Medicines for Children*) use a single dose convention and indicate the number of times the dose should be repeated in a 24-hour period. Other formularies indicate the total daily dose and the number of doses this is divided into. Confusing the total daily dose with the single dose to be repeated may have catastrophic consequences and the single dose convention has become the preferred convention.

While age, weight and height are the easiest parameters to measure, the changing requirement for drug dosage during childhood corresponds most closely with changes in body surface area (BSA). Nomograms which allow the surface area to be easily derived are available. The surface area can also be calculated using the following equation:

$$BSA = \sqrt{\frac{height\ (cm) \times weight\ (kg)}{3600}}$$

There are practical problems in using the surface area method for prescribing; accurate height and weight may be difficult to obtain in a sick child, and manufacturers rarely provide dosage information on a surface area basis. The surface area formula for children has been used to produce the percentage method, giving the percentage of adult dose required at various ages and weights (Table 8.5).

In selecting a method of dosage calculation the therapeutic index of the drug should be considered. For agents with a narrow therapeutic index, such as cytotoxic agents, where recommendations are quoted per square metre, dosing must be based on the calculated surface area. However, there may be exceptions in children less than 1 year of age who have a proportionally larger surface area than other age groups. In children less than 1 year, dosages of chemotherapeutic agents are often based on weight rather than surface area to prevent overestimation of the dose in this age group.

For drugs with a wide therapeutic index, such as penicillin, single doses may be quoted for a wide age range. Between these two extremes, doses are quoted in milligrams per kilogram, and this is the most widely used method of calculation. Whichever method is used, the resulting dosage should be modified according to response and adverse effects.

It is important to note that none of the available methods of dosage calculation account for the change in dosage interval that may be required because of age-related changes in drug clearance. Where possible, the use of therapeutic drug monitoring to confirm the appropriateness of a dose is recommended.

Table 8.5 Percentage of adult dose required at various ages and body weights

Age	Mean weight for age lb	Mean weight for age kg	Percentage of adult dose
Newborn (full term)	7.7	3.5	12.5
2 months	10	4.5	15
4 months	14	6.5	20
1 year	22	10	25
3 years	33	15	33.3
7 years	50	23	50
10 years	66	30	60
12 years	86	39	75
14 years	110	50	80
16 years	128	58	90
Adult	150	68	100

Choice of preparation

The choice of preparation and its formulation will be influenced by the intended route of administration, the age of the child, availability of preparations, other concomitant therapy and, possibly, underlying disease states.

Buccal route

Drugs may be absorbed rapidly from the buccal cavity (the cheek pouch) or they may dissolve when administered and be swallowed and absorbed from the stomach. 'Melt' technology (e.g. piroxicam, ondansetron), in which the drug and flavourings are freeze-dried into a rapidly dissolving pellet, can be very useful. The 'melt' dissolves instantly into a very small volume which is difficult for the child to reject. Gels, sprays and liquids can also be administered into the buccal cavity, using drugs such as midazolam to treat seizures.

Oral route

The oral route is usually the most convenient, but in an uncooperative child it can be the least reliable. Safe and effective drug therapy requires accurate administration, yet the 5 ml spoon is a difficult means of administering liquid medicines. Use of an oral syringe can provide controlled administration, ensure accurate measurement of the calculated dose and avoids the need for dilution of preparations with syrup. Concentrated formulations may be administered as oral drops in a very small volume. Although convenient there could be significant dosage errors if drops are not delivered accurately.

In general, liquid preparations are more suitable for children under 7 years of age, although some quite young children can cope with solid dose formulations. Some commercially available products contain excipients such as alcohol, propylene glycol and dyes that may cause adverse effects or be inappropriate for use in children with particular disease states. The osmolality and tonicity of preparations may be important; necrotizing enterocolitis (a disorder seen in the neonatal period) has been associated with many different factors including high-osmolality infant feeding formulae and pharmaceutical preparations, although a causal relationship has not been established. Oral liquids with high osmolality may irritate the stomach and should be diluted for administration. Sugar-free preparations may be necessary in the diabetic child or be desirable in other children for the prevention of dental caries. It is, however, important to be aware of the potential problems associated with substitutes for sucrose. The artificial sweetening agent aspartame, used in some preparations, should be used with caution in children with phenylketonuria because of its phenylalanine content. Other carbohydrates such as sorbitol and glycerol may not contribute to dental caries but produce diarrhoea if large doses are given. In these instances a specially formulated preparation containing a higher amount of the active drug in small volume may be preferable.

Injection solutions can sometimes be administered orally although their concentration and pH must be considered together with the presence of unsuitable excipients. Powders or small capsules may be prepared and used as an alternative. However, lactose is a common diluent in powders, and caution must be exercised in children with lactose intolerance as a result of an inborn error of metabolism, or temporarily following gastrointestinal diseases or gut surgery.

Parents must be discouraged from adding the dose of medicine to an infant's feed. Quite apart from potential interactions which may arise with milk feeds, if the entire feed is not taken a proportion of the dose will be lost. It is also important to advise parents when it is not appropriate to crush solid dosage forms (e.g. sustained-release preparations).

Nasogastric and gastrostomy administration

Medicines may be administered into the stomach via a nasogastric tube in the unconscious child or when swallowing is difficult. A gastrostomy tube may be placed into the stomach transcutaneously if the problem is long term, for example in some children with cerebral palsy. Enteral nutrition may also be administered through such tubes. Drugs such as phenytoin may adsorb to the plastic of the tubes and interact with enteral feeds requiring special administration techniques to ensure bioavailability (Yeung & Ensom 2000).

Intranasal routes

Several drugs, such as desmopressin and midazolam, have been shown to be absorbed from the nasal mucosa. This route may avoid the need for injections but administration may be difficult in the uncooperative child and drugs administered may irritate the mucosa or be painful.

Rectal route

Although the rectal route can be useful, it is limited by the range of products available and the dosage inflexibility associated with rectal preparations. Some oral liquid preparations such as chloral hydrate and carbamazepine can be administered rectally. The route is useful in the unconscious child in the operating theatre or intensive care unit and it is not uncommon to administer perioperative analgesics such as diclofenac and paracetamol and the antiemetic ondansetron using suppository formulations. Parents and teachers may express concerns about using this route, fearing accusations of child abuse, but it is an important route of administration for diazepam or paraldehyde enema in the fitting child.

When oral and rectal routes are inappropriate the parenteral route may be necessary.

Parenteral route

The problems associated with the administration of intramuscular injections in infants and children have been described earlier in this chapter. The route has a limited role in paediatric drug therapy and should not be used routinely. The intravenous route of administration is more widely used, but it is still associated with a number of potential problems that are outlined below.

Intravenous access. The practical difficulties of accessing small veins in the paediatric patient do not require explanation. However, these difficulties can often explain the sites of access that are chosen. Scalp veins, commonly used in newborn infants, are often very prominent in this age group allowing easy access. It is also more difficult for the infant to dislodge a cannula from this site than from a site on the arm or foot. Likewise the umbilical artery offers a useful route for monitoring the patient but can also be used for drug administration in some circumstances. Vasoconstrictive drugs, for example adrenaline (epinephrine), dopamine, isoprenaline, should not be given by this route.

Fluid overload. In infants and children the direct administration of intravenous fluids from the main infusion container is associated with the risk of inadvertent fluid overload. This problem can be averted by the use of a paediatric administration set and/or a volumetric infusion device to control the flow rate. A paediatric administration set incorporates a graduated volumetric chamber with a maximum capacity of 150 ml. Although this system is intended primarily as a safety device, the volume within the burette chamber can be readily adjusted, allowing its use for intermittent drug administration and avoiding the need for the 'piggy back system' commonly used in adult intravenous administration.

Dilution of parenteral preparations for infusion may also cause inadvertent fluid overload in children. In fluid-restricted or very young infants, it is possible that the volume of diluted drug can exceed the daily fluid requirement. In order to appreciate this problem, the paediatric practitioner should become familiar with the fluid volumes that children can tolerate. As a guide these volumes can be calculated using the following formula: 100 ml/kg for the first 10 kg, plus 50 ml/kg for the next 10 kg, plus 20 ml/kg thereafter. Worked examples are given in Table 8.6. It is important to remember that these volumes do not account for losses such as those caused

Table 8.6 Calculation of standard daily fluid requirements in paediatric patients

15 kg patient	35 kg patient
100 ml/kg × 10 kg = 1000 ml	100 ml/kg × 10 kg = 1000 ml
Plus 50 ml/kg × 5 kg = 250 ml	Plus 50 ml/kg × 10 kg = 500 ml
Total = 1250 ml/day	Plus 20 ml/kg × 15 kg = 300 ml
	Total = 1800 ml/day

by dehydration, diarrhoea or artificial ventilation. While the use of more concentrated infusion solutions may overcome the problem of fluid overload, stability data on concentrated solutions is often lacking. It may therefore be necessary to manipulate other therapy to accommodate the treatment or even to consider alternative treatment options.

Fluid overload may also result from excessive volumes of flushing solutions. This problem is described later in this section.

Lack of suitable paediatric formulations. A large number of parenteral products are only available in adult dose sizes. The concentrations of these products can make it difficult to measure the small doses required in paediatrics and may lead to errors.

Displacement volume. Reconstitution of powder injections in accordance with manufacturers' directions usually makes no allowance for the displacement volume of the powder itself. Hence the final volume may be greater than expected and the concentration will therefore be less than expected. This can result in the paediatric patient receiving an under-dose, which becomes even more significant in younger patients receiving smaller doses. Paediatric units usually make available modified reconstitution directions which take account of displacement volumes.

Rates of infusion. The slow infusion rates often necessary in paediatrics may influence drug therapy. The greater the distance between the administration port and the distal end of the delivery system, and the slower the flow rate, the longer the time required for the drug to be delivered to the patient. In very young infants and children it may take several hours for the drug to reach the patient, depending on the point of injection. This is an important consideration if dosage adjustments are being made in response to serum level monitoring. Bolus injections should always be given as close to the patient as possible.

Dead space. Following administration via an injection port, a residual amount of drug solution can remain trapped at the port. If dose volumes are small the trapped fluid may represent a considerable proportion of the intended dose. Similarly the volume of solution

required to prime the intravenous lines or the in-line filters (i.e. the dead space) can be a significant proportion of the intended dose. This problem can be minimized by ensuring that drugs are flushed into the main infusion line after administration via an injection port or through a filter, and by priming the lines initially with a compatible solution.

It is important to remember that flushing volumes can add a significant amount to the daily fluid and sodium intake, and it may be important to record the volume of flushing solutions used in patients susceptible to fluid overload.

Excipients. Analogous to oral preparations, excipients may be present in parenteral formulations and can be associated with adverse effects. Benzyl alcohol, polysorbates and propylene glycol are commonly used agents which may induce a range of adverse effects in children including metabolic acidosis, altered serum osmolality, central nervous system depression, respiratory depression, cardiac arrhythmias and seizures. Knowledge of the products that contain these ingredients may influence drug selection.

Many hospitals have established centralized intravenous additive services (CIVAS) that prepare single intravenous doses under sterile conditions, thus avoiding the need for preparation at ward level. Such services have not only significantly decreased the risks associated with intravenous therapy, particularly in the paediatric population, but can also produce considerable cost savings.

Pulmonary route

The use of aerosol inhalers for the prevention and treatment of asthma presents particular problems for children because of the coordination required. The availability of breath-activated devices and spacer devices has greatly improved the situation. The National Institute for Clinical Excellence has produced evidence-based guidance on the use of inhaler devices in children less than 5 years of age (NICE 2002a) and in older children (NICE 2002).

It must be remembered that drugs can be absorbed into the systemic circulation after pulmonary administration or may be absorbed by the enteral route when excess drug is swallowed. High dose corticosteroid inhalation may suppress the adrenal cortical axis and growth by this mechanism.

Counselling adherence and concordance

Parents or carers are often responsible for the administration of medicines to their children and therefore the concordance and adherence of both parties must be considered. Literature about non-adherence and concordance in children is limited, but the problem is considered to be widespread and similar to that reported in adults.

Non-adherence may be caused by several factors such as patient resistance to taking the medicine, complicated dosage regimens, misunderstanding of instructions and apparent ineffectiveness or side-effects of treatment. In older children and adolescents who may be responsible for their own medication, different factors may be responsible for non-adherence, for example they may be unwilling to use their medication because of peer pressure.

Several general principles should be considered in an attempt to improve adherence. Adherence is usually better when fewer medicines are prescribed. Attention should be given to the formulation, taste, appearance and ease of administration of treatment. The regimen should be simple and tailored to the child's waking day.

Many health professionals often counsel the parents/carer only, rather than involving the child in the counselling process. Where possible treatment goals should be set in collaboration with the child. Studies have shown that parents consider the 8–10 year age group the most appropriate at which to start including the child in the counselling process. As well as verbal instruction, parents often want written information. However, current patient information leaflets must reflect the Summary of Product Characteristics (SPC) and so are often inappropriate. If a drug is used in an 'off-label' manner, statements such as 'not recommended for use in children' may cause confusion and distress. Care needs to be taken, therefore, to ensure that the information provided, whether written or spoken, is appropriate for both the parent and the child.

Medicines in schools

Children who are acutely ill will be treated with medicines at home or in hospital, although during their recovery phase it may be possible to return to school. Children with chronic illness such as asthma or epilepsy, and children recovering from acute illnesses, may require medicines to be administered while at school. In addition, there are some medical emergencies which may occur at school or on school trips that require prompt drug administration before the arrival of the emergency services. These emergencies include anaphylaxis (associated with food allergy or insect stings), severe asthma attacks and seizures.

Policies and guidance

There is considerable controversy over the administration of medicines in schools. Policies and procedures are required to ensure that prescribed medicines are labelled, stored and administered safely and appropriately, and that teachers and care assistants are adequately trained and understand their responsibilities. Guidance has been issued by the Department of Education and Science (1990). NICE (2000b) has provided guidelines for the use of methylphenidate in the treatment of attention deficit/ hyperactivity disorder (ADHD, or hyperactivity). This requires a partnership between doctors, teachers, educational psychologists, parents and children to ensure appropriate diagnosis and treatment. Shared care guidelines should be developed to allow GPs to participate in management. Many children will require methylphenidate, a controlled drug, to be administered while at school unless sustained-release preparations are available. The administration of adrenaline (epinephrine) by injection and rectal diazepam cause particular and understandable concern to some teachers. The school should have a policy on the use by pupils of over-the-counter remedies and on possession of medicines. The school authority and teachers' unions must make clear statements about liability should problems occur.

Responsibility for common medicines

Responsible pupils should be allowed to administer their own medication. Asthmatics should carry their 'reliever' inhaler (e.g. salbutamol or terbutaline), a spare should be available in school, and easy access before and during sports assured. There should be no need to have 'preventer' inhalers at school since 2 or 3 times daily administration schedules are appropriate and can avoid school hours. Medicines with a 2 or 3 times daily administration schedule should be supplied wherever possible so that dosing during school hours is avoided. Sustained-release preparations or drugs with intrinsically long half-lives may be more expensive but avoid the difficulties of administration at school. When administration at school is unavoidable, the schooltime doses can be provided by the pharmacist in a separate, labelled container.

Special schools

Some children with severe, chronic illness will go to special rather than mainstream schools where their condition can receive attention from teachers and carers who have received appropriate training. Some special schools will be residential. Pupils may also attend another institution for respite care. Particular attention to communication of changes to drug treatment between parents, general practitioners, hospital doctors and school staff is required if medication errors are to be avoided.

Monitoring parameters

Paediatric vital signs (Table 8.7) and haematological and biochemical parameters (Table 8.8) change throughout childhood and differ from those in adults. The figures presented in the tables are given as examples and may vary from hospital to hospital.

Table 8.7   Paediatric vital signs

	Age		
	< 1 year	2–5 years	5–12 years
Heart rate (beats/min)	120–140	100–120	80–100
Blood pressure (systolic) (mmHg)	70–90	80–90	90–110
Respiratory rate (breaths/min)	90	80	80

Table 8.8   Biochemical and haematology reference ranges

	Neonate	Child	Adult
Albumin (g/l)	24–48	30–50	35–55
Bilirubin (μmol/l)	< 200	< 15	< 17
Calcium (mmol/l)	1.8–2.8	2.15–2.7	2.20–2.55
Chloride (mmol/l)	95–110	95–110	95–105
Creatinine (μmol/l)	28–60	30–80	50–120
Haemoglobin (g/dl)	18–19	11–14	13.5–18.0 (males) 12–16 (females)
Haematocrit	0.55–0.65	0.36–0.42	0.4–0.45 (males) 0.36–0.44 (females)
Magnesium (mmol/l)	0.6–1.0	0.6–1.0	0.7–1.0
Phosphate (mmol/l)	1.3–3.0	1.0–1.8	0.85–1.4
Potassium (mmol/l)	4.0–7.0	3.5–5.5	3.5–5.0
Sodium (mmol/l)	130–145	132–145	135–145
Urea (mmol/l)	1.0–5.0	2.5–6.5	3.0–6.5
White cell count ($\times 10^9$/l)	6–15	5–14	3.5–11

Assessment of renal function

There are a number of methods of measuring renal function in children. These include the use of ^{51}Cr-EDTA, ^{99m}Tc-DTPA and using plasma and urine creatinine concentrations over a timed period. However, despite some limitations, the use of plasma creatinine and estimated creatinine clearance are the most frequently used and most practical methods for day-to-day assessment of renal function.

In adults, several formulae and nomograms are available for calculating and estimating renal function. However, these cannot be extrapolated to the paediatric population; the Cockcroft and Gault equation, for example, is validated for patients aged 18 years and over.

A number of validated models are available for use in children. These equations use combinations of serum creatinine, height, weight, body surface area, age and sex to provide a simple estimate of creatinine clearance. A number of these equations (e.g. Schwartz equation) have been further modified to better predict creatinine clearance; however, the advantage of simplicity is thereby lost. Several examples with their validated age ranges are shown below:

- Traub and Johnson (age 1–18 years)

$$\text{Creatinine clearance (ml/min/1.73m}^2) = \frac{42 \times \text{height (cm)}}{\text{Serum creatinine (μmol/l)}}$$

- Counhahan (age 2 months to 14 years)

$$\text{Creatinine clearance (ml/min/1.73m}^2) = \frac{38 \times \text{height (cm)}}{\text{Serum creatinine (μmol/l)}}$$

- Schwartz et al

$$\text{Creatinine clearance (ml/min/1.73m}^2) = \frac{\kappa \times \text{height (cm)}}{\text{Serum creatinine (μmol/l)}}$$

Where κ varies dependent on the age of the patient:

Low birth weight infants $\kappa = 30$

Normal infants 0–18 months $\kappa = 40$

Girls 2–16 years $\kappa = 49$

Boys 2–13 years $\kappa = 49$

Boys 13–16 years $\kappa = 60$

Whichever equation is chosen, it should be borne in mind that there are several limitations to their use, for example they should not be used in rapidly changing renal function, anorexic or obese patients, and they should NOT be taken as an accurate measure, but as a guide to glomerular filtration rate.

Adverse drug reactions

The incidence of adverse drug reactions (ADRs) in children outside the neonatal period is thought to be less than at all other ages; however, the nature and severity of the ADRs that children experience may differ from those experienced by adults.

Studies have shown an incidence of ADRs in paediatric patients of between 0.2% to 22% of patients. The wide range reflects the limited number of formal prospective and retrospective studies examining the incidence and characteristics of adverse drug reactions in the paediatric age group and the variations in study setting, patient group and definition of adverse drug reaction used. One consistent finding is that the greater the number of medications the child is exposed to the greater the risk of adverse drug reactions.

ADRs in infants and older children typically occur at lower doses than in adults, and symptoms may be atypical. Examples include:

1. Enamel hypoplasia and permanent discolouration of the teeth with tetracyclines.
2. Growth suppression with long-term corticosteroids in prepubertal children.
3. Paradoxical hyperactivity in children treated with phenobarbital.
4. Hepatotoxicity associated with the use of sodium valproate. There are three major risk factors:
   - age under 3 years
   - children receiving other anticonvulsants
   - developmental delay.

   The mechanism is not fully understood but is thought to relate to abnormal metabolism.
5. Increased risk of Reye's syndrome with the use of salicylates in children with mild viral infection. Reye's syndrome is a life-threatening illness associated with drowsiness, coma, hypoglycaemia, seizures and liver failure. Mechanism of this toxicity remains unknown but aspirin is generally avoided in children under 12 years.

Many adverse drug reactions occur less frequently in the paediatric population, for example gastrointestional bleeds with NSAIDs, hepatotoxicity with flucloxacillin and severe skin reactions with trimethoprim/ sulfamethoxazole.

The reporting of ADRs is particularly important because the current licensing system not only deprives children of useful drugs because of the lack of clinical trials in children but also excludes them from epidemiological studies of ADRs to prescribed drugs. ADR reporting can ultimately be used to reduce the incidence of ADRs resulting in reduced patient morbidity and mortality.

Medication errors

In contrast to adverse drug reactions, medication errors occur as a result of human mistakes or system flaws.

Medication errors are now recognized as being an important cause of adverse drug events in paediatrics and should always be considered as a possible causative factor in any unexplained situation. They can produce a variety of problems ranging from minor discomfort to death. In the USA it is estimated that 100–150 deaths occur annually in children in hospitals due to medication errors. The actual reported incidence of errors varies considerably between studies, ranging from 0.15% to 17% of admissions. However, different reporting systems and criteria for errors make direct comparisons between studies difficult.

The incidence of medication errors and the risk of serious errors occurring in children are significantly greater than in adults. The causes are many and include the following:

- The heterogeneous nature of the paediatric population with the corresponding lack of standard dosage.
- Calculation errors by the prescriber, dispensing pharmacist, nurse or caregiver.
- Lack of available dosage forms and concentrations appropriate for administration to children, necessitating additional calculations and manipulations of commercially available products.
- Lack of familiarity with paediatric dosing guidelines.
- Confusion between adult and paediatric preparations.
- Limited published information.
- Need for precise dose measurement and appropriate drug delivery systems leading to administration errors and the inappropriate use of measuring devices.
- Ten-fold dosing errors are particularly important and potentially catastrophic; however, they appear regularly in the published literature.

The reporting and prevention of medication errors is an important aspect of the paediatric pharmacist's role. The causes of medication errors are usually multifactorial and it is essential that when investigating medication errors, particular focus should be made on system changes.

Licensing medicines for children
Medicines licensing process

All medicines marketed in the UK must have been granted a product license (PL) under the terms of the Medicines Act 1968, or a marketing authorization (MA) following more recent European legislation on the authorization of medicines. The aim of licensing is to ensure that medicines have been assessed for safety, quality and efficacy. In the UK, evidence submitted by a pharmaceutical company is assessed by the Medicines Control Agency (MCA) with independent advice from the Committee on Safety of Medicines (CSM) and the Medicines Commission.

The licensed indications for a drug are published in the summary of product characteristics (SPC). Many medicines granted a PL or MA for adult use have not been scrutinized by the licensing authorities for use in children. This is reflected by contraindications or cautionary wording in the SPC. There is a lack of commercial incentive to develop medicines for the relatively small paediatric market and perceived difficulties in carrying out clinical trials in this group. It is not illegal to use medicines for indications or ages not specified in the data sheet, but to ensure safe and effective treatment, health professionals should have adequate supporting information about the intended use before proceeding. Failure to ensure that the use of a medicine is reasonable could result in a suit for negligence if the patient comes to harm.

Unlicensed and 'off-label' medicines

Up to 35% of drugs used in a large children's hospital and 10% of drugs used in general practice may be used outside the terms of the approved, licensed indications (Turner et al. 1998, McIntyre et al. 2000). In the USA the term 'off-label' is often used to describe this. Because many of these medicines will have been produced in 'adult' dose forms, such as tablets, it is often necessary to prepare extemporaneously a suitable liquid preparation for the child. This may be made from the licensed dose form (by crushing tablets and adding suitable excipients) or from chemical ingredients. An appropriate formula with a validated expiry period and ingredients to approved standards should be used. Care must be taken to ensure accurate preparation, particularly when using formulae or ingredients, such as 'old-fashioned' galenicals, which are unfamiliar.

On some occasions the drug to be used has no PL or MA, perhaps because it is only just undergoing clinical trials in adults, has been imported from another country, has been prepared under a 'specials' manufacturing license, or is being used for a rare condition for which it has not previously been used. As with 'off-label' use, there must always be information to support the quality, efficacy and safety of the medicine as well as information on the intended use. There is always a risk to using such a medicine, which must be balanced against the seriousness of the child's illness and discussed with the parents if practicable.

Some authorities suggest that the patient should always be informed if the medicine prescribed is unlicensed or 'off label', and even suggest that written informed consent be obtained before treatment begins. In many situations in paediatrics this would be impractical, but if patients are not informed the patient information leaflet (PIL) included with many medicines may cause confusion since it may state that it is 'not for use in children'. Patient or parent information specific to the situation should be prepared and provided.

Recent legislation on medicines for children

The worldwide legislation on medicines for children is beginning to change. This is in recognition of the limited research and small number of licensed medicines brought about by a lack of incentive for commercial development. In the USA an Orphan Drugs Act has assisted the development of medicines for rare diseases, such as betaine for homocystinuria, and the FDA Modernization Act and Pediatric Rule have provided a 'carrot and stick' approach to paediatric drug development. Pharmaceutical companies can be required to research and submit appropriate drugs for paediatric licenses but can also receive patent extension worth many millions of dollars. In Europe a similar Orphan Drugs Act became law in January 2000.

Selecting a drug dosage regimen for paediatric patients

A summary of the factors to be considered when selecting a drug dosage regimen or route of administration for a paediatric patient is shown in Table 8.9.

Table 8.9   Factors to be considered when selecting a drug dosage regimen or route of administration for a paediatric patient

Factor	Comment
1. Age/weight/surface area	Is the weight appropriate for the stated age? If it is not, confirm the difference. Can the discrepancy be explained by the patient's underlying disease, e.g. patients with neurological disorders such as cerebral palsy may be significantly underweight for their age? Is there a need to calculate dosage based on surface area (e.g. cytotoxic therapy)? Remember heights and weights may change significantly in children in a very short space of time. It is essential to recheck the surface area at each treatment cycle using recent heights and weights
2. Assess the appropriate dose	The age/weight of the child may have a significant influence on the pharmacokinetic profile of the drug and the manner in which it is handled. In addition, the underlying disease state may influence the dosage or dosage interval
3. Assess the most appropriate interval	In addition to the influence of disease states and organ maturity on dosage interval, the significance of the child's waking day is often overlooked. A child's waking day is generally much shorter than that of an adult and may be as little as 12 hours. Instructions given to parents particularly should take account of this, e.g. the instruction 'three times a day' will bear no resemblance to 'every 8 hours' in a child's normal waking day. If a preparation must be administered at regular intervals, then the need to wake the child should be discussed with the parents or preferably an alternative formulation, such as a sustained-release preparation, should be considered.
4. Assess the route of administration in the light of the disease state and the preparations and formulations available	Some preparations may require manipulation to ensure their suitability for administration by a specific route. Even preparations which appear to be available in a particular form may contain undesirable excipients that require alternatives to be found, e.g. patients with the inherited metabolic disorder phenylketonuria should avoid oral preparations containing the artificial sweetner aspartame because of its phenylalanine content
5. Consider the expected response and monitoring parameters	Is the normal pharmacokinetic profile altered in children? Are there any age-specific or long-term adverse events such as on growth that should be monitored?
6. Interactions	Drug interactions remain as important in reviewing paediatric prescriptions as they are in adult practice. However, drug–food interactions may be more significant; particularly drug–milk interactions in babies having five to six milk feeds per day
7. Legal considerations	Is the drug licensed? If an unlicensed drug is to be used, the pharmacist should have sufficient information to support its use

CASE STUDIES

Case 8.1

M.K.
2 years old
Female
13 kg

Presenting condition:	PUO, 38.7°C, pain on passing urine
	Suspected UTI
PMH:	One previous UTI requiring Septrin®
Allergies:	Nil
Drug Hx:	Rx: Cefalexin 130 mg four times a day
	2/7 later patient was changed to ciprofloxacin 130 mg twice daily

Question

Comment on the above case.

Answer

Points to consider in this patient are:

- Risk of severe skin reactions with Septrin® is lower in children than adults. However, ideally use single agent trimethoprim.
- With cefalexin or other medicines given four times daily, administer during child's waking day, i.e. when at waking, lunch time, dinner time and before the child goes to bed.
- Consider frequency change to twice or three times a day to improve compliance.
- Use of 250 mg/5 ml rather than 125 mg/5 ml suspension to improve tolerability.
- Dose change to 125 mg from 130 mg to make it easier to measure.
- Use of quinolones in children is cautioned. They have been shown to cause erosion of cartilage of weight-bearing joints and other signs of arthropathy in immature animals and for this reason their use is restricted in children less than 12 years of age. However, there are few reported problems in children and there is a body of evidence to support their safety in children. Quinolones are the only orally active antipseudomonal agent and should be reserved for patients who have confirmed pseudomonas infection. Need to consider risk/benefit ratio.
- Recommended ciprofloxacin dose is 5–10 mg/kg per dose twice daily.
- Suggest changing dose to 125 mg twice daily for ease of administration. Could consider the use of half a tablet crushed and given in jam/topping if there are difficulties with the suspension, which has a bitter after-taste.
- Ciprofloxacin absorption is reduced by milk and therefore it should not be co-administered. The calcium ions chelate the quinolone molecule and reduce its absorption.
- Patient information leaflet states 'should not be given to pre-pubertal children'. Need for counselling.

Case 8.2

T.L.
4 years old
Male
Weight 12 kg
Well-known patient with cerebral palsy, epilepsy.

Presenting condition:	Fever, vomiting	
HPC:	Discharged from hospital 4/7 previously following admission for rotavirus	
	Had 1 vomit yesterday	
	Temperature 38.5°C	
	Increased seizure activity	
	Given p.r. diazepam	
PMHx:	Cerebral palsy	
	Epilepsy	
	Gastrostomy	
Drug history:	Diazepam oral	2.5 mg BD and 5 mg ON
	Sodium valproate	200 mg BD
	Lamotrigine	25 mg OM 50 mg ON
	Vigabatrin	500 mg daily
	Phenytoin	80 mg BD
	Omeprazole	20 mg daily
Allergies:	Rash with carbamazepine	
OE:	Rash – cause?	
	Chest clear	
	Afebrile	

Question

What issues would you need to consider if presented with a prescription for this patient?

Answer

Points to consider in this patient are as follows:

- Sodium valproate: there is increased risk of hepatotoxicity in children, particularly those less than 3 years. Use crushable tablets or solution. Blood levels are of limited value. There is need to have a modified dosage regimen if patients are started on lamotrigine and already on valproate. Valproate inhibits the metabolism of lamotrigine and leads to higher lamotrigine levels. Increased risk of rash.
- Lamotrigine has an increased risk of severe skin reactions in children such as Stevens–Johnson syndrome and toxic epidermal necrolysis (risk in adults is 1 in 1000, whereas risk in children may be as high as 1 in 100). It is therefore important to start with a low dose and increase gradually. This helps to reduce the incidence of rash.
- Vigabatrin. Use sachets and dissolve in water or a soft drink immediately before taking.
- Vigabatrin is associated with visual field defects. Visual field testing is advised before starting treatment and at 6 monthly intervals thereafter.
- Phenytoin absorption is reduced in the presence of milk or some feeds such as Osmolite®. If given via nasogastric or gastrostomy tubes phenytoin has been shown to bind to tubing. Suggested that phenytoin is diluted one to one with

water/saline and flushed before and after. Best to separate from milk feeds.

- Some phenytoin side-effects are more of a problem in children. Gingival hyperplasia occurs more frequently in children. Encourage regular brushing of teeth, which helps to reduce gum overgrowth. Also phenytoin leads to coarsening of the features and is therefore often not the drug of choice in children. Monitor blood levels. Levels can increase or decrease with sodium valproate.
- Omeprazole. Administration of omeprazole was a problem with the capsule formulation. Capsules could be opened;

however, the beadlets were enteric coated (omeprazole is acid labile) and therefore it is not recommended that beadlets are crushed. There were also problems with the beadlets blocking nasogastric and gastrostomy tubes. In practice capsules were often opened and beadlets sprinkled on food or similar. Some hospitals manufacture omeprazole suspensions (base solution is sodium bicarbonate). The new omeprazole tablets formulation (MUPS) are dispersible and so overcome many of these problems.

REFERENCES

Department of Education and Science 1990 Staffing for pupils with special educational needs. Department of Education and Science Circular 11/90

Department of Health 1996 Immunisation against infectious disease. HMSO, London

International Committee on Harmonization 2000 Note for guidance on Clinical Investigation of Medicinal Products in the Paediatric Population (CPMH/ICH/2711/99). European Agency for the Evaluation of Medicinal Products, London, July

Kaye J A, del Mar Malero-Montes M, Jick H 2001 Mumps, measles, and rubella vaccine and the incidence of autism recorded by general practitioners: a time trend analysis. British Medical Journal 322: 460–463.

McIntyre J, Conroy S, Avery A et al 2000 Unlicensed and off label prescribing of drugs in general practice. Archives of Disease in Childhood 83: 498–501

MRC Vitamin Study Research Group 1991 Prevention of neural tube defects: results of the Medical Research Council vitamin study. Lancet 338: 131–137

NICE 2000a Guidance on the use of inhaler systems (devices) in children under the age of 5 years with chronic asthma. National Institute for Clinical Excellence, London

NICE 2000b Guidance on the use of methylphenidate for attention deficit/hyperactivity disorder (ADHD) in childhood. National Institute of Clinical Excellence, London

NICE 2002 Asthma-inhaler devices for older children. Technology Appraisal No 38. National Institute for Clinical Excellence, London

Scott E, Swanton J, McElnay J et al 1995 Pharmacists and child health. Centre for Pharmacy Postgraduate Education/HMSO, London

Turner S, Longworth A, Nunn A J et al 1998 Unlicensed and off-label drug use in paediatric wards: prospective study. British Medical Journal 316: 343–345

Yeung S C, Ensom M H 2000 Phenytoin and enteral feedings: does evidence support an interaction? Annals of Pharmacotherapy 3(7–8): 896–905

FURTHER READING

Advanced Life Support Group 2000 Advanced paediatric life support. BMJ Books, London

British National Formulary 2002 BNF 43, March 2002. BMJ Books/Pharmaceutical Press, Oxford and London

Joint Working Party of the British Paediatric Association and the Association of the British Pharmaceutical Industry 1996 Licensing medicines for children. British Paediatric Association, London

Nelson W E 2000 Textbook of pediatrics, 16th edn. W B Saunders, Philadelphia

American Society of Health System Pharmacists 1996 Guidelines for the administration of intravenous medications to pediatric patients, 5th edn.

USEFUL PAEDIATRIC DOSAGE REFERENCE SOURCES

Royal College of Paediatrics and Child Health 1999 Medicines for children, 1st edn. RCPCH Publications, London

Royal College of Paediatrics and Child Health 2001 Pocket medicines for children, 1st edn. RCPCH Publications, London

Lewisham and North Southwark Health Authority 1999 Guy's, St Thomas's and Lewisham Hospitals paediatric formulary, 5th edn. Lewisham and North Southwarke Health Authority, London

Taketomo C, Hodding J H, Kraus D M 2000/2001 Paediatric dosage handbook, 7th edn. Lexi-comp, Hudson, Ohio, USA

Royal Children's Hospital, Melbourne 2002 Paediatric Pharmacopeia, 13th edn. Parville, Australia

Phelps S J 2001 Pediatric Injectable Drugs, 6th edn. American Society of Health-System Pharmacists, USA

Geriatrics 9

H. G. M. Shetty   K. Woodhouse

KEY POINTS

- The elderly form about 18% of the population and receive about one-third of health service prescriptions in the UK.
- Ageing results in physiological changes that affect the absorption, metabolism, distribution and elimination of drugs.
- Alzheimer's disease and multi-infarct dementia are the most important diseases of cognitive dysfunction in the elderly. Donepezil, rivastigmine and galantamine are inhibitors of acetylcholinesterase and improve cognitive function in Alzheimer's disease.
- The elderly patient with Parkinson's disease is more susceptible to the adverse effects of levodopa such as postural hypotension, ventricular dysrhythmias and psychiatric effects.
- Aspirin and clopidogrel reduce the reoccurrence of non-fatal strokes in the elderly.
- Treatment of elevated systolic and diastolic blood pressure in the elderly with a low dose thiazide diuretic, β-blocker, calcium antagonist or angiotensin-converting enzyme inhibitor have all been shown to be beneficial.
- Urinary incontinence can be classified as stress incontinence, overflow incontinence or due to detrusor instability. Stress incontinence is not amenable to drug therapy. The most common drugs used in detrusor instability are oxybutynin and tolterodine.
- Non-steroidal anti-inflammatory drugs are more likely to cause gastroduodenal ulceration and bleeding in the elderly.

There has been a steady increase in the number of elderly people, defined as those over 65 years of age, since the beginning of the 20th century. They formed only 4.8% of the population in 1901, increasing to 15.2% in 1981 and about 18% in 2001. In 1990, in England and Wales there were 8 million people aged over 65 years of which 784 000 were aged over 85 years. Between 1991 and 2031 the total population of England and Wales is expected to increase by 8%. However, the numbers of those aged between 60 and 74 years will rise by 43%, those aged between 75 and 84 by 48% and those aged over 85 years by 138%. The significant increase in the number of very elderly people will have important social, financial and health care planning implications.

The elderly have multiple and often chronic diseases. It is not surprising therefore that they are the major consumers of drugs. Elderly people receive about one-third of National Health Service (NHS) prescriptions in the UK. In most developed countries the elderly now account for 25–40% of drug expenditure.

A survey of drug usage in 778 elderly people in the UK showed that 70% had been on prescribed medication and 40% had taken one or more prescribed drugs within the previous 24 hours; 32% were taking cardiovascular drugs, and the other therapeutic categories used in decreasing order of frequency were for: disorders of the central nervous system (24%), musculoskeletal system (10%), gastrointestinal system (8%) and respiratory system (7%). The most commonly used drugs were: diuretics; analgesics; hypnotics, sedatives and anxiolytics; antirheumatic drugs; and β-blockers.

Institutionalized patients tend to be on larger numbers of drugs compared with patients in the community. One study has shown that patients in long-term care facilities are likely to be receiving on average eight drugs. Psychotropic drugs are used widely in nursing or residential homes.

For optimal drug therapy in the elderly, a knowledge of age-related physiological and pathological changes that might affect handling of and response to drugs is essential. This chapter discusses the age-related pharmacokinetic and pharmacodynamic changes which might affect drug therapy and the general principles of drug use in the elderly.

Pharmacokinetics

Ageing results in many physiological changes that could theoretically affect absorption, first-pass metabolism, protein binding, distribution and elimination of drugs. Age-related changes in the gastrointestinal tract, liver and kidneys are:

- reduced gastric acid secretion
- decreased gastrointestinal motility
- reduced total surface area of absorption
- reduced splanchnic blood flow
- reduced liver size
- reduced liver blood flow

- reduced glomerular filtration
- reduced renal tubular filtration.

Absorption

There is a delay in gastric emptying, reduction in gastric acid output and splanchnic blood flow with ageing. These changes do not significantly affect the absorption of the majority of drugs. Although the absorption of some drugs such as digoxin may be slower, the overall absorption is similar to that in the young.

First-pass metabolism

After absorption, drugs are transported via the portal circulation to the liver, where many lipid-soluble agents are metabolized extensively (more than 90–95%). This results in a marked reduction in systemic bioavailability. Obviously, even minor reductions in first-pass metabolism can result in a significant increase in the bioavailability of such drugs.

Impaired first-pass metabolism has been demonstrated in the elderly for several drugs, including clomethiazole, labetalol, nifedipine, nitrates, propranolol and verapamil. The clinical effects of some of these, such as the hypotensive effect of nifedipine, may be significantly enhanced in the elderly. In frail hospitalized elderly patients, i.e. those with chronic debilitating disease, the reduction in pre-systemic elimination is even more marked.

Distribution

The age-related physiological changes which may affect drug distribution are:

- reduced lean body mass
- reduced total body water
- increased total body fat
- lower serum albumin level
- α_1-acid glycoprotein level unchanged or slightly raised.

Increased body fat in the elderly results in an increased volume of distribution for fat-soluble compounds such as clomethiazole, diazepam, desmethyl-diazepam and thiopental. On the other hand, reduction in body water results in a decrease in the distribution volume of water-soluble drugs such as cimetidine, digoxin and ethanol.

Acidic drugs tend to bind to plasma albumin, while basic drugs bind to α_1-acid glycoprotein. Plasma albumin levels decrease with age and therefore the free fraction of acidic drugs such as cimetidine, furosemide (frusemide) and warfarin will increase. Plasma α_1-acid glycoprotein levels may remain unchanged or may rise slightly with ageing, and this may result in minimal reductions in free fractions of basic drugs such as

lidocaine (lignocaine). Disease-related changes in the level of this glycoprotein are probably more important than age per se.

The age-related changes in distribution and protein binding are probably of significance only in the acute administration of drugs because, at steady state, the plasma concentration of a drug is determined primarily by free drug clearance by the liver and kidneys rather than by distribution volume or protein binding.

Renal clearance

Although there is a considerable interindividual variability in renal function in the elderly, in general the glomerular filtration rate declines, as do the effective renal plasma flow and renal tubular function. Because of the marked variability in renal function in the elderly, the dosages of predominantly renally excreted drugs should be individualized. Reduction in dosages of drugs with a low therapeutic index, such as digoxin and aminoglycosides, may be necessary. Dosage adjustments may not be necessary for drugs with a wide therapeutic index, for example penicillins.

Hepatic clearance

Hepatic clearance (Cl_H) of a drug is dependent on hepatic blood flow (Q) and the steady state extraction ratio (E), as can be seen in the following formula:

$$Cl_H = Q \times \frac{C_a - C_v}{C_a}$$

$$= Q \times E$$

where C_a and C_v are arterial and venous concentrations of the drug, respectively. It is obvious from the above formula that when E approaches unity, Cl_H will be proportional to and limited by Q. Drugs which are cleared by this mechanism have a rapid rate of metabolism, and the rate of extraction by the liver is very high. The rate-limiting step, as mentioned earlier, is hepatic blood flow, and therefore drugs cleared by this mechanism are called 'flow limited'. On the other hand, when E is small, Cl_H will vary according to the hepatic uptake and enzyme activity, and will be relatively independent of hepatic blood flow. The drugs which are cleared by this mechanism are termed 'capacity limited'.

Hepatic extraction is dependent upon liver size, liver blood flow, uptake into hepatocytes, and the affinity and activity of hepatic enzymes. Liver size falls with ageing and there is a decrease in hepatic mass of between 20% and 40% between the third and tenth decade. Hepatic blood flow falls equally with declining liver size. Although it is recognized that the microsomal mono-oxygenase enzyme systems are significantly reduced in ageing male rodents, recent evidence suggests that this is not the case in ageing humans. Conjugation reactions have been reported to be unaffected in the elderly by some investigators, but a small decline with increasing age has been described by others.

Impaired clearance of many hepatically eliminated drugs has been demonstrated in the elderly. Morphological changes rather than impaired enzymatic activity appear to be the main cause of impaired elimination of these drugs. In frail debilitated elderly patients, however, the activities of drug-metabolizing enzymes such as plasma esterases and hepatic glucuronyltransferases may well be impaired.

Pharmacodynamics

Molecular and cellular changes that occur with ageing may alter the response to drugs in the elderly. There is, however, limited information about these alterations because of the technical difficulties and ethical problems involved in measuring them. It is not surprising therefore that there is relatively little information about the effect of age on pharmacodynamics.

Changes in pharmacodynamics in the elderly may be considered under two headings:

- those due to a reduction in homeostatic reserve
- those that are secondary to changes in specific receptor and target sites.

Reduced homeostatic reserve

Orthostatic circulatory responses

In normal elderly subjects there is blunting of the reflex tachycardia that occurs in young subjects on standing or in response to vasodilatation. Structural changes in the vascular tree that occur with ageing are believed to contribute to this observation, although the exact mechanism is unclear. Antihypertensive drugs, drugs with α receptor blocking effects (e.g. tricyclic antidepressants, phenothiazines and some butyrophenones), drugs which decrease sympathetic outflow from the central nervous system (e.g. barbiturates, benzodiazepines, antihistamines and morphine) and antiparkinsonian drugs (e.g. levodopa and bromocriptine) are therefore more likely to produce hypotension in the elderly.

Postural control

Postural stability is normally achieved by static reflexes, which involve sustained contraction of the musculature, and phasic reflexes, which are dynamic, short-term and involve transient corrective movements. With ageing, the frequency and amplitude of corrective movements increase and an age-related reduction in dopamine (D_2) receptors in the striatum has been suggested as the probable cause. Drugs which increase postural sway, for example hypnotics and tranquillizers, have been shown to be associated with the occurrence of falls in the elderly.

Thermoregulation

There is an increased prevalence of impaired thermoregulatory mechanisms in the elderly, although it is not universal. Accidental hypothermia can occur in the elderly with drugs that produce sedation, impaired subjective awareness of temperature, decreased mobility and muscular activity, and vasodilatation. Commonly implicated drugs include phenothiazines, benzodiazepines, tricyclic antidepressants, opioids and alcohol, either on its own or with other drugs.

Cognitive function

Ageing is associated with marked structural and neurochemical changes in the central nervous system. Cholinergic transmission is linked with normal cognitive function, and in the elderly the activity of choline acetyltransferase, a marker enzyme for acetylcholine, is reduced in some areas of the cortex and limbic system. Several drugs cause confusion in the elderly. Anticholinergics, hypnotics, H_2 antagonists and β-blockers are common examples.

Visceral muscle function

Constipation is a common problem in the elderly as there is a decline in gastrointestinal motility with ageing. Anticholinergic drugs, opiates, tricyclic antidepressants and antihistamines are more likely to cause constipation or ileus in the elderly. Anticholinergic drugs may cause urinary retention in elderly men, especially those who have prostatic hypertrophy. Bladder instability is common in the elderly, and urethral dysfunction more prevalent in elderly women. Loop diuretics may cause incontinence in such patients.

Age-related changes in specific receptors and target sites

Many drugs exert their effect via specific receptors. Response to such drugs may be altered by the number (density) of receptors, the affinity of the receptor, postreceptor events within cells resulting in impaired enzyme activation and signal amplification, or altered response of the target tissue itself. Ageing is associated with some of these changes.

α adrenoceptors

α_2 adrenoceptor responsiveness appears to be reduced with ageing while α_1 adrenoceptor responsiveness appears to be unaffected.

β adrenoceptors

β adrenoceptor function declines with age. It is recognized that the chronotropic response to isoprenaline infusion is less marked in the elderly. Propranolol therapy in the elderly produces less β adrenoceptor blocking effect than in the young. In isolated lymphocytes, studies of cyclic adenosine monophosphate (AMP) production have shown that on β adrenoceptor stimulation the dose–response curve is shifted to the right, and the maximal response is blunted.

An age-related reduction in β adrenoceptor density has been shown in animal adipocytes, erythrocytes and brain, and also in human lymphocytes in one study, although this has not been confirmed by other investigators. As maximal response occurs on stimulation of only 0.2% of β adrenoceptors, a reduction in the number by itself is unlikely to account for age-related changes. Some studies have shown a reduction in high-affinity binding sites with ageing, in the absence of change in total receptor numbers, and others have suggested that there may be impairment of postreceptor transduction mechanisms with ageing that may account for reduced β adrenoceptor function.

Cholinergic system

The effect of ageing on cholinergic mechanisms is less well known. Atropine produces less tachycardia in elderly humans than in the young. It has been shown in ageing rats that the hippocampal pyramidal cell sensitivity to acetylcholine is reduced. The clinical significance of this observation is unclear.

Benzodiazepines

The elderly are more sensitive to benzodiazepines than the young, and the mechanism of this increased sensitivity is not known. No difference in the affinity or number of benzodiazepine-binding sites has been observed in animal studies. Habituation to benzodiazepines occurs to the same extent in the elderly as in the young.

Warfarin

The elderly are more sensitive to warfarin. This phenomenon may be due to age-related changes in pharmacodynamic factors. The exact mechanism is unknown.

Digoxin

The elderly appear to be more sensitive to the adverse effects of digoxin, but not to the cardiac effects.

Common clinical disorders

This section deals in detail only with the most important geriatric diseases. Other conditions are mentioned primarily to highlight areas where the elderly differ from the young or where modifications of drug therapy are necessary.

Dementia

Dementia is characterized by a gradual deterioration of intellectual capacity. Alzheimer's disease (AD) and multi-infarct dementia (MID) are the most important diseases of cognitive dysfunction in the elderly. AD has a gradual onset, and it progresses slowly. Forgetfulness is the major initial symptom. The patient has difficulty in dressing and other activities of daily living. He or she tends to get lost in his or her own environment. Eventually the social graces are lost. MID is the second most important cause of dementia. It usually occurs in patients in their 60s and 70s, and is more common in those with a previous history of hypertension or stroke. Abrupt onset and stepwise progression of dementia is characteristic of MID. Mood changes and emotional lability are common. There may be focal neurological deficit. A number of drugs and other conditions cause confusion in the elderly, and their effects may be mistaken for dementia. These are listed in Table 9.1.

In patients with AD, damage to the cholinergic neurones connecting subcortical nuclei to the cerebral

Table 9.1 Causes of confusion in the elderly
Drugs
Antiparkinsonian drugs
Barbiturates
Benzodiazepines
Cimetidine
Diuretics
Hypoglycaemic agents
Monoamine oxidase inhibitors
Opioids
Steroids
Tricyclic antidepressants
Conditions
Hypothyroidism
Vitamin B_{12} deficiency
Chronic subdural haematoma
Normal pressure hydrocephalus
Alcoholism

cortex has been consistently observed. Postsynaptic muscarinic cholinergic receptors are usually not affected, but ascending noradrenergic and serotonergic pathways are damaged, especially in younger patients. Based on those abnormalities, several drugs have been investigated for the treatment of AD. Lecithin, which increases acetylcholine concentrations in the brain, 4-aminopyridine, piracetam, oxitacetam and pramiracetam, all of which stimulate acetylcholine release, have been tried, but have produced no, or unimpressive, improvements in cognitive function. Anticholinesterases block the breakdown of acetylcholine and enhance cholinergic transmission. Tetrahydroaminoacridine (THA, which is a longer-acting anticholinesterase) showed promise in non-blinded clinical studies. However, a controlled clinical trial did not show any benefit. The National Institute for Clinical Excellence (NICE 2001) has approved the use of three drugs, donepezil, rivastigmine and galantamine, for treatment of AD. Donepezil is a piperidine-based acetylcholinesterase inhibitor. It has been shown to improve cognitive function in patients with mild to moderately severe AD. However, it does not improve day-to-day functioning, quality-of-life measures or rating scores of overall dementia. It is well tolerated. Rivastigmine is a non-competitive cholinesterase inhibitor. It has been shown to slow the rate of decline in cognitive and global functioning in AD. It is associated with anorexia, nausea, vomiting and weight loss. Other adverse effects include agitation, confusion, depression and diarrhoea. Galantamine, a reversible and competitive inhibitor of acetylcholinesterase, has also been shown to improve cognitive function significantly and is well tolerated.

Deposition of amyloid (in particular the peptide β/A4) derived from the Alzheimer amyloid precursor protein (APP) is an important pathological feature of the familial form of AD that accounts for about 20% of patients. Point mutation of the gene coding for APP (located in the long arm of chromosome 21) is thought to be associated with familial AD. Future treatment strategies, therefore, might involve development of drugs which inhibit amyloidogenesis.

There have been few studies on the management of MID, although at least one report has shown that the progression of the illness may be delayed by aspirin therapy.

Parkinsonism

Parkinsonism is a relatively common disease of the elderly with a prevalence between 50 and 150 per 100 000. It is characterized by resting tremors, muscular rigidity and bradykinesia (slowness of initiating and carrying out voluntary movements). The patient has a mask-like face, monotonous voice and walks with a stoop and a slow shuffling gait.

The elderly are more susceptible than younger patients to some of the adverse effects of antiparkinsonian drugs. Because of the age-related decline in orthostatic circulatory responses, postural hypotension is more likely to occur in elderly patients with levodopa therapy. The elderly are more likely to have severe cardiac disease, and levodopa preparations should be used with caution in such patients because of the risk of serious ventricular dysrhythmias. Psychiatric adverse effects such as confusion, depression, hallucinations and paranoia occur with dopamine agonists and levodopa preparations. These adverse effects may persist for several months after discontinuation of the offending drug and may result in misdiagnosis (e.g. of AD) in the elderly. Bromocriptine and other ergot derivatives should be avoided in elderly patients with severe peripheral arterial disease as they may cause peripheral ischaemia. 'Drug holidays', which involve discontinuation of drugs, for example for 2 days per week, may reduce the incidence of adverse effects of antiparkinsonian drugs, but their role is questionable.

Stroke

Stroke is the third most common cause of death and the most common cause of adult disability in UK. About 110 000 people in England and Wales have their first stroke each year and about 30 000 people go on to have further strokes. The incidence of stroke increases by 100-fold from the fourth to the ninth decade. A number of important advances in the management of stroke have occurred in the past 10 years (Intercollegiate Working Party for Stroke 2000).

Treatment of acute stroke

About 85% of strokes are due to cerebral embolism or thrombosis resulting in ischaemia, and 15% are due to haemorrhage. A number of drugs have been investigated for treatment of ischaemic stroke (Brott & Bogousslavsky 2000).

Thrombolytic agents. The National Institute of Neurological Disorders and Stroke (1995) in the USA showed that, compared with placebo, thrombolysis with tissue plasminogen activator (rt-PA) within 3 hours of onset of ischaemic stroke improved clinical outcome at 3 months despite increased incidence (6%) of symptomatic intracranial bleeding. European co-operative acute stroke studies (ECASS I: Hacke et al 1995; ECASS II: Hacke et al 1998) of thrombolysis with rt-PA failed to show a significant benefit on an intention to treat primary analysis. A further trial, the alteplase thrombolysis for acute non-interventional therapy in acute stroke study (ATLANTIS: Clark et al 1999), which thrombolysed patients between 3 and 5 hours from onset of stroke, also did not show benefit. Clinical trials with streptokinase as the thrombolytic agent have shown worse outcomes and have been abandoned. Further studies are under way to study the efficacy of rt-PA in acute stroke although in some countries, such as the USA and Germany, it is currently being used in appropriately selected patients.

Antiplatelet therapy. Aspirin in doses of 150–300 mg commenced within 48 hours of onset of ischaemic stroke has been shown to reduce the relative risk of death or dependency by 2.7% up to 6 months after the event in two large studies (Chinese Acute Stroke Trial (CAST) and International Stroke Trial (IST): Chen et al 2000).

Anticoagulation. Use of intravenous unfractionated heparin and low molecular weight heparin have not been shown to be beneficial and are associated with increased risk of intracranial haemorrhage.

Neuroprotective agents. A large number of neuroprotective agents have been used for treatment of acute ischaemic stroke but none have been shown to have long-term beneficial effects.

Secondary prevention

Aspirin in doses of 75–1500 mg/day has been shown to reduce the risk of non-fatal strokes. This is likely to be due to its antiplatelet effect. There is some evidence that addition of dipyridamole to aspirin may enhance the protective effect against stroke (Redman & Ryan 2001). Clopidogrel, which inhibits ADP-induced platelet aggregation, has been shown to be as effective as aspirin in secondary stroke prevention. Clopidogrel is not associated with neutropenia, unlike ticlopidine which is no longer used for stroke prevention. However, thrombotic thrombocytopenic purpura has been reported very rarely with the use of clopidogrel. In patients with atrial fibrillation who have had a previous stroke or transient ischaemic attack, anticoagulation with warfarin (INR 1.5–2.7) has been shown to be significantly better than aspirin for secondary prevention. Anticoagulation has not been shown to be effective for secondary prevention in patients with sinus rhythm.

Adequate control of hypertension, diabetes, hyperlipidaemia, stopping smoking and reducing alcohol consumption are also important in secondary stroke prevention. Although there is no evidence to support the use of hypolipidaemic drugs in elderly patients aged over 75 years, the decision as to whether to treat or not should be based on appropriate risk assessment on an individual basis.

Primary prevention

A number of randomized controlled trials have shown that anticoagulation with warfarin compared with placebo reduces the risk of stroke in patients with atrial fibrillation (Benavente et al 2000). As with secondary prevention, control of risk factors such as hypertension, hyperlipidaemia, diabetes, smoking and ethanol abuse are important.

Osteoporosis

Osteoporosis is a progressive disease characterized by low bone mass and micro-architectural deterioration of bone tissue resulting in increased bone fragility and susceptibility to fracture. It is an important cause of morbidity in post-menopausal women. The most important complication of osteoporosis is fracture of the hip. Fractures of wrist, vertebrae and humerus also occur. In the UK over 200 000 fractures occur each year, costing the NHS £1.5 billion per year of which 87% is spent on hip fractures.

Prevention

As complications of osteoporosis have enormous economic implications, preventive measures are extremely important (Law et al 1991). Regular exercise has been shown to halve the risk of hip fractures. Stopping smoking before the menopause reduces the risk of hip fractures by 25%.

Treatment

Vitamin D and calcium. Vitamin D deficiency is common in elderly people. Treatment for 12 to 18 months with 800 IU of vitamin D plus 1.2 g of calcium given daily has been shown to reduce hip and non-vertebral fractures in elderly women (mean age 84 years) living in sheltered accommodation. It is not known whether vitamin D supplementation alone reduces hip fractures. Calcium supplementation on its own does not reduce fracture incidence and is no longer recommended for treatment of osteoporosis.

Calcitriol and alfacalcidol. Calcitriol (1,25-di-hydroxy vitamin D), the active metabolite of vitamin D), and alfacalcidol, a synthetic analogue of calcitriol, reduce bone loss and have been shown to reduce vertebral fractures, but not consistently. Serum calcium should be monitored regularly in patients receiving these drugs.

Bisphosphonates. The bisphosphonates, synthetic analogues of pyrophosphate, bind strongly to the bone surface and inhibit bone resorption. Currently three oral bisphosphonates are available for the treatment of osteoporosis: alendronate, etidronate and risedronate. Alendronate can be given either daily (10 mg) or weekly (70 mg) with equal efficacy. It is effective in reducing vertebral, wrist and hip fractures by about 50%. Etidronate is given cyclically with calcium supplements to reduce the risk of bone mineralization defects. It reduces the risk of vertebral fractures by 50% in postmenopausal women. There is no evidence to support its effectiveness in preventing hip fractures. Risedronate reduces vertebral fractures by 41% and non-vertebral fractures by 39%. It has been shown to significantly reduce the risk of hip fractures in postmenopausal women.

All bisphosphonates cause gastrointestinal side-effects. Alendronate and risedronate are associated with severe oesophageal reactions including oesophageal stricture. Patients should not take these tablets at bedtime and should be advised to stay upright for at least 30 minutes after taking them. They should avoid food for at least 2 hours before and after taking etidronate. Alendronate and risedronate should be taken 30 minutes before the first food or drink of the day. Bisphosphonates should be avoided in patients with renal impairment.

Hormone replacement therapy (HRT). Oestrogens increase bone formation and reduce bone resorption. They also increase calcium absorption and decrease renal calcium loss. HRT, if started soon after the menopause, is effective in preventing vertebral fractures but has to be continued lifelong if protection against fractures is to be maintained. It is associated with increased risk of endometrial cancer, breast cancer and venous thromboembolism. One study has shown that HRT may increase the risk of deaths due to myocardial disease in elderly women with pre-existing ischaemic heart disease.

Calcitonin. Calcitonin inhibits osteoclasts and decreases the rate of bone resorption, reduces bone blood flow and may have central analgesic actions. It is effective in all age groups in preventing vertebral bone loss. It is costly and has to be given parenterally or intranasally. It should not be given for more than 3–6 months at a time to avoid its inhibitory effects on bone resorption and formation, which usually disappear after 2–4 weeks. Antibodies do develop against calcitonin, but they do not affect its efficacy. Calcitonin is useful in treating acute pain associated with osteoporotic vertebral fractures.

Arthritis

Osteoarthrosis, gout, pseudogout, rheumatoid arthritis and septic arthritis are the important joint diseases in the elderly. Treatment of these conditions is similar to that in the young. If possible, non-steroidal anti-inflammatory drugs (NSAIDs) should be avoided in patients with osteoarthrosis. Total hip and knee replacements should be considered in patients with severe arthritis affecting these joints.

Hypertension

Hypertension is an important risk factor for cardiovascular and cerebrovascular disease in the elderly. The incidence of myocardial infarction is 2.5 times higher, and that of cerebrovascular accidents twice as high in elderly hypertensive patients compared with non-hypertensive subjects. Elevated systolic blood pressure is the single most important risk factor for cardiovascular disease and more predictive of stroke than diastolic blood pressure.

There is evidence that treatment of both systolic and diastolic blood pressure in the elderly is beneficial. One large study (EWPHE) has shown reductions in cardiovascular events, and mortality associated with cerebrovascular accidents in treated elderly patients with hypertension (Amery et al 1986). The treatment did not reduce the total mortality significantly. Another study (SHEP 1991), which used low dose chlortalidone to treat isolated systolic hypertension (systolic blood pressure 160 mmHg or more with diastolic blood pressure less than 95 mmHg), showed a 36% reduction in the incidence of stroke, with a 5-year benefit of 30 events per 1000 patients. It also showed a reduction in the incidence of major cardiovascular events with a 5-year absolute benefit of 55 events per 1000 patients. In addition, this study reported that antihypertensive therapy was beneficial even in patients over the age of 80 years. There is some data, although not conclusive, to support antihypertensive therapy in patients over 80 years of age. Subgroup meta-analysis of seven randomized controlled trials, which included 1670 patients over 80 years, showed that antihypertensive therapy for about 3.5 years reduces the risk of heart failure by 39%, strokes by 34% and major cardiovascular events by 22%.

Treatment of hypertension

Non-pharmacological. In patients with asymptomatic mild hypertension, non-pharmacological treatment is the method of choice. Weight reduction to within 15% of desirable weight, restriction of salt intake to 4–6 g/day, regular aerobic exercise such as walking, restriction of ethanol consumption and stopping smoking are the recommended modes of therapy.

Pharmacological.

Thiazide diuretics. Thiazides lower peripheral resistance and do not significantly affect cardiac output or renal blood flow. They are effective, cheap, well tolerated and have also been shown to reduce the risk of hip fracture in elderly women by 30%. They can be used in combination with other antihypertensive drugs. Adverse effects include mild elevation of creatinine, glucose, uric acid and serum cholesterol levels as well as hypokalaemia. They should be used in low doses, as higher doses only increase the incidence of adverse effects without increasing their efficacy.

β adrenoceptor blockers. Although theoretically the β-blockers are expected to be less effective in the elderly, they have been shown to be as effective as diuretics in clinical studies. Water-soluble β-blockers such as atenolol may cause fewer adverse effects in the elderly.

Calcium antagonists. Calcium antagonists act as vasodilators. Verapamil and, to some extent, diltiazem decrease cardiac output. These drugs do not have a significant effect on lipids or the central nervous system. They may be more effective in the elderly, particularly in the treatment of isolated systolic hypertension. Adverse effects include headache, oedema and postural hypotension. Verapamil may cause conduction disturbances and decrease cardiac output. The use of short-acting dihydropyridine calcium antagonists, for example nifedipine, is controversial. Some studies indicate adverse outcomes with these agents, particularly in those patients with angina or myocardial infarction.

Angiotensin-converting enzyme (ACE) inhibitors. ACE inhibitors and other vasodilators used for treatment of hypertension are discussed elsewhere. The ACE inhibitors should be used with care in the elderly, who are more likely to have underlying atherosclerotic renovascular disease that could result in renal failure. Excessive hypotension is also more likely to occur in the elderly. Losartan, a non-peptide angiotensin II type 1 receptor antagonist, has been shown to be better tolerated than captopril in elderly patients. In particular, the incidence of cough appears to be lower compared with captopril.

Myocardial infarction

The diagnosis of myocardial infarction in the elderly may be difficult in some patients because of an atypical presentation (Bayer et al 1986). In the majority of patients, chest pain and dyspnoea are the common presenting symptoms. Confusion may be a presenting factor in up to 20% of patients over 85 years of age. The diagnosis is made on the basis of history, serial electrocardiograms and cardiac enzyme estimations.

The principles of management of myocardial infarction in the elderly are similar to those in the young. Thrombolytic therapy has been shown to be safe and effective in elderly patients.

Cardiac failure

In addition to the typical features of cardiac failure, i.e. exertional dyspnoea, oedema, orthopnoea and paroxysmal nocturnal dyspnoea (PND), elderly patients may present with atypical symptoms. These include confusion due to poor cerebral circulation, vomiting and abdominal pain due to gastrointestinal and hepatic congestion, or insomnia due to PND. Dyspnoea may not be a predominant symptom in an elderly patient with arthritis and immobility. Treatment of cardiac failure

depends on the underlying cause and is similar to that in the young. Diuretics, ACE inhibitors, nitrates and digoxin are the important drugs used in the treatment of cardiac failure in the elderly. ACE inhibitors are valuable recent additions for the treatment of cardiac failure, and have been shown to reduce mortality in patients with moderate to severe heart failure. Treatment with some β-blockers, such as carvedilol, has been shown to increase left ventricular ejection fraction in patients with cardiac failure due to ischaemic or idiopathic aetiology. They do not appear to improve exercise tolerance, but some studies indicate that they may reduce mortality and the number of admissions to hospitals. The role of β blockers in treatment of cardiac failure in the elderly is unclear at present.

Leg ulcers

Leg ulcers are common in the elderly. They are mainly of two types: venous or ischaemic. Other causes of leg ulcers are blood diseases, trauma, malignancy and infections (Cornwall et al 1986), but these are less common in the elderly. Venous ulcers occur in patients with varicose veins who have valvular incompetence in deep veins due to venous hypertension. They are usually located near the medial malleolus and are associated with varicose eczema and oedema. These ulcers are painless unless there is gross oedema or infection. Ischaemic ulcers, on the other hand, are due to poor peripheral circulation, and occur on the toes, heels, foot and lateral aspect of the leg. They are painful and are associated with signs of lower limb ischaemia, such as absent pulse or cold lower limb. There may be a history of smoking, diabetes or hypertension.

Venous ulcers respond well to treatment, and over 75% heal within 3 months. Elevation of the lower limbs, exercise, compression bandage, local antiseptic creams when there is evidence of infection, with or without steroid cream, are usually effective. Antiseptics should not be used when there is granulation tissue. Topical streptokinase may be useful to remove the slough on the ulcers. Gell colloid occlusive dressings may also be useful in treating chronic ulcers. Skin grafting may be necessary for large ulcers. Ischaemic ulcers do not respond well to medical treatment, and the patients should be assessed by vascular surgeons.

Urinary incontinence

Urinary incontinence in the elderly may be of three main types:

1. *Stress incontinence:* due to urethral sphincter incompetence. It occurs almost exclusively in women and is associated with weakening of pelvic musculature. Involuntary loss of small amounts of

urine occurs on performing activities which increase intra-abdominal pressure, e.g. coughing, sneezing, bending, lifting, etc. It does not cause significant nocturnal symptoms.

2. *Overlow incontinence:* constant involuntary loss of urine in small amounts. Prostatic hypertrophy is a common cause and is often associated with symptoms of poor stream and incomplete emptying. Increased frequency of micturition at night is often a feature. Use of anticholinergic drugs and diabetic autonomic neuropathy are other causes.

3. *Detrusor instability:* causes urge incontinence where a strong desire to pass urine is followed by involuntary loss of large amounts of urine either during the day or night. It is often associated with neurological lesions or urinary outflow obstruction, e.g. prostatic hypertrophy, but in many cases the cause is unknown.

Stress incontinence is not amenable to drug therapy. In patients with prostatic hypertrophy α_1 blockers such as prazosin, indoramin, alfuzosin, terazosin, and tamsulosin have all been shown to increase peak urine flow rate and improve symptoms in about 60% of patients. They reduce outflow obstruction by blocking α_1-receptors and thereby relaxing prostate smooth muscle. Postural hypotension is an important adverse effect and occurs between 2% and 5% of patients.

5 α-reductase converts testerone to dihydrotesterone (DHT) which plays an important role in the growth of prostate. The 5 α-reductase inhibitor finasteride reduces the prostate volume by 20% and improves peak urine flow rate. The clinical effects, however, might not become apparent until after 3–6 months of treatment. Main adverse effects are reductions in libido and erectile dysfunction in 3–5% of patients.

The most commonly used drugs for detrusor instability are oxybutynin and tolterodine, both of which are antimuscarinic. Both drugs also cause antimuscarinic side-effects such as dry mouth, blurred vision and constipation. Tolterodine is better tolerated than oxybutynin by elderly people.

Constipation

The age-related decline in gastrointestinal motility and treatment with drugs which decrease gastrointestinal motility predispose the elderly to constipation. Decreased mobility, wasting of pelvic muscles and a low intake of solids and liquids are other contributory factors. Faecal impaction may occur with severe constipation, which in turn may cause subacute intestinal obstruction, abdominal pain, spurious diarrhoea and faecal incontinence. Adequate intake of dietary fibre, regular bowel habit and use of bulking agents such as bran or ispaghula husk may help to prevent constipation.

When constipation is associated with a loaded rectum, a stimulant laxative such as senna or bisacodyl may be given. Frail, ill elderly patients with a full rectum may have atonic bowels that will not respond to bulking agents or softening agents, and in such cases a stimulant is more effective. A stool-softening agent such as docusate sodium is effective when stools are hard and dry. For severe faecal impaction a phosphate enema may be needed. Long-term use of stimulant laxatives may lead to abuse and atonic bowel musculature.

Gastrointestinal ulceration and bleeding

Gastrointestinal bleeding associated with peptic ulcer is less well tolerated by the elderly. The clinical presentation may sometimes be atypical with, for example, patients presenting with confusion. *Heliocobacter pylori* infection is common and its treatment is similar to that in younger patients.

Non-steroidal anti-inflammatory drugs (NSAIDs) are more likely to cause gastroduodenal ulceration and bleeding in the elderly (Griffin et al 1988). Cyclo-oxygenase 2 (COX-2) inhibitors are associated with a lower incidence of gastrointestinal bleeding compared with NSAIDs.

Principles and goals of drug therapy in the elderly

A thorough knowledge of the pharmacokinetic and pharmacodynamic factors discussed is essential for optimal drug therapy in the elderly. In addition, some general principles based on common sense, if followed, may result in even better use of drugs in the elderly.

Avoid unnecessary drug therapy

Before commencing drug therapy it is important to ask the following questions:

- Is it really necessary?
- Is there an alternative method of treatment?

In patients with mild hypertension, for example, it may be perfectly justified to try non-drug therapies which are of proven efficacy. Similarly, unnecessary use of hypnotics should be avoided. Simple measures such as emptying the bladder before going to bed to avoid having to get up, avoidance of stimulant drugs in the evenings or night, or moving the patient to a dark, quiet room may be all that is needed.

Effect of treatment on quality of life

The aim of treatment in elderly patients is not just to prolong life but also to improve the quality of life. To achieve this, the correct choice of treatment is essential. In a 70-year-old lady with severe osteoarthrosis of the hip, for example, total hip replacement is the treatment of choice rather than prescribing NSAIDs with all their attendant adverse effects.

Treat the cause rather than the symptom

Symptomatic treatment without specific diagnosis is not only bad practice but can also be potentially dangerous. A patient presenting with 'indigestion' may in fact be suffering from angina, and therefore treatment with H_2 blockers or antacids is clearly inappropriate. When a patient presents with a symptom every attempt should be made to establish the cause of the symptom and specific treatment, if available, should then be given.

Drug history

A drug history should be obtained in all elderly patients. This will ensure the patient is not prescribed a drug or drugs to which they may be allergic, or the same drug or group of drugs to which they have previously not responded. It will help to avoid potentially serious drug interactions.

Concomitant medical illness

Concurrent medical disorders must always be taken into account. Cardiac failure, renal impairment and hepatic dysfunction are particularly common in the elderly, and may increase the risk of adverse effects of drugs.

Choosing the drug

Once it is decided that a patient requires drug therapy, it is important to choose the drug likely to be the most efficacious and least likely to produce adverse effects. It is also necessary to take into consideration coexisting medical conditions. For example, it is inappropriate to commence diuretic therapy to treat mild hypertension in an elderly male with prostatic hypertrophy. A calcium antagonist is more appropriate in this situation.

Dose titration

In general, elderly patients require relatively smaller doses of all drugs compared with young adults. It is recognized that the majority of adverse drug reactions in the elderly are dose related and potentially preventable. It is therefore rational to start with the smallest possible dose of a given drug in the least number of doses and then gradually increase both, if necessary. Dose titration should obviously take into consideration age-related pharmacokinetic and pharmacodynamic alterations that may affect the response to the chosen drug.

Choosing the right dosage form

Most elderly patients find it easy to swallow syrups or suspensions or effervescent tablets rather than large tablets or capsules.

Packaging and labelling

Many elderly patients with arthritis find it difficult to open child-resistant containers and blister packs. Medicines should be dispensed in easy-to-open containers that are clearly labelled using large print.

Good record keeping

Information about a patient's current and previous drug therapy, alcohol consumption, smoking and driving habits may help in choosing appropriate drug therapy when the treatment needs to be altered. It will help to reduce costly duplications and will also identify and help to avoid dangerous drug interactions.

Regular supervision and review of treatment

A UK survey showed that 59% of prescriptions to the elderly had been given for more than 2 years, 32% for more than 5 years and 16% for more than 10 years. Of all prescriptions given to the elderly, 88% were repeat prescriptions; 40% had not been discussed with the doctor for at least 6 months, especially prescriptions for hypnotics and anxiolytics. It also showed that 31% of prescriptions were considered pharmacologically questionable, and 4% showed duplication of drugs. It is obvious that there is a need for regular and critical review of all prescriptions, especially when long-term therapy is required.

Adverse drug reactions

It is recognized that ADRs occur more frequently in the elderly. A multicentre study in the UK in 1980 showed that ADRs were the only cause of admission in 2.8% of 1998 admissions to 42 units of geriatric medicine. It also showed that ADRs were contributory to a further 7.7% of admissions. On the basis of this study it can be estimated that up to 15 000 geriatric admissions per annum in the UK are at least partly due to an ADR. Obviously, this has enormous economic implications.

The elderly are more susceptible to ADRs for a number of reasons. They are usually on multiple drugs, which in itself can account for the increased incidence of ADRs. It is, however, recognized that ADRs tend to be more severe in the elderly, and gastrointestinal and haematological ADRs are more common than would be expected from prescribing figures alone. Age-related pharmacokinetic and pharmacodynamic alterations and impaired homeostatic mechanisms are the other factors which predispose the elderly to ADRs, by making them more sensitive to the pharmacological effects of the drugs. Not surprisingly, up to 80% of ADRs in the elderly are dose-dependent and therefore predictable.

Adherence

Although it is commonly believed that the elderly are poor compliers with their drug therapy, there is no clear evidence to support this. Studies in Northern Ireland and continental Europe have shown that the elderly are as adherent with their drug therapy as the young, provided that they do not have confounding disease. Cognitive impairment, which is not uncommon in old age, multiple drug therapy and complicated drug regimens may impair adherence in the elderly. Poor adherence may result in treatment failure. The degree of adherence required varies depending on the disease being treated. For treatment of a simple urinary tract infection, a single dose of an antibiotic may be all that is required and therefore compliance is not important. On the other hand, adherence of 90% or more is required for successful treatment of epilepsy or difficult hypertension. Various methods have been used to improve adherence. These include prescription diaries, special packaging, training by pharmacists and counselling.

Conclusion

The number of elderly patients, especially those aged over 75 years, is steadily increasing, and they are accounting for an ever-increasing proportion of health care expenditure in the West. Understanding age-related changes in pharmacodynamic factors, avoiding polypharmacy and regular and critical review of all drug treatment will help in the rationalization of drug prescribing, reduction in drug-related morbidity and also the cost of drug therapy for this important subgroup of patients.

CASE STUDIES

Case 9.1

An 80-year-old woman presented to an out-patient clinic with a history of severe giddiness and a few episodes of blackouts. She was being treated for angina and hypertension. She had been on bendroflumethiazide (bendrofluazide) 2.5 mg once daily, and slow-release isosorbide mononitrate 60 mg once daily for a few years. Her general practitioner had recently commenced nifedipine SR 20 mg twice daily for poorly controlled hypertension. On examination her blood pressure was 120/70 mmHg while supine and 90/60 mmHg on standing up.

Question

What is the underlying problem in this patient, and could it be caused by any of the medications that the patient is taking?

Answer

This patient obviously has significant postural hypotension. All her drugs have the potential to produce postural hypotension, and when used together they may produce symptomatic postural hypotension.

It is important to recognize that some drugs such as nifedipine and nitrates have impaired first-pass metabolism in the elderly and that their clinical effects are enhanced. In addition, orthostatic circulatory responses are also impaired in the elderly. The need for antihypertensive drugs should be carefully assessed in all elderly patients, and, if therapy is indicated, the smallest dose of drug should be commenced and increased gradually. Patients should also be told to avoid sudden changes of posture.

Case 9.2

An 85-year-old man was admitted to hospital with anorexia, nausea and vomiting. He was known to have atrial fibrillation, congestive cardiac failure and chronic renal impairment. He was on digoxin 250 micrograms once daily and furosemide (frusemide) 80 mg twice daily.

His serum biochemistry revealed the following (normal range in parentheses):

Potassium	4.5 mmol/l	(3.5–5)
Urea	40 mmol/l	(3.0–6.5)
Creatinine	600 μmol/l	(50–120)
Digoxin	3.5 micrograms/l	(1–2)

Question

What are the likely underlying problems in this patient and do they necessitate a change in therapy?

Answer

The patient's biochemical results confirm the presence of renal impairment and digoxin toxicity. As digoxin is predominantly excreted through the kidneys, the dose should be reduced in the presence of impaired renal function. In the presence of severe renal impairment, digitoxin, which is predominantly metabolized in the liver, can be used instead of digoxin.

Case 9.3

An 80-year-old woman with a previous history of hypothyroidism presented with a history of abdominal pain and vomiting. She had not moved her bowels for the previous 7 days. Two weeks earlier her general practitioner had prescribed a combination of paracetamol and codeine to control pain in her osteoarthritic hips.

Question

What are the likely underlying causes of this patient's bowel dysfunction?

Answer

This patient developed severe constipation after taking a codeine-containing analgesic. Ageing is associated with decreased gastrointestinal motility. Hypothyroidism, which is common in the elderly, is also associated with reduced gastrointestinal motility. Whenever possible, drugs that are known to reduce gastrointestinal motility should be avoided in the elderly.

Case 9.4

A 75-year-old lady who suffered from osteoarthritis of hip and knee joints presented with a history of passing black stools. Her drug therapy included diclofenac 50 mg three times daily and paracetamol 1 g as required.

Question

What is the likely cause of this patient's symptoms?

Answer

The likely cause is upper gastrointestinal bleeding due to diclofenac, which is a NSAID. Elderly people are more prone to develop ulceration in stomach and duodenum with NSAIDs compared with young patients.

Case 9.5

A 70-year-old man was found to have hypertension by his GP and was commenced on lisinopril 5 mg once a day. He had a previous history of peripheral vascular disease for which he had required angioplasty. Two weeks after commencing antihypertensive treatment he presented with lack of appetite, nausea and decreased urine output.

Question

What do you think has happened? What is the most likely underlying problem?

Answer

The patient is probably developing renal failure. With a previous history of peripheral vascular disease, he is likely to have bilateral renal artery stenosis. ACE inhibitors can cause renal failure in the presence of bilateral renal stenosis by reducing blood supply to the kidneys.

REFERENCES

Amery A, Birkenhager W, Brixko P et al 1986 Efficacy of antihypertensive drug treatment according to age, sex, blood pressure, and previous cardiovascular disease in patients over the age of 60. Lancet 2: 589–592.

Bayer A J, Chadha J S, Farag R R et al 1986 Changing presentation of myocardial infarction with increasing old age. Journal of the American Geriatrics Society 34: 263–266

Benavente O, Hart R, Koudstaal P et al 2000 Oral anticoagulants for preventing stroke in patients with non-valvular atrial fibrillation and no previous history of stroke or transient ischaemic attacks. Cochrane Review. Cochrane Library no. 3 Update Software, Oxford:

Brott T, Bogousslavsky J 2000 Treatment of acute ischaemic stroke. New England Journal of Medicine 343: 710–722.

Chen Z M, Sandercock P, Pan H C et al 2000 Indications for early aspirin use in acute ischaemic stroke: a combined analysis of 40,000 randomised patients from the Chinese acute stroke trial and the international stroke trial. On behalf of the CAST and IST collaborative groups. Stroke 31: 1240–1249

Clarke W M, Wissman S, Albert G W et al 1999 Recombinant tissue-type plasminogen activator (Alteplase) for ischaemic stroke 3 to 5 hours after symptom onset. The ATLANTIS study: a randomised controlled trial. Alteplase Thrombolysis for Acute Noninterventional Therapy for Ischaemic Stroke. Journal of the American Medical Association 282: 2019–2026

Cornwall J V, Dore C J, Lewis J D 1986 Leg ulcers: epidemiology and aetiology. British Journal of Surgery 73: 693–696

Griffin M R, Ray W A, Schaffner W 1988 Non-steroidal anti-inflammatory drug use and death from peptic ulcer in elderly persons. Annals of Internal Medicine 109: 359–363

Hacke W, Kaste M, Fieschi C et al, for the ECASS Study Group 1995 Intravenous thrombolysis with tissue plasminogen activator for acute hemispheric stroke: the European cooperative acute stroke study (ECASS). Journal of the American Medical Association 274: 1017–1025

Hacke W, Kaste M, Fieschi C et al 1998 Randomised double-blind placebo-controlled trial of thrombolytic therapy with intravenous alteplase in acute ischaemic stroke (ECASS II). Second European-Australasian acute stroke study investigators. Lancet 352: 1245–1251

Intercollegiate Working Party for Stroke 2000 National clinical guidelines for stroke. Royal College of Physicians, London

Law M R, Wald N J, Mead W 1991 Strategies for prevention of osteoporosis and hip fracture. British Medical Journal 303: 453–459

National Institute for Clinical Excellence 2001 Guidance on the use of donepezil, rivastigmine and galantamine for the treatment of Alzheimer's disease. Technology appraisal guidance no. 19. NICE, London

National Institute of Neurological Disorders on Stroke rt-PA Stroke Study Group 1995 Tissue plasminogen activator for acute ischaemic stroke. New England Journal of Medicine 333: 1581–1587

Redman A R, Ryan G J 2001 Analysis of trials evaluating combinations of acetylsalicylic acid and dipyridamole in the secondary prevention of stroke. Clinical Therapeutics 23: 1391–1408

SHEP Cooperative Research Group 1991 Prevention of stroke by antihypertensive drug treatment in older persons with isolated systolic hypertension: final results of the systolic hypertension in the elderly programme (SHEP) Journal of the American Medical Association 265: 3255–3264

FURTHER READING

Eastell R 1998 Treatment of post menopausal osteoporisis. New England Journal of Medicine 338: 736–746

Iqbal P, Castleden C M 1997 Management of urinary incontinence in the elderly. Gerontology 43: 151–157

Prisant L M, Moser M 2000 Hypertension in the elderly: can we improve results of therapy Archives of Internal Medicine 160: 283–289

Wardlaw J M 2001 Overview of Cochrane thrombolysis meta-analysis. Neurology 57(5 Suppl. 2): S69–76

THERAPEUTICS

Peptic ulcer disease

10

S. Ghosh   M. Kinnear

The term 'peptic ulcer' describes a condition in which there is a discontinuity in the entire thickness of the gastric or duodenal mucosa that persists as a result of acid and pepsin in the gastric juice (Fig. 10.1). Important advances in understanding the cause of peptic ulcer have occurred in the past 15 years, resulting in effective therapy, improved healing and fewer recurrences. Oesophageal ulceration due to acid reflux is generally classified under gastro-oesophageal reflux disease. This definition excludes carcinoma and lymphoma, which may also cause gastric ulceration, and also excludes other rare causes of gastric and duodenal ulceration such as Crohn's disease, viral infections and amyloidosis. About 10% of the population in developed countries is likely to be affected at some time by peptic ulcer, with the prevalence for active ulcer disease being about 1% at any particular point in time.

Peptic ulcer disease often presents to clinicians as dyspepsia. However, not all patients with dyspepsia have peptic ulcer disease. Dyspepsia is defined as persistent or recurrent pain or discomfort in the upper abdomen. About 50% of dyspeptic patients have a definite cause for their symptoms, for example peptic ulcer, gastric cancer or pancreatic or biliary disease; another 20% have abnormalities of uncertain relevance such as gastritis or upper gastrointestinal dysmotility; the remaining 30% have no recognizable abnormalities. The last two groups are commonly categorized as non-ulcer or functional dyspepsia. Dyspepsia is a common symptom and affects between 30% and 40% of people at some time in their lives. Dyspepsia is the reason for 5–10% of consultations with primary care physicians, and up to 70% of referrals to gastrointestinal units are patients with dyspepsia.

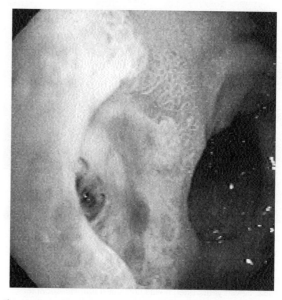

Figure 10.1 Duodenal ulcer seen at endoscopy. Note also a visible blood vessel that is a stigma of recent haemorrhage.

Epidemiology

There has been a decrease in uncomplicated duodenal ulcer and also, to a lesser extent, in gastric ulcer over the last two decades in the UK, Europe and the USA. In the past peptic ulcer was predominantly a disease of men, but this has now changed to a nearly equal sex distribution. Complex epidemiological factors, particularly changing patterns of smoking and non-steroidal anti-inflammatory drug (NSAID) use, may underlie these changes. Peptic ulcer is more common in unskilled labourers and other low socioeconomic groups. Geographical variations exist, such as the higher prevalence of duodenal ulcer in Scotland and the north of England compared with the south of England.

Infection by *Helicobacter pylori (H. pylori)*, a spiral bacterium of the stomach, is the most important epidemiological factor in causing peptic ulcer (Fig. 10.2). Most *H. pylori* infections are acquired by oral–oral and oral–faecal transmission. The prevalence of *H. pylori* is decreasing in most developed countries, and is paralleled by a decrease in the incidence of duodenal ulcer and gastric cancer. The most important risk factors for *H. pylori* infection are low social class, overcrowding and home environment during childhood (e.g. bed-sharing). Transmission may occur within a family, a fact demonstrated by the finding that family members, especially spouses, may have the same strain of *H. pylori*. *H. pylori* seropositivity increases with age. Subjects who become infected with *H. pylori* when young are more likely to develop chronic or atrophic gastritis with reduced acid secretion that may protect them from developing duodenal ulcer, but may promote development of gastric ulcer as well as gastric cancer. Duodenal ulcer seems to develop in those who are infected with *H. pylori* at the end of childhood or later. However, some epidemiological data are in conflict with this view of pathogenesis. Basal acid output and stimulated acid output are increased in people with duodenal ulcer. The high and low rates of *H. pylori* infection in, respectively, developing and developed countries are not reflected in the distribution of peptic ulcer, indicating that other host and environmental factors besides *H. pylori* may be needed for ulcer development.

Pathogenesis of peptic ulcer disease

There are two common forms of peptic ulcer disease, those associated with the organism *H. pylori* and those associated with the use of NSAIDs. Massive hypersecretion of acid occurs in the rare gastrinoma (Zollinger–Ellison) syndrome.

Helicobacter pylori (see Fig. 10.2)

This organism is a microaerophilic bacterium found primarily in the gastric antrum of the human stomach. Ninety-five per cent or more of duodenal ulcers and 80–85% of gastric ulcers are associated with *H. pylori*. The bacterium is located in the antrum, and the acid-secreting micro environment of the corpus of the stomach is less hospitable to the bacterium. In the developed world, reinfection rates are low – about 0.3–1.0% per year – whereas in the developing world reinfection rates are higher – approximately 20–30%. Ulcerogenic strains of *H. pylori,* ulcer-prone hosts, age of infection and interaction with other ulcerogenic factors such as NSAIDs determine peptic ulcer development following *H. pylori* infection. The effect of *H. pylori* in patients receiving NSAIDs is unclear. *H. pylori* causing peptic ulcer disease may be more virulent than in those without ulcers, and produces cytotoxin-associated gene A *(CagA)* proteins and vacuolating cytotoxins such as vac A to activate the inflammatory cascade. *CagA* status and one genotype of the vac A gene are predictors of ulcerogenic capacity of a strain. *H. pylori* expresses sialic acid-specific haemagglutinins and a lipid-binding adhesion that mediate binding to the mucosal surface. A number of enzymes produced by the bacteria may be involved in causing tissue damage, such as urease, haemolysins, neuraminidase and fucosidase. Gastrin is the main hormone involved in stimulating gastric acid secretion, and gastrin homeostasis is altered in *H. pylori* infection. The hyperacidity in duodenal

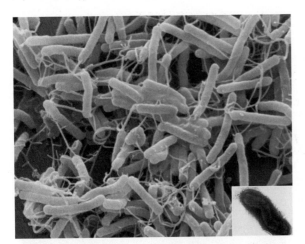

Figure 10.2 *Helicobacter pylori.* The Gram-negative spiral bacterium *Helicobacter pylori*, formerly known as *Campylobacter pylori*, was isolated serendipitously from patients with gastritis by Barry Marshall and Robin Warren in 1982. Seven years later, it was conceded that *Helicobacter pylori* is responsible for most cases of gastric and duodenal ulcer.

ulcer may result from *H. pylori*-induced hypergastrinaemia. The elevation of gastrin may be a consequence of bacterially mediated decrease of antral D cells that secrete somatostatin, thus losing the inhibitory modulation of somatostatin on gastrin, or direct stimulation of gastrin cells by certain cytokines liberated during the inflammatory process. Long-standing hypergastrinaemia leads to an increased parietal cell mass. High acid content in the proximal duodenum leads to metaplastic gastric-type mucosa, which provides a niche for *H. pylori* infection followed by inflammation and ulcer formation.

Non-steroidal anti-inflammatory drugs (NSAIDs)

Three patterns of mucosal damage are caused by NSAIDs. These include superficial erosions and haemorrhages, silent ulcers detected at endoscopy and ulcers causing clinical symptoms and complications. Weak acid NSAIDs (such as acetylsalicylic acid) are concentrated from the acidic gastric juice into mucosal cells, and may produce acute superficial erosions via inhibition of cyclo-oxygenase (COX) and by mediating the adherence of leucocytes to mucosal endothelial cells. Enteric coating may prevent this superficial damage, but does not reduce the ulcer risk. The major systemic action of NSAIDs in producing ulcers is the reduction of mucosal prostaglandin production. All NSAIDs share the ability to inhibit COX (Fig. 10.3). The presence of NSAID-induced ulcers does not correlate with abdominal pain and in fact NSAIDs themselves often mask ulcer pain. Approximately 20% of patients taking NSAIDs experience symptoms of dyspepsia but symptoms correlate poorly with the presence of mucosal

damage. Ulcers and ulcer complications occur in approximately 4% of NSAID users every year.

In the UK there are an estimated 1200 NSAID-related ulcer deaths each year. NSAIDs increase the risk of ulcer complications (Table 10.1), and the estimates of increase in risk vary from unity to greater than 10-fold (Hawkey 2000). NSAID-related ulcer complications increase with advancing age, particularly in those over 75 years; the risk being greatest within the first month of therapy. The risk of mucosal damage increases with even very low doses of NSAIDs, particularly aspirin. Corticosteroids alone are an insignificant ulcer risk, but potentiate the ulcer risk when added to NSAIDs, particularly in daily doses of at least 10 mg prednisolone.

Low dose aspirin alone increases the risk of ulcer bleeding and concomitant use with NSAIDs further increases the risk. There is no evidence that anticoagulants increase the risk of NSAID ulcers but they are associated with an increase in the risk of haemorrhage. Cardiovascular disease has also been

Table 10.1 Risk factors for NSAID ulcers	
Uncontroversial risk factors	Controversial risk factors
Age greater than 60 years	Smoking
Previous peptic ulceration	Alcohol
High dose of NSAID or more than one NSAID	Sex of patient
Concomitant corticosteroid use	*H. pylori*
NSAID, non-steroidal anti-inflammatory drug.	

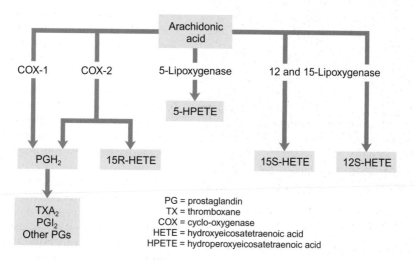

Figure 10.3   Arachidonic acid pathway.

identified as an independent risk factor (Schoenfeld et al 1999). Enteric coating does not reduce risk (Sorensen et al 2000) and a meta-analysis found no evidence that reduction in aspirin dose reduces the risk of gastrointestinal haemorrhage (Derry & Loke 2000).

Selective cyclo-oxygenase-2 (COX-2) inhibitors

Newer NSAIDs such as the COX-2 inhibitors (see Fig. 10.3) should reduce inflammation with minimal adverse effects. COX-1 stimulates synthesis of homeostatic prostaglandins while COX-2 is predominantly induced in response to inflammation. COX-2 inhibitors tend not to reduce the mucosal production of protective prostaglandins to the same extent as NSAIDs that also inhibit COX-1. Theoretically the degree of COX selectivity is associated with the safety profile in terms of gastric mucosal damage. Comparative studies of the COX-2 inhibitors currently available suggest that rofecoxib is more selective for COX-2 than celecoxib. Selectivity ratios of 36 for rofecoxib, 7 for celecoxib, 3 for diclofenac, 2 for meloxicam and 0.4 for indometacin have been reported (Hawkey et al 2001).

The relative roles of COX-1 and COX-2 inhibition in dyspepsia symptoms are unknown. In practice dyspepsia symptoms reduce drug tolerability but there is no correlation with mucosal damage. Large prospective, blinded, randomized trials have been completed looking at the toxicity and risk factors associated with COX-2 inhibitors compared with non-selective NSAIDs over a 6 month exposure period. The results show that celecoxib, at dosages greater than those indicated clinically, was associated with a lower incidence of symptomatic ulcers and ulcer complications compared with ibuprofen and diclofenac at standard dosages. The decrease in upper gastrointestinal toxicity was greatest among patients not taking aspirin concomitantly (Silverstein et al 2000). Another study in rheumatoid arthritis patients, none of whom took aspirin, shows that rofecoxib at a dose greater than recommended was also associated with a lower incidence of symptomatic ulcers and ulcer complications compared with naproxen at normal doses (Bombardier et al 2000). However, there was a higher rate of cardiovascular events in the rofecoxib group, a finding that requires further investigation. Caution should be exercised in patients with a history of cardiac failure or hypertension.

Further data are needed to establish the long-term safety of these agents.

Nitric oxide (NO) NSAIDs

Nitric oxide (NO) NSAIDs are being investigated to see if gastric mucosa protection associated with nitric oxide prevents ulceration when prostaglandins are inhibited by NSAIDs (Hawkey 2000). NO is coupled to the NSAID via an ester, resulting in prolonged release of nitric oxide. Nitric oxide itself has anti-inflammatory effects adding to the potency of the NSAID. Studies are needed to assess the efficacy and safety of these agents which may have the potential to overcome some of the theoretical disadvantages of COX-2 inhibition such as inhibition of vascular prostacyclin.

Clinical manifestations

Upper abdominal pain occuring 1–3 hours after meals and relieved by food or antacids is the classic symptom of peptic ulcer disease. The relationship to meals is more marked in duodenal ulcer than in gastric ulcer. However, the symptoms of peptic ulcer disease lack specificity; they do not distinguish between duodenal ulcer, gastric ulcer and non-ulcer or functional dyspepsia. Anorexia, weight loss, nausea and vomiting, heartburn and eructation can all occur with peptic ulcer disease. Patients with predominant symptoms of heartburn are likely to have gastro-oesophageal reflux disease. Complications of peptic ulcer disease may occur with or without previous dyspeptic symptoms. These are haemorrhage, chronic iron deficiency anaemia, pyloric stenosis and perforation. In the elderly the presentation is more likely to be silent. Physical examination is either negative or may reveal epigastric tenderness. Peptic ulcers in the past tended to relapse and remit, and 70–80% of ulcers relapse within 1–2 years after being healed by medical therapy such as antisecretory therapy. This tendency to relapse is dramatically reduced by eradication of *H. pylori*.

Patient assessment

Presenting symptoms of dyspepsia require careful assessment to judge the risk of serious disease or to provide appropriate symptomatic treatment. Symptom subgroups such as ulcer-type, reflux-type and dysmotility-type may be useful to identify the predominant symptom subgroup that a patient belongs to, although many patients have symptoms which fit more than one subgroup (Talley et al 1992; Table 10.2). Many patients seek reassurance, lifestyle advice and symptomatic treatment with a single consultation, others have chronic symptoms.

The National Institute for Clinical Excellence (NICE) recommends that all patients over the age of 55 with new symptoms of dyspepsia should be referred for endoscopic investigation, as should younger patients with alarm symptoms (Table 10.3). These groups of patients are at a higher risk of underlying serious disease such as cancer, ulcers or severe oesophagitis. Endoscopic investigation is not recommended in patients

Table 10.2 Dyspepsia symptom subgroups

Reflux-like dyspepsia
Heartburn plus dyspepsia
Acid regurgitation plus dyspepsia

Ulcer-like dyspepsia
Localized epigastric pain
Pain when hungry
Pain relieved by food
Pain relieved by antacids or acid reducing drugs
Pain that wakens the patient from sleep
Pain with remission and relapses

Dysmotility-like dyspepsia
Upper abdominal discomfort (pain not dominant)
Early satiety
Postprandial fullness
Nausea
Retching or vomiting
Bloating in the upper abdomen (no visible distension)
Upper abdominal discomfort often aggravated by food

Unspecified dyspepsia

Table 10.3 Alarm Symptoms

Dysphagia
Pain on swallowing
Weight loss
Bleeding or anaemia
Vomiting
On NSAIDs or warfarin
NSAID, non-steroidal anti-inflammatory drug

under the age of 45 unless alarm symptoms are present or the symptoms are refractory to empirical treatment. There is much debate about the need to refer patients without alarm symptoms between the ages of 45 and 55.

Patients with predominant reflux-like symptoms are likely to respond to acid suppressing therapy and a therapeutic trial with a greater than standard dose of proton pump inhibitor for 1–2 weeks may be used as a diagnostic test for gastro-oesophageal reflux disease. The sensitivity and specificity of this test is similar to a 24 hour oesophageal pH monitoring test, and more readily acceptable to patients. Eradication of *H. pylori* is not beneficial in gastro-oesophageal reflux. In those patients with ulcer-like dyspepsia, there is an argument to be made for testing for the presence of *H. pylori* and to giving eradication treatment to those who test positive and empirical acid suppression to those who test

negative. *H. pylori* testing is best applied to those likely to have an ulcer. A small but significant benefit of eradication treatment has been shown in non-ulcer or functional dyspepsia. It is suggested that a subset of patients with functional dyspepsia may benefit in the long term. Further research is needed to define this subset and cost-effectiveness studies are required to support a test and treat approach in this subgroup of patients.

Investigations

Endoscopy

Endoscopy is generally the investigation of choice for diagnosing peptic ulcer, and the procedure is sensitive, specific and safe. However, it is also invasive and expensive. A decision algorithm, as illustrated in Figure 10.4, may help to rationalize referrals for endoscopy. Biopsies may be taken to exclude malignancy and uncommon lesions such as Crohn's disease.

Radiology

Double-contrast barium radiography should detect 80% of peptic ulcers. A Gastrograffin meal is used to diagnose peptic perforation in patients presenting with an acute abdomen.

Helicobacter pylori detection

There are several methods of detecting *H. pylori* infection. They include non-invasive tests such as serological tests to detect antibodies and [^{13}C]- or [^{14}C]urea breath tests. Commercial serological tests are becoming increasingly available, but a critical evaluation is needed. Sensitivity is considered insufficient for routine incorporation into management policies. Serological tests do not allow conclusions about eradication until at least 6 months post-therapy. Urea breath tests have a sensitivity of 90–100% and a specificity of 80–100%, and are frequently used 4 weeks after completion of therapy to confirm eradication. An enzyme immunoassay can detect *H. pylori* antigen in stool.

Invasive tests needing gastric antral biopsies include urease tests, histology and culture. Of these, the biopsy urease test is widely used. Agar-based biopsy urease tests (CLO) are designed to be read at 24 hours, whereas the strip-based biopsy urease tests (Pyloritek) can be read at 2 hours following incubation with the biopsy material. Patients on proton pump inhibitors can have false-negative results for *H. pylori* when using the urea breath test or biopsy urease test and therefore these medicines should be discontinued at least 2 weeks before testing.

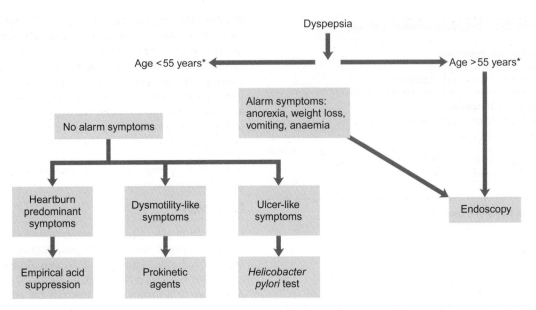

Figure 10.4 An algorithm approach to the diagnosis of peptic ulcer disease. (*The age cut-off , which is arbitrary, has been agreed by BSG, SIGN and NICE.)

The question of who should be tested for *H. pylori* is as yet unanswered. Patients with ulcer-like symptoms or those known to have had an ulcer should be tested, while individuals with predominant heartburn or dysmotility-like symptoms are less likely to benefit. The faecal occult blood test is neither specific for nor sensitive to detection of NSAID-induced gastric damage. A full blood count may provide evidence of blood loss from peptic ulcer.

Treatment

Complications of peptic ulcer disease

Bleeding peptic ulcer

Most patients with bleeding peptic ulcer stop bleeding without any intervention. A number of studies have shown that endoscopic injection therapy is an effective haemostatic procedure and is successful in reducing mortality. A number of pharmacological agents have been used such as 1:10 000 or 1:100 000 adrenaline (epinephrine), human thrombin and fibrin glue. Thermocoagulation and adrenaline (epinephrine) is routinely used in practice. Bleeding recurs in 15–20% of patients. A study of high dose infusion of omeprazole has demonstrated a decrease in the re-bleeding rate although acid suppression had not previously demonstrated a role in arresting haemorrhage (Lau et al 2000). After successful *H. pylori* eradication the rate of re-bleeding from peptic ulcers is markedly reduced. Omeprazole is superior to *H. pylori* eradication in preventing recurrent bleeding in patients taking non-

aspirin NSAIDs, and is equivalent to *H. pylori* eradication in those taking low dose aspirin (Chan et al 2001).

Pyloric stenosis

There is limited anecdotal evidence that incomplete gastric outlet obstruction may improve within several months of successful *H. pylori* eradication. Conventional treatment with acid-suppressive therapy may also help. If medical therapy fails to relieve the obstruction, endoscopic balloon dilatation or surgery may be required.

Late complications of peptic ulcer surgery

Few patients currently have peptic ulcer disease that is refractory to medical therapy. However, surgical operations were common in the 1960s and 1970s, with nearly half the patients surgically treated for peptic ulcer disease experiencing some resulting debility. Symptoms include early satiety with or without postcibal vomiting, reactive hypoglycaemia, diarrhoea, weight loss, anaemia, bone loss and vasomotor phenomena such as flushing, palpitations, sweating, tachycardia and postural hypotension. Medical treatment of these symptoms consists of the use of pectin or guar to slow gastric emptying, metoclopramide for gastric stasis, colestyramine for postvagotomy diarrhoea, somatostatin for reactive hypoglycaemia, antibiotics for bacterial colonization and antidiarrhoeal agents such as loperamide. Only a few of these treatments are supported by evidence from randomized controlled trials.

Zollinger–Ellison syndrome

This rare syndrome consists of a triad of non-β islet cell tumours of the pancreas that contain and release gastrin, gastric acid hypersecretion and severe ulcer disease. Extrapancreatic gastrinomas are also common and may be found frequently in the duodenal wall. A proportion of these patients have tumours of the pituitary gland and parathyroid gland (multiple endocrine neoplasia type I). Surgical resection of the gastrinoma may be curative. Medical management consists of greater than standard doses of proton pump inhibitors. The somatostatin analogue octreotide is also effective but has no clear advantage over proton pump inhibitors.

Stress ulcers

Severe physiological stress such as head injury, surgery or burns may induce superficial mucosal erosions or gastroduodenal ulcerations. These may lead to haemorrhage or perforation. Diminished blood flow to the gastric mucosa, decreased cell renewal, diminished prostaglandin production and, occasionally, acid hypersecretion are involved in causing stress ulceration. Intravenous histamine H_2 receptor antagonists (cimetidine, ranitidine, nizatidine), nasogastric tube administration of sucralfate (4–6 g daily in divided doses) and titrated doses of antacids have been used to prevent stress ulceration in the intensive care unit. However, there is no clear evidence of effectiveness of either of these strategies in comparison to placebo (Messori et al 2000).

Uncomplicated peptic ulcer disease

Treatment of endoscopically proven uncomplicated peptic ulcer disease has changed dramatically in recent years (Fig. 10.5). Cure of *H. pylori* infection and discontinuation of NSAIDs are key elements for the successful management of peptic ulcer disease.

Helicobacter pylori eradication

It is known that *H. pylori* infection is associated with over 90% of duodenal ulcers and 80% of gastric ulcers. Cure of this infection with antibiotic therapy and simultaneous treatment with conventional ulcer-healing drugs facilitates symptom relief and healing of the ulcer and reduces the ulcer relapse rate. Antibiotics alone, or acid suppressing agents alone, do not eradicate *H. pylori*. Both therapies act synergistically as growth of the organism occurs at elevated pH and antibiotic efficacy is enhanced during growth. Additionally, increasing intragastric pH may enhance antibiotic absorption.

Eradication treatment regimens that consistently achieve eradication rates above 90% should be chosen.

Studies have demonstrated that, currently, the highest eradication rates are achieved by 1 week of triple therapy consisting of a proton pump inhibitor and two specified antibiotics. The MACH-1 study was the first large randomized placebo controlled trial of *H. pylori* eradication. The most effective 1-week twice daily regimens in this trial were the following: *either* (1) OCA: omeprazole 20 mg, clarithromycin 500 mg and amoxicillin 1 g; *or* (2) OCM: omeprazole 20 mg, clarithromycin 250 mg and metronidazole 400 mg (Lind et al 1996). Omeprazole may be substituted with any of the other proton pump inhibitor drugs. The MACH-1 triple therapies are consistently effective in both active gastric and duodenal ulcer disease.

In the UK, resistance to metronidazole has been reported in 11–68% of *H. pylori* isolates, and to clarithromycin in 3–10%. Resistance to amoxicillin is rare. Sensitivity testing is of little value as in vitro resistance to either drug does not preclude eradication when those drugs are used as part of a triple-therapy regimen. The MACH-2 study showed that metronidazole resistance reduced the efficacy of OCM from 95% to 76%. The MACH-2 study also showed that the potent acid suppression of a proton pump inhibitor partially overcomes metronidazole resistance (Lind et al 1999). Tinidazole might be used in place of metronidazole. A lower dose of clarithromycin (250 mg twice daily) may be as effective, but consensus groups have recommended 500 mg twice daily to achieve consistency and avoid prescribing errors.

Ranitidine bismuth citrate (RBC) is a chemical entity which incorporates bismuth into the ranitidine molecule and which was designed for *H. pylori* eradication. There is no difference in the efficacy rate of *H. pylori* eradication between proton pump inhibitor-based and RBC-based triple therapies. Proton pump inhibitors are more effective in triple-therapy regimens than H_2 receptor antagonists in similar regimens. Failure of a first-line regimen to achieve eradication will necessitate treatment with another triple-therapy regimen or with a quadruple regimen. Most four-drug regimens contain bismuth subsalicylate, metronidazole, tetracycline or amoxicillin and a proton pump inhibitor. Future regimens of different drug combinations, shorter duration and fewer doses are being evaluated.

Successful eradication relies upon patients adhering to their medication regimen. Eradication rates have fallen from 94% to 65% in patients with poor adherence who are taking less than 60% of their medicines (Graham et al 1992). It is therefore important to educate patients about the principles of eradication therapy and also about common adverse effects associated with their regimen and how to cope with them. Diarrhoea is the most common adverse effect and should subside after treatment is complete. In rare cases this can be severe and continue after treatment. If this happens patients

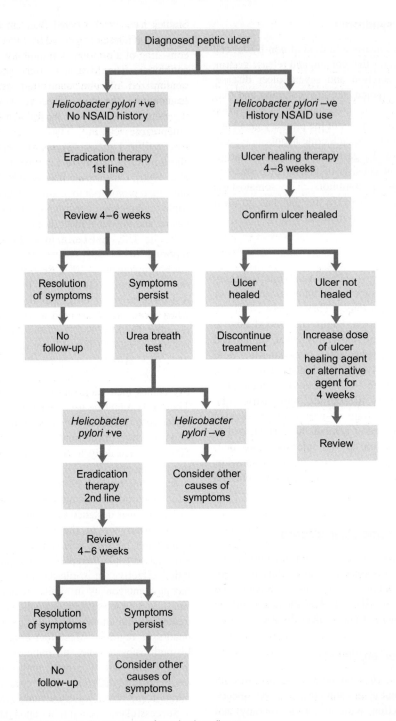

Figure 10.5 An algorithm approach to the treatment of peptic ulcer disease.

should be advised to return to their doctor as rare cases of antibiotic-associated colitis have been reported. Non-adherence may result in antibiotic resistance as there is a possibility that the concentration of antibiotic at the site of infection decreases to a level where resistance may emerge if drugs are not taken as intended.

Uncomplicated active duodenal ulcers heal without the need to continue ulcer healing drugs beyond the duration of eradication therapy. Active gastric ulcers may require continued acid suppression for an additional 3 weeks although evidence suggests in the future eradication alone may prove sufficient. If acid suppression is continued, the dose should be reduced to that recommended for ulcer healing. Patients with persistent symptoms after eradication therapy should have their *H. pylori* status rechecked. This should be carried out no sooner than 4 weeks after discontinuation of therapy to avoid false-negative results due to suppression rather than eradication of the organism. If the patient is *H. pylori*-positive, an alternative eradication regimen should be given. If eradication was successful but symptoms persist, gastro-oesophageal reflux or other causes of dyspepsia should be considered.

Patients who have had a previous gastrointestinal bleed from a gastric ulcer should continue ulcer-healing therapy until confirmation of eradication of *H. pylori*. H$_2$ receptor antagonists can be given after completion of the eradication regimen as they are less likely than proton pump inhibitors to result in a false-negative *H. pylori* test.

Other accepted indications for *H. pylori* eradication include mucosal-associated lymphoid tissue (MALT) lymphoma of the stomach, severe gastritis, and in patients with a high risk of gastric cancer such as those with family history of the disease.

Treatment of NSAID-associated ulcers

NSAID-associated ulcers may be *H. pylori*-positive. The effectiveness of eradicating *H. pylori* in these patients is unknown. Eradication of *H. pylori* decreases the rate of ulcer recurrence in patients not taking NSAIDs but does not seem to affect the rate of recurrence in NSAID users (Hawkey et al 1998a). In the same study, *H. pylori* eradication led to impaired ulcer healing in NSAID users. In contrast, another study suggested that successful eradication before NSAIDs are started could lessen the incidence of ulceration (Chan et al 1997). Long-term studies are needed to clarify these findings.

If NSAIDs are discontinued, most uncomplicated ulcers heal using standard doses of a proton pump inhibitor, H$_2$ receptor antagonist, misoprostol or sucralfate. Proton pump inhibitors are the drugs of choice for patients with large or complicated NSAID-induced ulcers because of their more rapid rate of ulcer healing. Healing is impaired if NSAID use is continued and proton pump inhibitors have shown similar healing rates to misoprostol and superior healing rates to H$_2$ receptor antagonists in this situation (Yeomans et al 1998, Hawkey et al 1998b, Agrawal et al 2000). The choice of ulcer-healing agent depends upon concurrent disease states and other drug therapy. Tables 10.4 and 10.5 list examples of adverse effects and drug interactions associated with conventional ulcer-healing agents.

Prophylaxis of NSAID ulceration

NSAIDs should be avoided in patients who are at risk of gastrointestinal toxicity (see Table 10.1). However, some patients with chronic rheumatological conditions may require long-term NSAID treatment, in which case the lowest effective dose should be used. Ulcer prophylaxis is indicated for 'at risk' patients who need to continue NSAID treatment. Future studies are required to compare the cost-effectiveness of cytoprotective prophylaxis with the potentially safer COX-2 inhibitors.

Omeprazole 20 mg daily is more effective and better tolerated than the prostaglandin analogue misoprostol 400 micrograms daily in the prevention of ulcer relapse after initial healing in patients who must continue an

Table 10.4   Adverse reactions to ulcer-healing drugs

Drug	Adverse reactions	
	Common	Rare
Omeprazole	Diarrhoea	Photosensitivity
Lansoprazole	Headache	Angio-oedema
Pantoprazole	Nausea	Alopecia
Rabeprazole	Constipation	Paraesthesia
Esomeprazole	Abdominal pain Skin rashes Dizziness Fatigue	Confusion Myalgia Taste disturbance Gynaecomastia Leucopenia Liver dysfunction
Cimetidine	Dizziness	Headache
Ranitidine	Fatigue	Liver dysfunction
Famotidine	Rash	Blood disorders
Nizatidine		Bradycardia Confusion Interstitial nephritis (cimetidine) Gynaecomastia (cimetidine)
Sucralfate	Constipation	Nausea Dry mouth Skin rashes Dizziness Headache
Bismuth chelate	Darkened tongue Blackened faeces Bismuth absorption	Nausea
Misoprostol	Diarrhoea Abdominal pain Menstrual disorders	

Table 10.5 Examples of drug interactions with ulcer-healing drugs

Drug	Interaction and effect		Mechanism
Omeprazole	Phenytoin	↑ effect	↓ clearance
Esomeprazole	Benzodiazepines	↑ effect	↓ clearance
	Warfarin	↑ effect	↓ clearance
	Tacrolimus	↑ effect	↓ clearance
Lansoprazole Pantoprazole Rabeprazole	To date no reports of clinical importance. Limited data		
Cimetidine	β-blockers	↑ effect	↓ clearance
	Calcium channel blockers	↑ effect	↓ clearance, ↑ absorption
	Benzodiazepines	↑ effect	↓ clearance
	Imipramine	↑ effect	↓ clearance
	Phenytoin	↑ effect	↓ clearance
	Theophylline	↑ effect	↓ clearance
	Warfarin	↑ effect	↓ clearance
Ranitidine	Theophylline	↑ effect (but little clinical importance)	↓ clearance
Famotidine Nizatidine	No reports of clinical importance		
Bismuth chelate	Tetracycline	↓ effect	↓ absorption
Sucralfate	Warfarin	↓ effect	↓ absorption
	Phenytoin	↓ effect	↓ absorption
	Thyroxine	↓ effect	↓ absorption
	Tetracycline	↓ effect	↓ absorption
Antacids	Tetracycline	↓ effect	↓ absorption

NSAID (Hawkey et al 1998b). Omeprazole 20 mg daily was also more effective than ranitidine 150 mg twice daily in prevention of ulcer relapse in patients who continued to take NSAIDs. There is evidence to suggest that lansoprazole 15 mg or 30 mg daily is similar to misoprostol 800 micrograms daily in preventing NSAID-induced ulceration (Rose et al 1999). The incidence of diarrhoea is problematic with misoprostol at doses of 800 micrograms. High dose famotidine, 40 mg twice daily, also appears effective in healing and preventing NSAID-induced ulcers (Hudson et al 1997). No studies have compared a proton pump inhibitor with high dose H$_2$ receptor antagonist for prevention of NSAID-induced ulcers. Gastroprotective agents licensed for prophylaxis of NSAID ulceration are listed in Table 10.6.

NICE recommends proton pump inhibitors for prophylaxis of NSAID ulceration in patients who must continue NSAIDs after a documented NSAID induced ulcer.

Gastro-oesophageal reflux disease (GORD)

Gastro-oesophageal reflux disease (GORD) is a term used to describe any symptomatic clinical condition or histopathological alteration resulting from episodes of reflux of acid, pepsin and, occasionally, bile into the oesophagus from the stomach. Heartburn is the characteristic symptom, and the patient may also complain of acid regurgitation and dysphagia. Complications include oesophageal stricture, oesophageal ulceration and formation of specialized columnar-lined oesophagus at the gastro-oesophageal junction (Barrett's oesophagus). The mechanism of acid reflux is multifactorial, and involves transient lower oesophageal sphincter relaxations, reduced tone of the lower oesophageal sphincter, hiatus hernia and abnormal oesophageal acid clearance. Strategies for initial treatment include lifestyle measures and self-treatment (over-the-counter antacids). Either a step-up or a step-down strategy may be adopted regarding initial medical

Table 10.6   Drugs licensed for prophylaxis for NSAID-induced ulceration

Drug	Indication	Prophylaxis dose
Omeprazole	Prophylaxis of further DU or GU	20 mg every day
Lansoprazole	Prophylaxis of DU or GU	15–30 mg every day
Misoprostol	Prophylaxis of DU or GU	200 micrograms twice a day to four times a day
Ranitidine	Prophylaxis of DU	150 mg twice a day

NSAID, non-steroidal anti-inflammatory drug; DU, duodenal ulcer; GU, gastric ulcer

therapy (Fig. 10.6). Both approaches have their proponents. The most effective therapy is standard dose proton pump inhibitor therapy. Long-term management should consist of the least expensive but effective drug. A selected group of patients may benefit from antireflux surgery rather than the escalation of acid-suppressing treatment. Patients with endoscopically severe oesophagitis should be kept on standard dose proton pump inhibitors long term and should not be stepped down.

Ulcer healing drugs

Proton pump inhibitors

The proton pump inhibitors are all benzimidazole derivatives that control gastric acid secretion by inhibition of gastric H^+,K^+1-ATPase, the enzyme responsible for the final step in gastric acid secretion from the parietal cell (Fig.10.7).

The proton pump inhibitors are inactive prodrugs that are carried in the bloodstream to the parietal cells in the gastric mucosa. The prodrugs readily cross the parietal cell membrane into the cytosol. These drugs are weak bases and therefore have a high affinity for acidic environments. They diffuse across the secretory membrane of the parietal cell into the extracellular secretory canaliculus, the site of the active proton pump (see Fig. 10.7). Under these acidic conditions the prodrugs are converted to their active form, which irreversibly binds the proton pump, inhibiting acid secretion. Since the 'active principle' forms at a low pH it concentrates selectively in the acidic environment of the proton pump and results in extremely effective inhibition

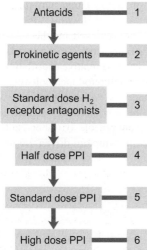

Figure 10.6   Ranking of the efficacy of drug treatment for gastro-oesophageal reflux (1, least effective; PPI, proton pump inhibitor).

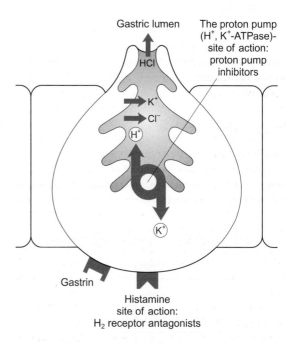

Figure 10.7   Receptor stimulation of acid secretion.

153

of acid secretion. The different proton pump inhibitors (omeprazole, esomeprazole, lansoprazole, pantoprazole and rabeprazole) bind to different sites on the proton pump, which may explain their differences in potency.

Proton pump inhibitors are rapidly absorbed, with a maximum plasma concentration after 2–3 hours and a half-life of 1–1.5 hours (Table 10.7). Since these drugs irreversibly bind to the proton pump they have a sustained duration of acid inhibition which does not correlate with the plasma elimination half-life. The apparent half-life is approximately 48 hours. This prolonged duration of action allows once daily dosing of proton pump inhibitors, although twice daily dosing is recommended in some cases. All proton pump inhibitors are most effective if taken about 30 minutes before a meal as they inhibit only actively secreting proton pumps. Meals are the main stimulus to proton pump activity.

Proton pump inhibitors are metabolized in the liver to various sulphate conjugates that are extensively (80%) eliminated by the kidneys. With the exception of severe hepatic dysfunction, no dose adjustments are necessary in liver disease or in renal disease.

Esomeprazole is the first proton pump inhibitor to be developed as a single optical isomer. It is the S-isomer from the racemic mixture that is omeprazole and is more potent on a mg per mg basis. Compared with omeprazole 20 mg, esomeprazole 40 mg provides greater and more sustained acid control. It is the first proton pump inhibitor to be licensed for symptom-driven on-demand therapy for GORD in patients who do not have endoscopically visible oesophagitis.

Adverse drug reactions

Experience suggests that proton pump inhibitors are a remarkably safe group of drugs, the risk of serious adverse reactions being approximately 1%. Diarrhoea, headache, dizziness and rash are the most commonly reported events.

Drug interactions

The cytochrome P450 enzyme system is classified into a number of subgroups, several of which are involved in drug metabolism. All proton pump inhibitors are metabolized by the same cytochrome P450 isoenzymes,

CYP2C19 and CYP3A, to varying degrees, and have the potential to interact with other drugs metabolized through this system although drug interactions involving CYP3A have not been identified. The affinity of individual proton pump inhibitors for these enzymes influences the incidence of clinically relevant drug interactions.

- Pantoprazole has lower affinity for the enzyme system than the other proton pump inhibitors and is also metabolized by a sulphotransferase which is non-saturable and not part of the cytochrome P450 system.
- Lansoprazole is a weak inducer of CYP1A2 and concurrent administration results in increased theophylline clearance.
- Omeprazole inhibits CYPs 2C9 and 2C19, the isoenzymes involved in the metabolism of, for example, phenytoin (2C9), S-warfarin (2C9), diazepam (2C19), R-warfarin (2C19). Omeprazole 40 mg daily has been shown to decrease the clearance of phenytoin, but phenytoin levels were unchanged after a dose of 20 mg of omeprazole daily. It is therefore recommended that phenytoin plasma concentrations should be monitored when omeprazole is taken concomitantly. Omeprazole may increase the coagulation time in patients receiving warfarin therapy, especially if doses higher than 20 mg daily are given. Changes in the plasma concentration of the less potent (R) enantiomer of warfarin have been observed, therefore monitoring of the international normalized ratio (INR) is recommended during concomitant therapy. The effects of benzodiazepines may be increased by omeprazole.
- Isolated case reports suggest lansoprazole may reduce the efficacy of the oral contraceptive pill.

Approximately 3% of the population are poor metabolizers of proton pump inhibitors due to genetic polymorphism associated with CYP2C19. High plasma concentrations are achieved and the relative capacity for metabolism by other isoenzymes may alter and result in drug interactions. The relative contribution of CYP2C19 to proton pump inhibitor metabolism is greatest with omeprazole and least with rabeprazole.

There have been no clinically significant interactions reported for pantoprazole or rabeprazole. The use of esomeprazole in symptom-driven on-demand therapy

Table 10.7 Comparison of proton pump inhibitors					
	Omeprazole	Lansoprazole	Pantoprazole	Rabeprazole	Esomeprazole
Bioavailability	65%	80%	77%	52%	89%
Elimination half-life	0.7 h	1.3 h	1.0 h	1.5 h	1.2 h
Protein binding	95%	97%	98%	96%	95%

may prove problematic if used concomitantly with warfarin or phenytoin. Careful monitoring should be undertaken. All acid-suppressing drugs potentially decrease the absorption of some drugs by increasing gastric pH. Reduction in absorption of ketoconazole and increased absorption of digoxin have been reported with proton pump inhibitors. The absorption of drugs formulated as pH dependent, controlled-release products may also be altered. Very few clinically important drug interactions have been reported despite the widespread use of these agents.

Clinical use

Proton pump inhibitors relieve symptoms and heal peptic ulcers faster than H_2 receptor antagonists. They also heal ulcers that are refractory to H_2 receptor antagonists. All proton pump inhibitors provide similar eradication rates and ulcer healing when used at their recommended doses. Only omeprazole and lansoprazole are currently licensed for healing and preventing NSAID-induced ulcers. In GORD, proton pump inhibitors heal oesophagitis and control symptoms more rapidly than H_2 receptor antagonists. Differences between proton pump inhibitors in terms of speed of symptom relief are observed only in the first few days of treatment. Patients with severe oesophagitis should continue long-term proton pump inhibitor therapy, whereas those with milder GORD should be stepped down in terms of acid suppression and therapy withdrawn if symptoms are controlled. Patients with non-ulcer or functional dyspepsia should not routinely be treated with proton pump inhibitors. The proton pump inhibitors differ in terms of their licensed indications (Table 10.8). NICE recommend that the least expensive appropriate proton pump inhibitor should be used.

H_2 receptor antagonists

The H_2 antagonists are all structural analogues of histamine. They competitively block the histamine receptors in gastric parietal cells, thereby preventing acid secretion. Pepsinogen requires acid for conversion to pepsin, and so when acid output is reduced, pepsin generation is, in turn, also reduced.

All the available drugs have similar properties (Table 10.9). They are all eliminated to a significant extent via the kidneys, and all require dosage reduction in renal failure. They are equally effective at suppressing daytime and nocturnal acid secretion while they do not cause total achlorhydria. The duration of acid suppression appears to be more important than the extent. The evening dose of an H_2 antagonist is particularly important because during the daytime gastric acid is buffered for long periods by food; however, during the night this is not the case and the intragastric pH may fall below 2.0 for several hours. For healing oesophagitis, intragastric pH must remain above 4.0 for 18 hours or more per day. H_2 receptor antagonists are therefore not effective in healing oesophagitis.

The role of H_2 receptor antagonists in the management of peptic ulcer disease has diminished. H_2 receptor antagonists are less effective than proton pump inhibitors in eradication regimens, in treating ulcers when NSAIDs are continued, and in prophylaxis of NSAID-induced ulcers. H_2 receptor antagonists do effectively heal ulcers in patients who discontinue their NSAID and they also have a role in continuing acid suppression following eradication therapy. Their main role is in the empirical management of dyspepsia symptoms. H_2 receptor antagonists can be purchased in doses lower than those prescribed for the management of heartburn and indigestion.

Table 10.8   Common licensed indications for proton pump inhibitors

	Omeprazole	Lansoprazole	Pantoprazole	Rabeprazole	Esomeprazole
H. pylori eradication	✓	✓	✓	✓	✓
Ulcer healing	✓	✓	✓	✓	
NSAID ulcer prophylaxis	✓	✓			
Healing of reflux oesophagitis	✓	✓	✓	✓	✓
Prevention of GORD relapse	✓	✓	✓	✓	✓
Symptomatic treatment in endoscopy-negative GORD					✓

GORD, gastro-oesophageal reflux disease

Table 10.9 Comparison of H₂ antagonists

	Cimetidine	Ranitidine	Famotidine	Nizatidine
Bioavailability	60%	50%	43%	98%
Elimination half-life	2 h	2–3 h	3 h	1.3 h
Non-renal clearance	70%	30% i.v. 70% oral	30%	40%
Duration of action	5–6 h	9–10 h	12 h	11 h

Adverse drug reactions

H₂ receptor antagonists are a remarkably safe group of drugs. The risk of any adverse reaction is below 3% and serious adverse reactions account for less than 1%.

Drug interactions

Much has been made of the drug interactions with cimetidine; however, many have only been demonstrated in vitro and are of doubtful clinical significance (see Table 10.5). Cimetidine inhibits the activity of cytochrome P450 and consequently retards oxidative metabolism of a number of drugs. This interaction is potentially important for drugs with a narrow therapeutic index. The clearance of theophylline is reduced to about 40% of normal, and raised plasma levels occur as a result. Phenytoin metabolism is reduced, and toxicity is theoretically possible. The metabolism of a number of benzodiazepines, including diazepam, flurazepam and triazolam, is impaired, and levels are raised.

The interaction with warfarin has frequently been cited as justification to change to an alternative H₂ antagonist; however, careful investigation has shown that this interaction is complex. The metabolism of (R)-warfarin is affected to a greater degree than that of (S)-warfarin. As the (S) enantiomer is the more potent, the pharmacodynamic effects of the interaction may be modest although the plasma warfarin concentrations may be increased. Current opinion suggests that warfarin may safely be added with appropriate monitoring when patients are already taking cimetidine in regular daily doses. Other H₂ antagonists should be used in patients who are difficult to stabilize on warfarin or for whom frequent monitoring is not feasible.

Bismuth chelate

Bismuth has been included in antacid mixtures for many decades but fell from favour because of its neurotoxicity. Bismuth chelate is a relatively safe form of bismuth that has ulcer healing properties comparable to those of H₂ antagonists. Its mode of action is not clearly understood but it is thought to have cytoprotective properties. Bismuth is toxic to *H. pylori* and was one of the first agents to be used to eradicate the organism and reduce ulcer recurrence. A combination of ranitidine and bismuth as ranitidine bismuth citrate in combination with two antibiotics results in *H. pylori* eradication rates greater than 90%. Bismuth is also included in quadruple therapy regimens for use in patients resistant to triple therapy.

Adverse drug reactions

Small amounts of bismuth are absorbed from bismuth chelate, and urinary bismuth excretion may be raised for several weeks after a course of treatment. The risks of bismuth intoxication are small if these products are used with the recommended dose and for short courses of treatment. Bismuth may accumulate in patients with impaired renal function. The most commonly reported events are nausea, vomiting, blackened tongue and dark faeces.

Sucralfate

Sucralfate is the aluminium salt of sucrose octasulphate. Although it is a weak antacid, this is not its principal mode of action in peptic ulcer disease. It has mucosal protective effects including stimulation of bicarbonate and mucus secretion and stimulation of mucosal prostanoids. At pH < 4.0 it forms a sticky viscid gel that adheres to the ulcer surface and may afford some physical protection. It is capable of adsorbing bile salts. These activities appear to reside in the entire molecular complex and are not due to the aluminium ions alone. Sucralfate can be used to treat ulcers but it is mainly used in the prophylaxis of stress ulceration.

Adverse drug reactions

Constipation appears to be the most common problem with sucralfate, and this is thought to be related to the aluminium content. About 3–5% of a dose is absorbed, and therefore there is a risk of aluminium toxicity with long-term treatment. This risk is correspondingly greater in patients with renal impairment. Caution is required to avoid oesophageal bezoar formation around a nasogastric tube in patients managed in the intensive care unit.

Antacids

Antacids have a place in symptomatic relief of dyspepsia, in particular symptoms associated with gastro-oesophageal reflux disease. They have a role in the management of symptoms which sometimes remain for a short time after *H. pylori* eradication of uncomplicated duodenal ulcer. The choice of antacid lies between aluminium-based and magnesium-based products, although many proprietary products combine the two. Calcium-based products are unsuitable as calcium stimulates acid secretion. Antacids containing sodium bicarbonate are unsuitable for regular use because they deliver a high sodium load and generate large quantities of carbon dioxide. It should be noted that magnesium trisilicate mixtures contain a large amount of sodium bicarbonate. Some products contain other agents such as dimeticone or alginates. Products containing sodium alginate with a mixture of antacids are effective in relief of symptoms in gastro-oesophageal reflux disease but are not particularly effectual antacids.

Aluminium-based antacids cause constipation, and magnesium-based products cause diarrhoea. When combination products are used, diarrhoea tends to predominate as a side-effect. Although these are termed 'non-absorbable', a proportion of aluminium and magnesium is absorbed, and the potential for toxicity exists, particularly with coexistent renal failure.

The H_2 receptor antagonists can be purchased without a prescription for short-term symptomatic relief of dyspepsia. The doses recommended are less than those used in peptic ulcer disease or gastro-oesophageal reflux disease.

Future treatment strategies

Animal models are raising the possibility that therapeutic immunization against *H. pylori* might be a future option in the management of peptic ulcer disease. Potentially the young could be protected against the infection and existing infection could be eradicated, radically changing the epidemiology of peptic ulcer disease.

Costs of treatment

Eradication of *H. pylori* infection has revolutionized the therapeutic management of peptic ulcer disease. After successful eradication, the risk of ulcer recurrence is virtually eliminated, removing the need for maintenance therapy.

Upper gastrointestinal endoscopy is relatively inexpensive in the UK. In a health care system in which endoscopy is expensive, there might well be economic advantages in empirical therapy, either antisecretory or *H. pylori* eradication. A study in the UK has shown that non-invasive testing for *H. pylori* is as effective and less expensive than endoscopy in patients with uncomplicated dyspepsia (McColl et al 2002). The economic importance of prescription of antisecretory therapy in the general practice is immense. Out of 1000 patients in general practice, 15–20 will have peptic ulcer disease and 30–35 will have gastro-oesophageal reflux disease, while only one patient will have upper gastrointestinal cancer. Only a minority of patients with functional dyspepsia benefit from *H. pylori* eradication and many continue to use acid suppressing therapy.

Cost-effectiveness studies need to compare the benefits of COX-2 inhibition with non-selective NSAIDs and concomitant cytoprotective agents. The rapidly increasing use of aspirin in prevention of cardiovascular disease also has economical considerations in terms of gastroprotection.

Patient care

Patient education

Patients who present with symptoms of dyspepsia should be assessed in terms of risk of serious disease. Their age should be established and if they are over 45 years or exhibit alarm features, referral for investigation is indicated. In younger patients symptom assessment should be undertaken to identify whether or not the patient has reflux-like symptoms and is likely to respond to antacid/alginate medicines. Lifestyle should be assessed as weight loss is known to improve reflux symptoms in obese patients. Smoking contributes to heartburn symptoms and delays ulcer healing. A drug history should also be undertaken to identify likely drug-induced causes of symptoms. Many drugs can give rise to symptoms of dyspepsia. Drugs that decrease lower oesophageal sphincter tone may give rise to gastro-oesophageal reflux, eventually leading to oesophagitis. Several drugs are known to cause this, including anticholinergics, tricyclic antidepressants and calcium channel blockers. Patients taking prescribed medication which may contribute to symptoms should be referred to the general practitioner. If symptoms persist after 2 weeks of over-the-counter medication, the patient should also be referred to the general practitioner. Before initiating NSAID or aspirin therapy, patients should be assessed in terms of gastrointestinal risk. Many patients present with ulcer complications and describe no prior symptoms. Benefits must outweigh risks when patients with risk factors receive NSAIDs. Appropriate prophylaxis should be prescribed. Misoprostol should not be used in pregnant women, and women of child-bearing age should be warned appropriately.

Patients should be advised to seek the pharmacist's advice when purchasing over-the-counter analgesic preparations. Aspirin- and ibuprofen-containing preparations should be avoided in patients with dyspepsia or in those with risk factors for peptic ulcer disease. Products containing paracetamol should be recommended.

Patients with diagnosed peptic ulcer disease need to be educated about the current principles of therapeutic management. This education should assure adherence to prescribed medication and should be directed at correcting any misunderstandings about previous ulcer healing management. In most patients a single treatment course only is required and there is no need for maintenance therapy.

Patients receiving eradication therapy for *H. pylori* should be advised of the need to treat the organism using a combination of three drugs for a short period of time. Patient adherence is necessary for successful ulcer treatment. Previous adverse reactions should be established; for example patients who are sensitive to penicillin need an eradication regimen which does not include amoxicillin. Patients should be warned of the specific side-effects to be expected from the regimen that has been chosen for them and advised what to do should they experience any of these effects. Patients taking metronidazole must avoid alcohol as they might have a disulfiram-like reaction with sickness and headache. Patients also need to know how their therapy will be followed up.

Patient monitoring

Treatment success in peptic ulcer disease is measured by review of the patient in terms of symptom control. Patients with complicated ulcers or those who continue to have symptoms will receive a urea breath test and/or an endoscopy (see Fig.10.4). Patients should be aware of what their review will entail and when their review will take place. If patients comply with their medication the review process may be kept to a minimum.

Following eradication therapy some patients continue to experience symptoms of abdominal pain. Patients should be reassured that these symptoms will resolve spontaneously, but if necessary an antacid preparation can be recommended to relieve symptoms until review. Patients receiving treatment for NSAID-induced ulceration should continue their ulcer-healing therapy until review. Only patients who continue to take an NSAID require continued prophylactic therapy.

Patients who are anaemic following a bleeding ulcer may be prescribed iron therapy. If patients suffer side-effects such as constipation or diarrhoea, the dose of iron should be reduced. Treatment with iron should be for at least 3 months. Iron preparations are best absorbed from an empty stomach but if gastric discomfort is felt, the preparation should be taken with food.

Some common therapeutic problems in the treatment of peptic ulcer disease are summarized in Table 10.10.

CASE STUDIES

Case 10.1

Mrs M. P., a 60-year-old unemployed woman, who smokes 20 cigarettes a day and drinks over 25 units of alcohol per week, had eradication therapy for *H. pylori*-associated duodenal ulcer 12 months ago. She was asymptomatic after treatment, but 6 months later had recurrence of epigastric pain. A [^{14}C]urea breath test was positive. Her haemoglobin level was 14.2 g/dl and mean cell volume (MCV) was 102 fl.

Questions

1. What further evaluation is needed?
2. What treatment will you recommend?

Answers

1. Eradication treatment for *H. pylori* has failed in this patient. The reasons for failure may be non-compliance with treatment, drug resistance or re-infection, which is uncommon in the West. Mrs M. P.'s circumstances and alcohol abuse may underlie poor adherence. Metronidazole interacts with alcohol and may lead to side-effects, especially nausea, facial flushing and headache. It is therefore essential to know the exact drugs she had received, whether she had abstained from alcohol during therapy and whether she complied with treatment.
   The MCV in this patient is high. This is likely to be due to alcohol, but folate and vitamin B$_{12}$ levels need to be measured. Epigastric pain may be due to pancreatitis or cholecystitis and needs further investigations. Abdominal ultrasonography is necessary.
2. Mrs M. P. needs another 7 day course of eradication therapy with clarithromycin, amoxicillin and a proton pump inhibitor. The need to comply with therapy needs to be emphasized. Her eradication therapy course can be taken at a convenient time to allow her to cope with the common adverse effects such as diarrhoea, should she experience them. She should be advised that smoking can delay ulcer healing and she should try to stop the habit. Her symptoms should be assessed 4 weeks after completing eradication therapy. If her symptoms persist, the breath test should be repeated.

Case 10.2

Mrs C. S. is a 72-year-old woman with osteoarthritis of the knees who has taken diclofenac 50 mg three times daily

Table 10.10   Common therapeutic problems in peptic ulcer disease

	Comments
Ulcer-like symptoms of dyspepsia are not specific for peptic ulcer disease and are often present in functional (non-ulcer) dyspepsia. Empirical therapy should be based on underlying pathology	Predominant heartburn differentiates gastro-oesophageal reflux disease (GORD) from dyspepsia. Patients with GORD benefit from a stepped approach to antisecretory therapy. Patients with ulcers benefit from early diagnosis and treatment of *Helicobacter pylori*
In uncomplicated patients with ulcer-like symptoms of dyspepsia there is controversy about whether to investigate or treat patients empirically with drug therapy	There is no clear evidence to support early endoscopy in the investigation of uncomplicated dyspepsia. There is emerging evidence to suggest a 'test and treat' policy is as effective and safe as endoscopy in patients with uncomplicated dyspepsia.
Patients with ulcer-like pain but no ulcer detected on endoscopy fall into the diagnostic category of 'functional dyspepsia'	Meta-analysis has shown that a very small proportion of *H. pylori*-positive patients with functional dyspepsia benefit from eradication therapy. There is no evidence to confirm the cost-effectiveness of widespread eradication of *H. pylori* in primary care
Patients on proton pump inhibitors can have false-negative results for *H. pylori*	Proton pump inhibitors should be withdrawn at least 2 weeks before urea breath test or biopsy urease testing (endoscopy)
Following a 7 day eradication therapy regimen, antisecretory therapy can normally be stopped	Antisecretory therapy is required for a further 3 weeks in patients with active gastric ulcers or in patients with ulcers complicated by NSAID use
Patients taking aspirin or other NSAIDs chronically and test positive for *H. pylori*	There is no clear evidence that eradication of *H. pylori* has any beneficial or detrimental effects in patients on long-term NSAIDs. Eradication of *H. pylori* reduces the effectiveness of acid suppression and may influence gastroprotection in high risk patients on NSAIDs and antisecretory agents
Patients with NSAID associated active peptic ulcer disease who test positive for *H. pylori*	The ulcer should be healed with a proton pump inhibitor (PPI) for 4 weeks. Eradication therapy after the ulcer has healed may prevent re-bleeding
Treatment of NSAID-associated ulcers; choice and duration	If NSAIDs are withdrawn, healing rates are similar between H_2 receptor antagonists and PPIs after 8 weeks although PPIs heal ulcers more rapidly. Once healed, antisecretory therapy can be stopped. Continued NSAID use impairs healing and and PPIs are superior to H_2 receptor antagonists after 8 weeks. PPIs should be continued for prophylaxis if NSAIDs must be continued
Patients in whom low dose aspirin is indicated but have risk factors for peptic ulcer disease	There is no evidence to compare the risk of gastrointestinal bleeding with the benefits of low dose aspirin for thromboprophylaxis. Enteric coating does not reduce this risk
NSAID use in elderly patients	Patients over 65 years of age are at increased risk of peptic ulcer disease associated with NSAIDs and often present with 'silent ulcers'. NSAIDs (prescription and non-prescription) should be avoided in the elderly
Patients who are candidates for COX-2 inhibitors	COX-2 inhibitors are associated with less gastrointestinal toxicity than non-selective NSAIDs. NICE recommend that COX-2 inhibitors should be reserved for patients with rheumatoid arthritis or osteoarthritis who are at high risk of developing serious gastrointestinal adverse events. Concomitant aspirin reduces any benefit of using COX-2 inhibitors. There is no evidence that gastroprotective agents further reduce the risk of adverse events. There is no evidence to compare the reduction in risk associated with COX-2 inhibitors with non-selective NSAIDs in combination with gastroprotective agents

for the past 2 years. She was admitted to hospital following an episode of 'coffee ground' vomit and melaena stool. She had no symptoms of abdominal pain. Endoscopy revealed a gastric ulcer which was negative for *H. pylori*. Her full blood count revealed an iron deficiency anaemia. The patient had no documented history of cardiovascular disease but admitted to taking low dose aspirin daily for primary prevention of cardiovascular disease.

Questions

1. Were any gastrointestinal risk factors for NSAID toxicity present?
2. What ulcer treatment strategy would you recommend?
3. Discuss the therapeutic options to control her arthritic pain.

Answers

1. This lady's age places her at risk of developing peptic ulcer disease associated with NSAID therapy and patients > 60 years are more likely to develop potentially life-threatening complications such as perforation and haemorrhage than their younger counterparts. There may not be any warning symptoms prior to haemorrhage in patients such as Mrs C. S., who had an asymptomatic (silent) ulcer. Low dose aspirin itself poses a risk of upper gastrointestinal bleeding and potentiates the risk associated with non-aspirin NSAIDs. Superficial damage to the gastric mucosa can occur over a long period of chronic NSAID therapy and cause minor haemorrhage. In time this can result in iron deficiency anaemia. Mrs C. S. was anaemic on admission, and the haematological findings showed this to be the result of iron deficiency from both an acute and chronic bleed.
2. Initial treatment of Mrs C. S.'s bleeding ulcer should be adrenaline (epinephrine) injection to arrest the bleed. The reversal of melaena to normal stool gives an indication of the effectiveness of this treatment, which can be confirmed by follow-up endoscopy. If necessary a blood transfusion should be given. Ulcer-healing therapy should then be commenced and her NSAID discontinued. Low dose aspirin should also be discontinued as the benefits in terms of prevention of cardiovascular disease do not outweigh the risks of gastrointestinal toxicity. Treatment with a conventional ulcer-healing agent is indicated. Since proton pump inhibitors heal ulcers faster, current practice is to use these agents in elderly patients with ulcer complications. After 4–8 weeks of proton pump inhibitor therapy, Mrs C. S. should have a follow-up endoscopy to confirm ulcer healing.
3. Simple analgesics are first-line therapy for the control of mild to moderate pain associated with osteoarthritis in elderly patients. Paracetamol, when given at full therapeutic doses, has comparable efficacy to ibuprofen in the management of this type of pain. Paracetamol should be prescribed and Mrs C. S.'s pain assessed after the ulcer has healed.

   If Mrs C. S.'s osteoarthritis pain is poorly controlled after ulcer healing, an anti-inflammatory agent may have to be considered. The Medicine Control Agency recommends initiating therapy with the drug that has the lowest risk. The relative safety of a non-specific NSAID in combination with a gastroprotective agent in comparison to one of the newer coxibs is unknown. Gastroprotective agents reduce but do not abolish the risk of ulcers associated with NSAID

treatment. Trials suggest the coxibs have an incidence of gastrointestinal events similar to placebo, although during its initial year on the market, gastrointestinal adverse events accounted for half the adverse reactions associated with rofecoxib and 12% of these were for peptic ulcer complications. Cost-effectiveness studies are required to establish the most rational management option for Mrs C. S. The combination of ibuprofen, currently the safest conventional NSAID, and a proton pump inhibitor is less expensive than a coxib in terms of drug costs. Until future studies are conducted, this combination is likely to be the option chosen in practice.

Case 10.3

Mr B. C., a 38-year-old man, presented to his GP with abdominal pain, weight loss, nausea and early satiety. He was referred to the open access endoscopy clinic where endoscopy revealed an ulcerated lesion in the antrum of the stomach with raised, rolled edges. Biopsies showed a low-grade non-Hodgkin's lymphoma. His haemoglobin concentration was 10.1 g/dl with an MCV of 72 fl.

Question

Did the GP take appropriate action?

Answer

Alarm symptoms that may indicate the presence of underlying malignancy in patients presenting with dyspepsia are weight loss, early satiety, anorexia and vomiting. It is imperative that these symptoms be investigated irrespective of age. Empirical therapy is unwise, and this patient should undergo an endoscopy. The microcytic anaemia is suggestive of iron deficiency and chronic blood loss.

It is important to investigate the extent (i.e. stage) of the disease using computed tomography (CT) and abdominal and endoscopic ultrasonography. Low-grade gastric lymphomas are associated with *H. pylori* infection, and eradication of *H. pylori* may lead to complete regression of these tumours. Hence, *H. pylori* status should be established. Otherwise surgical resection will probably be required. *H. pylori* is also regarded as a class 1 carcinogen for gastric carcinomas.

Case 10.4

Mrs M. B. is a 35-year-old overweight young professional who visits the pharmacy complaining of severe retrosternal pain. On enquiry she describes a 1 month history of milder symptoms occasionally after eating a heavy meal late at night. She does not take any medication but requests something to relieve these more severe symptoms.

Question

What advice should be given?

Answer

Gastro-oesophageal reflux disease is a very common cause of dyspepsia. Clearance of refluxed acid and pepsin relies primarily on oesophageal peristalsis induced by swallowing. Refluxed contents are neutralized by the alkaline saliva, while other protective mechanisms include gastric emptying and the tone of the lower oesophageal sphincter. A breakdown of any of these protective mechanisms allows acid to damage the oesophageal mucosa.

Direct mucosal irritation results in heartburn whereas more severe chest pain is the result of acid-induced oesophageal spasm that may radiate to the jaw or arm. These symptoms typically occur within 1 hour of a meal and tend to occur on stooping or lying in bed at night. Precipitating factors that weaken the normal protective mechanisms include eating large meals at night, especially fatty meals which delay gastric emptying, coffee, alcohol and wearing tight clothing.

Mrs M. B. may therefore appreciate some advice to help herself control her symptoms through altering her lifestyle. It is unlikely that Mrs M. B. is suffering from gastric or oesophageal cancer as she did not describe any other alarming symptoms such as weight loss, bleeding or dysphagia. The pain of a duodenal ulcer is more likely to be epigastric, radiating to the back. The retrosternal pain of oesophageal spasm does, however, resemble ischaemic heart disease, therefore Mrs M. B. should be advised to see her general practitioner, and to try a regular antacid/alginate preparation after meals and at bedtime. Alginates act by forming a viscous layer on top of the gastric contents, providing a barrier to reflux.

Case 10.5

Mr S. T. is a 63-year-old man with a history of angina and asthma. He takes diltiazem, aspirin, a beclometasone inhaler and theophylline to treat these conditions and uses a salbutamol inhaler when breathless. He was admitted to hospital with chest pain. Cardiovascular investigations indicated stable angina. He was referred for endoscopy, which revealed severe grade C oesophagitis.

Questions

1. What treatment strategy would you recommend for Mr S. T.'s oesophagitis?
2. Does his medication require review in light of this diagnosis?

Answers

1. Proton pump inhibitors are more effective than H_2 receptor antagonists in controlling symptoms and healing oesophagitis. In severe oesophagitis full treatment doses of proton pump inhibitors are required for 8 weeks to relieve symptoms and heal oesophagitis. Endoscopy is repeated to confirm healing, and maintenance therapy with a treatment dose of proton pump inhibitor is continued to prevent relapse in patients with grade C or D oesophagitis.
2. Drugs such as theophylline can contribute to oesophagitis. Review of Mr S. T.'s asthma management and assessment

of his inhaler technique to ensure maximum benefit from inhaled corticosteroid therapy may permit withdrawal of theophylline. If theophylline is necessary, then he should be instructed to take the medication with a full glass of water to minimize local mucosal damage.

Diltiazem has the potential to relax the smooth muscle of the oesophagus, allowing longer exposure of the mucosa to acid and pepsin. Mr S. T.'s angina appears to be well controlled and the alternative β-blockers are contraindicated in asthma and therefore it is likely that the benefits of diltiazem outweigh the potential harmful effects on the oesophagus.

The potential risk of peptic ulceration and bleeding associated with low dose aspirin therapy will be reduced with concomitant use of a proton pump inhibitor, prescribed to control Mr S. T.'s gastro-oesophageal reflux disease.

Case 10.6

Mr G. T., a 52-year-old lecturer, presented to his general practitioner complaining of recurrent but mild upper abdominal discomfort occurring on at least 5 days every week. This was associated with nausea. The symptoms did not respond to over-the-counter antacids and H_2-receptor antagonists and after 8 months of symptoms he decided to seek medical advice. His physical examination was normal apart from being overweight (body mass index (BMI) = 29 kg/m^2). He was a non-smoker and drank 10 units of alcohol per week on average. His only medication consisted of simvastatin 20 mg per day. An ultrasound scan of the abdomen showed a normal gallbladder. He was referred for an open-access endoscopy which showed Barrett's oesophagus, a sliding hiatus hernia, no oesophagitis and a slightly red gastric antral mucosa, which was positive for *Helicobacter pylori* on biopsy.

Question

What management measures should be taken?

Answer

Mr G. T. has non-ulcer dyspepsia. Simvastatin might give rise to abdominal symptoms. Acid suppressant therapy does not reverse columnar lined oesophagus with intestinal metaplasia (Barrett's oesophagus), though the metaplastic change might have been provoked by acid reflux. Patients with Barrett's oesophagus have an increased risk of developing oesophageal adenocarcinoma, and endoscopic surveillance to detect high grade dysplasia is undertaken by some but not all gastroenterologists. Eradication of *H. pylori* may improve symptoms of non-ulcer dyspepsia in approximately 10% of patients. Weight loss might improve general health but its effect on gastro-oesophageal reflux is minimal. Mr G. T. was treated with domperidone 10 mg three times daily half an hour before meals for 1 month; this improved his abdominal symptoms. Subsequently, reassurance, information regarding the link with simvastatin and recruitment into a Barrett's surveillance programme with endoscopy every 3 years was sufficient and he required no further drug therapy.

REFERENCES

Agrawal N M, Campbell D R, Safdi M A et al 2000 Superiority of lansoprazole vs ranitidine in healing nonsteroidal anti-inflammatory drug-associated gastric ulcers. Archives of Internal Medicine 160: 1455–1461

Bombardier C, Laine L, Reicin A et al 2000 Comparison of upper gastrointestinal toxicity of rofecoxib and naproxen in patients with rheumatoid arthritis. VIGOR Study Group. New England Journal of Medicine 343: 1520–1528

Chan F K, Sung J J, Chung S C et al 1997 Randomised trial of eradication of *Helicobacter pylori* before non-steroidal anti-inflammatory drug therapy to prevent peptic ulcers. Lancet 350: 975–979

Chan F K, Chung S C, Suen B Y et al 2001 Preventing recurrent upper gastrointestinal bleeding in patients with *Helicobacter pylori* infection who are taking low dose aspirin or naproxen. New England Journal of Medicine 344: 967–973

Derry S, Loke Y K 2000 Risk of gastrointestinal haemorrage with long term aspirin: meta-analysis. British Medical Journal 321: 1183–1187

Graham D Y, Lew G M, Malaty H M et al 1992 Factors influencing the eradication of *Helicobacter pylori* with triple therapy. Gastroenterology 102: 493–496

Hawkey C J, Tulassay Z, Szczepanski L et al 1998a Randomised controlled trial of *Helicobacter pylori* eradication in patients on non-steroidal anti-inflammatory drugs: HELP NSAIDs study. Lancet 352: 1016–1021

Hawkey C J, Karrasch J A, Szczepanski L et al 1998b Omeprazole compared with misoprostol for ulcers associated with nonsteroidal antiinflammatory drugs. The OMNIUM Study Group. New England Journal of Medicine 338: 727–734

Hawkey C J 2000 Nonsteroidal anti-inflammatory drug gastropathy. Gastroenterology 119: 521–535

Hawkey C J, Jackson L, Harper S E et al 2001 The gastrointestinal safety profile of rofecoxib, a highly selective inhibitor of cyclooxygenase-2, in humans. [Review article.] Alimentary Pharmacology and Therapeutics 15: 1–9

Hudson N, Taha A S, Russell R I et al 1997 Famotidine for healing and maintenance in non-steroidal anti-inflammatory drug-associated gastroduodenal ulceration. Gastroenterology 112: 1817–1822

Lau J Y, Sung J J, Lee K K et al 2000 Effect of intravenous omeprazole on recurrent bleeding after endoscopic treatment of bleeding peptic ulcers. New England Journal of Medicine 343: 310–316

Lind T, Veldhuyzen van Zanten S, Unge P et al 1996 Eradication of *Helicobacter pylori* using one-week triple therapies combining omeprazole with two antimicrobials: the MACH 1 study. Helicobacter 1: 138–144

Lind T, Megraud F, Unge P et al 1999 The MACH-2 study: role of omeprazole in eradication of *Helicobacter pylori* with 1-week triple therapies. Gastroenterology 116: 248–253

McColl K E L, Murray L S, Gillen D et al 2002 Randomised trial of endoscopy with testing for *Helicobacter pylori* compared with non-invasive *H. pylori* testing alone in the management of dyspepsia. British Medical Journal 324: 999–1006

Messori A, Trippoli S, Vaiani M et al 2000 Bleeding and pneumonia in intensive care patients given ranitidine and sucralfate for prevention of stress ulcer: meta-analysis of randomised controlled trials. British Medical Journal 321: 1103–1106

Rose P, Huang B, Lukasik N et al 1999 Evidence that lansoprazole is effective in preventing NSAID-induced ulcers. Gastroenterology 166: G1293

Schoenfeld P, Kimmey M B, Scheiman J et al 1999 Nonsteroidal anti-inflammatory drug-associated gastrointestinal complications-guidelines for prevention and treatment. [Review article.] Alimentary Pharmacology and Therapeutics 13: 1273–1285

Silverstein F E, Faich G, Goldstein J L et al 2000 Gastrointestinal toxicity with celecoxib vs nonsteroidal anti-inflammatory drugs for osteoarthritis and rheumatoid arthritis. The CLASS Study. Journal of the American Medical Association 284: 1247–1255

Sorensen H T, Mellemkjaer L, Blot W J et al 2000 Risk of upper gastrointestinal bleeding associated with use of low dose aspirin. American Journal of Gastroenterology 95: 2218–2224

Talley N J, Zinsmeister A R, Schleck C D et al 1992 Dyspepsia and dyspepsia subgroups: a population-based study. Gastroenterology 102: 1259–1268

Yeomans N D, Tulassay Z, Juhasz L et al 1998 A comparison of omeprazole with ranitidine for ulcers associated with nonsteroidal antiinflammatory drugs. The ASTRONAUT Study Group. New England Journal of Medicine 338: 719–726

FURTHER READING

British Society of Gastroenterology 1996 Dyspepsia management guidelines. British Society of Gastroenterology, London Revised version April 2002 available on BSG website www.bsg.org.uk

Dent J, Brun J, Fendrick A M et al 1999 An evidence-based appraisal of reflux disease management. The Genval Workshop Report. Gut 44(Suppl. 2): S1–S16

National Institute for Clinical Excellence 2000 Guidance on the use of proton pump inhibitors in the treatment of dyspepsia.

National Institute for Clinical Excellence (NICE) Technology Appraisal Guidance No 7. NICE, London, July 2000

Rubin G P, Hungin A P S 1998 Guidelines for the management of *Helicobacter pylori* in primary care. Digestion 59(Suppl. 3): 428

Scottish Intercollegiate Guidelines Network 1996 *Helicobacter pylori* eradication therapy in dyspeptic disease. Guideline No. 7. SIGN, Edinburgh

Inflammatory bowel disease

11

B. K. Evans

KEY POINTS

- Inflammatory bowel diseases are chronic relapsing conditions with a high morbidity and remain largely incurable. Routine treatment has not changed significantly over the last 40 years and still relies heavily on steroids and aminosalicylates. Epidemiology and aetiology of the diseases also remain consistent.
- Ulcerative colitis and Crohn's disease are in many respects similar but there are contrasting features, which relate to the site of involvement and extent of inflammation across the bowel wall.
- Both disease occur in adults and children. The differences between the diseases have a bearing on the therapeutic approach.
- Ulcerative colitis is limited to the large bowel and the mucosa, whereas Crohn's disease frequently involves the small intestine with inflammation extending through the bowel wall to the serosal surface.
- Although the mucosa is involved in both diseases, agents which target topical application of a drug to the inflamed mucosa might be expected to be more effective in colitis than in Crohn's disease where the systemic level of drug in blood supplying the bowel wall may be important.
- The only well-established therapies for colitis are mesalazine and steroids in their various formulations. Other potential alternatives do not yet have a clearly established role in clinical management.
- Original formulation designs to deliver mesalazine to the colon have led to their use for colonic delivery of other drugs including steroids. The systems have been based on coating materials which make delayed release possible when applied not only to the solid dose form but also to microgranules, microspheres and even powders.
- The development and use of humanized monoclonal antibodies to treat inflammatory bowel disease by inhibiting tumour necrosis factor-α (TNF-α), a key cytokine is a novel and effective approach to treatment.

Introduction

Crohn's disease and ulcerative colitis are chronic inflammatory conditions of the gut, characterized by periods of remission and relapse over many years. Although quite distinct pathologically, the treatment, including drug therapy, is often very similar.

Crohn's disease

Crohn's disease takes its name from one of the three physicians who first described the disease in 1932; Crohn's may affect any part of the gastrointestinal tract from the lips to the anal margin, but ileocolic disease remains the commonest presentation. The disease produces considerable morbidity, the cause remains unknown and current treatment is palliative not curative (Hanauer and Meyers 1997).

Epidemiology

Crohn's disease is very common in northern Europe and North America. It is occurring more frequently in southern Europe but is relatively uncommon in other areas of the world. The highest prevalence is in Scandinavia and Britain (26–75 per 100 000 population).

The incidence of Crohn's disease has risen during the last two decades, a rise which cannot solely be attributed to an increased differential diagnosis from ulcerative colitis. The condition is marginally more common in females and most commonly diagnosed in patients between the ages of 15 and 40 years.

Aetiology

Generally investigations have centred on the role of immunological mechanisms as a causative factor in Crohn's disease but all have been inconclusive.

Immunology

Normal humoral immune responses are seen in patients with Crohn's disease although a defect in the cell mediated immune functions may exist due to malnutrition. Improvement in nutritional status will often improve the immune response.

Genetic factors

A consistent genetic association has not been established although 10% of patients have a first degree relative with the disease while siblings are affected 30 times more often than the general population. Evidence confirms a tenfold familial risk for Crohn's disease and ulcerative colitis. Ankylosing spondylitis sufferers have a ninefold greater prevalence of Crohn's disease. It remains unclear whether Crohn's sufferers are more likely to develop atopic disease, although they are often from families with a history of atopic conditions.

Diet

Dietary intake has centred on milk, fibre and sugar. The role of fibre and milk consumption in Crohn's patients has not been clearly established although some work has confirmed a high refined carbohydrate intake by sufferers compared with controls.

Patients with Crohn's disease are more likely to be smokers than are controls, with the association being stronger for smoking habit prior to disease onset than current smoking habit.

The risk of developing the disease increases in women who use oral contraceptives.

Infective agents

Pathological similarities between Crohn's disease and tuberculosis have focused attention on *Mycobacterium* species, but again no consistent evidence is available. Crohn's disease sufferers have higher faecal counts of anaerobic Gram-negative rods and Gram-positive coccoid rods from *Coprococcus* subspecies and *Peptostreptococcus* subspecies but the implications of this are unclear.

Pathophysiology

Ileocolonic disease accounts for 60% of all cases of Crohn's disease, with only 20% having colonic involvement and the remainder having ileal or proximal small bowel disease.

Chronic inflammation of the bowel wall, often associated with granulomas and deep fissuring ulceration, is common. Patches of defined inflamed areas appear interdispersed by normal bowel. The relationship between pathological and clinical features is shown in Table 11.1.

Clinical manifestation

The major clinical features presented depend on the site, extent and severity of disease at presentation. Patients complain of ill health, lassitude and recurrent fever. Clinical features of intestinal involvement are abdominal pain, nausea, diarrhoea, anorexia, and abdominal tenderness. Quite often weight loss is the most striking feature as a consequence of anorexia. Considering the

Table 11.1 Relationship between pathological and clinical features (from Misiewicz et al 1994, with kind permission from Blackwell Scientific Publications Oxford)

Pathological features	Clinical features
Thickened bowel wall	Obstructive symptoms
Submucosal fibrosis	Proximal bowel distension
Narrow lumen and strictures	
Transmural fissures	Adhesions
Serosal inflammation	Inflammatory masses
	Abscesses
	Fistulae to adherent bowel, skin or other organs

chronic inflammatory nature of the condition, it is surprising that initial presentation may vary from a form of fulminant colitis or be relatively benign.

Terminal ileal disease causes localized abdominal pain associated with a palpable tender mass while some patients with extensive disease present with only weight loss. Children affected before puberty may suffer retarded growth and sexual development.

Anal and rectal pathology is the basis for diagnosis. Anal features frequently occur with ilecocolonic disease but not with isolated small bowel involvement. The most distressing aspect is sepsis from secondary abseses and perianal fistulae. Despite anal involvement the rectal mucosa is often unaffected except in severe cases when the mucosa appears thickened.

Intestinal obstruction due to a simple stricture is probably the most common complication in Crohn's disease. Resolution can occur spontaneously but severe attacks may require surgery. Perforations producing an abscess can be seen in patients with very active disease. In colonic disease rectal bleeding of the inflamed mucosa is likely, gradually causing iron deficiency anaemia. During active disease intra-abdominal abscesses discharge their contents through fistulae, which sometimes open to the skin and may also penetrate the bladder and vaginal wall, causing recurrent infections.

There appears to be an increased risk of gastrointestinal malignancy but this remains unproven. Systemic illnesses may accompany the condition and these are shown in Figure 11.1.

Investigations

Clinical, radiological and pathological investigations will confirm diagnosis and recurrent disease. Colonoscopy helps to assess the extent of disease and the nature of colonic strictures and polyps.

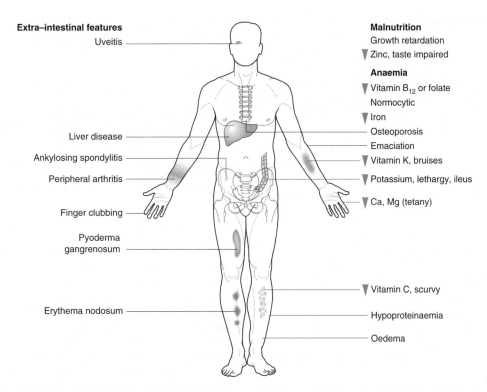

Figure 11.1 Some of the extra-intestinal illnesses and features of malnutrition found in patients with Crohn's disease (from Misiewicz et al 1994, with kind permission from Blackwell Scientific Publications, Oxford).

Radiology

Upper bowel radiology is performed using a conventional barium meal followed through the small intestine, while a double contrast barium enema is used in the colon. Narrowed segments of bowel with ulcerated mucosa are commonly seen in the small intestine, with proximal dilatation. Duodenal strictures may cause gastric dilatation and delayed gastric emptying. Distinguishing features include the appearance of aphthoid ulcers, lesions with predominantly right-sided involvement, strictures and fissures.

Histology

Histology confirms the diagnosis and prevents certain small bowel and colonic lesions being wrongly labelled Crohn's disease. Initial diagnosis is frequently established following rectal biopsies, identifying the presence of granulomas, patchy mucosal inflammation, well-preserved goblet cells and few crypt abscesses. This contrasts with the uniformally heavy lymphocytic infiltration of the mucosa in ulcerative colitis (Fig. 11.2). Biopsies taken during treatment provide an indication of patient response.

Crohn's	Features	Ulcerative colitis
Normal	Goblet cells	Depleted
Scanty	Crypt abcesses	Common
Preserved	Glandular architecture	Distorted atrophic
Patchy, heavy in places	Lymphocytic infiltrate	Uniformly heavy
Present	Granulomas	Absent
Normal	Muscularis mucosae	Thickened
Disproportionately heavy	Submucosal inflammation	Little

Figure 11.2 Histological features in the rectal biopsy that helps to distinguish between ulcerative colitis and Crohn's disease (from Misiewicz et al 1994, with kind permission from Blackwell Scientific Publications, Oxford).

Clinical assessment

A practical clinical index is valuable in assessing disease activity and response to medical treatment, and in evaluating surgical intervention. A suitable index would include general well-being, abdominal pain, diarrhoea, presence of an abdominal mass and intestinal or systemic complications.

Because abdominal pain and diarrhoea may be unrelated to disease activity the index should be supplemented with laboratory parameters, such as serum orosomucoids, C-reactive protein and faecal α_1-antitrypsin concentrations. Alternatively erythrocyte sedimentation rate, albumin concentration and platelet count are helpful.

Malnutrition is often a major problem and assessment of a patient's nutritional status using a mid-arm circumference is important in terms of the treatment programme.

Ulcerative colitis

Ulcerative colitis is a chronic relapsing inflammatory disorder affecting colonic and rectal mucosa. Its origin and cause remain unclear. The first definitive description of this condition was made in 1909 and in certain aspects it resembles Crohn's disease.

If ulcerative colitis affects only the rectal mucosa it is termed proctitis, if it involves the rectum and the sigmoid colon it is known as proctosigmoiditis. Involvement of other parts of the colon is termed colitis. The disease tends to progress proximally. Current therapy is palliative not curative (Hanauer 2000).

Epidemiology

Figures from north-western Europe, and the USA show similar prevalence rates of 79.9 and 87.0 per 100 000 population, respectively. Incidence rates based on hospitalized patients vary between 4.7 and 15.1 per 100 000 population for the USA and western Europe.

A twofold increase occurred during the 1950s and 1960s but incidence has remained steady over the last 20 years.

Contrary to the findings of earlier studies, there is no variation between men and women or between different socioeconomic groups. However, ulcerative colitis is more common in non-smokers, quite the opposite of Crohn's disease.

All age groups are at risk, and the peak age of onset is between 15 and 40 years.

Aetiology

Genetic factors

Familial or genetic incidence of ulcerative colitis shows a wide variation from 1% to 16% among immediate family members, with a possible tenfold increase in likelihood occurring when the parent has the disease.

Environmental factors

Infective agents, diet and psychosocial stress may be important but their present role remains ill defined and unconfirmed. Like Crohn's sufferers, urban dwellers appear to be more at risk than rural dwellers.

Similarly, evidence linking fibre, milk and food intake to ulcerative colitis is lacking although countries where fibre intake is high appear to have a low incidence.

Pathophysiology

Although scientific and clinical evidence linking immunology with disease pathogenesis is lacking, some patients suffering from proctitis have a higher serum IgG concentration than controls. Serum antibodies against intestinal bacteria and colon epithelial component antigens have also been found but are considered to be secondary to a damaged mucosa.

Complement found in the basement membrane of patients' colonic epithelium is evidence of deposition of immune complex in the mucosa. Monocyte stimulation by these complexes may explain the increased prostaglandin synthesis that occurs in active disease.

Water and electrolyte balance is affected in extensive ulcerative colitis as a result of reduction in the absorption of sodium, chloride and water. Daily faecal weights of patients are generally higher than in normal subjects with proctitis sufferers sometimes demonstrating a slightly raised potassium to sodium ratio. Malabsorption of salt and water in the colon occurs as a result of decreased permeability of the mucosa to chloride ions and a defect in active sodium transport.

Macroscopic examination of the rectum showing excoriated skin is often the first pathological evidence, and in acute active disease, blood, pus and mucus discharge from the colon to the rectum. Sigmoidoscopy will confirm the presence of granular haemorrhagic mucosa, and the extent of disease. With inactive disease the rectal mucosa appears quite normal but close macroscopical examination reveals an abnormal vessel pattern, together with a fine granularity.

Microscopic examination allows subdivision of the disease into active colitis, resolving colitis and colitis in remission. Active disease is characterized by dilatation of local blood capillaries and haemorrhages, reduction in goblet cell population and epithelial cell necrosis and the presence of crypt abscesses formed following polymorphonuclear cell infiltration of the lamina propria (see Fig. 11.2). Although generally confined to the mucosa if ulceration is present, inflammatory cells may infiltrate the submucosa. During treatment, microscopical examination reveals a reduction of cellular infiltration of the lamina propria and restoration of the goblet cell population. This phase is termed resolving colitis and disease remission is recognized by shortening of the crypts, with a defined gap between the crypt base and the muscularis mucosae.

Clinical manifestations

Depending on the severity and site of activity, patients can present with systemic and intestinal symptoms. A patient with proctitis may show only intestinal symptoms such as pain, diarrhoea and rectal bleeding but a patient suffering from proctosigmoiditis is likely to have more severe symptoms.

Abdominal pain is graded in degrees of severity relating to the extent of colonic involvement. Total colitis is usually accompanied by severe persistent pain whereas this rarely occurs in proctitis.

The majority of patients have diarrhoea, the severity relating to the extent of the disease. However, elderly patients suffering from proctosigmoiditis may complain of constipation. Blood coating a formed stool usually suggests proctitis and patients may display systemic symptoms such as anorexia, weight loss, lethargy and fever.

Active disease is classified as mild, moderate or severe and of short- or long-term duration. Number of bowel motions, macroscopic appearance of blood in stools, anaemia and erythrocyte sedimentation rates are used quantitatively to determine disease severity.

Investigations

Endoscopy

Sigmoidoscopy is used to confirm diagnosis of ulcerative colitis. Rectal biopsies support the diagnosis and are used to evaluate progress, assess the patient's response to treatment and differentiate between ulcerative colitis and other causes of proctitis such as Crohn's disease. Disease assessment takes note of the appearance of the mucosa, changes in the vascular pattern, and severity of spontaneous bleeding.

Examination further along the colon from the rectum requires colonoscopy, which allows assessment of extent of disease, and the taking of multiple biopsies.

Radiology

Double contrast barium enemas will detect early mucosal changes and the extent of the disease. The typical radiograph of the chronic stage of ulcerative colitis shows a narrowing of the lumen, the walls becoming more rigid and the bowel shortened (Fig. 11.3).

Plain abdominal radiographs, not barium enemas, are used when initial diagnosis indicates the presence of acute disease or toxic dilatation.

Laboratory

Haematological and biochemical values pointing to ulcerative colitis include iron deficiency anaemia, elevated white cell count, raised erythrocyte sedimentation rate and a low serum albumin. Microbiological examination of stool samples taken at initial diagnosis may provide evidence of infection as a cause of colonic inflammation.

Clinical assessment

Treatment is aimed at resolving the disease and maintaining the patient in remission although a small number of patients suffer continuous symptoms. Patient management revolves around the treatment of acute attacks, maintenance of remission and assessing the risk of colonic carcinoma.

Sudden deterioration in a patient's condition may occur as a consequence of toxic dilatation which, if untreated, can prove fatal following colonic perforation. Early diagnosis of inflammatory bowel disease is

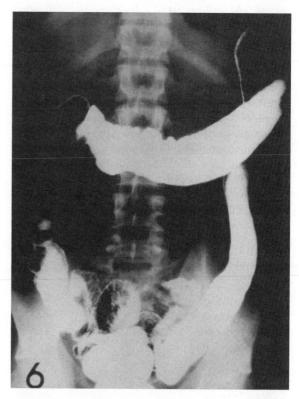

Figure 11.3 Ulcerative colitis showing total involvement with loss of haustral pattern and fine ulceration. (By courtesy of Professor John Rhodes.)

difficult and may delay treatment. This is particularly true in children and young adults (Winter 2000).

Treatment of inflammatory bowel disease

A wide range of drugs and nutritional supplements are available to maintain the patient in long periods of remission in both Crohn's disease and ulcerative colitis. However, surgical intervention will eventually become necessary when the patient relapses and fails to respond to drug therapy.

Nutritional needs

Although dietary control of the disease is usually inappropriate, some dietary refinements can be beneficial (Fernandes-Banares et al 1999). For example, patients with small intestinal strictures should avoid indigestible foods that may cause obstruction by aggregation at strictures (Table 11.2).

Carbohydrate intake is often higher than the population average but subsequent reduction is not associated with clinical improvement. Inadequate food intake is sometimes presented as a problem in Crohn's disease and patients with a poor appetite will often respond to supplemental enteral feeds.

Malnourished patients undergoing surgery should have their nutritional status improved, which may even render surgery unnecessary. Abnormal growth patterns in children with Crohn's disease can be corrected by concurrent enteral and medical therapy. Many nutritional deficiencies are associated with inflammatory bowel disease due to malabsorption following extensive small bowel resection. Iron depletion, hypoproteinaemia, deficiencies in water- and fat-soluble vitamins, trace elements and electrolytes can be corrected using a suitable replacement regimen.

Table 11.2 Foods to avoid in inflammatory bowel disease (from Misiewicz et al 1994, with kind permission from Blackwell Scientific Publications, Oxford)

Foods that may cause bolus obstruction if there is an intestinal stricture:

  Segments of any citrus fruit
  Sweetcorn
  Coleslaw or uncooked vegetables
  Raw fruits, unless chewed thoroughly
  Nuts
  Popcorn
  Tough or gristly meat

A total parenteral nutrition (TPN) regimen suitable for each patient can be established and maintained where appropriate. Often the most successful is one based on using partial parenteral and enteral nutrition.

Drug treatment

Current drug treatment aims to induce and then maintain the patient in remission and ameliorate the disease's secondary effects rather than modify or reverse the underlying pathogenic mechanism (Meyers & Sachar 1995). Corticosteroids, aminosalicylates and immunosuppressive agents such as azathioprine are routinely used. Other drugs such as metronidazole, ciclosporin, broad-spectrum antibiotics, nicotine and thalidomide are helpful in some cases, while colestyramine, sodium cromoglicate, bismuth and arsenical salts, methotrexate, lidocaine (lignocaine), sucralfate, new steroid entities, cytoprotective agents, fish oils and human growth hormone may well provide future alternative therapy. A new treatment approach using humanized monoclonal antibody preparations has so far produced encouraging results and may eventually provide a welcome alternative in that these drugs modify the affected biochemical inflammatory pathways.

Corticosteroids

The glucocorticoid properties of hydrocortisone and prednisolone are the mainstay of treatment. The preferred steroid is prednisolone, administered orally or rectally, and parenterally in emergency situations.

Corticosteroids can be used either alone or in combination with a suitable mesalazine formulation to induce and maintain remission in inflammatory bowel disease. Moderately ill patients require prednisolone in doses of 30–40 mg/day orally, in divided doses, for 2–3 weeks. Depending on the patient's response, a gradual dose reduction can be introduced to 10–20 mg/day for 4–6 weeks. Milder cases can be controlled by morning administration only, mimicking the diurnal rhythm of the body's cortisol secretion. Severe extensive or fulminant disease will require hospitalization and the use of parenteral therapy using hydrocortisone sodium succinate, administered intramuscularly or intravenously in doses of 100–500 mg three or four times a day. Oral prednisolone therapy should be introduced as soon as possible.

Abrupt withdrawal of steroids must be avoided. Maintenance doses are normally in the range of 6–15 mg daily or on alternate days.

The incidence of adverse effects appears to increase when prednisolone doses are higher than 40 mg/day. An alternate-day regimen is helpful, causing less adrenal suppression. Azathioprine, with its steroid-sparing property, may be introduced together with a lower dose of steroid or as an alternative.

Formulations. Oral administration will control moderate inflammatory bowel disease but proctitis, left-sided disease and Crohn's disease of the anus and rectum are more appropriately treated using topical preparations. The choice of locally applied formulations will depend on patient acceptability and preference (Table 11.3).

Prednisolone sodium phosphate and metasulpho-benzoate enemas, hydrocortisone acetate foam enema and hydrocortisone and prednisolone sodium phosphate suppositories are available. Pack presentation is important to the patient because the ease with which a patient can open a suppository pack or insert an enema will influence compliance. Self-administration of a short tube enema may be difficult for rheumatic patients who may cope using the long tube version. The enema's volume and viscosity must allow easy application and retention. Foam formulations, which adhere to the mucosa, may be preferred.

Following rectal administration, prednisolone metasulphobenzoate is poorly absorbed compared to prednisolone-21-phosphate but gives comparative therapeutic results. These factors must be considered when recommending a suitable preparation. Rectal administration should be performed just before bedtime when the supine position allows much longer retention times.

Uncoated steroid tablets are suitable for most patients while enteric-coated preparations do not offer any proven advantage. Patients with short bowel or strictures should avoid enteric-coated preparations because of poor absorption and bolus formation at strictures, respectively. Prednisolone steaglate appears to be more rapidly absorbed from the gut and is slowly metabolized to prednisolone.

Other steroids

New molecular configurations and formulations of steroids are being investigated. Methylprednisolone 40 mg enema appears as effective as hydrocortisone 100 mg in achieving remission. Similarly, betamethasone valerate enema, beclometasone diproprionate and budesonide enema 2 mg/100 ml compare favourably with hydrocortisone, prednisone and prednisolone, respectively. Budesonide treatment also has fewer side-effects. Oral formulations of budesonide and fluticasone appear beneficial to some patients (Thomsen et al 1998).

Tixocortol pivolate, a cortisol derivative, possesses anti-inflammatory activity equivalent to hydrocortisone, demonstrates a lower incidence of side-effects and like betamethasone and budesonide undergoes extensive first-pass metabolism.

Aminosalicylates

Aminosalicylates can be used in combination with steroids to induce and maintain remission in inflammatory bowel disease. Sulfasalazine is most effective in maintaining remission in ulcerative colitis. Its use in Crohn's disease is less well-established (Prantera et al 1999).

Sulfasalazine consists of sulfapyridine diazoized to 5-amino salicylic acid (5-ASA, mesalazine). When it reaches the colon the diazo bond is cleaved by bacterial azoreductase liberating mesalazine and sulfapyridine. Sulfapyridine is absorbed and metabolized by hepatic acetylation or hydroxylation followed by glucuronidation. Mesalazine is partly absorbed, metabolized by the liver and excreted via the kidneys as n-acetyl 5-amino-salicylic acid, although the majority is acetylated during passage through the intestinal mucosa Sulfasalazine itself is poorly absorbed. That which is absorbed is recycled back into the gut via the bile either unchanged or as the n-acetyl metabolite.

Table 11.3 Comparison of commercially available preparations for rectal administration in inflammatory bowel disease

Generic name	Formulation	Site of release
Sulfasalazine	Suppositories Retention enema	Descending colon and rectum
Mesalazine	Retention enema Foam enema Suppositories	Descending colon and rectum
Prednisolone sodium phosphate	Retention enema	Rectum and rectosigmoid colon
Prednisolone (metasulphobenzoate or 21-phosphate)	Retention enema	Ascending transverse and descending colon
Hydrocortisone (acetate)	Foam enema	Rectum and descending colon

Sulfasalazine metabolites are responsible for the yellow colouration of urine. Elimination of sulfapyridine depends on the patient's acetylator phenotype; those who inherit the 'slow' acetylator phenotype experience more side-effects. Mesalazine is the active component of sulfasalazine exerting a predominant local topical action independent of blood levels. Its effectiveness depends on the site of ulceration in relation to the drug's dissolution profile. This is very important when choosing aminosalicylate preparations, as illustrated in Figure 11.4.

The optimal dose of sulfasalazine to achieve and maintain remission is usually in the range of 2–4 g per day in four divided doses. Acute attacks require 4–8 g per day in divided doses until remission occurs, but at these doses associated side-effects begin to appear.

Of patients taking sulfasalazine, 30% experience adverse effects that are either dose-related, dependent on acetylator phenotype or idiosyncratic non-dose related reactions. The first group includes nausea, vomiting, headache, malaise, haemolytic anaemia, reticulocytosis, and methaemoglobulinaemia. The second includes skin rash, hepatic and pulmonary dysfunction, aplastic anaemia and reversible azoospermia. Adverse effects usually occur during the first 2 weeks of therapy, the majority being related to serum sulfapyridine levels.

Many of the adverse effects listed above can be avoided by using one of the aminosalicylate formulations now available (Table 11.4).

Formulations. As mesalazine is unstable in acid medium and rapidly absorbed from the gastrointestinal tract, the new preparations have been developed using three different approaches (see Fig. 11.4):

- a mesalazine tablet coated with a pH-dependent acrylic resin
- ethylcellulose-coated mesalazine granules
- diazotization of mesalazine to itself or to an inert carrier.

Asacol contains 400 mg of mesalazine coated with an acrylic resin, Eudragit-S, that dissolves at pH 7 and releases mesalazine in the terminal ileum and the colon. Salofalk tablets are a similar formulation containing 250 mg mesalazine with sodium carbonate-glycine and a cellulose ether, coated with Eudragit-L which dissolves at pH 6 and above, releasing mesalazine in the jejunum and ileum.

Pentasa tablets 250 mg and 500 mg comprise ethylcellulose-coated granules of mesalazine which are released when the tablet disintegrates in the stomach. Prolonged release granules 1 g are also available. Mesalazine is leached slowly from the granules

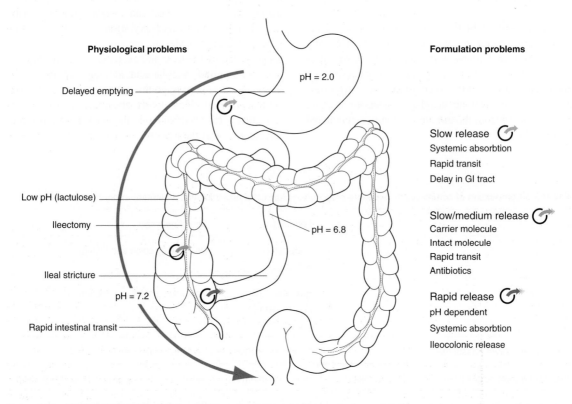

Figure 11.4 Physiological and formulation problems encountered with mesalazine oral delivery systems.

Table 11.4 Comparison of available oral aminosalicylate preparations for patients with inflammatory bowel disease

Generic (proprietary) name	Formulation	Release profile	Site of release
Sulfasalazine (Salazopyrin)	Compressed tablet. Plain and film coated	Azo-linked, independent of pH	Terminal ileum and colon
Mesalazine (Asacol)	Compressed tablet, acrylic coating	Acrylic coating dissolving at pH 7	Terminal ileum and colon
Mesalazine (Salofalk and generic forms)	Compressed tablet and/or capsule acrylic coating	Acrylic coating dissolving at pH 6	Mid-jejunum ileum and colon
Mesalazine (Pentasa)	Microgranules coated with ethylcellulose and compressed into tablets. Granules also available	Disintegration not dependent on pH. Slow dissolution rate	Stomach, duodenum, jejunum, ileum and colon
Olsalazine (Dipentum)	Hard gelatin capsules and tablets, uncoated	Azo-linked disintegration independent of pH	Terminal ileum and colon
Balsalazide (Colazide)	Hard gelatin capsules	Azo-linked disintegration in dependent of pH	Terminal ileum and colon
Polyasa	Compressed tablet and/or capsule	Azo-linked disintegration in dependent of pH	Terminal ileum and colon

throughout the gastrointestinal tract at all physiological pHs.

Dipentum 250 mg capsules and 500 mg tablets contain olsalazine sodium which is a dimer of mesalazine. Like sulphasalazine it remains intact until it reaches the colon where it undergoes bacterial cleavage releasing two molecules of mesalazine. Similarly, Colazide 750 mg capsules contain balsalazide sodium, a pro-drug of mesalazine, which also relies on bacterial cleavage in the lower bowel releasing mesalazine from 4-aminobenzoyl beta-alanine, its inert carrier molecule.

Clinical studies have shown all formulations to be as effective as sulfasalazine in maintaining remission in inflammatory bowel disease. Each preparation offers alternative therapy to sulfasalazine-intolerant patients if used as a new treatment. The dose range of mesalazine and olsalazine is 1–3 g daily in divided doses. For balsalazide a maximum daily dose of 6.75 g (equivalent to 1.575 g of mesalazine) in divided doses is recommended.

Mesalazine enemas (1 g in 100 ml), foam enemas (1 g per application) or suppositories (250 mg, 500 mg and 1 g) are also effective alternatives for treating localized Crohn's disease or proctitis.

An alternative to mesalazine is 4-amino salicylic acid (para-amino salicylic acid, PAS). It has been used as a 2 g enema in the treatment of distal ulcerative colitis. An oral 500 mg acrylic coated formulation is available in the USA.

Aminosalicylates appear to inhibit the production of cyclo-oxygenase, thromboxane synthetase, platelet-activating factor synthetase, and interleukin-1 by macrophages. Production of immunoglobulin by plasma cells is also decreased.

An alternative proposal is that it acts as a scavenger of super oxide radicals released by neutrophils at the inflammatory site. Hypochlorite, formed by this process, would react with the amino group in 5-ASA to produce a chloramine group-NHCl, high concentrations of mesalazine in the faecal stream would react with small concentrations of substrate and so neutralize the toxic potential of hypochlorite.

Immunosuppressants

Azathioprine and 6-mercaptopurine are used in patients unresponsive to steroids and aminosalicylates (Korelitz et al 1998). Azathioprine is metabolized to 6-mercaptopurine by the liver. Both possess steroid-sparing properties and are used either with prednisolone or alone in maintaining remission in Crohn's disease and occasionally in ulcerative colitis. Mercaptopurine is preferred although side-effects occur more frequently.

Maintenance doses for azathioprine and 6-mercaptopurine are usually 2 and 1.5 mg/kg body weight, respectively, with doses adjusted to the patient's response and tolerance and white cell and platelet counts. A low dose regimen of methotrexate appears to be effective in maintaining remission in patients with chronically active Crohn's disease (Feagan et al 2000). In early studies patients received weekly injections of methotrexate ranging from 15 mg to 25 mg. Overall incidence of side-effects was low, mainly nausea and vomiting.

Major concerns with immunosuppressive agents are their adverse effects. Skin rashes and nausea are common; raised liver enzymes and allergic hepatitis are less frequent and reversible. Thrombocytopenia and leucopenia have also been reported. Patients are monitored regularly for bone marrow depression, and have routine blood counts and liver function tests including serum bilirubin and alkaline phosphatase.

The increased incidence of lymphomas in patients receiving immunosuppressants compared with other treatments is of concern and there is evidence of a greater incidence in patients taking azathioprine compared to 6-mercaptopurine.

Although the action of immunosuppressive agents in inflammatory bowel disease is unclear their active metabolites do inhibit purine ribonucleotide which may in turn inhibit lymphocyte function, primarily that of T cells.

Metronidazole

Metronidazole has been used with some success in Crohn's patients using a dose of 10–20 mg/kg/day. Patients with severe perineal involvement have responded to metronidazole treatment, experiencing less pain and tenderness and eventually decreased erythema and swelling, and wound healing.

An 800 mg dose of metronidazole has proved as effective as 3 g sulfasalazine in treating Crohn's disease but is ineffective in ulcerative colitis. It is generally well tolerated with patients suffering only mild adverse effects such as metallic taste, glossitis, paraesthesia, darkening of urine and urticaria. Paraesthesia appears to be dose-related, occurring frequently with prolonged treatment. Doses should be gradually reduced during treatment.

Oral and rectal doses of metronidazole are partly metabolized by gut bacterial flora and, following rapid absorption, by the liver. The metabolite's free nitro group is thought to be responsible for its local activity. It also inhibits phospholipase A, contributing to a reduction in damage induced by polymorphonuclear leukocytes.

Ciclosporin

The effectiveness of ciclosporin in treating inflammatory bowel disease has been studied in patients refractory to conventional drug therapy using doses ranging from 10 to 15 mg/kg/day (Kornbluth et al 1997). Patient response to this treatment has varied, adverse effects causing withdrawal of treatment in some cases. However, some patients have been able to discontinue concurrent steroid therapy and remain in remission for some time. Abdominal pain, diarrhoea and weight gain are common non-dose-related side-effects while nephrotoxicity and hepatotoxicity are dose related, usually occurring when serum concentrations are greater than 400 ng/ml. Tremors and hirsutism occur at serum concentrations of 100–400 ng/ml.

Ciclosporin should be reserved for the treatment of severe refractory cases of ulcerative colitis and careful monitoring of patients is needed.

Ciclosporin acts at an early stage on precursors of helper cells by interfering with the release of interleukin-2, consequently inhibiting the formation of cytotoxic lymphocytes that cause tissue damage.

Sodium cromoglicate

Sodium cromoglicate reduces degranulation of mast cells by inhibiting the passage of calcium ions across cell membranes, a process essential for the release of inflammatory mediators from mast cells, Intestinal lesions contain mast cells, macrophages and eosinophils and rectal biopsies show large numbers of IgE plasma cells in the lamina propria. This points to a hypersensitivity response which may be inhibited by sodium cromoglicate stabilizing the mast cell. Some patients suffering from proctitis respond to 100 mg sodium cromoglicate three times a day orally and 200 mg twice daily as enemas. Its use in inflammatory bowel disease remains unproven but some patients may derive benefit.

Bismuth salts

Bismuth subsalicylate citrate and bismuth chelate administered as enemas are effective treatments for ulcerative colitis. Bismuth salts inhibit sulphatase and sialidase enzymes which are secreted by colonic bacteria and contribute to the process of mucus degradation. Bismuth also demonstrates cytoprotective properties through a mechanism, which increases tissue prostaglandin levels. A dose of 480 mg bismuth chelate suspension has been shown to be effective when administered nightly for 4 weeks. Similarly 700 mg of bismuth subsalicylate suspension administered twice daily for 8 weeks has also been shown to give good results.

Elemental bismuth (200 mg) complexed with an acrylic polymer (carbomers) and administered as an enema appears to be as effective as mesalazine enema in proctitis.

Arsenic salts

Arsenic salts, particularly acetarsol in the form of 250 mg suppositories, have been used successfully to treat ulcerative proctitis, but toxicity limits their use. Acetarsol is bactericidal and chemically similar to bismuth which may account for its mode of action.

Thalidomide

The use of thalidomide has been restricted to monitored refractory cases of Crohn's disease (Vasiliauskas et al 1999). It acts as a tumor necrosis factor (TNF-α) inhibitor and probably stabilizes lysosomal membranes, and at therapeutic doses inhibits the formation of superoxide and hydroxyl radicals, potent oxidants capable of causing tissue damage. Daily doses in the range of 50–400 mg have proved beneficial when used for periods of 1 week to several months. Adverse events during treatment include sedation, dry skin and reduced libido.

Antibiotics

With the exception of metronidazole, antibacterials are not routinely used because causative bacterial agents have not been identified. However, systemic complications such as toxic colitis may respond to metronidazole or vancomycin. Active Crohn's disease accompanied by fever complications may be alleviated by the administration of cefazolin, tetracycline or ampicillin. A study using anti-tuberculous drugs proved ineffective (Thomas et al 1998); ciprofloxacin has been used with limited success.

Antidiarrhoeals

Codeine, diphenoxylate and loperamide should be used cautiously to treat diarrhoea and abdominal cramping in inflammatory bowel disease, as their use may mask inflammation, infection, obstruction or colonic dilatation thereby delaying correct diagnosis.

Colestyramine

Following ileal resection, colestyramine has been used in Crohn's disease to decrease diarrhoea associated with bile-acid malabsorption caused by the decrease in small bowel absorptive surface area and the cathartic effect of bile salts on the colon. At doses of up to 4 g three times a day it inhibits bile-acid stimulated secretion of water and electrolytes.

Fish oils

Fish liver oils which contain eicosapentaenoic acid and docosahexaenoic acid have been used with some success in the treatment of both ulcerative colitis and Crohn's disease. Enteric coating of this product has reduced the unpleasant regurgitation, which previously made it unacceptable in long-term studies. It is postulated that fish oils might work by diverting fatty acid metabolism from leukotriene B4 to the formation of the less inflammatory leukotriene B5.

Monoclonal antibodies

The administration of humanized monoclonal antibodies is an entirely new and potentially highly successful concept in treating inflammatory bowel disease. The first such product, infliximab (Remicade), is available for treating refractory Crohn's disease (D'Haens et al 1999). It acts by inhibiting the functional activity of TNF-α. Following treatment histological evaluation of colonic biopsies revealed a substantial reduction in detectable TNF-α. Treatment was also associated with a reduction of the commonly elevated serum inflammatory maker C-reactive protein (CRP). Administered by intravenous infusion, a dose of 5 mg/kg is given over a 2 hour period in severe active disease; in fistulating disease an initial dose of 5 mg/kg is infused over a 2 hour period, repeated at 2 and 6 weeks after the first infusion, Infliximab can be re-administered within 14 weeks of the last infusion if symptoms recur. Infliximab has been associated with acute infusion effects, delayed hypersensitivity reactions and may also affect normal bodily immune responses in a significant number of patients. Patients receiving this therapy should be closely monitored

Other drugs

Alternative effective treatments for inflammatory bowel disease are still being sought. These have included sucralfate, nicotine, oxygen-derived free radical scavengers, somatostatin analogues, lidocaine (lignocaine), chloroquine, d-penicillamine, carbomers, antituberculous agents, specific monoclonal antibodies and bacterial interleukin-10.

Of these, nicotine is of interest in view of its relationship with smoking status. The addition of transdermal nicotine at doses ranging from 5 mg to 15 mg over a 24 hour period to conventional maintenance therapy improved symptoms in patients with ulcerative colitis although some of its side-effects became intolerable. A nicotine enema formulation has also proved beneficial (Green et al 1997). Similarly, lidocaine (lignocaine) given as enemas, at a dose of 200–800 mg daily has shown some benefit in patients with proctosigmoiditis, probably by inhibiting nervous reflexes with blockade of the neuro-immune interactions in the colonic mucosa.

Carbomers interact with mucus adhering to the mucosal surface, effectively increasing the mucus thickness. Since this layer of mucus is the interface between luminal content and the epithelium, this characteristic alone may be beneficial. Successful

Table 11.6 Pharmacological profile of drugs used in adults with inflammatory bowel disease

Pharmacological group	Daily dose	t $\frac{1}{2}$(h)	Metabolism
Steroids			
Hydrocortisone	125–250 mg as foam 100–400 mg in 0.9% w/v Sodium chloride i.v.	1.5	Hepatic metabolism 70% and 30% unchanged
Prednisolone	20–60 mg orally 20 mg as enema 5–10 mg as suppositories	3	Hepatic metabolism 70% and 30% unchanged
Budesonide	3–9 mg orally 2 mg rectally	2.8	90% hepatic metabolism
Aminosalicylates			
Mesalazine	150 mg–1.5 g as suppositories 1 g as enema 1.2–2.4 g orally	0.7–2.4	Local and systemic Hepatic acetylation, glucuronidation
Olsalazine	1–3 g orally	1.0	Local and systemic Hepatic acetylation, glucuronidation
Sulfasalazine	3 g as enema 1–2 g as suppositories 4–8 g orally	5–8	Colonic azo-reduction. Local and systemic acetylation Hepatic glucuronidation
4-Aminosalicylic acid	1–2 g orally 1–2 g as enema	0.75–1.0	Rapid absorption and distribution. Systemic acetylation
Balsalazide	3–6.75 g orally	1.0	Local and systemic hepatic acetylation
Antibiotics			
Metronidazole	600 mg–1.2 g orally 2 g i.v.	6–24	Hepatic metabolism
Immunosuppressants			
Azathioprine	2 mg/kg orally	3	Hepatic metabolism to 6-mercaptopurine
6-Mercaptopurine	2.5 mg/kg orally	1.5	Hepatic metabolism to inactive metabolite
Ciclosporin	10–15 mg/kg	19–27	Mainly hepatic metabolism
Monoclonal antibody			
Infliximab	5 mg/kg infusion as a single dose over 2 hours	8–9 days	Unknown
Miscellaneous			
Arsenic salts	250 mg–1 g rectally	72	Tissue deposition excreted unchanged
Bismuth salts	200 mg–1.2 g rectally	60–80	Tissue deposition excreted unchanged
Fish oils	3–4 g	None	Used in the arachidonic acid cycle
Sodium cromoglicate	200–800 mg orally 100–400 mg	Unknown	Poorly absorbed, excreted unchanged in urine and bile
Nicotine	5–15 mg transdermally	0.5–2.0	Hepatic oxidation to cotinine 5% excreted unchanged
Lidocaine (lignocaine)	200–800 mg rectally	1–2	Hepatic de-ethylation and hydrolysis 3% excreted unchanged
Methotrexate	15–25 mg by i.m. injection weekly	3–10	Insignificant metabolism at low doses Largely excreted unchanged
Human growth hormone	1.5–5 mg daily by subcutaneous injection	0.5–4	Unknown

Case 11.2

Mr B. is 35 years old and has a 12-year history of Crohn's disease. He has been maintained in remission, apart from three or four acute exacerbations, for the last 3 years. His current therapy is:

- mesalazine 400 mg three times a day
- prednisolone 5 mg once a day (increased during acute exacerbations)
- ferrous sulphate 200 mg three times a day.

At his last clinic visit he was found to have glycosuria and mildly elevated blood pressure which, in association with a noticeable change in his facial features, were considered characteristic side-effects of his long-term steroid therapy. It was decided to start him on azathioprine.

Questions

1. What is the rationale behind this change in drug treatment?
2. What precautions should be taken?
3. If azathioprine fails to allow adequate reduction in the dose of steroid, what alternative could be tried?

Answers

1. The steroid-sparing effects of azathioprine are being utilized.
2. High doses of azathioprine produce bone marrow suppression and so a maximum of 2 mg/kg/day should be used. Liver function and blood counts should be monitored regularly.
3. The immunosuppressant ciclosporin may be useful. It may be used in combination with steroids and azathioprine but gradual withdrawal of the azathioprine is preferred to reduce combined toxicity.

Case 11.3

Mrs C., 45 years old, was admitted to hospital for an ileostomy. Ulcerative colitis was diagnosed 15 years ago and since then she has had a number of hospital admissions with profuse diarrhoea, rectal bleeding and generalized symptoms such as reduced appetite, nausea and weight loss. She is no longer able to retain her prednisolone enemas for longer than a few minutes and needs oral prednisolone 40 mg a day with codeine phosphate 15 mg tablets taken as required.

Question

What prescription and over-the-counter drugs should Mrs C. avoid following her ileostomy?

Answer

Drugs altering fluid and electrolyte balance should be avoided. Laxatives and magnesium-containing antacids in particular can increase fluid loss through the stoma and lead to dehydration. Diuretics may aggravate dehydration. There may be reduced release of drug from sustained-release and enteric-coated preparations.

Case 11.4

Mr D. is 53 years of age and has suffered from ulcerative colitis for 25 years. Until recently he has been maintained in remission on a low dose oral prednisolone and sulfasalazine regimen but relapses are now occurring frequently. He has subsequently developed rheumatoid arthritis. Mr D. is found to be suffering from predominantly left-sided colitis and radiographic evidence reveals that a proximal stricture has formed.

Questions

1. What alternative therapy, in terms of (a) the formulation and (b) the drug should be considered for this patient?
2. Why should Mr D. be followed up at a hospital out-patient clinic?

Answers

1a. The use of an enema foam, or suppository formulation should be considered for left-sided colitis. The stricture may prevent complete tablet disintegration, especially in the case of enteric-coated sulfasalazine formulations.
1b. The choice of mesalazine formulation, which disintegrates proximally to the stricture, may be helpful. Alternative drugs worth considering would be bismuth or nicotine enemas.
2. Because he has rheumatoid arthritis it may be difficult, depending on how the disease progresses, for Mr D. to self-administer enema preparations. Adherence failure may then cause further relapses.

Case 11.5

Mr E., a young married man of 26 years, has suffered from ulcerative colitis for many years and has remained in remission by taking oral maintenance doses of sulfsalazine and prednisolone. He has appeared to be free of any untoward side-effects of these drugs, and apart from ulcerative colitis is fit and in good health. His wife has no clinical problems. On a routine annual check-up at his local hospital he mentions to the gastroenterologist that he and his wife have been unsuccessful in their attempts to start a family.

Questions

1. Could Mr E.'s drug therapy be in any way contributing to the couple's problem?
2. If his drug treatment is in any way responsible, what alternative drug(s) would you prescribe?

Answers

1. There is well-documented evidence that long-term therapy using sulfasalazine can cause oligospermia in a small number of male patients. Refer patient for sperm count for case confirmation.
2. Discontinue the sulfasalazine and use one of the mesalazine formulations. Choose the one that is most compatible with the patient's sites of disease (see Table 11.4 and Fig. 11.4).

Case 11.6

Mrs K. is middle aged and a long-term sufferer from Crohn's disease. She has once again relapsed and been admitted to hospital for assessment and to re-establish remission. She currently takes:

- mesalazine 800 mg four times a day
- prednisolone 10 mg daily
- ciclosporin 250 mg daily.

Questions

1. Mrs K.'s current medication has failed to maintain remission. What new approach in her treatment could be made while she is hospitalized?
2. What adjustments would be made to her current therapy?
3. What could be a long-term problem for patients treated with this new therapeutic approach?

Answers

1. Because Mrs K. has suffered from Crohn's disease for may years, her existing drug treatment reflects the limited availability of drugs to treat this condition. In these situations it is worth considering the use of a monoclonal antibody such as infliximab. This would be administered in the hospital environment under close medical supervision.
2. Existing conventional drug therapy could continue if necessary during this period. Dose adjustments could be made if the infliximab treatment were to prove successful.
3. The re-administration of infliximab following a drug free interval of between 2 and 4 years has been associated with a delayed hypersensitivity reaction in a significant number of Crohn's sufferers.

REFERENCES

D'Haens G, van Deventer S, van Hogezand R et al 1999 Endoscopic and histological healing with infliximab anti-tumor necrosis factor antibodies in Crohn's disease. Gastroenterology 116: 1029–1034

Feagan B G, McDonald J, Hopkins M et al 2000 A randomised controlled trial of methotrexate (MTX) as a maintenance therapy for chronically active Crohn's disease (CD). New England Journal of Medicine 342 (May): 1627–1632

Fernandes-Banares F, Hinojoso J, Sanchez-Lombrana J L et al 1999 Randomised clinical trial of *Plantago ovata* seeds (dietary fiber) as compared with mesalazine in maintaining remission in ulcerative colitis. American Journal of Gastroenterology 2: 427–433

Green J T, Thomas G A O, Rhodes J et al 1997 Nicotine enemas for active ulcerative colitis: a pilot study. Alimentary Pharmacology and Therapeutics 11: 859–863

Hanauer S B 2000 Medical therapy of ulcerative colitis. In: Kirsner J B (ed) Inflammatory bowel disease 5th ed. W B Saunders, Philadelphia, PP. 529–577

Hanauer S B, Meyers S 1997 Management of Crohn's disease in adults. American Journal of Gastroenterology 92: 559–566

Korelitz B I, Hanauer S, Rutgeerts P et al 1998 Post-operative prophylaxis with 6-MP, 5-ASA, or placebo in Crohn's disease: a 2-year multicenter trial. Gastroenterology 114: A4141

Kornbluth A, Present D H, Lichtiger S et al 1997 Ciclosporin for severe ulcerative colitis: a user's guide. American Journal of Gastroenterology 92: 1424–1428

Meyers S, Sachar D B 1995 Medical therapy of Crohn's disease.

In: Kersnar J B, Shorter R G (eds) Inflammatory bowel disease, 4th ed. Williams and Wilkins, Baltimore, pp. 695–714

Misiewicz J J, Pounder R E, Venables C W (eds) 1994 Diseases of the gut and pancreas, 2nd edn. Blackwell Scientific Publications, Oxford

Prantera C, Cottone M, Pallone F et al 1999 Mesalamine in the treatment of mild to moderate active Crohn's ileitis: results of a randomised multicenter trial. Gastroenterology 116: 521–526

Rhodes J, Thomas G, Evans B K 1997 Inflammatory bowel disease management: some thoughts on future drug development. Drugs 53: 189–194

Schreiber S, Nikolaus S, Hampe J et al 1999 Tumor necrosis factor alpha and interleukin 1 beta in relapse of Crohn's disease. Lancet 353: 459–461

Thomas G A, Swift G L Green J T et al 1998 Controlled trial of anti-tuberculous chemotherapy in Crohn's disease: a five year follow up study. Gut 42: 497–500

Thomsen O O, Cortot A, Jewell D et al 1998 A comparison of budesonide and mesalazine for active Crohn's disease. New England Journal of Medicine 339: 370–374

Vasiliauskas E A, Kam L Y, Abreu M T et al 1999 An open-label, step-wise dose-escalating pilot study of low-dose thalidomide in chronically active, steroid-dependent Crohn's disease. Gastroenterology 117: 1278–1287

Winter H S 2000 Management of ulcerative colitis in children. In: Bayliss T M, Hanauer S B (eds) Advanced therapy of inflammatory bowel disease 2nd eds. Decker Ontario BC, pp. 153–155

FURTHER READING

British Society of Gastroenterology 1996 Inflammatory bowel disease: BSG guidelines in gastroenterology. British Society of Gastroenterology, London

Kornbluth A, Sachar D B 1997 Ulcerative colitis practice guidelines in adults. American Journal of Gasteroenterology 92: 204–211

Lofberg R 1998 New data on inflammatory bowel disease treatment with topical steroids. Resident Clinical Forum 20: 179–186

Marshall J K, Irvine E J 1997 Rectal corticosteroids versus alternative treatments in ulcerative colitis: a meta-analysis. Gut 40: 775–781

Sandborn W J 1996 A review of immune modifier therapy for inflammatory bowel disease: azathioprine, 6-mercaptopurine, ciclosporin and methotrexate. American Journal of Gastroenterology 91: 423–433

Stein R B, Hanauer S B 1999 Medical therapy for inflammatory bowel disease. Gasroenterology Clinics of North America 828: 297–321

Sutherland L, Roth D, Beck P et al 1998 Oral 5-aminosalicylic acid for maintenance of remission in ulcerative colitis. Cochrane Review. Cochrane Library. Update Software, Oxford, p. 3

Constipation and diarrhoea

12

R. Walker

KEY POINTS

Constipation

- About 90% of people defaecate between three times a day and once every 3 days.
- Constipation is considered as infrequent bowel action of twice a week or less that involves straining to pass hard stools accompanied by a sensation of pain or incomplete evacuation.
- Diagnosis requires an accurate history and identification of associated disorders and circumstances.
- Over 700 medicinal products, including some eye drops, have been reported to cause constipation.
- Non-drug treatment involves increasing fibre intake, increasing fluid intake and encouraging exercise.
- Drugs used to treat constipation may be grouped into four main groups: bulk forming, stimulant, osmotic and faecal softener.

Diarrhoea

- Diarrhoea is the passage of loose or watery stools, at least three times in a 24 hour period, which may be accompanied by anorexia, nausea, vomiting, abdominal cramps or bloating.
- It is not a disease but a sign of an underlying problem such as an infection or gastrointestinal disorder.
- In the UK rotavirus and small round structured virus (SRSV) are the most common causes of gastroenteritis in children.
- In adults *Campylobacter* followed by rotavirus are the most common cause.
- Blood in diarrhoea is classed as dysentery and indicates the presence of an invasive organism such as *Camplylobacter, Salmonella, Shigella* or *Escherichia coli* O157.
- Over 1200 medicinal products are known to cause diarrhoea. Broad-spectrum antibiotics are probably the commonest cause.
- Diarrhoea results in fluid and electrolyte loss which may progress to dehydration.
- Correction of fluid and electrolyte loss with an oral rehydration solution is generally the mainstay of treatment, particularly in children and the elderly.
- Antimotility agents, e.g. loperamide, diphenoxylate, codeine, may give symptomatic control in mild to moderate diarrhoea. They are not recommended for use in children.

Constipation and diarrhoea are two of the most common disorders of the gastrointestinal tract. Most adults will suffer from these disorders at some time in their life and while they are often self-limiting, they can cause significant morbidity or occur as a secondary feature to a more serious disorder. For example, constipation may be secondary to hypothyroidism, hypokalaemia, diabetes, multiple sclerosis or gastrointestinal obstruction by a tumour. Likewise, diarrhoea may be secondary to ulcerative colitis, Crohn's disease or bowel carcinoma. Both constipation and diarrhoea can also be drug-induced and this should be considered when trying to identify a likely cause and determine effective management.

CONSTIPATION

In Western populations, 90% of people defaecate between three times a day and once every three days. It is clear, therefore, that to base a definition of constipation on frequency alone is problematic. What is perceived to be constipation by one individual may be normal to another. Most definitions of constipation include infrequent bowel action of twice a week or less that involves straining to pass hard faeces and which may be accompanied by a sensation of pain or incomplete evacuation. A pragmatic definition would simply be the passage of hard stools less frequently than the patient's own normal pattern.

The Rome criteria (Thompson et al 1999) set out a number of symptoms of which two or more must be present for at least 12 weeks before the diagnosis of constipation can be made in adults (Table 12.1). Different criteria (Rasquin-Weber et al 1999) are used to define constipation in children (Table 12.2).

Incidence

Each year over 10 million prescriptions are written for laxatives in England alone. Constipation appears to be more common in the elderly: up to 20% of elderly people, compared to 8% of middle-aged and 3% of young people, seek medical advice for constipation. In the

Table 12.1   Rome II criteria for the diagnosis of functional constipation

Two or more of the following criteria should be present for at least 12 weeks, which need not be consecutive, in the preceding 12 months:

- Straining at defaecation on at least a quarter of occasions
- Lumpy and/or hard stools for at least a quarter of defaecations
- Sensation of incomplete evacuation in at least a quarter defaecations
- Sensation of anorectal obstruction/blockade in at least a quarter of defaecations
- Manual manoeuvres to facilitate at least a quarter of defaecations, e.g. digital evacuation, support of the pelvic floor

Table 12.2   Rome II criteria for diagnosis of functional constipation in children

In infants and pre-school children, at least 2 weeks of:

- Scybalous, pebble-like, hard stools for a majority of stools; or
- Firm stools two or less times per week; and

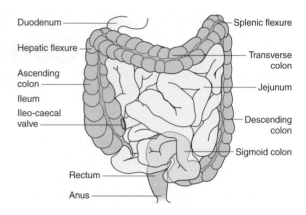

Figure 12.1   The lower gastrointestinal tract.

elderly, poor diet, insufficient intake of fluids, lack of exercise, concurrent disease states and use of drugs that predispose to constipation have all been identified as contributory factors.

Women are often reported to have a higher incidence of constipation than men although this probably reflects the greater likelihood that they seek medical advice. Constipation is, however, common in late pregnancy due to reduced gastrointestinal motility and delayed bowel emptying caused by the pressure of the uterus. It has also been reported that between 5% and 10% of children have constipation.

Aetiology

The digestive system can be divided into the upper and lower gastrointestinal tract. The upper gastrointestinal tract starts at the mouth and includes the oesophagus and stomach and is responsible for the ingestion and digestion of food. The lower gastrointestinal tract consists of the small intestine, large intestine (colon), rectum and anus (Fig. 12.1) and is responsible for the absorption of nutrients, conserving body water and electrolytes, drying the faeces, and elimination.

The remains of undigested food are swept along the gastrointestinal tract by waves of muscular contractions called peristalsis. These peristaltic waves eventually move the faeces from the colon to the rectum and induce the urge to defaecate. By the time stool reaches the rectum it generally has a solid consistency because most of the water has been absorbed.

Normally there is a net uptake of fluid in the intestine in response to osmotic gradients involving the absorption and secretion of ions, and the absorption of sugars and amino acids. This process is under the influence of the autonomic nervous system (sympathetic and parasympathetic). In those situations where absorption increases this will generally lead to constipation, whereas a net secretion will result in diarrhoea.

Agents that alter intestinal motility, either directly or by acting on the autonomic nervous system, affect the transit time of food along the gastrointestinal tract. Since the extent of absorption and secretion of fluid from the gastrointestinal tract generally parallels transit time, a slower transit time will lead to the formation of hard stools and constipation. Motility is largely under parasympathetic (cholinergic) control, with stimulation bringing about an increase in motility while antagonists such as anticholinergics, or drugs with anticholinergic side-effects, decrease motility and induce constipation. This mechanism is distinct from that of the other major group of drugs that induce constipation, the opioids. Opioids cause constipation by maintaining or increasing the tone of smooth muscle, suppress forward peristalsis, raise sphincter tone at the ileocaecal valve and anal sphincter and reduce sensitivity to rectal distension. This delays passage of faeces through the gut, with a resultant increase in absorption of electrolytes and water in the small intestine and colon.

It is normally the lower section of the gastrointestinal tract that becomes dysfunctional during constipation. Constipation is, however, a symptom and not a disease and can be caused by many different conditions (Table 12.3). Knowledge of the underlying cause of constipation helps in both prevention and treatment (Fig. 12.2).

Table 12.3 Common causes of constipation

Cause	Comment
Poor diet	Diets high in animal fats, e.g. meats, dairy products, eggs, and refined sugar, e.g. sweets, but low in fibre predispose to constipation
Imaginary constipation	Misconception as to what is normal bowel habit
Irritable bowel syndrome	Spasm of colon delays transit of intestinal contents
Poor bowel habit	Ignoring urge to have a bowel movement
Laxative abuse	Habitual consumption of laxatives necessitates increase in dose over time until intestine becomes insensitive and fails to work
Travel	Changes in lifestyle, daily routine, diet and drinking water may all contribute to constipation
Hormone disturbances	E.g. hypothyroidism, diabetes
Pregnancy	Mechanical pressure of womb on intestine and hormonal changes, e.g. high levels of progesterone
Fissures and haemorrhoids	Painful disorders of the anus produce spasm of anal sphincter muscle and delay bowel movement
Diseases	E.g. scleroderma, lupus, multiple sclerosis, depression, Parkinson's disease, stroke
Loss of body salts	Loss through vomiting or diarrhoea, e.g. hypokalaemia
Mechanical compression	Scarring, inflammation around diverticula and tumours can produce mechanical compression of intestine
Nerve damage	Spinal cord injuries and tumours pressing on the spinal cord affect nerves that lead to intestine
Colonic motility disorders	Peristaltic activity of intestine may be ineffective resulting in colonic inertia
Medication	See Table 12.4
Dehydration	Insufficient fluid intake or excessive fluid loss. Water and other fluids add bulk to stools, making bowel movements soft and easier to pass
Immobility	Prolonged bed rest after an accident, during an illness or general lack of exercise
Electrolyte abnormalities	E.g. hypercalcaemia, hypokalaemia

For convenience, many classify constipation as originating from within the colon and rectum, or externally. Causes directly attributable to the colon or rectum include obstruction from neoplasm, Hirschsprung's disease, outlet obstruction due to rectal prolapse or damage to the pudendal nerve, typically during childbirth. Causes of constipation outside the colon include poor diet, inadequate fibre intake, inadequate water intake, excessive intake of coffee, tea or alcohol, use of medicines with constipating side-effects or systemic disorders such as hypothyroidism, diabetic autonomic neuropathy, spinal cord injury, cerebrovascular accident, multiple sclerosis or Parkinson's disease.

Treatment

Before appropriate treatment can commence, an accurate history is required and associated disorders must be identified. Questions need to be asked about the frequency and consistency of stools, nausea, vomiting, abdominal pain, distension, discomfort, mobility, diet and other concurrent symptoms or disorders the patient may be suffering. It may also be necessary to ask about access to a toilet or commode. The individual with limited mobility may suppress the urge to defaecate because of difficulty in getting to the toilet. Likewise, lack of privacy or dependency on a nurse or carer for

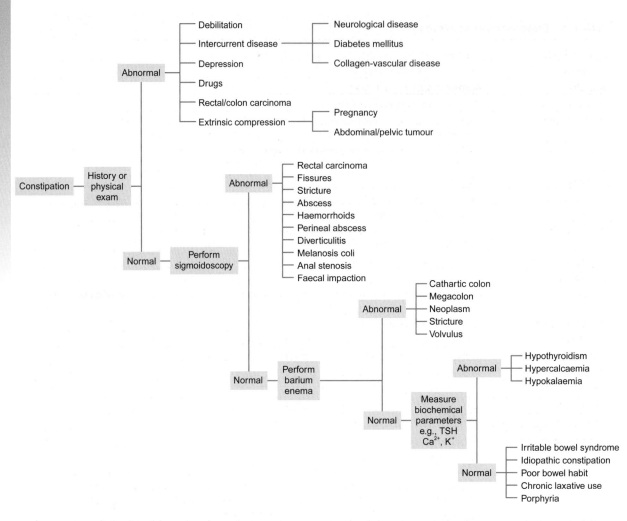

Figure 12.2 A diagnostic algorithm for constipation.

toileting may result in urge suppression that precipitates constipation or exacerbates an underlying predisposition.

General management

In uncomplicated constipation, education and advice on diet and exercise are the mainstay of management and may adequately control symptoms in many individuals. Typically this advice will include reassurance that the individual does not have cancer, that the normal frequency of defaecation varies widely between individuals, and that mild constipation is not in itself harmful. It may also be of value to reassure the patient that in most people there is often no obvious cause for the constipation.

If the patient is taking medication for a concurrent disorder this must be assessed for its propensity to cause constipation. In the UK over 700 medicinal products, including ophthalmic preparations, have constipation listed as possible side-effect. Examples of the drugs involved are presented in Table 12.4.

Most cases of constipation can be readily managed with non-drug or drug treatment, those where further investigation is required include:

- symptoms of sudden onset
- long-standing constipation that has not responded to treatment
- change of bowel habit in a middle-aged or elderly individual
- individual at high risk of neoplasia
- presence of rectal bleeding at any age
- new, severe symptoms unresponsive to treatment.

Non-drug treatment

Non-drug treatment often includes advising an increase in fluid intake at the same time as reducing strong or excessive intake of tea or coffee, since these act as a

Table 12.4 Drugs known to cause constipation

ACE inhibitor	Enalapril, imidapril, lisinopril, moexipril, ramipril, trandolapril
α-blocker	Prazosin, tamsulosin, terazosin
Antacid	Aluminium salts, calcium salts
Antiarrhythmic	Disopyramide, mexiletine, propafenone
Anticholinergic	Atropine, benzatropine, trihexyphenidyl (benzhexol), biperiden, dicycloverine (dicyclomine), distigmine, hyoscine, ipratropium, oxybutynin, procyclidine, propiverine, tolterodine
Antidepressant	Amitriptyline, amoxapine, clomipramine, dosulepin (dothiepin), doxepin, fluvoxamine, imipramine, maprotiline, nefazodone, paroxetine, reboxetine, venlafaxine, viloxazine
Antidiabetic	Glipizide
Antiepileptic	Carbamazepine, phenytoin
Antifungal	Itraconazole
Antihistamine	Alimemazine, brompheniramine, chlorphenamine (chlorpheniramine), cyproheptadine, diphenhydramine, promethazine
Antihypertensive	Clonidine, diazoxide, losartan, methyldopa
Antiplatelet	Clopidogrel
Antipsychotic	Amisulpride, chlorpromazine, fluphenazine, haloperidol, loxapine, olanzapine, pericyazine, pimozide, pipothiazine, quetiapine, risperidone, thioridazine, zotepine
Antispasmodic	Mebeverine, peppermint oil
Antiviral	Foscarnet, ganciclovir, itraconazole, saquinavir, stavudine, tribavirin, zalcitabine
Antibiotic	Azithromycin, cinoxacin, clindamycin, clofazimine, isoniazid, metronidazole
Benzodiazepine	Clobazam, diazepam, midazolam
β-blocker	Atenolol, carvedilol, timolol, oxprenolol, propranolol
Bisphosphonate	Alendronic acid, disodium etidronate, disodium pamidronate
Calcium channel blocker	Diltiazem, felodipine, nifedipine, nimodipine, nisoldipine, verapamil
Catecholaminergic	Phentermine
Corticosteroid	Hydrocortisone, methylprednisolone
Cytotoxic	Bicalutamide, buserelin, carboplatin, cladribine, docetaxel, doxorubicin, etoposide, exemestane, flutamide, formestane, gemcitabine, hydroxycarbamide (hydroxyurea), ifosfamide, irinotecan, letrozole, methotrexate, mitoxantrone (mitozantrone), pentostatin, raltitrexed, temozolomide, topotecan, tretinoin, vinblastine, vincristine, vindesine, vinorelbine
Diuretic	Chlortalidone, furosemide (frusemide), hydrochlorothiazide, indapamide, polythiazide
Dopaminergic	Amantadine, bromocriptine, carbegolide, entacapone, levodopa, lisuride, pergolide, pramipexole, quinagolide, selegiline
Ganglion-blocking	Trimetaphan
G-CSF stimulating factor	Filgrastim
Immunosuppressant	Basiliximab, mycophenolate mofetil, tacrolimus
Lipid lowering agents	Atorvastatin, colestipol, colestyramine, gemfibrozil, simvastatin
Iron	Ferrous sulphate
MAO inhibitor	Moclobemide
Muscle relaxant	Baclofen, dantrolene
NSAID	Acemetacin, aspirin, benorilate, celecoxib, diclofenac, diflunisal, fenbufen, fenoprofen, indometacin, ketoprofen, ketorolac, meloxicam, nabumetone, naproxen, phenylbutazone, piroxicam, rofecoxib, sulindac, tenoxicam, tiaprofenic acid
Ophthalmic	Apraclonidine, cyclopentolate, tropicamide
Opioid	Buprenorphine, codeine, dextropropoxyphene, diamorphine, dihydrocodeine, fentanyl, hydromorphone, loperamide, morphine, naltrexone, oxycodone, pentazocine, phenazocine, pholcodine, remifentanil, tramadol
Phenothiazine	Chlorpromazine, prochlorperazine
Serotonin antagonist	Granisetron, ondansetron, pizotifen, tropisetron
SSRI	Citalopram
Ulcer healing	Esomeprazole, famotidine, lansoprazole, omeprazole, pantoprazole, rabeprazole, sucralfate
Vitamin	Calcitriol, ergocalciferol

diuretic and serve to make constipation worse. It is generally recommended that fibre intake in the form of fruit, vegetables, cereals, grain foods, wholemeal bread, etc. be increased to about 30 g per day. Such a diet should be tried for at least 1 month to determine if it has an effect. Most will notice an effect within 5 days. Unfortunately a high fibre diet is not without problems with patients complaining of flatulence, bloating and distension, although these effects should diminish over a period of several months. Patients who increase their fibre intake must also be advised to ingest 2 litres of water a day. Where an intake of this volume cannot be ingested it will be necessary to avoid increasing dietary fibre. An increased level of exercise should also accompany the raised fibre intake as this is thought to help relax and contract the abdominal muscles and help food move more efficiently through the gut.

A high fibre diet is not recommended in those with megacolon or hypotonic colon/rectum because they do not respond to bulk in the colon. Similarly, a high fibre diet may not be appropriate in those with opioid-induced constipation.

Drug treatment

Drug treatment is indicated where there is faecal impaction, constipation associated with illness, surgery, pregnancy, poor diet, where the constipation is drug-induced, where bowel strain is undesirable, and as part of bowel preparation for surgery. The various laxatives available can be classified as bulk forming, stimulant, osmotic, and faecal softeners. Overall there would appear to be little difference in efficacy between many of the laxatives.

In general the fit, active, elderly person should be treated as a younger adult. In contrast, management of constipation in children is often complex. Early treatment is required in children to avoid developing a megarectum, faecal impaction and overflow incontinence. Encouraging the child to use the toilet after meals and increasing dietary fibre have a role alongside oral drug treatment. Depending on circumstances, behavioural therapy may be indicated.

Bulk forming agents

Ispaghula, methylcellulose, sterculia and bran are typical bulk forming agents, and are usually taken as granules, powders or tablets. Their use is most appropriate in situations where dietary intake of fibre cannot be increased and the patient has small hard stools, haemorrhoids or an anal fissure.

The mechanism of action for bulk forming agents involves polysaccharide and cellulose components that are not digested and which retain fluid, increase faecal bulk and stimulate peristalsis. They may also encourage the proliferation of colonic bacteria and this helps further increase faecal bulk and stool softness. Following ingestion it usually takes 12–36 hours before any effect is seen, but may take longer. An adequate volume of fluid should also be ingested to avoid intestinal obstruction. Bulk forming agents can be used safely long term, during pregnancy or breastfeeding but many users will experience problems with flatulence and distension. The use of bulk forming agents is not recommended in patients with colonic atony, intestinal obstruction or faecal impaction and they are less effective, or may even exacerbate constipation, in those who lack mobility.

Stimulant laxatives

Drugs in this group include bisacodyl, senna and dantron. They directly stimulate colonic nerves that cause movement of the faecal mass, reduce transit time and result in the passage of stool within 8–12 hours. As a consequence of their time to onset, oral dosing at bedtime is generally recommended. For a rapid action (within 20–60 minutes) suppositories can be used. Abdominal cramps are common as an immediate side-effect of stimulant laxatives, while electrolyte disturbances and an atonic colon may result from chronic use.

In the elderly, long-term adverse effects are of less concern and prolonged use may be appropriate in a few cases. However, dantron alone, or in combination with a faecal softener, is restricted for use in constipation in terminally ill patients of all ages.

Osmotic laxatives

Osmotic laxatives include magnesium salts, polyethylene glycol, phosphate enemas, sodium citrate enemas, lactulose and lactitol. These agents retain fluid in the bowel by osmosis or change the water distribution in faeces to produce a softer, bulkier stool. Their ingestion should be accompanied by an appropriate fluid intake.

Rectal preparations of phosphates and sodium citrate are useful for quick relief, within 30 minutes, and bowel evacuation before abdominal radiological procedures, sigmoidoscopy, and surgery. Oral magnesium salts such as the sulphate are also indicated for rapid bowel evacuation and have an effect within 2–5 hours.

Lactulose and lactitol are semi-synthetic disaccharides which are not absorbed from the gut. They increase faecal weight, volume and bowel movement and must be taken regularly. It may take 48 hours or longer for them to work and they are probably no more effective than fibre or senna. Both agents are useful in the treatment of hepatic encephalopathy since they produce an osmotic diarrhoea of low faecal pH that discourages the growth of ammonia-producing organisms.

Faecal softeners/emollient laxatives

Docusate sodium is a non-ionic surfactant that has stool-softening properties. It reduces surface tension, increases the penetration of intestinal fluids into the faecal mass and has weak stimulant properties. While useful in the management of constipation in a patient with haemorrhoids or anal fissure, short-term use for up to 7 days only is advised. Rectal docusate has a rapid onset of action but should not be used in individuals with haemorrhoids or anal fissure.

The classical lubricant, liquid paraffin, has no place in modern therapy. It seeps from the anus, is associated with granulomatous reactions following absorption of small quantities and lipoid pneumonia following aspiration, and malabsorption of fat soluble vitamins.

DIARRHOEA

Diarrhoea can be defined as the passage of loose or watery stools, usually at least three times in a 24 hour period. It may be accompanied by anorexia, nausea, vomiting, abdominal cramps or bloating. It is not a disease but a sign of an underlying problem such as an infection or gastrointestinal disorder. The following section primarily focuses on acute infective gastroenteritis but also includes reference to drug-induced diarrhoea. Diarrhoea associated with ulcerative colitis, Crohn's disease and irritable bowel syndrome will not be covered here. Similarly, functional diarrhoea, i.e. diarrhoea which is present for at least 12 weeks (not necessarily consecutive) in the preceding 12 months, will also not be covered.

Acute gastroenteritis is most common in children but the precise incidence is difficult to determine because many cases are self-limiting and not reported. It has been estimated that children under the age of 5 years have between one and three bouts of diarrhoea per year. Children in the same age range account for over 5% of consultations to primary care doctors, with 18 000 children a year in England and Wales being admitted to hospital with rotavirus infection.

The incidence of diarrhoea in adults is, on average, just under one episode of diarrhoea per person each year. Many of these cases are thought to be food related with 22% of those consulting a docotor claiming to have 'food poisoning'. Traveller's diarrhoea is another common cause of diarrhoea, occurring in 8–50% of travellers, depending on destination. The highest incidence is seen in those visiting Egypt, Mexico and India. Over recent years *Escherichia coli* O157 has gained prominence because of a number of outbreaks in different communities associated with severe disease and even death. It is, however, an uncommon cause of diarrhoea, accounting for only 0.1% of cases.

Aetiology

In the UK rotavirus and small round structured virus (SRSV) are the most common identified causes of gastroenteritis in children. In adults, *Campylobacter* followed by rotavirus are the most common causes. Other identified causes include: the bacteria *E. coli*, *Salmonella*, *Shigella*, *Clostridium perfringens* enterotoxin; viruses such as adenovirus and astrovirus; and the protozoa *Cryptosporidium*, *Giardia* and *Entamoeba*. These pathogens produce diarrhoea: by producing enterotoxins that affect gut function with secretion and loss of fluids, for example enterotoxigenic *E. coli*; by interfering with normal mucosal function, for example adherent enteropathogenic *E. coli*; or by causing injury to the mucosa and deeper tissues, for example enteroinvasive *E. coli* or enterohaemorrhagic *E. coli* such as *E. coli* O157. Other organisms, for example *Staphylococcus aureus* and *Bacillus cereus*, produce preformed enterotoxins which on ingestion induce rapid onset diarrhoea and vomiting that usually lasts less than 12 hours.

So-called traveller's diarrhoea frequently affects people travelling from developed to developing countries. It is caused by bacterial gastroenteritis in over 80% of cases and associated with ingestion of contaminated food or water. The organisms usually involved, in descending order, are the enterotoxigenic bacteria *E. coli*, *Shigella*, *Salmonella*, *Campylobacter*, *Vibrio* and *Yersinia* species. Viruses and parasites, such as *Giardia*, *Cryptosporidium* and *Entamoeba*, account for the remainder.

Many drugs, particularly broad-spectrum antibiotics such as ampicillin, erythromycin and neomycin, induce diarrhoea secondary to therapy (Table 12.5). With these antibiotics the mechanism involves the overgrowth of antibiotic-resistant bacteria and fungi in the large bowel after several days of therapy. The diarrhoea is generally self-limiting. However, when the overgrowth involves *Clostridium difficile* and the associated production of its bacterial toxin, life-threatening pseudomembranous colitis may be the outcome. Diarrhoea may also be a symptom of drug withdrawal from alcohol and opioids.

Symptoms and signs

Acute onset diarrhoea is associated with loose or watery stools that will probably be accompanied by anorexia, nausea, vomiting, abdominal cramps, flatulence or bloating. When there is blood in the diarrhoea this is classed as dysentery and indicates the presence of an invasive organism such as *Campylobacter*, *Salmonella*, *Shigella* or *E. coli* O157.

The history of symptom onset is important. The duration of diarrhoea, whether other members of the

Table 12.5 Examples of drug-induced diarrhoea and the different underlying mechanisms (adapted from Chassany et al 2000)

Osmotic
Lactulose, sorbitol, fructose, mannitol (laxatives, sugar-free products)
Magnesium (laxatives, antacids)
Maldigestion of carbohydrates
    Antibacterials
    Acarbose

Secretory
Antibacterials
Antineoplastics
Auranofin
Biguanides (metformin)
Calcitonin
Chenodeoxycholic acid
Colchicine
Digoxin
Non-steroidal anti-inflammatory drugs
Olsalazine
Prostaglandins (misoprostol, carboprost, dinoprostone, gemeprost)
Stimulant laxatives (bisacodyl, senna)
Ticlopidine

Motility
Colchicine
Macrolides (erythromycin) and other antibacterials
Levothyroxine (thyroxine)
Ticlopidine

Exudative
Antibacterials
Antineoplastics
Non-steroidal anti-inflammatory drugs
Simvastatin
Stimulant laxatives
Ticlopidine

Malabsorption of fat
Aminoglycosides
Auranofin
Biguanides
Colestyramine
Colchicine
Laxatives
Methyldopa
Octreotide
Orlistat
Tetracyclines

Microbial proliferation
Antibacterials
Antineoplastics
Immunosuppressive agents
Non-steroidal anti-inflammatory drugs

Histological colitis
Antineoplastics
Auranofin
Ciclosporin
Non-steroidal anti-inflammatory drugs
Carbamazepine
Cimetidine, ranitidine
Ferrous sulphate
Levodopa-benserazide
Simvastatin
Ticlopidine

family and contacts are ill, recent travel abroad, food eaten, antibiotic use and weight loss are all important factors to elucidate. The possibility of underlying diseases such as AIDS or infective proctitis in homosexual men must also be considered.

Dehydration is a common problem in the very young and frail elderly and the signs and symptoms must be recognized. In mild dehydration tiredness, anorexia, nausea and lightheadedness may be the only symptoms present. Symptoms become more prominent in moderate dehydration and include thirst along with tiredness, apathy and dizziness. Decreased skin turgor, dry mucous membranes, sunken eyes, absence of tears on crying and postural hypotension are common additional findings. In severe dehydration hypovolaemic shock, oliguria or anuria, cool extremeties, a rapid and weak pulse and low or undetectable blood pressure may all be present.

Investigations

Before any investigations are undertaken a detailed drug history is required to eliminate antibiotic and other drug-induced diarrhoeas, or the possibility of a laxative (overuse) induced diarrhoea. Testing for *Clostridium difficile* induced pseudomembranous colitis is indicated in those with severe symptoms or where hospitalization or antibiotic therapy with lincomycins, broad-spectrum β-lactams or cephalosporins has occurred within the preceding 6 weeks.

In general, stool culture is required in patients with bloody diarrhoea, severe symptoms or where there is no improvement within 48 hours. If there is a history of recent overseas travel stool should be examined for ova, cysts and parasites. Rotavirus should be looked for in those under 5 years.

Where the diarrhoea persists for more than 10 days further investigation should be undertaken to exclude parasites such as *Giardia*, *Entamoeba* and *Cryptosporidium*. Acute, severe or persistent diarrhoea in a homosexual male or patient with AIDS warrants referral for specialist advice. The onset of what appears to be acute diarrhoea may in fact be the first presentation of gastrointestinal pathology such as diverticulitis, colitis or inflammatory bowel disease.

Treatment

Acute infective diarrhoea, including traveller's diarrhoea, is usually a self-limiting disorder. However, depending on the causative agent a number of complications may have to be dealt with. Dehydration and electrolyte disturbance can be readily treated but may, if severe, progress to acidosis and circulatory failure with hypoperfusion of vital organs, renal failure and death. Toxic megacolon due to infective colitis has been documented, associated arthritis or Reiter's syndrome may complicate the invasive diarrhoeas of *Campylobacter* and *Yersinia*, *Salmonella* species may infiltrate bones, joints, meninges and the gallbladder and *E. coli* infection may, for example, be complicated by haemolytic uraemic syndrome.

General measures

Patients should be advised on handwashing and other hygiene related issues to prevent transmission to other family members. Exclusion from work or school until the patient is free of diarrhoea is advised. In acute, self-limiting diarrhoea, health care workers and food handlers should be symptom free for 48 hours before returning to work. More exacting criteria for return to work, such as testing for negative stool samples, are rarely required.

In both children and adults normal feeding should be restarted as soon as possible. In children with gastroenteritis early feeding after rehydration has been shown to result in higher weight gain, no deterioration or prolongation of the diarrhoea and no increase in vomiting or lactose intolerance (Sandhu et al 1997). Breastfeeding infants should continue to feed as cessation may reduce milk supply. Avoidance of milk or other lactose containing food is seldom justified.

Dehydration treatment

Since diarrhoea results in fluid and electrolyte loss it is important to ensure the effected individual maintains adequate fluid intake. Most patients can be advised to increase their intake of fluids, particularly fruit juices with their glucose and potassium content, and soups because of their sodium chloride content. High carbohydrate foods such as bread and pasta can also be recommended because they promote glucose and sodium co-transport.

Young children and the frail elderly are prone to diarrhoea-induced dehydration and use of an oral rehydration solution is recommended. The formula (Table 12.6) recommended by the World Health Organization (WHO) contains glucose, sodium, potassium, chloride and bicarbonate in an almost isotonic fluid. A number of similar preparations are available commercially in the form of sachets that require reconstitution in clean water before use. Glucose concentrations between 80 and 120 mmol/l are needed to optimize sodium absorption in the small intestine. Glucose concentrations in excess of 160 mmol/l will cause an osmotic gradient that will result in increased fluid and electrolyte loss. High sodium solutions in excess of 90 mmol/l may lead to hypernatraemia, especially in children, and should be avoided.

The WHO oral rehydration solution contains 90 mmol/l sodium. However, commercially available solutions in the UK contain no more that half this concentration because patients in the UK generally suffer less severe sodium loss. The risk of hypernatraemia from using the WHO formula is therefore avoided. The presence of potassium prevents hypokalaemia occurring in the elderly, especially in those taking diuretics. For healthy adults an appropriate substitute for a rehydration sachet is 1 level teaspoonful of table salt plus 1 tablespoon of sugar in 1 litre of drinking water. The volume of oral rehydration solution to be taken in treating mild to moderate diarrhoea is dependent on age. In adults 2 litres of oral rehydration fluid should be given in the first 24 hours, followed by unrestricted normal fluids with 200 ml of rehydration solution per loose stool or vomit. For children, 30–50 ml/kg of an oral rehydration solution should be given over 3–4 hours. This can be followed with unrestricted fluids, either with normal fluids alternating with oral rehydration solution or normal fluids with 10 ml/kg rehydration solution after each loose stool or vomit (Murphy 1998). The solution is best sipped every 5–10 minutes rather than drunk in large quantities less frequently.

Care is required in diabetic patients who may need to monitor blood glucose levels more carefully.

Drug treatment

Antimotility agents

In acute diarrhoea, antimotility agents such as loperamide, diphenoxylate and codeine are occasionally useful for symptomatic control in adults who have mild to moderate diarrhoea and require relief from associated abdominal cramps. Management should initially focus on prevention or treatment of fluid and electrolyte depletion before antimotility agents are considered.

Table 12.6 The World Health Organization's recommended oral rehydration solution for use in the treatment of diarrhoea (to be made up in clean water)

Ingredient	Concentration (mmol/l)	Ingredient in 1.0 l water
Glucose	111	20 g (glucose)
Sodium	90	3.5 g (NaCl)
Potassium	20	1.5 g (KCl)
Chloride	80	–
Bicarbonate	30	2.5 g ($NaHCO_3$)

Antimotility agents should be avoided in severe gastroenteritis or dysentry because of the possibility of precipitating ileus or toxic megacolon. Of the various agents available loperamide is the drug of choice because of its low incidence of CNS effects. Antimotility agents are not generally recommended for use in children.

Diphenoxylate

Diphenoxylate is a synthetic opioid available as co-phenotrope in combination with a subtherapeutic dose of atropine. The atropine is present to discourage abuse but may cause atropinic effects in susceptible individuals. Administration of co-phenotrope at the recommended dosage carries minimal risk of dependence. However, prolonged use or administration of high doses may produce a morphine-type dependence. Its adverse effect profile resembles that of morphine.

In cases of suspected overdose signs may be delayed for up to 48 hours. Young children are particularly susceptible to diphenoxylate overdose where as few as 10 tablets of co-phenotrope may be fatal.

Concurrent use of diphenoxylate with monoamine-oxidase inhibitors can precipitate a hypertensive crisis while the action of CNS depressants such as barbiturates, tranquillizers and alcohol are enhanced

Loperamide

Loperamide is also a synthetic opioid analogue that exerts its action by binding to opiate receptors in the gut wall, reducing propulsive peristalsis, increasing intestinal transit time, enhancing the resorption of water and electrolytes, reducing gut secretions and increasing anal sphincter tone. In uncomplicated diarrhoea it may have an effect within 1 hour of oral administration. Due to high first pass metabolism and the affinity for gut wall receptors, very little loperamide reaches the systemic circulation. It is relatively free of CNS effects at therapeutic doses although CNS depression may be seen in overdose, particularly in children. Because it undergoes hepatic metabolism it should be used with caution in patients with hepatic dysfunction. Co-trimoxazole increases the bioavailability of loperamide by inhibiting first-pass metabolism.

Codeine

The constipating side-effect of the opioid analgesic codeine may be used to treat diarrhoea and it can be found in a number of anti-diarrhoeal preparations. Codeine is susceptible to misuse and, given in large doses, may induce tolerance and psychological and physical dependence.

Morphine

The fact that opioid analgesics induce constipation was discussed at the start of this chapter. This effect may be employed in the management of diarrhoea. However, dependence and associated problems of misuse limit its usefulness. Morphine may still be obtained in combination with agents such as the adsorbent kaolin. Evidence of efficacy in the treatment of diarrhoea is limited and these combination products cannot be recommended.

Bismuth subsalicylate

Bismuth subsalicylate is an insoluble complex of trivalent bismuth and salicylate that has been shown to be effective in reducing stool frequency. It possesses antimicrobial activity on the basis of its bismuth content while the salicylate is considered to confer antisecretory properties. At therapeutic doses it is relatively free from side-effects although it may cause blackening of the tongue and stool. The relatively large quantity of the liquid preparation that has to be consumed is seen as a disadvantage.

Antimicrobials

Antibiotics are generally not recommended in diarrhoea associated with acute infective gastroenteritis. Inappropriate use will only contribute further to the problem of resistant organisms. There is, however, a place for antibiotics in patients with positive stool culture where the symptoms are not receding. In patients presenting with dysentery or suspected exposure to bacterial infection, treatment with a quinolone, for example ciprofloxacin, may be appropriate. However, quinolones are not without their problems: they may cause tendon damage, induce convulsions in epileptics and in situations that predispose to seizures, or in patients taking NSAIDs. Their use in adolescents is also not recommended because use has been associated with arthropathy.

Where *Campylobacter* is the suspect causative organism, patients with severe symptoms or dysentery should receive early treatment with erythromycin or ciprofloxacin. Severe symptoms or dysentery associated with *Shigella* can also be treated with ciprofloxacin. Nalidixic acid can be used in children and trimethoprim may be appropriate in pregnant women where resistance is not a problem.

The use of antibiotics in patients with *Salmonella* is not generally recommended because of the likelihood that excretion is prolonged. Antibiotics may, however, be indicated in the very young and the immunocompromised. The benefit of antibiotic use in enterohaemorrhagic infection, for example *E. coli* O157, is even less clear. In this situation there is evidence that antibiotics cause toxins to be released which may lead to haemolytic uraemic syndrome.

In both amoebic dysentery and giardiasis, metronidazole is the drug of choice. Diloxanide is also used in amoebic dysentery to ensure eradication of the intestinal disease. Antibiotics are not indicated in the treatment of cryptosporidiosis in immunocompromised individuals.

Table 12.7 outlines some of the common therapeutic problems in constipation and diarrhoea.

Table 12.7   Common therapeutic problems in constipation and diarrhoea

Problem	Comment
Constipation	
Bulk laxative, e.g. ispaghula taken at bedtime	Drugs such as ispaghula should not be taken before going to bed because of risk of oesophageal blockage
Urine changes colour	Anthraquinone glycosides, e.g. senna, are excreted by kidney and may colour urine yellowish-brown to red colour, depending on pH
Patient claims dietary and fluid advice expect ineffective in resolving constipation	May find high fibre diet difficult to adhere to, socially unacceptable, and result in less than 4 weeks
Patient taking docusate complains of unpleasant aftertaste or burning sensation	Advise to take with plenty of fluid after ingestion
Diarrhoea	
Antimotility agent requested for a young child	Antimotility agents must be avoided in young children or patients with severe gastroenteritis or dysentery
Antimotility agent requested by patient with persistent diarrhoea (> 10 days)	Antimotility agent inappropriate. Stool culture required to exclude parasitic infection such as *Giardia, Entamoeba* and *Cryptosporidium*
Mother stops breastfeeding to allow baby's diarrhoea to settle	Breastfeeding should continue
Adult with diarrhoea stops eating and drinking to allow diarrhoea to settle	Patient should eat and drink as normally as possible. Plenty of fluids required to prevent dehydration. Fruit juice (glucose and potassium), soup (salt), bread and pasta (carbohydrate) are of particular benefit

CASE STUDIES

Case 12.1

Mr A.'s mother has recently moved in with his family following the death of his father 4 month ago. Although she was formerly a sprightly 78-year-old she is now withdrawn, eats little of the meals prepared for her and no longer goes for her daily walks. Mr A. knows she is taking medicine for a long-standing heart complaint and has recently started taking antidepressants. She is complaining of constipation.

Question

Mr A. would like to know if there is any medicine suitable to help his mother.

Answer

Constipation is a common problem in the elderly. Activity levels often diminish and many also suffer from medicine-induced constipation exacerbated by reduced muscle tone. Pain on defaecation associated with haemorrhoids is also a common contributory factor. The elderly often have poor dental status or false teeth and consequently avoid high fibre foods because they are more difficult to chew.

In the case of Mr A.'s mother, the history provides little insight into the underlying problem although there are a number of factors that warrant further investigation. Clearly a reduction in physical activity has occurred and her diet and fluid intake may have changed. The identity of her 'heart medicine' may reveal a drug-induced factor that could have been enhanced by the recent prescription for antidepressants. It is also unclear whether she has been constipated previously.

The elderly often want to take laxatives, not only to restore normal bowel function, but also to prevent constipation. This in turn may lead to laxative abuse that can result in chronic constipation and damage bowel muscle tone. The death of her husband and loss of independence are significant lifestyle issues for Mr A.'s mother that cannot readily be addressed. Appropriate exercise, proper diet and sufficient fluid may be the only key actions that need to be taken.

Case 12.2

Mr B. is a busy 45-years-old executive who works for a large multinational company. He has noted blood in his stools over the past 2 weeks and for 3 days has had

continuous abdominal discomfort. He has discussed his symptoms with his wife and they suspect haemorrhoids are the cause. Mr B. is going away on business in 6 days and seeks your advice on a suitable treatment.

Question

What advice should be given to Mr B.?

Answer

Blood in the stool is not necessarily serious. If the blood appears fresh and can only be seen on the surface of the stool it is likely the source is the anus or distal colon. It is probably caused by straining and bleeding from haemorrhoids. Similarly if the blood appears as specks or as a smear on the toilet paper after defacation it too is likely to indicate haemorrhoids, particularly if such a diagnosis has been made previously following clinical examination.

If the blood is mixed with the faeces and has a dark or 'tarry' appearance a more serious underlying cause such as diverticulosis, a bleeding peptic ulcer, or, in rare cases, a carcinoma is possible. If this is the case the patient should have a proper clinical examination.

If Mr B. is taking iron or bismuth tablets these may cause darkened stools and in this situation the signs are of no clinical consequence and reassurance should suffice.

However, given the presence of continuous or severe abdominal pain accompanying constipation, and of recent onset, a thorough clinical examination is required. Underlying factors include bowel obstruction caused by a tumour, diverticular disease or irritable bowel syndrome. The constellation of symptoms presented by Mr B. warrants a thorough clinical investigation as soon as possible.

Case 12.3

A 7-year-old boy in previous good health was admitted to hospital with bloody diarrhoea and dehydration 4 days after attending a children's birthday party. He was treated with intravenous fluids and given nothing by mouth. The day after admission to hospital a colonoscopy revealed haemorrhagic colitis. His diarrhoea seemed to be improving up to day 5 when he experienced a generalized convulsion following which he was transferred to a children's intensive care bed. He was irritable and pale, hypertensive and an emergency laboratory report revealed thrombocytopenia, hyponatraemia and hyperkalaemia.

Questions

1. What is the likely diagnosis in this child?
2. What specific therapy is required?

Answers

1. This patient probably has haemolytic uraemic syndrome caused by *E. coli* O157. Haemolytic uraemic syndrome is the most common form of acquired renal insufficiency in young children. It is characterized by nephropathy, thrombocytopenia, and microangiopathic haemolytic anaemia. Although there are a number of potential

causative factors the most common is the toxin producing O157 strain of *E. coli*. In 1996, 21 people died from *E. coli* O157 after eating contaminated meat from a butcher's shop in Scotland. In 2001, 13 girl guides and their leader contracted *E. coli* O157 after camping in a field in Inverclyde, Scotland, previously grazed by sheep.

The syndrome typically has a prodrome of bloody diarrhoea occurring 5–7 days before onset of renal insufficiency. Colonoscopy is usually non-specific and shows haemorrhagic colitis. At diagnosis most children are pale and very irritable. Hypertension and hyponatraemia may be associated with convulsions and are generally a consequence of a disorder of fluid and salt balance. Laboratory findings may include anaemia and thrombocytopenia, hyponatraemia, hyperkalaemia, hypocalcaemia and metabolic acidosis. The kidney typically shows signs of glomerular endothelial injury. Capillary thrombosis is quite prominent but with no evidence of immune complex deposition. Similar findings can usually be seen in all other organs including the brain, liver, and intestine.

2. Treatment is usually supportive. Fluid and electrolyte balance need to be corrected and the hypertension controlled. In cases with prolonged oliguria or anuria, peritoneal dialysis may be used. Approximately 85% of patients recover normal renal function.

Case 12.4

Mr G. is planning to travel to Mexico on business. He was last there 6 months ago but was incapacitated with diarrhoea for 3 of 6 days in a busy work schedule. He does not want a repeat experience on his forthcoming visit and seeks advice about taking a course of antibiotics with him to use as empirical treatment should the need arise.

Questions

1. Is there any evidence that antibiotics are of benefit in travellers' diarrhoea?
2. Are there any problems associated with empirical use of antibiotics in traveller's diarrhoea?

Answers

1. The empirical use of antibiotics has been shown to increase the cure rate in individuals suffering from traveller's diarrhoea. Studies in travellers including students, package tourists, military personnel and volunteers have compared antibiotic use against placebo (De Bruyn et al 2000). The antibiotics studied have included aztreonam, ciprofloxacin, co-trimoxazole, norfloxacin, ofloxacin and trimethoprim given for durations varying form a single dose to a 5 day treatment course. Overall antibiotics increased the cure rate at 72 hours (defined as cessation of unformed stools, or less than one unformed stool/24 hours) without additional symptoms.
2. The use of antibiotics in the treatment of traveller's diarrhoea do have problems. Adverse effects in up to 18% of recipients have been reported with gastrointestinal (cramp, nausea, anorexia), dermatological (rash) and respiratory (cough, sore throat) symptoms the most frequently reported. Antibiotic resistant isolates have also been reported following the use of ciprofloxacin, co-trimoxazole and norfloxacin.

REFERENCES

Chassany O, Michaux A, Bergman J F 2000 Drug-induced diarrhoea. Drug Safety 22: 53–72

De Bruyn G, Hahn S, Borwick A 2000 Antibiotic treatment for travellers' diarrhoea. Cochrane Review. Cochrane Library, issue 3. Update Software, Oxford.

Murphy M S 1998 Guidelines for managing acute gastroenteritis based on a systematic review of published research. Archives of Disease in Childhood 79: 279–284

Rasquin-Weber A, Hyman P E, Cucchiara S et al 1999 Childhood functional gastrointestinal disorders. Gut 45(Suppl. 2): 60–68

Sandhu B K, Isolauri E, Walker-Smith J A et al 1997 A multicentre study on behalf of the European Society of Paediatric Gastroenterology and Nutrition Working Group on Acute Diarrhoea: early feeding in childhood gastroenteritis. Journal of Pediatric Gastroenterology and Nutrition 24: 522–527

Thompson W G, Longstreth G F, Drossman D A et al 1999 Functional bowel disorders and functional abdominal pain. Gut 45(Suppl. 2): 43–47

FURTHER READING

Anon. 2000 Managing constipation in children. Drug and Therapeutics Bulletin 38: 57–60

Bartlett J G 2002 Antibiotic-associated diarrhoea. New England Journal of Medicine 346: 334–339

Borum M L 2001 Constipation: evaluation and management. Primary Care 28: 577–590

Cope D G 2001 Management of chemotherapy-induced diarrhoea and constipation. Nursing Clinics of North America 36: 695–707

Elawad M A, Sullivan P B 2001 Management of constipation in children with disabilities. Developmental Medicine and Child Neurology 43: 829–832

Pappagallo M 2001 Incidence, prevalence and management of opioid bowel dysfunction. American Journal of Surgery 182(Suppl. 5A): 115–185

Sellin J H 2001 The pathophysiology of diarrhoea. Clinical Transplantation 15(Suppl. 4): 2–10

Xing J H, Soffer E E 2001 Adverse effects of laxatives. Diseases of the Colon and Rectum 44: 1201–1209

Adverse effects of drugs on the liver

13

B. E. Cadman   B. Featherstone

KEY POINTS

- Approximately 2–5% of jaundice cases, 10% of hepatitis cases and 20–30% of acute liver failure cases are attributed to drugs.
- Risk of drug-induced liver disorders increases with age and is generally more common in women.
- Generally drug induced liver damage can be categorized into cytotoxic (necrotic or steatic) or cholestatic. The reaction may be intrinsic or idiosyncratic.
- Drugs can cause all types of liver disorder and should always be considered during diagnosis.
- The clinical features of drug-induced hepatotoxicity vary widely, depending upon the type of liver damage caused.
- Treatment of drug-induced hepatotoxicity relies on correct diagnosis, prompt withdrawal of the causative agent and supportive therapy.
- Patients given potentially hepatotoxic drugs should be informed how to recognize signs of liver dysfunction and advised to report symptoms immediately.
- Any new drug released onto the market may have the potential to cause hepatotoxicity. Post-marketing surveillance is extremely important to highlight any new potential hepatotoxic effects.

An adverse drug reaction (ADR) is an effect that is unintentional, noxious and occurs at doses used for diagnosis, prophylaxis and treatment. A hepatic drug reaction is an ADR which predominantly affects the liver.

Drugs can induce almost all forms of acute or chronic liver disease, with some drugs producing more than one type of hepatic lesion. Although not a particularly common form of adverse drug reaction, drugs should always be considered as a possible cause of liver disease.

Epidemiology

The incidence of drug-induced liver disease has continued to rise steadily since the late 1960s, although the incidence for most drugs remains low. In studies from the 1960s and 1970s, the incidence of drug-induced disease was between 2% and 5% of patients presenting with jaundice as hospital in-patients, approximately 10% of cases of hepatitis, and up to 20–30% of acute liver

failure cases. More recent studies have suggested 15–40% of acute liver failure cases may be attributable to drugs.

In the early 1990s, acute overdose with paracetamol accounted for 30–40 000 hospital admissions and over half the cases of acute liver failure referred to liver units. It was the definite cause of at least 150 deaths a year in the UK. Acute liver failure induced by paracetamol has become an important indication for liver transplantation. Hepatotoxicity induced by such drugs as halothane, the antituberculous agents isoniazid and rifampicin, psychotropics, antibiotics and cytotoxic drugs still continues to cause concern.

Many drugs cause elevated liver enzymes with apparently no clinically significant adverse effect, although in a few patients there may be significant hepatotoxicity. For example, isoniazid causes elevated liver enzymes in 10–36% of patients taking the drug as a single agent. However, only 1% suffer significant hepatotoxicity, with the liver function tests of the majority returning to normal if therapy is discontinued. Other examples of drugs that elevate liver enzymes are shown in Table 13.1.

Although it is not possible to identify patients who will suffer adverse drug reactions manifesting in hepatic toxicity, a number of risk factors have been identified.

Risk factors

Pre-existing liver disease

Pre-existing liver disease does not in general increase the risk of developing drug-induced hepatic injury although exceptions have been noted with methotrexate, other cytotoxic agents, aspirin and sodium valproate. Patients with liver disease are more likely to suffer ADRs in general.

Age

It is generally accepted that the elderly have an increased risk of adverse drug reactions. There are multiple reasons for this including higher exposure rates and decreased metabolism. Drug-induced hepatic injury is more likely to

Table 13.1 Examples of drugs that elevate liver enzymes	
Drug	Percentage of patients with increases in transaminases
Cefaclor	11%
Cefixime	0.7%
Ciprofloxacin	5%
Diclofenac	15%
Donepezil	CSM reports
Isoniazid	10–36%
Naproxen	4%
Norfloxacin	0.1%
Rifampicin	15–30%
Rofecoxib	CSM reports
Sodium valproate	11%
SSRIs	CSM reports
Sulphonamides	10%

occur in elderly patients than in those under 35 years of age. Similarly, halothane hepatitis and isoniazid or chlorpromazine hepatotoxicity is more likely in patients over 40 years of age. The severity of the reactions also appears to increase with age, especially in those over 60 years. Sodium valproate toxicity, on the other hand, demonstrates an increased risk of developing serious or fatal hepatotoxicity in those under 3 years, with risk decreasing as age advances. Aspirin is an example of another drug causing hepatotoxicity specifically in children. Reye's syndrome in children has been linked to the use of aspirin following a viral illness; it is life-threatening and associated with coma, seizures and liver failure.

Gender

The frequency of drug-induced hepatotoxicity is more common in females than males, particularly with halothane, isoniazid, nitrofurantoin and flucloxacillin. There is weak evidence of a gender difference in toxicity of sodium valproate, being more common in boys before puberty and in females after puberty. Cholestatic jaundice associated with co-amoxiclav has been reported to be more common in males than females.

Genetics

Genetic differences that affect an individual's ability to metabolize certain drugs may predispose to drug-induced liver disease. For example, both fast and slow acetylators may be more susceptible to isoniazid-induced liver damage. The conventional view is that rapid acetylators are at risk of increased toxic reactions due to transformation of acetylhydrazine by cytochrome P450 into a reactive metabolite; other studies suggest slow acetylation may result in toxicity due to formation of hydrazine, which is toxic in itself. Monitoring of liver function tests (LFTs) is recommended monthly for the first 3 months, as toxicity is most likely to occur early in therapy.

Halothane-induced injury has been reported for multiple family members in one study.

It is thought that a genetic predisposition to allergic forms of drug hypersensitivity could be a factor in some types of liver disease.

Enzyme induction

Alcohol, rifampicin and other drugs that induce cytochrome P450 isoenzyme 2El potentiate the risk of hepatotoxicity with other drugs such as paracetamol, isoniazid and halothane.

Concomitant therapy with other anticonvulsants, particularly phenytoin and phenobarbital, is a risk factor for toxicity with sodium valproate, where 90% of cases of liver injury are associated with combination therapy.

Polypharmacy

A typical example of this is seen with NSAIDs. The risk of liver disease with NSAIDs is normally extremely low but is increased when NSAIDs are used with other hepatotoxic drugs.

Concurrent diseases

Pre-existing renal disease, diabetes, pregnancy and poor nutrition may all affect the ability of the liver to metabolize drugs effectively and may put the patient at risk of developing liver damage.

Aetiology

Drug-induced hepatotoxicity may present as an acute insult that may or may not progress to chronic disease, or it can present as an insidious development of chronic disease. The type of lesion may be cytotoxic (cellular destruction) or cholestatic (impaired bile flow). Cytotoxic damage may be further classified as necrotic (cell death) or steatic (fatty degeneration). The liver damage resulting from drug toxicity often presents as a mixed picture of cytotoxic and cholestatic injury. The mechanisms of drug-induced hepatic damage can be divided into intrinsic (type A) and idiosyncratic (type B) hepatotoxicity. Intrinsic hepatotoxicity is predictable, dose-dependent, and usually has a short incubation period ranging from hours to weeks. The majority of individuals who take a toxic dose are affected and exhibit the same type of injury that can be reproduced in experimental animals. Examples are paracetamol, salicylates, methotrexate and tetracycline. Other examples are presented in Table 13.2. Toxicity may be avoided by ensuring the doses listed are not exceeded.

Idiosyncratic reactions occur at a low frequency, typically less than 1%, in individuals who are exposed to the drug. The incubation period is variable but is typically weeks or months, and the type of injury is less predictable and not dose related. This type of reaction may be due to either drug hypersensitivity or a metabolic abnormality. The reactions are difficult to reproduce in experimental animals. Examples of drugs that induce idiosyncratic reactions are chlorpromazine, halothane and isoniazid.

Table 13.2. Examples of dose-related drug-induced hepatotoxicity

Drug	Toxic dose
Paracetamol	Single dose > 10 g
Tetracycline	> 2 g daily (oral) (increased risk of toxicity in pregnancy and renal failure)
Methotrexate	Weekly dose > 15 mg Cumulative dose > 2 g in 3 years (increased risk of toxicity in pre-existing liver disease, alcohol, diabetes)
6-Mercaptopurine	> 2.5 mg/kg
Vitamin A	Chronic use of 40 000 units daily
Cyclophosphamide	Daily dose > 400 mg/m^2
Salicylates	Chronic use > 2 g daily
Anabolic steroids	High dose > 1 month
Oral contraceptive steroids	Increased risk with higher oestrogen content seen in earlier preparations Duration of treatment also a risk factor
Iron	Single dose > 1 g

The precise mechanisms resulting in drug-induced liver disease are often not completely understood, although injury to the hepatocytes may result directly from interference with intracellular function, membrane integrity or indirectly by immune-mediated damage to cells.

Necrosis

Necrosis is characterized by cytotoxic cellular breakdown (hepatocellular destruction).

Paracetamol causes hepatic necrosis when its normal metabolic pathway is saturated. Subsequent metabolism occurs by an alternative pathway that produces a toxic metabolite which covalently binds to liver cell proteins and causes necrosis.

Steatosis

In steatosis hepatocytes become filled with small droplets of lipid (microvesicular fatty liver), or occasionally with lipid droplets that are much larger (macrovesicular fatty liver). Tetracyclines are thought to cause steatosis by interfering with synthesis of lipoproteins that normally remove triglycerides from the liver.

Cholestasis

Some drugs injure bile ducts and cause partial or complete obstruction of the common bile duct resulting in retention of bile acids and the condition known as cholestasis.

Cholestasis caused by anabolic and contraceptive steroids is due to inhibition of bilirubin excretion from the hepatocyte into the bile.

The penicillins, although commonly associated with allergic drug reactions, are a very rare cause of liver disease. The isoxazoyl group present in the synthetic β-lactamase-resistant oxypenicillins has been implicated as a cause of liver injury. Acute cholestatic hepatitis has increasingly been reported during treatment with flucloxacillin, and in some countries it has become the most important cause of drug-induced cholestatic hepatitis. The incidence appears to be about twice that of the related isoxazoyl penicillins cloxacillin and dicloxacillin. Moreover, there is likely to be under-reporting due to a delay in onset of up to 42 days after stopping treatment. Female sex, age over 55 years, longer courses and high daily doses also seem to be associated with a higher risk of liver reaction to flucloxacillin.

Rifampicin causes hyperbilirubinaemia by inhibiting uptake of bilirubin by the hepatocyte as well as inhibiting bilirubin excretion into bile. Other therapeutic agents affect sinusoidal or endothelial cells, which may result in veno-occlusive disease or fibrosis. Vitamin A affects the fat-storing cells, causing toxicity that leads to fibrosis.

Pathophysiology

The range of drug-induced liver diseases is illustrated in Table 13.3. Increased serum levels of hepatobiliary enzymes without clinical liver disease occurs with variable frequency between drugs but for some agents it may occur in up to half the patients who receive it. This may reflect subclinical liver injury.

Hepatocellular necrosis

In severe cases acute hepatocellular necrosis presents with jaundice and liver function test (LFT) abnormalities including a modestly raised alkaline phosphatase and a markedly elevated alanine aminotransferase level of up to 200 times the upper limit of the reference range. Prolongation of the prothrombin time occurs but depends on the severity of the injury, increasing dramatically in severe cases. Microscopy reveals necrosis of the hepatocytes in a characteristic pattern.

Steatosis

Steatosis (fatty liver) is the accumulation of fat droplets within liver cells and is associated with abnormal LFTs, although the elevation of alanine aminotransferase is not as high as that seen in acute hepatocellular necrosis. Hyperammonia, hypoglycaemia, acidosis and clotting factor deficiency may also be present. Histologically, the liver damage resembles the acute fatty liver of pregnancy. Fat distribution within the hepatocyte is either microvesicular, as occurs with tetracycline, aspirin and sodium valproate, or macrovesicular where the hepatocyte cell nucleus is displaced to the periphery by a single large fat droplet. This type of damage occurs typically with steroids, methotrexate, alcohol and amiodarone.

A less severe, more chronic form of fatty liver steatohepatitis also occurs. Steatohepatitis differs from diffuse fatty change. Notably the clinical symptoms and biochemisty resemble chronic parenchymal disease and the histology is similar to that seen in alcoholic hepatitis. Amiodarone is an example of a drug that can cause chronic steatohepatitis associated with phospholipidosis.

Cholestasis

Cholestasis without hepatitis is associated with a raised bilirubin and a normal or minimally raised alanine aminotransferase level. No inflammation or

Table 13.3 Examples of adverse drug reactions on the liver

Adverse reaction	Drugs associated with reaction
Hepatocellular necrosis	Paracetamol Propythiouracil Salicylates Iron salts Allopurinol Dantrolene Halothane Ketoconazole Isoniazid Mithramycin Cocaine 'Ecstasy'
Fatty liver	Amiodarone Tetracyclines Steroids Sodium valprotate L-Asparaginase
Cholestasis	Oral contraceptives Carbimazole Anabolic steroids Ciclosporin
Cholestasis with hepatitis	Chlorpromazine Tricyclics Erythromycin Flucloxacillin Co-amoxiclav ACE inhibitors Sulphonamides Sulphonylureas Phenytoin NSAIDs Cimetidine Ranitidine
Granulomatous hepatitis	Phenytoin Allopurinol Carbamazepine Clofibrate Hydralazine Sulphonamides Sulphonylureas
Acute hepatitis	Dantrolene Isoniazid Phenytoin
Chronic active hepatitis	Methyldopa Nitrofurantoin Isoniazid
Fibrosis and cirrhosis	Methotrexate Methyldopa Vitamin A (dose related)
Vascular disorders	Azathioprine Dactinomycin Dacarbazine

hepatocellular necrosis is seen. In contrast, cholestasis associated with hepatitis presents with raised bilirubin, alanine aminotransferase and alkaline phosphatase levels and a certain amount of liver damage.

Granulomatous hepatitis

Granulomatous hepatitis occurs with modestly elevated LFTs, and usually normal synthetic liver function. Histology reveals granulomas and tissue eosinophilia.

Acute hepatitis

Acute hepatitis resembles viral hepatitis with LFTs raised in proportion to the severity of the hepatocellular damage. The best indicator of severity is the prothrombin time. Histologically, necrosis and cellular degeneration in combination with an inflammatory infiltrate are seen.

Chronic active hepatitis

Chronic active hepatitis may present as an acute injury or progress to cirrhosis. Serum transaminases are usually raised and albumin is low. The histology resembles that of autoimmune chronic active hepatitis and is associated with circulating autoantibodies. Methyldopa is an example of a drug that can cause chronic active hepatitis.

Fibrosis

In patients with fibrosis, the serum transaminase levels may be only slightly raised, and are not good predictors of hepatic damage. Microscopy shows deposition of fibrous tissues. Fibrosis may proceed to cirrhosis. Such damage may be seen with long-term methotrexate use.

Vascular disorders

A variety of drugs can cause veno-occlusive disease, which is characterized by non-thrombotic narrowing of small centrilobular veins, and is typically caused by cytotoxic agents and some herbal remedies. Use of oral contraceptives or cytotoxic agents may exacerbate an underlying thrombotic disorder and increase the risk of the Budd–Chiari syndrome (obstruction of the large veins) developing.

Tumours

Drugs have been associated with a variety of hepatic tumours. The drugs most commonly linked to malignancy are the oral contraceptives, anabolic steroids and danazol.

Clinical manifestations

The clinical features of drug-induced hepatotoxicity vary widely, depending on the type of liver damage caused.

In acute hepatocellular necrosis caused by paracetamol, early symptoms include anorexia, nausea and vomiting, malaise and lethargy. Abdominal pain may be the first indication of liver damage, and is not usually apparent for 24–48 hours. A period of apparent recovery precedes the development of jaundice and production of dark urine. If the liver injury is severe, deterioration follows, with repeated vomiting, hypoglycaemia, metabolic acidosis, bruising and bleeding, drowsiness and hepatic encephalopathy. Oliguria (diminished urine output) and anuria (complete cessation of urine production) may result from acute tubular necrosis. Renal failure may occur even in the absence of severe liver disease. In addition to acute renal failure, myocardial injury and pancreatitis have also been reported. In fatal cases, death from acute hepatic failure occurs between 4 and 18 days after ingestion.

A patient presenting with steatosis generally shows fatigue, nausea, vomiting, hypoglycaemia and confusion. Jaundice is present in severe cases.

Acute hepatitis may present with a prodromal illness with non-specific symptoms or include features of drug allergy followed by anorexia, nausea and vomiting, dark urine, pale stools and jaundice. Jaundice tends to be present in severe cases. Weight loss may also be a feature of acute hepatitis. Fatalities occur in 5–30% of jaundiced patients. Acute hepatitis is second only to paracetamol self-poisoning as a cause of drug-induced liver disease.

Drug-induced chronic active hepatitis may present with tiredness, lethargy and malaise, in a manner similar to other types of chronic liver disease; the symptoms may evolve over many months. Gastrointestinal symptoms are usually present, and patients may show one or more complications of severe liver disease, including ascites, bleeding oesophageal varices or hepatic encephalopathy. If the adverse drug reaction has an allergic component, a skin rash and other extrahepatic features of a drug allergy such as lymphadenopathy, evidence of bone marrow suppression (particularly petechial haemorrhages) may be present.

The main clinical feature of pure cholestasis is severe pruritus, with or without other features, according to the severity, such as dark urine, pale stools and jaundice.

Drug-induced cholestatic hepatitis usually presents with gastrointestinal symptoms following an influenza-like illness. Abdominal pain with typical features of cholestasis then occurs. The pruritus is generally less severe than with pure cholestasis.

Veno-occlusive disease may present with painful hepatomegaly, ascites and jaundice along with other features of liver insufficiency. It has been reported following chemotherapy with drugs such as cyclophosphamide, doxorubicin and dacarbazine. It has also been reported as a common complication of bone marrow transplantation.

Patients with hepatic tumours in general present in a similar manner. Abdominal pain may or may not be reported, together with a feeling of fullness after eating. Weight loss, fatigue, anorexia, nausea and, occasionally, vomiting can occur, especially in advanced cases.

Investigations

Various types of investigation are used in the diagnosis of drug-induced hepatotoxicity, with the number and type of tests depending on the clinical presentation.

Routine LFTs are measured, which generally include total bilirubin, alanine transaminase and alkaline phosphatase. Impairment of the synthetic function of the liver is detected by total protein, albumin and the prothrombin time. Other biochemical tests may include measurement of γ-glutamyl transpeptidase which may be elevated in all forms of liver disease, including drug-induced disease. α-Fetoprotein may be measured to exclude malignancy. Conjugated bilirubin may be measured to establish if there is biliary obstruction.

Serological markers for hepatitis A, B and C and other viruses such as the Epstein–Barr virus should be determined in patients with symptoms of hepatitis with appropriate risk factors to exclude an infective cause.

Attention should be directed to exclude autoimmune chronic active hepatitis, acute severe cholestasis, ischaemic hepatic necrosis, pregnancy-related liver disease, the Budd–Chiari syndrome, Wilson's disease and other rare metabolic disorders. Alcoholic liver disease must also be excluded.

Radiological investigations, such as ultrasound, computed tomography, percutaneous cholangiograms and endoscopic retrograde cholangiopancreatography, are used to look for physical obstruction of bile ducts by gallstones, masses or strictures.

Liver biopsy and histological evaluation are useful in the diagnosis of acute hepatocellular dysfunction where a drug-induced cause is implicated. Certain drugs can cause characteristic lesions, such as the distribution of microvesicular fat droplets seen with tetracyclines. Specific diagnostic tests for drug-induced disease exist for few drugs, with halothane being a notable exception.

Treatment

The aim of treatment for drug-induced hepatotoxicity is complete recovery. This relies on correct diagnosis, withdrawal of the causative agent, and supportive therapy that may include liver transplantation where appropriate.

Diagnosis

Drug-induced hepatic injury should be suspected in every patient with jaundice while ruling out other causes of liver disease by the clinical history and the results of investigations. Figure 13.1 illustrates the typical process.

Drugs that are commonly prescribed such as non-steroidal anti-inflammatory drugs (NSAIDs), anti-microbials and antihypertensive agents are more likely to be implicated in drug-induced liver disease, although the frequency for the individual agents is low. Identifying the causative agent and stopping it is important in reducing the morbidity and mortality associated with drug-induced liver disease. Recovery normally follows discontinuation of a hepatotoxic drug. Serious toxicity or acute liver failure may result if the drug is continued after symptoms appear or the serum transaminases rise significantly. Failure to discontinue the drug may give grounds for claims of negligence.

A detailed and thorough drug history, including use of oral contraceptives, over-the-counter medicines, vitamins, herbal preparations and illicit drug use, should be obtained. Examples of herbal preparations implicated in causing liver damage are listed in Table 13.4. Attention to the duration of treatment with a specific drug and the relationship to the onset of symptoms is important. The likelihood of a drug-related disease is greatest when the abnormality begins between 5 and 90 days after taking the first dose and within 15 days of taking the last dose. The latent period (the time between

Table 13.4 Examples of herbal remedies implicated in hepatotoxicity (Shaw et al 1997)
Borage oil
Chapparal
Chinese herbal preparations for skin disorders
Garcinia (*Garcinia camboge*)
Germander (*Teucrium chamaedrys*)
Khat (*Catha edulis*)
Passion flower (*Passiflora incarnata*)
Ubiquinone
Valerian (*Valeriania officinalis*)

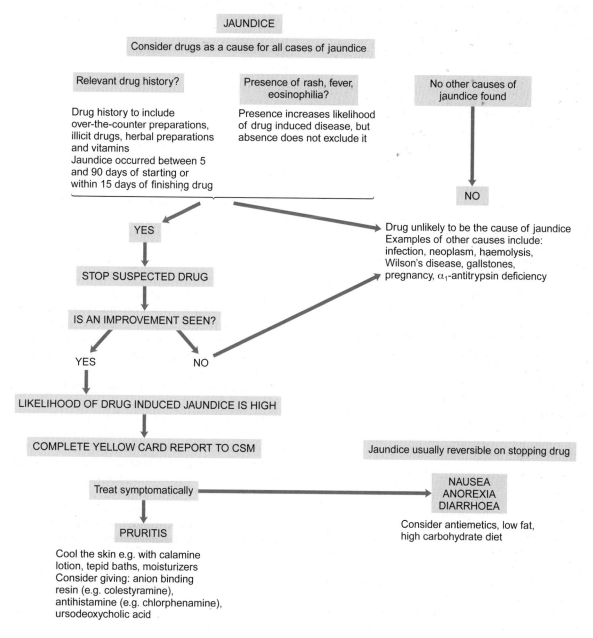

Figure 13.1 General approach to the diagnosis and management of drug-induced jaundice.

starting therapy and the appearance of symptoms) may vary but for many drugs is sufficiently reproducible to be of some diagnostic value.

Predisposing factors for liver toxicity should also be noted. If the liver injury is accompanied by fever, rash and eosinophilia, the likelihood of drug-induced disease increases, although lack of these features does not exclude it. Unequivocal diagnosis cannot be made in most circumstances, and improvement on withdrawal of the implicated drug may provide the strongest evidence for drug-induced disease. Time for resolution of the abnormalities is dependent on the individual drug and type of liver disease. In some cases several months may elapse.

Idiosyncratic reactions may also need to be considered and the literature consulted for previous reports. A key component of secondary prevention is the reporting of all suspected hepatic drug reactions to the appropriate monitoring agency, particularly for newer agents with fewer published cases.

Withdrawal

Once drug-induced hepatotoxicity has been recognized as a possibility, therapy should be stopped. If the patient is receiving more than one potentially hepatotoxic drug, all drugs should be stopped. Withdrawal of the agent usually results in recovery that begins within a few days. The LFTs may take many months to return to normal. Co-amoxiclav and phenytoin are examples of drugs that have been associated with a worsening of the patient's condition for several weeks after withdrawal, and a protracted recovery period of several months.

Rechallenge

When drug-induced hepatotoxicity has been confirmed by improvement on drug withdrawal, subsequent use in the patient is generally contraindicated. Rechallenge is not normally justified as this is potentially dangerous for the patient although a positive rechallenge is the most definitive evidence of drug-induced disease. Inadvertent rechallenge may occur. If the rechallenge is negative, this is usually taken to indicate the patient may resume using the drug. Another adverse reaction on re-exposure to the drug precludes any further use.

Management

If clinical or laboratory signs of hepatic failure appear, hospitalization is mandatory.

After withdrawal of the drug, attempts to remove it from the body are only relevant for acute hepatotoxins such as paracetamol, metals or toxic mushrooms such as *Amanita phalloides* (death cap).

If patients present a few hours post-ingestion, any unabsorbed drug may best be removed by gastric lavage, rather than by use of emetics.

Antidotes

Specific antidotes are acetylcysteine and methionine for paracetamol, and desferrioxamine for iron overdose. Desferrioxamine 5–10 g in 50–100 ml of water is administered orally as soon as possible after ingestion for acute iron poisoning. Parenteral desferrioxamine is indicated in addition to oral administration, to chelate absorbed iron where the plasma levels exceed 89.5 µmol/l, where the plasma levels exceed 62.6 µmol/l and there is evidence of free iron, and in patients with signs and symptoms of acute iron poisoning.

Corticosteroids

Immunosuppression with corticosteroids has been used in the management of drug-induced hepatotoxicity, but evidence indicates their use does not affect survival of patients with acute liver failure. There have, however, been anecdotal reports of impressive responses to corticosteroids that are persuasive, and it may be appropriate for a short trial in rare types of drug-induced disease.

Supportive treatment

For most patients there is no specific treatment available. General supportive treatment is necessary in liver failure, with appropriate attention to fluid and electrolyte balance.

Nutritional support should be along conventional medical lines. Some patients find that a low-fat, high-carbohydrate diet provides relief from the anorexia, nausea and diarrhoea that may accompany cholestasis.

Pruritis

The main symptom of drug-induced cholestasis is pruritus due to high systemic concentrations of bile acids deposited in tissues. General measures include light clothing (avoid wool) and cooling the skin with tepid baths or calamine lotion, and a general moisturizing agent such as aqueous cream. The management of liver-induced pruritus is discussed in more detail in Chapter 14.

Coagulation disorders

Coagulation disorders should be treated by correcting vitamin K deficiency with intravenous phytomenadione injection. This should correct the prothrombin time within 3–5 days. Anaphylaxis may occur following intravenous injection of the polyethoxylated castor oil formulation, but can be avoided by use of the mixed-micelle formulation. Oral phytomenadione is ineffective in cholestasis. Menadiol sodium phosphate, the water-soluble vitamin K analogue, may be effective in an oral dose of 10 mg daily. If bleeding occurs, infusion of fresh frozen plasma or clotting factor concentrates will be indicated. The administration of other fat-soluble vitamins may also be necessary. Liver transplantation is often considered the treatment of choice for patients with acute hepatic failure induced by drugs.

Long-term treatment

When the drug-induced liver disease is under control, consideration will have to be given to the treatment of the original condition for which the implicated drug was prescribed. In many cases, drug therapy will still be required, and caution must therefore be exercised, as drugs with similar chemical structures may cause similar hepatotoxicity (Table 13.5).

Hepatotoxicity may occur with different derivatives of a drug. Erythromycin-induced cholestatic hepatitis has

Table 13.5 Examples of cross-sensitivity within drug groups

	Problem	Action
Phenothiazine	Cross-sensitivity	Avoid
Tricyclic	Cross-sensitivity	Avoid
NSAID	Cross-sensitivity	Avoid
Isoniazid, pyrazinamide	Chemically related	Avoid
Halothane	Avoid enflurane	Isoflurane appears safe

been most frequently reported with the estolate preparation than with other erythromycin esters (ethylsuccinate, stearate, propionate and lactobionate). It is not clear which part of the drug is responsible for hypersensitivity.

Paracetamol-induced hepatotoxicity

Paracetamol causes a dose-related toxicity resulting in centrilobular necrosis. It normally undergoes the phase 2 reactions of glucuronidation and sulphation. However, paracetamol is metabolized by cytochrome P450 2E1 to N-acetyl-p-benzoquinoneimine (NABQI) if the capacity of the phase 2 reactions are exceeded or if cytochrome P450 2E1 is induced. After normal doses of paracetamol, NABQI is detoxified by conjugation with glutathione to

produce mercaptopurine and cysteine conjugates. Following overdose, tissue stores of glutathione are depleted, allowing NABQI to accumulate and cause cell damage. Illness, starvation and alcohol deplete glutathione stores and increase paracetamol toxicity, while acetylcysteine and methionine provide a specific antidote by replenishing glutathione stores.

Ingestion of doses as low as 10–15 g of paracetamol have been reported to cause severe hepatocellular necrosis. Removal of unabsorbed paracetamol by gastric lavage may be worthwhile if more than 150 mg/kg body weight has been taken and the patient presents within 4 hours of ingestion. Activated charcoal may also be administered to reduce further absorption of paracetamol and facilitate removal of unmetabolized paracetamol from extracellular fluids. This may lessen the effect of any methionine given. A plasma paracetamol concentration should be taken as soon as possible, but not within 4 hours of ingestion due to the fact that a misleading and low level may be obtained because of continuing absorption and distribution of the drug. The plasma concentration measured should be compared with a standard nomogram reference line of a plot of plasma paracetamol concentration against time in hours after ingestion. This may be a semilogarithmic (Figure 13.2) or linear (Fig. 13.3) plot. Generally, administration of intravenous acetylcysteine is the treatment of choice for paracetamol overdose when the blood paracetamol level is in the range predictive of possible or probable liver injury (Fig. 13.2). Patients allergic to acetylcysteine may receive oral methionine.

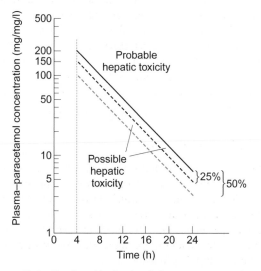

Figure 13.2 Semilogarithmic plot of plasma paracetamol concentration versus time in hours after ingestion.

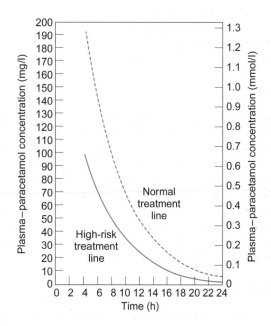

Figure 13.3 A linear plot of plasma paracetamol concentration versus time in hours after ingestion.

Acetylcysteine is most effective within 8 hours of overdose. However, late administration in patients who present more than 16–24 hours post-ingestion may be appropriate. Acetylcysteine administered at this stage will not counteract the oxidative effects of paracetamol but it may have a cytoprotective role in hepatic failure, and has been shown to reduce morbidity and mortality in patients who have already developed acute liver failure.

Patient care

Patients may be at risk of drug-induced hepatotoxicity from prescribed drugs or from purchased drugs. Additionally, children may be at risk from medicines that are not stored properly. Parents should be reminded to store all medicines in child-resistant containers and out of reach. Deaths from liver failure have occurred in children following overdose with drugs commonly available such as iron tablets.

Patient counselling

Patients who purchase preparations containing paracetamol should be made aware of the danger of overdosing, which may occur if they take other paracetamol-containing preparations simultaneously. Since 1994 the European guidelines on package labelling have required products containing paracetamol to warn patients of the need to avoid other paracetamol-containing products. The pack size of paracetamol sold from general sales outlets has been limited to 16 tablets or capsules (32 where paracetamol is sold under the supervision on a pharmacist) with the aim of limiting availability and reducing residual stocks in the home. To reduce the risk associated with inadvertent overdose, paracetamol preparations containing the antidote methionine have been manufactured but are more expensive. In addition, there have been concerns regarding the long-term safety of methionine when taken for chronic conditions. It is therefore unlikely to be the answer to the morbidity and mortality associated with paracetamol overdose to include methionine in all paracetamol formulations.

All patients should be advised of potential side-effects. This information needs to be reinforced with the use of patient information leaflets.

Patients and their carers should be helped to recognize signs of liver disorder and know to report immediately symptoms such as malaise, nausea, fever and abdominal discomfort that may be significant although non-specific during the first few weeks of any change of therapy. If these are accompanied by elevated LFTs, the drug should be discontinued.

Patients who recover from drug-induced hepatotoxicity should be informed of the causative agent, warned to avoid it in the future, and advised to inform their doctor, dentist, nurse and pharmacist about the occurrence of such an event.

Parents of children commenced on sodium valproate should be warned to report side-effects that may be suggestive of liver injury such as the onset of anorexia, abdominal discomfort, nausea and vomiting. Early features include drowsiness and disturbed consciousness. Fever may also be present. The time to onset is between 1 and 4 months in the majority of cases.

The challenge for all members of the health care team is to alert patients to the potentially toxic effects of drugs without creating so much concern they fail to comply with vital medication. For the limited number of drugs presented in Table 13.6, careful monitoring of LFTs during the first 6 months of treatment is advisable, although not always practical. Thereafter, regular monitoring of LFTs is appropriate in patients who are at greater risk of hepatotoxicity. Such patients would include those with known liver disease, those taking other hepatotoxic drugs, those aged over 40 years, and heavy alcohol consumers. Surveillance should be particularly frequent in the first 2 months of treatment. In patients with no risk factors and normal pre-treatment liver function, LFTs need only be repeated if fever, malaise, vomiting, jaundice or unexplained deterioration during treatment occurs. Since many drugs cause elevation of LFTs there may be difficulty in assessing when to stop a drug, particularly when treating an individual for tuberculosis or epilepsy. An empirical guideline is that the drug should be stopped if the levels of alanine transaminase exceed three times the upper limit of the reference range. Any clinical features of liver disease or drug allergy would require immediate discontinuation of the drug. Conversely, a raised γ-glutamyl transpeptidase level and elevated alanine transaminase level in the absence of symptoms often reflect microsomal induction and would not indicate drug-induced injury.

It should be noted that monitoring of LFTs is not a complete safeguard against hepatotoxicity, as some drug reactions develop very quickly, and the liver enzymes are an unreliable indicator of fibrosis.

Minimizing the risk of drug-induced liver disease

Cholestatic jaundice has been reported to occur in about 1 in 6000 patients treated with co-amoxilav. The risk of acute liver injury with co-amoxiclav is approximately six times that of amoxicillin and increases with treatment courses above 14 days (Garcia Rodriguez et al 1996). Hence the indications for co-amoxiclav have been restricted to cover infections caused by amoxicillin-resistant β-lactam producing infections.

Patients admitted for procedures requiring a general anaesthetic should be questioned about past exposure

Table 13.6 Examples of drugs where regular monitoring of liver function tests is recommended

Drug	Baseline measurement*	Frequency of monitoring
Isoniazid	Yes	
Rifampicin		LFTs checked weekly for the first 2 months then every 2 weeks
Pyrazinamide		LFTs checked weekly for the first 2 months then every 2 weeks
Amiodarone	Yes	LFTs checked every 6 months
Cyproterone	Yes	Recheck if any symptoms
Methotrexate	Yes	LFTs checked every 2 weeks for the first 2 months, then monthly for 4 months, then every 3 months
Methyldopa	Yes	Check LFTs at intervals during the first 6–12 weeks of treatment
Sodium valproate	Yes	Check LFTs regularly during the first 6 months of therapy
Dantrolene	Yes	Repeat LFTs after first 6 weeks of therapy
Sulfasalazine	Yes	LFTs checked every 2 weeks for the first 2 months, then monthly for 4 months then every 3 months

* Baseline and subsequent LFTs difficult to interpret in critically ill patients as LFTs will be affected by multiple factors.

and any previous reactions to halothane. Halothane is well known to be associated with hepatotoxicity, particularly if patients are re-exposed. Repeated exposure to halothane within a period of less than 3 months should be avoided, while some increase in risk persists regardless of the time interval since last exposure (Ray & Drummond 1991). Unexplained jaundice or delayed-onset postoperative fever in a patient who has received halothane is an absolute contraindication to future use in that individual. Patients with a family history of halothane-related liver injury should also be treated with caution.

The individuals at greatest risk of halothane hepatitis are obese, postmenopausal women. Halothane may be present in detectable amounts even in theatres equipped with scavenging devices, and it is possible for these small concentrations to provoke a reaction in a highly sensitized individual. If electing to avoid halothane, a halothane-free circuit and operating theatre should be used. Cross-hepatotoxicity with other haloalkanes is a possibility, and enflurane should also be avoided. Isoflurane appears to be safe, as no reports of cross-sensitivity have been published. Some anaesthetists would prefer to use total intravenous anaesthesia in patients who have had a reaction to halothane.

Although hepatic adverse drug reactions are rare for most drugs, when they do occur they can cause significant morbidity and mortality.

Over 600 drugs have been associated with hepatotoxicity, and any new drug released on to the market may have the potential to cause hepatotoxicity. Pemoline, troglitazone and tolcapone are examples of drugs withdrawn from the market due to reports of serious hepatic reactions. These cases help to highlight the importance of post-marketing surveillance and yellow card reporting.

Appropriate selection of drugs, an awareness of predisposing factors and avoidance of toxic dose thresholds and potentially hepatotoxic drug–drug interactions will minimize the risk to patients.

CASE STUDIES

Case 13.1

Miss R.S. is a 17-year-old female student who presented with jaundice and a rising bilirubin and prothrombin time. There was no previous family history of liver disease and no history of alcohol intake. She had never had an operation or received a blood transfusion and denied using illicit drugs.

She had initially developed pain in her right foot 5 weeks previous for which she was prescribed ibuprofen. Seven days before admission she started diclofenac. Two days after starting diclofenac she became increasingly tired and nauseated, and was treated with a course of ampicillin.

On examination she was jaundiced with no encephalopathy and had a blood pressure of 160/84 mmHg. There were no cardiac murmurs, hepatosplenomegaly or ascites.

Initial investigations

Albumin	24 g/l
Alanine transaminase	635 units/l
Bilirubin	331 μmol/l
Alkaline phosphatase	213 units/l
Haemoglobin	12.4 g/dl
WCC	11.7×10^9/l
Platelets	172×10^9/l
Prothrombin time	61 seconds
α_1 antitrypsin	Normal
Immunoglobulins	All normal
Creatinine clearance	127 ml/min
Urinary copper	1.4 μmol/24 hours (normal)
Serum copper	7 μmol/l (normal)
Caeruloplasmin	0.6 g/l (normal)

Slit lamp examination of the eyes: no evidence of Kayser–Fleischer rings. No evidence of infection with cytomegalovirus or Epstein–Barr virus.

Management

Despite treatment with acetylcysteine, Miss R. S.'s prothrombin time continued to rise and she developed encephalopathy. She was listed for a liver transplant with a diagnosis of acute liver failure possibly related to drugs. She successfully underwent orthotopic liver transplantation.

....

Questions

1. What is the significance of the clinical history?
2. What type of liver disease do the signs and symptoms indicate?
3. Which drug is most likely to be responsible and why?
4. What advice should the patient be given concerning medication use after a liver transplantation?

....

Answers

1. The patient was a student and was unlikely to be exposed to an excessive risk of infection with hepatitis A or a tropical disease as she had not travelled abroad in the recent past. The fact that Miss. R. S. had not received a general anaesthetic recently also excludes postoperative jaundice. A negative transfusion and illicit drug use history made infections such as hepatitis B and C unlikely.

   Her alcohol consumption was minimal, and this excluded alcoholic liver disease. Many possible causes of liver disease could be excluded from the clinical history alone. The results from the investigations exclude other causative factors such as cytomegalovirus or Epstein–Barr virus. α_1-Antitrypsin deficiency, an inherited disorder that may be associated with liver disease in some patients, was excluded. Wilson's disease, a disorder of copper metabolism, was excluded by the negative Kayser–Fleisher rings and measurement of serum caeruloplasmin and urinary copper excretion.

2. The patient's elevated LFTs indicate an acute hepatocellular injury. The prolonged prothrombin time also indicates a severe reaction. The fact that albumin is on the low side is also an indicator of severity. The albumin level would also be expected to be low in chronic disease, because it reflects loss of synthetic function. In this case there is clearly no evidence to support a diagnosis of chronic disease. The rapid deterioration is not unusual in a severe drug reaction.

3. The evidence from the drug history suggests only two causative agents as the ampicillin was commenced after the initial symptoms appeared. The relationship of symptoms to the administration of drugs implicates diclofenac as the most likely cause.

   Ibuprofen is a very commonly used NSAID and is available without prescription. Hepatotoxicity with ibuprofen appears to be very rare although cases of hepatocellular injury exist and cholestasis without hepatitis has been observed. A single case of fatal liver failure associated with fatty changes has been reported. Most reported cases of hepatotoxicity have had an onset within 3 weeks of commencing ibuprofen treatment.

   There have been several reports of diclofenac-induced hepatitis published in the literature, and a considerable number reported to the regulatory authorities. A frequency of 5 cases per 100 000 patients exposed to diclofenac has been described. Females appear to be more susceptible, and there is some evidence for increased risk in patients over 65 years of age. The onset of action is usually within the first 3 months of treatment.

   Ampicillin has rarely been involved with liver injury. Reports of systemic hypersensitivity with hepatic involvement, granulomatous hepatitis and cholestasis with vanishing bile duct syndrome have been reported.

   Diclofenac appears to be the most likely candidate. All drug therapy was stopped on admission.

4. Following a liver transplant the patient will require counselling about the immunosuppressive drugs she has to take long term. Information about all aspects of drug therapy including advice on what to do if doses are missed and advice on any potential side-effects should be covered for all drugs, which may include ciclosporin, azathioprine, prednisolone, ranitidine, antifungals and co-trimoxazole.

   Over time the number of drugs and doses will be reduced. Future use of NSAIDs and diclofenac are contraindicated for this patient.

Case 13.2

A 50-year-old man was admitted with a 2-week history of general malaise, anorexia and jaundice. His drug history was as follows:

Metoprolol for hypertension
Isosorbide mononitrate for ischaemic heart disease
Thioridazine for schizophrenia.

All drugs had been taken by the patient for many years.
One month previously he had been prescribed diclofenac 50 mg three times a day for joint pains.

Initial biochemical tests revealed LFTs, bilirubin, ALT, AST and alkaline phosphatase were all raised but his coagulation tests were normal.

A liver biopsy showed hepatitis consistent with a drug reaction. All drugs were stopped on admission and the LFTs improved over the next few weeks.

Questions

1. Is diclofenac the most likely causative agent?
2. What are the implications for the future management of this patient?

Answers

1. The timing of the reaction suggests that the addition of diclofenac to the regimen is responsible. Most drug-induced liver disease occurs within the first 2 months of treatment. The other drugs had been taken by the patient for several years.

   Diclofenac has been reported to cause hepatic toxicity. The earliest reaction date recorded by the CSM was 1978.

   The incidence is very low for NSAIDs in general and is relatively unimportant compared with the risk of peptic ulcer disease and gastrointestinal bleeding. Reports of hepatic injury range from increased LFTs in about 15% of patients, with values up to 3 times the upper limit of the reference range, to acute liver failure.

   With diclofenac the reaction occurs within the first 6 months of therapy and most patients recover their liver function after stopping the drug (Purcell et al 1991). There is a suggestion that it is a dose-related reaction and impaired clearance may be the mechanism of injury.

   Considering the other drugs the patient was receiving, significant hepatotoxicity is extremely rare for β adrenergic receptor antaonists, with an isolated case of hepatitis reported with metoprolol (Larrey et al 1988). Cholestasis is an infrequent complication with phenothiazines other than chlorpromazine. There have been anecdotal reports of cholestasis with thioridazine.
2. The reaction should be documented in the patient's medical records and future use of NSAIDs is contraindicated.

   There have been reports in the literature of patients re-exposed to diclofenac developing recurrent liver disease. It would also seem prudent to avoid NSAIDs in general as there have been reports of cross-sensitivity, although this is rare.

Case 13.3

A 76-year-old man with a history of COPD was prescribed a course of co-amoxiclav 375 mg three times a day for 7 days. He presented to his GP with general malaise, vomiting and pruritis.

Questions

1. Do the clinical signs in this patient suggest liver disease?
2. Is co-amoxiclav a possible cause of liver disease? What other information is required?
3. What treatment is appropriate?

Answers

1. General malaise, tiredness and nausea and vomiting are possible signs of liver disease. Abdominal pain may also be a feature. Pruritis is associated with cholestatic jaundice as the bile salts are deposited in the skin and cause itching.
2. A full drug history including use of over-the-counter drugs and herbal drugs to is required.

   The onset of liver disease caused by co-amoxiclav is usually within 10 days of commencing therapy but has been reported a few weeks after completing a course of treatment (Garcia Rodriguez et al 1996). Co-amoxiclav is a likely culprit here, although a complete history is required to exclude other drugs or causes of illness or pre-existing liver disease.
3. Symptomatic treatment of the itch with antihistamines is appropriate. Colestyramine may be added if necessary but is poorly tolerated. Topical treatment with menthol in aqueous cream may provide relief for some patients.

   The reaction should be documented in the patient's medical records and an ADR report completed.

Case 13.4

A patient presents with increasing jaundice, nausea, vomiting and right subcostal pain and tenderness after taking 80 tablets of paracetamol 36 hours ago. The patient had vomited soon after taking the overdose and had not called the GP. Laboratory results were as follows:

	Day 1 morning	Day 1 evening	Day 2	Day 3	Day 6
Sodium (mmol/l)	144	134	135	133	
Potassium (mmol/l)	4.1	3.1	3.6	3.8	
Urea (mmol/l)	6.7	5.4	8	11.9	33
Creatinine (μmol/l)	98	84	132	334	990
ALT (units/l)	1161	1848	Unrecordable	8435	5520
Bilirubin (μmol/l)	50	42			
Alk Phosphatase (units/l)					
INR	1.88	4.2	71.8		
PT				48.8	
pH			7.45		
Paracetamol (mg/l)	12				
Salicylate (mg/l)	0.5				
Urine output (ml/hour)	40–50			Nil	Nil

Questions

1. What treatment should be initiated for this patient?
2. What syndrome is likely to be developing?
3. How is the efficacy of acetylcysteine monitored?
4. What other treatment is appropriate?
5. What is the prognosis?

Answers

1. A toxic screen should be performed to exclude overdose with any other drug. A paracetamol level is required, although the prognostic value after 15 hours is uncertain. A plasma paracetamol concentration above the relevant treatment line should be regarded as carrying serious risk of liver disease. As the patient has overt clinical signs of liver disease, therapy with acetylcysteine should be commenced. Acetylcysteine has been shown to increase cardiac output, oxygen delivery, oxygen extraction and consumption, and these effects might account for the improved survival associated with the delayed administration of acetylcysteine in patients with paracetamol-induced acute liver failure (Harrison et al 1991).
2. This patient has developing renal failure secondary to acute tubular damage and necrosis. This usually occurs in association with hepatocellular necrosis, and rarely in the absence of major liver damage.

3. Monitoring PT, LFTs, creatinine and blood pH levels indicate whether the acetylcysteine is being effective.
4. Other treatment options are shown below:

Problem	Treatment
Cardiovascular system	Expand circulating volume Inotropes
Respiratory support	Mechanical ventilation
Renal support	Intermittant haemodiafiltration
Cerebral oedema	Mannitol Furosemide (frusemide)
Encephalopathy	Correct precipitating factors Avoid sedatives if possible Lactulose
Hypoglycaemia	Continuous glucose infusions
Bleeding	Vitamin K Fresh frozen plasma (FFP) Platelets H_2 antagonist
Fluids and electrolytes	Hydration Potassium Restrict sodium to 50 mmol per day
Infection	Antifungals Broad-spectrum antibiotics

Transplantation may be considered but this patient does not meet the criteria for transplantation (Wendon & William 1995), which are:

- Arterial pH < 7.3

OR

- The presence of the following together:
  Prothrombin time > 100 s
  Grade III/IV encephalopathy
  Creatinine > 300 μmol/l.

5. In acute liver failure, where time from onset of jaundice to encephalopathy is 0–7 days, the incidence of cerebral oedema is frequent and the predicted survival route is 36% (O'Grady et al 1989).

The prolonged prothrombin time is suggestive of a poor prognosis (O'Grady et al 1993).

Presentation more than 36 hours after an overdose with the following:

- PT > 36
- Creatinine > 200 μmol/l
- Blood pH below 7.3
- Encephalopathy

also suggests a poor prognosis.

A patient who develops severe liver disease and recovers does not usually suffer any long term sequelae.

REFERENCES

Garcia Rodriguez L A, Stricker B H, Zimmerman H J 1996 Risk of acute liver injury associated with the combination of amoxycillin and clavulanic acid. Archives of Internal Medicine 156: 1327–1333

Harrison P M, Wendon J A, Gimson A E et al 1991 Improvement by acetylcysteine of hemodynamics and oxygen transport in fulminant liver failure. New England Journal of Medicine 324: 1852–1857

Hebbard G C, Smith K G, Gibson P R et al 1992 Augmentin induced jaundice with a fatal outcome. Medical Journal of Australia 156: 285–286

Larrey D, Henrion J, Heller F et al 1988 Metoprolol-induced hepatitis: rechallenge and drug oxidation phenotyping. Annals of Internal Medicine 108: 67–68

Lee W M 1993 Acute liver failure. New England Journal of Medicine 329: 1862–1872

Mankouvian A V, Carson J L 1996 Non steroidal anti inflammatory drug induced hepatic disorders: incidence and prevention drug safety. 15(1): 64–71

O'Grady J, Schalm S W, Williams R 1993 Acute liver failure redefying the syndromes. Lancet 342: 273–275

O'Grady J G, Alexander G J M, Hayllar K M et al 1989 Early indicators of prognosis in fulminant hepatic failure. Gastroenterology 97(2): 439–445

Purcell P, Henry D, Melville G 1991 Diclofenac hepatitis. Gut 32(11): 1381–1385

Ray D C, Drummond B G 1991 Halothane hepatitis. British Journal of Anaesthesia 67: 84–99

Shaw D, Leon C, Koler S et al 1997 Traditional remedies and food supplements. Drug Safety 17(5): 342–356

Thorax Editorials 1996 Hepatotoxicity of antituberculous drugs. Thorax 51: 111–113

Wendon J, Williams R 1995 Acute liver failure. In: Williams R, Partman B, Tan K (eds.) The practice of liver transplantation. Churchill Livingstone, London, 93–103

FURTHER READING

Farrell G C (ed) 1994 Drug-induced liver disease. Churchill Livingstone, London

Kaplowitz N 2001 Drug-induced liver disorders: implications for drug development and regulation. Drug Safety 24(7): 483–490

Lee W M 2000 Assessing causality in drug-induced liver injury. Journal of Hepatology 33(6): 1003–1005

Lewis J H 2000 Drug-induced liver disease. Medical Clinics of North America 84(5): 1275–1311

Lewis J H, Zimmerman H J 1999 Drug- and chemical-induced cholestasis. Clinics in Liver Disease 3(3): 433–464

Ryan M, Desmond P 2001 Liver toxicity: could this be a drug reaction? Australian Family Physician 30(5): 427–431

Zimmerman H J 2000 Drug-induced liver disease. Clinics in Liver Disease 4(1): 73–96

Liver disease 14

F. M. Ward   M. J. Daly

Blood is supplied to the liver via the hepatic artery and the portal system which collects venous blood draining from the abdominal viscera. The portal vein, hepatic artery and the bile duct system (which drains bile from the liver to the intestine) enter the liver through the porta hepatis, and branch repeatedly until they lie in the portal tracts, which carry the finest branches of the vessels and ducts. From these portal tracts, columns of liver cells and blood-filled sinusoids extend towards hepatic venules, which collect blood draining from the liver tissue into central veins that form the large hepatic veins discharging into the inferior vena cava (Bircher et al 1999).

There are two main types of liver disease, namely acute and chronic.

Acute liver disease

Acute liver disease is usually a self-limiting episode of liver cell (hepatocyte) inflammation or damage which in most cases resolves without clinical sequelae. In some cases, however, the hepatocyte damage is so severe that it affects the whole liver, leading to hepatic failure with an associated high mortality. Alternatively, the patient can develop chronic liver disease.

The liver is the largest organ in the body weighing 1200–1500 g. It is a key organ in regulating homeostasis within the body. Functions undertaken include protein synthesis, storage and metabolism of fats and carbohydrates, detoxification of drugs and other toxins, excretion of bilirubin and metabolism of hormones, as summarized in Figure 14.1. The liver has considerable reserve capacity, can often maintain function in spite of significant disease and is one of the few human organs capable of regeneration. However, in cases of severe injury or disease of the liver, a diverse range of physiological roles are impaired, with potentially serious consequences for the individual concerned.

In order to understand the changes that can occur in patients with liver disease, it is first necessary to understand the normal liver architecture. This is shown diagrammatically in Figure 14.2.

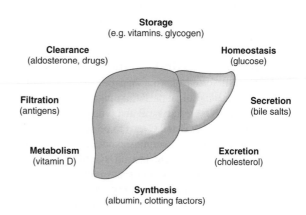

Figure 14.1 Normal physiological functions of the liver, with examples of each.

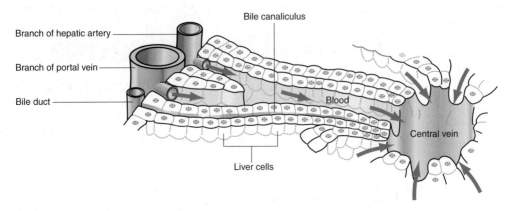

Figure 14.2 Illustration of the relationship between the three structures that comprise the portal tract, with blood from both the hepatic artery and portal vein perfusing the hepatocytes before draining away towards the hepatic veins (central veins). Each hepatocyte is also able to secrete bile via the network of bile ducts. (Reproduced with permission of McGraw-Hill from Vander 1980, Figure 14.23, p. 431).

Chronic liver disease

Chronic liver disease occurs when permanent structural changes within the liver occur secondary to long-standing cell damage, with the consequent loss of normal liver architecture. In most cases this progresses to cirrhosis, where fibrous scars divide the liver cells into areas of regenerative tissue called nodules (Fig. 14.3). This process is irreversible and eventually leads to liver failure. Cirrhosis may follow an attack of acute viral hepatitis, may be secondary to autoimmune hepatitis, or may result from chronic alcohol ingestion.

Causes of liver disease

Viral infections

Many viruses affect liver function, but only a few are truly infectious to the liver itself, leading to clinically significant hepatitis. The term 'viral hepatitis' refers to the diseases caused by this subgroup.

Five human viruses have been identified, including hepatitis A (HAV), B (HBV), C (HCV), D (HDV) and E (HEV). All forms of viral hepatitis have a similar pathology, causing an acute inflammation of the entire liver. In general, type A, type B and type C run the same clinical course. Type B and C tend to be more severe and may be associated with a serum sickness-like syndrome. In mild attacks, the patient has no symptoms and the only marker is a rise in serum transaminases. In other cases, increasing grades of severity can occur from a patient feeling generally unwell for a couple of weeks, from which recovery is usual, through to chronic hepatitis or, in extreme cases, fatal acute liver failure.

Hepatitis A

Hepatitis A (HAV) is the major cause of acute hepatitis worldwide, accounting for 20–25% of clinical hepatitis in the developed world. Most attacks are mild and often pass unnoticed by the patient. HAV is spread via the

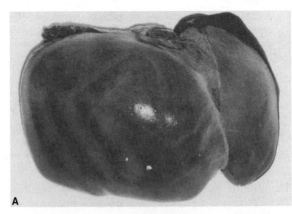

A

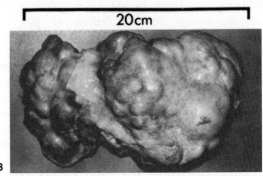

B

Figure 14.3 The gross post-mortem appearance of **A** a normal and **B** a cirrhotic liver demonstrating scarring and nodule formation in part B.

faecal–oral route, and is therefore particulary prevalent in areas of poor sanitation, and often associated with water- and food-borne epidemics. The 5–14 age group is most commonly affected, and adults are often infected by contact with their children. Within the body, there is a short incubation period of between 2 and 7 weeks, during which time the virus replicates and liver function tests become progressively more abnormal. HAV is usually mild, particularly in younger age groups, where it may be subclinical or mistaken for gastroenteritis. The disease is more serious and prolonged in adults, although fulminant cases are rare.

Hepatitis B

The prevalence of hepatitis B (HBV) is low in the USA and Britain, with approximately 0.1–0.2% of the population having markers that indicate that they are chronic carriers. However, in Africa and the Far East, 15–20% of the population are chronic carriers while the majority of the population may have had a discrete acute HBV infection at some time in their life. In the Far East, chronic HBV infection is the leading cause of liver cirrhosis.

HBV is parenterally transmitted, occurring during birth in babies born to HBV infected mothers, after transfusion of blood and blood products from infected donors, after intravenous drug use, and after sexual contact. The outcome of HBV infection depends on the age of the patient and genetic factors. Acute HBV infection has an incubation period of 3–6 months, which is generally self-limiting and does not require antiviral therapy, with most patients recovering 1–2 months after the onset of jaundice. Chronic HBV is defined as viraemia and hepatic inflammation continuing for more than 6 months following infection. The majority of patients with chronic HBV have a relatively benign outcome, although approximately 15–20% of patients acquiring this infection in adulthood will develop cirrhosis over a 5–20 year period. Infection in childhood may have a different prognosis, with a higher percentage developing cirrhosis and hepatocellular carcinoma.

Hepatitis C

Hepatitis C (HCV) is a blood borne virus with greater infectivity than the human immunodeficiency virus (HIV). The global prevalence of HCV infection is estimated at around 3% in the general population, with more than 150 million carriers worldwide (Malnick et al 2000).

HCV is transmitted parenterally, commonly via intravenous drug abuse and the sharing of needles. It was also spread through blood transfusion prior to the introduction of screening in 1991. There is a small risk of HCV infection associated with tattooing, electrolysis,

ear piercing, acupuncture and sexual contact. The transmission rate from mother to child if the mother is a HCV carrier is about 6%.

After exposure to HCV, patients are often asymptomatic, although about 20% will develop acute hepatitis and may experience malaise, weakness and anorexia. Up to 85% of people exposed to the virus develop chronic disease, which can lead to progressive liver damage. Approximately 20–30% of patients with chronic HCV infection progress to end-stage liver disease within 20 years and a small percentage develop hepatocellular carcinoma. Patients with end-stage liver disease require a liver transplant to prevent death from the complications of cirrhosis. HCV infection is now the leading indication for liver transplantation worldwide.

Hepatitis D

Hepatitis D (HDV) can establish infection only in patients simultaneously infected by HBV. It is acquired in the same way as HBV infection, and can cause both acute and chronic hepatitis.

Hepatitis E

Hepatitis E (HEV) is endemic in areas of poor sanitation, where it is transmitted enterically and leads to acute hepatitis. The symptoms of HEV are similar to those of other acute viral illnesses, with an average incubation period of 40 days. In most cases, resolution of abnormal liver function tests occurs within 3 weeks.

Alcohol

The ingestion of ethanol in alcoholic beverages is the commonest cause of cirrhosis in the Western world. In general, deaths from alcoholic liver disease in a particular country correlate with the consumption of alcohol per head of population, although additional factors can influence this trend.

Alcoholic liver cirrhosis illustrates the changes that occur in chronic liver disease. Prolonged and excessive exposure to alcohol induces inflammatory activity within the liver tissue, and the hepatocytes accumulate large droplets of fat as inclusion bodies within swollen cells. This process is generally reversible if the patient stops drinking, but with continued insult the fibrosis will develop further and become widespread.

A fine network of collagen fibres develops around the liver cells near the hepatic venule, and gradually the liver cells die and the extent of fibrosis increases. Eventually, the hepatic venules are obliterated and the areas of fibrosis around them link to form bands of fibrous tissue. While areas of living cells between the fibrous bands regenerate, the destruction of the normal intergrity of the portal tracts and the draining hepatic venules causes the cells to divide haphazardly, and islands of liver tissue (nodules) develop. This disordered anatomy prevents blood from the portal system flowing efficiently through the liver, thereby causing an increase in blood pressure within the portal system, leading to portal hypertension, one of the major complications of cirrhosis. As the number of normally functioning liver cells reduces further, this leads to eventual liver cell failure, where the number of hepatocytes becomes insufficient to maintain the essential synthetic, metabolic and excretory roles of the organ.

Immune disorders

Autoimmune disease occurs when the immune system develops autoantibodies to tissues within the body.

Autoimmune hepatitis

Autoimmune hepatitis is a liver disease associated with auto-antibodies in the serum, and is usually a chronic, progressive disease which may occasionally present acutely. Typically, autoimmune hepatitis occurs in young women, with age at onset between 20 and 40 years.

Primary biliary cirrhosis. Primary biliary cirrhosis (PBC) is characterized by progressive destruction of the small and intrahepatic bile ducts, leading to fibrosis and cirrhosis. It primarily affects women between 40 and 60 years of age. There is no cure, and in the long term many patients will require a liver transplant. The end stages of the disease are characterized by uncontrollable pruritus, severe jaundice and extreme lethargy.

Primary sclerosing cholangitis. Primary sclerosing cholangitis (PSC) occurs mainly in young men aged 25–40 years, and is a cholestatic liver disease caused by diffuse inflammation and fibrosis which can involve the entire biliary tree. The progressive pathological process leads to biliary cirrhosis, portal hypertension and hepatic failure. Cholangiocarcinoma develops in between 10% and 30% of patients.

Vascular abnormalities

The Budd–Chiari syndrome occurs when obstruction of the major hepatic veins leads to cell destruction and cirrhosis. In approximately 75% of affected patients the cause is a thrombosis secondary to a thrombophilic disorder. Veno-occlusive disease occurs when the smaller veins of the liver become obliterated as a result of exposure to toxins, irradiation or cytotoxic drugs.

Inherited metabolic disorders

There are various inherited metabolic disorders that can affect the functioning of the liver.

Haemochromatosis is a genetically recessive error of metabolism that results in excess iron absorption and deposition throughout the body. With sufficient iron accumulation, fibrosis occurs leading to eventual cirrhosis.

Wilson's disease is characterized by copper overload, caused by a recessive genetic defect that leads to excessive absorption and deposition of dietary copper in the liver, brain, kidneys and other tissues.

α_1-**antitrypsin** deficiency is a dominant genetic defect that leads to a reduction in a specific protein which protects tissues from attack by digestive enzymes, such as trypsin. This reduction leads to emphysematous lung disease or liver disease.

Glycogen storage disease is a recessive genetic disease which usually presents in childhood. It is characterized by deranged homeostasis of glucose and glycogen leading to an accumulation of metabolites that damage hepatocytes.

Biliary tract diseases

Obstruction of bile outflow from the liver can cause inflammation, scarring and eventual cirrhosis. The obstruction may be due to gallstones or a tumour, or may alternatively be secondary to surgical or traumatic damage to the common bile duct. Primary malignant tumours of the liver and biliary tract are relatively rare in developed countries, with secondary metastatic tumours being around 40 times more common than primary malignancies.

Gilbert's syndrome

Gilbert's syndrome, otherwise known as hereditary non-haemolytic unconjugated hyperbilirubinaemia, is most frequently recognized in adolescents and young adults with an incidence of between 5% and 7% in the general population. Serum bilirubin levels usually exceed 50 μmol/l, but may be higher. Patients usually complain of non-specific symptoms such as hyperpyrexia, fatigue, nausea and abdominal discomfort, but Gilbert's syndrome is otherwise a benign condition and requires no active treatment.

Infectious diseases

In the tropics, liver disease secondary to infection by blood and liver flukes (schistomes) is a major cause of morbidity and mortality in local populations.

Drugs and toxins

Many drugs and toxins have been implicated in causing liver disease, usually as a consequence of direct toxicity of the parent drug or the indirect toxicity of metabolites (see Chapter 13).

Clinical manifestations of liver disease

Symptoms of liver disease

Patients frequently complain of being easily fatigued and generally run down, with loss of appetite and weight loss. In chronic liver disease there may be loss of muscle from the arms and legs and swelling of the abdomen and lower body due to fluid retention. Individuals with enlarged livers may complain of abdominal pain and tenderness. A distressing symptom for many patients is intractable pruritus secondary to jaundice. Patients with chronic liver disease and associated abnormal clotting of the blood or low platelet counts often complain of increased bleeding from the gums and nose, and easy bruising.

Signs of liver disease

Many of the signs associated with chronic liver disease are related to the failure of the liver to carry out normal synthetic, metabolic and excretory functions. The most common signs are summarized in Table 14.1.

Cutaneous signs

There are a number of cutaneous signs that indicate the presence of chronic liver disease, although none are entirely specific. They include finger clubbing (swelling of the finger ends), spider naevi (small vascular malformations in the skin) and palmar erythema (reddening of the palm of the hand). These changes are thought to be related to alterations in the vascular system that cause the development of arterial venous shunts in the skin and hands. Additional features include white nails (associated with low serum albumin), Dupuytren's contracture (abnormal fibrous tissue in the palms of the hands causing retraction of one or more fingers) and easy bruising secondary to deficiency of clotting factors and a reduction in the number of platelets due to hypersplenism.

Abdominal signs

Various changes may be detectable on examination of the abdomen. An enlarged liver (hepatomegaly) is a common finding in acute liver disease, indicating inflammation and regeneration of the liver tissue. In cirrhotic patients the liver may be large or small depending on the stage of the chronic disease. An enlarged spleen (splenomegaly) may be caused by increased pressure in the portal venous system, and indicates portal hypertension secondary to cirrhosis. Allied with this may be distended abdominal wall veins, secondary to portal hypertension, as the portal blood joins other veins to drain around the liver.

Jaundice

Jaundice indicates impaired liver cell function, and is a common finding in acute liver disease, but may be absent in chronic liver disease until the terminal stages of cirrhosis are reached. The causes of jaundice are shown in Figure 14.4.

Portal hypertension

Portal hypertension occurs when there is increased pressure within the portal venous system secondary to increased resistance to flow through the damaged liver. Collateral veins develop, and these can bleed due to the increased flow and pressure within. Portal hypertension is an important contributory factor to the formation of ascites and the development of encephalopathy due to bypassing of blood from the liver to the systemic circulation. The major, potentially life-threatening complication of portal hypertension is torrential venous haemorrhage from the thin-walled veins in the oesophagus and stomach. Many patients with portal hypertension are often asymptomatic, while others may present with bleeding varices, ascites and/or encephalopathy.

Table 14.1 Physical signs of chronic liver disease

Common findings	End-stage findings
Jaundice	Ascites
Gynaecomastia	Dilated abdominal blood vessels
Hand changes:	Fetor hepaticus
Liver palms	Hepatic flap
Clubbing	Neurological changes:
Dupuytren's contracture	Disorientation
Xanthoma	Changes in consciousness
Liver mass reduced or	Oedema
increased	
Parotid enlargement	
Scratch marks on skin	
Purpura	
Spider naevi	
Splenomegaly	
Testicular atrophy	
Xanthelasma	
Hair loss	

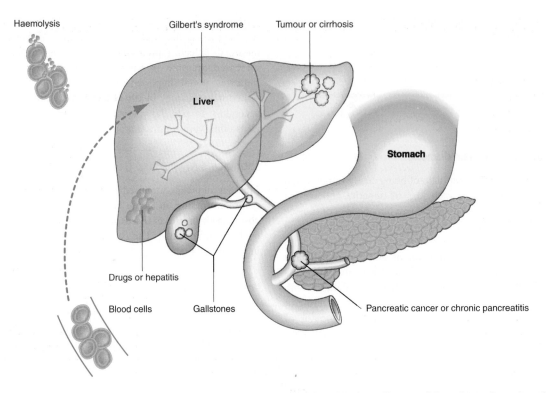

Figure 14.4 Common causes of jaundice: Obstructive – due to blockage of the bile ducts; Hepatocellular – due to drugs, hepatitis, chronic liver disease or tumour formation; Prehepatic – due to increased blood breakdown such as occurs in haemolysis.

Ascites

A swollen abdomen (ascites) is caused by the accumulation of fluid within the abdominal cavity, and may occur due to several factors, including:

- A reduction in the excretion of sodium by the kidney, due to the enhanced activity of the renin–angiotensin–aldosterone system secondary to central hypovolaemia. There may also be a decrease in aldosterone metabolism due to reduced liver metabolizing capacity and this again will increase retention of fluid in the body.
- A reduction in serum albumin leads to osmotic changes and allows fluid to leak out of blood vessels. Swollen lower limbs and peripheral oedema may occur due to a combination of these two factors.
- Portal hypertension, which tends to drive fluid out of the capillaries and into the abdominal cavity.

Gynaecomastia

Hormonal changes may occur in patients with liver disease, partly due to the inability of the cirrhotic liver to metabolize oestrogen, which may even lead to the development of gynaecomastia in males. In females of reproductive age, there may be a reduction in fertility.

Investigations

Most of the investigations to determine the cause and extent of liver disease are similar for both acute and chronic liver disease, and are summarized in Table 14.2.

Imaging techniques

Visualization of liver texture and of the bile ducts is important to exclude an obstructive cause for impaired liver function. Ultrasound is the investigation of first choice, allowing investigation of possible liver tumours and the extent of splenomegaly and portal hypertension. Computed tomography is used to enable more detailed examinations.

Liver biopsy

Liver biopsy may be helpful in establishing the severity of chronic liver disease, and especially whether or not cirrhosis is present. In acute hepatic dysfunction, a liver biopsy is not usually needed if the condition is clearly self-limiting, but may be useful if the diagnosis is in doubt, such as where there is a suspected drug reaction.

Table 14.2   Comparison of changes in liver function tests and diagnostic tests in acute and chronic liver disease

Test	Acute	Chronic	Remarks
Liver function tests			
Bilirubin	↑	↑	Marker of excretory function
Transaminases (e.g. ALT, AST)	↑	↔ or ↑	Indicate cell destruction
Alkaline phosphatase	↔	↔ or ↑	Indicates biliary obstruction
Albumin	↔	↓	Indicates synthetic function
Prothrombin time	↔ or ↑	↑	Indicates synthetic function
Diagnostic tests			
Autoantibodies	–	+	Positive in: autoimmune primary biliary cirrhosis chronic active hepatitis diseases
Hepatitis B	+/–	+/–	Present if infected
Hepatitis C	+/–	+/–	Present if infected
Hepatitis A	+/–	–	Only in acute liver disease
α-Fetoprotein	–	+/–	Present if hepatoma (liver cancer)
Serum caeruloplasmin	↔ or ↓	↔ or ↓	Only reduced in Wilson's disease

↑ = increased; ↔ = normal or unchanged; ↓ = decreased; +/– = present/absent.

Hepatitis serology

Tests for hepatitis A, B, and C are mandatory in unexplained liver disease.

Biochemical liver function tests

Biochemical liver function tests (LFTs) are simple, inexpensive and easy to perform, but provide a relatively crude measure of liver function which cannot be used in isolation to make a diagnosis. They are most useful in monitoring disease progression and response to treatment. Serum elevations greater than twice the upper limit of the reference range are usually considered significant changes. Usually more than one LFT tends to be raised in patients with liver disease. Biochemical liver function tests are not specific to the liver, and clinicians should consider other possible causes of deranged values, especially if only one value appears to be abnormal.

Bilirubin

An increase in bilirubin concentration in body fluids results in jaundice and is usually clinically apparent when the serum bilirubin level exceeds 35 μmol/l. Hepatocellular damage, cholestasis and haemolysis can all cause elevations in the serum bilirubin concentration.

Transaminases

Aspartate transaminase (AST) and alanine transaminase (ALT) enzymes are present in hepatocytes and may enter the blood in patients with liver cell damage. The highest values (up to 20 times the upper normal limit) occur in acute liver disease, such as viral hepatitis.

Alkaline phosphatase

This enzyme is present in the canalicular and sinusoidal membranes of the liver and many other tissues, such as bone. The serum alkaline phosphatase level may be raised by up to four to six times the normal limit in intrahepatic or extrahepatic cholestasis. It can also be raised in conditions associated with infiltration of the liver, such as metastases and cirrhosis.

Albumin

Plasma albumin is synthesized in the liver, and has a half-life of approximately 20 days. Changes in the serum concentration of albumin can be a useful guide to the synthetic function of the liver and to the extent of chronic liver disease.

Prothrombin time

Prothrombin time is a measure of clotting factor synthesis, and is a sensitive indicator of both acute and chronic liver disease. It is a useful marker for determining the synthetic capacity of the liver.

Patient care

Pruritus

Pruritus is one of the most common and distressing symptoms associated with liver disease. It can be of variable severity tending to be more severe in cholestatic conditions. In general it is thought to be due to the deposition of bile salts within the skin, although their concentration in the skin does not appear to correlate with the intensity of itching. Management depends upon severity and on the nature of the underlying condition. For example, if a bile duct is blocked by gallstones, then these should be removed surgically, endoscopically or by using a supplementary bile acid such as ursodeoxycholic acid. In patients where this is either not possible or the cause of the pruritus is unknown, then medical thereapy is appropriate.

Anion exchange resins

In patients, with obstructive jaundice, anion exchange resins may be effective. Colestyramine and colestipol act by binding bile acids within the intestinal lumen, thereby preventing their absorption. Colestyramine is usually initiated at a dose of 4 g once or twice daily, and the dose titrated to give adequate relief without causing gastrointestinal upset. Adverse effects are common but usually mild, including constipation, diarrhoea, fat and vitamin malabsorption and an unpleasant taste. Consequently, adherence is often a problem.

Colestyramine can be mixed with drinks and incorporated into special recipies to help improve patient palatability. To facilitate good compliance patients should be reassured that the benefits of therapy may take up to a week to become apparent.

Anion exchange resins can reduce the absorption of many co-administered drugs, such as digoxin, levothyroxine (thyroxine) and propranolol. To avoid this, other oral medicines should be taken at least 1 hour before or 4–6 hours after a dose of colestyramine or colestipol.

Antihistamines

For symptomatic relief of itching, antihistamines may be effective, but they are contraindicated in severe liver disease. A non-sedating antihistamine such as cetirizine (10 mg once daily) or loratidine (10 mg once daily) is preferred to avoid precipitating or masking encephalopathy. Antihistamines such as chlorphenamine (chlorpheniramine) or hydroxyzine have traditionally been avoided because of their sedative properties, although they may be useful at night if the severity of pruritus is sufficient to prevent a patient from sleeping.

Ursodeoxycholic acid

The bile acid ursodeoxycholic acid (10 mg/kg daily in two divided doses) is frequently used in cholestatic liver disease, where long-term use has been shown to improve pruritus.

Topical preparations

Topical therapy with calamine lotion or menthol 2% in aqueous cream may benefit some patients.

Ondansetron

The 5-HT$_3$ antagonist ondansetron has been shown to reduce pruritus in some patients when given intravenously. Oral administration of ondansetron gives more variable results.

Rifampicin and phenobarbital

Rifampicin and phenobarbital induce hepatic microsomal enzymes, which may benefit some patients, possibly by improving bile flow. Rifampicin should be used cautiously due to its hepatotoxicity and potential to interact with many drugs.

Opioid antagonists

Endogenous opioids in the central nervous system are potential mediators of itch. The opioid antagonists naloxone and naltrexone, which are thought to reverse the actions of these endogenous opioids, have been shown to be effective (Wolfhagen et al 1997). Table 14.3 summarizes the drugs commonly used in the management of pruritus.

Clotting abnormalities

The liver is the principal site for the synthesis of factors involved in coagulation, anticoagulation and fibrinolysis. Haemostatic abnormalities develop in approximately 75% of patients with chronic liver disease, and the most frequently used indicator of defective clotting factor synthesis is the prothrombin time. This is a very useful and sensitive marker of the synthetic capacity of the liver. In patients with acute liver failure prothrombin time is used as a prognostic indicator to identify patients potentially requiring a liver transplant. The relationship of liver disease to clotting abnormalities is shown diagrammatically in Figure 14.5.

While the normal prothrombin time is between 12 and 16 seconds, prolongation of more than 3 seconds (or

Table 14.3   Drugs commonly used in the management of pruritus

Drug	Indication	Daily dose	Advantage	Disadvantage
Colestyramine	Cholestasis Jaundice Itching (first-line)	4–16 g (in two or three divided doses)	Reduce systemic bile salt levels	Poor patient compliance due to unpalatability Diarrhoea/constipation Increased flatulence Abdominal discomfort
Ursodeoxycholic acid	Cholestatic jaundice Itching	10 mg/kg (in two divided doses)		Variable response
Menthol 2% in aqueous cream	Itching	As required	Local cooling effect	Variable response
Chlorphenamine (chlorpheniramine)	Itching	4–16 mg (in three or four divided doses)	Sedative effects may be useful for night-time itching	May precipitate/aggravate encephalopathy
Hydroxyzine	Itching	25–100 mg (in three or four divided doses)	Sedative effects may be useful for night-time itching	May precipitate/aggravate encephalopathy
Cetirizine	Itching	10 mg (once daily)	Antihistamine with low incidence of sedation	Variable response
Loratidine	Itching	10 mg (once daily)	Antihistamine with low incidence of sedation	Variable response

international normalized ratio (INR) greater than 1.2) is usually considered abnormal. Patients with liver disease who develop deranged blood clotting should receive intravenous doses of phytomenadione (vitamin K), usually 10 mg daily for 3 days. In patients with significant liver disease, administration of vitamin K does not usually improve the prothrombin time as the liver is unable to utilize the vitamin for the synthesis of clotting factors. Oral vitamin K is less effective than the parenteral form because it is a fat-soluble vitamin which may not be adequately absorbed if there is a reduction in bile salt production due to cholestasis. This may be addressed by administering oral menadiol sodium phosphate, a water-soluble preparation of vitamin K. However, this is a provitamin, which requires activation in the liver before it can exert vitamin K-like effects.

Aspirin, non-steroidal anti-inflammatory drugs (NSAIDs) and anticoagulants should be avoided in patients with liver disease because of the risk of altering platelet function and causing gastric ulceration and bleeding. NSAIDs have also been implicated in precipitating renal dysfunction in patients with end-stage liver disease. Although COX-2 inhibitors cause a lower incidence of bleeding complications, current practice is

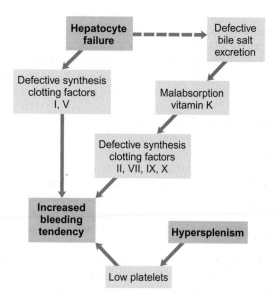

Figure 14.5   Mechanisms of deranged clotting in chronic liver disease.

to avoid these agents in patients with liver disease as their use still poses a risk.

Ascites

Ascites is one of the earliest and most common complications of cirrhosis, occurring within 10 years of diagnosis in about 50% of patients. The aim of treatment is to mobilize the intra-abdominal fluid by reducing sodium intake and increasing renal excretion so that approximately 0.5 kg of body weight is lost per day (1 kg per day if peripheral oedema is present). Aggressive body weight reduction in the absence of oedema should be avoided as it may cause intravascular fluid depletion and renal dysfunction. General measures in the management of ascites include bed rest, to improve renal perfusion, fluid restriction and reduction in dietary sodium. A low-sodium diet, providing 40–60 mmol of sodium per day, will usually be enough to initiate net sodium loss in approximately 20% of patients. Table 14.4 outlines the sequential approach to the management of ascites, with the mainstay of medical management being diuretics and/or paracentesis.

Diuretics

The usual doses of diuretics employed for the treatment of ascites are shown in Table 14.5. The diuretic of choice is the aldosterone antagonist spironolactone, which blocks sodium reabsorption in the collecting tubules of the kidney. Spironolactone is usually initiated at 100 mg per day, depending on the patient's clinical status and other drug therapy. The dose can usually be increased gradually at 4–5 day intervals if required. The addition of furosemide (frusemide) 40 mg per day enhances the natriuretic activity of spironolactone, and should be used when spironolactone alone does not produce acceptable diuresis.

Occasionally, single doses of more potent diuretics such as metolazone may confer additional benefit. Urea and electrolytes should be monitored regularly to detect impending hyperkalaemia and hyponatraemia, which can commonly occur during therapy with spironolactone. Care should also be taken to avoid overdiuresis, since this may precipitate the hepatorenal syndrome. Dose escalation of diuretics should generally be stopped if the serum sodium level decreases to less than 130 mmol/l or if creatinine levels rise to greater than 130 μmol/l. All diuretics may cause side-effects, and common complications include encephalopathy, hypokalaemia, hyponatraemia, azotaemia, gynaecomastia and muscle cramps.

Ascites is considered to be diuretic-resistant once daily doses of spironolactone of between 300 and 600 mg and furosemide (frusemide) at doses of 120–160 mg

are ineffective, in which case alternative therapeutic measures will be required.

Paracentesis

In patients with refractory ascites, or acute tense ascites, paracentesis is the treatment of choice. Paracentesis provides rapid relief of symptoms by draining fluid from the abdomen in conjunction with intravenous colloid replacement to prevent adverse effects on the renal and systemic circulation. Colloid replacement is in the form of 6–8 g albumin/l of ascites removed (1 unit (100 ml) of 20% human albumin solution (HAS) for every 2.5 l of ascitic fluid removed).

Transjugular intrahepatic portosystemic shunting (TIPSS)

TIPSS is a minimally invasive technique, carried out under radiological guidance to control variceal bleeding or manage refractory ascites. An expandable metal stent is placed within the liver to create a shunt between the portal and hepatic venous systems (Fig. 14.6), thereby reducing portal pressure. There is a high incidence of hepatic encephalopathy, between 30% and 75%, with this procedure.

Spontaneous bacterial peritonitis

Some 15–20% of patients with ascites develop spontaneous bacterial peritonitis (SBP), with an associated mortality rate of up to 40%. If there is a clinical suspicion of SBP, treatment with appropriate antibiotics should be commenced as soon as possible after a diagnostic ascitic tap. An ascitic neutrophil count greater than 250 cells/mm^3 confirms a diagnosis of SBP.

Table 14.4 The sequential approach to the management of cirrhotic ascites

Bed rest and sodium restriction (60–80 mmol/day)

▼

Spironolactone (or other potassium-sparing diuretic)

▼

Spironolactone and loop diuretic

▼

Large-volume paracentesis and colloid replacement

Other measures

Transjugular intrahepatic portosystemic shunt

Peritonovenous shunt

Extracorporeal ascites concentration

Consider orthotopic liver transplantation

Table 14.5   Diuretics used for ascites

Drug	Indication	Daily dose	Advantage	Disadvantage
Spironolactone	Fluid retention	100–600 mg	Aldosterone antagonist Slow diuresis	Painful gynaecomastia Variable bioavailability Hyperkalaemia
Furosemide (frusemide)	Fluid retention	40–160 mg	Rapid diuresis, sodium excretion	Nephrotoxic Dehydration Hypokalaemia Hyponatraemia Caution in prerenal uraemia
Bumetanide	Fluid retention	1–4 mg	Rapid diuresis, sodium excretion ?Better oral bioavailability than furosemide (frusemide)	Nephrotoxic Dehydration Hypokalaemia Hyponatraemia Caution in prerenal uraemia
Amiloride	Mild fluid retention	5–10 mg	As K$^+$-sparing agent or weak diuretic if spironolactone contraindicated	Not potent
Metolazone	Unresponsive fluid retention	5 mg stat. Repeated daily as required with caution	Useful in inducing diuresis in resistant cases	Severe electrolyte disturbances Hyponatraemia/hypokalaemia

The causative organism is of enteric origin in approximately three-quarters of infections, and originates from the skin in the remaining one-quarter. Cefotaxime is commonly used as the first-line treatment in the empiric management of SBP. Other antibiotics that have been used include co-amoxiclav and ceftriaxone.

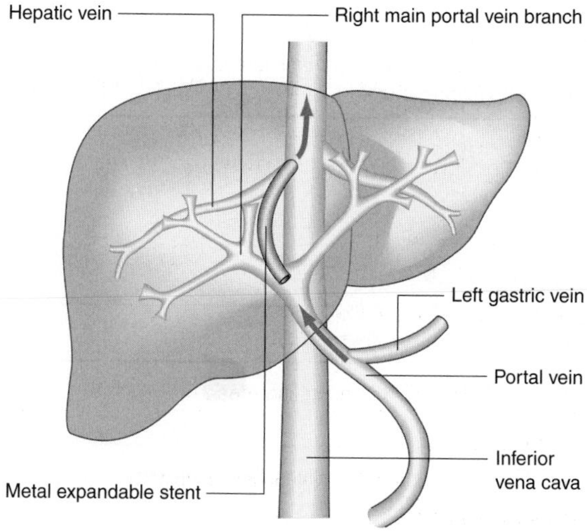

Hepatic encephalopathy

Hepatic encephalopathy is a neuropsychiatric syndrome that occurs with significant liver dysfunction, but which has the potential for full reversibility. The precise cause of encephalopathy remains unclear, but three factors are known to be implicated, namely portosystemic shunting, metabolic dysfunction and an alteration of the blood–brain barrier. It is thought that intestinally-derived neuroactive and neurotoxic substances such as ammonia pass through the diseased liver or bypass the liver through shunts directly to the brain, resulting in cerebral dysfunction. Ammonia is thought to increase the permeability of the blood–brain barrier, enable other neurotoxins to enter the brain, and indirectly alter neurotransmission in the brain. Other substances that have been implicated in causing hepatic encephalopathy include free fatty acids, gamma-aminobutyric acid (GABA) and glutamate.

Clinical features of hepatic encephalopathy include altered mental state, fetor hepaticus (development of a sweetish, pungent odour to the breath) and asterixis (flapping tremor of the hands). During the early phase of

Figure 14.6   Intrahepatic stent shunt links the hepatic vein with the intraheptic portal vein.

encephalopathy, the altered mental state may present as a slight derangement of judgement, personality or change of mood. Drowsiness, confusion and, finally, coma can ensue (Table 14.6).

Although hepatic encephalopathy has a wide range of presentations, it is important to differentiate between two common types which differ in progression, severity and management. In acute liver failure, the shorter the interval between jaundice and encephalopathy, the more likely cerebral oedema, a major cause of death in fulminant hepatic failure, may occur. In this situation encephalopathy can progress from grade 1 or 2 to 4 in a few hours. Alternatively, encephalopathy complicating cirrhosis and portosystemic shunting often develops as a result of specific precipitating factors (Table 14.7) or an acute deterioration of liver function. The patient usually improves after correction of the precipitating cause.

After identifying and removing precipitating causes, therapeutic management is aimed primarily at reducing the amount of ammonia or nitrogenous products in the circulatory system. Protein restriction may reduce the production of ammonia, but the merits of protein restriction must be balanced against the potential adverse effects on nutritional status. Treatment with a laxative should be started to increase the throughput of bowel contents. The most common drug therapies for encephalopathy are summarized in Table 14.8.

Lactulose, a disaccharide molecule broken down by gastrointestinal bacteria to form lactic, acetic and formic acids, is usually the drug of choice. This preparation acidifies the colonic contents and leads to the ionization of nitrogenous products within the bowel, with a consequent reduction in their absorption from the gastrointestinal tract. If a patient is unable to take oral medication then enemas, for example phosphate enema, should be administered to empty the bowels regularly (Jalan & Hayes 1997).

Antibiotics such as metronidazole or neomycin may also be used to reduce ammonia production from gastrointestinal bacteria. Metronidazole is the preferred option as approximately 2–3% of an oral dose of neomycin may be absorbed and result in renal impairment and ototoxicity. Other therapies that have been investigated to treat encephalopathy include branched-chain amino acids, levodopa, bromocriptine and flumazenil.

Table 14.6	Grading of hepatic encephalopathy
Grade 0	Normal
Subclinical	Abnormal psychometric tests for encephalopathy (e.g. number correction test)
Grade 1	Euphoria or depression, abnormal sleep pattern, impaired handwriting +/– asterixis
Grade 2	Drowsiness, grossly impaired calculation ability, asterixis
Grade 3	Confusion, disorientation, somnolent but arousable, asterixis
Grade 4	Stupor to deep coma, unresponsive to painful stimuli

Table 14.7 Precipitating causes of hepatic encephalopathy

- Gastrointestinal bleeding
- Infection (spontaneous bacterial peritonitis, other sites of sepsis)
- Hypokalaemia, metabolic alkalosis
- High-protein diet
- Constipation
- Sedative drugs
- Uraemia after diuretic therapy
- Deterioration of liver function
- Post-surgical portosystemic shunt or transjugular portosystemic shunt

Table 14.8 Drugs commonly used in the management of encephalopathy

Drug	Dose	Comment	Side-effects
Lactulose	15–30 ml orally 2–4 times daily	Aim for 2–3 soft stools daily	Bloating, diarrhoea
Metronidazole	400–800 mg orally daily in divided doses	Metabolism impaired in liver disease	Gastrointestinal disturbance
Neomycin	2–4 g orally daily in divided doses	Maximum duration of 48 h	Potential for nephro- and ototoxicity

Oesophageal varices

Massive upper gastrointestinal bleeding from ruptured oesophageal varices is the main complication of portal hypertension and one of the leading causes of death in patients with liver cirrhosis. About 50% of patients presenting with their first variceal bleed will die within 6 weeks, and each subsequent bleed carries a 30% mortality. Subsequent management of cases is difficult and complex. Variceal bleeding should therefore be managed in a centre with appropriate facilities as soon as the haemorrhage has been controlled.

The aims of treatment are to stop or slow down immediate blood loss, treat hypovolaemic shock if it develops, and prevent recurrent bleeding. Immediate measures include prompt resuscitation, obtaining intravenous access, carrying out an endoscopy to confirm diagnosis and making an attempt to reduce blood loss. Fluid replacement is usually required, and should be in the form of colloid or packed red cells. Saline should be avoided as it may exacerbate the development of ascites.

Over-zealous expansion of the circulating volume may precipitate further bleeding by raising portal pressure, and should therefore be avoided. A suggested flow chart for the management of bleeding oesophageal varices is shown in Figure 14.7.

Endoscopic management

Until recently, sclerotherapy was regarded as the treatment of choice for bleeding oesophageal varices, with sclerosants such as ethanolamine, sodium tetradecyl sulphate (STD) or ethanol controlling variceal bleeding in up to 95% of patients. Although sclerotherapy is usually effective at arresting haemorrhage, complications such as oesophageal ulceration occur in 10–30% of patients. Variceal ligation, or 'banding', is a newer technique whereby prestretched rubber bands are attached around the base of a varix that has been sucked into a cylinder attached to the front of an endoscope. Variceal ligation controls bleeding in approximately 90% of cases; is at least as effective as sclerotherapy and is associated with fewer side-effects. Balloon tamponade with a Sengstaken-Blakemore balloon or Linton balloon may be used to stabilize a patient with actively bleeding varices by directly compressing the bleeding varices until more definitive therapy can be undertaken.

Pharmacological therapy

Several pharmacological agents are available for the emergency control of variceal bleeding (Table 14.9). Most act by lowering portal venous pressure. They are

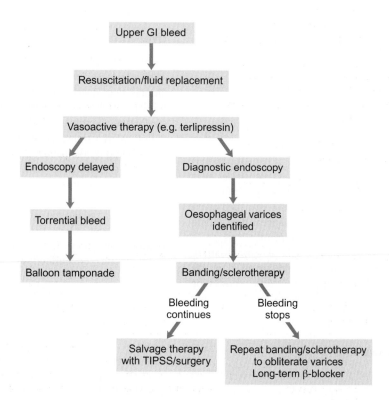

Figure 14.7 Management of oesophageal variceal haemorrhage.

Table 14.9 Drugs used in the treatment of acute bleeding varices

Drug	Dosage and administration
Somatostatin	250 microgram/hour i.v. infusion for 48 hours or longer if patient re-bleeds
Octreotide	50 microgram/hour i.v. infusion for 48 hours or longer if patient re-bleeds
Terlipressin +/− glyceryl trinitrate 10 mg patch replaced every 24 hours	1–2 mg bolus 4–6 hourly for 48 hours
Vasopressin + glyceryl trinitrate 10 mg patch replaced every 24 hours	20 units over 15 minutes, 0.4 units per minute i.v. infusion until bleeding stopped for 12 hours

generally used in addition to balloon tamponade and emergency endoscopic techniques to control bleeding. Vasopressin was the first preparation to be used in this way, but was found to be associated with systemic vasoconstrictive side-effects. Terlipressin, a synthetic analogue of vasopressin, effectively controls bleeding in about 80% of patients. It is convenient to administer in bolus doses every 4–6 hours. In a meta-analysis of trials (D'Amico et al 1995), terlipressin was shown to control bleeding and reduce overall mortality.

Somatostatin infusion and octreotide (a somatostatin analogue) have also been found to be effective in controlling bleeding, although terlipressin is currently the agent of choice.

Transjugular intrahepatic portosystemic stent shunt (TIPSS)

TIPSS is particularly useful in patients who continue to bleed after endoscopic therapy (see Fig. 14.7).

Prevention of re-bleeding

Banding (ligation) can be performed at regular intervals (1–2 weeks) to obliterate the varices. Once varices have been eradicated, endoscopic follow-up should be undertaken every 3 months for the first year then every 6–12 months thereafter. If varices re-appear they should be banded regularly until eradicated again.

Non-selective β-blockers, such as propranolol, decrease portal venous pressure and are used in the prophylaxis of further bleeds. The dose should be adjusted until the heart rate is reduced by 25% but not less than 55 beats per minute.

Acute liver failure

Acute liver failure (ALF) occurs when there is a sudden cessation of normal hepatic function associated with encephalopathy, development of a coagulopathy and subsequent jaundice. ALF is a rare condition but may lead to cerebral oedema, renal impairment and multiorgan failure. Drug toxicity and viral hepatitis account for 95% of cases, with overall mortality ranging from 7% to 100%, depending on the cause. Management is complicated, involving the central nervous system, cardiovascular system and renal system. All ALF patients are at risk of infection, and prophylactic administration of broad-spectrum antibiotics and anti-fungal agents is recommended.

Coagulopathy and bleeding are serious complications of acute liver failure which require careful monitoring and treatment, as appropriate, with fresh frozen plasma.

Liver transplantation

Liver transplantation is the established treatment for selected patients with acute liver failure, decompensated chronic liver disease, inherited metabolic disorders and primary liver cancer, with a 1 year post-transplant survival of about 80%.

Following transplantation, the main problems encountered by the patient are rejection of the graft and opportunistic infection. Patients receive a combination of immunosuppressants such as tacrolimus or ciclosporin, azathioprine and prednisolone, and therapy is monitored and titrated carefully according to the needs of the patient. Over time, doses of the immuno-suppressants may be reduced or even stopped. Prophylactic anti-infectives are administered to minimize the risk of infection.

Hepatitis A

There is at present no specific therapy for hepatitis A (HAV) infection, and management of patients is generally supportive. Passive immunization with the appropriate immunoglobulin is advised in high-risk patients.

Hepatitis B

The primary approach to the management of hepatitis B (HBV) infection should be conservative, with education of the patient, the avoidance of further injury, and the protection of contacts. Specific therapies have been developed for chronic hepatitis, but these are of no apparent benefit in acute hepatitis.

In chronic HBV, treatment is aimed at reducing or abolishing the replication of the virus and thereby preventing the development of complications. Interferon alfa-2a is effective in seroconverting to an anti-hepatitis B antibody (anti-HBAb) status in 20–40% of patients after 4–6 months of therapy. Of those who respond, approximately two-thirds will go on to lose their anti-HBAb within 4 years, and can then be considered to be cured of their hepatitis. Treatment with interferon alfa-2a can cause worsening of liver function in some patients. Patients with a low serum hepatitis B virus DNA titre, those with IgM anti-HBAb indicative of recent infection, and those with high transaminase levels have been shown to have more favourable overall response rates. Other agents under investigation include cytokines and lamivudine.

Hepatitis C

The primary aim of treating patients with chronic hepatitis C (HCV) is to achieve clearance of the virus, sustained for at least 6 months after treatment has stopped, thereby improving quality of life for patients and reducing the risk of cirrhosis and hepatocellular carcinoma.

Ribavirin (tribavirin) in combination with interferon alfa-2b is the treatment of choice in managing moderate to severe HCV (defined as histological evidence of significant fibrosis and/or significant necrotic inflammation). Patients receive 3 megaunits of interferon alfa-2b three times a week along with ribavirin (tribavirin) orally at a dose of 1000 mg per day (for patients weighing less than 75 kg) or 1200 mg per day (for patients weighing more than 75 kg). Treatment is continued for 6 months, with a further 6 months recommended in patients infected with hepatitis C virus of genotype 1. Adverse effects of combination treatment include influenza-like symptoms, decrease in haematological parameters such as haemoglobin, neutrophils, white blood cell count and platelets, gastrointestinal complaints, psychiatric disturbances, for example anxiety and depression, and hypo- or hyper-thyrodism.

Pegylated interferon alfa-2b is a new formulation of interferon, the use of which is likely to supersede conventional interferon alfa-2b. It is produced by the addition of a polyethylene glycol molecule to standard interferon and results in prolongation of the half-life so that only one dose per week (1.5 micrograms/kg) is required. This sustained action reduces the incidence of viral replication and leads to a prolonged virological response in a greater proportion of patients than standard interferon therapy. Doses of tribavirin used in combination with pegylated interferon tend to be lower than those used with standard interferon therapy (Schafer & Sorrell 2000).

Autoimmune hepatitis

Corticosteroids and/or azathioprine are the mainstay of therapy for autoimmune hepatitis. Prednisolone is usually the corticosteroid of choice at an initial dose of 60 mg/day, reduced after about 2 weeks to 40 mg/day. Subsequent reduction of corticosteroid dose depends on the clinical response, with a maintenance dose of 10–20 mg/day usually required for several months before reduction to less than 10 mg/day. Azathioprine at a dose of 1–1.5 mg/kg per day is used as an adjunct to corticosteroid therapy. Azathioprine alone is ineffective in treating the acute phase of autoimmune hepatitis, but is useful in maintaining remission.

Patients intolerant of azathioprine, or those who do not respond to combined prednisolone and azathioprine, may be treated with ciclosporin at a dose of 3–6 mg/kg/day. Ultimately, liver transplantation is the treatment of choice in patients with end-stage autoimmune hepatitis and cirrhosis.

Primary biliary cirrhosis

Several therapies have been associated with short-term symptomatic improvements in liver function tests. Ursodeoxycholic acid reduces the retention of bile acids, increases their hepatic excretion, and is effective if used early in the management of primary biliary cirrhosis at a dose of 10–15 mg/kg/day. Immunosuppressive agents such as ciclosporin, azathioprine and methotrexate have also been assessed, but the benefits of treatment are usually limited. Liver transplantation remains the only effective option in patients with end-stage disease.

Primary sclerosing cholangitis

There is no effective treatment for this condition. Anion-exchange resins and/or ursodeoxycholic acid can be used to manage the associated cholestasis, but studies with various immunosuppressive agents have been disappointing. Transplantation is the only real solution.

Wilson's disease

This rare condition is usually managed with chelation therapy using penicillamine, administered at a dose of 1–2 g per day before food in divided doses, followed by a maintenance dose of 0.75–1 g per day. Penicillamine generally improves symptomatic patients over a period of several weeks, but is relatively slow acting and has a number of potentially serious adverse effects. These include worsening of neurological symptoms, renal dysfunction and haematological abnormalities. Regular monitoring of the full blood count and electrolytes is required, as well as the co-administration of small doses of pyridoxine to counteract neurological toxicity.

Patients who are unable to tolerate penicillamine may respond to trientine, a chelating agent that is less potent than penicillamine but has fewer adverse effects.

Drug selection in patients with liver disease

The effects of hepatic insufficiency on the pharmacokinetics of drugs are not consistent or predictable. Unfortunately, there are no sensitive and specific clinical criteria that can accurately assess the extent of liver disease and determine metabolic capacity of the diseased liver. For this reason, drug doses cannot be predicted with the same precision that can be applied to doses of drugs for patients with renal impairment.

Two issues need to be considered when using drugs in patients with liver disease, namely the pharmacokinetics of the drug concerned and the pharmacodynamic response of the diseased liver.

Pharmacokinetics

Pharmacokinetic predictions of drug handling in the presence of liver disease depend on several factors including hepatic blood flow, portosystemic shunting, hepatic cell mass and protein binding.

Hepatic blood flow

In patients with significant cirrhosis of the liver, hepatic blood flow is reduced. As a result there is an increase in the systemic bioavailability of oral drugs which are usually removed by the liver during first pass metabolism. When the clearance of a drug is highly dependent on liver blood flow it is known as a high extraction drug. Many drugs undergo extensive first-pass metabolism, including clomethiazole, lidocaine (lignocaine), morphine and propranolol. Drugs with a high hepatic extraction ratio are generally used at between 10% and 50% of the dose that would be used in the absence of liver disease. All dose modifications should be monitored closely for clinical effects, with therapeutic drug monitoring wherever possible. For low-extraction drugs, where elimination of these drugs is not dependent on liver blood flow, dose reductions do not need to be as great.

Portosystemic shunting

In cirrhotic patients, up to 60% of the blood supply reaching the liver in the portal vein may be diverted into collateral vessels. This has a similar effect to the reduction in blood flow through the liver, and leads to increased bioavailabilty of many drugs, particularly those which have a high extraction ratio during first pass metabolism.

Reduced hepatic cell mass

In patients with severe liver disease there can be as little as 30% metabolic capacity of the liver remaining. This is an important consideration for those drugs that are primarily metabolized by the liver.

Reduction in protein binding

Patients with liver disease tend to have low serum albumin due to a reduction in the synthetic capacity of the liver. A reduction in protein binding is important for drugs that are highly protein bound, such as phenytoin or warfarin. In these situations the free drug concentration (which is pharmacologically active) will increase, although clearance may also increase correspondingly.

Pharmacodynamics

The pharmacodynamic response to various drugs is altered in patients with liver cirrhosis. Patients with cirrhosis are more sensitive to sedative drugs, such as benzodiazepines and opiates, and drugs with the potential to cause sedation should generally be avoided in patients with significant cirrhosis due to the risk of precipitating or masking encephalopathy.

Where liver disease has reduced or impaired the production of clotting factors, patients are at increased risk of bleeding. Drugs associated with causing haemorrhage or alterations in platelet function, such as aspirin, NSAIDs and warfarin, should therefore be avoided. Drugs that are known to affect liver enzymes are best avoided in patients who have deranged liver function tests. Similarly, drugs that alter the concentration of liver enzymes may increase the toxicity of concurrent therapy. For example, rifampicin may increase the hepatotoxicity of isoniazid by increasing the production of hepatotoxic metabolites of the latter.

Table 14.10 summarizes some of the common indications, and the choice of drugs, for use in patients with liver disease with different conditions.

Table 14.11 summarizes the common therapeutic problems that can arise in the treatment of patients with liver disease.

Table 14.10 Common indications and drugs of choice in patients with liver disease

Therapeutic use	Drugs	Comments
Analgesia	Paracetamol	Use in standard doses Use low doses (max 2 g/day) in alcoholic patients or those taking enzyme-inducing drugs Avoid following paracetamol overdose
	NSAIDs	Avoid Risk of gastric mucosal bleeding Can precipitate/exacerbate renal impairment
	Opioids	Can mask/precipitate encephalopathy Use small doses at greater dosage intervals Monitor patient carefully Titrate according to patient response
Anxiety	Short-acting benzodiazepine	Can mask/precipitate encephalopathy Use small doses
Convulsions	Phenytoin	Anti-epileptic of choice Reduce dose in patient with low serum albumin
Depression	Paroxetine	Use doses at lower end of range
Diabetes	Insulin	Sulphonylureas can cause hepatotoxicity
Gastrointestinal disease	Antacids	Avoid high-sodium containing products – can worsen fluid retention
	Ranitidine	Few reports of hepatotoxicity
	Omeprazole	Few reports of hepatotoxicity
Infection – low-grade	Penicillins/cephalosporins	Care with high-sodium containing preparations
Nausea/vomiting	Domperidone Metoclopramide (second-line)	Use lowest clinically-effective dose
Psychosis	Haloperidol	Rarely associated with hepatotoxicity Caution – sedative potential
Gout	Colchicine	Use with caution at standard doses Mild elevation of liver enzymes reported

Table 14.11 Common therapeutic problems in liver disease

Patient problem	Drug	Therapeutic problem
Ascites	Diuretic	Aggressive dosing and inadequate monitoring can precipitate renal dysfunction
Encephalopathy	Lactulose	Inadequate dosing of lactulose is common; need doses of 30 ml three times a day to give 2–3 loose motions per day
Acute variceal bleed	Terlipressin	Inappropriate choice of agent: acid suppressing agents are ineffective; need to prescribe agents to lower portal pressure e.g. terlipressin
Pain	Paracetamol	Standard dose (4 g per day) can be hepatotoxic in patients on enzyme inducing agents e.g. alcohol, phenytoin, rifampicin
	Aspirin and NSAIDs	Avoid. Patient has impaired clotting and can precipitate renal dysfunction
	Opiates	May mask or precipitate encephalopathy; dose cautiously
Depression	Tricyclic antidepressants	Can mask or precipitate encephalopathy. Use SSRI instead
Agitation	Haloperidol	Can precipitate encephalopathy. Start with small dose only

CASE STUDIES

Case 14.1

A 56-year-old man is admitted to hospital following haematemesis and melaena. He has a known history of alcoholic liver disease (stopped drinking alcohol 1 year ago) with marked ascites. A provisional diagnosis of bleeding oesophageal varices is made.

A Sengstaken-Blakemore tube is inserted and the balloon inflated as a temporary measure to arrest bleeding. The patient is transferred 8 hours later to a specialist regional centre for further management.

Laboratory data on admission are:

Na	124	(133–143 mmol/l)
K	3.0	(3.5–5.0 mmol/l)
Creatinine	131	(80–124 µmol/l)
Urea	14.3	(2.7–7.7 mmol/l)
Bili	167	(3.15 µmol/l)
ALT	24	(0–35 IU/l)
PT	18.9	(13 second)
Alb	24	(35–50 g/dl)
Hb	8.9	(13.5–18 g/dl)

Drugs on admission:

Spironolactone 200 mg one each morning.

Questions

1. What other action would you have recommended before the patient was transferred to the regional centre?
2. What options (drug and/or non-drug) are likely to be available at the regional centre for managing the patient's bleeding varices?
3. What further long-term measures would you recommend for this patient?

Answers

1. Initial restoration of circulating blood volume with colloid, followed by cross-matched blood. Fluid replacement is necessary to protect renal perfusion. In view of the patient's ascites, saline should be avoided. Dextrose 5% with added potassium (hypokalaemia present), would be a reasonable choice. A pharmacological agent to reduce portal pressure, such as terlipressin 1–2 mg every 4–6 hours or octreotide 50 micrograms/h, should be started. Current evidence supports terlipressin over octreotide. Broad-spectrum antibiotics such as cefuroxime and metronidazole should be started intravenously if there is suspicion of abdominal infection or sepsis. There is no evidence that gastric acid suppression is beneficial, but if the bleeding is caused by a gastric mucosal lesion, a proton pump inhibitor such as lansoprazole or omeprazole, or a histamine type-2 receptor antagonist such as ranitidine can be administered.

   Spironolactone is likely to be either causing or exacerbating the low sodium and should be discontinued.

   Vitamin K, 10 mg intravenously once daily for 3 days, should be administered to try to correct the raised prothrombin time. As the patient has severe liver disease with varices and ascites there is a possibility he may develop encephalopathy. It would be advisable to start lactulose or, if the patient is unable to take medicines orally, administer an enema such as a phosphate enema.

2. Specialist endoscopy facilities will allow the following:

   Sclerotherapy: 1–2 ml of sodium tetradecyl sulphate or 3–5 ml of ethanolamine injected directly into the oesophageal varices to arrest bleeding. This achieves haemostasis in up to 95% of patients.

   Banding/ligation: this has a similar efficacy to sclerotherapy but fewer complications. It involves mechanical strangulation of variceal channels by small elastic plastic rings mounted on the tip of the endoscope.

Transjugular intrahepatic portosystemic stent shunt (TIPSS): this can be used to reduce portal pressure, but beware of precipitating encephalopathy.

Banding, and to a lesser extent sclerotherapy: these tend to be the first-line options for managing bleeding oesophageal varices. Patients who continue to bleed after two endoscopic treatments should be considered for TIPSS. Surgery involving portal-systemic shunts, devascularization or transplantation are possible options if the above alternatives repeatedly fail. Extrahepatic portal-systemic shunts are situated outside the liver and divert portal blood flow into the systemic circulation bypassing the liver. Devascularization involves obliteration of the collateral vessels supplying blood to the varices.

3. Banding/ligation can be performed at regular intervals of 1–2 weeks to obliterate the varices. Once varices have been eradicated, endoscopic follow-up should be undertaken every 3 months for the first year then every 6–12 months thereafter. If varices re-appear they should be banded regularly until eradicated again.

Non-selective β-blockers such as propranolol are used in the prophylaxis of further bleeds, with the dose adjusted until the heart rate is reduced by 25%, but to not less than 55 beats per minute.

Case 14.2

A 68-year-old woman with a long-standing history of alcoholic liver disease is admitted to hospital with a 2 week history of vomiting, confusion, increased abdominal distension and worsening jaundice.

On admission laboratory data are as follows:

Na	116	(133–143 mmol/l)
K	3.8	(3.5–5 mmol/l)
Urea	8.5	(3.3–7.7 mmol/l)
Cr	119	(80–124 µmol/l)
Bili	459	(3–17 µmol/l)
Alb	23	(35–50 g/l)
ALT	23	(0–35 iu/l)
Alk P	524	(70–300 iu/l)
PT	18.6	(13 seconds)

Drugs on admission are as follows:

Spironolactone 300 mg each morning
temazepam 10 mg at night.
lactulose 10 ml twice daily.

Questions

Discuss the initial treatment plan for the management of:

1. Ascites
2. Nausea and vomiting
3. Confusion.

Answers

From the presenting features and LFTs on admission it is apparent that the patient's liver disease is getting progressively worse, probably as a result of continued alcohol intake. She is confused on admission and this suggests encephalopathy, a common complication of chronic liver disease.

1. Ascites management. The patient has increased abdominal distension on admission suggestive of worsening ascites. This might be due to poor adherence with spironolactone, or alternatively her ascites may have become diuretic-resistant.

The patient should be sodium restricted and confined to bed. Spironolactone therapy should be stopped in view of the low sodium and confusion, as over-use of diuretics can precipitate encephalopathy. Fluid restriction is necessary to reduce the ascites, but sufficient fluid is required to rehydrate the patient following vomiting.

Paracentesis should be used to manage the ascites. Every litre of ascitic fluid removed should be replaced with 6–8 g of albumin. A diagnostic ascitic tap should be taken to ensure there is no infection in the ascites.

2. Nausea/vomiting management. Urea is slightly raised, indicating possible dehydration as a result of vomiting. The patient should be rehydrated with dextrose 5%, not saline, as this will worsen the ascites. Additional potassium should be given to correct the low serum potassium. Note that if the patient has been taking the spironolactone there would normally be an increase in potassium, but in this case the vomiting has probably reduced this. The patient's nausea can be managed with a suitable antiemetic such as domperidone 10 mg four times a day initially and then titrated according to the response.

3. Confusion. Confusion may be an early sign of encephalopathy in this patient. Temazepam should be stopped. The patient is on an inadequate dose of lactulose for the management of encephalopathy, so this should be increased to produce 2–3 loose motions per day. A typical dose would be 20 ml three or four times daily. In view of the patient's confusion it may be worth considering other agents in the management of the encephalopathy, such as metronidazole, 400 mg twice daily.

Case 14.3

A 54-year-old woman with primary biliary cirrhosis has been complaining of increasing backache over the last 3 months. Her general condition has deteriorated over the past year during which she has suffered from ascites and encephalopathy. Her main complaint is of continuous back pain, which disturbs her sleep.

Question

How would you manage this patient's back pain?

Answer

Back pain secondary to osteoporosis-related vertebral fractures is common in patients with chronic liver disease, such as PBC. This is due to the fact that most patients with PBC are postmenopausal women in their late fifties where bone thinning is likely, secondary to both menopausal and liver changes. Once the diagnosis has been confirmed, the patient should be counselled that the bone pain is chronic, tends to be intermittent, and takes several months to settle after each new fracture. Bed rest is useful in the acute situation, but prolonged bed rest can accelerate bone loss.

Although there have been rapid advances in recent years in the treatment of postmenopausal osteoporosis, very few studies have addressed the problems of treating osteoporosis in patients with chronic liver disease. Hormone replacement therapy has not been evaluated in patients with chronic liver disease, and oestrogen therapy is widely believed to be contraindicated in such patients, although there is little evidence to support this. Transdermal oestrogen preparations that avoid the first-pass metabolic effect may be a possible future option.

The patient should be advised to take adequate calcium supplementation of 1–1.5 g/day in addition to her normal diet. Vitamin D deficiencies are common in chronic liver disease and it would be advisable to administer 300 000 units intramuscularly every 3 months.

For symptomatic management of the pain a variety of analgesics are available. The choice of drug is influenced by both the severity of the pain and the degree of liver impairment.

For mild pain, paracetamol is the mainstay of treatment, and may be used in standard doses in the majority of patients with liver dysfunction. Patients pretreated with cytochrome P450-inducing drugs or patients with a history of alcohol abuse are at increased risk of paracetamol-induced liver injury and should receive only short courses at low doses (maximum of 2 g per day for an adult).

Opioid analgesics should usually be avoided in liver disease because of their sedative properties and the risks of precipitating or masking encephalopathy. If a patient has stable mild to moderate liver disease then short-term use of opioids can be considered. Moderate potency opioids, such as dihydrocodeine and codeine, are eliminated almost entirely by hepatic metabolism. Therapy should be initiated at a low dose, and the dosage interval titrated according to the response of the patient. Despite their low potency, these preparations may still precipitate encephalopathy.

In severe pain, the use of potent opioids is usually unavoidable. They undergo hepatic metabolism, and are therefore likely to accumulate in liver disease. To compensate for this it is important to increase the dosage interval when using these drugs. Morphine, pethidine or diamorphine should be administered at doses at the lower end of the dosage range at intervals of 6–8 hours. The patient should be regularly observed and the dose titrated according to patient response. In any patient with liver disease receiving an opioid it is advisable to coprescribe a laxative as constipation can increase the possibility of developing encephalopathy.

NSAIDs should be avoided in patients with liver disease. All NSAIDs can prolong bleeding time via their effects on platelet function. Impaired liver function itself can lead to a reduced synthesis of clotting factors and an increased bleeding tendency. NSAIDs may also be dangerous due to the increased risk of gastrointestinal haemorrhage and potential to preciptate renal dysfunction.

Acknowledgements

The authors thank Mr R. Swallow and Dr P. Bramley for permission to reproduce material originally included in their chapter that appeared in the first edition of this book.

REFERENCES

Bircher J, Benhamou J P, McIntyre N et al (eds) 1999 Oxford textbook of clinical hepatology; 2nd edn. Oxford University Press, Oxford, vols I and II

D'Amico G, Pagliaro L, Bosch J 1995 The treatment of portal hypertension: a meta-analytic review. Hepatology 22: 332–354

Jalan R, Hayes P 1997 Hepatic encephalopathy and ascites. Lancet 350: 1309–1315

Malnick S, Beergabel M, Lurie Y 2000 Treatment of chronic hepatitis C infection. Annals of Pharmacotherapy 34: 1156–1163

Schafer D F, Sorrell M F 2000 Conquering hepatitis C, step by step. New England Journal of Medicine 343(23): 1723–1724

Vander A 1980 Human physiology: mechanisms of body functions, 3rd edn. McGraw-Hill Education

Wolfhagen F, Sternieri E, Hop W et al 1997 Oral naltrexone treatment for cholestatic pruritus: a double blind, placebo controlled trial. Gastroentrology 113: 1264–1269

FURTHER READING

Karnik A, Freeman J 1998 Acute liver failure. Care of the Critically Ill 14(5): 148–154

Magee C, Denton M, Milford E 1999 Immunosuppressive agents in organ transplantation. Hospital Medicine 60(5): 364–369

Acute renal failure 15

J. Marriott   S. Smith

KEY POINTS

- Acute renal failure (ARF) is diagnosed when the excretory function of the kidney declines rapidly over a period of hours or days.
- A wide range of factors can precipitate ARF, including trauma, obstruction of urine flow or any event that causes a reduction in renal blood flow, including surgery and medical conditions (e.g. sepsis, diabetes, acute liver disease).
- Drug involvement in the development of ARF is possible.
- There are no specific signs and symptoms of ARF. The condition is typically indicated by raised blood levels of urea and creatinine.
- The clinical priorities in ARF are to manage life-threatening complications, correct intravascular fluid balance and establish the cause of the renal failure, reversing factors causing damage where possible.
- The aim of medical treatment is to remove causative factors and maintain patient well-being so that the kidneys have a chance to recover.
- Creatinine clearance (Cl_{Cr}) provides a useful guide to renal function although most measures of Cl_{Cr} are inaccurate when renal function deteriorates or improves rapidly.
- Treatment of ARF is essentially preventative and supportive with control of serum biochemistry, prevention of infection and early use of renal replacement therapies as support where necessary.
- ARF is a serious condition with mortality rates ranging from 5% to 90%, varying according to cause; the average mortality rate is approximately 40% despite improvements in management.

Definition and incidence

Acute renal failure (ARF) manifests as an abrupt decline in glomerular filtration rate occurring over a period of days or weeks. This results in an accumulation of nitrogenous waste products and other toxins. In patients with pre-existing renal impairment a rapid decline in renal function is termed 'acute on chronic renal failure'.

Estimates indicate that ARF affects about 5% of hospitalized patients and up to 15% of those who are critically ill. This process may be reversed with appropriate intervention. However, severe ARF is associated with multiple organ failure and mortality rates of up to 90% (Dishart & Kellum 2000).

Classification

ARF is not a single disease state with a uniform aetiology. Rather it is a syndrome that results from a range of different diseases and conditions. However, it is often useful to classify ARF as a start point for the diagnostic and treatment process. The most common classification into prerenal (functional), intrarenal (intrinsic) and postrenal forms is outlined in Table 15.1.

Pre-renal ARF

The causes of prerenal ARF are summarized in Figure 15.1. These all produce a reduction in renal perfusion resulting in renal ischaemia. Prerenal failure is the most common form of renal dysfunction seen in hospitalized patients (see Table 15.1). It may progress to acute tubular necrosis (ATN) thus blurring the distinction between these conditions.

Intrarenal ARF

Any form of damage to the renal infrastructure, usually involving some form of ischaemic or nephrotoxic insult, may result in ARF. Intrarenal ARF may therefore be classified according to the renal structures principally affected.

Table 15.1	Classification of acute renal failure (ARF)	
ARF type	Typical % cases	Common aetiology
Prerenal	40–80	↓ renal perfusion – through ↓ in effective extracellular volume
Intrarenal	10–50	Renal parenchymal injury
Postrenal	< 10	Urinary tract obstructions

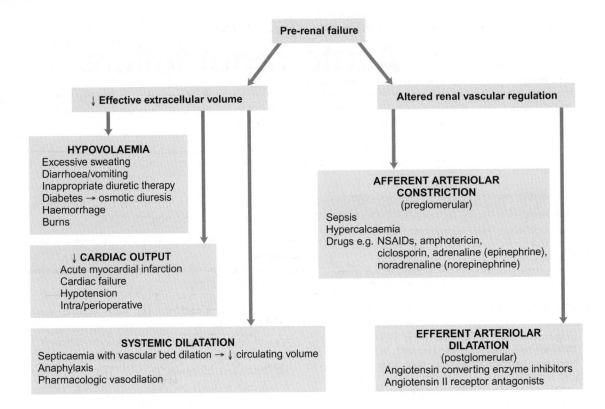

Figure 15.1 Causes of prerenal failure.

Acute tubular necrosis (ATN)

The most common form of intrarenal damage encountered is acute tubular necrosis (ATN) resulting from ischaemia and/or direct toxin action.

The healthy kidney is a vascular organ well supplied with oxygenated blood. This renal blood flow is maintained at approximately 20% of cardiac output. However, regional blood flow within the kidney varies, resulting in relatively hypoxic regions such as the outer medulla. This area is also the site of highly metabolically active parts of the nephron. Owing to the relatively poor oxygen supply and high metabolic demands, the outer medulla is at risk of ischaemia, even under normal conditions. The regulation of regional blood flow in the kidney, and therefore oxygen supply, relies upon vasomotor mechanisms mediated in part by adenosine. Adenosine appears to exert either vasoconstrictor or dilator effects within the kidney depending upon the relative distribution of A_1 and A_2 receptors.

Clearly, any circumstance that interferes with the delicate balance of oxygen supply within the kidney can result in ATN because of ischaemia or through greater vulnerability to nephrotoxins. The likelihood of ATN is increased by underlying conditions that predispose to ischaemia such as development of a prerenal state, sepsis, diabetes, or atherosclerosis.

Common clinical precipitants of ATN. Table 15.2 shows some of the common factors encountered clinically that may cause ATN.

Interstitial nephritis

Interstitial damage (interstitial nephritis) is thought to be a nephrotoxin-induced hypersensitivity reaction with inflammation affecting those cells lying between the nephrons. There is usually secondary involvement of the tubules. Drugs that have been shown to be responsible include the penicillins (particularly methicillin), cephalosporins, allopurinol and azathioprine.

Glomerulonephritis

Glomerular lesions (glomerulonephritis) are thought to be caused by the deposition of immune complexes in the glomerular tuft which elicit an inflammatory response. The antigens responsible for the immune complexes may be exogenous, precipitating a hypersensitivity reaction, or endogenous, resulting in an autoimmune condition. Specific aetiological factors can rarely be identified, although some drugs have been implicated, including gold, penicillamine and phenytoin. Glomerulonephritis is a relatively rare cause of ARF.

Table 15.2   Common clinical factors known to cause acute tubular necrosis (ATN)

Clinical factor	mechanism
Hypoperfusion	Reduced oxygen/nutrient supply
Radiocontrast media	Medullary ischaemia may result from contrast media induced renal vasoconstriction. The high ionic load of contrast media may produce ischaemia
Sepsis	Infection produces endotoxaemia and systemic inflammation in combination with a prerenal state and nephrotoxins. The immunological response to sepsis involves release of vasoconstrictors and vasodilators (e.g. eicosanoids, nitric oxide) and damage to vascular endothelium with resultant thrombosis
Rhabdomyolysis	Damaged muscles release myoglobin, which can cause ATN through direct nephrotoxicity and by a reduction in blood flow in the outer medulla
Renal transplantion	The procedures and conditions encountered during renal transplantation can induce ischaemic ATN, which can be difficult to distinguish from the nephrotoxic effects of immunosuppressive drug therapy used in these circumstances
Hepatorenal syndrome	Renal vasoconstriction is frequently seen in patients with end stage liver disease. The cause appears complex and progression to ATN common
Nephrotoxins	
Aminoglycosides	Aminoglycosides are transported into tubular cells where they exert a direct nephrotoxic effect. Current dosage regimens recommend once daily doses to minimize total uptake of aminoglycoside
Amphotericin	Amphotericin appears to cause direct nephrotoxicity by disturbing the permeability of tubular cells. The nephrotoxic effect is dose dependent and minimized by limiting total dose used, rate of infusion and by volume loading. These precautions also apply to newer liposomal formulations
Immunosuppressants	Ciclosporin and tacrolimus cause intrarenal vasoconstriction that may result in ischaemic ATN. The mechanism is unclear but enhanced by hypovolaemia and other nephrotoxic drugs
NSAIDs	Vasodilator prostaglandins, chiefly E_2, D_2 and I_2 (prostacyclin) produce an increase in blood flow to the glomerulus and medulla. In normal circumstances they play no part in the maintenance of the renal circulation. However, increased amounts of vasoconstrictor substances arise in a variety of clinical conditions such as volume depletion, congestive cardiac failure or hepatic cirrhosis associated with ascites. Maintenance of renal blood flow then becomes more reliant on the release of vasodilatory prostaglandins. Inhibition of prostaglandin synthesis by NSAIDs may cause unopposed arteriolar vasoconstriction, leading to renal hypoperfusion

Renal vascular damage (intrarenal/renal artery or vein)

Occlusion of either the renal arterial or venous supply can lead to intrinsic renal damage, as can disturbances of the intrarenal vasculature, for example vasculitis.

Intrarenal obstruction

Debris deposited within the renal architecture may lead to intrinsic renal failure.

Postrenal ARF

Postrenal ARF results from obstruction of the urinary tract by a variety of mechanisms including urinary stones, prostatic hypertrophy, blood clots and neoplasms. It is extremely unusual for drugs to be responsible for postrenal ARF. Practolol-induced retroperitoneal fibrosis resulting in postrenal ARF is a rare example.

Clinical manifestations

The signs and symptoms of ARF are often non-specific and the diagnosis can be confounded by coexisting clinical conditions. The patient may exhibit signs and symptoms of either volume depletion or overload, depending upon the precipitating conditions, course of the disease and prior treatment.

ARF with volume depletion

In those patients with volume depletion a classic pathophysiological picture is likely to be present, with tachycardia, postural hypotension, reduced skin turgor and cold extremities (see Table 15.3). The most common sign in ARF is oliguria, where the 24-hour urine production falls to 200–400 ml. The oliguric kidney is unable to concentrate urine sufficiently to excrete products of metabolism. Inevitably, the serum concentration of those substances normally excreted by the kidney will rise. Diagnosis can be assisted by detecting elevated levels of creatinine, urea, potassium, hydrogen ion (acidosis) and phosphate in blood. The accumulation of urea and other waste products leads to uraemia, which describes the accumulation of excess blood metabolites together with the other signs and symptoms associated with renal failure, such as nausea, vomiting, diarrhoea, gastrointestinal haemorrhage, muscle cramps and a declining level of consciousness.

ARF with volume overload

In those patients with ARF who have maintained a normal or increased fluid intake as a result of oral or intravenous administration, it is possible to find the pulmonary and systemic signs and symptoms of fluid overload (Table 15.3).

Diagnosis and clinical evaluation

In hospitalized patients, ARF is usually diagnosed incidentally, often by the detection of elevated serum creatinine or urea levels or by a reduction in urine output, including oliguria.

Creatinine is a by-product of normal muscle metabolism and is formed at a rate proportional to muscle mass. It is freely filtered by the glomerulus, with little secretion or reabsorption by the tubule. When muscle mass is stable, any change in serum creatinine levels reflects a change in its clearance by filtration. Consequently, measurement of creatinine clearance gives an estimate of the glomerular filtration rate (GFR). One method of calculating creatinine clearance (Cl_{Cr}) is by performing an accurate collection of urine over 24 hours and taking a serum sample midway through this period. The following equation may then be used:

$$Cl_{Cr} = \frac{(U \times V)}{S}$$

where U is the urine creatinine concentration (μmol/l), V is the urine flow rate (ml/min) and S is the serum creatinine concentration (μmol/l).

A more convenient method to estimate GFR involves measurement of the serum creatinine concentration at a given time, compensating for those factors that affect creatinine levels, including age, sex and weight (preferably ideal body weight). Figure 15.2 shows a range of factors, including drugs that may affect creatinine levels in serum and urine.

An estimation of creatinine clearance can be made from average population data. The equation of Cockroft & Gault (1976) is a useful way of making such an estimation:

$$Cl_{Cr} = \frac{F\,(140 - \text{age (years)}) \times \text{weight (kg)}}{\text{serum creatinine (}\mu\text{mol/l)}}$$

where $F = 1.04$ (females) or 1.23 (males).

When the patient is malnourished and debilitated, the equation developed by Sanaka et al. (1996) should be used.

In men:

$$Cl_{Cr} \text{ (ml/min)} = \frac{0.0884 \times (19 \times \text{serum albumin (g/l)} + 320) \times \text{weight (kg)}}{\text{serum creatinine (}\mu\text{mol/l)}}$$

Table 15.3 Factors associated with acute renal failure

	Volume depletion	Volume overload
History	Thirst	Weight increase
	Excessive fluid loss (sweating, diarrhoea)	Orthopnoea/nocturnal dyspnoea
	Oliguria	
Physical examination	Dry mucosae	Ankle swelling
	↓ skin elasticity	Oedema
	Tachycardia	Jugular venous distension
	↓ blood pressure	Pulmonary crackles
	↓ jugular venous pressure	Pleural effusion

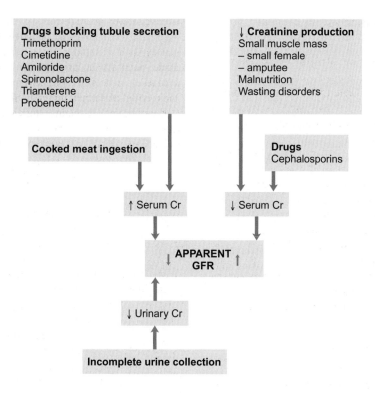

Figure 15.2 Factors that influence serum and urinary creatinine levels.

In women:

$$Cl_{Cr} \text{ (ml/min)} = \frac{0.0884 \times (13 \times \text{serum albumin (g/l} + 290) \times \text{weight (kg)}}{\text{serum creatinine (μmol/l)}}$$

Assuming a normal creatinine clearance of 120 ml/min, renal impairment can be classified as shown in Table 15.4.

Equations such as that of Cockroft & Gault (1976) are based on population statistics but have been validated in all but the very young and the very elderly.

Unless a patient is at steady state, measurement of serum creatinine does not provide a reliable guide to renal function. For example, serum creatinine levels will usually rise by only 50–100 μmol/l per day following complete loss of renal function in a previously normal

Table 15.4   Classification of renal impairment

Degree of impairment	Glomerular filtration rate (ml/min)	Urine production	Symptoms
Decreased renal reserve	< 120	Possible polyuria	–
Mild	50–20	Usually polyuria	+
Moderate	20–10	Oliguria	++
Severe	< 10	Oliguria	+++ Patient usually uraemic requiring dialysis
End stage	< 5	Oliguria/anuria	Death will ensue unless renal replacement therapy instigated rapidly

patient. These changes in serum creatinine are not sufficiently responsive to serve as a practical indicator of deteriorating renal function, particularly in critical care scenarios.

Urea is also commonly used in the assessment of renal function despite its variable production rate and diurnal fluctuation in response to the protein content of the diet. Levels of urea may also be elevated by dehydration or an increase in protein catabolism such as that accompanying gastrointestinal haemorrhage, severe infection, trauma (including surgery) and high-dose steroid therapy. Serum urea levels are therefore an unreliable measure of renal function, but can be often used as an indicator of the patient's general condition and state of hydration. A rapid elevation of serum urea (before any rise in corresponding creatinine levels) is often an indication that the patient is progressing into a prerenal state.

In the hospital situation, when the condition is detected incidentally, the cause(s) of the condition, such as fluid depletion, infection or the use of nephrotoxic drugs, are often apparent on close examination of the clinical history. In some patients, however, or in those discovered outside hospital practice, more extensive investigation is required to determine the cause. Although the majority of patients have ATN, other rare causes such as rapidly progressive glomerulonephritis, acute nephritis or urinary tract obstruction must be excluded. Specific longer-term treatment for the underlying cause may be required.

Possible steps in the investigation of ARF are outlined in Figure 15.3

Various other parameters should be monitored through the course of ARF. Fluid balance charts are frequently used, but are often inaccurate and should not be relied upon exclusively. Records of daily weight are more reliable, but are dependent on the mobility of the patient.

Central venous pressure (CVP) is one of a number of haemodynamic measurements that can be made following insertion of a central venous catheter, and is a measure of the pressure in the large systemic veins and the right atrium produced by venous return. Although the insertion of a central catheter carries the risks of any invasive procedure, CVP provides the best assessment of circulating volume and therefore the degree of fluid deficit, and reduces the risk of pulmonary oedema following over-rapid transfusion.

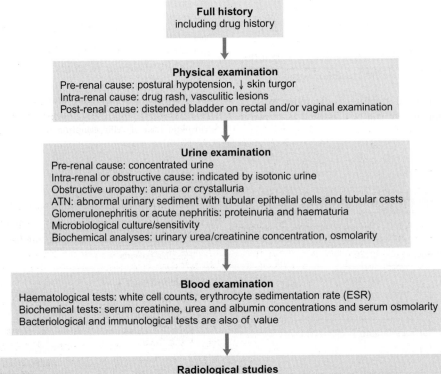

Full history
including drug history

Physical examination
Pre-renal cause: postural hypotension, ↓ skin turgor
Intra-renal cause: drug rash, vasculitic lesions
Post-renal cause: distended bladder on rectal and/or vaginal examination

Urine examination
Pre-renal cause: concentrated urine
Intra-renal or obstructive cause: indicated by isotonic urine
Obstructive uropathy: anuria or crystalluria
ATN: abnormal urinary sediment with tubular epithelial cells and tubular casts
Glomerulonephritis or acute nephritis: proteinuria and haematuria
Microbiological culture/sensitivity
Biochemical analyses: urinary urea/creatinine concentration, osmolarity

Blood examination
Haematological tests: white cell counts, erythrocyte sedimentation rate (ESR)
Biochemical tests: serum creatinine, urea and albumin concentrations and serum osmolarity
Bacteriological and immunological tests are also of value

Radiological studies
Plain abdominal radiography, renal arteriography and venography, ultrasonography and biopsy may be performed

Figure 15.3 Investigations and possible causes in acute renal failure.

CVP should usually be maintained within the normal range of 5–12 cm H_2O.

Serum electrolytes including potassium, bicarbonate, calcium, phosphate and acid–base balance should similarly be monitored.

Course and prognosis

The course of ARF caused by ATN may be divided into three phases. The first is the oliguric phase in which uraemia and hyperkalaemia occur inevitably unless adequate management is initiated. The oliguric phase is usually no longer than 7–14 days but may last for 6 weeks. If death does not ensue the patient with ARF will enter the diuretic phase, which is characterized by a urine output that rises over a few days to several litres per day. The diuretic phase lasts for up to 7 days and corresponds to the recommencement of tubular function. Patients who survive into this phase have a relatively good prognosis and progress to the recovery phase. Recovery of renal function where tubule cells regenerate takes place slowly over the following months, although the GFR rarely returns completely to its initial level. The elderly recover renal function more slowly and less completely.

The mortality rate of ARF varies accordingly to the cause but is typically 10–15% for an isolated episode (Dishart & Kellum 2000). Mortality rates are much higher when ARF is complicated by other factors such as multiple organ dysfunction and may be in the range 50–90%. High mortality rates are more common in patients aged over 60 years.

Death resulting from uraemia and hyperkalaemia is now less common. Consequently, the major causes of death associated with ARF are septicaemia and, to a lesser extent, gastrointestinal haemorrhage. High circulating levels of uraemic toxins that occur in ARF result in general debility. These, together with the significant number of invasive procedures such as bladder catheterization and intravascular cannulation which are necessary in the management of ARF, render such patients prone to infection and septicaemia. Uraemic gastrointestinal haemorrhage is a recognized consequence of ARF, probably as a result of reduced mucosal cell turnover.

Management

The aim of the medical management of a patient with ARF is to prolong life in order to allow recovery, either partial or complete, of kidney function. Effective management of ARF depends upon rapid diagnosis. If the underlying acute deterioration in renal function is detected early enough, it is often possible to prevent progression. If the condition is advanced, however, management consists of mainly preventive and supportive strategies, with close monitoring and appropriate correction of metabolic, fluid and electrolyte disturbances. Specific therapies that promote recovery of ischaemic renal damage remain under investigation.

Early preventive and supportive strategies

Initial treatment should include rapid correction of fluid and electrolyte balance. A diagnosis of acute deterioration of renal function caused by renal underperfusion implies that restoration of renal perfusion would reverse impairment by improving renal blood flow, reducing renal vasoconstriction and flushing nephrotoxins from the kidney. Sodium chloride 0.9% is an appropriate choice of intravenous fluid since it replaces both water and sodium ions in a concentration approximately equal to serum. The effect of fluid replacement on urine flow and, whenever possible, CVP should be carefully monitored. However, fluid loading with 1–1.5 l saline at < 0.5 l/h is unlikely to cause harm in most patients who do not show signs of fluid overload.

If the kidneys do not respond to fluid replacement therapy, other measures taken have included:

- loop diuretics
- mannitol
- dopamine
- atrial natriuretic peptide analogues
- adenosine antagonists
- calcium channel blockers.

The conversion of oliguria or anuria to non-oliguric ARF indicates fluid overload and electrolyte disturbances are likely to be at least partially reversed. It is unclear, however, whether survival is improved.

Loop diuretics

In addition to producing a substantial diuresis, loop diuretics reduce renal tubular cell metabolic demands and increase renal blood flow by stimulating the release of renal prostaglandins, a haemodynamic effect inhibited by NSAIDs. It is thought the use of loop diuretics may thereby help salvage renal tissue. The associated increased urine flow will also reduce the likelihood of intrarenal obstruction.

Diuretic therapy should only be initiated after the circulating volume has been restored. If not, any diuresis might produce a negative fluid balance and precipitate or exacerbate a prerenal state.

Doses up to 1–2 g of furosemide (frusemide) in 24 hours can be given by continuous intravenous infusion at a rate of not more than 4 mg/min. Higher infusion rates may cause transient deafness. The use of continuous infusions of loop diuretics has been shown to produce a more effective diuresis with a lower incidence of side-effects than seen with bolus administration. Bolus doses of loop diuretics may induce renal vasoconstriction and be detrimental to function.

The addition of small oral doses of metolazone may also be considered. Metolazone is a weak thiazide diuretic alone but produces a synergistic action with loop diuretics.

Mannitol

The rationale for using mannitol in ARF arises from the concept that tubular debris may contribute to oliguria. The tubular debris causes mechanical intrarenal obstruction and the use of an osmotic diuretic will wash it out. A dose of 0.5–1.0 g/kg as a 10–20% infusion has therefore been recommended. However, intravenous mannitol will, before producing a diuresis, cause a considerable increase in the extracellular fluid volume by drawing water from the intracellular compartment. This expansion of the intravascular volume is potentially dangerous for patients with cardiac failure, especially if a diuresis is not produced. It is also possible that mannitol exacerbates renal medullary hypoxia (i.e. the partial pressure of oxygen (Po_2) is further reduced in the renal medulla) since increased glomerular filtration raises medullary oxygen consumption; these effects might also offset any positive benefits of mannitol in ARF. The evidence for mannitol producing benefit in ARF over and above aggressive hydration is not clear. Consequently, mannitol is now less widely used.

Dopamine

Dopamine (DA) at low doses (e.g. 1–3 micrograms/kg/min) has a direct vasodilator effect in the kidney mediated by DA_1-receptors. At slightly higher doses (e.g. 4–10 micrograms/kg/min) inotropic effects on the heart produce an increase in cardiac output by an action on β_1-receptors. These effects might increase renal perfusion and thus improve urine output. Dopamine might also exert a diuretic and natriuretic action by DA_1-receptors mediated inhibition of sodium-potassium ATPase within the tubular epithelium. However, at higher doses still (e.g. >10 micrograms/kg/min) dopamine also acts on α_1-receptors and β_1 receptor mediated renin release causing peripheral and renal vasoconstriction, resulting in impairment of renal perfusion. Consequently, an initial dose of 2 micrograms/kg/min increasing to a maximum of 10 micrograms/kg/min with careful monitoring of CVP is often employed in an attempt to selectively improve ARF. However, the clinical response to dopamine can vary markedly between patients and conditions. Firm evidence for the use of dopamine in the treatment or prevention of ATN is lacking and some studies have indicated dopamine is of little benefit (ANZICS 2000). Consequently, alternatives should be considered carefully, as the vasoconstrictor effects of dopamine could be detrimental in ARF.

Dobutamine does not produce renal vasodilation but may occasionally be added at an initial dose of 2.5 micrograms/kg/min for its inotropic effects. Dopexamine has also been used as it produces both a positive inotropic effect via its action on β_2 receptors in the heart and an increase in renal perfusion via its effect on peripheral dopamine receptors; it is reported not to induce vasoconstriction.

Other drug therapies

Atrial natriuretic peptide is secreted by cardiac atria and produces dilation of preglomerular arterioles and constriction of postglomerular arterioles. The result is an increase in GFR independent of renal blood flow. A related peptide (ularitide) is secreted from renal tubule cells and produces similar effects but with less systemic hypotension. Despite the potential benefits of these peptides in improving renal function, further evidence is required to determine their place in the treatment of ARF.

Blockade of adenosine receptors using theophylline might be of value in some types of ATN and this is being investigated.

Calcium channel blockers of all classes dilate preglomerular arterioles and also induce a natriuresis. These agents also appear to block processes associated with cell injury such as intracellular Ca^{2+} influx and angiotensin-induced cytokine production. The use of calcium channel blockade has therefore been proposed in ARF, but as yet evidence has only been partially confirmed in renal transplant patients.

Drug therapy and renal autoregulation

Intrarenal blood flow is controlled by an autoregulatory mechanism unique to the kidney called tubuloglomerular feedback (TGF). This mechanism produces arteriolar constriction in response to an increased solute load to the distal nephrons. GFR and kidney workload are thus reduced. It has been proposed that oliguria is an adaptive response to renal ischaemia and therapy geared to improve GFR that increases solute load on the nephrons might increase kidney workload and worsen ARF. Clearly, reversal of a prerenal state with fluids is a logical therapeutic manoeuvre. However, care should be exercised in the choice of therapy in intrarenal ARF to avoid detrimental effects on the kidney.

Non-dialysis treatment of established acute renal failure

Uraemia and intravascular volume overload

In renal failure, the symptoms of ureaemia include nausea, vomiting and anorexia, and result principally from accumulation of toxic products of protein metabolism such as urea. It is often possible to reduce these symptoms by restricting protein intake to about 0.6 g/kg body weight per day. However, care should be taken to ensure the diet provides all the essential amino acids and sufficient nutrition to prevent protein catabolism. A higher intake of protein, by exceeding the body's basic requirements, permits its use as an energy source, resulting in increases in blood urea concentration; further reduction in protein intake brings about endogenous protein catabolism and again causes the blood urea concentration to increase. Fat and carbohydrate should also be given to maintain a high energy intake of about 2000–3000 kcal, or more in hypercatabolic patients, to prevent protein catabolism and promote anabolism. It should be noted, however, that excessive amounts of carbohydrate could increase production of carbon dioxide and induce respiratory acidosis in these patients.

Unfortunately, since uraemia causes anorexia, nausea and vomiting, many severely ill patients are unable to tolerate any kind of diet. In these patients and those who are catabolic, the use of enteral or parenteral nutrition should be considered at an early stage.

Intravascular fluid overload must be managed by restricting NaCl intake to about 1–2 g/day if the patient is not hyponatraemic and total fluid intake to less than 500 ml/day plus the volume of urine and/or loss from dialysis. Care should be taken with so-called 'low salt' products, as these usually contain KCl, which will exacerbate hyperkalaemia.

Hyperkalaemia

This is a particular problem in ARF, not only because urinary excretion is reduced but also because intracellular potassium may be released. Rapid rises in extracellular potassium are to be expected when there is tissue damage, as in burns, crush injuries and sepsis. Acidosis also aggravates hyperkalaemia by provoking potassium leakage from healthy cells. The condition may be life-threatening by causing cardiac arrhythmias and, if untreated, can result in asystolic cardiac arrest.

Dietary potassium should be restricted to less than 40 mmol/day and potassium supplements and potassium-sparing diuretics removed from the treatment schedule. Emergency treatment is necessary if the serum potassium level reaches 7.0 mmol/l (normal range 3.5–5.0 mmol/l) or if there are the progressive changes in the electrocardiogram (ECG) associated with hyperkalaemia. These include tall, peaked T waves, reduced P waves with increased QRS complexes or the 'sine wave' appearance that often presages cardiac arrest.

Emergency treatment of hyperkalaemia consists of the following:

1. 10–30 ml (2.25–6.75 mmol) of calcium gluconate 10% intravenously over 5–10 minutes; this improves myocardial stability but has no effect on the serum potassium levels. The effect is short lived, but the dose can be repeated.
2. 50 ml of 50% glucose together with 10–20 units of soluble insulin. Endogenous insulin, stimulated by a glucose load or administered intravenously, stimulates intracellular potassium uptake, thus removing it from the serum. The effect lasts for 2–3 hours.
3. Calcium polystyrene sulphonate (calcium resonium) 15–30 g two to four times a day, either orally or by enema. This ion exchange resin binds potassium in the gastrointestinal tract, releasing calcium in exchange. Rectal administration will reduce potassium over a period of 2–6 hours, while oral administration is most effective at 10–12 hours.

Ion exchange resins will not produce dramatic reductions in serum potassium alone when the starting level is dangerously high. Rather they are used as a method of sustaining potassium reduction because the effect of glucose/insulin is only temporary. Both the oral and rectal routes of administration have disadvantages. Administration of large doses by mouth may result in faecal impaction. The oral dose can be mixed with lactulose in an attempt to prevent constipation. The manufacturers recommend that an enema should be retained for 9 hours; this is not usually a problem, rather the reverse. Constipation resulting from the use of resins may necessitate the use of laxatives.

Acidosis

The inability of the kidney to excrete hydrogen ions may result in a metabolic acidosis. This in itself is not usually a serious problem although it may contribute to hyperkalaemia. It may be treated orally with sodium bicarbonate 1–6 g/day in divided doses, or 50–100 mmol of bicarbonate ions (50–100 ml of sodium bicarbonate 8.4%) intravenously may be used. If calcium gluconate is being used to treat hyperkalaemia, care should be taken not to mix it with the sodium bicarbonate as the resulting calcium bicarbonate forms an insoluble precipitate. If elevations in serum sodium preclude the use of sodium bicarbonate, extreme acidosis (serum bicarbonate of less than 10 mmol/l) is best treated by dialysis.

Hypocalcaemia

Calcium malabsorption, probably secondary to disordered vitamin D metabolism, often occurs in ARF. Hypocalcaemia usually remains asymptomatic, as tetany of skeletal muscles or convulsions do not normally occur until serum concentrations are as low as 1.6–1.7 mmol/l (normal 2.20–2.55 mmol/l). Should it become necessary, oral calcium supplementation with calcium gluconate or lactate is usually adequate, and although vitamin D may be used to treat the hypocalcaemia of ARF, it rarely has to be added. Effervescent calcium tablets should be avoided as they invariably contain a high sodium or potassium load.

Hyperphosphataemia

As phosphate is normally excreted by the kidney, hyperphosphataemia may occur in ARF but rarely requires treatment. Should it become necessary to treat, phosphate-binding agents may be used to retain phosphate ions in the gut. The most common agents are calcium carbonate with glycine tablets (Titralac) or aluminium hydroxide in the form of mixture or capsules (Aludrox).

Infection

Patients with ARF are prone to infection and septicaemia, which can ultimately cause death. Bladder catheters, central catheters and even peripheral intravenous lines should be used with care to reduce the chance of bacterial invasion. Leucocytosis is sometimes seen in ARF and does not necessarily imply infection; but any unexplained pyrexia must be immediately treated with appropriate antibiotic therapy, especially if accompanied by toxic symptoms such as disorientation or hypotensive episodes. Samples from blood, urine and any other material such as catheter tips should be sent for culture before antibiotics are started and therapy should cover as wide a spectrum as possible until a causative organism is identified.

Other problems

Uraemic gastrointestinal erosions. These are a recognized consequence of ARF, probably as a result of reduced mucosal cell turnover owing to high circulating levels of uraemic toxins. H_2 receptor antagonists are effective and it is unlikely that any one is more advantageous than another.

Muscle cramps. These are common in patients with renal failure, probably as a result of electrolyte imbalances. Patients are generally prescribed quinine salts 200–300 mg at night. The efficacy of quinine has been questioned since few comparative trials have been performed. Fortunately, at the doses used in the management of muscle cramps, toxicity is not a problem. Alternatives that have been suggested for the treatment of cramps include benzodiazepines such as clonazepam (0.5–1 mg at night) or calcium channel blockers such as verapamil (120 mg at night).

Nutrition

There are two major constraints concerning the nutrition of patients with ARF:

- patients are frequently anorexic, vomiting and too ill to eat
- oliguria associated with renal failure limits the volume of enteral or parenteral nutrition that can be given safely.

The introduction of dialysis or haemofiltration allows fluid to be removed easily and therefore makes parenteral nutrition possible. Large volumes of fluid may be administered without producing fluid overload. Factors that should be considered when formulating a parenteral nutrition regimen include fluid balance, calorie/protein requirements, electrolyte balance/requirements, and vitamin and mineral requirements.

The basic calorie requirements are similar to those in a non-dialysed patient, although the need for protein may occasionally be increased in haemodialysis and haemofiltration because of amino acid loss. A similar loss may also occur in patients undergoing peritoneal dialysis. In all situations protein is usually supplied as 12–20 g/day of an essential amino acid formulation, although individual requirements may vary. Similarly, although lipid emulsions may theoretically reduce the efficiency of haemofiltration by blocking the filter, in practice their use does not have any noticeable effect. It is useful, however, to infuse parenteral nutrition solutions into blood as it is returned to the body after haemofiltration or haemodialysis, thereby ensuring that it is available to the patient before being presented to the filter.

Electrolyte-free amino acid solutions should be used in parenteral nutrition formulations for patients with ARF as they allow the addition of electrolytes as appropriate. Potassium and sodium requirements can be calculated on an individual basis depending on serum levels. There is usually no need to try to normalize serum calcium and phosphate levels as they will stabilize with the appropriate therapy, or, if necessary, with haemofiltration or dialysis. Water-soluble vitamins are removed by dialysis and haemofiltration but the standard daily doses normally included in parenteral nutrition fluids more than compensate for this. Magnesium and zinc supplementation may be required, not only because tissue repair often increases requirements but also because they may be lost during dialysis or haemofiltration.

It is necessary to monitor the serum urea, creatinine and electrolyte levels daily in order to make the appropriate alterations in the nutritional support. The glucose concentration should also be checked at least every 6 hours as patients in renal failure sometimes develop insulin resistance. The plasma pH should be checked initially to see whether the addition of amino acid solutions is causing or aggravating metabolic acidosis. It is also valuable to check calcium, phosphate and albumin levels regularly, and when practical, daily weighing gives a useful guide to fluid balance.

Renal replacement therapy

Renal replacement therapy is indicated in a patient with ARF when kidney function is so poor that life is at risk. However, it is desirable to introduce renal replacement therapy early in ARF, as complications and mortality are reduced if the serum urea level is kept below 35 mmol/l. Generally, replacement therapy is used in ARF to:

1. remove toxins when severe symptoms are apparent (e.g. impaired consciousness, seizures, pericarditis)
2. remove fluid resistant to diuretics (e.g. pulmonary oedema), to facilitate parenteral nutrition
3. correct electrolyte and acid–base imbalances, e.g. hyperkalaemia > 6.5 mmol/l or 5.5–6.5 where there are ECG changes, increasing acidosis (pH < 7.1 or serum bicarbonate < 10 mmol/l) despite bicarbonate therapy, or where bicarbonate is not tolerated because of fluid overload
4. control the effects of sepsis (e.g. to reduce temperature).

Forms of renal replacement therapy

The common types of renal replacement therapy used in clinical practice are:

- haemodialysis
- peritoneal dialysis
- haemofiltration
- haemodiafiltration.

Although the basic principles of these replacement therapies are similar, clearance rates, i.e. extent of solute removal, vary.

In all types of renal replacement therapy blood is presented to a dialysis solution across some form of semi-permeable membrane that allows free movement of low molecular weight compounds. The processes by which movement of substances occur are:

- *Diffusion.* Diffusion depends upon concentration differences between blood and dialysate and molecule size. Water and low molecular weight solutes (up to a molecular weight of about 5000) move through pores in the semi-permeable membrane to establish equilibrium. Smaller molecules can be cleared from blood more effectively as they move more easily through pores in the membrane.
- *Ultrafiltration.* A pressure gradient (either +ve or –ve) across a semi-permeable membrane will produce a net directional movement of fluid from relative high to low pressure regions. The quantity of fluid dialysed is the ultrafiltration volume.
- *Convection.* Any molecule carried by ultrafiltrate may move passively with the flow by convection. Larger molecules are cleared more effectively by convection.

Haemodialysis

In haemodialysis, blood is heparinized and diverted out of a large central venous cannula line and actively pumped through the lumen of an artificial kidney (dialyser) returning to the patient by a venous line (Fig. 15.4). In those at high risk of haemorrhage when heparinized, such as post-surgical patients, epoprostenol (prostacyclin), a prostaglandin with a short plasma half-life of 2–3 minutes that inhibits platelet aggregation, may be used to prevent extracorporeal clotting.

The dialyser consists of a cartridge comprised of either a bundle of hollow tubes (hollow fibre dialyser) or a series of parallel flat plates (flat-plate dialyser) made of a synthetic semi-permeable membrane. Dialysis fluid is perfused around the membrane in a countercurrent to the flow of blood in order to maximize diffusion gradients. The dialysis solution is essentially a mixture of electrolytes in water with a composition approximating to

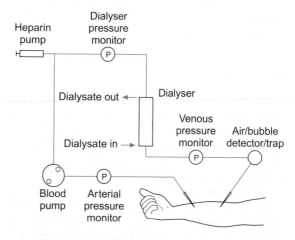

Figure 15.4   Typical haemodialysis circuit.

extracellular fluid into which solutes diffuse. The ionic concentration of the dialysis fluid can be manipulated to control the rate and extent of electrolyte transfer. Calcium and bicarbonate concentrations can also be increased in dialysis fluid to promote diffusion into blood as replacement therapy. By manipulating the hydrostatic pressure of the dialysate and blood circuits, the extent and rate of water removal by ultrafiltration can be controlled.

Haemodialysis can be performed in either intermittent or continuous schedules. The latter regimen is preferable in the critical care situation, providing 24-hour control, minimizing swings in blood volume and electrolyte composition that are found using intermittent regimens.

The capital cost of haemodialysis is considerable, requires specially trained staff, and is seldom undertaken outside a renal unit. It does, however, treat renal failure rapidly and is therefore essential in hypercatabolic renal failure where urea is produced faster than, for example, peritoneal dialysis could remove it. Haemodialysis can also be used in patients who have recently undergone abdominal surgery in whom peritoneal dialysis would be ill advised.

Peritoneal dialysis

A semi-rigid catheter is inserted into the abdominal cavity. Warmed sterile peritoneal dialysis fluid (typically 1–2 litres) is instilled into the abdomen, left for a period of about 30 minutes (dwell time) and then drained into a collecting bag (Fig. 15.5). This procedure may be performed manually or by semiautomatic equipment. The process may be repeated up to 20 times a day, depending on the condition of the patient.

Peritoneal dialysis is relatively cheap and simple, does not require specially trained staff nor the facilities of a renal unit. It does, however, have the disadvantages of being uncomfortable and tiring for the patient, producing a high incidence of peritonitis and permitting protein loss, as albumin crosses the peritoneal membrane.

Haemofiltration

Haemofiltration is an alternative technique to dialysis whose simplicity of use, fine control of fluid balance and low cost have ensured its widespread use in the treatment of ARF.

A similar arrangement to haemodialysis is employed but dialysis fluid is not used. The hydrostatic pressure of the blood drives a filtrate similar to interstitial fluid across a high permeability dialyser (passes substances of molecular weight up to 30 000) by ultrafiltration. Solute clearance occurs by convection. Commercially prepared haemofiltration fluid may then be introduced into the filtered blood in quantities sufficient to maintain optimal fluid balance. As with haemodialysis, haemofiltration can be intermittent or continuous. In continuous arteriovenous haemofiltration (CAVH), blood is diverted, usually from the femoral artery, and returned to the femoral vein. In continuous venovenous haemofiltration (CVVH), blood is taken from a vein, usually the femoral, jugular or subclavian, and returned via a double linear catheter, the process being assisted by a blood pump. In slow continuous ultrafiltration (SCU or SCUF) the process is performed so slowly that no fluid substitution is necessary. In addition to avoiding the expense and complexity of haemodialysis, this system enables continuous but gradual removal of fluid, thereby allowing very fine control of fluid balance in addition to electrolyte control and removal of metabolites. This control of fluid balance often facilitates the use of parenteral nutrition. Because of the advantages of haemofiltration over peritoneal dialysis and haemodialysis, continuous haemofiltration is now generally agreed to be the most appropriate form of dialysis in the majority of patients with ARF.

Haemodiafiltration

Haemodiafiltration is a technique that combines the ability to clear small molecules, as in haemodialysis, with the large molecule clearance of haemofiltration. It is, however, more expensive than traditional haemodialysis.

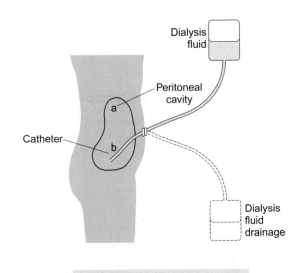

1. Connect bag to catheter
2. Drain dialysis fluid into abdomen
3. Dwell time
4. Drain fluid out
   a. perirotoneal cavity
   b. catheter

Figure 15.5 Procedure for peritoneal dialysis.

Drug dosage in renal replacement therapy

Whether a drug is significantly removed by dialysis or haemofiltration is an important clinical problem. Drugs that are not removed may well require dose reduction to avoid accumulation and minimize toxic effects. Alternatively, drug removal may be significant and require a dosage supplement to ensure an adequate therapeutic effect is maintained. In general, since haemodialysis, peritoneal dialysis and haemofiltration depend on filtration, the process of drug removal can be considered analoguous to glomerular filtration. Table 15.5 gives an indication of approximate clearances of common renal replacement therapies, which for continuous regimens provide an estimate for the creatinine clearance of the system.

Drug characteristics that favour clearance by the glomerulus are similar to those that favour clearance by dialysis or haemofiltration. These include:

- low molecular weight
- high water solubility
- low protein binding
- small volume of distribution
- low metabolic clearance.

Unfortunately, a number of other factors inherent in the dialysis process affect clearance; they include:

- duration of dialysis procedure
- rate of blood flow to dialyser
- surface area and porosity of dialyser
- composition and flow rate of dialysate

For peritoneal dialysis other factors come into play and include:

- rate of peritoneal exchange
- concentration gradient between plasma and dialysate.

In view of the above, it is usually possible to predict whether a drug will be removed by dialysis, but it is very difficult to quantify the process except by direct measurement, which is rarely practical. Consequently, a definitive, comprehensive guide to drug dosage in dialysis does not exist. However, limited data for specific drugs are available in the literature, while many drug manufacturers have information on the dialysability of their products and some now even include dosage recommendations in their summaries of product characteristics. The most practical method for treating patients undergoing dialysis is to assemble appropriate dosage guidelines for a range of drugs likely to be used in patients with renal impairment and attempt to restrict use to these.

Because drug clearance by haemofiltration is more predictable than in dialysis, it is possible that standardized guidelines on drug elimination may become available. In the interim, a set of individual drug dosage guidelines similar to those described above would be useful in practice.

Factors affecting drug use

How the drug to be used is absorbed, distributed, metabolized and excreted, and whether it is intrinsically nephrotoxic are all factors that must be considered. The pharmacokinetic behavior of many drugs may be altered in renal failure.

Absorption

Oral absorption in ARF may be reduced by vomiting or diarrhoea, although this is frequently of limited clinical significance.

Metabolism

The main hepatic pathways of drug metabolism appear unaffected in renal impairment. The kidney is also a site of metabolism in the body, but the effect of renal impairment is clinically important in only two situations. The first involves the conversion of 25-hydroxycholecalciferol to 1,25-dihydroxycholecalciferol (the active form of vitamin D) in the kidney, a process that is impaired in renal failure. Patients in ARF occasionally require vitamin D replacement therapy, and this should be in the form of 1α-hydroxycholecalciferol (alfacalcidol) or 1,25-dihydroxycholecalciferol (calcitriol). The latter is the drug of choice in the presence of concomitant hepatic impairment. The second situation involves the metabolism of insulin. The kidney is the major site of insulin metabolism, and the insulin requirements of diabetic patients in ARF are often reduced.

Distribution

Changes in drug distribution may be altered by fluctuations in the degree of hydration or by alterations in tissue or serum protein binding. The presence of oedema or ascites increases the volume of distribution

Table 15.5 Approximate clearances of common renal replacement therapies

Renal replacement therapy	Clearance rate (ml/min)
Intermittent haemodialysis	150–200
Intermittent haemofiltration	100–150
Acute intermittent peritoneal dialysis	10–20
Continuous haemofiltration	5–15

while dehydration reduces it. In practice these changes will only be significant if the volume of distribution of the drug is small, i.e. less than 50 litres. Serum protein binding may be reduced owing to either protein loss or alteration in binding caused by uraemia. For certain highly bound drugs the net result of reduced protein binding is an increase in free drug, and care is therefore required when interpreting serum concentrations. Most analyses measure the total serum concentration, i.e. free plus bound drug. A drug level may therefore fall within the accepted concentration range but still result in toxicity because of the increased proportion of free drug. However, this is usually only a temporary effect. Since the unbound drug is now available for elimination, its concentration will eventually return to the original value, albeit with a lower total bound and unbound level. The total drug concentration may therefore fall below the therapeutic range while therapeutic effectiveness is maintained. It must be noted that the time required for the new equilibrium to be established is about four of five elimination half-lives of the drug, and this may be altered itself in renal failure. Some drugs that show reduced serum protein binding include diazepam, morphine, phenytoin, levothyroxine (thyroxine), theophylline and warfarin. Tissue binding may also be affected, for example the displacement of digoxin from skeletal muscle binding sites by metabolic waste products that accumulate in renal failure result in a significant reduction in digoxin's volume of distribution.

Excretion

Alteration in renal clearance of drugs in renal impairment is the most important parameter to consider when considering dosage. Generally, a fall in renal drug clearance indicates a decline in the number of functioning nephrons. The GFR, of which creatinine clearance is an approximation, can be used as an estimate of the number of functioning nephrons. Thus, a 50% reduction in the GFR will suggest a 50% decline in renal clearance.

Renal impairment therefore often necessitates drug dosage adjustments. Loading doses of renally excreted drugs are often necessary in renal failure because of the prolonged elimination half-life leading to an increased time to reach steady state. The equation for a loading dose is the same in renal disease as in normal patients, thus:

$$\text{loading dose (mg)} = \text{target concentration (mg/l)} \times \text{volume of distribution (l)}$$

The volume of distribution may be altered but generally remains unchanged.

It is possible to derive other formulae for dosage adjustment in renal impairment. One of the most useful is:

$$DR_{rf} = DR_n \times [(1-F_{eu}) + (F_{eu} \times RF)]$$

where DR_{rf} is the dosing rate in renal failure, DR_n is the normal dosing rate, RF is the extent of renal impairment = patient's creatinine clearance (ml/min)/ideal creatinine clearance (120 ml/min) and F_{eu} is the fraction of drug normally excreted unchanged in the urine. For example, when RF = 0.2 and F_{eu} = 0.5, 60% of the normal dosing rate should be given.

An alteration in dosing rate can be achieved by either altering the dose itself or the dosage interval, or a combination of both as appropriate. Unfortunately it is not always possible to obtain the fraction of drug excreted unchanged in the urine. In practice, it is simpler to use the guidelines for prescribing in renal impairment found in the British National Formularly. These are adequate for most cases, although the specialist may need to refer to other texts.

Nephrotoxicity

The list of potentially nephrotoxic drugs is long. Although the commonest serious forms of renal damage are interstitial nephritis and glomerulonephritis, the majority of drugs cause damage by hypersensitivity reactions and are safe in many patients. Some drugs, however, are directly nephrotoxic, and their effects on the kidney are more predictable. Such drugs include aminoglycosides, amphotericin, colistin, the polymixins and ciclosporin. The use of any drug with recognized nephrotoxic potential should be avoided where possible. This is particularly true in patients with pre-existing renal impairement or renal failure. Figure 15.6 summarizes the most important and common adverse effects of drugs on renal function, indicating the likely regions of the nephron in which damage occurs. Additional information on adverse effects can be found in Hems (2001).

Inevitably, occasions will arise when the use of potentially nephrotoxic drugs become necessary, and on these occasions constant monitoring of renal function is essential. In conclusion, when selecting a drug for a patient with renal failure, an agent should be chosen that approaches the ideal characteristics listed in Table 15.6.

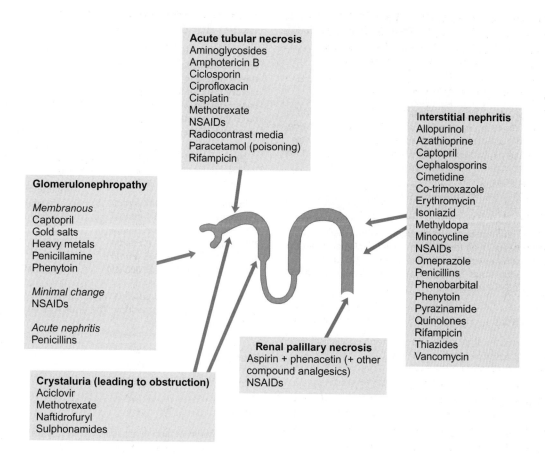

Acute tubular necrosis
Aminoglycosides
Amphotericin B
Ciclosporin
Ciprofloxacin
Cisplatin
Methotrexate
NSAIDs
Radiocontrast media
Paracetamol (poisoning)
Rifampicin

Interstitial nephritis
Allopurinol
Azathioprine
Captopril
Cephalosporins
Cimetidine
Co-trimoxazole
Erythromycin
Isoniazid
Methyldopa
Minocycline
NSAIDs
Omeprazole
Penicillins
Phenobarbital
Phenytoin
Pyrazinamide
Quinolones
Rifampicin
Thiazides
Vancomycin

Glomerulonephropathy

Membranous
Captopril
Gold salts
Heavy metals
Penicillamine
Phenytoin

Minimal change
NSAIDs

Acute nephritis
Penicillins

Renal palillary necrosis
Aspirin + phenacetin (+ other compound analgesics)
NSAIDs

Crystaluria (leading to obstruction)
Aciclovir
Methotrexate
Naftidrofuryl
Sulphonamides

Figure 15.6   Common adverse effects of drugs on the kidney. The likely sites of damage to the nephron (stylized) are indicated.

Table 15.6   Characteristics of the ideal drug for use in a patient with renal failure

No active metabolites

Disposition unaffected by fluid balance changes

Disposition unaffected by protein binding changes

Response unaffected by altered tissue sensitivity

Wide therapeutic margin

Not nephrotoxic

CASE STUDIES

Case 15.1

Mrs J. a 60-year-old widow, had long-standing hypertension that was unsatisfactorily controlled on a variety of agents. Her drug therapy included furosemide (frusemide) 40 mg once a day, verapamil SR 240 mg twice daily and a salt restricted diet. Following a routine review of her therapy, losartan 50 mg once daily was added to her treatment regimen in an attempt to improve blood pressure control.

The following day Mrs J. noticed that she did not produce as much urine as usual and her ankles had started to swell. Later that evening she presented to her local hospital accident and emergency unit, where her blood pressure was found to be 100/60 mmHg and serum biochemistry revealed creatinine levels of 225 μmol/l (50–120 μmol/l, Na$^+$ 125 mmol/l (135–145 mmol/l) and K$^+$ 5.2 mmol/l (3.5–5.0 mmol/l).

Questions

1. What was the likely cause and underlying mechanism to this patients's problem?
2. What treatment should be given?

Answers

1. Angiotensin II receptor antagonists can precipitate renal failure under a variety of circumstances in a similar manner to ACE inhibitors. This generally occurs following blockade of angiotensin II mediated vasoconstriction of the efferent arterioles that contributes to the high-pressure gradient across the glomerulus necessary for filtration. It is not usually a problem in the majority of individuals; however, in patients with pre-existing compromised renal blood flow, such as renal artery stenoses, the kidney relies more heavily on angiotensin mediated vasoconstriction of the preglomerular arterioles to maintain renal function. Hypovolaemia caused, for example, by diuretic use would tend to exacerbate this problem. Moreover, it is likely that sodium depletion would render the kidney even more dependent upon vasoconstriction of efferent arterioles through activation of the tubuloglomerular feedback system, further sensitizing the kidney to the effects of angiotensin antagonists.

   Mrs J. might well have been suffering from incipient renal failure, but remained asymptomatic until her renal reserve diminished.
2. The inappropriate use of an angiotensin II receptor antagonist should be stopped, as should the diuretic temporarily. Mrs J. should be rehydrated using sodium chloride 0.9% and kidney function markers monitored in the hope that recovery will occur.

Case 15.2

Mr B. a known intermittent heroin and cocaine abuser, was discovered comatose in his room early in the morning. He was admitted to hospital as an emergency. An indirect history from an acquaintance indicated that Mr B. had been drinking very heavily prior to the incident (probably more than a bottle of whisky in a 24-hour period) and had smoked both heroin and cocaine of unknown source and purity.

On examination he was found to be dehydrated and serum biochemistry revealed the following:

		Reference range
Sodium	147 mmol/l	(135–145)
Potassium	6.1 mmol/l	(3.5–5.0)
Calcium	1.72 mmol/l	(2.20–2.55)
Phosphate	2.0 mmol/l	(0.9–1.5)
Creatinine	485 μmol/l	(50–120)
Creatinine kinase	120 000 IU/l	(< 200 IU/l)

Urine dipstick reacted positive for blood with no signs of red blood cells on microscopy. The urine was faintly reddish-brown in colour.

Question

What is likely to have occurred and how should it be treated?

Answer

Cocaine, heroin or alcohol abuse sometimes cause muscle damage resulting in rhabdomyolysis. The mechanism is unclear, but includes vasoconstriction, an increase in muscle activity, possibly because of seizures, self-injury, adulterants in the drug (e.g. arsenic, strychnine, amphetamine, phencyclidine, quinine) or compression (associated with long periods of inactivity). ATN may ensue from a direct nephrotoxic effect of the myoglobin released from damaged muscle cells, microprecipitation of myoglobin in renal tubules or a reduction in medullary blood flow. The presence of myoglobin is suggested by the urine dipstick test, which reacts not only to red cells but also to free haemoglobin and myoglobin. Extremely high levels of myoglobinuria may result in urine the colour of Coca-Cola. High serum creatinine kinase levels are indicative of rhabdomyolysis together with the presence of free myoglobin in serum and urine. Serum levels of potassium and phosphate are elevated partly by the effects of incipient renal failure but also through tissue breakdown and intracellular release. Creatinine levels are often higher than expected because of muscle damage.

Treatment should involve fluid replacement with normal saline to reverse dehydration. If an adequate urine output is not achieved, the use of intravenous furosemide (frusemide) may be required to stimulate diuresis. In cases where urine pH is less than 6, administration of intravenous isotonic sodium bicarbonate may be of use, since acidic urine favours myoglobin nephrotoxicity. The patient's ECG should be monitored, because of the risks involved with rapid elevation in serum potassium. Timely, appropriate corrective therapy must be instigated where necessary. In 50–70% of cases with rhabdomyolysis, dialysis is required to support recovery.

Case 15.3

Mr D. is a patient who has been admitted to an intensive care unit with ARF, which developed following a routine cholecystectomy. His electrolyte picture shows the following:

		Reference range
sodium	138 mmol/l	(135–145)
potassium	7.2 mmol/l	(3.5–5.0)
bicarbonate	19 mmol/l	(22–31)
urea	32.1 mmol/l	(3.0–6.5)
creatinine	572 μmol/l	(50–120)
pH	7.28	(7.36–7.44)

The patient was connected to an ECG monitor and the resultant trace indicated absent P waves and a broad QRS complex.

Question

Explain the biochemistry and ECG abnormalities and indicate what therapeutic measures must be implemented?

Answer

Hyperkalaemia is one of the principal problems encountered in patients with renal failure. The increased levels of potassium arise from failure of the excretory pathway and also from intracellular release of potassium. Attention should also be paid to pharmacological or pharmaceutical processes that might lead to potassium elevation (e.g. inappropriate potassium supplements, ACE inhibitors, etc.). The acidosis noted in this patient, which is common in ARF, also aggravates hyperkalaemia by promoting leakage of potassium from cells. A serum potassium level greater than 7.0 mmol/l indicates that emergency treatment is required as the patient risks life-threatening ventricular arrhythmias and asystolic cardiac arrest. If ECG changes are present, as in this case, emergency treatment should be initiated when serum potassium rises above 6.5 mmol/l.

The emergency treatment should include:

1. Stabilization of the myocardium by intravenous administration of 10–30 ml calcium gluconate 10% over 5–10 minutes. The effect is temporary but the dose can be repeated.
2. Intravenous administration of 10–20 units of soluble insulin with 50 ml of 50% glucose to stimulate cellular potassium uptake. The dose may be repeated. The blood glucose should be monitored for at least 6 hours to avoid hypoglycaemia.
3. Intravenous salbutamol 0.5 mg in 100 ml 5% dextrose administered over 15 minutes has been used to stimulate the cellular sodium-potassium ATPase pump and thus drive potassium into cells. This may cause disturbing muscle tremors at the doses required to reduce serum potassium levels.
4. Acidosis may be corrected with an intravenous dose of 50–100 ml of sodium bicarbonate 8.4%. Correction of acidosis stimulates cellular potassium re-uptake. Hypertonic bicarbonate solutions (8.4%) can cause volume expansion and should be used with extreme caution.

REFERENCES

Australian and New Zealand Intensive Care Society Clinical Trials Group (ANZICS) 2000 Low dose dopamine in patients with early renal dysfunction: a placebo-controlled randomized trial. Lancet 356: 2139–2143

Cockcroft D, Gault M 1976 Prediction of creatinine clearance from serum creatinine. Nephron 16: 31–34

Dishart M K, Kellum J A 2000 An evaluation of pharmacological strategies for the prevention and treatment of acute renal failure. Drugs 59: 79–91

Hems S 2001 Renal disorders. In: Lee A. (ed) Adverse drug reactions. Pharmaceutical Press, London

Sanaka M, Takano K, Simakura K et al 1996 Serum albumin for estimating creatinine clearance in the elderly with muscle atrophy. Nephron 73: 137–144

FURTHER READING

Firth J 1999 Acute renal failure. Medicine 27(5): 24–29

Gaskin G 1999 Signs and symptoms of renal disease. Medicine 27(5): 1–4

Gokal R, Mallick N P 1999 Peritoneal dialysis. Lancet 353: 823–827

Mallick N P, Gokal R 1999 Haemodialysis. Lancet 353 737–742

Short A, Cumming A 1999 ABC of intensive care: renal support. British Medical Journal 319: 41–44

Chronic renal failure 16

J. Marriott   S. Smith

KEY POINTS

- The need for renal replacement therapy continues to increase, with attendant resource implications.
- The incidence of chronic renal failure (CRF) increases with age and is greater in some ethnic populations.
- In CRF virtually all body systems are adversely affected.
- Clinical signs and symptoms of CRF include nocturia, oedema, anaemia, electrolyte disturbances, hypertension, bone disease, neurological changes, disordered muscle function and uraemia.
- The aims of treatment are to reverse or arrest the process responsible for CRF and relieve symptoms.
- To prevent further renal damage, adequate control of blood pressure is essential.
- Renal anaemia is almost inevitable when the glomerular filtration rate (GFR) falls below 30 ml/min but can be corrected by epoetin in 90–95% of cases.
- CRF invariably reaches a point at which life can only be sustained by dialysis or transplantation. This may occur soon after presentation or after several years.
- There are traditionally two principal types of dialysis: haemodialysis and peritoneal dialysis. In both, toxic metabolites are transferred from the patient's blood across a semi-permeable membrane to a dialysis solution.
- Renal transplantation remains the treatment of choice for end-stage renal disease. However, up to 50% of patients on dialysis programmes are not fit enough to be put on the transplant list.

Chronic renal failure (CRF) may be defined as a condition characterized by uraemia, anaemia, acidosis, osteodystrophy, neuropathy and general debility frequently accompanied by hypertension, oedema and susceptibility to infection resulting from a significant reduction in the excretory, homeostatic, metabolic and endocrine functions of the kidney that occur over a period of months or years. The symptoms of CRF generally manifest when the glomerular filtration rate (GFR) has fallen to about 15 ml/min.

Chronic renal disease generally progresses through four stages:

1. renal reserve reduction
2. renal insufficiency
3. CRF
4. end-stage renal failure (ESRF).

Reduction in renal reserve

The kidney usually has greater capacity to function than is required under normal conditions. This extra capacity is termed 'renal reserve'. In the early stages of chronic renal disease, damage to the kidney eradicates this reserve. Normal renal function is maintained, but responses to conditions that place additional demands upon the kidney, such as pregnancy or increased dietary protein, cannot adequately be met.

Renal insufficiency

In this stage, toxins such as creatinine and urea that are normally excreted by the kidney begin to accumulate, although electrolyte levels often remain within normal limits as a result of homeostatic adaptations. Compensation will inevitably result in imbalances elsewhere, such as acidaemia, bone disease and changes in hormone levels, for example, parathyroid hormone.

CRF

A progressive decline in renal function produces a wide range of both biochemical and hormonal abnormalities. Symptoms may still be insignificant despite severe disturbance of homeostasis.

ESRF

ESRF is characterized by uraemia and a wide spectrum of gastrointestinal, dermatological and CNS symptoms. Figure 16.1 outlines the range of signs and symptoms associated with CRF/ESRF.

Incidence

Accurate information on the incidence of CRF is difficult to obtain but some data are available from community-based studies and registries of patients entering renal replacement programmes. Recent estimates indicate that in the UK population, CRF occurs in approximately 58 patients per million per year in the 20–49-year-old group,

247

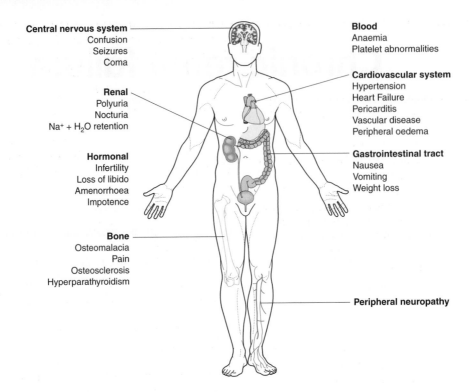

Figure 16.1 Typical signs and symptoms of chronic renal failure.

rising to 588 per million per year in the over 80s. The incidence of CRF in men is at least 1.5 times greater than in women and this difference becomes more pronounced with age. The increasing incidence of CRF with age is attributable to non-immunological causes including vascular disease and undiagnosed prostatic disease in men. There are also racial differences in the incidence of CRF, with treatment required 3–5 times more often in Afro-Caribbean and Asian populations in comparison with comparable white populations. These differences might result from the greater severity of hypertension in Afro-Caribbeans and diabetic nephropathy in Asian groups, but other factors, such as social deprivation may also contribute.

Causes

The reduction in renal function observed in CRF results from damage to the infrastructure of the kidney. It is thought that nephrons are lost as complete units with all functions lost simultaneously. The remaining nephrons cope initially with the increased demand upon them. The patient remains well until so many nephrons are lost that the glomerular filtration rate (GFR) can no longer be maintained despite activation of compensatory mechanisms. As a consequence the GFR progressively

declines. The patient may well remain symptom free until the GFR falls as low as 15–20 ml/min.

CRF arises from a variety of causes (Table 16.1). The difficulty in establishing a diagnosis of CRF increases in patients aged over 65. However, establishing a cause is useful in the identification and elimination of reversible factors, in planning for likely outcomes and treatment

Table 16.1.   Common causes of CRF in dialysis patients in the UK (UK Renal Registry 1999)

Cause of CRF	Approximate % of CRF patients
Diabetes	10
Chronic glomerulonephritis	15
Pyelonephritis and obstructive uropathy	15
Polycystic kidney disease	9
Hypertension	5
Renovascular disease	6
Other	15
Unknown	25

needs, and for appropriate counselling when a genetic basis is established.

Chronic glomerulonephritis

Glomerulonephritis should not be regarded as a single disease as there are many forms, which may be either idiopathic or part of systemic disease. The precise aetiology is unknown but it is thought to be mediated by deposition of immune complexes in the glomerular tuft with subsequent development of an inflammatory response. Responsible antigens include certain strains of streptococci, other infections such as malaria, endogenous antigens from, for example neoplastic lesions, DNA, for example in systemic lupus erythematosus, and certain drugs, including non-steroidal anti-inflammatory agents, gold and penicillamine.

Hypertension

Hypertension is both a common result and a frequent cause of CRF. It may be prevented by adequate treatment, thereby preventing a further decline in renal function.

Chronic pyelonephritis

Chronic pyelonephritis refers to chronic inflammation of the renal parenchyma with scarring of the kidney. It is generally caused by recurrent urine infection, which may be secondary to outflow obstruction or reflux nephropathy.

Metabolic diseases

Diabetes mellitus is the most common metabolic disease that may lead to chronic glomerulonephritis.

Urinary obstruction

Urinary obstruction may develop insidiously and the classical symptoms of oliguria or pain may even be absent. Causes include:

- prostate hypertrophy
- renal calculi
- congenital abnormalities
- vesicoureteric reflux.

Interstitial nephritis

Inflammation of the interstitium of the kidney with secondary involvement of the tubules is often caused by toxins. Drugs such as penicillins, analgesics and diuretics are typical toxins. Interstitial nephritis is more common in those patients aged over 65, possibly because people in this age group are prescribed greater numbers of drugs.

Congenital abnormalities

The principal congenital abnormality encountered is adult polycystic kidney disease. This is an autosomal dominant inherited condition which results in the formation of multiple cysts in both kidneys throughout life. The kidneys becomes enlarged and frequently fail in middle age.

Diagnosis, investigations and monitoring

The diagnosis may be suspected because of signs and symptoms of renal disease. More often CRF is discovered during investigation of other medical problems or following routine screening.

Family, drug and social histories are all important in elucidating the causes of renal failure, since genetics or exposure to toxins, including prescription, over-the-counter and herbal drugs, might be implicated.

The history of CRF often includes a long period of polyuria (excessive urine production), usually with nocturia (waking at night to pass urine). The symptoms of uraemia are usually non-specific and include lethargy, breathlessness, anorexia and nausea. When these symptoms occur they are often exacerbated by anaemia resulting from a reduction in erythropoetin production. Other typical symptoms include an excruciating itch, poor sleep patterns, lack of concentration and 'restless legs', that may be particularly troublesome at night. Patients may also present with pigmented skin or hypertension.

Functional assessment of the kidney may be performed by testing serum and urine. The serum creatinine level is a more reliable indicator of renal function than the serum urea level though both are normally measured. Hyperkalaemia, acidosis with a correspondingly low serum bicarbonate level, hypocalcaemia and hyperphosphataemia may also be present.

Urine should be examined visually and microscopically, tested with dipsticks, cultured and a 24 hour collection made for determination of GFR.

The patient may report a change in urine colour, which might result from blood staining by whole cells or haemoglobin, drugs or metabolic breakdown products. Urine may also appear milky after connection with lymphatics, cloudy following infection, contain solid material such as stones, crystals casts, or froth excessively in proteinuria.

Dipstick tests enable simple, rapid estimation of a wide range of urinary parameters including pH, specific gravity, glucose, blood and protein. Positive results should, however, be quantified by more specific methods.

Urinary creatinine excretion and the serum creatinine concentration may be used to calculate creatinine clearance, which approximates to GFR.

As the serum creatinine is determined partially by muscle bulk as well as renal function, corrections for muscle mass using the patient's weight, age and sex yield estimates of the GRF from the serum creatinine. This can be determined using methods such as that of Cockcroft and Gault (described in Chapter 15) which are as accurate as those of formal urine and blood methods.

In some patients the kidneys may be palpable. Large irregular kidneys are indicative of polycystic disease, whereas smooth, tender enlarged kidneys are likely to be infected or obstructed. However, in most cases of CRF, the kidneys appear shrunken.

Structural assessments of the kidney may be performed using a number of imaging procedures, including:

- ultrasonography
- intravenous urography (IVU)
- plain abdominal radiography
- computed tomography (CT), magnetic resonance imaging (MRI) and magnetic resonance angiography (MRA).

Ultrasonography

This method produces two dimensional images using sound waves and is used as the first line investigational tool in many hospitals. The technique is harmless, non-invasive, quick, inexpensive, enables measurements to be made and produces images in real time. The latter feature allows accurate and safe positioning of biopsy needles. Ultrasonography is particularly useful in the differentiation of renal tumours from cysts and in the assessment of renal tract obstruction. Doppler ultrasonography is a development that enables measurement of flow rate and direction of the intra- and extrarenal blood supply.

Intravenous urography (IVU)

IVU is used less often nowadays than in the past because it uses high doses of radiation and contrast media.

Timed serial radiographs are taken of the kidneys and the full length of the urinary tract following an intravenous injection of an iodine-based contrast medium that is filtered and excreted by the kidney. IVU will show the following:

- the presence, length and position of the kidneys; in CRF the kidneys generally shrink in proportion to nephron loss, the exception being the enlarged kidneys seen in polycystic disease
- the presence or absence of renal scarring and the shape of the calices and renal pelvis; renal cortical scarring and caliceal distortion indicate chronic pyelonephritis
- obstruction to the ureters, for example by a stone, tumour or retroperitoneal fibrosis; these require surgical intervention
- the shape of the bladder and the presence of residual urine; enlargement and a postmicturition residue suggest urethral obstruction such as prostatic hypertrophy.

Plain abdominal radiography

Plain radiography must be used with IVU as contrast media can obscure some lesions. Calcification, renal outlines and evidence for renal osteodystrophy may be observed.

Computed tomography (CT) and magnetic resonance imaging (MRI)

The newer techniques of CT and MRI provide excellent structural information about the kidneys and urinary tract. They use less radiation (none in the case of MRI) and less contrast media, although the machinery required is more expensive than needed for traditional imaging methods. Magnetic resonance angiography (MRA) can also give information about renal blood supply.

Renal biopsy

If imaging techniques fail to give a cause for the reduction in renal function, a renal biopsy may be performed, although in advanced disease scarring of the renal tissue may render diagnosis difficult. Also, the small shrunken kidneys usually encountered in CRF can be difficult to biopsy and may well subsequently bleed. In patients whose creatinine is above 400 μmol/l, injection of vasopressin (DDAVP) might minimize bleeding following renal biopsy.

Reciprocal creatinine plots

All patients with CRF should have their serum biochemistry and haematology monitored regularly to detect any of the sequelae of the disease. In many forms of CRF the decline in renal function progresses at a constant rate and may be monitored by plotting the reciprocal of the serum creatinine concentration against time (Fig. 16.2). The decline in renal function is usually linear in most patients (Fig. 16.2A). The intercept with the x-axis indicates the time at which renal function will fall to zero and can be used to predict when the

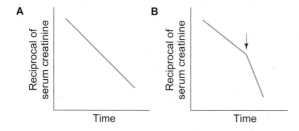

Figure 16.2 Stylized reciprocal creatinine plots. **A** Linear, uniform progression in the decline in renal function. **B** Sudden decline in renal function (arrow).

glomerular filtration rate will reach approximately 10 ml/min – i.e. when renal replacement therapy should be initiated. If an abrupt decline in the slope of a reciprocal plot is noted (Fig. 16.2B), this indicates a worsening of the condition or the presence of an additional renal insult. The cause should be detected and remedied if possible.

Clinical manifestations

Urinary symptoms

Polyuria, where the patient frequently voids high volumes of urine, is often seen in CRF and results from medullary damage and the osmotic effect of high plasma urea levels (> 40 mmol/l). The ability to concentrate urine is also lost in CRF, which together with failure of physiological nocturnal antidiuresis, results almost invariably in nocturia, where the patient will be wakened two or three times a night with a full bladder.

Proteinuria

A degree of proteinuria invariably occurs in CRF and can result from glomerular leaks, infection, failure of protein reabsorption in the tubules or overflow of excess plasma proteins as seen in myeloma.

Pronounced proteinuria (> 2 g of protein in a 24-hour collection) usually indicates a glomerular aetiology.

Fluid retention

As the GFR falls to very low levels the kidneys are unable to excrete salt and water adequately, resulting in the retention of extra vascular fluid, which may manifest as both peripheral and pulmonary oedema and ascites. Oedema may be seen around the eyes on waking, the sacral region in supine patients and from the feet upwards in ambulatory patients. Volume dependent hypertension occurs in about 80% of patients with CRF and becomes more prevalent as the GFR falls.

Uraemia

Many substances including urea, creatinine and water are normally excreted by the kidney and accumulate as renal function decreases. Some of the substances responsible for the toxicity of uraemia are intermediate in size between small, readily dialysed molecules and large non-dialysable proteins. These are described as 'middle molecules' and include phosphate, guanidines, phenols and organic acids. Clearly, there are a wide range of uraemic toxins but it is the blood level of urea that is often used to estimate the degree of toxin accumulation in uraemia.

The symptoms of uraemia are many and various and include anorexia, nausea, vomiting, constipation, foul taste and skin discoloration that is presumed to be due to pigment deposition compounded by the pallor of anaemia. The characteristic complexion is often described as 'muddy', and is frequently associated with severe pruritus without an underlying rash. In extremely severe cases crystalline urea is deposited on the skin (uraemic frost).

Anaemia

Anaemia is an almost inevitable consequence of chronic renal failure and is generally noticeable when the GFR falls to less than 30 ml/min (the serum creatinine is likely to be > 300 μmol/l at this point). The fall in haemoglobin level is a slow, insidious process accompanying the decline in renal function. A normochromic, normocytic pattern is usually seen with haemoglobin levels falling to between 6 and 8 g/dl in ESRF.

Several factors are thought to contribute to the pathogenesis of anaemia in CRF, including shortened red cell survival, marrow suppression by uraemic toxins and iron or folate deficiency associated with poor dietary intake or increased losses, for example from gastrointestinal bleeding. However, the principal cause results from damage of peritubular cells leading to inadequate secretion of erythropoietin. This hormone, which is produced mainly, though not exclusively, in the kidney, is the main regulator of red cell proliferation and differentiation in bone marrow. Hyperparathyroidism also reduces erythropoiesis by damaging bone marrow and therefore exacerbates anaemia associated with CRF.

Clinical findings

Anaemia in CRF is the major cause of fatigue, breathlessness at rest and on exertion, lethargy and angina often seen in patients with CRF. These patients will also complain of a sensation of feeling cold, poor concentration and reduced appetite and libido. Compensatory haemodynamic changes occur in patients with anaemia associated with CRF. Cardiac output is increased to improve oxygen delivery to tissues although this may result in tachycardia and palpitations. As a consequence many patients cope relatively well with profoundly low haemoglobin concentrations but benefit from corrective therapy.

Electrolyte disturbances

Since the kidneys play such a crucial role in the maintenance of volume, extracellular fluid composition and acid–base balance, it is not surprising that disturbances of electrolyte levels are seen in CRF.

Sodium

Serum sodium levels can be relatively normal even when creatinine clearance is very low. However, patients may exhibit hypo- or hypernatraemia depending upon the condition and therapy employed (Table 16.2).

Potassium

Potassium levels are generally elevated in CRF. Hyperkalaemia is a potentially dangerous condition as the first indication of elevated potassium levels may be life-threatening cardiac arrest. Potassium levels of over 7.0 mmol/l are life-threatening and should be treated as an emergency. Hyperkalaemia may be exacerbated in acidosis as potassium shifts from within cells.

ECG changes accompany any rise in serum potassium and become more pronounced as levels increase. T waves peak ('tenting'), there is a reduction in the size of P waves, an increase in the PR interval and a widening of the QRS complex. P waves eventually disappear and the QRS complex becomes even wider. Ultimately the ECG assumes a sinusoidal appearance prior to cardiac arrest.

Hydrogen ions

Hydrogen ions (H^+) are a common end-product of many metabolic processes and about 40–80 mmol are normally excreted via the kidney each day. In renal failure H^+ is retained, causing acidosis; the combination of H^+ with bicarbonate (HCO_3^-) results in the removal of some hydrogen as water, the elimination of carbon dioxide via the lungs, and a reduction in plasma bicarbonate level.

Hypertension and CRF changes

The vast majority of patients with CRF will have hypertension. Furthermore, raised blood pressure may exacerbate renal damage and precipitate or worsen CRF.

Severe renal impairment leads to sodium retention, which in turn produces circulatory volume expansion with consequent hypertension. This form of hypertension is often termed 'salt-sensitive', as it may be exacerbated by salt intake, or 'wet', as it results from fluid retention. Lesser degrees of renal impairment reduce kidney perfusion, which activates renin production, with subsequent angiotensin mediated vasoconstriction. Hypertension of this form may be termed 'salt-resistant', as it is not generally salt sensitive, or 'dry' hypertension owing to its dependence upon vasoconstriction. The wet and dry forms of hypertension may coexist under certain circumstances.

Treatment of blood pressure, irrespective of choice of therapy, generally improves the course of CRF.

Eye damage in the form of hypertensive retinopathy may be found in those patients whose blood pressure has not been adequately controlled. Appropriate and timely antihypertensive therapy can help prevent this.

In uraemia there is also an increased tendency to bleed. This is further exacerbated by anaemia because of impaired platelet adhesion and modified interaction between platelets and blood vessels resulting from altered blood rheology.

Consideration should also be given to the lipid profile of the patient and where appropriate, treatment with HMG CoA reductase inhibitors (statins) commenced.

Table 16.2.   Causes and mechanism of plasma sodium abnormalities in CRF

	Mechanism	Cause/effect
Hypernatraemia	Sodium overload	Drugs e.g. antibiotic sodium salts
	Hypotonic fluid loss	Osmotic diuresis Sweating
	↓ water intake	Unconsciousness
Hyponatraemia	Dilution by intracellular water movement	Mannitol Hyperglycaemia
	Water overload	Acute dilution by intravenous fluids, e.g. 5% dextrose infusion Excessive intake Congestive cardiac failure Nephrotic syndrome

The clearance of statins is less affected by renal failure than other lipid lowering therapies.

Bone disease (renal osteodystrophy)

Renal osteodystrophy describes the four types of bone disease associated with CRF:

- secondary hyperparathyroidism
- osteomalacia (reduced mineralization)
- mixed renal osteodystrophy (both hyperparathyroidism and osteomalacia)
- adynamic bone disease (reduced bone formation and resorption).

Cholecalciferol, the precursor of active vitamin D, is both absorbed from the gastrointestinal tract and produced in the skin by the action of sunlight.

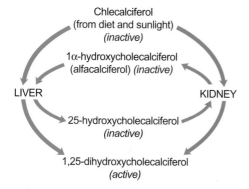

Figure 16.3 Renal and hepatic involvement in vitamin D metabolism.

Production of 1,25-dihydroxycholecalciferol (calcitriol) requires the hydroxylation of the colecalciferol molecule at both the 1α and the 25 position (Fig. 16.3).

Hydroxylation at the 25 position occurs in the liver, while hydroxylation of the 1α position occurs in the kidney; this latter process is impaired in renal failure. The resulting deficiency in vitamin D leads to defective mineralization of bone, and osteomalacia.

The deficiency in vitamin D with the consequent reduced calcium absorption from the gut in combination with the reduced renal tubular reabsorption results in hypocalcaemia (Fig. 16.4).

These disturbances are compounded by hyperphosphataemia caused by reduced phosphate excretion, which in turn reduces the concentration of ionized serum calcium by sequestering calcium phosphate in bone or, eventually, in soft tissue. Hypocalcaemia and a reduction in the direct suppressive action of 1,25-dihydroxycholecalciferol on the parathyroid glands results in an increased secretion of parathyroid hormone (PTH).

Since the failed kidney is unable to respond to PTH by increasing renal calcium reabsorption, the serum PTH levels remain persistently elevated, and hyperplasia of the parathyroid glands occurs. The resulting secondary hyperparathyroidism produces a disturbance in normal architecture of bone termed osteosclerosis (hardening of the bone). Bone pain is the main symptom, and distinctive appearances on radiography may be observed, such as 'rugger-jersey' spine, where there are alternate bands of excessive and defective mineralization in the vertebrae (Fig. 16.5).

A further possible, though by no means inevitable, consequence of the secondary hyperparathyroidism

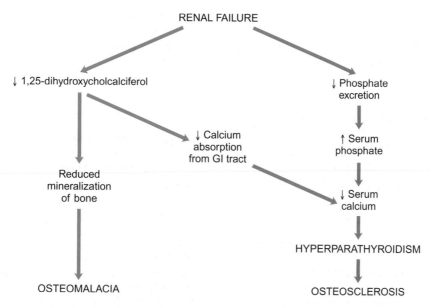

Figure 16.4 Disturbance of calcium and phosphate balance in chronic renal failure.

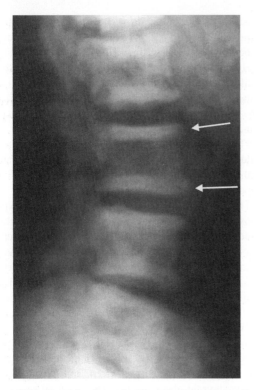

Figure 16.5 Lateral radiograph of the spine in a patient with chronic renal failure. Characteristic endplate sclerosis (arrows) are referred to as 'rugger-jersey spine'. (Reproduced by kind permission of Dr M. J. Kline, Department of Diagnostic Radiology, Cleveland Clinic Foundation; from 'Osteomalacia and renal osteodystrophy', www.emedicine.com/radio/topic5000.htm)

produced in response to hypocalcaemia is that sufficient bone resorption may be caused to maintain adequate calcium levels. This, in combination with the hyperphosphataemia, may result in calcium phosphate deposition and soft tissue calcification.

Neurological changes

The most common neurological changes are non-specific and include inability to concentrate, memory impairment, irritability and stupor probably caused by uraemic toxins. Fits owing to cerebral oedema or hypertension may occur. Most patients have evidence of peripheral neuropathy, although this is usually asymptomatic.

Muscle function

Muscle cramps and restless legs are common and may be major symptoms causing distress to patients, particularly at night. These conditions are probably caused by general nutritional deficiencies and electrolyte disturbances, notably of divalent cations and especially by hypocalcaemia. A proximal myopathy of shoulder and pelvic girdle muscles may rarely develop.

Prognosis

When the GFR has declined to about 20 ml/min, a continuing deterioration in renal function to end-stage renal failure appears inevitable in most pateints even when the initial cause of the kidney damage has been removed and appropriate treatment instigated. The mechanism for the relentless decline in renal function is obscure, but hypertension, deposition of calcium phosphate or urate crystals in the kidney and damage resulting from an increased blood flow through the remaining intact nephrons have been suggested. Serum creatinine levels and creatinine clearance should be monitored to ensure the detection of the most appropriate point at which to commence renal replacement therapy.

Treatment

The aims of the treatment of CRF may be summarized as follows:

- reverse or arrest the process causing the renal damage (this is rarely possible)
- avoid conditions that might worsen renal failure (Table 16.3)
- relieve symptoms
- implement regular dialysis treatment and/or transplantation at the most appropriate time.

Reversal or arrest of primary disease

As indicated above, reversal or arrest of the primary cause of renal failure is rarely possible. However, early

Table 16.3. Factors that might exacerbate established chronic renal failure

Reduced renal blood flow
Hypotension
Hypertension
Nephrotoxins including drugs
Renal artery disease
Obstruction, e.g. prostatic hypertrophy

detection of some causes may enable remedial action to be taken. A postrenal obstructive lesion such as a ureter obstructed by a stone or a ureteric tumour may be successfully treated surgically. Glomerulonephritis may respond to immunosuppressants and/or steroids. Clearly, when drug-induced renal disease is suspected the offending agent should be stopped.

Relief of symptoms

Hypertension

Adequate control of blood pressure is one of the most important therapeutic measures since there is a vicious cycle of events whereby hypertension causes damage to the intrarenal vasculature resulting in thickening and hyalinization of the walls of arterioles and small vessels. This damage effectively reduces renal perfusion, leading to stimulation of the renin–angiotensin–aldosterone system. Sodium conservation and vasoconstriction result, which in turn exacerbates the degree of hypertension.

Antihypertensive therapy might produce a transient reduction in GFR over the first 3 months of treatment as the blood pressure drops. However, it is possible that control of blood pressure will ultimately lead to an improvement in renal function. This can be sufficiently dramatic that suspension of renal replacement therapy can occasionally be warranted in patients with ESRF.

The drugs used to treat hypertension in renal disease are generally the same as those used in other forms of hypertension although allowances must be made for the effects of renal failure on drug disposition. A logical choice of antihypertensive agent might be made if the predominant mechanism responsible for the elevation of blood pressure is known. In predominantly dry forms of hypertension, raised levels of renin and angiotensin are expected and therefore agents such as angiotensin-converting enzyme inhibitors, angiotensin II antagonists and β-blockers are considered appropriate. In wet forms of hypertension, salt restriction, diuretics, selective α_1-blockers and calcium entry blockers might be of greater benefit.

Diuretics. Diuretics are of use in patients with volume overload, which is usually indicated by the presence of oedema. This type of hypertension may be particularly difficult to treat. The choice of agent is generally limited to a loop diuretic. Potassium sparing diuretics are usually contraindicated owing to the risks of developing hyperkalaemia, and thiazides become ineffective as renal function progresses.

As loop diuretics need to be filtered to exert an action progressively higher doses are required as CRF worsens. Doses of 500–1000 mg of furosemide (frusemide) or higher may be required in severe failure. Patients who do not respond to oral loop diuretic therapy alone may benefit from concomitant administration of metolazone, which acts synergistically to produce a profound diuresis. Alternatively, the loop diuretic may be given intravenously. Care must be taken to avoid hypovolaemia (monitor body weight) and electrolyte disturbances such as hypokalaemia and hyponatraemia.

Thiazide diuretics, with the notable exception of metolazone, are ineffective at a low GFR and may accumulate, causing an increased incidence of side-effects.

Calcium channel blockers. These agents produce vasodilation principally by reducing Ca^{2+} influx into vascular muscle cells. Calcium channel blockers also appear to promote sodium excretion in wet hypertension. The mechanism is unclear but may revolve around the finding that high sodium levels can cause vaso-constriction by interfering with calcium transport.

Both verapamil and diltiazem block conduction across the atrioventricular node and should not be used in conjuction with β-blockers. By contrast, dihydro-pyridines such as nifedipine produce less cardiac depression but only dilate afferent arterioles. High systemic blood pressures can therefore cause intraglomerular hypertension and damage.

Calcium channel blockers can produce headache, facial flushing and oedema. The latter can be confused with the symptoms of volume overload but is resistant to diuretics.

Selective α_1-blockers. These vasodilators produce a variety of actions that might be of benefit in hypertension associated with CRF. Sympathetic adrenergic activity can lead to sodium retention. Blockade of α_1-mediated vasoconstriction might therefore be of use in wet forms of hypertension. These agents have also been shown to produce improvements in insulin sensitivity, adverse lipid profiles and obstruction caused by hypertrophy of the prostate, all of which might be associated with some forms of CRF.

Angiotensin-converting enzyme (ACE) inhibitors and angiotensin II receptor antagonists. The role of ACE inhibitors in hypertensive patients with renal insufficiency is complicated. ACE inhibitors reduce the amount of circulating angiotensin II, which results in vasodilatation and reduced sodium retention.

They can produce a reduction in renal function by preventing the angiotensin II-mediated vasoconstriction of the efferent glomerular arteriole, which contributes to the high-pressure gradient across the glomerulus. This problem is important only in patients with renal vascular disease, particularly those with bilateral renal artery stenoses. However, as ACE inhibitors preferentially dilate efferent glomerular arterioles they lower intraglomerular pressure, thus reducing proteinuria and further development of glomerulosclerosis. Increases in

GFR in hypertensive patients with renal insufficiency have been shown following ACE inhibitor therapy. Clearly, ACE inhibitors exert beneficial intrarenal haemodynamic effects in addition to actions on systemic blood pressure.

For long-term managment, it is usually preferable to use an agent with a duration of action that permits once-daily dosing. There is little to choose clinically between the ACE inhibitors currently on the market; however, consideration should be given to the cost benefits of choosing an agent that does not require dose adjustment in renal failure.

It has been reported that ACE inhibitors may reduce thirst, which may be useful in those patients who have a tendency to fluid overload as a result of excessive drinking. ACE inhibitors are potassium sparing and therefore plasma potassium should be monitored carefully. A low-potassium diet may be necessary.

Angiotensin II receptor antagonists have properties similar to the ACE inhibitors with the advantage that, since they do not inhibit the breakdown of kinins such as bradykinin, they do not cause the dry cough associated with the ACE inhibitors.

β-blockers. β-blockers are commonly used in the treatment of hypertension in CRF. They exhibit a range of actions including a reduction of renin production. Consequently, β-blockers have a particular role in the rational therapy of dry hypertension. However, the β-blockers reduce cardiac output and cause peripheral vasoconstriction they can exacerbate peripheral vascular disease.

It is advisable to use the more cardioselective β-blockers atenolol or metoprolol. Given that atenolol is excreted renally, it should require dosage adjustment in renal failure. In practice, however, it is effective and tolerated well by renal patients at standard doses. Nevertheless, metoprolol would theoretically be a better choice since it is cleared hepatically and needs no dosage adjustment, although small initial doses are advised in renal failure since there may be increased sensitivity to its hypotensive effects.

Vasodilators. The vasodilators hydralazine and minoxidil have been used to treat hypertension in CRF with varying degrees of success but are usually only used when other measures inadequately control blood pressure. The sensitivity of patients to these drugs is often increased in renal failure so, if used, therapy should be initiated with small doses. These agents cause direct peripheral vasodilation with resultant reflex tachycardia, which may require suppression with co-prescription of a β-blocker.

Centrally acting drugs. Methyldopa and clonidine are not commonly used as antihypertensives in CRF because of their adverse side-effect profiles. If they are used in renal failure, initial doses should be small because of increased sensitivity to their effects.

Management of uraemia

Dietary modifications

Although urea is only one of the toxins encountered in uraemia, many patients experience a symptomatic improvement when dietary protein intake is reduced, presumably through a reduction in the output of nitrogenous waste. There is some evidence that, as well as reducing the symptoms of uraemia, protein restriction slows the progression of CRF, but this remains controversial. The optimal time to initiate protein restriction is also not clear, but many consider it appropriate when the GFR falls to about 50 ml/min.

Protein restricted diets are designed to provide all the essential amino acids in a total protein intake of 40 g/day. A higher intake of protein stimulates its use as an energy source, resulting in increases in blood urea concentrations, whereas further reduction in protein intake brings about endogenous protein catabolism, which also cause blood urea levels to rise. Fat and carbohydrate should also be given to maintain a high-energy intake of about 2000–3000 kcal/day, or more in hypercatabolic patients, as this will help to prevent protein catabolism and promote anabolism. Lower protein diets can also be used while minimizing catabolism by supplementing the patient with ketoacid analogues of essential amino acids, which may provide substrates for protein synthesis without additional nitrogen intake.

Other dietary precautions include sodium restriction to reduce the risk of fluid overload, potassium restriction to reduce the risk of hyperkalaemia and vitamin supplementation.

Fluid retention

Oedema may occur as a result of sodium retention and the resultant associated water retention. Patients with CRF also often have hypoalbuminaemia following renal protein loss, and this can result in an osmotic extravasation of fluid and its retention. Pulmonary and peripheral oedema is best controlled with dialysis but diuretics can be useful. The daily fluid intake should be restricted to 300–500 ml in addition to the volume of urine produced (if any). It is important to note that the fluid allowance must include fluids ingested in any form, including sauces, medicines and fruits in addition to drinks. The fluid restriction is very difficult to maintain. Sucking ice cubes may relieve an unpleasantly dry mouth, but the melted water must not be swallowed.

Sodium restriction. Sodium intake may often be reduced to a satisfactory level of 80 mmol/day by avoiding convenience foods and snacks or the addition of salt to food at the table. This is usually tolerable to patients. It is important to be aware of the contribution of sodium-containing medications, including some antibiotics, soluble or effervescent preparations, magnesium trisilicate mixture, Gaviscon, sodium bicarbonate and the plasma expanders hetastarch and gelatin.

Potassium restriction. Hyperkalaemia often occurs in CRF and may cause life-threatening cardiac arrhythmias. If untreated, asystolic cardiac arrest and death may result. Patients are often put on a potassium-restricted diet by avoiding potassium-rich foods such as fruit and fruit drinks, vegetables, chocolate, beer, instant coffee and ice cream. Many medicines have a high potassium content, for example potassium citrate mixture, Sandocal tablets, some antibiotics and ispaghula husk sachets. The use of these drugs is less of a problem in dialysed patients. Emergency treatment is necessary if the serum potassium level is above 7.0 mmol/l or if there are ECG changes. The most effective treatment is dialysis but if this is not available other measures may be tried, as discussed in Chapter 15.

Vitamin supplementation. Vitamin supplementation is sometimes necessary as water-soluble vitamins may be lost during dialysis. This is becoming less of a problem as dialysis techniques and dietary control improve.

The rationale and necessity for a renal diet and fluid restriction can be difficult for a patient to understand and adherence may be a problem. Consequently, involvement with a specialist renal dietician can be invaluable in optimizing dietary therapies.

Gastrointestinal symptoms

Nausea and vomiting may persist after starting a low-protein diet. In this situation, metoclopramide is useful, but sometimes accumulation of the drug and its metabolites may occur, leading to a high incidence of extrapyramidal side-effects. Patients should be started on a low dose, which should then be increased slowly. Prochlorperazine or cyclizine may also be useful. The 5-HT$_3$ antagonists such as ondansetron have also been shown to be effective, but cost–benefit factors should be considered. The anaemic patient often becomes less nauseated when treated with epoetin.

Constipation is a common problem in patients with renal disease, partly as a result of fluid restriction and anorexia and partly as a consequence of drug therapy with agents such as aluminium supplements used as phosphate binders. It is particularly important that patients controlled by peritoneal dialysis do not become constipated, as this can reduce the efficacy of dialysis and predispose to peritonitis. Conventional laxative therapy may be used, such as bulk-forming laxatives or increased dietary fibre for less severe constipation, or a stimulant such as senna with enemas or glycerine suppositories for severe constipation. Higher doses of stimulant laxatives such as 2–4 tablets of senna at night may be required. It should be noted that certain brands of ispaghula husk preparations may contain significant quantities of potassium, and should be avoided in renal failure because of the risk of hyperkalaemia. Sterculia preparations are an effective alternative.

Pruritus

Itching associated with renal failure can be extremely severe and can often be distressing, disfiguring as a result of over-enthusiastic scratching and difficult to treat. The exact mechanism responsible is not clear and several possibilities have been suggested. Xerosis (dry skin) associated with renal failure, skin micro-precipitation of divalent ions, elevated parathyroid hormone levels and increased dermal mast cell activity are all possible. Generally, however, no underlying cause is found and it is likely that a multifactorial process is responsible.

Sometimes correction of serum phosphate or calcium levels improves the condition, as does para-thyroidectomy. Conventionally, oral antihistamines are used to treat pruritus; however, topical versions should not be used owing to the risks of allergy. Non-sedating antihistamines such as loratidine are generally less effective than sedating antihistamines such as chlorphenamine (chlorpheniramine). Alimemazine (trimeprazine) may be useful, particularly at night. Topical crotamiton lotion and creams are also reported to be useful in some patients. Other non-drug therapies include either warming or cooling the skin using baths, three times weekly UVB phototherapy and modified electrical acupuncture.

Anaemia

The normochromic, normocytic anaemia of CRF does not respond to iron or folic acid unless there is a coexisting deficiency. Traditionally the only treatment available was to give red blood cell transfusions, but this is time-consuming, may lead to fluid and iron overload and promotes antibody formation, which may give problems if transplantation is subsequently attempted. The introduction of recombinant human erythropoietins (epoetin alfa and beta), genetically engineered forms of the hormone, have rendered treatment safer and at least as effective. Epoetin alfa and beta are indistinguishable in practical terms, and are immunologically and biologically indistinguishable from physiological erythropoietin. Both forms of epoetin may be given by either the intravenous or the subcutaneous route; the latter route is preferred as it provides equally effective clinical results while using similar or smaller dose (up to 30% less) when given three times a week. Most patients report a dramatically improved quality of life.

Novel erythropoiesis stimulating protein (NESP) is a recombinant hyperglycosylated analogue of epoetin that stimulates red blood cell production by the same mechanism as the endogenous hormone. The terminal half-life of NESP in man is three times longer than that of epoetin and consequently requires a once weekly dosing schedule.

Iron and folate deficiencies must be corrected before therapy is initiated, while patients receiving epoetin generally require concurrent iron supplements because of increased marrow requirements. Supplemental iron is often given intravenously owing to bioavailability problems with oral forms. Maintaining iron stores ensures the effect of epoetin is optimized for minimum cost.

Epoetin therapy should aim to achieve a slow rise in the haemoglobin concentration to avoid cardiovascular sides-effects resulting from a rapidly increasing red cell mass, such as hypertension, increased blood viscosity/volume, seizures and clotting of vascular accesses. Blood pressure should be closely monitored.

An initial subcutaneous or intravenous epoetin dose of 50 units/kg body-weight three times weekly, increased as necessary in steps of 25 units/kg every 4 weeks, should be given to produce a haemoglobin increase of not more than 2 g/dl per month. The target haemoglobin concentration is commonly 10–13 g/dl, and, once this has been reached, a maintenance dose of epoetin in the region of 33–100 units/kg three times a week or 50–150 units/kg twice weekly should maintain the level.

Correcting anaemia usually helps control the symptoms of lethargy and myopathy, and often greatly reduces nausea. Improved appetite on epoetin therapy can, however, increase potassium intake, and may necessitate dietary control.

Acidosis

Since the kidney is the main route for excreting H^+ ions, CRF may result in a metabolic acidosis. This will cause a reduction in serum bicarbonate that may be treated readily with oral doses of sodium bicarbonate 1–6 g/day. As the dose of bicarbonate is not critical, it is easy to experiment with different dosage forms and strengths to suit individual patients. If acidosis is severe and persistent then dialysis may be required.

Neurological problems

Neurological changes are generally caused by uraemic toxins and improve on the treatment of uraemia by dialysis or diet. Muscle cramps are common and are often treated with quinine sulphate (see Chapter 15). Restless legs may respond to low doses of clonazepam or co-careldopa.

Osteodystrophy

The osteodystrophy of renal failure is due to three factors: hyperphosphataemia, vitamin D deficiency and hyperparathyroidism.

Hyperphosphataemia

The management of hyperphosphataemia depends initially upon restricting dietary phosphate. This can be difficult to achieve effectively, even with the aid of a specialist dietician, because phosphate is found in many palatable foods such as dairy products, eggs, chocolate and nuts. Phosphate-binding agents can be used to reduce the absorption of orally ingested phosphate in the gut, by forming insoluble, non-absorbable complexes. Phosphate-binders are usually salts of a di- or trivalent metallic ion, such as aluminium, calcium or occasionally magnesium.

Aluminium hydroxide has been widely used as a phosphate binder owing to the avid binding capacity of aluminium ions. Unfortunately, a small amount of aluminium may be absorbed by patients with CRF owing to poor clearance of this ion, which can produce toxic effects including encephalopathy, osteomalacia, proximal myopathy and anaemia. Dialysis dementia was a disease observed among haemodialysis patients associated with aluminium deposition in the brain and exacerbated by aluminum in the water supply and the use of aluminium cooking pans. Desferrioxamine (4–6 g in 500 ml of saline 0.9% per week) has been used to treat this condition by removing aluminium from tissues by chelation. The tendency of aluminium to constipate is an added disadvantage. The use of aluminium as a phosphate binder in CRF should therefore be approached with caution.

Calcium carbonate has been used as a phosphate binder in the form of Titralac or Calcichew. Unfortunately, it is less effective as a phosphate binder than aluminium, and sometimes requires doses of up to 10 g daily. Calcium carbonate has advantages, however, in that correction of concurrent hypocalcaemia can be achieved.

Calcium acetate is now also available for use as a phosphate binder. The capacity of calcium acetate and calcium carbonate to control serum phosphate appears similar. However, phosphate control is achieved using between half and a quarter of the dose of elemental calcium when calcium acetate is used. Whether this translates to a decreased likelihood of producing unwanted hypercalcaemia with calcium acetate therapy is as yet unclear.

Recently, sevelamer, a hydrophilic but insoluble polymeric compound has been licensed as a phosphate binder for use in haemodialysis patients. Sevelamer binds phosphate with an efficacy similar to calcium acetate but with a decreased likelihood of hypercalcaemia. Since sevelamer does not contain either calcium or aluminium, intoxication with these metals does not limit its use as a phosphate binder. Mean levels of total and low-density cholesterol are also reduced with sevelamer use. This compound does not appear to present any risk of toxicity but may cause bowel obstruction and is relatively expensive when compared to other phosphate binders.

Vitamin D deficiency

Vitamin D deficiency may be treated with the synthetic vitamin D analogues 1α-hydroxycholecalciferol (alfacalcidol) at 0.25–1 microgram/day or 1,25-dihydroxycholecalciferol (calcitriol) at 1–2 micrograms/day. The serum calcium level should be monitored, and the dose of alfacalcidol or calcitriol adjusted accordingly. Hyperphosphataemia should be controlled before starting vitamin D therapy since the resulting increase in the serum calcium concentration may result in soft tissue calcification.

Hyperparathyroidism

The rise in plasma 1,25-dihydroxycholecalciferol and calcium levels that results from starting vitamin D therapy usually suppresses the production of parathyroid hormone by the parathyroids. If vitamin D therapy does not correct parathyroid hormone levels then parathyroidectomy to remove part or most of the parathyroid glands may be needed. This surgical procedure was once commonly performed on CRF patients, but is now less frequent owing to effective vitamin D supplementation.

Implementation of regular dialysis treatment and/or transplantation

End-stage renal failure is the point at which, despite the conservative measures discussed above, the patient will die without the institution of renal replacement by dialysis or transplantation. This may occur very rapidly after presentation or after a period of several years.

The principle of dialysis is simple. The patient's blood is on one side, and a dialysis solution on the other side of a semi-permeable membrane across which exchange of metabolites occurs. There are traditionally two main types of dialysis, haemodialysis and peritoneal dialysis, both of which are discussed in detail in Chapter 15. Neither has been shown to be superior to the other in any particular group of patients and so the personal preference of the patient is important when selecting dialysis modality.

Because patients with CRF may require dialysis treatment for many years, adaptations to the process of peritoneal dialysis have been made that enable the patient to follow a lifestyle as near normal as possible. Continuous ambulatory peritoneal dialysis (CAPD) involves a flexible non-irritant silicone rubber catheter (Tenckhoff catheter) that is surgically inserted into the abdominal cavity. Dacron cuffs on the body of the catheter become infiltrated with scar tissue during the healing process, causing the catheter to be firmly anchored in place. Such catheters may remain viable for many years. During the dialysis process thereafter, a bag typically containing 2.5 litres of warmed dialysate and a drainage bag are connected to the catheter using aseptic techniques. Used dialysate is drained from the abdomen under gravity into the drainage bag, fresh dialysate is run into the peritoneal cavity and the giving set is disconnected. The patient continues his or her activities until the next exchange some hours later. The procedure is repeated regularly so that dialysate is kept in the abdomen 24 hours a day. This is usually achieved by repeating the process four times a day with an average dwell time of 6–8 hours.

Since CAPD is by definition continuous and corrects fluid and electrolyte levels constantly, dietary and fluid restrictions are less stringent. Blood loss is also avoided, making the technique safer in anaemic patients.

Unfortunately, peritoneal dialysis is not an efficient process; it only just manages to facilitate excretion of the substances required and, as albumin crosses the peritoneal membrane, up to 10 g of protein a day may be lost in the dialysate. It is also uncomfortable and tiring for the patient, and is contraindicated in patients who have recently undergone abdominal surgery.

Peritonitis is the most frequently encountered complication of peritoneal dialysis. Its diagnosis usually depends on a combination of abdominal pain, cloudy dialysate or positive microbiological culture. Empirical antibiotic therapy should therefore be commenced as soon as peritonitis is clinically diagnosed. Gram-positive cocci (particularly *Staphylococcus epidermidis*) and Enterobacteriaceae are the causative organisms in the majority of cases, while infection with *Pseudomonas* species is also well recognized. Fungal infections are also seen, albeit less commonly.

Most centres have their own local protocol for antibiotic treatment of peritonitis. In one example, ceftazidime, a broad-spectrum cephalosporin with good Gram-negative activity, and vancomycin, which has excellent activity against Gram-positive bacteria, are administered in combination via the intraperitoneal route. As in all situations, the antibiotic regimen should be adjusted appropriately after the results of microbiological culture and sensitivity have been obtained.

Oral ciprofloxacin in a dose of 500 mg four times a day for 14 days has been shown to be effective in the treatment of CAPD peritonitis (it should be noted that this dose is above the manufacturer's recommended dose). When this regimen is used it is important that any oral aluminium preparations are discontinued, as they reduce the absorption of ciprofloxacin by chelation.

Haemodialysis is particularly suitable for patients producing large amounts of metabolites, such as those with high nutritional demands or a large muscle mass, where these substances are produced faster than peritoneal dialysis can remove them. It also provides a back-up for those patients in whom peritoneal dialysis has failed.

The various techniques of haemofiltration, a technique related to haemodialysis, are discussed in detail in Chapter 15.

Renal transplantation

Renal transplantation remains the treatment of choice for patients with end-stage renal failure, as a relatively normal lifestyle is usually re-established. Expensive dialysis procedures are not needed, dietary restrictions are lifted and improvements are seen in anaemia and bone disease. However, there is a shortage of suitable organs for transplantation and up to 50% of patients on the dialysis programme are not physically fit enough to undergo the surgery and postoperative treatment.

Except in those rare cases where a genetically identical donor is available, the most important therapeutic aspect of transplantation is immuno-suppression to prevent rejection. The major disadvantage of all immunosuppressive agents is their relative non-specificity, in that they cause a general depression of the immune system. This exposes the patient to an increased risk of malignancy and infection, which remains an important cause of morbidity and mortality.

Immunosuppressants

The major pharmacological groups of immuno-suppressive agents are summarized in Table 16.4.

Most transplant centres have their own regimens involving combinations of the agents outlined in Table 16.4 for prophylaxis against rejection and for reversal of acute and chronic episodes of rejection.

Immunosuppression is usually commenced immediately before the grafting procedure on induction of anaesthesia and is continued for as long as the transplanted kidney remains in situ. In order to minimize side-effects, doses of immunosuppressants are gradually reduced over a 2–6 month period to the lowest that will maintain effective immunosuppression. In addition, transplants appear to become less immunogenic over a period of time so lower prophylactic levels of immunosuppression are required.

One of the most common immunosuppressant regimens is the so-called 'triple therapy' involving ciclosporin, azathioprine and prednisolone. However, the drugs and doses employed vary widely between individual transplant centres. Many tend to gradually withdraw the steroid, maintaining patients on dual therapy, while some commonly use monotherapy for prophylaxis.

Steroids. Prednisolone is the oral agent commonly used for immunosuppression after renal transplantation, while methylprednisolone is used intravenously in regimens to reverse acute rejection. The maintenance dose of prednisolone is about 10–20 mg/day given as a single dose in the morning to minimize adrenal suppression. The use of steroid therapy often leads to complications, particularly if high doses are given for long periods. In addition to a cushingoid state there may be gastrointestinal bleeding, hypertension, dyslipid-aemia, diabetes, osteoporosis and mental disturbances. Patients who are temporarily unable to take oral prednisolone should be given an equivalent dose of hydrocortisone intravenously.

Azathioprine. Azathioprine should be given in a dose of 2.5 mg/kg/day either orally or intravenously; the two routes have the same bioavailability. There is no advantage in giving it in divided doses. Since azathioprine interferes with nucleic acid synthesis, it may be mutagenic, and pharmacy and nursing staff should avoid handling the tablets. Azathioprine has a significant drug interaction with allopurinol causing fatal marrow suppression and this combination should be avoided.

Mycophenolate mofetil. Mycophenolate mofetil is a pro-drug of mycophenolic acid that has a more selective mode of action than azathioprine. It is licensed for prophylaxis against acute renal transplant rejection when used in combination with ciclosporin and steroids, and is given in a dose of 1 g twice daily. There is evidence that, compared to similar regimens incorporating azathioprine, it reduces the risk of acute rejection episodes; however, the risk of opportunistic infections and the occurrence of blood disorders such as leucopenia may be higher.

Ciclosporin. The discovery and development of ciclosporin immunosuppression regimens have greatly increased transplant survival rates. The action of ciclosporin is partially selective in that it suppresses T cytotoxic cell production and to some extent spares B lymphocyte activity, permitting a greater response to infection than can normally be mounted by patients using older forms of immunosuppression. Thus, there is a relatively low incidence of severe infection associated with ciclosporin therapy, although the incidence of malignancies appear to be similar to that found with other immunosuppressants.

Table 16.4   Mechanism of action of immunosuppressants commonly used following renal transplantation

Drug	Mechanism	Comment
Steroids	Bind to steroid receptors and inhibit gene transcription and function of T cells, macrophages and neutrophils	Prophylaxis against and reversal of rejection
Ciclosporin	Forms complex with intracellular protein cyclophilin → inhibits calcineurin. Ultimately inhibits interleukin-2 synthesis and T cell activation	Long-term maintenance therapy against rejection
Tacrolimus	Forms complex with an intracellular protein → inhibits calcineurin	Long-term maintenance therapy against rejection Rescue therapy in severe or refractory rejection
Sirolimus	Inhibits interleukin-2 cell signalling → blocks T cell cycling and inhibits B cells	Usually used in combination with ciclosporin ± steroids
Mycophenolate	Inhibits inosine monophosphate dehydrogenase → reduces nucleic acid synthesis → inhibits T and B cell function	Usually used in combination with ciclosporin/tacrolimus ± steroids
Azathioprine	Incorporated as a purine in DNA → inhibits lymphocyte and neutrophil proliferation	Usually used in combination with ciclosporin/tacrolimus ± steroids
Muromonab (OKT3, mouse monoclonal anti-CD3)	Binds to CD3 complex → blocks, inactivates or kills T cell. Short $T_{1/2}$	Prophylaxis against rejection Reversal of severe rejection
Polyclonal horse/rabbit antithymocyte globulin (ALG, ATG)	Antibodies against lymphocycte proteins → alter T and B cell activity	Prophylaxis against rejection Reversal of severe rejection
Humanized or chimeric anti-CD25 (basiliximab and daclizumab)	Monoclonal antibodies that bind CD25 in interleukin-2 complex → prevent T cell proliferation	Prophylaxis against acute rejection in combination with ciclosporin and steroids

The earliest formulation of ciclosporin, Sandimmun is currently only available on a named-patient basis for patients who cannot be transferred to a newer formulation such as Neoral.

Neoral is a formulation of ciclosporin that undergoes microemulsification in the presence of water. It was developed to reduce the bioavailability problems associated with Sandimmun. Since Neoral's absorption is more predictable, blood levels are easier to control although careful monitoring is still essential.

None of the formulations of ciclosporin should be administered with grapefruit juice, which should also be avoided for at least an hour pre dose, as this can result in marked increases in blood concentrations. This effect appears to be due to inhibition of enzyme systems in the gut wall resulting in transiently reduced ciclosporin metabolism.

Ciclosporin carries a high risk of side-effects, including nephrotoxicity, hypertension, fine muscle tremor, gingival hyperplasia, nausea and hirsutism. Serum biochemistry can also be adversely affected with dose-dependent increases in creatinine and urea occurring in the first few weeks of treatment. Hyperkalaemia, hyperuricaemia, hypomagnesaemia and hypercholestraemia may also occur. Nephrotoxicity is a particularly serious side-effect and occasionally necessitates the withdrawal of ciclosporin. There is tremendous inter- and intra-patient variation in absorption of ciclosporin. Blood level monitoring is essential to achieve the maximum protection against rejection with the minimum risk of side-effects. The range regarded as acceptable varies between centres, but is commonly taken as 100–200 ng/ml.

Ciclosporin is known to interact with a number of drugs that either lead to a reduction in ciclosporin levels (increased risk of rejection) or cause and elevation in ciclosporin levels (increased toxicity). Some drugs enhance the nephrotoxicity of ciclosporin (Table 16.5).

Table 16.5   Examples of drug interactions involving ciclosporin

Reduce ciclosporin serum levels (hepatic enzyme inducers):
Phenytoin, phenobarbital, rifampicin, isoniazid

Increase ciclosporin serum levels (hepatic enzyme inhibitors):
Diltiazem, erythromycin, corticosteroids, ketoconazole

Enhance ciclosporin nephrotoxicity:
Aminoglycosides, amphotericin, co-trimoxazole, melphalan

Tacrolimus.   Tacrolimus is not chemically related to ciclosporin, but acts by a similar mechanism. The side-effect profile also appears to be similar to that of ciclosporin with some subtle differences. Neurotoxicity is more common with tacrolimus, which also causes disturbances of glucose metabolism. In contrast, hirsutism is less of a problem. Tacrolimus appears to be particularly useful in attempts to reverse acute rejection episodes.

Anti-T-cell sera.   Anti-T-cell sera are used perioperatively as prophylaxis against rejection and in some cases to reverse episodes of severe rejection. The main preparations are antithymocyte globulin (ATG), antilymphocyte globulin (ALG) and OKT3.

Antithymocyte globulin (ATG) is an antilymphocyte globulin produced from rabbit serum immunized with human T cells. It contains antibodies to human T lymphocytes, which on injection will attach to, neutralize and eliminate most T lymphocytes, thereby weakening the immune response. Antilymphocyte globulin (ALG) is similar to ATG, but is of equine origin, and is not specific to T lymphocytes, acting on B lymphocytes also.

The main drawback to the use of anti-T-cell sera is the relatively high incidence of side-effects, notably anaphylactic reactions including hypotension, fever and urticaria. These reactions are more frequently observed with the first dose and may require supportive therapy with steroids and antihistamines. Severe reactions may necessitate stopping the treatment. Steroids and antihistamines may be given prophylactically to prevent or minimize allergic reactions. Pyrexia often occurs on the first day of treatment but usually subsides without requiring treatment. Tolerance testing by administration of a test dose is advisable, particularly in patients such as asthmetics who commonly experience allergic reactions. ALG and ATG can be substituted for each other, should adverse reactions occur.

Table 16.6   Common therapeutic problems in chronic renal failure

Problem	Comment
Drug choice	Care with choice/dose of all drugs. Care to avoid renotoxic agents pre-dialysis to preserve function. Beware herbal therapies as some contain immune system boosters (reverse immunosuppressant effects) and some are nephrotoxic
Drug excretion	CRF will lead to accumulation of drugs and their active metabolites if they are normally excreted by the kidney
Dietary restrictions	Restrictions on patient often severe. Fluid allowance includes foods with high water content, e.g. gravy, custard, and fruit
Hypertension	Frequently requires complex multiple drug regimens. Calcium channel blockers can cause oedema that might be confused with fluid overload
Analgesia	Side-effects are increased. Initiate with low doses and gradually increase. Avoid pethidine as metabolites accumulate. Avoid NSAIDs unless specialist advice available
Anaemia	Epoetin requires sufficient iron stores to be effective. Absorption from oral iron supplements may be poor and i.v. iron supplementation might be required. Care required to make sure that epoetin use does not produce hypertension
Immunosuppression	Use of live vaccines should be avoided (BCG, MMR, mumps, oral polio, oral typhoid, smallpox, yellow fever)
Pruritis (itching)	Can be severe. Treat with chlorphenamine (chlorpheniramine); less sedating antihistamines often less effective. Some relief with topical agents, e.g. crotamiton
Restless legs	Involuntary jerks can prevent sleep. Clonazepam 0.5 mg–1 mg at night may help

Monoclonal antibodies. Muromonab (OKT3) is a monoclonal antibody directed against the CD3 complex associated with human T cell receptors. It blocks the function and generation of the T cytotoxic cells responsible for kidney transplant rejection. Muromonab has a short half-life and is eventually neutralized by an antibody response. As with other anti-T-cell sera, the main drawbacks to the use of muromonab are its side-effects, which include nausea, vomiting and diarrhoea, marked pyrexia (often over 40°C), chills, dyspnoea, chest pain and rigors. It is common practice to prescribe agents prophylactically against these side-effects, especially with the early doses of the course.

The humanized or chimeric anti-CD25 monoclonal antibodies basiliximab and daclizumab bind to CD25 in the interleukin-2 complex. This renders all T cells resistant to interleukin-2 and therefore prevents T cell proliferation. They are used as prophylaxis against acute rejection in combination with ciclosporin and steroids.

Other precautions

Transplant patients will be given prophylactic antibiotic therapy for varying periods postoperatively owing to the risks of infection associated with immunosuppression. Treatment with co-trimoxazole to prevent *Pneumocystis carinii*, isoniazid and pyridoxine to prevent tuberculosis, aciclovir or ganciclovir to prevent cytomegalovirus, and nystatin or amphotericin to prevent oral candidiasis are commonly used. Vaccination with live organisms (e.g. BCG, MMR, oral poliomyelitis, oral typhoid) must be avoided in the immunosuppressed patient.

CASE STUDIES

Case 16.1

Mr D., a 19-year-old undergraduate student, visited his university health centre complaining of a 3-month history of fatigue, weakness, nausea and vomiting that he had attributed to 'examination stress'. His previous medical history indicated an ongoing history of bed wetting from an early age. Laboratory results from a routine blood screen showed:

		Reference range
Sodium	137 mmol/l	(135–145)
Potassium	4.8 mmol/l	(3.5–5.0)
Phosphate	2.5 mmol/l	(0.9–1.5)
Calcium	1.6 mmol/l	(2.20–2.55)
Urea	52 mmol/l	(3.0–6.5)
Creatinine	620 μmol/l	(50–120)
Haemoglobin	7.5 g/dl	(13.5–18.0)

Subsequent referral to a specialist hospital centre established a diagnosis of chronic renal failure secondary to reflux nephropathy.

Question

Explain the signs and symptoms experienced by Mr D. and the likely course of his disease?

Answer

Mr D. is suffering from the signs and symptoms of uraemia resulting from chronic renal failure. Mechanical reflux damage to his kidneys has compromised renal function and resulted in an accumulation of toxins, including urea and creatinine that, in turn, have contributed to his nausea, vomiting and general malaise. His biochemical results indicate other typical features of uraemic syndrome associated with chronic renal failure. The low haemoglobin is indicative of reduced erythropoetin production following progressive kidney damage. Renal osteodystrophy is also present, as inadequate vitamin D production and the raised serum phosphate have contributed to the hypocalaemia.

This patient is likely to have remained symptom free for a period of years despite progressively worsening renal function. The kidney operates with a substantial functional reserve under normal conditions. Patients generally remain asymptomatic as their renal reserve diminishes. Eventually there is a failure in the ability of the damaged kidney to compensate and symptoms appear late in the condition.

Case 16.2

Mr K., a 43-year-old male with established CRF, had been maintained for 3 years on continuous ambulatory peritoneal dialysis. He was admitted to hospital for cadaveric renal transplantation. On examination he was found to have slight ankle oedema. He weighed 60 kg and his blood pressure was 135/90 mmHg and pulse rate 77/min. He was administered the following immunosuppressants preoperatively: ciclosporin 150 mg i.v. (approximately 3 mg/kg), azathioprine 50 mg i.v. (approximately 1 mg/kg). Methylprednisolone 1 g was given intravenously immediately after grafting.

Question

How should the intravenous immunosuppressants be administered in this patient and how should immunosuppression be managed postoperatively?

Answer

In a patient with CRF consideration should be given to the use of dextrose 5% as a vehicle rather than normal saline in order to reduce the sodium load and therefore minimize the risks of fluid overload. Ciclosporin should be diluted at least 1:20 and, ideally, administered over 2 hours. With cadaveric transplants, time is usually limited and the inevitable rapid administration of ciclosporin will increase the likelihood of side-effects. Ciclosporin injection can precipitate severe allergic reactions and the patient should be checked regularly. Azathioprine is very irritant and the intravenous line should be flushed following administration. Intravenous triple therapy can be continued postoperatively until the patient can manage oral medication.

Typically, ciclosporin 5 mg/kg/day, azathioprine 1 mg/kg/day and methylprednisolone 300 micrograms/kg/day are used intravenously. However, in practice regimens vary considerably from centre to centre.

Oral therapy should be initiated as soon as the patient can practically manage. Predisolone should replace methylprednisolone according to the potency ratio 5:4, resulting in a daily oral dose of 22.5 mg. Azathioprine absorption can be variable; however, in most patients the oral dose is the same as that given intravenously. Ciclosporin absorption is subject to inter-patient variability, although the microemulsion formulation of Neoral has led to improvements, as absorption from the gastrointestinal tract is not bile salt-dependent. Generally the initial oral dose of ciclosporin should be about three times the intravenous dose, i.e. 450 mg twice daily in this patient. The dose should be individualized by measuring plasma levels after 3 days with appropriate adjustment.

Case 16.3

Mr A. is a patient with CRF secondary to chronic interstitial nephritis. He complains of chronic fatigue, lethargy and breathlessness on exertion, palpitations and poor concentration. His recent haematological results were found to be:

		Reference range
Haemoglobin	5.6 g/dl	(13.5–17.5)
Red cell count	$2.92 \times 10^9/l$	$(4.5–6.5 \times 10^9/l)$
Haematocrit	0.208	(0.40–0.54)
Serum ferritin	88.0 micrograms/l	(15–300)

Question

Explain this patient's symptoms and haematological results and outline the optimal treatment.

Answer

Mr A.'s symptoms are most likely to result from a normochromic, normocytic anaemia caused by renal failure. Levels of erythropoetin produced by the kidney are reduced in renal failure. Production of erythropoetin from extra-renal sites, e.g. liver, are not sufficient to maintain erythropoesis, which is also inhibited by uraemic toxins and hyperparathyroidism. The anaemia associated with renal failure is further compounded by a reduction in red cell survival through low-grade haemolysis, bleeding from the gastrointestinal tract and blood loss through dialysis, aluminium toxicity which interferes with haem synthesis, and iron deficiency, usually through poor dietary intake.

Therapy with epoetin is the treatment of choice. However, iron and folate deficiencies should be corrected if epoetin therapy is to be successful. Iron demands are generally raised during epoetin treatment and iron status should be regularly monitored. If serum ferritin falls below 100 micrograms/l then iron supplementation should be started. Often intravenous iron is required to provide an adequate supply, despite the dangers associated with administration of iron by this route.

REFERENCE

UK Renal Registry 1999 Second annual report, Renal Association, Bristol

FURTHER READING

Cassidy M J D 1999 Renal osteodystrophy. Medicine 27(6): 37–40

Macdougall I C 1999 Anaemia of chronic renal failure. Medicine 27(6): 41–43

Masterson T M, Kimmel P L 1999 Management of chronic renal failure. Medicine 27(6): 33–37

O'Callaghan C A, Brenner B M 2000 The kidney at a glance. Blackwell Science, Oxford

Ready A R 1999 Renal transplantation. Medicine 27(6): 50–52

Walker R 1997 Recent advances: general management of end stage renal disease. British Medical Journal 315: 1429–1432

Hypertension 17

S. H. L. Thomas

KEY POINTS

- Hypertension can be defined as a condition in which blood pressure is elevated to an extent where benefit is obtained from blood pressure lowering. There is no clear-cut blood pressure threshold separating normal from hypertensive individuals. The risk of complications is related to the extent that blood pressure is elevated.
- The complications of hypertension include stroke, myocardial infarction, heart failure, renal failure and dissecting aortic aneurysm. Small reductions in blood pressure result in substantial reductions in the relative risks of these complications.
- For correct diagnosis, careful measurement of blood pressure is necessary on several occasions using well-maintained and validated equipment.
- Non-pharmacological interventions are important and include weight reduction, avoidance of excessive salt and alcohol, increased intake of fruit and vegetables and regular dynamic exercise. Other cardiovascular risk factors such as smoking, hyperlipidaemia and diabetes should be addressed.
- A large selection of antihypertensive drugs is available. It is important to use a drug that is free from adverse effects.
- Most patients should start with a thiazide diuretic, but the choice of drug therapy will also be determined by other medical conditions that are present.
- Many people need combinations of drugs to achieve adequate blood pressure control. Medication should be convenient to take and adverse effects should be avoided.

evidence from clinical trials to demonstrate that treatment of subjects with blood pressures above the thresholds currently used in clinical practice results in important clinical benefits.

The cardiovascular complications associated with hypertension are shown in Table 17.1. The most common and important of these are stroke and myocardial infarction. An increase of 5 mmHg in usual diastolic blood pressure is associated with a 35–40% increased risk of stroke. There is a similar but less steep association for coronary heart disease risk. The risk of heart failure is increased sixfold in hypertensive subjects. Meta-analysis of clinical trials has indicated that a 38% reduction in stroke and a 16% reduction in coronary events results from drug therapy which reduces blood pressure by approximately 10/6 mm of mercury (Collins et al 1990). A 5 mmHg reduction in blood pressure is associated with a 25% reduction in risk of renal failure.

The absolute benefits of blood pressure lowering achieved as a result of these relative risk reductions depend on the underlying level of risk in an individual subject. High-risk subjects gain more benefit in terms of events saved per year of therapy. Absolute risk is increased for those who already have evidence of cardiovascular disease, such as previous myocardial infarction, transient ischaemic attack, stroke, etc., or who

Hypertension (high blood pressure) is not a disease but an important risk factor for cardiovascular complications. It can be defined as a condition where blood pressure is elevated to an extent where clinical benefit is obtained from blood pressure lowering. Blood pressure measurement includes systolic and diastolic components, and both are important in determining an individual's cardiovascular risk.

Blood pressure is continuously distributed in the population and there is no clear cut-off point between hypertensive and normotensive subjects. Blood pressure values that are used as treatment thresholds or targets are therefore arbitrary. Nevertheless, there is considerable

Table 17.1 Complications of hypertension
- Myocardial infarction

- Stroke
   Cerebral/brainstem infarction
   Cerebral haemorrhage
   Lacunar syndromes
   Multi-infarct disease

- Hypertensive encephalopathy/malignant hypertension
- Dissecting aortic aneurysm
- Hypertensive nephrosclerosis
- Peripheral vascular disease

have other evidence of cardiovascular dysfunction such as electrocardiogram (ECG) or echocardiographic abnormalities. Risk is also increased in the elderly and in people with diabetes or renal failure and is further enhanced by other risk factors such as smoking, hyperlipidaemia, obesity and sedentary lifestyle. In those under the age of 75, men are at greater risk than women. Cardiovascular risk in an individual who has no current cardiovascular disease can be estimated from tables or nomograms such as the Joint British Societies coronary risk prediction chart (Ramsay et al 1999a) or the revised Sheffield tables (Wallis et al 2000).

Genetic factors account for about one-third of the blood pressure variation between individuals although no single gene appears to be responsible except in some rare disease processes (Beevers et al 2001). The remaining 5–10% of cases are secondary to some other disease process (Table 17.2).

Blood pressure increases with age in Westernized societies and hypertension is therefore substantially more common in elderly subjects. It is also more common in people of African Caribbean origin, who are also at particular risk of stroke and renal failure. Hypertension is exacerbated by other factors, for example high salt or alcohol intake or obesity.

Epidemiology

Between 10% and 25% of the population are expected to benefit from drug treatment of hypertension, the exact figure depending on the cut-off value for blood pressure and the age group considered for active treatment.

In 90–95% of cases of hypertension there is no underlying medical illness to cause high blood pressure. This is termed 'essential' hypertension. The aetiology of essential hypertension is currently unknown. Genetic factors clearly play a part and essential hypertension tends to run in families, with hypertension being twice as common in subjects who have a hypertensive parent.

Regulation of blood pressure

The mean blood pressure is the product of cardiac output and total peripheral resistance. In most hypertensive individuals cardiac output is not increased and high blood pressure arises as a result of increased total peripheral resistance caused by constriction of small arterioles.

Control of blood pressure is important in evolutionary terms and a number of homeostatic reflexes have

---

Table 17.2 Causes of hypertension

Primary hypertension (90–95%)
· Essential hypertension

Secondary hypertension (5–10%)

● Renal diseases

● Endocrine diseases
Steroid excess	– hyperaldosteronism (Conn's syndrome)
	– hyperglucocorticoidism (Cushing's syndrome)
Growth hormone excess	– acromegaly
Catecholamine excess	– phaeochromocytoma
Others	– pre-eclampsia

● Vascular causes
Renal artery stenosis	– fibromuscular hyperplasia
	– renal artery atheroma
Coarctation of the aorta	

● Drugs
Sympathomimetic amines
Oestrogens (e.g. combined oral contraceptive pills)
Ciclosporin
Erythropoietin
Non-steroidal anti-inflammatory drugs (NSAIDs)
Steroids

evolved to provide blood pressure homeostasis. Minute-to-minute changes in blood pressure are regulated by the baroreceptor reflex, while the renin–angiotensin aldosterone cascade is important for longer term salt, water and blood pressure control. Increases in blood pressure are also attenuated by local release of nitric oxide from vascular endothelium in response to increased sheer stresses in the blood vessel wall, and endothelial dysfunction is implicated in the pathogenesis of hypertension. Other mechanisms that also play a part in controlling blood pressure include secretion of atrial natiuretic peptide, endothelins, bradykinin and antidiuretic hormone (Beevers et al 2001).

Clinical presentation

Hypertension itself causes no symptoms. Although headache may be present, it is usually unclear if this is caused by hypertension or is an incidental finding. Hypertension is often an incidental finding when subjects present with unrelated conditions. It may be discovered as a result of systematic population screening. In the UK, all patients under 80 years of age should have their blood pressure checked at least every 5 years, with an annual review for those with high normal values in the range 135–139 systolic or 85–89 diastolic. Hypertension may also come to light for the first time when the individual suffers a hypertension-related complication such as myocardial infarction (MI) or stroke.

Malignant (accelerated) hypertension

Malignant or accelerated hypertension is an uncommon condition characterized by greatly elevated blood pressure associated with evidence of ongoing small vessel damage. This is evident in the optic fundus, where papilloedema, haemorrhages and/or exudates may be present. Renal damage, including haematuria, proteinuria and impaired renal function, is also characteristic. The condition may be associated with hypertensive encephalopathy, which is caused by small vessel changes in the cerebral circulation associated with cerebral oedema. The clinical features are confusion, headache, visual loss and coma.

Malignant hypertension is a medical emergency that requires hospital admission and rapid control of blood pressure over 12–24 hours towards normal levels. In the absence of treatment, malignant hypertension is usually fatal with a 1-year survival of less than 20%. Fortunately, the condition has become much less common since the advent of effective antihypertensive therapy, although there is still substantial long-term morbidity and patients require careful follow-up.

Management of hypertension

In the UK the management of hypertension is guided by consensus guidelines produced by the British Hypertension Society (BHS). The guidelines are available in both detailed (Ramsay et al 1999a) and summary (Ramsay et al 1999b) forms and also via the internet (www.hyp.ac.uk/bhs/).

Diagnosis of hypertension

Blood pressure should be measured using a well-maintained sphygmomanometer of validated accuracy. The subject should be relaxed and, at least at the first presentation, blood pressure should be measured in both the sitting and the standing positions. It is important to use an appropriate sized cuff since one that is too small will result in an overestimation of the patient's blood pressure. As a result a person may be falsely diagnosed as having hypertension and may receive unnecessary treatment with antihypertensive drugs. The arm should be supported level with the heart. It is important that the patient does not hold the arm out since isometric exercise increases blood pressure. Blood pressure is measured using the Korotkov sounds which appear (the first phase) and disappear (the fifth phase) over the brachial artery as pressure in the cuff is released. Cuff deflation should occur at approximately 2 mmHg per second to allow accurate measurement of the systolic and diastolic blood pressures. The fourth Korotkov phase (muffling of sound) has previously been used for diastolic blood pressure measurement but is not currently recommended.

Having established that the blood pressure is increased, the measurement should be repeated several times over several weeks, unless the initial measurement is at dangerously high levels, in which case several measurements should be made during the same clinic attendance.

Some people develop excessive and unrepresentative blood pressure when attending the doctors surgery, so called 'white coat' hypertension. When the blood pressure is checked at home, it is normal. These patients can be diagnosed if they use a blood pressure machine themselves at home or by 24-hour ambulatory blood pressure monitoring. Home blood pressure measurement is inexpensive but it is important to have a machine of validated accuracy that the patient can use properly. Ambulatory blood pressure monitoring over 24 hours is also useful for patients who have unusual variability in blood pressure, resistant hypertension or symptoms suggesting hypotension. Home or ambulatory blood pressure measurements are usually lower than clinic recordings, on average by 12/7 mm of mercury.

Assessment of the hypertensive patient

For possible secondary causes

It is important to take a careful history for features that might suggest a possible secondary cause. Examples would be symptoms of renal disease (e.g. haematuria, polyuria, etc.) or the paroxysmal symptoms that suggest the rare diagnosis of phaeochromocytoma. A careful physical examination should be performed for abdominal bruits (suggesting possible renal artery stenosis), radiofemoral delay (suggesting coarctation of the aorta) and palpable kidneys (suggesting renal disease). Laboratory analysis should include a full blood count, electrolytes, urea, creatinine and urinalysis. In some patients further investigations may be appropriate, for example ultrasound of the abdomen or isotope renogram where renal disease is expected, a renin–angiotensin ratio to investigate for possible hyperaldosteronism and 24-hour or overnight urinary catecholamines for phaeochromocytoma.

For contributing factors

The patient should also be assessed for possible contributory factors to hypertension such as obesity, excess alcohol or salt intake and lack of exercise. Occasionally, hypertension may be provoked by the use of drugs (see Table 17.2), including over-the-counter medicines. Other risk factors should also be documented and addressed, for example smoking, diabetes and hyperlipidaemia. It is important to establish whether there is a family history of cardiovascular disease.

For evidence of end organ damage

The patient should also be examined carefully for evidence of end organ damage from hypertension. This should include examination of the optic fundi to detect retinal changes. An ECG should be performed to detect left ventricular hypertrophy or subclinical ischaemic heart disease.

Treatment

Non-pharmacological approaches

Non-pharmacological management of hypertension is important, although the effects are often disappointing. In order to maximize potential benefit, patients should receive clear and unambiguous advice, including written information that they can digest in their own time. Written advice for patients can be downloaded from the BHS website (www.hyp.ac.uk/bhs/).

Weight loss results in reduction in blood pressure of about 2.5/1.5 mmHg per kilogram. Subjects should reduce their salt intake, for example by not adding salt to food on the plate. A diet high in fruit and vegetables, legumes and wholegrain cereal improves cardiovascular risk. Most subjects will need to control their intake of calories and saturated fat. Regular dynamic exercise, at a level appropriate to the individual subject, should occur at least three times weekly for maximum benefit. This results in improved physical fitness as well as a reduction in blood pressure. Alcohol intake should be restricted to 2 or 3 units per day.

Unless hypertension is severe, it is appropriate to observe the subject over several months while instituting non-pharmacological interventions. However, if there is a more urgent need for drug treatment non-pharmacological interventions should occur in parallel.

Drug treatment

Treatment thresholds. Treatment thresholds are summarized in Table 17.3. Patients with severe hypertension (> 200/110 confirmed on several readings on the same occasion) should be treated immediately. Patients whose initial blood pressure is in the range 160–199/100–110 should be observed over a few weeks and then treated if the blood pressure persists at this level. Patients whose blood pressure is in the range 140–159/90–99 should be observed annually unless they have evidence of target organ damage, cardiovascular complications, diabetes or a calculated cardiovascular risk > 15% over 10 years, in which case drug treatment should be offered. Patients with blood pressure in the range 135–139/85–89 should be reassessed annually, while those with blood pressure lower than this can be rechecked every 5 years.

Target blood pressures. Evidence from the hypertension optimal treatment study (Hansson et al 1998) suggested that the optimum target blood pressure was 139/83 for patients whose initial diastolic blood pressure was between 100 and 115. Although no harm was demonstrated by reducing blood pressure further, patients are little disadvantaged provided their blood pressure is controlled below 150/90. Diabetic patients are an exception and benefit from more aggressive blood pressure reduction. Target blood pressures for diabetic and non-diabetic subjects are summarized in Table 17.4. It should be emphasized that the audit standard will not be achieved in all patients.

Choice of drugs. As in other clinical situations, drugs should be chosen on the basis of efficacy, safety, convenience to the patient and cost. For assessing efficacy, it is more important to use evidence from large-scale clinical 'end point' trials than smaller scale studies looking at the effects of drugs on blood pressure. When considering safety, it is important to recognize that these drugs will be taken in the long term and there are

Table 17.3   Threshold blood pressures for intervention

Initial blood pressure		Management
Systolic	Diastolic	
Malignant hypertension		Admit and treat immediately
> 200	> 110	Repeat several times at the same attendance and treat if blood pressure persists in this range
160–169	100–109	Repeat over several weeks, institute non-pharmacological measures and treat if blood pressure persists in this range
140–159	90–99	Repeat over several weeks. Institute non-pharmacological measures. Treat if remains in this range and patient has target organ damage, cardiovascular complications or an estimated 10 year coronary heat disease risk > 15%. Otherwise reassess annually
135–139	85–89	Reassess annually
< 135	< 85	Reassess in 5 years

Table 17.4   Target blood pressures according to British Hypertension Society guidelines 1999 (Ramsay et al 1999a and 1999b)

	Clinic blood pressure		Home/ambulatory blood pressure	
	No diabetes	Diabetes	No diabetes	Diabetes
Optimal	< 140/85	< 140/80	< 130/80	< 130/75
Audit standard	< 150/90	< 140/85	< 140/85	< 140/80

advantages to using drugs which have long established safety records. It is also important to recognize the importance of symptomatic adverse effects since these may reduce compliance. Patients should feel as well during treatment of their blood pressure as they did before drug treatment was instituted. Patient convenience is another important factor and use of once or twice daily preparations will result in better compliance than more frequent regimens. Since the hypertensive population is very large it is necessary to be conscious of the cost of individual preparations. Combinations of low doses of antihypertensive drugs are often better tolerated than single drugs taken in high dose.

The choice of drugs available for treating hypertension is shown in Table 17.5, and common therapeutic problems are noted. Most evidence of benefit in placebo-controlled clinical trials comes from studies that primarily involved thiazide diuretics or β-blockers (Table 17.6). However, there is increasing evidence of clinical benefit from newer drug classes including angiotensin-converting enzyme (ACE) inhibitors and calcium channel blockers. There is no convincing evidence that any drug group is more effective than any other in reducing clinical end points, although there may be advantages for particular patient subgroups (Table 17.7). Unless there are compelling reasons (e.g. contraindications or intolerance with other drugs), most patients, and particularly the elderly, should receive a low dose of a thiazide diuretic as first line therapy. The majority of hypertensives are not adequately controlled by a single drug and more than a third will require three or more drugs to produce ideal blood pressure control.

Diuretics

There is substantial clinical trial evidence that benefit is obtained from the use of thiazide diuretics in hypertension, and these drugs are both inexpensive and well tolerated by most patients. They initially reduce blood pressure by reducing circulating blood volume. However, in the longer term blood volume is restored towards normal and the fall in blood pressure is associated with a reduction in total peripheral resistance,

Table 17.5 Summary of antihypertensive drugs and common therapeutic problems

Class	Examples	Major adverse effects	Notes
Diuretics	Thiazides – bendroflumethiazide (bendrofluazide) Loops – furosemide (frusemide)	Hypokalaemia Gout Glucose intolerance Hyperlipidaemia Uraemia Dehydration Impotence	Cheap, effective. Efficacy proven in clinical trials. Concerns about long term metabolic effects. First-line Especially for patients with cardiac failure and the elderly
β-blockers	Atenolol Propranolol Metoprolol Labetalol Celiprolol	Tiredness Reduced exercise tolerance Bradycardia Cold peripheries Claudication Wheezing Cardiac failure Impotence	Cheap, effective. Adverse effects common, especially in young. Efficacy proven in clinical trials First-line Especially for patients with ischaemic heart disease
Calcium antagonists – dihydropyridine	Nifedipine Amlodipine	Flushing Oedema Postural hypotension Headache	More expensive. Not well tolerated (especially early in treatment). Recent trials confirm reductions in stroke and myocardial infarction. Similar efficacy to thiazides. Especially for patients with ischaemic heart disease or diabetes
Calcium ischaemic antagonists – rate limiting	Verapamil Diltiazem	Bradycardia/heart block Constipation (verapamil only)	Well tolerated. Suitable for patients with heart disease who are unable to tolerate β-blockers Caution needed when used in combination with β-blockers
ACE inhibitors	Captopril Enalapril Lisinopril Perindopril Ramipril	Cough Rash, taste disturbance Renal failure Angioedema	More expensive. Cough very common Efficacy appears no better than conventional therapy Limit use to those with cardiac failure or diabetes, and those with resistant hypertension
α-blockers	Prazosin Doxazosin Terazosin	Oedema Postural hypotension	More expensive. Adverse effects common. No evidence to date of long-term efficacy. Less effective than thiazides at preventing heart failure and combined cardiovascular outcomes (ALLHAT study) Second-line
Angiotensin II antagonists	Losartan Valsartan Irbesartan	Renal failure Oedema Headache	More expensive Especially for patients in whom ACE inhibitor indicated but not tolerated due to cough More effective in preventing vascular events than atenolol in patients with LVH
Centrally acting vasodilators	Methyldopa Moxonidine	Tiredness Depression	Poorly tolerated. Only use in severe hypertension or hypertension of pregnancy Third-line
Direct acting vasodilators	Diazoxide Minoxidil Nitroprusside	Oedema Postural hypotension Headache	Poorly tolerated. Only use in severe hypertension

Table 17.6 Placebo-controlled trials of antihypertensive drug therapy

Trial	Reference	Drugs – first-line (second-line)
Veterans administration study	Veterans Administration (1970)	Thiazide (reserpine, hydralazine)
Joint National Committee on Detection, Evaluation, and Treatment of High Blood Pressure	Anon (1977)	Thiazide (rauwolfia)
Australian therapeutic trial in mild hypertension	Anon (1980)	Thiazide (methyldopa, propranolol, pindolol, hydralazine, clonidine)
Medical Research Council trial of treatment of mild hypertension	MRC (1985)	Thiazide and propranolol
European working party on high blood pressure in the elderly trial	Amery et al (1985)	Thiazide (methyldopa)
Systolic hypertension in the elderly program (SHEP)	SHEP (1991)	Thiazide (atenolol)
Swedish trial of old patients with hypertension (STOP – hypertension).	Dahlöf et al (1991)	Thiazide (amiloride, atenolol, metoprolol, pindolol)
Medical Research Council trial of treatment of hypertension in older adults	MRC (1992)	Thiazide and atenolol
Shanghai trial of nifedipine in the elderly (STONE)	Gong et al (1996)	Nifedipine
Systolic hypertension in Europe (SYST-EUR) trial	Staessen et al (1997)	Nitrendipine (thiazide, enalapril)
Systolic hypertension in China (SYST-CHINA) trial	Liu et al (1998)	Nitrendipine (thiazide, captopril)

suggesting a direct vasodilatory action. Thiazide diuretics are appropriate for most patients. Loop diuretics are no more effective at lowering blood pressure unless renal function is significantly impaired or the patient is receiving agents that inhibit the renin–angiotensin system. Most blood pressure lowering occurs with very low doses of thiazide diuretics. Increasing the dose substantially increases the risk of metabolic disturbance without causing further blood pressure reduction. For bendroflumethiazide (bendrofluazide), it is rarely (if ever) appropriate to use doses greater than 2.5 mg per day and a dose of 1.25 mg daily is often effective.

β-adrenoreceptor antagonists

β-blockers also have substantial clinical trial evidence of benefit and are relatively inexpensive. Their mode of action in hypertension is uncertain. Beta blockade reduces cardiac output in the short term and during exercise. They also reduce renin secretion by antagonizing secretion by antagonizing β-receptors in the juxtaglomerular apparatus. Central actions may also be important for some agents. Non-selective β-blockers may give rise to adverse effects as a result of antagonism of β_2 adrenoceptors, i.e. asthma and worsened intermittent claudication. However, so-called 'cardioselective' (β_1-selective) β-blockers are not free of these adverse effects. Patients who develop very marked bradycardia and tiredness may tolerate a drug with partial agonist activity such as pindolol.

Renin–angiotensin–aldosterone antagonists

ACE inhibitors block the conversion of angiotensin I to angiotensin II, while angiotensin II antagonists block the action of angiotensin II at the $AT2_1$ receptor. Since angiotensin II is a vasoconstrictor and stimulates the

Table 17.7 Use of antihypertensive drugs adapted from British Hypertension Society guidelines. Strong indications and contraindications are shown, with weak/possible indications or contraindications in parentheses

Class	Indications	Contraindications
Diuretics	Elderly	Gout (Dyslipidaemia)
β-blockers	Myocardial infarction Angina (Heart failure)	Asthma/chronic obstructive pulmonary disease (COPD) Heart block (Heart failure) (Dyslipidaemia) (Peripheral vascular disease)
Calcium antagonists – dihydropyridine	Elderly isolated systolic hypertension (Elderly) (Angina)	
Calcium antagonists (rate limiting)	Angina (Myocardial infarction)	Combination with β-blocker (Heart block) (Heart failure)
ACE inhibitors	Heart failure Left ventricular (LV) dysfunction Type 1 diabetic nephropathy (Chronic renal disease) (Type 2 diabetic nephropathy)	Pregnancy Renovascular disease (Renal impairment) (Peripheral vascular disease)
α-blockers	Prostatism (Dyslipidaemia)	Urinary incontinence (Postural hypotension)
Angiotensin II antagonists	Cough with ACE inhibitors (when ACE inhibitors indicated)	As ACE inhibitors
Centrally acting vasodilators	Pregnancy (methyldopa only) Resistant hypertension unresponsive to first-line therapy	
Direct acting vasodilators	Resistant hypertension, unresponsive to first-line therapy	

release of aldosterone, antagonism results in vasodilatation and potsassium retention as well as inhibition of salt and water retention. ACE inhibitors also block kininase and thus prevent the break down of bradykinin. This appears to be important in the aetiology of cough, which is a troublesome side-effect of these drugs. Angiotensin II antagonists do not inhibit kininase, and are an appropriate choice for patients who are intolerant of ACE inhibitors because of cough.

The recent captopril prevention project (CAPPP) (Hansson et al 1999b) demonstrated that captopril was as effective as diuretics or β-blockers for preventing cardiovascular morbidity. However, captopril was associated with a 25% higher stroke risk, perhaps because it did not reduce blood pressure as effectively as conventional therapy in this particular study.

The recently published Losartan For Endpoint reduction in hypertension study (LIFE) (Dahlöf et al 2002) demonstrated that iosartan was more effective at preventing vascular events, especially stroke, than atenolol in hypertensive patients with LVH.

Calcium channel blockers

These agents block slow calcium channels in the peripheral blood vessels and/or the heart. The dihydropyridine group work almost exclusively on peripheral arterioles and reduce blood pressure by reducing total peripheral resistance. In contrast, verapamil's effects are primarily on the heart, reducing heart rate and cardiac output. Dihydropyridines that are long acting are preferred because they are more convenient for patients and avoid the large fluctuations in plasma drug concentrations that may be associated with adverse effects.

Concerns have previously been raised by observational studies (Psaty et al 1995) and meta-analysis (Furberg et al 1995) that there may be an increased risk of coronary heart disease in recipients of dihydropyridine calcium channel blockers. However, recent randomized clinical trials have not confirmed these observations (Gong et al 1996, Staessen et al 1997, Liu et al 1998) and have indicated that dihydropyridines are of similar efficacy to thiazide diuretics in preventing cardiovascular events (Brown et al 2000).

α adrenoreceptor blockers

Drugs of this class antagonize α adrenoceptors in the blood vessel wall and thus prevent noradrenaline (norepinephrine) induced vasoconstriction. As a result, they reduce total peripheral resistance and blood pressure. Prazosin was originally used but has the disadvantage of being short-acting and causing first dose hypotension. Newer agents such as doxazosin and terazosin have a longer duration of action. There are concerns about the first-line use of α-blockers since the Antihypertensive and Lipid Lowering treatment to prevent Heart Attack Trial (ALLHAT) study has indicated doxazosin is more often associated with heart failure and stroke than thiazide diuretics (ALLHAT 2000). However, they are an appropriate choice as add-in therapy for patients inadequately controlled using other agents.

Centrally acting agents

Methyldopa and moxonidine inhibit sympathetic outflow from the brain resulting in a reduction in total peripheral resistance. Methyldopa is not widely used because it has pronounced central adverse effects including tiredness and depression. It continues to be used in pregnancy, since it has a very good safety record. It is also sometimes needed for people with resistant hypertension. Moxonidine is a newer agent that blocks central imidazoline and α_2 adrenoceptors. It appears to have fewer central adverse effects than methyldopa. Other centrally acting agents such as clonidine and reserpine are almost never used in modern practice because of their pronounced adverse effects.

Other agents

Several other drugs are available for use for people with more resistant hypertension. Minoxidil is a powerful antihypertensive drug but its use is associated with severe peripheral oedema and reflex tachycardia. It should be restricted to patients with severe hypertension who are also taking β-blockers and diuretics. It causes pronounced hirsutism and is not a suitable treatment for women. Hydralazine can be used as add on therapy for patients with resistant hypertension but is not well tolerated and may occasionally be associated with drug-induced systemic lupus erythematosus. Sodium nitroprusside is a direct acting arterial and venous dilator that is administered as an intravenous infusion for treating hypertensive emergencies and for the acute control of blood pressure during anaesthesia. Hypertension has previously been treated with ganglion blockers such as guanethidine but these drugs are now of historical interest only.

Special patient groups

Race

People of African Caribbean origin have an increased prevalence of hypertension and left ventricular hypertrophy. They are at high risk of stroke and renal failure. They obtain particular benefit from reduced salt intake and are also sensitive to diuretic and calcium channel blockers, while β-blockers appear less effective, at least when used as monotherapy. African Caribbean people have reduced plasma renin activity and, as a result, ACE inhibitors and angiotensin antagonists are also less effective.

British Asians also have an increased prevalence of hypertension, diabetes and insulin resistance and a particularly high risk of coronary heart disease. There is currently no evidence of a difference in drug response when compared with white Europeans.

Elderly

The elderly have a high prevalence of hypertension and are also at high absolute risk of cardiovascular events. Therefore the absolute benefits of blood pressure treatment are particularly large in this group. Antihypertensive therapy may also reduce the risk of heart failure and dementia (Seux et al 1999). However, the elderly may be at risk of certain adverse effects of treatment such as postural hypotension. Nevertheless, the benefits of therapy are so great that treatment should be offered at any age unless the patient is very frail or their life expectancy is very short. Isolated systolic hypertension (systolic > 160, diastolic < 90 mmHg) is common in the elderly and there is irrefutable evidence that drug treatment is beneficial in this group (SHEP 1991, Staessen et al 1997, Liu et al 1998).

Low dose thiazide diuretics are a safe and effective treatment for elderly hypertensive people and their use is endorsed by large-scale clinical trials. Calcium channel blockers are a suitable alternative. β-blockers may be less effective at reducing blood pressure and preventing clinical end points. The Swedish trial in old patients with hypertension-2 (STOP-2) study compared the effects of conventional (β-blocker or thiazide) and newer drugs (ACE inhibitors or calcium channel blockers) on cardiovascular morbidity in older subjects and did not detect significant differences (Hansson et al 1999a).

Diabetes

In type I diabetes, the presence of hypertension often indicates the presence of diabetic nephropathy. In this group, blood pressure reduction and ACE inhibition slow the rate of decline in renal function. To achieve adequate blood pressure control combinations of drugs will be needed. Thiazides, β-blockers, calcium channel blockers, and α-blockers are all suitable as add on treatments to ACE inhibitors which should be first-line therapy. Target blood pressure should be < 130/80, or < 125/75 if there is diabetic nephropathy.

In type II (non-insulin dependent) diabetes, hypertension is particularly common, affecting 70% of people in this group. It is strongly associated with obesity and insulin resistance and control of blood pressure is more important for preventing complications than tight glycaemic control. There is particular evidence of benefit for tight blood pressure control to a target of < 140/80, and this will usually need combinations of drugs (UKPDS 1998a). There is no evidence that one group of drugs is more or less effective than any other and it is not clear if ACE inhibitors have a specific renoprotective effect in this group over and above their blood pressure lowering actions. In the UKPDS (United Kingdom Prospective Diabetes Study Group) 39 study, no differences were observed between atenolol and captopril in terms of preventing cardiovascular complications in hypertensive patients with diabetes, although the study and its statistical power was comparatively small (UKPDS 1999b). In the appropriate blood pressure control in diabetes (ABCD) trial (Estacio et al 1998) and the fosinopril versus amlodipine cardiovascular events randomized trial (FACET) (Tatti et al 1998), an ACE inhibitor was more effective than a dihydropyridine calcium channel blocker in preventing cardiovascular events. However, in both studies this was a secondary end point and the observation needs to be confirmed in a suitably designed prospective clinical trial.

Renal disease

In patients with chronic renal impairment, good blood pressure control slows the progression of renal dysfunction. ACE inhibition reduces the incidence of end stage renal failure but it is not clear if this is a specific effect or non-specific action as a result of blood pressure lowering. ACE inhibitors also reduce 24 hour protein loss and should be used in patients with 24 hour protein excretion of > 3 g or rapidly progressive renal dysfunction. ACE inhibitors may worsen renal impairment in patients with renal vascular disease and careful monitoring of electrolytes and creatinine is mandatory. Salt restriction is particularly important in managing hypertension in renal disease. Thiazide diuretics are ineffective in patients with significant renal dysfunction and loop diuretics should be used when a diuretic is needed.

Pregnancy

An increased blood pressure before 20 weeks gestation usually indicates pre-existing chronic hypertension that may not have been previously diagnosed. As in all younger hypertensive patients, a careful assessment is needed to exclude possible secondary causes, although radiological and radionuclide investigations should usually be deferred until after pregnancy. Hypertension diagnosed after 20 weeks gestation may also indicate chronic hypertension, which may have been masked during early pregnancy by the fall in blood pressure that occurs at that time. Patients with elevated blood pressure in pregnancy are at increased risk of pre-eclampsia and intrauterine growth retardation. They need frequent checks of their blood pressure, urinalysis and fetal growth.

Pre-eclampsia is diagnosed when the blood pressure increases by 30/15 from measurements obtained in early pregnancy or if the diastolic blood pressure exceeds 110 mmHg and proteinuria is present. There is consensus that blood pressure should be treated with drugs if it exceeds 170/110 and some clinicians use a lower threshold, for example 140/90. Methyldopa is the most suitable drug choice for use in pregnancy because of its long-term safety record. Calcium channel blockers, hydralazine and labetalol are also used. β-blockers, particularly atenolol, are used less often as they are associated with intrauterine growth retardation. Although diuretics reduce the incidence of pre-eclampsia they are little used in pregnancy because of concerns about decreasing maternal blood volume. ACE inhibitors and angiotensin II antagonists are contraindicated, as they are associated with oligohydramnios, renal failure and intrauterine death.

Oral contraceptives

Use of combined oral contraceptives results, on average, in an increase of 5/3 mmHg in blood pressure. However severe hypertension may occur in a small proportion of recipients and this may occur months or years into treatment. Progesterone-only preparations do not cause hypertension so often. Combined oral contraceptives are not absolutely contraindicated in hypertension unless other risk factors for cardiovascular disease, such as smoking, are present.

Hormone replacement therapy

There is little evidence that hormone replacement therapy is associated with an increase in blood pressure and women with hypertension should not be denied access to these agents. Large increases in blood pressure have occasionally been reported in individuals and it is important to monitor blood pressure during the first few weeks of therapy and 6-monthly thereafter. In women with resistant hypertension during treatment with HRT, the effectiveness of discontinuing hormone replacement should be assessed.

Ancillary drug treatment

Aspirin

The use of aspirin reduces cardiovascular events at the expense of an increase in gastrointestinal complications. Its use should be restricted to patients who have no contraindications and either:

- have evidence of established vascular disease, or
- have no evident cardiovascular disease but who are over 50 years of age and have either evidence of target organ damage or a 10 year coronary heart disease risk of > 15%.

Blood pressure should be controlled before aspirin is instituted.

Lipid lowering therapy

Lipid lowering drug treatment should be prescribed to patients under 75 years of age who have pre-existing vascular disease and whose total cholesterol is greater than 5 mmol/l. Primary prevention is appropriate for patients under 70 years of age who have familial hyperlipidaemia or who have a calculated 10 year coronary risk of > 30%.

CASE STUDIES

Case 17.1

A 55-year-old woman of African Caribbean origin is found to have consistently elevated blood pressure over several weeks, her lowest reading being 155/98. She is overweight and has diabetes, and is being treated with metformin. Her renal function and urinalysis are both normal.

Questions

1. Should drug therapy be initiated for her hypertension?
2. If her hypertension was treated with drugs, which agents offer particular advantages, and which should be avoided?

Answers

1. Provided her blood pressure has been measured accurately over several weeks, it should be treated, since her diabetes is an important additional risk factor. It is important to ensure that an appropriately sized blood pressure cuff is being used, in view of her obesity. Non-pharmacological interventions should also take place in parallel. Restriction of salt intake may be particularly helpful in people of African Caribbean race and weight reduction would benefit her hypertension and her diabetes.
2. ACE inhibitors are an attractive choice for diabetic patients who have nephropathy. However, there is no evidence of nephropathy in this patient and ACE inhibitors are less effective antihypertensives in people of African Caribbean origin. β-blockers reduce hypoglycaemic awareness; this is not a contraindication in this case since metformin does not cause hypoglycaemia. However, β-blockers are also less effective in those of African Caribbeans descent. Diuretics work well in African Caribbean hypertensives, but may worsen glucose tolerance and may not therefore be the most appropriate first choice. Calcium channel blockers do not have adverse metabolic effects and are effective in people of this origin, and would therefore be an appropriate choice. Tight blood pressure control is important and several agents may be required, including diuretics, ACE inhibitors, β-blockers and α-blockers.

Case 17.2

A 35-year-old man is overweight and has a blood pressure of 178/114. He smokes 25 cigarettes daily and drinks 28 units of alcohol per week. He has a sedentary occupation. He eats excessive quantities of saturated fat and salt.

Questions

1. How should this patient be managed?
2. What pharmacological treatment for blood pressure would be appropriate if non-pharmacological treatment was unsuccessful?

Answers

1. Since he is a young man, his absolute risk of cardiovascular events is low, at least for the time being. However, he has several additional risk factors that need to be addressed, including his sedentary lifestyle and his smoking. Non-pharmacological methods have the potential of reducing his blood pressure considerably, including reduction in weight and salt intake. Measurement of plasma cholesterol may help him modify his diet although he is unlikely to qualify for lipid lowering therapy in view of his young age.
2. If drug treatment was appropriate, any class of antihypertensive drug could be used since no

contraindications are present. It would be reasonable to start with a thiazide diuretic or β-blocker, since these are inexpensive and have a long safety record. Other drugs could be added or substituted if he was intolerant to initial therapy or it did not reduce his blood pressure to target levels.

Case 17.3

The patient described above in Case 17.2 stopped smoking and lost a little weight but remained hypertensive. He was treated with atenolol 50 mg daily. His blood pressure fell to 136/84 but he developed tiredness and bradycardia and complained of erectile impotence.

Question

What are the treatment options for this patient?

Answer

The options are to change him to a different class of drug or to use a β-blocker with special properties. It is possible that he would feel less tired using a β-blocker with intrinsic sympathomimetic activity (e.g. pindolol) but this is by no means guaranteed. The effects on his sexual function are unpredictable. It would probably be better to change him to a drug of a different class such as a thiazide diuretic (although these also commonly cause impotence), a calcium channel blocker or an ACE inhibitor.

Case 17.4

A 24-year-old woman with a family history of hypertension is prescribed an oral contraceptive. Six months after starting this, she is noted to have a blood pressure of 148/96.

Question

How should this patient be managed?

Answer

If her blood pressure is consistently raised she may have either essential hypertension or hypertension induced by the oral contraceptive, or a combination. Her blood pressure may fall if her oral contraceptive is discontinued. She will, however, need advice on adequate contraceptive methods. A progesterone-only preparation would be one possibility. She would need careful counselling about the methods available and how successful they are. If her blood pressure remained elevated after discontinuing her oral contraceptive, she is likely to have underlying hypertension. This may be essential in nature, in view of the family history; however, because of her age she should undergo some investigations to exclude possible secondary causes of hypertension. She is at low risk of complications and there is no urgency to consider drug treatment.

Case 17.5

A lady of 73 has a long-standing history of hypertension and intolerance to antihypertensive drugs. Bendroflumethiazide (bendrofluazide) was associated with acute attacks of gout, she developed breathlessness and wheezing while taking atenolol, nifedipine caused flushing and headache, and doxazosin was associated with intolerable postural hypotension. Four weeks earlier she had been started on enalapril but was now complaining of a dry persistent cough. Her blood chemistry has remained normal.

Questions

1. Is the patient's cough likely to be an adverse effect of enalapril?
2. What other options are available for controlling her blood pressure?

Answers

1. Yes it is. A dry cough is a common adverse effect of ACE inhibitors. It affects approximately 20% of recipients and is more common in women. Some patients are able to tolerate the symptom but in many the drug has to be discontinued.
2. Angiotensin II antagonists can be used in patients intolerant of ACE inhibitors due to cough. They are unlikely to produce this symptom since they do not inhibit the metabolism of pulmonary bradykinin. Centrally acting agents such as methyldopa or moxonidine could also be considered. However, these are not well tolerated and side-effects are quite likely in this patient. A non-dihydropyridine calcium channel blocker such as verapamil is another alternative. Measurement of plasma uric acid could also be considered followed by prophylactic treatment with allopurinol before introducing a diuretic.

Case 17.6

A 23-year-old woman has a normal blood pressure (118/82) when reviewed at 8 weeks of pregnancy. In the 24th week of pregnancy she is reviewed by her midwife and found to have a blood pressure of 148/96. Urinalysis is normal.

Questions

1. What is the likely diagnosis?
2. What complications does the patient's high blood pressure place her at increased risk of?
3. Should she receive drug treatment? If so with which drug? If not, how should she be managed?

Answers

1. She may have gestation-induced hypertension or chronic hypertension that had previously been masked by the fall in blood pressure that happens in early pregnancy.
2. She is at increased risk of pre-eclampsia and intrauterine growth retardation.

3. There are differences of opinion between specialists as to whether blood pressure should be treated at this level during pregnancy. In favour of treatment is the substantial rise over the earlier blood pressure recording. Some specialists would not treat unless the blood pressure was >170/110 or other complications were present. If she were treated, methyldopa would be a suitable choice. In any event, she needs close monitoring of her blood pressure, urinalysis and fetal growth.

Case 17.7

An elderly patient comes to the pharmacy with a prescription for the following medications: salbutamol inhaler 200 micrograms as required, beclometasone inhaler 200 micrograms twice daily, bendroflumethiazide (bendrofluazide) 2.5 mg daily, Dilzem XL 180 mg once daily and atenolol 50 mg daily. The atenolol was being started by the patient's GP, apparently because of inadequate blood pressure control.

Question

What action should the pharmacist take?

Answer

There are two reasons to be concerned about the addition of atenolol to this patient's drug regimen. First, there is a potentially hazardous interaction with diltiazem (Dilzem XL) which may result in severe bradycardia or heart block. Second, the patient is receiving treatment for obstructive airways disease and this may be worsened by the atenolol. The prescription should be discussed with the prescriber.

REFERENCES

ALLHAT Collaborative Research Group 2000 Major cardiovascular events in hypertensive patients randomised to doxazosin vs. chorthalidone. Antihypertensive and lipid lowering treatment to prevent heart attack trial (ALLHAT). Journal of the American Medical Association 283: 1967–1975

Amery A, Birkenhâger W, Brixko P et al 1985 Mortality and morbidity results from the European working party on high blood pressure in the elderly trial. Lancet i: 1349–1354

Anon 1977 Report of the Joint National Committee on Detection, Evaluation, and Treatment of High Blood Pressure: A cooperative study. Journal of the American Medical Association 237: 255–261

Anon 1980 Australian therapeutic trial in mild hypertension: report by the management committee. Lancet 1: 1261–1267

Beevers G, Lip G Y H, O'Brien E 2001 The pathophysiology of hypertension. British Medical Journal 322: 912–916

Brown M J Palmer C R, Castaigne A et al 2000 Morbidity and mortality in patients randomised to double blind treatment with a long aching calcium channel blocker or diuretic in the international nifedipine GITS study: intervention as a goal a hypertension treatment (INSIGHT). Lancet 356: 366–372

Collins R, Petro R, MacMahon S et al 1990 Blood pressure, stroke and coronary heart disease. Part 2. Short-term reductions in blood pressure: overview of randomised drugs trials in their epidemiological context. Lancet 335: 827–838

Dahlöf B, Lindholm L H, Hansson L et al 1991 Morbidity and mortality in the Swedish trial of old patients with hypertension (STOP-Hypertension). Lancet 338: 1281–1285

Dahlöf B, Devereux R, Kjeldsen S E et al 2002 Cardiovascular morbidity and mortality in the Losartan For Endpoint reduction in hypertension study (LIFE): a randomised trial against atenolol. Lancet 359: 995–1003

Estacio R O, Barrett M D, Jeffers W et al 1998 The effect of nisoldipine as compared with enalapril on cardiovascular outcomes in patients with non-insulin dependent diabetes and hypertension. New England Journal of Medicine 338: 645–681

Furberg C D, Psaty B M, Meyer J V 1995 Nifedipine: dose-related increase in mortality in patients with coronary heart disease. Circulation 92: 1326–1331

Gong L, Zhang W, Zhu Y et al 1996 Shanghai trial of nifedipine in the elderly (STONE). Journal of Hypertension 14: 1237–1245

Hansson L, Zanchetti A, Carruthers S G et al for the HOT Study Group 1998 Effects of intensive blood-pressure lowering and low-dose aspirin in patients with hypertension; principal results of the hypertension optimal treatment (HOT) randomised trial. Lancet 351: 1755–1762

Hansson L, Lindholm L H, Ekbom T et al 1999a Randomised trial of old and new antihypertensive drugs in elderly patients: cardiovascular mortality and morbidity in the Swedish trial in old patients with hypertension – 2 study. Lancet 354: 1751–1756

Hansson L, Lindholm L H, Niskanen L et al 1999b Effect of angiotensin-converting-enzyme inhibition compared with conventional therapy on cardiovascular morbidity and mortality in hypertension. The captopril prevention project (CAPPP). Lancet 353: 611–616

Liu L, Wang J G, Gong L et al for the Systolic Hypertension in China (Syst-China) Collaborative Group. Comparison of active treatment and placebo for older Chinese patients with isolated systolic hypertension. Journal of Hypertension 16: 1823–1829

Medical Research Council Working Party 1985 MRC trial of treatment of mild hypertension: principal results. British Medical Journal 291: 97–104

Medical Research Council Working Party 1992 Medical Research Council trial of treatment of hypertension in older adults: principal results. British Medical Journal 304: 405–412

Psaty B M, Heckbert S R, Kocpsell T D et al 1995 The risk of myocardial infarction associated with antihypertensive drug therapies. Journal of the American Medical Association 274: 620–625

Ramsay L E, Williams B, Johnson G D et al 1999a Guidelines for management of hypertension: report of the third working party of the British Hypertension Society. Journal of Human Hypertension 319: 630–635

Ramsay L E, Williams B, Johnson G D et al 1999b British Hypertension Society guidelines for hypertension management 1999: summary. British Medical Journal 319: 630–635

Seux M-L, Forette F, Staessent J A et al 1999 Treatment of isolated systolic hypertension and dementia prevention in older patients. European Society of Cardiology 1 (Suppl. M): M6–M12

SHEP Co-operative Research Group 1991 Prevention of stroke by antihypertensive drug treatment in older persons with isolated systolic hypertension: final results of the systolic hypertension in the elderly program (SHEP). Journal of the American Medical Association 265: 3255–3264

Staessen J A, Fagard R, Thijs L et al for the Systolic Hypertension in Europe (Syst-Eur) Trial Investigators 1997 Randomised double-blind comparison of placebo and active treatment for older patients with isolated systolic hypertension. Lancet 350: 757–764

Tatti P, Pahor M, Byington R P et al 1998 Outcome results of the fosinopril versus amlodipine cardiovascular events randomised trial (FACET) in patients with hypertension and NIDDM. Diabetes Care 21: 597–603

UK Prospective Diabetes Study Group. 1998a Tight blood pressure control and risk of macrovascular and microvascular complications in type 2 diabetes: UKPDS 38. British Medical Journal 317: 703–713

UK Prospective Diabetes Study Group. 1998b Efficacy of atenolol and captopril in reducing risk of macrovascular and microvascular complications in type 2 diabetes: UKPDS 39.

British Medical Journal 317: 713–726

Veterans Administration Co-operative Study Group on Antihypertensive Agents 1970 Effects of treatment on morbidity in hypertension II. Results in patients with diastolic blood pressure averaging 90 through 114 mm Hg. Journal of the American Medical Association 213: 1143–1152

Wallis E J, Ramsay L E, Ul Haq I et al 2000 Coronary and cardiovascular risk estimation for primary prevention: validation of a new Sheffield table in the 1995 Scottish health survey population. British Medical Journal 320: 671–676

Wilhelmsen L, Berglund G, Elmfeldt D et al 1987 Beta-blockers versus diuretics in hypertensive men: main results from the HAPPHY trial. Journal of Hypertension 5: 561–572

FURTHER READING

Oates J A, Brown N J 2001 Antihypertensive agents and the drug therapy of hypertension. In: Hardman J G, Limbard L E, Goodman A G (eds) Goodman and Gillman's The pharmacological basis of therapeutics, 10th edn. McGraw-Hill, New York, pp. 871–900

Swales J D 1996 Essential hypertension. In: Weatherall D J, Ledingham L G G, Warrell D A (eds) Oxford textbook of medicine, 3rd edn. Oxford University Press, Oxford, pp. 2527–2543

Beevers G, Lip G Y H, O'Brien E 2001 ABC of hypertension, 4th edn. BMJ Publications, London

McGregor G A, Kaplan N M 1998 Fast facts: hypertension. Health Press, Oxford

Grahame-Smith D G, Aronson J K 2002 The drug therapy of cardiovascular disorders: hypertension. In: Oxford textbook of clinical pharmacology and drug therapy, 3rd edn. Oxford University Press, Oxford, pp. 226–233

Coronary heart disease 18

D. Scott

KEY POINTS

- Coronary heart disease (CHD) is common, often fatal and frequently preventable.
- High dietary fat, smoking and sedentary lifestyle are risk factors for CHD and require modification if present.
- Hypertension, hypercholesterolaemia and diabetes mellitus are also risk factors and require optimal management.
- Stable angina should be managed with nitrates for pain relief and β-blockers, unless contraindicated, for long term prophylaxis. Where β-blockers are inappropriate, the use of calcium channel blockers and/or nitrates may be considered.
- Unstable angina should be treated with aspirin and heparin to reduce thombus formation and nitrates to reduce vasospasm. Glycoprotein IIb/IIIa antagonists may also be beneficial.
- Patients with acute myocardial infarction should receive an opioid analgesic, rapid thrombolysis, aspirin, a β-blocker and an ACE inhibitor.

Coronary heart disease (CHD), sometimes described as coronary artery disease (CAD), is a condition where the vascular supply to the heart is impeded by atheroma, thrombosis or spasm of coronary arteries. This may impair the supply of oxygenated blood to cardiac tissue sufficiently to cause myocardial ischaemia which, if severe or prolonged, may cause the death of cardiac muscle cells (myocardial infarction). Less commonly, myocardial ischaemia can also arise if oxygen demand is abnormally increased, as may occur in severe ventricular hypertrophy due to hypertension, or where the oxygen carrying capacity of blood is impaired, as in iron deficiency anaemia. The term ischaemic heart disease (IHD) may be used to include all causes of myocardial ischaemia. CHD kills over 6.5 million people worldwide each year.

Epidemiology

The epidemiology of CHD has been studied extensively and has led to much debate concerning the associated risk factors. Absence of established risk factors does not guarantee freedom from CHD for any individual, and some individuals with several major risk factors seem perversely healthy. None the less, there is evidence that in developed countries, education and publicity about the major risk factors has led to changes in social habits, particularly with respect to a reduction in smoking and fat consumption, and this has contributed to a decrease in the incidence of CHD. The UK has had a steady decline in CHD deaths of about 4% per annum since the late 1970s. This improvement has been chiefly among those with higher incomes, however, and the less prosperous social classes continue to have almost unchanged levels of CHD. Better treatment has also contributed to a decrease in cardiac mortality although CHD still accounted for some 132 000 deaths in 1999 in the UK including 70% of sudden natural deaths. In most developed countries, CHD is the leading cause of adult death, but in the UK the poor outcome of lung cancer treatments makes that the leading cause. In the UK, in comparison with Caucasians, people of South Asian descent have a 40% higher death rate from CHD and Afro-Caribbeans have a 25–50% lower rate. The location of deaths from coronary heart attacks in the UK is summarized in Table 18.1.

About 3.5% of UK adults have symptomatic CHD. One-third of 50–59-year-old men have evidence of CHD, and this proportion increases with age. In the UK, there are over 1 million people who have survived a myocardial infarction and about 1.4 million who have

Table 18.1 Location of death from coronary heart attacks in UK

Home	55%
Hospital	26%
Other health care sites	5.5%
Public places	12%
Work	1.5%

These data apply to people up to 75 years of age; the proportion dying in hospital increases with age. (Adapted from Norris 1998.)

angina. About 300 000 experience a myocardial infarction in any year, of whom about 140 000 die.

The increase in mortality with age is probably not due to a particular age-related factor but the cumulative effect of risk factors that lead to atheroma and thrombosis and hence to coronary artery disease. In the USA, age-related death rates for CHD have fallen by 25% over a decade, but the total number of CHD deaths has fallen by only 10% because the population is aging. The main risk factors are family history, hypertension, cigarette smoking and raised serum cholesterol. Of these, the determining factor appears to be serum cholesterol, because hypertension and smoking have little effect on the incidence of CHD in populations with low average cholesterol concentrations but a major effect in populations such as the UK with high cholesterol levels.

Other lipid-related risk factors include elevated serum triglyceride concentrations, high saturated fat intake and a high saturated:polyunsaturated dietary fat ratio. These and other dietary factors, including energy intake and obesity, are difficult to separate out since they are all interrelated. However, it is clear that obese people have a higher risk of CHD, whatever the prime cause, and all dietary factors should be addressed simultaneously in an attempt to decrease risk. Low fat diets are recommended. Some dietary studies have suggested a benefit from diets containing large quantities of fruit, vegetables and antioxidants (vitamins C and E and β-carotene). Prevention studies with pharmacological doses of these antioxidants have not shown the same benefit, and therefore dietary supplements cannot be justified although most authorities recommend at least five portions of fruit and vegetables each day. High serum homocysteine levels are associated with, but not proven to cause, CHD and this is of particular interest because levels may be reduced very easily by oral folic acid supplements.

Women appear to be less susceptible to CHD than men although they seem to lose this protection after the menopause, presumably because of hormonal changes. Race has not proved to be a clear risk factor since the prevalence of CHD seems to depend much more strongly on location and lifestyle than on ethnic origin or place of birth. A 1998 UK survey found that lower social or economic class was associated with increased obesity, poor cholesterol indicators, higher blood pressure, less use of hormone replacement therapy, and higher C-reactive protein measurements (CRP, an indicator of inflammatory activity); it is not therefore surprising that there is increased cardiac morbidity and mortality in those classes.

Diabetes mellitus is a positive risk factor in developed countries with high levels of CHD but not in countries with little CHD. Insulin resistance, as defined by high fasting insulin concentrations, is an independent risk factor for CHD in men. While unusual physical exertion is associated with an increased risk of infarction, an active lifestyle that includes regular, moderate exercise is beneficial, although the optimum level has not been determined and its beneficial effect appears to be readily overwhelmed by the presence of other risk factors. A family history of CHD is a positive risk factor, independent of diet and other risk factors. Hostility, anxiety or depression are associated with increased coronary heart disease and death, especially after myocardial infarction when mortality is doubled by anxiety and quadrupled by depression. Several studies have shown associations between CHD and prior infections with several common micro-organisms, including *Chlamydia pneumoniae* and *Helicobacter pylori*, but a causal connection has not been shown. The influence of fetal and infant growth conditions, and their interaction with social conditions in childhood and adult life, has been debated strongly for decades but it is clear that lower socio-economic status and thinness in very early life are linked to higher incidences of CHD (Barker et al 2001).

Aetiology

The vast majority of CHD occurs in patients with atherosclerosis of the coronary arteries that starts before adulthood. The cause of spontaneous arteriosclerosis is unclear, although it is thought that in the presence of hypercholesterolaemia a non-denuding form of injury occurs to the endothelial lining of coronary arteries and other vessels. This injury is followed by subendothelial migration of monocytes and the accumulation of fatty streaks containing lipid rich macrophages and T cells. Almost all adults, and 50% of children aged 11–14 years, have fatty streaks in their coronary arteries. Thereafter, there is migration and proliferation of smooth muscle cells into the intima with further lipid deposition. The smooth muscle cells, together with fibroblasts, synthesize and secrete collagen, proteoglycans, elastin and glycoproteins that make up a fibrous cap surrounding cells and necrotic tissue, together called a plaque. The presence of atherosclerotic plaques results in narrowing of vessels and a reduction in blood flow and this may become manifest as angina. Associated with the plaque is a loss of endothelium, which can serve as a stimulus for the formation of a thrombus and result in more acute manifestations of CHD, including unstable angina and myocardial infarction. Plaque rupture caused by physical stresses or plaque erosion may precipitate an acute reaction. Other pathological processes are probably involved, including endothelial dysfunction which alters the thrombosis–thrombolysis balance and the vasoconstriction–vasodilatation balance. There is interest in the possible role of statins and angiotensin-converting enzyme (ACE) inhibitors in modifying endothelial function. There is also great interest in the role of inflammation, especially in acute episodes. At post-mortem, many plaques are found to contain inflammatory cells. Signs of inflammatory damage are found consistently at the sites of plaque rupture. Measures of acute phase inflammatory markers, such as fibrinogen and C-reactive protein, have demonstrated a predictive association with coronary events and may possibly become useful in stratifying patients into high and low risk groups. There is also evidence that brief periods of ischaemia, followed by reperfusion, confer a protective effect on myocardial tissue and reduce the extent of subsequent infarctions. This process, ischaemic preconditioning, may involve adenosine and potassium channel activation, but the consequences for therapy are unclear (Ferrari et al 1999)

Clinical manifestations

CHD may present with the death of cardiac tissue (an infarction) or as a painful but reversible ischaemia (angina). There are three main branches of the coronary artery that supply blood to the heart. A major thrombus in one of these arteries can lead to a regional infarction, which may be transmural and affect the full thickness of the myocardium, or non-transmural in which only the subendocardial layer is affected. A more diffuse subendocardial infarction may be produced by a general reduction in perfusion, perhaps as a result of widespread arteriosclerosis, or perhaps as a result of myocardial hypertrophy or increased ventricular diastolic pressures. Perfusion of the subendocardium occurs only during diastole, and any increase in ventricular wall tension, as could arise in congestive cardiac failure, or a reduction in the length of diastole during a tachyarrhythmia, will reduce the oxygen supply. Ventricles are affected more than atria because of their higher workload. Infarcted areas begin to heal rapidly and collateral vessels develop to supply the tissue but the process may take several months and will not permit regeneration of a fully functioning myocardium. The thrombus which caused the infarction is broken down by t-PA (tissue plasminogen factor) from the endothelium; one-third of vessels regain patency within 6–12 hours of the event and about 75% within 2 weeks.

Unstable angina, sometimes called crescendo angina if progression is rapid, with its variable intensity and generally progressive nature, is thought to be caused by thrombosed plaques that may occlude vessels intermittently. Alternatively, platelets or small particles may break from the thrombus and occlude other small vessels. Because of difficulty distinguishing these syndromes and non-Q wave or ST-elevation infarction,

especially during the clinical event, the general term acute coronary syndrome is used.

Stable or exercise-induced angina is caused by a narrowing of the vessels which becomes critical at a certain level of demand.

Variant or Prinzmetal's angina is caused by spasm of the coronary arteries and may occur even at rest.

Prognosis

Many patients with CHD experience no clinical symptoms, and up to one-third of patients who have had angina-type chest pains deny it at a later examination when it appears to have resolved spontaneously. CHD is not necessarily fatal despite the large number of deaths it causes, but proven coronary artery disease has an annual mortality rate of 3% (single vessel disease) to 10% (triple vessel disease). Only about 20% of infarctions are preceded by angina.

The prognosis of an individual who has suffered a myocardial infarction is improving as thrombolytic therapy becomes more widely used and its use refined. Figure 18.1 shows the outcome of heart attacks in a London suburb, and indicates that some 25% of individuals will die before any medical intervention occurs. The most dangerous time after a myocardial infarction is the first few hours when ventricular fibrillation (VF) is most likely to occur; it is estimated that 225 000 Americans die of VF each year without reaching hospital, although not all of these will have had an infarction. Higher death rates occur in patients who are older, have had a previous infarction, suffer an anterior infarction, develop hypertension, heart failure or tachycardia, or who fail to stop smoking. Mortality is proportional to the size of the infarction which may be estimated by measuring the extent of release of cardiac enzymes into blood from damaged myocardial cells. The varying prognosis in patients treated with thrombolytic agents, in relation to the time of treatment after the infarction, is described later.

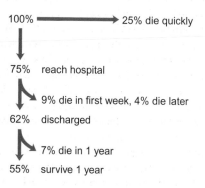

Figure 18.1 Prognosis of heart attacks in the community.

Signs, symptoms and investigations

CHD is very variable in presentation, and there are three main diagnostic factors in the evaluation of suspected CHD: the patient's symptoms and history, the electrocardiogram (ECG) and blood marker assays (Lee & Goldman 2000).

The patient with a classical presentation of CHD complains of pain of a gripping or tight nature that occurs in the retrosternal region of the chest and may radiate to the neck, back or left shoulder with possible involvement of the jaw, teeth or epigastrium. The pain is typically brought on by exertion, a heavy meal or a change in temperature, and is relieved by stopping the exertion. Sweating, pallor and anxiety are common but non-specific signs after an infarction. Fever may follow within 12 hours and last for several days while pericarditis or heart failure may also occur. CHD is very variable in presentation, and while classically associated with the symptoms described above, chest pain in particular is not always present and the physiological initiator of the pain is not clear. It has been reported that 25% of non-fatal infarcts are 'silent' and pain-free. Such patients may just feel non-specifically 'unwell' for a while and not seek medical attention or they may not remember the incident at all. Patients with or without angina may also have episodes of silent ischaemia without infarction.

The history of the pain is important because of the differing prognoses and the implications for treatment. Stable (exercise-induced) angina does not normally occur at rest, is generally predictable in relation to activities that induce pain, resolves on cessation of the causative activity and worsens only slowly. Unstable angina occurs unpredictably, including at rest, worsens rapidly over hours or days (crescendo angina) and has a 10% 1 year mortality rate.

The ECG is of considerable value in identifying ischaemia or infarction. It is, however, not unambiguous and may be difficult to interpret, especially after a previous infarction. In general, ECG changes are seen in three-quarters of patients with significant coronary artery disease but a resting ECG is normal in 50–75% of patients presenting for the first time with unequivocal angina. An ECG recorded during an episode of pain is more likely to be diagnostic, and an ECG during an exercise tolerance test may be useful.

A standard 12-lead electrocardiograph that records the electrical activity of the heart from different aspects can identify the region of the heart affected. In leads facing an infarcted area there will usually be S–T segment elevation early on, perhaps within seconds, followed within days by inversion of the T wave and then within weeks or months by a return to normal. S–T segment depression may occur in the opposite leads and in subendocardial infarctions. The only definitive ECG change, however, is the development of a Q wave within a few days of the infarction. Q waves generally persist, and their presence gives no real clue as to the time of an infarction without a clinical history or enzyme studies. In ischaemia without infarction there are no QRS changes but there are many possible changes in the S–T segment and T wave (see Fig. 20.3).

The most conclusive retrospective evidence that an individual has suffered an infarction is an increase in cardiac muscle components in the blood. Several cardiac muscle enzymes are assayed routinely, including aspartate transaminase (AST), lactate dehydrogenase (LDH) and creatine kinase (CK). Serial estimations of these enzymes are of greatest diagnostic value since their rate and extent of release varies, as does their serum half life (Fig. 18.2). All three enzymes can originate from sites other than the heart, and therefore it may be necessary to type the enzyme (isoenzyme) by electrophoresis to identify its site of origin. For example, CK of cardiac origin (CK-MB) may be distinguished from the isoenzymes found in the brain (CK-BB) and skeletal muscle (CK-MM). Other proteins, notably troponins I and T, are more specific and more sensitive for cardiac necrosis, false positives are rare and levels rise within 4 hours of an infarction, peak at about 12 hours and remain detectable for up to 7 days. They are increasingly the test of choice. Smaller rises are seen in acute coronary syndromes (described below) which do not have ECG evidence of infarction and the test is useful in deciding which patients need hospital or coronary care unit admission, and which do not.

More elaborate and invasive tests may be used to determine cardiac function in appropriate patients. A catheter may be introduced into a peripheral vein and passed through to the heart and lungs where pressures and flow rate can be measured in different chambers and vessels of the heart. A radiopaque dye may be used to outline the coronary circulation (angiography) and identify blockages (see Fig. 18.3). Radioisotopes such as technetium-99m are used to label blood cells and plasma for studying blood flow, while thallium-201 is used for studying perfusion in myocardial tissue to identify infarcted or non-functioning areas of muscle. Echocardiography by ultrasound is non-invasive and is used to examine the gross structure and function of the myocardium and valves. An area of poorly contracting muscle associated with an infarct may be identified.

Treatment

As in most diseases, the aim of treatment is to decrease mortality and morbidity. However, while mortality is easy to measure, morbidity is not. Several measures of

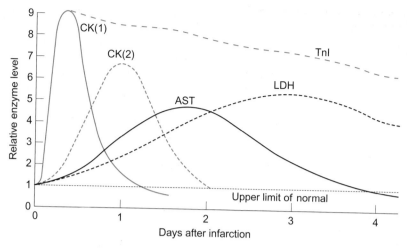

Figure 18.2 Typical enzyme activity in serum following myocardial infarction. CK(1), CK with thrombolytic therapy; CK(2), CK without thrombolytic therapy; TnI, Troponin I.

quality of life have been used to assess the outcome of CHD treatment, combining indicators of pain, breathlessness, exercise tolerance and ability to perform normal daily activities with duration of survival. A minimum aim for treatment would therefore be to prevent myocardial infarction and associated mortality and to increase the length of pain-free survival with a lifestyle acceptable to the patient.

This article describes drug therapy but many patients undergo coronary artery bypass grafting (CABG) or arterial dilatation by angioplasty. The latter technique usually involves using a balloon on the end of a catheter to forcibly dilate an arterial constriction from inside the artery. It may be accompanied by the insertion of a metal

meshwork (a stent) to line the artery and prevent re-constriction; in these and other cases drugs may be helpful in preventing the formation of thrombus in the area and this therapy is described below. Research on substances that promote the development of new blood vessels to bypass blocked ones, angiogenesis, is moving from animal models to humans.

The HOPE study, a secondary prevention trial which investigated the effect of an ACE inhibitor, ramipril, on patients over 55 years old who had known atherosclerotic disease, or else diabetes plus another cardiovascular risk factor, but who did not have any evidence of heart failure or left ventricular dysfunction, found that ramipril decreased the combined end point of stroke, myocardial infarction or cardiovascular death by about 22% compared to placebo (Yusuf et al 2000). Similar differences were found in all individual outcomes and in diabetics as well as non-diabetics. The benefits were greater than would be expected from simple blood pressure reduction. This has major implications for the management of CHD patients, both for the decision to treat at all, and the choice of treatment. Further studies to clarify the effect of ACE inhibitors as a class, the appropriate dosage, and the categories of patient who would benefit are needed. It is not known if these benefits might also be found in angiotensin II blockade.

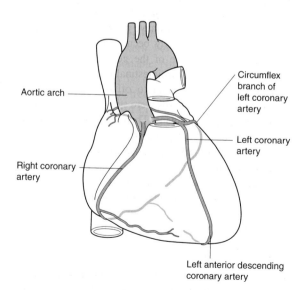

Figure 18.3 Main coronary arteries.

Modification of risk factors

Common to all stages of treatment of CHD is the need to reduce risk factors (Table 18.2). The patient needs to appreciate the value of the proposed strategy in terms of lifestyle and to be highly committed to a plan for changing

Table 18.3 β-blockers: properties and pharmacokinetics

	Blockade	Lipophilicity	ISA	Oral absorption	Elimination
Acebutolol renal)	β_1 (some β_2)	+	+	90%[a]	Active metabolite ($t_{1/2}$ 11–13 h, Gut 50% $t_{1/2}$ 3–4 h
Atenolol	β_1	−	−	50%	Renal $t_{1/2}$ 5–7 h
Betaxolol	β_1	+	−	100%	Hepatic + renal $t_{1/2}$ 15 h
Bisoprolol	β_1	+	−	90%	Hapatic + renal $t_{1/2}$ 10–12 h
Carteolol	$\beta_1\ \beta_2$	−	++	80%	Hepatic + renal $t_{1/2}$ 3–7 h
Carvedilol	$\beta_1\ \beta_2\ \alpha_1$	+	−	80%[a]	Hepatic + renal $t_{1/2}$ 4–8 h
Celiprolol	$\beta_1\ \alpha_2$	−	β_2+	30–70%	Renal + gut $t_{1/2}$ 5–6 h
Esmolol	β_1	−	−	i.v.	Blood enzymes $t_{1/2}$ 9 min
Labetalol	$\beta_1\ \beta_2\ \alpha_1$	−	−	100%[a]	Hepatic $t_{1/2}$ 6–8 h
Metoprolol	β_1	+	−	95%[a]	Hepatic $t_{1/2}$ 3–4 h
Nadolol	$\beta_1\ \beta_2$	−	−	30%	Renal $t_{1/2}$ 16–18 h
Nebivolol	β_1	+	−	12–96%[b]	Hepatic $t_{1/2}$ 8–27 h[b]
Oxprenolol	$\beta_1\ \beta_2$	+	++	90%[a]	Hepatic $t_{1/2}$ 1–2 h
Pindolol	$\beta_1\ \beta_2$	+	+++	90%	Hepatic + renal $t_{1/2}$ 3–4 h
Propranolol	$\beta_1\ \beta_2$	+	−	90%[a]	Hepatic $t_{1/2}$ 3–6 h
Sotalol	$\beta_1\ \beta_2$	−	−	70%	Renal $t_{1/2}$ 15–17 h
Timolol	$\beta_1\ \beta_2$	+	−	90%[a]	Hepatic + renal $t_{1/2}$ 3–4 h

All figures are approximate and subject to interpatient variability. Therapeutic ranges are not well defined.
ISA, intrinsic sympathomimetic activity; $t_{1/2}$, elimination half-life.
[a] Extensive first-pass metabolism may result in a significant decrease in bioavailability.
[b] Genetically-determined groups of slow and fast metabolizers have been identified.

production of nitric oxide from nitrates is probably mediated by intracellular thiols, and it has been observed that when tolerance occurs to the action of nitrates, a thiol donor (such as N-acetylcysteine) may partially restore the effectiveness of the nitrate. Antioxidants such as vitamin C have also been used. Tolerance is one of the main limitations to the use of nitrates, which remain the most useful class of agents in all forms of angina. While it was formerly thought that it was important to have high blood levels of nitrate at all times, it is now recognized that tolerance develops rapidly, and a 'nitrate free' period of a few hours in each 24-hour period is beneficial in maintaining the effectiveness of treatment.

The nitrate free period should coincide with the period of lowest risk, and this is usually night time, but not early morning which is a high risk period for infarction. Many patients receiving short-acting nitrates two or three times a day would do well to have their doses between 7 a.m. and 6 p.m. (say, 8 a.m. and 2 p.m. for isosorbide mononitrate), but this is generally not practised in unstable angina where there is no low-risk period and where continuous dosing is used, with increasing doses if tolerance develops. There are many nitrate preparations available, including intravenous infusions, conventional or slow release tablets and capsules, transdermal patches and ointments, sublingual tablets and sprays and adhesive buccal tablets. The majority of stable angina patients should be controlled by conventional tablets or capsules, which are cheap, can usually be administered two or three times daily and which permit a nitrate free period at night. There is no advantage in using more than one preparation. Slow release preparations and transdermal patches are expensive, do not generally offer such flexible dosing rates and may not permit a nitrate free period. Ointments are messy, and buccal tablets are expensive and offer no real therapeutic advantage in regular therapy. Like sublingual sprays and tablets, however, they have a rapid onset of action and the drug bypasses the liver, which has an extensive first-pass metabolic effect on oral nitrates. The sublingual preparations (sprays, suckable or chewable tablets) are used for the prevention or relief of acute attacks of pain but may elicit the two principal side-effects of nitrates, hypotension (with dizziness and fainting) and a throbbing headache. To minimize these effects, patients should be advised to sit down, and to spit out (or swallow) the tablet once the angina is relieved. Sublingual glyceryl trinitrate tablets have a very short shelf life on exposure to air and should be stored carefully and replaced frequently. All nitrates may also induce tachycardia.

Three main nitrates are used: glyceryl trinitrate (mainly for sublingual, buccal, transdermal and intravenous routes), isosorbide dinitrate and isosorbide mononitrate. All are effective if given in appropriate doses at suitable dose intervals (Table 18.4). Since isosorbide dinitrate is metabolized to the mononitrate, there is a preference in some quarters for using the more predictable mononitrate, but this is not a significant clinical factor. A more relevant feature may be that whereas the dinitrate is usually given three or four times a day, the mononitrate is given once or twice a day. More expensive slow release preparations exist for both drugs.

Nicorandil

Nicorandil is a compound that exhibits the properties of a nitrate but which also activates ATP-dependent potassium channels. The IONA study compared nicorandil with placebo as 'add-on' treatment in 5126 high-risk patients with stable angina. The main benefit

Table 18.4 Properties of commonly used nitrates

Drug	Speed of onset	Duration of action	Notes
Glyceryl trinitrate (GTN)			
Intravenous	Immediate	Duration of infusion	
Transdermal	30 min	Designed to release drug steadlly for 24 h	Tolerance develops if applied continuously
SR tablets and capsules	Slow	8–12 h	
Sublingual tablets	Rapid (1–4 min)	Less than 30 min	Inactivated if swallowed. Less effective if dry mouth
Spray	Rapid (1–4 min)	Less than 30 min	
Buccal tablets	Rapid (1–4 min)	4–8 h	Nearly as rapid in onset as sublingual tablets
Isosorbide dinitrate			
SR tablets	Similar to GTN		
Intravenous			
Sublingual	Slightly slower than GTN	As for GTN	
Chewable tablets	2–5 min	2–4 h	Less prone to cause headaches than sublingual tablets
Oral tablets	30–40 min	4–8 h	
Isosorbide mononitrate			
Oral tablets	30–40 min	6–12 h	
SR tablets or capsules	Slow	12–24 h	Some brands claim a nitrate-free period if given once daily

SR sustained-release.

for patients in the nicorandil group was a reduction in unplanned admission to hospital with chest pain. The study did not tell us when to add nicorandil to combinations of antianginals such as β-blockers, calcium channel blockers and long-acting nitrates.

Calcium channel blockers

Calcium channel blockers act on a variety of smooth muscle and cardiac tissues and there are a large number of agents which have differing specificities for different body tissues. Those of importance in angina are arterial vasodilators (Table 18.5), but some also possess antiarrhythmic activity, and most are myodepressants. Nifedipine and nicardipine (and other dihydropyridines) have no effect on the conducting tissues and are very effective arterial dilators, decreasing afterload and improving coronary perfusion but also causing flushing, headaches and reflex tachycardia. The tachycardia is overcome by use of a β-blocker. They have a particular role in the management of Prinzmetal's (variant) angina which is thought to be due to coronary artery spasm. Nicardipine has a smaller effect on myocardial contractility but neither drug has the myodepressant effect of diltiazem or verapamil, both of which also have significant effects on conducting fibres and are not suitable for use in ventricular failure. Caution should be exercised in considering their use with β-blockers because of the additive effects on bradycardia and myodepression. Verapamil is suitable for patients in whom β-blockers are contraindicated on grounds of respiratory or peripheral vascular disease; the most important non-cardiovascular side-effect is marked constipation.

There is concern over the use of dihydropyridine compounds because rapid onset, short acting drugs such as nifedipine stimulate the sympathetic nervous system by reflex mechanisms, and this may exacerbate heart failure or provoke CHD. Use of these compounds is now rare in heart failure and subject to caution in hypertension in the absence of β-blockade. It is not clear whether the same should apply to slow release preparations of nifedipine or to slower onset compounds such as amlodipine or felodipine although they also stimulate reflex activity. Many efficacy trials have used surrogate markers such as blood pressure or occurrence of myocardial infarction instead of mortality as their end point. This practice has been called into question by the recent suggestion of increased mortality despite improvement in other markers (Sleight 1996).

Treatment of unstable angina and non-Q wave infarction (acute coronary syndromes)

Whereas stable angina can be managed by a general practitioner, acute coronary syndromes have a high

Table 18.5 Properties of calcium antagonists used in angina

Drug	Absorption	Protein binding	Elimination route and half-life ($t_{1/2}$)	Effective serum concentrations
Amlodipine	60–65% available after first pass Peak 6–9 h	95%	Hepatic plus 5–10% renal $t_{1/2}$ = 35–50 h	5–15 ng/ml
Diltiazem	45% available after first pass Very rapid	80–85%	Hepatic (active metabolite) + gut $t_{1/2}$ = 4–7 h	50–300 ng/ml
Felodipine	10–20% available after first pass Peak 2–5 h	99%	60% hepatic, 30% renal, 10% gut $t_{1/2}$ 10–16 h	
Nicardipine	Rapid, well absorbed Extensive first-pass effect	> 90%	Hepatic $t_{1/2}$ = 4–5 h	
Nifedipine	60–70% available after first pass Rapid[a]	> 90%	Hepatic $t_{1/2}$ = 3–5 h (capsules)[a]	
Nisoldipine	4–8% available after first pass Peak 1–2 h	99%	90% hepatic, 10% gut $t_{1/2}$ = 7–12 h	
Verapamil	10–20% available after first pass Slow	90%	75% renal, 25% hepatic $t_{1/2}$ = 3–7 h	80–400 ng/ml

[a] Apparent $t_{1/2}$ and time to onset of action are greater after tablets because of slow absorption.

adverse outcome rate and should be treated in hospital with complete bed rest and vigorous management; the death or infarction rate at one month is about 15–20% in some series and about 8% in unstable angina alone. Several agents are given simultaneously, rather than by stepwise addition, including oxygen, nitrate infusions and possibly a sedative, such as diazepam.

A 2–5 day course of either unfractionated or low molecular weight heparin confers additional benefit over aspirin in unstable angina, but there is little evidence to support the subsequent use of oral warfarin because of the increased risk of bleeding. Thrombolysis with, for example, alteplase increases mortality. The anti-platelet agents ticlopidine or clopidogrel are expensive but effective alternatives to aspirin and clopidogrel showed a small advantage over aspirin in one study. A greater advantage was observed in the CURE study when clopidogrel was given with aspirin for 3–12 months (CURE Trial Investigators 2001). Low molecular weight heparins have the advantage over unfractionated heparin of greater predictability of effect, reduced monitoring, and possibly enhanced survival. Coronary angiography or angioplasty may be performed once the acute episode has settled or when medical management has failed. There is controversy over the use of routine early angioplasty in acute coronary syndromes: most trials have been done in North America where the use of angioplasty is high, even among conservatively managed patients, and the contradictory outcomes have not provided clear answers. Likewise, the use of glycoprotein IIb-IIIa inhibitors such as abciximab, eptifibatide or tirofiban is confused by the concomitant use of angioplasty, or not, and the choice of outcome measures. If unacceptable bleeding episodes are tightly defined, then the use of abciximab or other inhibitors appears beneficial; if a looser definition is used then the benefit is at best marginal (Cusack et al 2000, Sabatine & Jang 2000, Yeghiazarians et al 2000).

Treatment of myocardial infarction

Treatment of infarction may be divided into three categories:

- immediate care that is designed to remove pain, prevent deterioration and improve cardiac function
- management of complications, notably heart failure and arrhythmias
- prevention of a further infarction or death (secondary prophylaxis).

The management of heart failure and arrhythmias are covered in Chapters 19 and 20. The remaining therapeutic aims are pain relief, thrombolysis, minimization of infarct size, prophylaxis of arrhythmias and secondary prevention.

The timing of treatment is vital, since myocardial damage after onset of an acute ischaemic episode is progressive and there are pathological data to suggest that it is irreversible at 6 hours. Clinical data from large studies of thrombolysis (see below) have shown that the sooner treatment is started after the onset of pain, the better, although there is still some benefit up to 12 hours after infarction. Sixty per cent of post-infarction deaths occur within 1 hour, but while treatment within 1 hour has been found to be particularly advantageous it is extremely difficult to achieve for logistic reasons in anyone who has an infarct outside hospital.

Pain relief should be administered rapidly with intravenous diamorphine or morphine together with an antiemetic such as prochlorperazine or cyclizine, and oxygen. There is no benefit in leaving a patient in pain while the diagnosis is considered. The rhythm and blood pressure should be stabilized and diagnostic tests performed. Several large studies have shown the benefit of an aspirin tablet (usually 162 mg) chewed as soon after the infarct as possible and followed by a daily enteric-coated dose for at least 1 month. Follow-up of those studies shows additional benefit in continuing to take daily aspirin, probably for life. Enteric-coated preparations are not proven to reduce the risk of gastrointestinal bleeding which is increased in patients taking even small doses of aspirin. Doses in UK practice tend to be in the range 75–150 mg daily after an initial 300 mg. The reduction in mortality is additional to that obtained from thrombolytic therapy (Table 18.6) (Willard et al 1992).

Thrombolysis

Studies such as ISIS-3 and GISSI-2 demonstrated great benefit from thrombolytics given soon after the onset of pain, and the lack of a discernible difference between streptokinase and the more expensive tissue plasminogen activator (rt-PA, duteplase, alteplase) and anistreplase (anisoylated plasminogen streptokinase activated complex, APSAC, now discontinued) in reducing mortality. Further studies have generated controversy over the optimum method of administration, over adjunct therapy, and over other measures of benefit. Since mortality studies require a large number of patients and long-term follow-up, other studies have used coronary artery patency (as measured by

Table 18.6 Vascular deaths at 35 days in the ISIS-2 study	
Placebo	13.2%
Aspirin	10.7%
Streptokinase	10.4%
Aspirin + streptokinase	8.0%

angiography) or left ventricular function as outcome measures. The patency studies suggest that tissue plasminogen activator produces earlier and more frequent recanalization of the arteries, especially if intravenous heparin is administered. Heparin also seems to reduce the incidence of re-occlusion after tissue plasminogen activator but has no effect on streptokinase. Those findings are consistent with data on the relative clot specificity of the agents, but whether they lead to measurable differences in mortality is controversial. The GUSTO study compared four thrombolytic regimens in a non-blinded trial and concluded that fast injection of rt-PA was better than slower infusion of streptokinase, especially in younger patients with anterior infarcts. Although the trial was large, its conduct lead to controversy because of differences between results in North American centres and elsewhere. The trial did confirm that rapid treatment is important and speed has a greater effect than the choice of drug; several studies indicate that giving thrombolytics an average 30–60 minutes earlier can save 15 lives per 1000 treated. Hospitals need to maintain fast-track systems to ensure maximum benefit. Further benefit is obtained if trained and appropriately equipped paramedics or general practitioners administer thrombolytics before the patient goes to hospital, especially if the journey time is great. Tenecteplase has been marketed more recently with the advantage that it can be administered by bolus injection.

The ASSENT 2 study demonstrated benefits and risks equivalent to alteplase when tenecteplase was administered with aspirin and heparin. All agents cause haemorrhage, which may present as a stroke or a gastrointestinal bleed, and there is an increased risk with regimens that use intravenous heparin. The increased mortality from heparin-associated bleeding is of similar magnitude to the decrease in cardiac mortality in the same studies, and there is no advantage in the use of heparin in addition to aspirin, with the exception of rapid rt-PA regimens. Hirudin has greater specificity for thrombus but the increased risk of bleeding counteracts the benefits of increased vessel patency. Trials since those listed in Table 18.8 have used many newer thrombolytics and various dosing schedules but have not found a regimen that increases overall survival (Hannah & Smalling 1998). Recent strokes, bleeds, pregnancy and surgery are contraindications to thrombolysis. Streptokinase induces cross-reacting antibodies that reduce its potency and may cause an anaphylactoid response. Patients with exposure to streptokinase, or with a history of rheumatic fever or recent streptococcal infection, should not receive the drug. The use of hydrocortisone, to reduce allergic responses, has fallen out of favour, but patients should be carefully observed for hypotension during the administration of streptokinase. Old age is no longer considered to be a contraindication to thrombolysis. All the major trials

Table 18.7   ACE inhibitor trials in myocardial infarction

Trial	Drug and duration	Patient selection and number	Main outcomes
SAVE	Captopril > 2 years	LV dysfunction, 2231	↓ Death, ↓ HF
CONSENSUS II	Enalapril 6 months	All MI, 6090	No change in mortality ↑ HF (stopped early)
AIRE	Ramipril > 6 months	HF, 2006	↓ Death
TRACE	Trandolapril > 2 years	LV dysfunction 1749	↓ Death, ↓ HF
SMILE	Zofenopril 6 weeks	non-thrombolysed, 1556	↓ Death, ↓ HF
GISSI-3	Lisinopril 6 weeks	All MI, 19 394	↓ Death
ISIS-4	Captopril 1 month	All MI, 58 050	↓ Death

All trials used placebo control and excluded patients for whom ACE inhibitors were contraindicated.
SAVE, AIRE and TRACE started therapy several days after infarction, others started within 1 day.
LV dysfunction, abnormal left ventricular function but no overt heart failure; HF, heart failure; MI, myocardial infarction.

References
SAVE, 1992, New England Journal of Medicine 327:669–677
AIRE, 1993 Lancet 342: 821–828
SMILE, 1995 New England Journal of Medicine 332: 80–85
ISIS-4, 1995 Lancet 345: 669–685

CONSENSUS II, 1992 New England Journal of Medicine 327:678–684
TRACE, 1994 American Journal of Cardiology 73: 44c–50c
GISSI-3, 1994 Lancet 343: 115–122

(see Table 18.8) used specific ECG criteria for entry (usually ST elevation in adjacent leads or left-bundle branch block) and eliminated patients with major contraindications to thrombolysis. One survey found that in general hospital practice, about two-thirds of all myocardial infarction patients did not receive thrombolysis because of exclusions or uncertainties in diagnosis (24%), time delays (21%) and other unaccountable reasons (20%). The use of glycoprotein IIb-IIIa inhibitors (e.g., abciximab) as an adjunct to thrombolytics results in increased early blood flow in blocked coronary arteries, which may translate into increased survival, but also increases the incidence of major bleeding.

β-blockers and calcium channel blockers

β-blockers have been the subject of many studies because of their antiarrhythmic potential and because they permit increased subendocardial perfusion. In pre-thrombolysis studies, the early administration of an intravenous β-blocker was shown to limit infarct size and to reduce mortality from early cardiac events. Long-term use of a β-blocker has been shown in several studies to decrease mortality in patients in whom there is no contraindication. β-blockade should be avoided in heart block, bradycardia, asthma, obstructive airways disease and peripheral vascular disease. The most convincing trial evidence concerns timolol at 5–10 mg

Table 18.8 Major trials of management of acute myocardial infarction

Trial and number of patients (date)	Intervention	Control	Main outcomes
MIAMI, 5778 (1985)	Intravenous metoprolol then oral	Placebo	↓ Mortality
ISIS-1, 16 027 (1986)	Intravenous atenolol then oral	Placebo	↓ Mortality
TIMI, 1390 (1989)	Intravenous metoprolol then oral	Later oral metoprolol	↓ Reinfarction
ISIS-2, 17 187 (1988)	Aspirin for 1 month Streptokinase	Placebo Placebo	↓ Mortality ↓ Mortality
GISSI, 11 806 (1986)	Streptokinase	Open control	↓ Mortality
GISSI-2, 12 381 (1990)	rt-PA Subcutaneous heparin	Streptokinase Placebo	No difference No benefit
ISIS-4, 41 229 (1992)	rt-PA vs. streptokinase vs. Subcutaneous heparin	Anistreplase Placebo	No difference No benefit
GISSI-3, 19 394 (1994)	Glyceryl trinitrate patch Lisinopril	Placebo Placebo	No benefit ↓ mortality
ISIS-4, 58 050 (1995)	Isosorbide mononitrate Intravenous magnesium Captopril	Placebo Open control placebo	No benefit No benefit ↓ Mortality
GUSTO, 41 021 (1993)	Fast rt-PA + intravenous heparin	Slow rt-PA or streptokinase + s/c or intravenous heparin	↓ Mortality
GUSTO, 1000 (1996)	Primary angioplasty	Thrombolysis	Equivalence or small benefit
ASSENT 2, 16 949 (1999)	Bolus tenecteplase	Fast rt-PA	Equivalence

References
ASSENT 2, 1999 Lancet 354: 710–722
MIAMI, 1985 European Heart Journal 6: 199–226
TIMI, 1989 New England Journal of Medicine 320: 618–627
GISSI, 1987 Lancet 2: 871–874
ISIS-3, 1992 Lancet 339: 753–770
GUSTO, 1993 New England Journal of Medicine 329: 673–682

ISIS-4, 1995 Lancet 345: 669–685
ISIS-1, 1986 Lancet 2: 56–66
ISIS-2, 1990 Lancet 336: 71–75
GISSI-2, 1990 Lancet 336: 65–71
GISSI-3, 1994 Lancet 343: 1115–1122

For other trials, as well as most of the above, see Fibrinolytic Therapy Trialists' Collaboration Group 1994.

twice a day, but other agents have been used successfully. Fears of inducing heart failure, especially in the elderly, have lead to a low usage of β-blockers or to the use of doses lower than those in the major trials. One large cohort study compared low and high doses of β-blockers with no therapy and found benefit in all treated patients with similar survival rates in the treated groups but a lower heart failure rate in the low dose group (Rochon et al 2000). If a β-blocker is contraindicated because of respiratory or vascular disorders, verapamil may be used, since it has been shown to reduce late mortality and reinfarction in patients without heart failure, although it showed no benefit when given immediately after an infarct. Diltiazem is less effective but may be used as an alternative. This is clearly not a class effect. Other calcium channel blockers have produced different results and nifedipine increases mortality in patients following a myocardial infarction.

ACE inhibitors

ACE inhibitors have been tried in various doses and durations and have proved beneficial in reducing the incidence of heart failure and mortality. Current practice would be to give all patients an ACE inhibitor for 4–6 weeks and then to continue treatment in patients with signs or symptoms of heart failure or left ventricular dysfunction. Contraindications include hypotension or intractable cough (see Chapter 19). The HOPE study (Yusuf et al 2000) found that ramipril improved survival in all groups of patients with CHD and this may lead clinicians to continue ACE inhibitors in all infarction patients. Current research is focusing on the possible benefits of combining ACE inhibition with angiotensin II blockade. Angiotensin II blockade alone may be suitable in patients who cannot tolerate an ACE inhibitor but does not cause the accumulation of bradykinins that may be part of the benefit of ACE inhibitors.

The relative benefits of ACE inhibitors and other treatments are shown in Table 18.9.

Insulin

Patients with infarctions have high serum and urinary glucose levels, usually described as a stress response, while diabetics are known to do poorly after infarction. The DIGAMI trial involved patients with diabetes and showed that an intensive insulin regimen, both during admission and for 3 months afterwards, saved lives. The risk of dying was halved in patients who had not previously required insulin and who had few cardiovascular risk factors (Malmberg 1997). Further work is required on defining the criteria for treatment, especially in patients who have a glucose stress response

but no known diabetic history, since the presence of a stress response in a broader group of intensive care patients is itself associated with a poor outcome which is improved by intensive insulin therapy.

Antidepressants and rehabilitation

A quarter of patients with infarctions experience marked depression and this is associated with poor medication compliance, a lower quality-of-life score, and quadrupled mortality (Januzzi et al 2000). Anti-depressant treatments have not been subjected to formal trials but it seems reasonable to try to prevent such a risk. Rehabilitation programmes, which include some measure of social interaction and education, are of proven benefit.

Nitrates, anticoagulation and other therapies

Studies on nitrates in myocardial infarction were mostly completed before thrombolysis was widely used. Nitrates improve collateral blood flow and aid reperfusion, thus limiting infarct size and preserving functional tissue. ISIS-4 (1993) and GISSI-3 (1994) demonstrated that nitrates did not confer a survival advantage in patients receiving thrombolysis. Sublingual nitrates may be given for immediate pain relief, and the

Table 18.9   Relative benefits of treating 1000 patients for myocardial infarction (MI)

Intervention	Events prevented
Intravenous β adrenoceptor blocker	6 deaths
ACE inhibitor	6 deaths
Aspirin	20–25 deaths
Streptokinase (in hospital)	20–25 deaths
Alteplase (rt-PA) (in hospital)	35 deaths
Streptokinase (before hospital)	35–40 deaths
Thrombolysis $4\frac{1}{2}$–1 hour earlier	15 deaths
Long-term aspirin	16 deaths/MI/strokes
Long-term β blockade	18 deaths/MI
Long-term ACE inhibitor	21–45 deaths/MI
10% reduction in serum cholesterol	7 deaths/MI
Stopping smoking	27 deaths
Adapted from McMurray & Rankin (1994).	

use of intravenous or buccal nitrates considered in patients whose infarction pain does not resolve rapidly or who develop ventricular failure.

Anticoagulation with warfarin is not generally recommended, despite promising results in some trials conducted in the pre-thrombolysis era. This is partly because of the success of aspirin therapy, which does not have the same need for expensive and time consuming follow-up and is associated with fewer drug interactions. Routine use of dipyridamole and sulfinpyrazone is not recommended after infarction.

Magnesium infusions looked highly promising when given very early in medium sized trials (2000 patients). However, in ISIS-4 (41 000 patients), where the average delay to injection was longer, there was no reduction in mortality. Antiarrhythmics generally increase mortality and arrhythmias in post-myocardial infarction patients. They should only be used for symptomatic arrhythmias (see Ch. 20).

Mechanical intervention

The role of early coronary artery bypass grafting and percutaneous transluminal angioplasty (PCTA, the expansion of constricted vessels by a balloon device) in comparison to thrombolysis is highly controversial. These techniques work better in well-equipped and experienced centres where both cardiac and surgical staff are available. In such circumstances PCTA is as good as thrombolysis at decreasing 30 day mortality, and better as regards some other end points (Gersh 1999, Ryan et al 1999).

Angioplasty and stenting. Balloon angioplasty and insertion of metal stents (Fig. 18.4) cause damage to the vessel intima that exposes the thrombogenic subendothelium and promotes restenosis. This leads to a bad outcome (death, myocardial infarction or refractory angina) in about 15% of patients. There are several putative mechanisms but the formation of a layer of activated platelets, and consequent thrombosis, is important. Pharmacotherapy aimed at inhibiting the activation of platelets is thought to work because it allows time for a layer of intimal cells to grow over the damaged area and hide pro-thrombotic material underneath. In addition to long-term aspirin, 1 month of oral clopidogrel or ticlopidine is prescribed to inhibit ADP-induced platelet activation, together with perioperative intravenous abciximab, an inhibitor of the platelet glycoprotein IIb-IIIa receptor. Ticlopidine is less commonly used because of leucocytopenia, while oral IIb-IIIa blockers, including tirofiban and eptifibatide, may prove beneficial. An increased risk of thrombocytopenia and bleeding complicates all these therapies.

A treatment algorithm for coronary heart disease is shown in Figure 18.5.

Patient care

Patients with CHD range from those who have investigational evidence of CHD but no symptoms to those who have major pain and exercise limitation. All need counselling on preventive measures including diet, smoking and exercise. Prophylactic medication is important and for most patients will include aspirin and a statin. Doses of some statins need to be titrated against

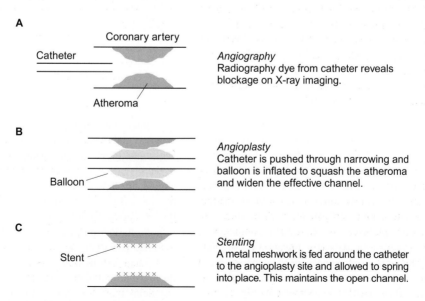

A

Coronary artery

Catheter

Atheroma

Angiography
Radiography dye from catheter reveals blockage on X-ray imaging.

B

Balloon

Angioplasty
Catheter is pushed through narrowing and balloon is inflated to squash the atheroma and widen the effective channel.

C

Stent

Stenting
A metal meshwork is fed around the catheter to the angioplasty site and allowed to spring into place. This maintains the open channel.

Figure 18.4 Procedures to overcome narrowing in atheromatous coronary vessels. The catheter is inserted from the femoral, radial or brachial arteries into the aorta and then into the coronary arteries.

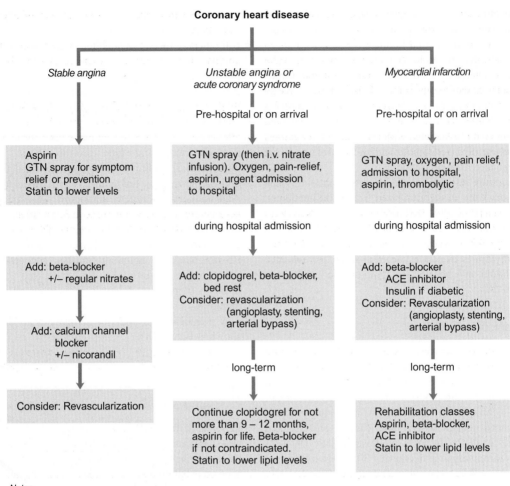

Coronary heart disease

Stable angina

Aspirin
GTN spray for symptom
relief or prevention
Statin to lower levels

Add: beta-blocker
+/– regular nitrates

Add: calcium channel
blocker
+/– nicorandil

Consider: Revascularization

*Unstable angina or
acute coronary syndrome*

Pre-hospital or on arrival

GTN spray (then i.v. nitrate
infusion). Oxygen, pain-relief,
aspirin, urgent admission
to hospital

during hospital admission

Add: clopidogrel, beta-blocker,
bed rest
Consider: revascularization
(angioplasty, stenting,
arterial bypass)

long-term

Continue clopidogrel for not
more than 9 – 12 months,
aspirin for life. Beta-blocker
if not contraindicated.
Statin to lower lipid levels

Myocardial infarction

Pre-hospital or on arrival

GTN spray, oxygen, pain relief,
admission to hospital,
aspirin, thrombolytic

during hospital admission

Add: beta-blocker
ACE inhibitor
Insulin if diabetic
Consider: Revascularization
(angioplasty, stenting,
arterial bypass)

long-term

Rehabilitation classes
Aspirin, beta-blocker,
ACE inhibitor
Statin to lower lipid levels

Notes
All patients should have lifestyle advice and regular follow-up.
Aspirin and a statin are indicated in most patients.
Consider ACE inhibitor in most patients.
Hypertension, heart failure and arrhythmias should be treated as required.
Revascularization requires assessment by angiography before possible angioplasty, stenting or bypass surgery.
Other drugs are prescribed only of there are no specific contraindications.
Verapamil or diltiazem may be suitable if beta-blockers are not tolerated.
Angiotensin II blockers may be suitable if ACE inhibitors are not tolerated because of cough.
Duration of clopidogrel treatment unclear.
Clopidogrel may be suitable if aspirin is not tolerated.

Figure 18.5   Treatment algorithm for coronary heart disease.

effect, by a GP. Patients need advice on how to reduce the risk of gastrointestinal bleeding by taking aspirin with food and dissolved in water when the soluble preparation is prescribed. Patients should be encouraged to adopt a lifestyle that makes the most of their abilities without undue hazard to their health. Most of the guidelines on prevention of CHD apply to all stages of the disease although the degree of exercise taken must be tailored according to the patient's threshold for angina. In general, although some patients are too cavalier, most are likely to err on the cautious side and may need to be encouraged to do more. Many centres now run cardiac rehabilitation classes to encourage patients to exercise and to adopt a suitable lifestyle.

A diary of anginal attacks is very useful as a record of progress and may be used to adjust treatment. The use of sublingual glyceryl trinitrate should be recorded as well as details of the activities or circumstances that provoke angina. In view of the success of early thrombolysis in myocardial infarction, patients should be encouraged if they experience chest pain that is similar to a previous infarction, or worse than their usual angina, to call for an ambulance without summoning a general practitioner first. There is little that general medical practitioners can do that the ambulance and casualty service cannot and any delay may worsen the patient's prognosis.

Patients should avoid over-the-counter preparations containing sympathomimetic drugs (e.g. cold cures) but occasional aspirin for analgesia does not affect the antiplatelet action of low dose aspirin.

Many patients will find the lifestyle changes burdensome or contrary to their wishes and it is essential they have support from their GP, practice nurse, pharmacist or cardiology centre. This is particularly so when drugs are prescribed that may further diminish quality of life. Nitrates may cause headaches and hypotensive episodes and β-blockers can be associated with bad dreams, difficulty sleeping, cold extremities, fatigue, etc. Patients requiring glyceryl trinitrate should be counselled on the best way to administer sublingual doses, i.e. while sitting, not standing or lying. Nitrate tablets should be placed under the tongue only until relief is obtained (to avoid headaches), and a fresh supply should be kept in a convenient place (pocket, handbag, etc.) at all times. Oral nitrates and transdermal patches should be taken or applied at the appropriate times to ensure a low nitrate period at night and a high nitrate period soon after rising.

Patients also need up-to-date advice when faced with difficult choices regarding medical treatment, angiographic procedures or surgery. Patients have good reason to be anxious at times but some patients restrict their activities unnecessarily out of fear of angina and infarction.

Common therapeutic problems in the management of coronary heart disease are described in Table 18.10.

CASE STUDIES

Case 18.1

A 55-year-old man presents to his GP complaining of tightness in his chest when he digs the garden. It eases when he has a rest. On investigation he has a raised serum glucose concentration and is considered to be a newly-diagnosed non-insulin dependent diabetic.

Question

What cardiovascular investigations and treatments should this patient receive?

Answer

The patient's blood pressure and electrocardiogram should be checked and he should be examined for signs of hypertensive

---

Table 18.10   Common therapeutic problems in coronary heart disease

Problem	Comment
Used incorrectly, nitrates may cause hypotensive episodes or collapse	Advise to sit down when using nitrate sprays or sub-lingual tablets
A daily nitrate-free period is required to maintain efficacy of nitrates	Avoid long-acting preparations and prescribe, asymmetrically (e.g., 8 a.m. and 2 p.m.)
Non-steroidal anti-inflammatory drugs are associated with renal failure when given with ACE inhibitors	Warn patients to use paracetamol as their analgesic of choice
Speed is essential when patients need fibrinolytic drugs after infarction	Arrange emergency admission to hospital where fast-track systems should exist
Aspirin may cause GI bleeding	Advise on taking with food and water. Consider use of prophylactic agents in high-risk patients
β-blockers are often considered unpleasant to take	Encourage patient to use regularly. Change the time of day. Consider a vasodilator if cold extremities are a problem. Consider verapamil or diltiazem
β-blockers are contraindicated in respiratory and peripheral vascular disease	Consider verapamil or diltiazem. Pay strict attention to other treatments and removal of precipitating factors
Patients often receive multiple drugs for prophylaxis and for treatment of coexisting disorders	Use once-daily preparations, dosing aids and intensive social and educational support. Avoid all unnecessary drugs
ACE inhibitors are contraindicated in pregnancy, especially the first trimester	Advise women of childbearing years to avoid conception or seek specialist advice first

or diabetic target organ damage, including albuminuria. His serum lipid profile should be measured.

He should receive GTN spray or sub-lingual tablets for the chest symptoms that are almost certainly angina. He should take aspirin daily and a statin if his lipid profile is abnormal. Some prescribers would give a statin in almost all diabetic, CHD patients and likewise an ACE inhibitor. Certainly any hypertension should be treated aggressively so that the diastolic pressure is less than 80 mmHg. A β-blocker may also be useful to control blood pressure and prevent further episodes of angina, but many prescribers would wait until there was evidence of failure of the other therapies. In view of his relatively young age, a referral to a cardiologist for possible angiography would be considered. Dietary advice and help to stop smoking, if needed, would be given. Diabetic treatments should be given (see Ch. 42).

Case 18.2

The following patients are admitted for treatment of myocardial infarction:

1. **an asthmatic**
2. **a man previously treated for infarction**
3. **a patient with rheumatoid arthritis.**

Question

What contraindications, or possible contraindications, are there to standard treatments in the above people?

Answers

1. An asthmatic should not receive a β-blocker without careful consideration and supervision because of the risk of bronchoconstriction; there is also a small risk of bronchoconstriction with aspirin.
2. A previous infarct may have been treated with streptokinase and a repeat dose should be avoided. Tissue plasminogen activator should be used instead.
3. Thrombolytics are contraindicated if there is a serious risk of bleeding. A patient with rheumatoid arthritis may be receiving non-steroidal anti-inflammatory drugs (NSAIDs) or steroids and enquiries must be made into any history of gastrointestinal bleeding. NSAIDs would also not be prescribed with ACE inhibitors because of the risk of impaired renal function. Aspirin is not contraindicated with NSAIDs, and may be useful, but will increase the risk of gastrointestinal bleeding.

REFERENCES

ACC/AHA/ACP-ASIM 1999 ACC/AHA/ACP-ASIM guidelines for the management of patients with chronic stable angina: executive summary and recommendations. Circulation 99: 2829–2848

Antiplatelet Trialists Collaboration 1991 Collaborative overview of randomised trials of antiplatelet therapy. British Medical Journal 308: 81–106

Barker D J, Forsen T, Uutela A et al 2001 Size at birth and resilience to effects of poor living conditions in adult life: longitudinal study. British Medical Journal 323: 1273

Clopidogrel in Unstable Angina to Prevent Recurrent Events (CURE) Trial Investigators 2001 Effects of clopidogrel in addition to aspirin in patients with acute coronary syndromes without ST-segment elevation. New England Journal of Medicine 345: 494–502

Cusack M, Redwood S, Coltart J 2000 Recent advances in ischaemic heart disease. Postgraduate Medical Journal 76: 542–546

Ferrari R, Ceconi C, Curello S et al 1999 Ischemic preconditioning, myocardial stunning, and hibernation: basic aspects. American Heart Journal 138: S61–S68

Fibrinolytic Therapy Trialists' Collaboration Group 1994 Indications for fibrinolytic therapy in suspected acute myocardial infarction: collaborative overview of early mortality and major morbidity results from all randomized trials of more than 1000 patients. Lancet 343: 311–322

Gersh B J 1999 Optimal management of acute myocardial infarction at the dawn of the next millenium. American Heart Journal 138: S188–S202

Hannah G P, Smalling R W 1998 Therapy with thrombolytic agents in coronary artery disease. Current Opinion in Cardiology 13: 267–273

Iona Study Group 2002 Effect of nicorandil on coronary events in patients with stable angina: the Impact Of Nicorandil in Angina (IONA) randomised trial. Lancet 349: 1269–1275

Januzzi J L, Stern T A, Pasternak R C et al 2000 The influence of anxiety and depression on outcomes of patients with coronary artery disease. Archives of Internal Medicine 160: 1913–1921

Kuller L H 2000 Hormone replacement and coronary heart disease. Medical Clinics of North America 84 (1): 181–197

Lavie C J, Milani R V 2000 Benefits of cardiac rehabilitation and exercise training. Chest 117: 5–6

Lee T H, Goldman L 2000 Evaluation of the patient with acute chest pain. New England Journal of Medicine 342: 1187–1195

McMurray J J V, Rankin A C 1994 Treatment of myocardial infarction, unstable angina and angina pectoris. British Medical Journal 309: 1343–1350.

Malmberg K 1997 Prospective randomised study of intensive insulin treatment on long term survival after acute myocardial infarction in patients with diabetes mellitus. DIGAMI (diabetes mellitus, insulin glucose infusion in acute myocardial infarction) Study Group. British Medical Journal 314: 1512–1515

Manson J E, Tosteson H, Ridker P M et al 1992 The primary prevention of myocardial infarction. New England Journal of Medicine 326: 1406–1416

Marchioli R, Valagussa F 2000 The results of the GISSI-Prevenzione trial in the general framework of secondary prevention. European Heart Journal 1: 949–952

Norris R M 1998 Fatality outside hospital from acute coronary events in three British health districts 1994–95. British Medical Journal 316: 1065–1070

Pearson T A 2000 Population benefits of cholesterol reduction: epidemiology, economics, and ethics. American Journal of Cardiology 85: 20E–23E

Rochon P A, Tu J V, Anderson G M et al 2000 Rate of heart failure and 1-year survival for older people receiving low-dose β-blocker therapy after myocardial infarction. Lancer 356: 639–644

Ryan T J, Ryan T J Jr, Jacobs A K 1999 Primary PTCA versus

thrombolytic therapy: an evidence-based summary. American Heart Journal 138: S96–S104

Sabatine M S, Jang I-K 2000 The use of glycoprotein IIb-IIIa inhibitors in patients with coronary artery disease. American Journal of Medicine 109: 224–237

Sleight P 1996 Calcium antagonists during and after myocardial infarction. Drugs 51: 216–225

Willard J E, Lange R A, Hillis L D 1992 The use of aspirin in ischaemic heart disease. New England Journal of Medicine 327: 175–181

Yeghiazarians Y, Braunstein J B, Askari A et al 2000 Unstable angina pectoris. New England Journal of Medicine 342: 101–114

Yusuf S, Sleight P, Pogue J et al 2000 Effects of an angiotensin-converting-enzyme inhibitor, ramipril, on cardiovascular events in high-risk patients. The Heart Outcomes Prevention Evaluation Study Investigators. New England Journal of Medicine 342: 145–153

FURTHER READING

Collins R, Peto R, Baigent C et al 1997 Aspirin, heparin and fibrinolytic therapy in suspected acute myocardial infarction. New England Journal of Medicine 336: 847–860

Hennekens C H, Albert C M, Godfried C M et al 1996 Adjunctive drug therapy of acute myocardial infarction – evidence from clinical trials. New England Journal of Medicine 335: 1660–1667

Orford J L, Selwyn A P, Ganz P et al 2000 The comparative pathobiology of atherosclerosis and restenosis. American Journal of Cardiology 86(Suppl.): 6H–11H

Task Force of the European Society of Cardiology and the European Resuscitation Council 1998 The pre-hospital management of acute heart attacks. European Heart Journal 19: 1140–1164

Zeymer U, Neuhaus K-L 1999 Clinical trials in acute myocardial infarction. Current Opinion in Cardiology 14: 392–402

Congestive heart failure 19

S. A. Hudson   J. McAnaw   F. Reid

Congestive heart failure occurs when the heart fails to sustain an adequate delivery of blood, and therefore oxygen and nutrients, to the tissues. It is associated with a number of symptoms arising from defects in left ventricular filling and/or emptying, including shortness of breath and exertional fatigue. The symptoms of heart failure are due to inadequate perfusion, venous congestion and disturbed water and electrolyte balance. In chronic heart failure, normal body compensatory mechanisms become counter-productive, and the resulting maladaptive secondary physiological effects contribute to the progressive nature of the disease. Treatment is aimed at improving left ventricular function, controlling the secondary effects that lead to the occurrence of symptoms and delaying progression of the condition. Drug therapy is indicated in all patients with heart failure to control symptoms where present, improve quality of life and prolong survival. Patients with heart failure can be classified according to their functional status using the New York Heart Association (NYHA) classification system shown in Table 19.1.

Epidemiology

Heart failure is a common condition with a prevalence ranging from 0.3% to 2% in the population at large, 3–5% in the population over 65 years old, and between 8% and 16% of those aged over 75 years. It accounts for 5% of adult medical admissions to hospital. There is a loss of cardiac reserve with age, and heart failure may often complicate the presence of other conditions in the elderly. More than 10% of patients with heart failure also have atrial fibrillation as a contributory factor. This combination presents a risk of thromboembolic complications, notably stroke; the risk is 2% in patients in sinus rhythm, but may exceed 10% a year in patients with atrial fibrillation who are not anticoagulated and have attendant risk factors.

Table 19.1   New York Heart Association (NYHA) classification of functional status of the patient with heart failure

I	No symptoms with ordinary physical activity (such as walking or climbing stairs)
II	Slight limitation with dyspnoea on moderate to severe exertion (climbing stairs or walking uphill)
III	Marked limitation of activity, less than ordinary activity causes dysponea (restricting walking distance and limiting climbing to one flight of stairs)
IV	Severe disability, dyspnoea at rest (unable to carry on physical activity without discomfort)

Heart failure is a progressive condition with a median survival of about 5 years after diagnosis, although mortality varies according to aetiology and severity. The prognosis can be predicted according to severity of the disease. The annual mortality rate for patients with chronic heart failure is estimated at 10%. Main causes of death are progressive pump failure, sudden cardiac death and recurrent myocardial infarction.

Aetiology

Heart failure is often gradual in onset, with symptoms arising insidiously and without any specific cause over a number of years. The common underlying aetiologies in patients with cardiac failure are coronary artery disease and hypertension, and therefore the appropriate management of these predisposing conditions is also an important consideration in controlling cardiac failure in the community. Identifiable causes of cardiac failure include aortic stenosis, cardiomyopathy, mechanical defects such as cardiac valvular dysfunction, hyperthyroidism or severe anaemia. Conditions that place increased demands on the heart can create a shortfall in cardiac output. In hyperthyroidism the tissues place a greater metabolic demand, and in severe anaemia there is an increased circulatory demand on the heart. Systolic contraction may also be compromised by bradycardia or tachycardia, or by a sustained arrhythmia such as that experienced by patients in atrial fibrillation. Atrial fibrillation often accompanies hyperthyroidism and mitral valve disease, where a rapid and irregular ventricular response may compromise cardiac efficiency. Improved management of the underlying causes, where appropriate, may alleviate the symptoms of heart failure, whereas the presence of mechanical defects may require the surgical insertion of prosthetic valve(s). The most common cause of heart failure is left ventricular systolic dysfunction (LVSD), and most of the available evidence from clinical trials regarding the pharmacological treatment of heart failure relates to the treatment of those patients with LVSD.

Pathophysiology

In health, cardiac output at rest is approximately 5 l/min with a mean heart rate of 70 beats per minute and stroke volume of 70 ml. Since the filled ventricle has a normal volume of 130 ml, the fraction ejected is over 50% of the ventricular contents, with 60 ml remaining as the residual volume. In LVSD the ejection fraction is reduced to below 45%, and symptoms are common when the fraction is below 35%. When the ejection fraction falls below 10%, patients also become at risk of thrombus formation within the left ventricle and in most cases anticoagulation with warfarin is indicated.

LVSD may be due to defects in systolic contraction, diastolic relaxation or both. Systolic dysfunction arises from impaired contractility, and is reflected in a low ejection fraction and cardiac dilatation. Normal filling requires active diastolic expansion of the ventricular volume. Diastolic dysfunction arises from impairment of the filling process due to impaired relaxation or reduced compliance of the left ventricle during diastole. Diastolic filling is determined by the rate of venous return. The tension on the ventricular wall at the end of diastole is called the preload, which is the volume of blood available to be pumped, and which contributes to the degree of stretch on the myocardium. Sustained diastolic dysfunction, which is a feature in a minority of patients with cardiac failure, may lead to systolic dysfunction associated with disease progression and left ventricular remodelling (structural changes and/or deterioration).

During systolic contraction, the tension on the ventricular wall is determined by the degree of resistance to outflow at the exit valve and that within the arterial tree – the systemic vascular resistance. Arterial hypertension, aortic narrowing and disorders of the aortic valve increase the afterload on the heart by increasing resistance against which the contraction of the ventricle must work. This results in an increased residual volume and leads to an increased preload as the ventricle overfills, and a greater tension on the ventricular wall. In the normal heart, a compensatory increase in performance would occur as the stretched myocardium responds through an increased elastic recoil. In the failing heart, this property of cardiac muscle under stretch is diminished, with the consequence that the heart dilates to accommodate the increased ventricular load. With continued dilatation of cardiac muscle the elastic recoil property becomes further diminished or absent. Failure of the heart to handle the increasing ventricular load leads to pulmonary and systemic venous congestion. At the same time, the increased tension on the ventricular wall in cardiac failure raises myocardial oxygen requirements with the risk of myocardial ischaemia and arrhythmias.

The failing heart may show cardiac enlargement due to dilatation, which is reversible with successful treatment. An irreversible increase in cardiac muscle mass – cardiac hypertrophy – occurs with progression of heart failure and is a consequence of longstanding hypertension. While hypertrophy may initially alleviate heart failure it ultimately increases workload and oxygen consumption.

A reflex sympathetic discharge caused by the diminished tissue perfusion in cardiac failure exposes the heart to catecholamines whose positive inotropic and chronotropic effects help to sustain cardiac output and produce a tachycardia. Arterial constriction diverts blood to the organs from the skin and gastrointestinal tract but also raises systemic vascular resistance and increases the afterload on the heart.

Renin is released from the kidney in response to reduced renal perfusion. Circulating renin leads to the formation of angiotensin I and angiotensin II, a vasoconstrictor, which in turn prompts adrenal aldosterone release. Aldosterone retains salt and water at the distal renal tubule and so expands blood volume and increases preload. Arginine vasopressin released from the posterior pituitary adds to the vasoconstriction and has an antidiuretic effect by retaining water at the renal collecting duct. These secondary effects become increasingly detrimental as cardiac failure progresses since the vasoconstriction adds to the afterload and the expanded blood volume adds to the preload. The expanded blood volume promotes the release of a natural vasodilator, atrial natriuretic peptide (ANP), from the atrial myocytes to counteract the increased preload by way of attenuation.

Emergence of clinical signs and symptoms of heart failure result from the compensatory mechanisms for the maintenance of the circulation becoming overwhelmed or counterproductive. The long-term consequences are for the myocardium of the failing heart to undergo biochemical and histological changes leading to remodelling of the left ventricle and further complicating disease progression. In those patients where the disease is severe and has progressed to an end-stage, heart transplantation may be the only remaining treatment option.

Clinical manifestations

The reduced cardiac output, impaired oxygenation and diminished blood supply to muscles causes fatigue. Shortness of breath occurs on exertion (dyspnoea) or on lying (orthopnoea). When the patient lies down, the postural change causes abdominal pressure on the diaphragm to redistribute oedema to the lungs, and thereby causing the breathlessness. At night the pulmonary symptoms give rise to cough and an increase in urine production (nocturia) prompts micturition, which adds to the sleep disturbance. The patient wakens at night as gradual accumulation of fluid in the lungs provokes attacks of gasping (paroxysmal nocturnal dyspnoea, PND). Characteristically the patient describes the need to sit or stand up to seek fresh air and requires to be propped up by three or more pillows to remedy the sleep disturbances.

Patients with heart failure may appear pale and the hands cold and sweaty. Reduced blood supply to the brain and kidney contributes to confusion and renal failure. Hepatomegaly occurs from congestion of the gastrointestinal tract, which is accompanied by abdominal distension, anorexia, nausea and abdominal pain. Oedema affects the lungs, ankles and abdomen. Signs in the lungs include crepitations heard at the lung bases. In acute cardiac failure symptoms of pulmonary oedema are prominent and may be life-threatening. The sputum may be frothy and tinged red from the leakage of fluid and blood from the capillaries. Severe dyspnoea may be complicated by cyanosis and shock. The clinical manifestations of heart failure are presented in Table 19.2.

Investigations

Patients with chronic congestive heart failure are diagnosed and monitored on the basis of signs and symptoms from physical examination, history and exercise tolerance test. On physical examination of the patient, a lateral and downward displacement of the apex beat is evidence of cardiac enlargement. Additional third and/or fourth heart sounds are typical of heart failure and arise from valvular dysfunction. Venous congestion can be demonstrated in the jugular vein of the upright reclining patient by an elevated jugular venous pressure (JVP), which reflects the central venous pressure. The JVP is measured by noting the visible distension above the sternum and may be accentuated in heart failure by the application of abdominal compression. Echocardiography is important when investigating patients with a suspected diagnosis of heart failure. An echocardiogram allows visualization of the heart in real time and will identify whether heart failure is due to LVSD and/or diastolic dysfunction, or to valvular defects. With the provision of direct access echocardiography services to general practitioners in primary care, an increasing number of patients can be referred for confirmation of suspected heart failure. A number of investigations are routinely performed in the diagnosis of heart failure; these are shown in Table 19.3.

Table 19.2 Clinical manifestations of heart failure

Venous (congestion)	Cardiac (cardiomegaly)	Arterial (peripheral hypoperfusion)
Dyspnoea	Dilatation	Fatigue
Oedema	Tachycardia	Pallor
Hypoxia	Regurgitation	Renal impairment
Hepatomegaly	Cardiomyopathy	Confusion
Raised venous pressure	Ischaemia Arrhythmia	Circulatory failure

Table 19.3   Clinical and laboratory investigations routinely performed in the diagnosis of heart failure

Investigation	Comment
Blood test	The following assessments are usually performed: • Blood gas analysis to assess respiratory gas exchange • Serum creatinine and urea to assess renal function • Serum alanine- and aspartate-aminotransferase plus other liver function tests • Full blood count to investigate possibility of anaemia • Thyroid function tests to investigate possibility of thyrotoxicosis
12-lead electrocardiogram	A normal electrocardiogram (ECG) usually excludes the presence of left ventricular systolic dysfunction. An abnormal ECG will require further investigation
Chest radiograph	A chest radiograph (X-ray) is performed to look for an enlarged cardiac shadow and consolidation in the lungs
Echocardiograph	An echocardiogram is used to confirm the diagnosis of heart failure and any underlying causes, e.g. valvular heart disease

More specialized, invasive methods are used on coronary and intensive care units, allowing haemodynamic measurements to be made. A Swan–Ganz balloon-tipped catheter is directed via a suitable vein into the right atrium through and out of the right ventricle, to wedge in the pulmonary artery. Inflation of the balloon briefly blocks pulmonary artery flow and the distal catheter tip at that point is able to monitor what is effectively the filling pressure in the left ventricle, from a position on the right side of the heart. In acute heart failure, haemodynamic monitoring from the Swan–Ganz catheter and a simultaneous arterial line allow measurement of the extent of pulmonary congestion and systemic vascular resistance.

Treatment of heart failure

The goals of treatment are to relieve symptoms, delay progression of the disease and reduce hospitalization and mortality. Effective therapy can considerably improve the quality of life and, ultimately, improve survival.

In patients with co-morbidity where one of the existing conditions is known to contribute to heart failure, such as hyperthyroidism, anaemia, atrial fibrillation and valvular heart disease, there is a need to ensure the coexisting conditions are effectively managed. Patients with persistent atrial fibrillation and resultant tachycardia usually require control of their ventricular rate through suppression of atrioventricular node conduction. The use of either digoxin or amiodarone is common in such circumstances. Consideration of the use of either anticoagulant or antiplatelet agents will also be necessary. In those patients with diagnosed diastolic dysfunction, there is

very little evidence to help select treatment other than the use of diuretics to control symptoms. Figure 19.1 illustrates how therapeutic intervention affects not only cardiac function but also the complex haemodynamic and neurohormonal reflex mechanisms.

Drug treatment of heart failure due to LVSD

An evidence base for reducing mortality in patients with LVSD is available for angiotensin-converting enzyme inhibitors (ACE inhibitors), β-blockers, spironolactone, angiotensin II antagonists (AII antagonists) and hydralazine/nitrate combinations. Digoxin has been shown to improve morbidity and reduce the number of hospital admissions in patients with heart failure, although its effect on mortality is still controversial. Table 19.4 describes the treatment of acute heart failure in the hospital setting, while Figure 19.2 shows a suggested treatment algorithm for the chronic treatment of patients with heart failure due to LVSD

Diuretics

In chronic heart failure, diuretics are used to relieve pulmonary and peripheral oedema by increasing sodium and chloride excretion through blockade of sodium reabsorption in the renal tubule. Normally about 70% of sodium is reabsorbed, along with water, in the proximal tubule. In mild heart failure, thiazide or loop diuretics may be chosen depending on the symptoms experienced by the patient or the degree of diuresis required. Thiazides are described as low-ceiling agents because maximum diuresis occurs at low doses. They act mainly on the cortical diluting segment, where the ascending limb merges with the distal renal tubule, at which 5–10% of sodium is normally removed. Although thiazides have

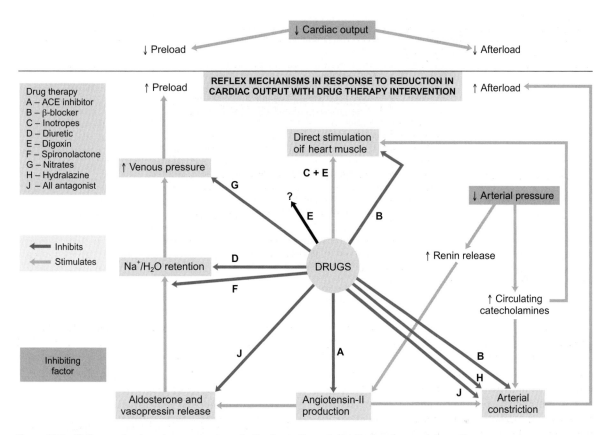

Figure 19.1 Reflex mechanisms in response to reduction in cardiac output with drug therapy intervention.

Table 19.4	Treatment of acute heart failure due to left ventricular systolic dysfunction in patients requiring hospitalization
Problem	**Drug therapy indicated**
Anxiety	Use of intravenous opiates reduce anxiety and reduce preload through venodilation
Breathlessness	High flow oxygen (60–100%) may be required in conjunction with i.v. furosemide (frusemide) as either direct injection or 24-hour infusion (5–10 mg/h). Venodilation with i.v. GTN is also effective at doses titrated every 10–20 min against systolic BP ≤ 110 mmHg
Arrhythmia	Digoxin useful in control of AF. Amiodarone is the drug of choice in ventricular arrhythmias
Expansion of blood volume after blood transfusion	An elevation in preload, such as can occur acutely by expansion of blood volume after a transfusion, can exacerbate the degree of systolic dysfunction. Therefore it is necessary to continue or increase diuretic dosage during this time

a minor action at this site they fail to produce a marked diuresis since a compensatory increase in sodium reabsorption occurs in the loop of Henle, and they are ineffective in patients with moderate to severe renal impairment (creatinine clearance < 25 ml/min) or persisting symptoms. Additionally, doses above the equivalent of bendroflumethiazide (bendrofluazide) 5 mg have an increased risk of adverse metabolic effects with no additional symptomatic benefit.

Loop diuretics are indicated in the majority of symptomatic patients and most patients will be prescribed one of either furosemide (frusemide), bumetanide or torasemide in preference to a thiazide. These agents are known as high-ceiling agents because their blockade of sodium reabsorption in the loop of Henle continues as the dose is increased. They produce less hypokalaemia than thiazides but in high doses their intensity of action may produce hypovolaemia with risk

Functional status of patient (NYHA)			Drug therapy indicated
Asymptomatic	I		ACE-inhibitor If contraindicated or poorly tolerated, consider **AII antagonist**, or either **digoxin** or **hydralazine + isosorbide dinitrate**
Symptomatic	II		Addition of **Diuretic (usually loop diuretic)** Where appropriate, consider **Carvedilol or bisoprolol** (both licensed for use in heart failure in the UK)
	III/IV		Where appropriate, consider further addition of • **Carvedilol or bisoprolol** • **Spironolactone** • **Digoxin** • **Metolazone** • **Hydralazine + isosorbide dinitrate**

Figure 19.2 Typical drug therapy indicated during the progression of chronic heart failure caused by left ventricular systolic dysfunction.

of postural hypotension, worsening of symptoms and renal failure. However, in practice high doses of furosemide (frusemide) (up to 500 mg/day) may be required to control oedema in patients with poor renal function. In the acute situation doses of loop diuretics are titrated to produce a weight loss of 0.5–1 kg per day.

Metolazone is a thiazide-like agent that is a useful adjunct to a loop diuretic in cases where the patient has severe heart failure or resistant oedema. Metolazone has a pronounced effect over 12–24 hours on the proximal tubule, even at low glomerular filtration rates. The sodium reabsorption in the loop of Henle that normally compensates for the proximal tubular action of metolazone is antagonized by the combination with a loop diuretic. Although the combination with a loop diuretic is synergistic, there are risks posed by inducing profound diuresis such as dehydration and hypotension, and therefore the patient must be carefully monitored to allow dosing adjustments to be made where necessary. In practice patients may undertake a degree of self-management by being instructed to make upward adjustments of doses of their loop diuretics or to add metolazone therapy on particular days, for example when they self-record a gain of 2 kg or over in their ideal weight over a short period of time.

Diuretics also have a mild vasodilator effect that helps improve cardiac function and the intravenous use of loop diuretics reduces preload acutely by locally relieving pulmonary congestion before the onset of the diuretic effect. Effective diuretic therapy is indicated by normalization of filling pressure. Therefore continued elevation of the jugular venous pressure suggests a need for more diuretic unless otherwise contraindicated. Intravenous furosemide (frusemide) must be administered at a rate not exceeding 4 mg/min to patients with renal failure, since it can cause ototoxicity when administered at a faster rate. Details of diuretic therapy used in LVSD are summarized in Table 19.5.

ACE inhibitiors

ACE inhibitors are indicated as first-line treatment for all grades of heart failure due to LVSD, including asymptomatic patients. They exert their effects by reducing both the preload and afterload on the heart, thereby increasing cardiac output.

ACE inhibitors act upon the renin–angiotensin–aldosterone system, and they reduce afterload by reducing the formation of angiotensin II, a potent vasoconstrictor in the arterial system. These drugs also have an indirect effect on sodium and water retention by inhibiting the release of aldosterone and vasopressin, thereby reducing venous congestion and preload. The increase in cardiac output leads to an improvement in renal perfusion, which further helps to alleviate oedema. ACE inhibitors may also potentiate the vasodilator bradykinin and intervene locally on ACE in cardiac and renal tissues.

ACE inhibitors are well tolerated by most patients and have been shown to improve the quality of life and survival in patients with mild to severe systolic dysfunction (Captopril Multicentre 1983, CONSENSUS I 1987, V-HeFT II 1991, SOLVD-T 1991,

Table 19.5   Diuretics used in the treatment of heart failure

Class and agent	Onset and duration of effect		Comment
Thiazide and related	*Oral:* Onset 1–2 h		Thiazides effective in the treatment of sodium and water retention, although there is generally a loss of action in renal failure (GFR < 25 ml/min). Metolazone has an intense action when added to a loop diuretic and is effective at low GFR.
Bendroflumethiazide (bendrofluazide)	Duration 12–18 h		
Metolazone	Duration 12–24 h		
Loop	*Oral*	*Parenteral*	Loops are preferred in the treatment of sodium and water retention where renal dysfunction is evident or more severe grades of heart failure present. Agents can be given orally or by infusion, and all are effective at low GFR
Furosemide (Frusemide)	Onset 0.5–1 h Duration 4–6 h	Onset 5 min Duration 2 h	
Bumetanide	As above	As above	
Torasemide	Onset < 1 h Duration < 8 h	Onset 10 min Duration < 8 h	
Potassium-sparing	*Oral:* Onset 12 h		Can enhance diuretic effect of loop and/or thiazide. Due to slow onset of action needs 2–3 days before maximum diuretic effect reached. Improves survival when given as an adjunt to ACE inhibitor and diuretic at a recommended dose of 25 mg daily
Spironolactone	Duration 12–18 h		

CONSENSUS II 1992, SOLVD-P 1992), including those patients who have suffered a myocardial infarction (SAVE 1992, AIRE 1993, TRACE 1995). When an ACE inhibitor is prescribed, it is important to ensure either that the dose is increased gradually to a target dose that represents the dose used in clinical trials, or that it is individually titrated and represents the maximum dose tolerated by the patient. There is some evidence to suggest that high doses of ACE inhibitor are more effective than low doses in relation to mortality reduction, although it is uncertain whether this is a class effect (ATLAS 1999). In clinical practice patients may be being treated with ACE inhibitors at doses below those used in trials. As a consequence outcomes in heart failure treatment may not be as good as expected.

The introduction of an ACE inhibitor may produce hypotension, which is most pronounced after the first dose and sometimes severe. Patients at risk include those already on high doses of loop diuretics, where they cannot be stopped or reduced, and patients who may have a low circulating fluid volume. In the primary care setting treatment must be started with a low dose administered at bedtime. In patients at particular risk of hypotension, a test dose of the shorter-acting agent captopril is usually given to assess suitability for treatment before commencing long-term treatment with a preferred ACE inhibitor. Once it has been established that the ACE inhibitor can be initiated safely, the preferred option is to switch to a longer-acting agent that requires twice or once daily dosing.

ACE inhibitors are potentially hazardous in those with pre-existing renal disease. Blockade of the renin–angiotensin system may lead to reversible deterioration of renal function. ACE inhibitors are contraindicated in patients with bilateral renal artery stenosis, in whom an activated renin–angiotensin system maintains renal perfusion. Since most ACE inhibitors or their active metabolites rely on elimination via the kidney, the risk of other forms of dose-related toxicity is also increased in the presence of renal failure. Fosinopril, which is partially excreted by metabolism, may be the preferred agent in patients with renal failure. ACE inhibitors are also contraindicated in patients with severe aortic stenosis because their use can result in a markedly reduced cardiac output due to decreased filling pressure within the left ventricle. The most common adverse effect seen with ACE inhibitors is a dry cough that is reported to occur in at least 10% of patients. Since a cough can occur naturally in patients with cardiac failure it is sometimes difficult to attribute the cause to the ACE inhibitor, and reports of the incidence of the adverse effect can vary. The activity and use of ACE inhibitors is summarized in Table 19.6.

Angiotensin II receptor antagonists

In patients suffering from a cough secondary to ACE inhibitors, angiotensin II antagonists such as losartan in a dosage of 25–50 mg daily can be used as an alternative,

Table 19.6   Vasodilators used in the treatment of heart failure

Class and agent		Pharmacological half-life	Comment
ACE inhibitors	(Target dose)		First-dose hypotension may occur. May worsen renal failure. Adjust dose in renal failure. Hyperkalaemia, cough, taste disturbance and allergies may occur particularly with captopril. Shown to improve survival
Captopril	(50–100 mg three times daily)	8 h	
Cilazapril		9 h	
Enalapril	(10–20 mg twice daily)	11 h	
Fosinopril		11–14 h	
Lisinopril	(30–35 mg daily)	12 h	
Perindopril		25 h	
Quinapril		3 h	
Ramipril	(5 mg twice daily)	13–17 h	
Trandolapril	(4 mg daily)	16–24 h	
β-blockers	(Target dose)		At present initial prescription by cardiologist only. May initially exacerbate symptoms but improves long-term mortality
Carvedilol	(25–50 mg twice daily)	6–10 h	
Bisoprolol	(5–10 mg daily)	10–12 h	
Nitrates			ISDN metabolized to ISMN. High doses needed. Tolerance can be prevented by overnight dose interval > 8 h. Protective effect against cardiac ischaemia. GTN given i.v. for sustained effect in acute/severe cardiac failure but limited by tolerance
Glyceryl trinitrate (GTN)		1–4 min	
Isosorbide dinitrate (ISDN)		1 h	
Isosorbide mononitrate (ISMN)		5 h	
Nitroprusside		2 min	Light sensitive. Acts on veins and arteries. Cyanide accumulation and acidosis limit treatment duration
Angiotensin II antagonists			Useful where intractable cough with ACE inhibitor. Not as effective as ACE inhibitors but with similar effects on renal function and blood pressure
Losartan		6–9 h	
Hydralazine		2–3 h	Hydralazine has a direct action on arteries. Tolerance occurs. May cause drug-induced lupus and sodium retention

although this is currently an unlicensed indication in the UK. Nevertheless, losartan has been shown to be effective in reducing mortality and alleviating symptoms in patients with symptomatic heart failure (ELITE I 1997, ELITE II 2000), although angiotensin II antagonists appear to be less effective than ACE inhibitors. Losartan has been shown to be better tolerated, but it must only be considered as a second-line treatment for ACE inhibitor intolerant patients. It is of no theoretical or practical benefit in patients who have renal failure secondary to ACE inhibitors (See Table 19.6).

β-blockers

The use of β-blockers in patients with heart failure was previously considered to be contraindicated. However, evidence has accumulated from clinical trails to support the effect of β-blockers in reducing mortality among patients with mild to moderate symptomatic heart failure (MDC 1993, CIBIS I 1994, US Carvedilol 1996, ANZ

Carvedilol 1997, CIBIS II 1999, MERIT-HF 1999, CAPRICORN 2001). Patients with severely symptomatic heart failure also appear to benefit (COPERNICUS 2001). In heart failure due to LVSD, β-blockers are thought to act by reducing the sympathetic neurohormonal overactivity, which occurs in response to the failing heart, and minimize the abnormal structural and physiological changes in the cardiac muscle. Carvedilol and bisoprolol are currently indicated for use as adjunctive therapy for patients with mild to moderate heart failure but require careful initiation and titration of the dose under specialist supervision. It is likely that the patient will experience a worsening of symptoms during initiation and so patients are commenced on very low doses of the β-blocker with the dose titrated upwards over a number of weeks of careful monitoring. Bisoprolol is started at a dose of 1.25 mg and slowly titrated to a target of 5–10 mg daily. Carvedilol is started at a dose of 3.125 mg twice daily and titrated to a target dose of 25–50 mg twice daily over a period of 2–3 months depending on the weight of the patient (50 mg twice daily if weight > 50 kg). The activity and use of β-blockers is summarized in Table 19.6.

Spironolactone therapy

The use of spironolactone, an aldosterone antagonist, as an adjunct to standard treatment (diuretic, ACE inhibitor +/– digoxin) has been shown to reduce mortality in patients with moderate to severe heart failure (RALES 1999). Aldosterone has been associated with sodium and water retention, sympathetic activation and parasympathetic inhibition, all of which are associated with harmful effects in the patient with heart failure. Spironolactone counteracts these effects by directly antagonizing the activity of aldosterone and provides a more complete blockade of the renin–angiotensin–aldosterone system when used in conjunction with an ACE inhibitor. Although the combination of spironolactone (at a dose of 50 mg daily or more) and an ACE inhibitor is associated with an increased risk of developing hyperkalaemia, the use of a 25 mg daily dose has been shown to have little effect on serum potassium and provides a significant reduction in mortality. The use of spironolactone is, however, contraindicated in those patients with a serum potassium > 5.5 mmol/l or serum creatinine > 200 μmol/l. The activity and use of spironolactone is summarized in Table 19.5.

Digoxin

Although digoxin has an established role in the control of atrial fibrillation, its place in the treatment of heart failure is still the subject of debate. There is evidence to show that when digoxin has been used to treat heart failure in patients in sinus rhythm, as an adjunct to ACE inhibitor and diuretic therapy, then worsening of symptoms occurs on withdrawal of digoxin (RADIANCE 1993, PROVED 1993). While the use of digoxin in heart failure in patients in sinus rhythm has no measurable impact on mortality it reduces the number of hospital admissions (DIG 1997). Consequently digoxin is currently recommended for use as add on therapy at low doses in patients with moderate to severe heart failure who remain symptomatic despite adequate doses of ACE inhibitor and diuretic treatment.

Digoxin is a positive inotrope, and acts by increasing the availability of calcium within the myocardial cell through an inhibition of sodium extrusion, thereby increasing sodium–calcium exchange and leading to enhanced contractility of cardiac muscle. Digoxin increases cardiac output in patients with coexisting atrial fibrillation by suppressing atrioventricular conduction and controlling the ventricular rate. In patients with atrial fibrillation, the plasma digoxin concentration usually needs to be at the higher end of the reference range (0.8–2

micrograms/litre) or in some cases higher to control the arrhythmia. However, a high serum digoxin concentration is not necessarily required to achieve an inotropic effect in patients in sinus rhythm. Digoxin is also associated with both vagal stimulation and a reduction in sympathetic nerve activity, and these may play important roles in the benefits experienced by those patients in sinus rhythm receiving lower doses. These considerations question the value of routine monitoring of serum digoxin concentrations in clinical decision making, other than in helping to confirm suspected toxicity. In practice the dose prescribed will be judged by the clinical response expressed as relief of symptoms and ventricular rate.

Digoxin treatment is potentially hazardous due its low therapeutic index and so all patients receiving this drug should be regularly reviewed to exclude the presence of adverse effects. Digoxin may cause bradycardia and lead to potentially fatal cardiac arrhythmias. Other symptoms associated with digoxin toxicity include nausea, vomiting, confusion and visual disturbances. Digoxin toxicity is more pronounced in the presence of metabolic or electrolyte disturbances and in patients with cardiac ischaemia. Those patients who develop hypokalaemia, hypomagnesaemia, hypercalcaemia, alkalosis, hypothyroidism or hypoxia are at particular risk of toxicity. Treatment may be required to restore serum potassium and in emergency situations, intravenous digoxin-specific antibodies fragments can be used to treat life-threatening digoxin toxicity. The activity and use of digoxin is summarized in Table 19.7.

Nitrates/hydralazine

Nitrates exert their effects predominantly on the venous system where they cause venodilation, thereby reducing the symptoms of pulmonary congestion. The preferred use of nitrates is in combination with an arterial vasodilator such as hydralazine, which reduces the afterload, to achieve a balanced effect on the venous and arterial circulation. The combined effects of these two drugs lead to an increase in cardiac output, and there is evidence to show that the combination is effective and associated with a reduction in mortality in patients with heart failure (V-HeFT I 1986). Although the effects are linked to improved survival, the reduction in mortality is much smaller than that seen with ACE inhibitors (V-HeFT II 1991). The evidence supports the use of hydralazine 300 mg daily with isosorbide dinitrate 160 mg daily (although in practice an equivalent dose of isosorbide mononitrate is used). With the emergence of ACE inhibitors and their superior effects on morbidity and mortality, the combination is only recommended in patients intolerant to an ACE inhibitor or where ACE inhibitor therapy is contraindicated.

Organic nitrate vasodilators work by interacting with sulphydryl groups found in the vascular tissue. Nitric

Table 19.7   Inotropic agents used in the treatment of heart failure

Class and agent	Pharmacological half-life	Comment
Cardiac glycosides		
Digoxin	39 h	In renal failure, half-life of digoxin prolonged. Dosage individualization required. Serum drug concentration monitoring used to confirm or exclude toxicity or effectiveness. Dose of digitoxin unaffected by renal failure. CNS, visual and GI symptoms linked to digoxin toxicity. No benefit in terms of mortality, but use associated with improved symptoms and reduced hospitalization for heart failure. Risk of arrhythmias, although beneficial in AF. If given i.v. must be administered slowly (20 min) to avoid cardiac ischaemia.
Digitoxin	5–8 days	
Phosphodiesterase inhibitors		
Enoximone	4.2 h	Used only in severe heart failure as adjunctive therapy. Associated with arrhythmias and increased mortality with chronic use
Milrinone	2.4 h	
Sympathomimetics		
Dobutamine	2 min	Continuous i.v. only. Require close monitoring in critical care setting
Dopamine	2 min	
Dopexamine	6–7 min	
Isoprenaline	> 1 min	

oxide is released from the nitrate compound and this in turn activates soluble guanylate cyclase in vascular smooth muscle leading to the vasodilatory effect. Serum nitric oxide concentrations are not clearly related to pharmacological effects because of their indirect action on the vasculature. Depletion of tissue sulphydryl groupings can occur during continued treatment with nitrates, and is partly responsible for the development of tolerance in patients with sustained exposure to high nitrate doses. Restoration of sulphydryl groupings occurs within hours of treatment being interrupted, therefore nitrate tolerance can be prevented by the use of an asymmetric dosing regimen to ensure that the patient experiences a daily nitrate-free period of more than 8 hours.

In the acute setting, glyceryl trinitrate (GTN) is frequently administered intravenously, along with a loop diuretic, to patients with heart failure to relieve pulmonary congestion. When using this route of administration, it is important that a Teflon© coated catheter is used to avoid adsorption of the GTN onto the intravenous line.

Isosorbide dinitrate (ISDN) can be given orally and is completely absorbed; however, only 25% of a given dose appears as ISDN in serum with 60% of an oral dose being rapidly converted to isosorbide mononitrate. Isosorbide mononitrate is longer acting and therefore most of the accumulated effects of a dose of ISDN are attributable to the 5-ISMN metabolite. Consequently, a 20 mg dose of ISDN is approximately equivalent to a 10 mg dose of ISMN. In practice, nitrate preparations are usually given orally in the form of isosorbide mononitrate, and intravenously in the form of GTN.

Hydralazine has a direct action on arteriolar smooth muscle to produce arterial vasodilation. Its use is associated with the risk of causing drug-induced systemic lupus erythematosus (SLE). SLE is an uncommon multisystem connective tissue disorder that is more likely to occur in patients classified as slow acetylators of hydralazine, which accounts for almost half the UK population. The activity and use of nitrates is summarized in Table 19.6.

Inotropic agents

The use of inotropic agents (except digoxin) is almost exclusively limited to hospital practice, where acute cardiac failure may require the use of one or more inotropic agents, particularly the sympathomimetic agents dobutamine and dopamine, in an intravenous continuous infusion. These agents have inotrope–vasodilator effects which differ according to their action on alfa, $beta_1$, $beta_2$ and dopamine receptors ($beta_1$ agonists increase cardiac contractility, $beta_2$ agonists produce arterial vasodilatation, dopamine agonists enhance renal perfusion). With dopamine, low doses (0–2 micrograms/kg/min) have a predominant effect on dopamine receptors within the kidneys to improve urine output, intermediate doses (2–5 micrograms/kg/min) effect $beta_1$ receptors producing an inotropic effect, and high doses (10 micrograms/kg/min) have a predominant action on alfa adrenoreceptors. Dobutamine has a predominantly inotropic and vasodilator action due to the action of the (+) isomer selectively on beta adrenoreceptors. Tolerance to sympathomimetic inotropic agents may develop on prolonged administration, particularly in patients with underlying ischaemia, and is also associated with a risk of precipitating arrhythmias. Noradrenaline (norepinephrine) is an alfa adrenoreceptor agonist where its vasoconstrictor action limits its usefulness in severely hypotensive patients such as those in septic shock. Adrenaline (epinephrine) has $beta_1$, $beta_2$ and alfa adrenoreceptor agonist effects and is used in patients with low vascular resistance. However, it is more arrhythmogenic than dobutamine and should be used with caution. Phosphodiesterase inhibitors are rarely used in clinical practice as a consequence of trials showing an increased risk of mortality (PROMISE 1991).

Other agents

Direct-acting vasodilators such as sodium nitroprusside are rarely used, and when they are it is in the acute setting when they are given by continuous infusion. Vasodilation occurs as a result of the catalysis of nitroprusside in vascular smooth muscle cells to produce nitric oxide. The fact that nitric oxide production in this instance is via a different route when compared to the catalysis of glyceryl trinitrate (where there is a need for sulphydryl groups) may explain why there is little tolerance seen with nitroprusside. In impaired renal function thiocyanate, a metabolic product of nitroprusside, accumulates over several days, causing nausea, anorexia, fatigue and psychosis.

Patients with coronary artery disease may be candidates for calcium-blocking anti-anginal vasodilators. However, some of these agents can exacerbate coexisting heart failure, since their negative inotropic effects offset the potentially beneficial arterial vasodilatation. Amlodipine and felodipine have a more selective action on vascular tissue and therefore a less pronounced effect on cardiac contractility than other calcium antagonists.

In hospitalized patients in whom compromised respiratory function remains despite medical management of heart failure, the treatment options include mechanical ventilation, continuous positive airway pressure ventilation and the use of intra-aortic balloon pumping.

Guidelines

Several sources have produced evidence-based clinical guidelines through the achievement of consensus among experts. The focus of the various guidelines tends to be on chronic medication use (Heart Failure Society of America 1999; Scottish Intercollegiate Guidelines Network 1999). Both sets of guidelines confirm the recommendation that ACE inhibitors should be given to all patients with all grades of heart failure (symptomatic and asymptomatic) in the absence of contraindication. Suggested alternatives to ACE inhibitor treatment include the use of hydralazine/nitrate combination, angiotensin II antagonists and digoxin, although these are considered to be inferior. For patients with symptomatic heart failure treatment with a loop diuretic is recommended to treat oedema and control symptoms. Digoxin is recommended for use in patients with atrial fibrillation, in those with predominantly systolic dysfunction and in those with an incomplete response to vasodilators. Other recommended adjuncts to ACE inhibitor and diuretic treatment are β-blockers (bisoprolol, carvedilol or metoprolol) and spironolactone. With regard to diastolic dysfunction, there is debate about distinguishing this as a specific diagnosis and so particular recommendations for treatment are often lacking.

Patient care

Patients with heart failure are often elderly with co-morbidity such as coronary heart disease, with or without hypertension. Other complications include renal impairment, polypharmacy and adherence to the prescribed medication regimen. Where renal function is compromised, careful attention to dosage selection is required for drugs excreted largely unchanged in the urine. Patients with heart failure are at particular risk of fluid or electrolyte imbalance, adverse effects and drug interactions. Consequently, careful monitoring is indicated to help detect problems associated with suboptimal drug therapy, unwanted drug effects and poor patient compliance.

A number of therapeutic problems may be encountered by the patient with heart failure. Notably, it often complicates other serious illness, and is a common cause of hospital admission. In addition to monitoring clinical signs and symptoms in the acute setting, other parameters monitored should include fluid and electrolyte balance, assessment of renal and hepatic function, chest radiograph, electrocardiograph and haemodynamic measurements where appropriate.

Patient education and self-monitoring

To encourage participation in their care, and gain concordance with the treatment plan, the patient must be in a position to understand the need for treatment and the benefits and risks offered by prescribed medication. Appropriate patient education is necessary to encourage an understanding of their condition, inform them as to the extent of their condition and how prescribed drug treatment will work and affect their daily lives. Specific advice should reinforce the timing of doses and how each medication should be taken. Patients also need to be advised of potentially troublesome symptoms that may occur with the medication, and whether the effects are avoidable, self-limiting, or a cause for concern.

Patients must be made aware that diuretics will increase urination, and that doses are usually timed for the morning to avoid inconvenience during the rest of the day or overnight. However, there are cases where patients alter the timing of the dose(s) to suit their lifestyle or commitments with the agreement of their doctor. There are also some patients who use a flexible diuretic dosing regimen, where they take an extra dose of diuretic in response to worsening signs or symptoms as part of an agreed self-management protocol. To use such a regimen, the patient has to monitor and record their weight on a daily basis, and have clear instructions to either take an extra dose of diuretic when a notable increase in weight is detected due to fluid retention, or to seek medical attention. It is also important for patients to be aware of signs and symptoms of drug toxicity with medicines such as digoxin, for example anorexia, diarrhoea, nausea and vomiting, and be aware of the action they should take if symptoms are experienced.

Timing of doses is also important. If a nitrate regimen is being used, then patients must be made aware that the last dose of the nitrate should be taken mid to late afternoon to ensure that a nitrate-free period occurs overnight, thus reducing the risk of nitrate tolerance. However, patients with prominent nocturnal symptoms require separate consideration. Where β-blockers are used in patients with heart failure, it is important they are aware of the need for gradual dose titration because of the risk of aggravating heart failure symptoms. They should also know what action to take if their symptoms become progressively worse, and whom to contact. Table 19.8 provides a general patient education and self-monitoring checklist.

Monitoring effectiveness of drug treatment

Therapeutic effectiveness is confirmed by assessing the patient for improvements in reported symptoms such as shortness of breath and oedema, and for noticeable changes in exercise tolerance. Oedema is often visible and remarked upon by patients, especially in the feet (ankles) and hands (wrists and fingers). Increased oedema may be reflected by an increase in the patient's body-weight, and can be more easily assessed if the patient records daily weight and reviews measurements routinely. Questions about tolerance to exercise are also useful in identifying patients who may be experiencing difficulties with their condition or medication. Onset or deterioration of symptoms is often slow and patients are inclined to adapt their lifestyle gradually by moderating daily activities to compensate. The identification of loss of control is complicated by many factors, and the presence of conditions such as arthritis and parkinsonism in a patient may also affect mobility. Therefore, consideration of these and other factors is necessary as any deterioration in symptoms may not be solely due to heart failure. The presence of respiratory disease complicates the identification of increased shortness of breath, and the exacerbation of symptoms may or may not be attributable to worsening heart failure or ineffective heart failure medication.

Dietary factors may also lead to loss of control, where failure to restrict sodium intake may contribute to the problem of fluid retention. Simple dietary advice to avoid processed foods and adding salt to food should be reinforced. The effectiveness of treatment can also be undermined by drug therapy used for other conditions, or even by certain remedies that can be purchased without prescription to treat minor ailments, for example ibuprofen. Captopril absorption may be slowed by food or antacids, perhaps decreasing its intensity of action advantageously when initiating therapy; however, differences in absorption between other ACE inhibitors are not clinically significant on long-term treatment.

Many patients with heart failure do not receive the preferred choice of drug treatment recommended in evidence-based guidelines, nor the doses associated with the benefits attributed to particular medications, for example ACE inhibitors. Those at risk of suboptimal treatment need to be identified. This will require the involvement of patients and health care professionals in the monitoring of symptoms and the tailoring of each patient's therapeutic plan to ensure he or she receives the most appropriate evidence-based treatments. Table 19.9 provides a summary of monitoring activity required to confirm the effectiveness of drug use.

Monitoring safety of drug treatment

A number of safety issues surround drug treatment, especially in those patients with co-morbidity and a large number of prescribed medicines. In these patients there is a risk of drug–drug and drug–disease interactions (Tables 19.10A and 19.10B). Not only does the practitioner need to be aware of these clinically important interactions and investigate potentially problematic combinations, but they also have to be vigilant when monitoring patients and regularly assess drug safety to confirm or exclude the presence of drug-related problems. This involves clinical monitoring for signs and symptoms of drug therapy problems such as negative inotropic effects, excessive blood pressure reduction, and salt and fluid retention. This monitoring for symptoms should also be accompanied, where appropriate, by laboratory measurement of serum drug

Table 19.8   Patient education and self-monitoring in the treatment of heart failure

Topic	Advice	Comment
Diuretics	Timing of dose Flexible dosing (where indicated)	Monitor for incontinence, muscle weakness, confusion, dizziness, gout, unusual gain in weight within very short time-period (few days) where an agreed extra dose is taken by the patient. Patient able to adjust time of dose to suit lifestyle
ACE inhibitors	Avoid standing rapidly	Monitor for hypotension, dizziness, cough, taste disturbance, sore throat, rashes, tingling in hands, joint pain
β-blockers	Avoid standing rapidly	Monitor for hypotension, dizziness, headache, fatigue, gastrointestinal disturbances, bradycardia
Cardiac glycosides	Report toxic symptoms	Monitor for signs or symptoms of toxicity, such as anorexia, nausea, visual disturbances, diarrhoea, confusion, social withdrawal
Nitrates	Timing of dose Avoid standing rapidly	Monitor for headache, hypotension, dizziness, flushing (face or neck), gastrointestinal upset. Ensure asymmetric dosing pattern for nitrates to provide nitrate-free period and reduce risk of tolerance developing
Potassium salts	Administration of dose (soluble + non-soluble)	Monitor for gastrointestinal disturbances, swallowing difficulty, diarrhoea, tiredness, limb weakness. Ensure patient knows how to take their medication safely, e.g. swallow whole immediately after food, or soluble forms to be taken with appropriate amount of water/fruit juice and allow fizzing to stop
Purchased medicines	Choice of medicines	Ensure patient is aware of need to seek advice when purchasing medicines for minor ailments. Advise to ask the pharmacist when unsure
Understanding the condition	What heart failure is Impact on lifestyle Treatment goals	Ensure patient understands their condition, treatment goals and complications that may impact on their quality of life. Important to motivate the patient with respect to lifestyle modification and achievement of agreed treatment goals relative to the degree of heart failure present (asymptomatic, mild, moderate or severe)
Health issues	Diet – sodium intake Alcohol intake Smoking Exercise Other risk factors	Issues related to diet, alcohol consumption, smoking habit, regular gentle exercise (walking). Other associated risk factors, e.g. hypertension, ischaemic heart disease, need to be addressed where appropriate

levels (e.g. digoxin) and monitoring of physiological markers such as potassium and creatinine.

Potential problems with diuretic therapy

The use of a diuretic is essential in the symptomatic treatment of heart failure, but it is not without its problems. Elderly patients in particular are at risk from the unwanted effects of diuretics. The increase in urine volume can worsen incontinence or precipitate urinary retention, while overuse can lead to a loss of control of heart failure and worsening of symptoms. Rapid diuresis with a loop diuretic leading to more than a 1 kg loss in body weight per day may exacerbate heart failure due to an acute reduction in blood volume, hypotension and diminished renal perfusion with a consequent increase in renin release. Therefore caution must be exercised with excessive use of diuretic therapy. Prolonged and excessive doses of diuretics can also worsen heart failure and contribute to symptoms of fatigue because of electrolyte disturbance and dehydration. The biochemical effects of excessive diuresis include uraemia, hypokalaemia and alkalosis. Diuretic-induced glucose intolerance may affect diabetic control in type II diabetes, but more commonly diuretics reveal glucose intolerance in patients who are not diagnosed as being diabetic. Diuretics also increase serum urate leading to hyperuricaemia, but this may not require a change in drug therapy if symptoms of gout are absent (estimated incidence of 2%).

Table 19.9   Monitoring the effectiveness of drug treatment in patients with heart failure

Consider	Monitor for	Comment
Clinical markers	Poor symptom control Achievement of agreed treatment goals	Signs or symptoms of undertreatment or advancing disease need to be addressed (dyspnoea, breathlessness and or fatigue). The aim is for good symptom control and either maintenance or improvement in quality of life. Persisting symptoms or hospitalization may indicate a revision of drug therapy or the addition of other agents where appropriate (see Fig. 19.2)
Interactions	Drug–drug interactions	Some interactions may result in reduced effectiveness and require dosage adjustment or change in choice of drug (see Table 19.8)
Compliance	Formulation acceptability Dose timing and interval Unusual time interval between requests for prescription medication	Poor compliance can result from drug being ineffective (over- or under-use), experience of side-effects, a complicated drug regimen being prescribed or patient behaviour (intentional or unintentional). Reasons need to be identified and addressed, e.g. adjusting frequency and timing of doses, review choice of formulation, education, etc. Introduction of compliance aids may be considered where appropriate
Evidence-based prescribing	Implementation of evidence-based guidelines	The drug of choice for a particular patient may not reflect the evidence base for treatment for patients with heart failure. It is important to ensure that these treatment choices are confirmed or changed where appropriate
Multidisciplinary working	Input from other health care professionals	It is important to be aware of what care has already been provided to minimize the risk of giving conflicting advice to the patient, or duplicating work already done. It may also allow reinforcement of key information

Table 19.10A   Common drug–drug interactions with prescribed heart failure medication

Drug	Interacts with	Result of interaction
Diuretics +	NSAIDs Carbamazepine Lithium	Decreased effect of diuretic Increased risk of hyponatraemia Excretion of lithium impaired (thiazides worse than loop diuretics)
ACE inhibitor + or Angiotensin II antagonis +	NSAIDs Ciclosporin Lithium Diuretics	Antagonism of hypotensive effect. Increased risk of renal impairment Increased risk of hyperkalaemia Excretion of lithium impaired Enhanced hypotensive effect. Increased risk of hyperkalaemia with potassium sparing drugs
Digoxin +	Amiodarone Propafenone Quinidine Verapamil Diuretics Amphotericin	Increased digoxin level (need to halve maintenance dose of digoxin) Increased risk of AV block Increased risk of hypokalaemia and therefore toxicity
Nitrates +	Sildenafil Heparin	Increased hypotensive effect Increased excretion of heparin
Spironolactone +	Digoxin	Spironolactone may interfere with measurement of digoxin serum levels resulting in inaccurate interpretation
β-blocker +	Amiodarone Diltiazem Verapamil	Increased risk of bradycardia Increased risk of hypotension, heart failure and asystole

Table 19.10B   Common drug–disease interactions with prescribed heart failure medication

Drug	Concurrent disease	Potential outcome
Diuretic +	Prostatism	Urinary retention/incontinence
	Hyperuricaemia	Exacerbation of gout
	Liver cirrhosis	Encephalopathy
ACE inhibitor +	Renal artery stenosis	Renal failure
	Severe aortic stenosis	Exacerbation of heart failure
	Renal impairment	Renal failure
	Hypotension	Hypotension and cardiogenic shock
β-blocker	Asthma	Bronchoconstriction/respiratory arrest
	Bradyarrhythmias	Exacerbation of heart failure
	Hypotension	Further hypotension and cardiogenic shock
Digoxin +	Bradyarrhythmias	Exacerbation of heart failure
	Renal impairment	Exacerbation of cardiac failure and digoxin toxicity leading to cardiac arrhythmias

Hyponatraemia may occur with diuretics, and is usually due to water retention rather than sodium loss. Severe hyponatraemia (serum sodium concentration of less than 115 mmol/l) causes confusion and drowsiness. It commonly arises when potassium–sparing agents are used in diuretic combinations.

Diuretics may also lead to hypokalaemia as a result of urinary sodium increasing the rate of K^+/Na^+ exchange in the distal tubule. Serum potassium concentrations below 3.0 mmol/l occur in less than 5% of patients receiving diuretics. The occurrence of hypokalaemia is hazardous for patients receiving digoxin and also for those with ischaemic heart disease or conduction disorders. It is more commonly found with thiazide diuretics than loop agents, and is more likely to occur when diuretics are used for heart failure than for hypertension, probably because higher doses are used and associated activation of the renin–angiotensin system. Patients with a serum potassium level of less than 3.5 mmol/l require treatment with potassium supplements or the addition of a potassium-sparing diuretic, which is considered to be more effective at preventing hypokalaemia than supplementing potassium. Prevention of hypokalaemia requires at least 25 mmol of potassium, while treatment requires 60–120 mmol of potassium daily. Since proprietary diuretic–potassium combination products usually contain less than 12 mmol in each dose, their use is often inappropriate. Potassium supplements are poorly tolerated at the high doses often needed to treat hypokalaemia. Liquid forms are preferable to solid forms, because they can cause local high concentrations of potassium salts and damage the gastrointestinal tract in patients with swallowing difficulties or delayed gastrointestinal transit. In patients with deteriorating renal function or renal failure, the use of potassium supplements or potassium-sparing diuretics can cause hyperkalaemia and therefore careful monitoring of these agents is necessary.

Potential problems with ACE inhibitor therapy

ACE inhibitors are the cornerstone of the treatment of heart failure, but there are risks associated with their use. These agents can predispose patients to hyperkalaemia through a reduction in circulating aldosterone, therefore potassium supplements or potassium-retaining agents should be avoided when using an ACE inhibitor unless careful monitoring of plasma potassium is to be undertaken. However, the use of spironolactone is recommended as an adjunct to ACE inhibitor and diuretic therapy, although the dose used must be 25 mg daily. The use of spironolactone at this dose alongside an ACE inhibitor has been shown to have little effect on the serum potassium concentration. Although this is supported by evidence from clinical trials, laboratory monitoring is mandatory. Potassium retention can be a problem with ACE inhibitors, although it can also be an advantage by helping to counteract the potassium loss that results from the use of diuretic therapy. However, since this effect on potassium cannot be assumed to be balanced, laboratory monitoring is still necessary to confirm the impact of the drug combination on serum potassium. Heparin therapy has also been shown to increase the risk of hyperkalaemia when used alongside an ACE inhibitor, and therefore similar caution must be exercised.

When initiating an ACE inhibitor, volume depletion due to prior use of a diuretic increases the risk of a large drop in blood pressure occurring following the first dose. As a consequence diuretic treatment is usually withheld during the initiation of ACE inhibitor therapy, to minimize this effect.

A dry cough, which may be accompanied by a voice change, occurs in about 10% of patients receiving an ACE inhibitor. It is more common in women and is associated with a raised level of kinins. Rashes, loss or disturbances of taste, mouth ulcers and proteinuria may also occur with ACE inhibitor therapy, particularly with captopril. These unwanted effects tend to be more common in patients with connective tissue disorders.

A number of ACE inhibitors are administered as prodrugs therefore close monitoring is advised in patients with liver dysfunction, as this could reduce the benefits associated with their use. Most ACE inhibitors are dependent on the kidney for excretion, and require careful dosage titration in those with existing renal dysfunction. Differences in the pharmacokinetic characteristics do not fully explain the differences in duration of action seen with the ACE inhibitors, as this is also related to ACE-binding affinity. Throughout treatment the dose must be individualized to obtain maximum benefit in relation to symptom relief and survival, with minimum side-effects. When the experience of adverse effects requires a review of therapeutic alternatives, angiotensin II receptor selective antagonists may be used, although their effect on morbidity and survival is less than for ACE inhibitors.

Potential problems associated with digoxin therapy

Although digoxin has been shown to reduce the hospitalization of patients with heart failure, its use is associated with a range of adverse effects including non-specific signs and symptoms such as nausea, anorexia, tiredness, weakness, diarrhoea, confusion and visual disturbances. Digoxin also has the potential to cause fatal arrhythmias. It slows atrioventricular conduction and produces bradycardia, but it may also cause various ventricular and supraventricular arrhythmias. Digoxin toxicity typically causes conduction disturbances with enhanced automaticity leading to premature ventricular contractions. Patients at particular risk are those with myocardial ischaemia, hypoxia, acidosis or renal failure.

The appropriateness of digoxin dosage should be guided by assessment of the patient's renal function, from serum creatinine and creatinine clearance determinations, and from the pulse rate observed in the patient. Renal function may also be affected by drug therapy or loss of control of heart failure, therefore any change in digoxin clearance will have an impact on the serum digoxin concentration. The possibility of a high serum digoxin concentration should also be considered in any patient whose health deteriorates or who shows signs and symptoms of digoxin toxicity.

Potential problems with β-blocker therapy

Until recently, the use of β-blockers in heart failure was contraindicated in patients with heart failure due to negative inotropic and chronotropic effects. However, bisoprolol and carvedilol have been shown to be effective in patients with heart failure when used as adjunctive therapy to ACE inhibitors and diuretic agents. Initiation of treatment and titration of dose must be under the supervision of a specialist, with very small dose increments used to minimize transient worsening of heart failure symptoms resulting from dose increases. Titration of carvedilol or bisoprolol to the target dose is normally performed over a number of months. Therefore close patient monitoring is required to ensure safety is not compromised. The maximum tolerable dose for a patient may be below the target dose and so limit further dose titration. Monitoring for excessive bradycardia or rapid deterioration of symptoms is necessary to ensure patient safety, while also monitoring the patient's prescribed dose to ensure that dosage increments are gradual and the patient is not subjected to an overall worsening of symptoms.

Potential problems with other drugs

There are a number of other cardiovascular drugs that may be prescribed for patients with diseases or conditions other than heart failure, with some agents capable of worsening or aggravating symptoms. Patients with coronary artery disease may be candidates for calcium-blocking anti-anginal vasodilators. However, some of these agents can exacerbate coexisting heart failure, since their negative inotropic effects offset the potentially beneficial arterial vasodilatation, for example diltiazem and verapamil. Second generation dihydropyridines such as amlodipine and felodipine have a preferential action on the vasculature. They have less pronounced effects on cardiac contractility than other calcium antagonists, and this makes them the agents of choice where a limitation of the heart rate is not required.

Symptoms of fainting or dizziness on standing may indicate a need to review diuretic or vasodilator therapy. Patients should be reassured about mild postural effects and given advice to avoid standing from the chair too quickly. The patient and the health care team need to confirm the safety of the patient's treatment plan regularly, and be vigilant for any signs or symptoms suggesting otherwise. Table 19.11 provides a summary of monitoring activity required to ensure the safety of drug use.

Table 19.11 Monitoring the safety of drug treatment in patients with heart failure

Consider	Monitor	Comment
Clinical markers	Side-effects Toxicity Adverse drug reactions	There is a need to monitor for signs/symptoms of overtreatment with prescribed medication, such as diuretics (dehydration) and digoxin (nausea and vomiting). Look for signs of patient intolerance, allergy, serious adverse effects or troublesome side-effects. Document any unexpected adverse drug reactions
Laboratory markers	Changes in organ function Biochemical changes Haematological changes Digoxin toxicity if suspected	Renal function assessment and implications for drug choice and dosage individualization required, especially in the elderly and for initiation or titration of ACE inhibitor therapy (creatinine, potassium, urea). Hypokalaemia can lead to digoxin toxicity, and serum drug concentration measurement may be performed to confirm or exclude toxicity. Haematological side-effects with some drugs have been reported, e.g. ACE inhibitors, therefore laboratory checks may be required in response to clinical signs/symptoms
Interactions	Drug–drug interactions Drug–disease interactions	Some interactions may result in harm to the patient (see Table 19.8)
Co-morbidity	Drug selection for concomitant conditions	The presence of heart failure may influence treatment choice for coexisting diseases or conditions, e.g. coronary artery disease, thyroid disease, respiratory disease. Where possible, ensure drugs known to worsen heart failure are avoided or used with caution, e.g. non-steroidal anti-inflammatory agents or corticosteroids in rheumatoid arthritis

CASE STUDIES

Case 19.1 – part one

Mrs E. L., a 53-year-old woman weighing 60 kg, has recently been discharged from hospital and is receiving digoxin 0.375 mg, carbimazole 10 mg three times daily, furosemide (frusemide) 40 mg daily, and propranolol 40 mg three times daily.

Questions

1. What information is required to confirm the appropriateness of treatment for this patient? Is Mrs. E. L. receiving a rational treatment regimen?
2. Once Mrs E. L.'s thyroid problem has resolved, why will the medication regimen on which she was discharged need to be reviewed?

Answer

1. There is a need to obtain as much background information as possible from the patient to confirm the purpose and duration of drug therapy and the reason for the recent hospital admission. Information relating to current symptoms, past medical and drug history, renal function, thyroid status, body weight, serum electrolyte and digoxin determinations would help complete the picture.

Mrs E. L. is receiving the antithyroid agent carbimazole to treat thyrotoxicosis, diuretic therapy possibly to treat the signs and symptoms of fluid retention associated with heart failure, and digoxin to treat atrial fibrillation (AF). Although digoxin has been used in combination with diuretics to treat heart failure, it has been largely superseded by the use of ACE inhibitors. Propranolol is probably being used to improve the symptoms of tremor and anxiety that accompany thyrotoxicosis, and is considered to be the drug of choice for this indication. Once a patient is diagnosed with thyrotoxicosis, antithyroid treatment will lead to gradual attainment of the euthyroid state over about 6 weeks (Ch. 41). In such patients a relative resistance to the pharmacological effects of digoxin occurs, therefore the dosage requirement in thyrotoxicosis is higher than would normally be expected. High serum digoxin concentrations are needed to suppress atrioventricular conduction in AF and to counteract the increased rate of digoxin elimination also seen in the thyrotoxic patient. Propranolol may also be beneficial in AF as it helps to control tachycardia and provide symptomatic treatment of thyrotoxicosis. Propranolol, as with all β-blockers, has a negative inotropic effect that can aggravate heart failure, although the positive inotropic action of digoxin may afford some protection against this. Overall, the choice of medication for this patient would appear rational, but there are a number of issues that merit further inquiry and clarification.

2. Once Mrs E. L.'s thyroid status has returned to normal, inquiry into the persistence of AF and the possible existence of heart failure is required. Where heart failure is confirmed,

consideration must be given to the initiation of ACE inhibitor treatment in the absence of contraindication or intolerance. The use of β-blocker treatment must also be reviewed in relation to need and its potential to aggravate symptoms of any underlying heart failure. Mrs E. L. is also receiving furosemide (frusemide) and is potentially at risk of developing hypokalaemia, which is particularly hazardous in a patient receiving digoxin. Signs and symptoms of digoxin toxicity may include a loss of appetite, nausea, a change in bowel habit or general malaise. Visual disturbances such as haloes or yellow/green colour blindness are characteristic of digoxin toxicity but are infrequently volunteered by patients.

Case 19.1 – part two

Two weeks after discharge Mrs E. L. seeks advice on what tonic preparation would be suitable for her to take with her medication. During your discussion you discover that she complains of tiredness, increased breathlessness and malaise.

Question

3. What medications/conditions might be responsible for the occurrence of these symptoms? What investigations are required?

Answer

3. There are a number of possibilities to consider when assessing the symptoms experienced by Mrs E. L. Persisting hyperthyroidism or the negative inotropic effects of propranolol could be contributory factors. Alternatively, the symptoms may be due to poor control of heart failure, bradycardia or any of a variety of arrhythmias (in particular heart block and ventricular extrasystoles). The presence of anaemia may also be contributing to the symptoms reported. When considering the side-effects or toxic effects of prescribed medication, it is possible that propranolol and/or digoxin may be implicated. Propranolol is associated with fatigue, while digoxin toxicity can be associated with malaise. The acute symptoms of digoxin toxicity include nausea and vomiting and are caused by an action on the chemoreceptor trigger zone. This emetic effect can occur independent of cardiotoxicity and other gastrointestinal disturbances such as anorexia, diarrhoea or constipation. The risk of digoxin toxicity is increased in patients prescribed a diuretic because of possible/concurrent hypokalaemia.

There are a number of clinical and laboratory investigations required for Mrs E.L. Checking the pulse would allow an assessment of heart rate to confirm or exclude bradycardia. If necessary the propranolol should be discontinued and its place in the treatment plan re-evaluated. Laboratory tests required include the confirmation or exclusion of digoxin toxicity through measurement of the serum digoxin concentration, and the determination of serum potassium, urea and creatinine to investigate the possibility of hypokalaemia, dehydration or compromised renal function. If an ECG was available then the presence of bigeminy (coupling of QRS complexes) is a

characteristic feature of digoxin toxicity. Where hypokalaemia is identified as a precipitant of digoxin toxicity, potassium supplementation should be administered orally, or intravenously if there is extreme hypokalaemia and life-threatening digoxin toxicity. Alternatively, high serum digoxin (> 5 micrograms/litre) with renal impairment will require immediate treatment with intravenous digoxin antibody fragments in a single or repeated dose.

Case 19.2

Mrs A. B., a 72-year-old, has been receiving digoxin 0.25 mg and furosemide (frusemide) 80 mg daily for her heart failure for the past 6 months. She now presents with a prescription for enalapril 10 mg twice daily, furosemide (frusemide) 80 mg in the morning, and potassium chloride (slow release) two 600 mg tablets three times daily.

Question

What issues are of concern with this medication regimen?

Answer

The introduction of an ACE inhibitor to the treatment plan is welcomed, although combination with a potassium supplement carries a risk of hyperkalaemia due to the fact that ACE inhibitors are potassium-conserving. It is unclear whether this patient has previously received an ACE inhibitor and if renal function and blood pressure checks have been scheduled. ACE inhibitors are usually introduced under close supervision, especially in elderly patients since large doses of furosemide (frusemide) (80 mg or more) place them at risk of first-dose hypotension. The history of digoxin treatment and its omission from the current prescription raises the question of whether it has been replaced by the ACE inhibitor or if it will be continued.

If the patient has not already started an ACE inhibitor (i.e. they are about to take enalapril for the first time), the risk of hypotension and the need for the administration of a low initial dose of 2.5 mg at bedtime may need to be highlighted. The use of the shorter-acting captopril in a dose of 6.25 mg is a safer option in this case. Captopril could be substituted for enalapril in an equivalent daily dosage (enalapril 5–10 mg to replace captopril 25–50 mg) beyond the first dose. If the patient has poor renal function then the dose of ACE inhibitor on initiation must be low and the use of potassium supplements or potassium-sparing diuretics monitored closely if their use is appropriate.

Case 19.3

Mrs F. M., a 70-year-old with chronic asthma and mild heart failure has been prescribed naproxen 250 mg three times daily. On inspection of her medication record you discover that she is also receiving.

Furosemide (frusemide) 40 mg each morning
ramipril 5 mg in the morning

prednisolone 5 mg daily
salbutamol inhaler two puffs four times daily when required
salmeterol 50 microgram inhaler one puff twice daily
beclometasone 250 microgram inhaler two puffs twice daily
magnesium hydroxide mixture 10 ml when required.

When you ask her about symptom control she tells you that she is still breathless at night which, in addition to her painful knee, is keeping her awake.

Questions

1. Do you think Mrs F. M. should be taking naproxen?
2. What other aspects of this patient's medication regimen could be improved?
3. What is the likely effect of the prescribed therapy on serum potassium concentrations?

Answers

1. NSAIDs such as naproxen can exacerbate asthma and heart failure by inducing bronchospasm and by causing fluid retention, respectively. They can also lead to upper gastrointestinal problems, particularly when co-prescribed with oral steroids. If the painful knee is responsive to a simple analgesic such as paracetamol, this would be the preferred option. Alternatively, if a NSAID is necessary, one such as ibuprofen in low dosage should be used as it is less likely to have an effect on respiratory and renal function although it may still aggravate symptoms of heart failure. Further investigation into the persistence of respiratory symptoms is required as it is unclear whether the patient's breathlessness is due to an exacerbation of her asthma or a worsening of her heart failure, and therefore the interpretation of this symptom is difficult.
2. It is important to establish whether the patient is receiving maximum benefit from inhaled treatment. Inhaler technique must be checked and improved if necessary and the dose of beclometasone optimized. A regular regimen of salbutamol is not advisable since it may impair control of asthma by masking the onset of exacerbations. A review of the need for an oral steroid should be undertaken, as any reduction in the use of an oral steroid must be done gradually to avoid exacerbation of the asthma and ensure that the patient does not experience adrenal insufficiency. Reduction of the oral steroid dose may benefit the heart failure and possibly reduce the need for an antacid.

   When considering the treatment of heart failure, there is scope to increase the dose of ramipril to 5 mg twice daily if tolerated, or increase the dose of furosemide (frusemide) if the breathelessness is due to heart failure.
3. Mrs F. M. is receiving a number of medications with the potential to affect serum potassium. Diuretics, oral and inhaled steroids (high-dose) and β-blockers can reduce potassium, while ACE inhibitors can increase potassium. It is impossible to predict the extent to which each agent will affect potassium, especially with inhaled treatments as the dose normally needs to be high before there is any significant systemic absorption. Determination of serum potassium is necessary and if it remains low under the current treatment plan, or is at risk of being altered due to changes in drug dosage, then close observation will be required.

Case 19.4

Mr H. L., a 72-year-old man, is admitted to hospital with increasing shortness of breath at rest. He has a previous medical history of severe left ventricular systolic dysfunction (confirmed by echocardiography), and angina. On admission he is taking the following medication:

lisinopril 10 mg daily
furosemide (frusemide) 80 mg in the morning
digoxin 62.5 micrograms in the morning
isosorbide mononitrate 60 mg daily
GTN spray 1–2 doses as required
aspirin 75 mg dispersible in the morning.

His chest X-ray shows severe pulmonary oedema and bisoprolol 5 mg daily is prescribed. Blood pressure is 110/70 mmHg and urea and electrolytes are within the normal range.

Questions

1. What therapeutic options would you choose to treat the acute symptoms presented by Mr H. L.?
2. Is the addition of bisoprolol appropriate in this patient?
3. What other drug treatment options might be considered for this patient in the longer term?

Answers

1. The administration of furosemide (frusemide) by the intravenous route is necessary as there is decreased absorption of oral furosemide (frusemide) secondary to gastrointestinal oedema in acute heart failure. Only after the oedema has resolved should the patient revert back to oral administration of diuretics. At this time, the dosage can be adjusted to maintain an appropriate fluid balance. Where inadequate diuresis is achieved with an oral loop diuretic alone, the addition of metolazone should be considered (initially at 2.5 mg daily). Care must be taken to ensure that hypotension and/or renal failure secondary to rapid fluid depletion does not occur when metolazone is added.
2. Although there is recent evidence that carvedilol may be used in NYHA stage IV heart failure, carvedilol is not currently recommended in patients with acute symptoms of heart failure. Where β-blocker therapy is indicated, initiation should occur when the patient's heart failure has been stable for at least 2 weeks and at a very low dose (i.e. bisoprolol 1.25 mg). The dose should be titrated gradually over a period of months towards the dose used in the relevant clinical trial, provided the patient tolerates previous increments. In Mr H. L.'s case, it is inappropriate to prescribe 5 mg bisoprolol at this time, but treatment with bisoprolol 1.25 mg daily could be considered once his heart failure had been stable for at least 2 weeks.
3. Spironolactone 25 mg daily could be added to Mr H. L.'s existing drug therapy, since it has significant benefits on morbidity and mortality in patients with NYHA stage III or IV heart failure who are prescribed a diuretic plus an ACE inhibitor and/or digoxin. There is also scope to increase the dose of lisinopril to 30–35 mg daily provided the patient can tolerate the higher dose, as this is associated with greater benefit on morbidity and mortality. Based on his systolic

blood pressure and assuming satisfactory renal function, there is no reason why this option cannot be explored and it would be reasonable to delay any titration of dosage until the symptoms become more stable. This is important since the use of large doses of loop diuretics in acutely ill patients may predispose to ACE inhibitor-induced renal impairment.

Case 19.5

Mrs T. D., a 65-year-old woman, is referred to a hospital out-patient clinic for initiation of hydralazine and isosorbide mononitrate therapy. She has been admitted to hospital recently for exacerbation of heart failure and was intolerant of ACE inhibitor therapy. She has a longstanding history of hypertension. She is currently receiving the following medication:

furosemide (frusemide) 80 mg in the morning and 40 mg at lunchtime (recent increase from 40 mg daily)
digoxin 62.5 micrograms daily
bendroflumethiazide (bendrofluazide) 2.5 mg daily
amlodipine 5 mg daily.

On presentation at the clinic you note that serum urea and creatinine are 11.2 mmol/l and 131 µmol/l respectively. Blood pressure is 105/60 mmHg.

Question

What does intolerance of ACE inhibitor mean? Describe how you would define true intolerance in this patient and how this will inform treatment choice?

Answer

Patients are found to be intolerant of ACE inhibitors for three main reasons: dry cough, hypotension or impairment of renal function. It is important to note that heart failure can produce symptoms of a dry cough and it can therefore be difficult to ascertain whether the ACE inhibitor is responsible for causing this adverse effect. Cough occurs secondary to inhibition of bradykinin metabolism and is generally identified shortly after initiation of an ACE inhibitor, so inquiry into the timing of symptoms is important. ACE inhibitor intolerance is frequently misdiagnosed in practice, and the patient can usually be successfully rechallenged with therapy once their condition is more stable. In some patients titration to the maximum tolerated dose will be a compromise between effectiveness and the occurrence of adverse effects. The occurrence of excessive hypotension on intiation of an ACE inhibitor can result where the patient is particularly sensitive to the agent, if they are hypovolaemic, and if the ACE inhibitor has been initiated at too high a dose or the dose has been increased too quickly. Renal function can deteriorate in patients due to reduction in renal perfusion that occurs due to worsening heart failure, hypovolaemia or hypotension. Examination of fluid balance, clinical chemistry and blood pressure readings are essential during initiation of therapy and future dose titration to ensure the safe use of ACE inhibitors. All of these circumstances have the ability to present as ACE inhibitor intolerance, therefore the next step in the treatment of Mrs T. D. should be another trial of an ACE inhibitor and not initiation of a hydralazine–nitrate combination.

Once reintroduced, careful monitoring of the patient during the initiation and titration of ACE inhibitor treatment is required to the 'target' dose or maximum tolerated dose. If the patient's serum creatinine increases by 50% on taking the first dose of the ACE inhibitor then treatment with an angiotensin II antagonist or hydralazine–nitrate combination may be considered as alternative options.

REFERENCES

AIRE 1993 Acute Infarction Ramipril Efficacy (AIRE) study investigators. Effect of ramipril on mortality and morbidity of survivors of acute myocardial infarction with clinical evidence of heart failure. Lancet 342: 821–828

ANZ Carvedilol 1997 Australia/New Zealand Heart Failure Research Collaborative Group. Randomised, placebo-controlled trial of carvedilol in patients with congestive heart failure due to ischaemic heart disease. Lancet 349: 375–380

ATLAS 1999 Packer M, Poole-Wilson P A, Armstrong P W et al 1999 Comparative effects of low and high doses of the angiotensin-converting enzyme inhibitor, lisinopril, on morbidity and mortality in chronic heart failure. ATLAS Study Group. Circulation 100: 2312–2318

CAPRICORN 2001 CAPRICORN Investigators. Effect of carvedilol on outcome after myocardial infarction in patients with left-ventricular dysfunction: the CAPRICORN randomised trial. Lancet 357: 1385–1390

Captopril Multicenter 1983 Captopril Multicenter Research Group. A placebo-controlled trial of captopril in refractory chronic congestive heart failure. Journal of the American College of Cardiology 2: 755–763

CIBIS I 1994 CIBIS Investigators and Committees. A randomised trial of beta-blockade in heart failure. The cardiac insufficiency bisoprolol study (CIBIS). Circulation 90: 1765–1773

CIBIS II 1999 CIBIS-II Investigators Committees. The cardiac insufficiency bisoprolol study II (CIBIS-II): a randomised trial. Lancet 353: 9–13

CONSENSUS-I 1987 CONSENSUS Trial Study Group. Effects of enalapril on mortality in severe congestive heart failure. New England Journal of Medicine 316: 1429–1435

CONSENSUS-II 1992 Swedberg K, Held P, Kjekshus J et al 1992 Effects of the early administration of enalapril on the mortality in patients with acute myocardial infarction. Results from the co-operative new Scandinavian enalapril survival study II. New England Journal of Medicine 327: 678–684

COPERNICUS 2001 Packer M, Coats A J, Fowler M B et al for the Carvedilol Prospective Randomized Cumulative Survival Study Group 2001 Effect of carvedilol on survival in severe chronic heart failure. New England Journal of Medicine 334: 1651–1658

DIG 1997 Digitalis Investigation Group. The effect of digoxin on mortality and morbidity in patients with heart failure. New England Journal of Medicine 336: 525–533

ELITE I 1997 Pitt B, Segal R, Martinez F A et al 1997 Randomised trial of losartan versus captopril in patients over 65 with heart failure (evaluation of losartan in the elderly study, ELITE). Lancet 349: 747–752

ELITE II 2000 Pitt B, Poole-Wilson P A, Segal R et al 2000 Effect of losartan compared with captopril on mortality in patients with symptomatic heart failure: randomised trial – the losartan heart failure survival study, ELITE II. Lancet 355: 1582–1587

Heart Failure Society of America (HFSA) 1999 HFSA guidelines for management of patients with heart failure caused by left ventricular systolic dysfunction: pharmacological approaches. Minneapolis, USA

MDC 1993 Waagstein F, Bristow M R, Swedberg K et al 1993 Beneficial effects of metoprolol in idiopathic dilated cardiomyopathy. Metoprolol in Dilated Cardiomyopathy (MDC) Trial Study Group. Lancet 342: 1441–1446

MERIT-HF 1999 MERIT-HF Study Group. Effect of metoprolol CR/XL in chronic heart failure: metoprolol CR/XL randomised intervention trial in congestive heart failure (MERIT-HF). Lancet 353: 2001–2007

PROMISE 1991 Packer M, Carver J R, Rodeheffer R J et al for the PROMISE Study Research Group 1991 Effect of oral milrinone on mortality in severe chronic heart failure. New England Journal of Medicine 325: 1468–1475

PROVED 1993 Uretsky B F, Young J B, Shahidi F E et al for the PROVED Investigative Group 1993 Randomized study assessing the effect of digoxin withdrawal in patients with mild to moderate chronic congestive heart failure: results of the PROVED trial. Journal of the American College of Cardiology 22: 955–962

RADIANCE 1993 Packer M, Gheorghiade M, Young J B et al 1993 Withdrawal of digoxin from patients with chronic heart failure treated with angiotensin-converting-enzyme inhibitors. RADIANCE study. New England Journal of Medicine 329: 1–7

RALES 1999 Pitt B, Zannad F, Remme W J et al for the Randomized Aldactone Evaluation Study Investigators 1999 The effect of spironolactone on morbidity and mortality in patients with severe heart failure. New England Journal of Medicine 341: 709–717

SAVE 1992 Pfeffer M A, Braunwald E, Moye L A et al 1992 Effect of captopril on mortality and morbidity in patients with left ventricular dysfunction after myocardial infarction. Results of the survival and ventricular enlargement trial (SAVE). New England Journal of Medicine 327: 669–677

Scottish Intercollegiate Guidelines Network (SIGN) 1999. Diagnosis and treatment of heart failure due to left ventricular systolic dysfunction. No. 35. Edinburgh, UK

SOLVD-P 1992 SOLVD Investigators. Effect of enalapril on mortality and the development of heart failure in asymptomatic patients with reduced left ventricular ejection fractions. New England Journal of Medicine 327: 685–691

SOLVD-T 1991 SOLVD Investigators. Effect of enalapril on survival in patients with reduced left ventricular ejection fractions and congestive heart failure. New England Journal of Medicine 325: 293–302

TRACE 1995 Trandolapril Cardiac Evaluation (TRACE) Study Group. A clinical trial of the angiotensin-enzyme inhibitor trandolapril in patients with left ventricular dysfunction after myocardial infarction. New England Journal of Medicine 333: 1670–1676

US Carvedilol 1996 Packer M, Bristow M R, Cohn J N et al 1996 The effect of carvedilol on morbidity and mortality in patients with chronic heart failure. U.S. Carvedilol Heart Failure Study Group. New England Journal of Medicine 334: 1349–1355

VHeFT-I 1986 Cohn J, Archibald D, Ziesche S et al 1986 Effect of vasodilator therapy on mortality in chronic congestive heart failure. Results of a Veterans Administration cooperative study. New England Journal of Medicine 314: 1547–1552

VHeFT-II 1991 Cohn J N, Johnson G, Ziesche S et al for the V-HeFT II study 1991 A comparison of enalapril with hydralazine-isosorbide dinitrate in the treatment of chronic congestive heart failure. New England Journal of Medicine 325: 303–310

Cardiac arrhythmias 20

D. Scott

KEY POINTS

- Arrhythmias are common.
- Arrhythmias should only be treated if they cause poor circulation, or threaten to do so.
- All antiarrhythmic drugs are pro-arrhythmic in some circumstances.
- Treating arrhythmias after acute myocardial infarction may increase death rates even though the arrhythmias are successfully controlled.
- Electrical treatments for arrhythmias are becoming more commonly used, especially for nodal rhythms.
- β-blockers and amiodarone are the most commonly used antiarrhythmic drugs.
- Atrial fibrillation is the most common arrhythmia and is associated with a high risk of stroke. Antithrombotic treatment is important.

An arrhythmia is an abnormal cardiac rhythm, usually involving a change in rate or regularity, and is monitored by an electrocardiograph. The term 'dysrhythmia' is probably better since arrhythmia implies 'without rhythm' but it is not in general use in the UK.

Physiology

The heart contains many different types of cell, including muscle cells and some specialized cells that generate or conduct electrical stimuli and cause the muscles to contract. Several types of cardiac cell are capable of generating impulses (automaticity) and the overall heart rhythm is determined by the cells that do so most rapidly. When a cell is stimulated it passes on the impulse to adjacent cells and then enters a latent phase (refractory period) during which it cannot be restimulated. Cells that possess automaticity depolarize steadily until they reach a threshold potential at which they depolarize rapidly and generate an impulse (Fig. 20.1). In the normal heart (Fig. 20.2), sinoatrial (SA) node cells depolarize quickest and thus control the heart rhythm. The impulses are conducted from the SA node across the atria to the atrioventricular (AV) node and then down the bundle of

His to the Purkinje fibres and the ventricles. This is termed sinus rhythm.

The activity of the heart is controlled by the sympathetic nervous system, which stimulates the SA node and penetrates most cardiac tissue, and the parasympathetic vagus nerve, which reduces conduction through the AV node and slows the SA node. When functioning normally, the AV node prevents the

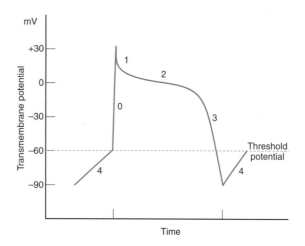

Figure 20.1 Cardiac cell potential (see Table 20.9 for dominant ion movement in each phase 0–4).

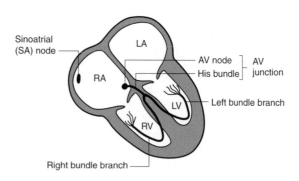

Figure 20.2 Heart conduction system.

321

conduction of excess atrial beats (such as occur in atrial fibrillation) to the ventricles but permits the passage of beats from a normal sinus rhythm. Excessive vagal stimulation results in bradycardia. This may occur in abdominal surgery, following oesophageal intubation or even in some very fit athletes when they stop exercise. Anticholinergic drugs such as tricyclic antidepressants or atropine may remove vagal control and cause tachycardia.

If the SA node is prevented from operating normally the AV node will usually take over as pacemaker or, if both are disabled, the ventricular conducting tissues will serve as pacemaker. Whenever the SA node is not the controlling pacemaker the heart beat is less well coordinated. This may result in inefficient pumping with an increase in energy expenditure to maintain an adequate circulation or ineffective pumping with an inadequate circulation.

Aetiology and epidemiology

It is estimated that 3.9 million people in USA have a cardiac rhythm disturbance and that this results in 730 000 hospital admissions each year. About 45 000 death certificates cite an arrhythmia as the main cause of death each year but about 500 000 (a quarter of all deaths) mention arrhythmias. Arrhythmias result from abnormal impulse formation or abnormal impulse conduction and these changes may be brought about in several ways:

1. An infarction may cause the death of pacemaker cells or conducting tissue.
2. A cardiac tissue disorder (e.g. fibrosis or rheumatic fever), or a multisystem connective tissue disorder (e.g. sarcoidosis) disrupts the conduction network.
3. Sympathetic or parasympathetic control changes (e.g. stress, anxiety, exercise or smoking).
4. Circulating drugs (e.g. antiarrhythmics or inotropes) or other substances (e.g. caffeine, alcohol or bile salts) affect the heart directly or via the nervous system.
5. Hypothyroidism, hyperthyroidism, hypoadrenalism, hyperkalaemia and hypokalaemia or other electrolyte disturbances may predispose to arrhythmias.

Patients who have pre-existing cardiac disorders including heart failure, hypertension, or a recent infarction are at greater risk of arrhythmias. Older age is an independent risk factor and arrhythmias are also more common in pregnancy and following surgery. Some patients have occasional arrhythmias that may be attributed to temporary ischaemia (angina), physical activity or stress but others have paroxysmal arrhythmias for no discernible reason. Most apparently normal adults have occasional ectopic beats, while in some studies up to 20% have brief periods of atrial fibrillation, and nearly half have both ventricular and supraventricular arrhythmias. In general, these arrhythmias are asymptomatic, and treatment is not recommended. Many young adults have resting sinus rhythms of as little as 40 beats per minute, which would be defined as bradycardia in an older or active patient.

Atrial arrhythmias are more common than ventricular arrhythmias and atrial fibrillation (AF) is the commonest chronic arrhythmia. The 2-year incidence of AF increases with age from less than 0.1% in the 30–39 year age group to above 1% in 70–79-year-old men. The prevalence in men aged over 70 years is about 10% and the hospital stay required for treating AF exceeds the total for all ventricular and junctional rhythms. Among emergency medical admissions to UK general hospitals, 7% of patients have AF. While 85% of chronic AF and 40% of paroxysmal AF has an identifiable cause, mostly valve disease, hypertension or ischaemic heart disease. Women have a lower risk of AF but respond less well to treatment and have a higher risk of dying. Women also have a lower risk of sudden cardiac death (defined as death within 1 hour of symptom onset in the absence of another probable cause, and presumed to be due to arrhythmia) but have a higher risk of drug-induced arrhythmias.

Description of arrhythmias

All cardiac rhythms can be described by a phrase which includes terms that relate to rate, origin and pattern.

Table 20.1 lists terms that may be combined into a single phrase. For example, 'atrial flutter' denotes a fast, regular rhythm originating in the atria. The term 'flutter' includes both rate and pattern. Even complex phrases can be broken down into the same three elements, for example 'paroxysmal atrial tachycardia with block' denotes a fast rhythm that originates from a single atrial focus and which occurs in bursts with some other rhythm in between. There is also a delay in conducting the beat from the atria to the ventricles.

Traditional names are still used for a few arrhythmias, such as 'torsades de pointes', a fast ventricular rhythm with polymorphic QRS complexes and a characteristic electrocardiogram (ECG) pattern. Some terms, for example 'supraventricular', have a general meaning such as 'originating above the ventricles', but can commonly denote something more specific, 'from the AV node'. This terminology arises partly because all descriptions depend on an indirect measure of the function of the heart, namely the electrocardiogram (ECG) recording. The ECG records patterns of electrical activity in the heart; it does not refer to how well the heart is

Table 20.1 Nomenclature for describing arrhythmias

Term	Notes
Rate	
Tachycardia Bradycardia	Both terms imply an SA node rhythm unless otherwise stated Often a regular rhythm Normal limits for rate vary according to the age and activity of the patient Bradycardia is slow, tachycardia is fast
Origin	
Sinus	SA node
Atrial	From the atria but not the SA node
Nodal	Atrioventricular node
Supraventricular	Usually, but not necessarily, from the AV node
Re-entrant	A circuit involving retrograde, (backward) conduction and an accessory pathway whereby impulses travel in a loop e.g. the Wolff–Parkinson–White syndrome
Ventricular	From the ventricular tissue
Pattern	
Ectopic Premature contraction	From a focus other than the SA node May be isolated or repeated
Paroxysmal	Occurs in bursts
Flutter	A fast, regular rhythm from a single ectopic focus
Fibrillation	A fast, chaotic rhythm from multiple foci
Block	A delay in, or absence of, conduction through the AV node
Mobitz Wenckebach	Terms used to describe particular varieties of second degree block
Torsades de pointes	A form of ventricular tachycardia with complexes of varying amplitude
Electromechanical dissociation	Electrical impulses (as recorded on an ECG) do not lead to mechanical activity (as detected by pulse)

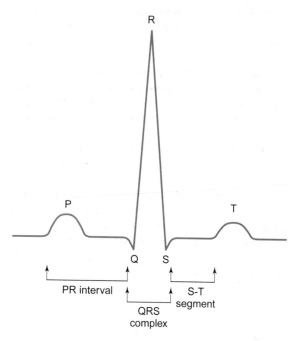

Figure 20.3 The electrocardiogram (ECG).

interval between the two (PR interval) is the time taken to conduct the beat through the AV node, and is lengthened in AV block. The QRS complex is generally narrow when the ventricles are controlled from above and wide when they are not. The T wave denotes ventricular repolarization, and the QT interval, the time between depolarization and polarization of the ventricles, may be altered by drugs such as tricyclic antidepressants and antiarrhythmics (Table 20.2). Some of these drugs, such as the antihistamines, are more likely to cause changes if given together with drugs that inhibit their metabolism, including erythromycin and the antifungal drugs fluconazole, itraconazole, ketoconazole and miconazole (Moss 1999). The QT interval varies with heart rate and a corrected figure (QTc) is used. A prolonged QTc predisposes to torsade de pointes; this may be drug-induced or, more rarely, an inherited characteristic.

functioning as a pump nor to the physical state of heart tissues. The pumping ability of the heart may be measured by pulse and blood pressure, and it is important that patients are treated on the basis of their heart function and not just on the basis of an electrical recording.

The ECG is useful, however, in providing clues to the nature and cause of an arrhythmia (Fig. 20.3). The P wave represents atrial depolarization and the QRS complex represents ventricular depolarization. The

Table 20.2 Drugs associated with prolonged QT intervals

Astemizole	Phenothiazines
Clarithromycin	Pimozide
Erythromycin	Sertindole
Halofantrine	Terfenadine
Haloperidol	Tizanidine
Lithium	Tricyclic antidepressants
Mizolastine	Class IA or III antiarrhythmics

Signs and consequences of arrhythmias

Arrhythmias are associated with increased morbidity and mortality but good data are available only for common varieties. AF roughly doubles the risk of a person having a stroke, triples the risk of heart failure and doubles mortality risk. Signs and symptoms of arrhythmias may include: dizziness or collapse because of a poor blood supply to the brain; shortness of breath because of poor oxygenation; angina associated with a poor coronary circulation and/or increased cardiac workload arising from a tachycardia; and weakness (Table 20.3). Palpitations are the awareness of one's heart beat and may be due to extra beats or the absence of a beat; they may range from a minor sensation to a distressing problem. Since these signs are not unique to arrhythmias, intermittent arrhythmias are not always easy to diagnose and 24-hour recordings of the ECG, or implantable recording devices activated when the patient has symptoms, may be used.

It is estimated that 80% of an individual's cardiac output comes from ventricular action, even when that is not coordinated with the atria. Thus, many patients with an abnormal rhythm but a regular ventricular rate experience little difficulty in normal daily living; indeed, only one in 12 patients with paroxysmal AF has symptoms. AF is sometimes described as 'slow' or 'fast' depending on the ventricular rate which can vary between 50 and 200 beats per minute, depending on the degree of AV conduction. A patient with slow AF in which an effective AV node block permits only a small proportion of impulses to pass from the atria to the ventricles may not need treatment. In contrast, fast AF, which occurs in patients with an ineffective AV node block, features rapid and irregular ventricular beats and consequent inefficient filling of the ventricles and inefficient circulation.

Treatment

Criteria for treatment

Suitable criteria for treatment of an arrhythmia include:

1. The arrhythmia causes haemodynamic failure (poor circulation).
2. Haemodynamic failure has not occurred but the present arrhythmia is known to be a predictor of a more serious arrhythmia. For example, patients who experience an episode of ventricular tachycardia following myocardial infarction have a 30% risk of dying within 1 year, probably from ventricular fibrillation.
3. The patient is distressed by an awareness of extra or missed beats (palpitations).

The aim of treatment is to restore a satisfactory circulation and to prevent further episodes of poor circulation or distress.

While it is thought that arrhythmias are implicated in many cases of sudden death, the main evidence comes from patients who died while having their ECG recorded continuously on a tape (Holter monitoring). Such patients may not represent the general population but confirm a general impression that ventricular tachyarrhythmias are a more common cause of death than bradyarrhythmias (Table 20.4). Patients who have heart failure, or have already been admitted to hospital for another reason, have a greater risk of dying from asystole or a muscle rupture.

Hazards of treatment

Since arrhythmias can occur without apparent ill effect, it follows that their presence does not automatically mandate treatment; indeed, the use of an antiarrhythmic agent may generate a worse arrhythmia. Such pro-arrhythmic effects are common to all antiarrhythmics but are probably less common in class II and class IV. The arrhythmias generated are many and varied and range from a rate change to a life-threatening pattern such as torsades de pointes. Table 20.5 lists some of the more common features of drug-induced arrhythmias.

Ten per cent of patients with postinfarction ventricular ectopics deteriorate if treated. The cardiac arrhythmia suppression trials (CAST) in the USA (CAST Investigators 1989, 1992) showed that the use of class IC drugs in such patients increased the risk of sudden death, and a meta-analysis of the use of lidocaine (lignocaine)

Table 20.3 Symptoms present at the emergency presentation of atrial fibrillation

Shortness of breath	52%
Pain (including angina)	34%
Palpitations	22%
Collapse or dizziness	19%

Table 20.4 Analysis of fatal arrythmias in monitored patients

Ventricular tachycardia leading to fibrillation	50%
Ventricular fibrillation	11%
Torsades de pointes	18%
Bradycardia	21%

Table 20.5   Common features of drug-induced arrhythmias

Incessant tachyarrhythmias
Bizarre arrhythmias
Cardiac arrest
New VT in a patient with SVT
Torsades de pointes
Acceleration of original rhythm

in myocardial infarction (Hine et al 1989) and a study of d-sotalol (Sanderson 1996) also demonstrated increased mortality when these drugs were used prophylactically, despite a reduction in arrhythmias. Table 20.6 shows estimates for the number of Americans who may have died as a result of misguided therapy with class I agents, in comparison to other causes.

Atrial and supraventricular arrhythmias are common in pregnancy; if treatment is required, then amiodarone should be avoided because of its effects on the fetus but β-blockers and adenosine are thought to be safer options. Long-established drugs such as digoxin and quinidine are probably safe but may not be effective.

Bradyarrhythmias

Bradyarrhythmias are generally caused by tissue damage, a decrease in sympathetic autonomic tone or an increase in parasympathetic tone mediated by the vagus nerve. Such changes in autonomic function may be caused or mimicked by drugs such as hyoscine, β-blockers, digoxin and verapamil or by deficiencies in thyroid or corticosteroid hormones. Increased vagal tone causes AV block of varying degree which reduces the rate of impulses reaching the ventricules. A ventricular escape rhythm involving ectopics, an idioventricular rhythm or even a tachycardia may then result, which should be recognized as secondary to the fault at the AV node and not treated as a primary disorder.

AV block may be classified into three types. First-degree block describes instances where all beats are

Table 20.6   Deaths in US citizens, 1965–75

Vietnam war	55 000
Road accidents	100 000
Homicide	200 000
Class i antiarrhythmics	1 000 000

conducted through the AV node, but with some delay. This does not require treatment but may be a warning to avoid drugs that would worsen the block, such as β-blockers and class IV agents.

Second-degree block implies that some, but not all, beats are conducted through the AV node, and there are further subdivisions of this class, e.g. Mobitz and Wenckebach. The need for treatment depends upon whether a satisfactory ventricular rate and output can be maintained.

Third-degree block implies that there is no conduction of sinus or atrial beats through the AV node, and treatment is usually required.

The treatment of bradycardia should include identification and treatment of the cause, such as treatment of jaundice or hypothyroidism, and removal of causative drugs. Immediate treatment is normally to decrease vagal tone with intravenous atropine, which will decrease AV block and increase the SA rate. It is important to note that it will take a minute or longer to see initial signs of benefit and at least 5 minutes to observe maximum effect. Doses of 300–600 micrograms of atropine may be given up to six times at 1-minute intervals until benefit is observed. If atropine is ineffective, intravenous adrenaline (epinephrine) or isoprenaline may be used.

Ultimately a pacemaker may be required to pace the heart from the right ventricle or from both the right atrium and ventricle. This approach may also be used where the patient has bouts of tachycardia and bradycardia (as seen in the sick sinus syndrome). In such cases the tachycardia may be controlled by β-blockers, amiodarone or class IV drugs, but an undesirable consequence may be the worsening of the bradycardia for which the only suitable treatment is a pacemaker.

Tachyarrhythmias

The primary treatment of any tachyarrhythmia is to remove the cause. Removal of arrhythmogenic drugs or stimulants such as caffeine, alcohol and smoking may solve the problem, and investigation of other medical causes, including abnormal thyroid function and abnormal serum electrolyte concentrations, is essential. Behavioural modifications to avoid stress and anxiety may help, and physical procedures such as the Valsalva manoeuvre have been useful in terminating re-entrant tachycardias.

Tachyarrhythmias that compromise cardiac output will require rapid control by direct-current (DC) electric shock, antiarrhythmic drugs or radiofrequency electric currents that destroy the aberrant conducting tissue. This last method is applied by a catheter passed through the great veins until the tip is close to the conducting pathways. It is of greatest value in junctional arrhythmias, where drug therapy is generally much less successful. Drugs may be used to convert an abnormal rhythm to sinus rhythm (cardioversion), to control the ventricular rate (e.g. digoxin) or as prophylaxis of further arrhythmias after electrical cardioversion. In some cases, where there is no immediate danger to the patient, drugs may be used to prepare a patient for electrical cardioversion (e.g. amiodarone for AF). Paroxysmal supraventricular tachyarrhythmias are usually easily converted to sinus rhythm by adenosine, flecainide or verapamil with success rates of between 70% and 100%. Flecainide also works well for atrial fibrillation, better than class IA drugs, which in turn are better than class III. β-blockers, calcium antagonists and digoxin work poorly. Atrial flutter responds less well, and generally only to class III drugs; class IC may convert the flutter to a worse rhythm by removing the AV block that protects the ventricles. Ventricular tachyarrhythmias are harder to terminate with drugs. Despite years of use, lidocaine (lignocaine) is effective in less than a quarter of patients, whereas sotalol and amiodarone have higher success rates.

In chronic tachyarrhythmias, the class of drug to be used, based on the Vaughan–Williams system (see below), must be selected. That choice is based upon the origin of the arrhythmia, regardless of its pattern. Table 20.7 lists the classes of drug considered useful for arrhythmias of various origin. Whatever the origin, the preference of one class to another may vary, depending on a clinician's experience with particular drugs, on the presentation of the arrhythmia and on patient characteristics. Such factors also govern the choice of drug within a class. The drug chosen should have the dosing schedule and adverse-effect profile that best suit the patient (or inconvenience the patient least, see Tables 20.11 and 20.14). Thus, for example, a patient with glaucoma or prostatism should not be given

disopyramide which possesses marked anticholinergic properties, and a patient with obstructive airways disease should preferably not have a β-blocker (class II), though if considered essential they could have a cardioselective agent.

Table 20.8 illustrates some of the factors affecting the choice of drug to treat atrial fibrillation.

It should be noted that it is not necessary to cure all arrhythmias to satisfy the criteria for treatment. Atrial arrhythmias may be well tolerated provided the ventricular rate is controlled and the patient is not distressed. Thus, digoxin may provide satisfactory control of the number of impulses that pass through the AV node to the ventricles without converting the patient to sinus rhythm.

Most patients who have episodes of ventricular tachycardia (VT) have coronary artery disease or cardiomyopathy, are at high risk of recurrence of VT, and require secondary prophylaxis. Those who have non-sustained VT or ventricular ectopics, without overt heart disease, have an entirely different prognosis that is no different from the normal population and they should not automatically have treatment (Landers & Reiter 1997). Prophylaxis against ventricular tachyarrhythmias is difficult and patients at high risk may have a DC defibrillator implanted in the same way as a pacemaker. The device monitors the ECG, and is programmed to recognize ventricular fibrillation or ventricular tachycardia and deliver an electric shock through electrodes sewn into the heart. A β-blocker is often given at the same time to reduce the risk of sympathetically driven arrhythmias and decrease the number of shocks delivered. Defibrillators have proved to be more successful than class I drugs but only a little better than amiodarone. Combinations of amiodarone and β-blockers are being tested with some promise. The

Table 20.7	Drug classes used in chronic tachyarrhythmias				
	SA node	Atria	AV node	Accessory pathway	Ventricles
Commonly used	II	II III	IV (for urgent cardioversion)	IC	II III
Also used		Digoxin IV IC IA	Digoxin IC	II IA	I

Class I drugs are not generally used in the context of acute illness (e.g. acute myocardial infarction, sepsis, etc.) or heart failure because of myodepression and increased proarrhythmic properties. Digoxin is most often used to control ventricular rate. AV-nodal and accessory pathway arrhythmias respond poorly to drugs in the long term but respond well to radiofrequency catheter ablation in which the aberrant pathway is destroyed.

Table 20.8   Drug choice in treating chronic or persistent atrial fibrillation

Associated factors	First choice	Second choice	Avoid
Acute systemic illness	Nothing or II	IV, III	I
Paroxysmal			
Exercise induced	II	Sotalolol, IC	Digoxin
Vagal origin	Disopyramide	Sotalol, IC	
Elderly	Sotalol/amiodarone		
Sustained AF			
Ventricular rate control	II	Digoxin, IV	
Cardioversion	IC	IA, III	II, IV, digoxin
Respiratory disorders			II, sotalol
Ischaemic heart disease	Sotalol	Amiodarone	I
Heart failure	Amiodarone	Digoxin	I
Hypertension	Sotalol	Amiodarone	

cardioverting shock, while life-saving, is unpleasant for the patient and there are often complications that necessitate hospital admission. Similar devices for atrial fibrillation have not been as successful because of difficulty in detecting fibrillation and patients' objections to repeated shocks.

Antithrombotic therapy

Atrial fibrillation is associated with a high incidence of stroke, about 5% per year, regardless of its impact on circulation. This is thought to be related to thrombus formation in the disorganized blood flow in the atrium. Nearly all patients with AF should be given oral anticoagulants or, if that is contraindicated, aspirin. The exceptions are young patients with no coexistent cardiovascular disease ('lone AF') when the risk of stroke is low and the patient is judged to have a high risk of bleeding on warfarin. Older patients were formerly excluded from warfarin therapy because of increased bleeding, but it is now recognized that old age, diabetes, hypertension, heart failure, thyrotoxicosis and previous strokes or transient ischaemic attacks (TIAs) are strong independent risk factors for stroke in AF; some groups have an annual incidence of 15%. Warfarin, adjusted to give an international normalized ratio (INR) in the range 2.0–3.0, reduces stroke rate by two-thirds in all patient groups, with little risk of excess bleeding. Patients with valvular disorders may require a higher INR but this carries a greater risk of bleeding. In comparison, aspirin reduces stroke risk by one fifth (Atrial Fibrillation Investigators 1994, Benavente et al 2000). There is a

small amount of evidence for adding dipyridamole to aspirin in patients who have already had a TIA or stroke (Diener et al 1996), but the role of newer agents such as clopidogrel is unclear.

DC cardioversion may lead to strokes, especially in patients with an established arrhythmia, and so elective cardioversion for AF that has lasted more than 48 hours is usually preceded by 3 weeks anticoagulation and followed by 4 weeks of further treatment.

Emergency treatment of arrhythmias in adults

Acute life-threatening arrhythmias may result in haemodynamic failure, the so-called cardiac arrest. Fast, but careful, management is required to prevent permanent damage or death. The emergency treatment options are set out in Figure 20.4 which is simplified from guidelines issued by the European Resuscitation Council.

Adrenaline (epinephrine), atropine and lidocaine (lignocaine) can be administered by endotracheal tube at double the intravenous dose in 10 ml of isotonic saline. The use of lidocaine (lignocaine) or bretylium as an adjunct to electrical defibrillation is controversial but common.

Acidosis may cause widespread problems, including serious arrhythmias, and sodium bicarbonate (50 mmol) may be given to counteract acidosis after prolonged resuscitation. Overdose is hazardous, however, and arterial blood gas measurements should be made where possible, before giving repeat doses.

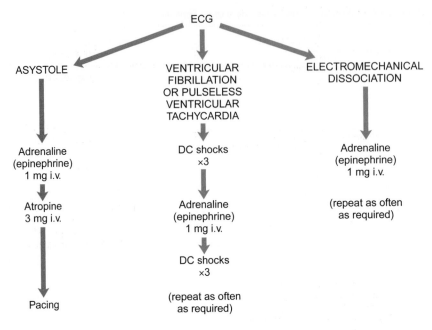

Figure 20.4 Emergency treatment options for arrhythmias in adults.

Severe bradycardia should be managed with atropine first and adrenaline (epinephrine) second.

A more general approach to the management of an arrhythmia is presented in Figure 20.5.

Treatment of arrhythmias after myocardial infarction

Despite the increased risk of death from arrhythmias post infarction, trials of antiarrhythmics have generally demonstrated that they increase the death rate still further. Presumably this arises because of their pro-arrhythmic properties although many drugs are known to act differently in normal compared to ischaemic tissue. Trials have shown increased risks from class I drugs and from d-sotalol (class III) but marginal benefit from amiodarone. β-blockers are useful in most patients, not only because they are antiarrhythmics but also because of their hypotensive and sympatholytic properties (Hjalmarson and Olsson 1991; see also Chapter 18). Approximately one-third of patients have non-sustained ventricular tachycardia that lasts less than 30 seconds in the acute postinfarction phase and the appropriate treatment is either reassurance or a β-blocker. Some will die early due to left ventricular failure but those who survive to leave hospital have the same prognosis as patients who did not have VT.

Classification of antiarrhythmic drugs

The most widely accepted classification is the Vaughan–Williams system based on electrophysiological data illustrated in Tables 20.9 and 20.10 and Figure 20.1. It is not only physiologically acceptable but it provides a good basis for clinical choices since drugs in the same class have similar therapeutic effects. Table 20.9 and Figure 20.1 relate to His–Purkinje fibres ('fast fibres'), which have a sodium-dependent phase 0. Other fibres have different characteristics, notably in the SA node and upper AV node, where phase 0 is calcium-dependent and overlaps phase 1 and 2 ('slow fibres'). The clinical consequences are that class I drugs (especially IB) have less effect on SA or AV nodal arrhythmias than those which originate from ventricular cells, while class IV drugs have major effects on the SA and AV nodes.

Most drugs have several modes of action, and their effectiveness as antiarrhythmic agents depends upon the summation of these effects. For example, class IB agents

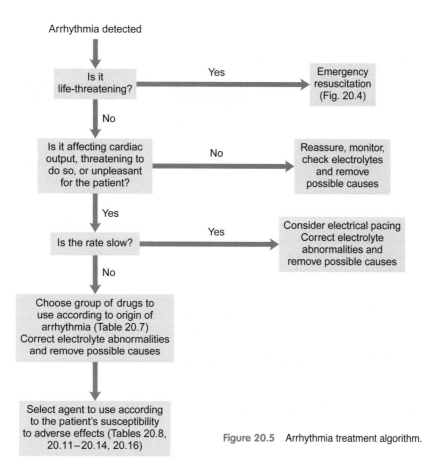

Figure 20.5 Arrhythmia treatment algorithm.

shorten the duration of the action potential thereby decreasing the refractory period and increasing the risk of sustaining a tachyarrhythmia. In contrast, they also slow phase 4, which increases the overall refractory period. The net result is a decrease in the risk of sustaining a tachyarrhythmia.

Table 20.9   Effect of different drug classes on phases of action potential in His–Purkinje fibres

Phase	Dominant ion movement	Drug class	Effect
0	Sodium inward	IA IB IC	Block ++ Block + Block +++
2	Calcium inward	IV	Block
3	Potassium outward	III	Marked slowing
4	Sodium inward Potassium outward	I, II, IV	Slows

Table 20.10   Electrophysiological effects of some antiarrhythmics

Class	Antiarrhythmic agents	Effects on duration of QRS	Effects on duration of QT	Sinus rate
IA	Quinidine, procainamide, disopyramide	+	+	+
IB	Lidocaine (lignocaine), mexiletine, tocainide, phenytoin, aprindine	0/–	0	0
IC	Flecainide, encainide, lorcainide, propafenone, moracizine	++	+	0
II	Atenolol, metoprolol, sotalol, esmolol	0	++	– –
III	Amiodarone, bretylium sotalol	0	+++	–
IV	Verapamil, diltiazem, adenosine	0	0	– –

+, increased; –, decreased; 0, no change.

It is important to note that all antiarrhythmics are also pro-arrhythmic.

Class I

All class I agents slow down sodium currents in phases 0 and 4 of the action potential but vary in their effects on phases 2 and 3. All may be used in ventricular tachyarrhythmias, but class IB are of no value in atrial disorders and are more effective in ischaemic tissue than in normal tissue. The use of class I agents is diminishing in favour of classes II and III. Lidocaine (lignocaine) may be used for prophylaxis of ventricular tachycardia or ventricular fibrillation and for management of ventricular ectopics and ventricular tachycardia, although it should be reserved for symptomatic patients. While it is also indicated in the management of VF, it is only an adjunct to DC electric shock. Lidocaine (lignocaine) is not available orally and is usually administered by an intravenous infusion regimen in which the dose is decreased with time, for example:

- 4 mg/minute for 30 minutes then
- 2 mg/minute for 2 hours then
- 1 mg/minute to continue.

It is unusual to continue for longer than 24–48 hours, after which an oral agent should be used if required.

Class IA agents are all potentially toxic but have a role as reserve agents in patients who have no contraindication to their use (Table 20.11). They may be used on their own or combined cautiously with digoxin for atrial arrhythmias. Quinidine and disopyramide are particularly prone to cause torsades de pointes but disopyramide is valuable in treating the Wolff–Parkinson–White syndrome, in which it inhibits both anterograde and retrograde conduction. All three class IA agents may be used in VT but individual variation in response to these agents is probably greater than in any other class. It may be useful, therefore, to try a second class IA agent if the first is not successful.

Class IC agents are effective in atrial and ventricular tachyarrhythmias but they also cause arrhythmias in a significant number of patients. The CAST (1989, 1992) studies demonstrated that flecainide, moracizine and encainide increased mortality when used in the management of ventricular ectopics after myocardial infarction. These agents are usually restricted to the management of ventricular arrhythmias resistant to other drugs although single-dose intravenous flecainide may be used to terminate atrial or supraventricular tachycardias. Longer-term use in AF is more common in the USA but is usually accompanied by a β-blocker to minimize the risk of pro-arrhythmia.

Class II

β-blockers are useful for treating arrhythmias that are provoked or exacerbated by sympathetic autonomic

Table 20.11 Adverse effects of antiarrhythmic drugs (class I)

Drug	Cardiac	Non-cardiac	Caution or avoid in
Disopyramide	Torsades de pointes Myodepressant	Anticholinergic (urinary retention, constipation, dry mouth, blurred vision)	Glaucoma, prostatism, hypotension
Procainamide		Lupus, nausea, diarrhoea	Myasthenia gravis, slow acetylators (increased risk of lupus)
Quinidine	Torsades de pointes Vasodilatation (i.v.)	Diarrhoea, nausea, tinnitus, headache, deafness, confusion, visual disturbances, blood dyscrasias	Myasthenia gravis
Lidocaine (lignocaine)		Convulsions in overdose, paraesthesiae	Liver failure (reduce dose)
Mexiletine		Nausea, paraesthesiae	2nd- or 3rd-degree heart block
Tocainide		Thrombocytopenia, nausea, pulmonary fibrosis, paraesthesiae	Use only if other agents have failed
Flecainide	Pro-arrhythmic Myodepressant	Paraesthesiae, tremor	Use only if other agents have failed
Propafenone	Pro-arrhythmic Myodepressant	Gastrointestinal disturbances	Use only if other agents have failed

nervous stimulation or by circulating catecholamines. They are valuable in arrhythmias originating from the SA or AV nodes that are provoked by anxiety, stress or exercise. They are also useful, along with α receptor blockers, in the arrhythmias of phaeochromocytoma. β-blockers are contraindicated in patients with extensive infarcts because of their myodepressant actions, but have a cardioprotective effect in uncomplicated acute myocardial infarction (see Chapter 18). For use in heart failure see Chapter 19.

β-blockers are contraindicated in patients with asthma or chronic obstructive airway disease. However, if other agents have been tried and failed, a cardioselective β-blocker may be used at low doses. It should be noted that cardioselectivity is a relative term and no agent is free from respiratory effects. Membrane-stabilizing activity and intrinsic sympathomimetic activity have no impact upon the choice of drug for arrhythmias. The risk of bradycardia is a threat with all β-blockers, especially in patients with myocardial disease, heart block or a mixed tachycardia–bradycardia (sick sinus syndrome). β-blockers with partial agonist activity have not proved useful in such cases despite theoretical promise. In general, β-blockers may also exacerbate peripheral vascular disease and cause nightmares or depression. There is little value in changing to a second β-blocker if the first agent has not been successful.

Atenolol, metoprolol and esmolol are available for intravenous use, and esmolol, with its short duration of action, is the most appropriate β-blocker for urgent use in SA, atrial or atrioventricular arrhythmias. Verapamil and adenosine (class IV) are also suitable, however, and esmolol has an even shorter duration of action. Care must be taken if both class II and IV agents are to be used since they have additive effects in suppressing the AV node and in depressing contractility. The combination is most dangerous if intravenous verapamil follows intravenous or oral β-blockers that have a prolonged action.

Sotalol has some class III activity as well as class II effects and bretylium is considered to have class II activity in addition to class III.

Class III

Class III drugs (amiodarone, bretylium, sotalol) prolong the action potential and bring greater uniformity among different cell types, thus reducing the means for generation of arrhythmias. Although they are all powerful antiarrhythmics, there the similarities end. Each drug has a different side-effect profile (Table 20.12) and other electrophysiological properties. Amiodarone can cause sodium channel blockade and has powerful class I activity and ancillary class II activity, bretylium is an

Table 20.12   Adverse effect of antiarrhythmic drugs (classes II–IV)

Drug	Cardiac	Non-cardiac	Caution or avoid in
β-blockers (general)	Myodepressant Heart block	Bronchoconstriction ($β_2$) Vasoconstriction Hallucinations/vivid dreams (lipophilic compounds) Decreased renal blood flow Changes in serum lipid profile Drowsiness, fatigue	Asthma, COAD, Raynaud's disease, gangrene, diabetes mellitus, depression
Azimilide Dofetilide Ibutilide Sotalol	Torsades de pointes		Combination with disopyramide or amiodarone or drugs in Table 20.2
Amiodarone	Torsades de pointes	Hyper-/hypothyroidism Pneumonitis, myopathy, neuropathy, hepatitis, corneal deposits, photosensitivity	Thyroid disease
Bretylium	Hypotension	Initial sympathomimetic response Nausea	
Verapamil and diltiazem	Heart block	Constipation, headaches, flushing, ankle oedema, lightheadedness	
Adenosine	Heart block	Bronchoconstriction, flushing, chest pain	Asthma, COAD, combination with dipyridamole

adrenergic neurone blocking agent, while sotalol is a β-blocker. Sotalol is a racemic mixture of which the d-isomer has class III activity and the l-isomer is a β-blocker. This combination is more successful than either element alone and d-sotalol alone has increased mortality in postinfarction patients. Amiodarone has an extensive range of side-effects, both trivial and fatal, that prevent its wider use. It is commonly restricted to serious ventricular arrhythmias that have proved resistant to other therapy, although it is increasingly being used in atrial arrhythmias and has a role in re-entrant rhythms such as the Wolff–Parkinson–White syndrome. A significant disadvantage to its use is its long half-life (about 1 month), which necessitates intensive oral loading, for example 200 mg three times daily for a week, then 200 mg twice daily for a week followed by 200 mg daily. The long half-life results in a slow onset of action and very prolonged effects after discontinuing therapy. Intravenous doses are effective immediately but there are hazards associated with rapid intravenous doses and incompatibility problems with common infusion fluids.

In contrast to amiodarone, bretylium has a rapid onset of action and short half-life, is only available parenterally and is not effective in atrial arrhythmias. It has been used mostly in emergency resuscitation for ventricular tachycardia or fibrillation, either to aid electric defibrillation or to cardiovert patients on its own. The major problem has been severe hypotension although, paradoxically, there may be an initial sympathetic stimulation that precedes the sympathetic block and causes hypertension and arrhythmias. Whereas amiodarone and bretylium have minimal myodepressant activity, sotalol is a significant myodepressant and also has the standard side-effect profile of a β-blocker. It is less effective than amiodarone but, despite its problems, a lot safer; it is available orally and it may be of particular benefit in treating arrhythmias in hypertension, in angina and after acute myocardial infarction. It is rarely used for non-antiarrhythmic purposes.

All three agents, by virtue of their class III activity, prolong the QT interval and increase the risk of torsades de pointes, especially in hypokalaemia or when combined with a bradycardic drug such as a class IA agent. Newer agents with a more pure class III action include ibutilide, dofetilide and azimilide.

Class IV

Verapamil and diltiazem inhibit slow channel conduction through the AV node and are referred to by a number of terms, including the general name 'calcium antagonists'. Other calcium antagonists such as nifedipine and other 4,5-dihydropyridines have no antiarrhythmic effect. The potassium channel opener adenosine and its prodrug ATP act as indirect calcium antagonists and resemble verapamil in their antiarrhythmic scope. The ultra-short duration of action of intravenous adenosine makes it very suitable as a diagnostic aid and for interrupting supraventricular arrhythmias without the myosuppressant effects of verapamil. Adenosine is, however, a bronchoconstrictor and causes dyspnoea, flushing, chest pain and further transient arrhythmias in a high proportion of patients, and its metabolism is inhibited by dipyridamole (see Table 20.12). All class IV agents should be avoided in second- or third-degree heart block and sick sinus syndrome, unless the patient has a pacemaker to overcome bradycardia. Likewise, combined therapy with a β-blocker is hazardous because of the risk of excessive AV block, although in some cases it may be useful to treat chronic atrial fibrillation or flutter with digoxin and a calcium antagonist where either agent alone has failed. Calcium antagonists may cause conversion to sinus rhythm but are used chiefly to control ventricular rate. Verapamil has a greater dilatatory effect on systemic arteries than diltiazem and may be especially useful in patients with hypertension or angina. Both agents cause myocardial suppression and are thus contraindicated in heart failure although their depressant actions on the SA node are usually offset by the reflex response to arterial vasodilatation. Side-effects are mostly predictable, and include ankle oedema, flushing, dizziness, light-headedness and headache. Constipation is common in patients receiving verapamil.

Digoxin

Digoxin is one of a group of cardiac (digitalis) glycosides with a well-defined role in the management of atrial tachyarrhythmias, in the presence of congestive heart failure. Digoxin inhibits conduction through the AV node and thus protects the ventricles from rapid atrial rhythms. In addition, some patients with established atrial fibrillation may convert to sinus rhythm although this is unusual in atrial flutter and in atrial fibrillation of recent origin (less than 1 week). It is ineffective in the presence of high sympathetic nervous activity, such as in exercise, and its use is diminishing as the use of amiodarone, sotalol and class II drugs increases. Digoxin also causes both atrial and ventricular ectopic beats and is a potent cause of arrhythmias (Table 20.13). Both beneficial and toxic effects are enhanced by hypokalaemia and hypercalcaemia, and the AV block is enhanced by β-blockers and calcium antagonists. There are numerous other drug interactions (Table 20.14), some of which are pharmacokinetic and some of which are pharmacological. Digoxin is the only antiarrhythmic for which therapeutic drug monitoring is widely used. It has a narrow therapeutic range of 1–2 ng/ml. This range is modified by serum electrolyte concentrations and by the concurrent use of other drugs, but the extent of the modification is not defined. Since digoxin is excreted by the liver and the kidney (70% renal elimination in normal renal function), reduced renal function increases digoxin levels and necessitates reduced doses, notably in the elderly.

Table 20.15 summarizes the pharmacokinetics of antiarrhythmics, Table 20.16 lists some common interactions, and Table 20.17 lists common therapeutic problems in the management of arrhythmias.

Patient care

Patients with arrhythmias may experience considerable anxiety about the possibility that they will have a serious arrhythmia at any moment and they may need considerable reassurance. This anxiety will not be helped by the fact that most antiarrhythmic drug treatments work in only a proportion of patients and several treatment options may be tried before satisfaction is obtained. Encouragement and realistic reassurance are required, with regular follow-up. The patient's family and friends may need to be advised on what to do in the event of an acute arrhythmia.

Stressful situations, smoking, cocaine and amphetamine use, alcohol binges and excessive caffeine intake should all be avoided.

Patients should give informed consent for all interventions, but their response to treatment options may not be the same as that of prescribers. A study of patients' and prescribers' attitudes to the use of aspirin and warfarin for stroke prevention in atrial fibrillation (Devereaux et al 2001) demonstrated not only that prescribers differ markedly on the balance of risks between stroke prevention and bleeding caused by treatment but also that patients feared stroke more then doctors did. This affected their decisions about taking warfarin or aspirin. Prescribers should seek and respect patients' views on such treatment choices, rather than assume all patients are the same or that they will agree with the prescriber's own views.

Table 20.13 Adverse effects of digoxin

Cardiac
Ventricular ectopics including bigeminy
Ventricular tachycardia
AV junctional beats or tachycardia
2nd- or 3rd-degree heart block
Atrial tachycardia (often paroxysmal) with block
SA node arrest

Non-cardiac
Anorexia, nausea, vomiting
Diarrhoea (less common)
Fatigue, confusion
Abnormal colour vision (excess yellow/green)

Table 20.14 Interactions involving digoxin

Serum levels increased by:	Amiodarone, verapamil, diltiazem, quinidine, propafenone, clarithromycin, broad-spectrum antibiotics (erythromycin, tetracyclines), decreased renal blood flow (β-blockers, NSAIDs), renal failure, heart failure
Serum levels decreased by:	Colestyramine, sulfasalazine, neomycin, rifampicin, antacids, improved renal blood flow (vasodilators), levothyroxine (thyroxine)
Effects of digoxin increased by:	Hypokalaemia, hypercalcaemia, hypomagnesaemia Antiarrhythmic classes IA, II, IV Diuretics that cause hypokalaemia, corticosteroids Myxoedema, hypoxia (acute or chronic), acute myocardial ischaemia or myocarditis
Effects of digoxin decreased by:	Hyperkalaemia, hypocalcaemia, thyrotoxicosis

Table 20.15 Pharmacokinetics of antiarrhythmics

	Oral absorption	% protein-binding	Approx. therapeutic range	Elimination, metabolism, half-life
Amiodarone	Slow, variable	> 95	0.5–2.5 mg/l	Extensive metabolism, very variable rate, $t_{1/2}$ 2 days initially increasing to 40–60 days
Bretylium	Intravenous/intramuscular only	Unbound	1–3 mg/l	Renal, $t_{1/2}$ 5–10 h
Digoxin	Variable, 70%	25	0.8–2 ng/ml	70% renal, variable, $t_{1/2}$ 36 h
Diltiazem	40% absorbed	80	0.05–0.3 mg/l	Hepatic, $t_{1/2}$ 3 h
Disopyramide	Rapid, > 80%	30–90	2–4 mg/l (depends on extent of binding)	50% renal, 15% bile, active metabolite, $t_{1/2}$ 4–10 h
Flecainide	Complete, slow	40	0.2–1 mg/l	30% renal, $t_{1/2}$ 20 h
Lidocaine (lignocaine)	Intravenous/intramuscular only	60–80	1.5–5 mg/l	10% renal, rapid hepatic metabolism to CNS-toxic products, $t_{1/2}$ 8–100 min increases with duration of dosing
Mexiletine	> 90%	60–70	0.5–2 mg/l	10% renal, $t_{1/2}$ 10–12 h, hepatic metabolites mostly inactive
Moracizine	Rapid	95%	0.2–3.6 mg/l	Hepatic metabolism to active metabolites, $t_{1/2}$ 2–6 h, metabolite >80 h
Phenytoin	Variable rate and extent	> 90	10–20 mg/l	Capacity-limited hepatic metabolism, $t_{1/2}$ 10–60 h but variable because of non-first-order elimination
Procalinamide	Rapid, > 75%	15–20	3–10 mg/l	50% renal, 25–40% converted to *N*-acetylprocainamide (active, $t_{1/2}$ 6 h), procainamide $t_{1/2}$ 2.5–4.5 h
Propafenone	Complete, rapid	> 95	0.06–1 mg/l	Extensive first-pass metabolism, capacity-limited, $t_{1/2}$ 2–12 h
Quinidine	Rapid, > 80%	80–90	2–6 mg/l	Mixed renal and hepatic, $t_{1/2}$ 6 h
Tocainide	Complete, rapid	> 10	4–10 mg/l	40% renal, 60% hepatic, $t_{1/2}$ 15 h
Verapamil	Rapid, > 90%	90	0.1–0.4 mg/l	Hepatic, $t_{1/2}$ 4–12 h, marked first-pass effect
Dofetilide	Rapid, > 92%		Not determined	60% renal, 40% oxidation, $t_{1/2}$ 7.1–9.7 h
Azimilide	Complete	94%	Not determined	> 90% hepatic, $t_{1/2}$ 4–5 d
Ibutilide	Extensive first-pass metabolism, not used directly	40%	Not determined	95% hepatic, $t_{1/2}$ 5.7–8.8 h

All values quoted are subject to marked interindividual variability. Most therapeutic ranges are poorly defined. Oral absorption does not account for drug lost by first-pass hepatic metabolism. Rapid absorption indicates a peak plasma concentration in less than 2 hours.

$t_{1/2}$ elimination half-life at normal renal function.

For the pharmacokinetics of β-blockers and other calcium channel blockers see Chapter 18.

Table 20.16 Common interactions involving antiarrhythmic agents (excluding digoxin)

Antiarrhythmic	Other drug	Effect
Disopyramide	Anticholinergics	Increased anticholinergic effects
	Pyridostigmine	Decreased anticholinergic effects of disopyramide
		Decreased cholinergic effects of pyridostigmine
	Class II, IV	Increased hypotension
	Class III	Torsades de pointes
Procainamide	Class III	Torsades de pointes
	Cimetidine	Decreased renal clearance
Quinidine	Class II, IV	Increased hypotension
	Class III	Torsades de pointes
	Warfarin	Increased anticoagulation
	Enzyme inducers	Decreased serum levels
	Enzyme inhibitors	Increased serum levels
Lidocaine (lignocaine)	β-blockers, cimetidine	Decreased elimination of lidocaine
	Enzyme inducers	Increased elimination of lidocaine
Mexiletine	Theophylline	Increased theophylline levels
Propafenone	Warfarin	Enhanced anticoagulation
Amiodarone	Warfarin	Enhanced anticoagulation

Additive antiarrhythmic or myosuppressant effects are not included.
Interactions between antiarrhythmics are listed under the first named drug only.
Enzyme inducers include barbiturates, rifampicin, smoking.
Enzyme inhibitors include cimetidine.

Table 20.17 Common therapeutic problems in the management of arrhythmias

Problem	Comment
Narrow therapeutic range of digoxin	Encourage compliance and check serum electrolytes regularly
β-blockers are generally contraindicated in bronchial and peripheral vascular disease	Consider verapamil or diltiazem
Verapamil-induced constipation	If it occurs, give regular osmotic laxatives
All antiarrhythmics are pro-arrhythmic too	Prevention is better than cure. Minimize the requirement for drugs by careful attention to precipitating factors. Consider use of pacemakers or electrical therapies if appropriate
Amiodarone is commonly associated with an increased tendency to sunburn	Warn all patients to stay covered up when outdoors, use sun block or stay indoors
Diagnosis of paroxysmal arrhythmias is difficult	Use continuous monitoring by tapes or implantable event recorders
Torsades de pointes may be precipitated by taking other medication with amiodarone or disopyramide	Patients should remind members of health care team that they are taking antiarrhythmic drugs

CASE STUDIES

Case 20.1

A middle-aged man with a medical history of stable angina treated with GTN (glyceryl trinitrate) spray when necessary and verapamil 80 mg three times daily presents to his GP with complaints of a fluttering sensation in his chest from time to time. It is a bit disconcerting but not painful. It occurs mainly in the morning after coffee. It does not limit him in his activities.

Question

What should the GP do?

Answer

This sounds like typical atrial fibrillation but needs an ECG investigation and a careful history. Coffee may be a precipitant, and if so should be avoided, but if the verapamil is a recent prescription then that too should be withdrawn. Dependent upon the nature of the angina and any risk of bronchoconstriction or peripheral vascular disease, the verapamil could be replaced by sotalol, or another β-blocker, even if the prescription is long-term. If the palpitations are only short-lived and do not trouble the patient unduly, he may be reassured and no treatment offered, but a thorough review of the management of his angina and fibrillation is probably indicated.

Case 20.2

A patient who is in intensive care with septicaemia following a bacterial chest infection is on permanent bedside ECG monitoring. She is febrile, has tachycardia, and is observed to have ventricular ectopic beats occasionally. She then develops atrial ectopics and short runs of atrial fibrillation. Her cardiac output decreases by about 10% during the fibrillatory episodes.

Question

How should this patient be managed?

Answer

Acutely ill patients often develop arrhythmias, especially atrial ectopics and fibrillation. These are usually not a significant problem and do not merit treatment unless the cardiac output is seriously compromised. Ventricular ectopics are also normal in all adults and only if they occur frequently or occur in runs of three or more consecutive beats are they an indicator of a possible poor outcome. In an intensive care unit patient, a 10% decrease in cardiac output, which is reversed when the rhythm is back to normal, is not a serious problem. If it becomes worse, the normal treatment would be a β-blocker but this lady has a respiratory problem and amiodarone or verapamil may be preferred. Since she is in intensive care, however, there is some protection against the risk of bronchoconstriction because intravenous access is probably in place and ventilators should be readily available. Other causes of arrhythmias should be sought, especially amongst her other prescribed medication (Table 20.2).

REFERENCES

Atrial Fibrillation Investigators 1994 Risk factors for stroke and efficacy of antithrombotic therapy in atrial fibrillation: analysis of pooled data from five randomised controlled trials. Archives of Internal Medicine 154: 1449–1457

Benavente O, Hart K, Koudstaal P et al 2000 Antiplatelet therapy for preventing stroke in patients with non-valvular atrial fibrillation and no previous history of stroke or transient ischaemic attacks. Cochrane Review. Cochrane Library (Issue 4), Update Software, Oxford

Cardiac Arrhythmia Suppression Trial (CAST) Investigators 1989 Preliminary report: effect of encainide and flecainide on mortality in a randomised trial of arrhythmias suppression after myocardial infarction. New England Journal of Medicine 321: 406–412

Cardiac Arrhythmia Suppression Trial II Investigators 1992 Effect of the antiarrhythmic agent moricizine on survival after myocardial infarction. New England Journal of Medicine 327: 227–233

Devereaux P J, Anderson D R, Gardner M J et al 2001

Differences between perspectives of physicians and patients on anticoagulation in patients with atrial fibrillation: observational study. British Medical Journal 323: 1218

Diener H C, Cunha L, Forbes C et al 1996 European stroke prevention study, 2: Dipyridamole and acetylsalicylic acid in the secondary prevention of stroke. Journal of the Neurological Sciences 143: 1–13

Hine L K, Laird N, Hewitt P et al 1989 Meta-analytic evidence against prophylactic use of lidocaine in acute myocardial infarction. Archives of Internal Medicine 149: 2694–2698

Hjalmarson A, Olsson G 1991 Myocardial infarction: effects of beta-blockade. Circulation 84: VI101–VI107

Landers M D, Reiter M J 1997 General principles of antiarrhythmic therapy for ventricular tachyarrhythmias. American Journal of Cardiology 80(8A): 31G–44G

Moss A J 1999 The QT interval and torsades de pointes. Drug Safety 21(Suppl. 1): 5–10

Sanderson J 1996 The SWORD of Damocles. Lancet 348: 2–3

FURTHER READING

Guerra P G, Talajic M, Roy D et al 1998 Is there a future for antiarrhythmic drug therapy? Drugs 56(5): 767–781

Joglar J A, Page R L 1999 Treatment of arrhythmias during pregnancy: safety considerations. Drug Safety 20(1): 85–94

Lévy S, Breithardt G, Campbell R W F et al 1998 Atrial fibrillation: current knowledge and recommendations for management. European Heart Journal 19: 1294–1320

Nattel S 1991 Antiarrhythmic drug classifications: a critical appraisal of their history, present status and clinical relevance. Drugs 41: 672–701

Roden D M 1994 Risks and benefits of antiarrhythmic therapy. New England Journal of Medicine 331: 785–791

Prystowsky E N 2000 Management of atrial fibrillation: therapeutic options and clinical decisions. American Journal of Cardiology 85(10A): 3D–11D

Sager P T 2000 New advances in class III antiarrhythmic drug therapy. Current Opinion in Cardiology 15: 41–53

Singh B N 1999 Overview of trends in the control of cardiac arrhythmia: past and future. American Journal of Cardiology 84(9A): 3R–10R

Van Gelder I C, Brügemann J, Crijns H J G M 1998 Current treatment recommendations in antiarrhythmic therapy. Drugs 55(3): 331–346

Thrombosis 21

P. A. Routledge   H. G. M. Shetty

KEY POINTS

Venous thromboembolism

- Venous thromboembolism has an incidence of 2–5%.
- Combinations of sluggish blood flow and hypercoagulability are the commonest causes of venous thromboemboembolism. Vascular injury is also a recognized causative factor.
- Proteins C and S are vitamin K-dependent antithrombotic factors that can be suppressed during the induction phase of warfarin administration and predispose individuals with a deficiency to venous thromboembolism and warfarin skin necrosis.
- Treatment of venous thromboembolism involves the use of anticoagulants and, in severe cases, thrombolytic drugs.
- Anticoagulant therapy usually involves an immediate-acting agent such as heparin followed by maintenance treatment with warfarin.
- Unfractionated heparins increase the rate of interaction of thrombin with antithrombin III 1000-fold and prevent the production of fibrin from fibrinogen.
- Low molecular weight heparins inactivate factor Xa, they have a longer half-life and produce a more predictable response than unfractionated heparins.
- Warfarin is the most widely used coumarin because of potency and more reliable bioavailability.
- Warfarin consists of an equal mixture of two enantiomers, (R)- and (S)-warfarin, that have different anticoagulant potencies and routes of metabolism.

Arterial thromboembolism

- Arterial thromboembolism is normally associated with vascular injury and hypercoagulability.
- Acute myocardial infarction is the commonest form of arterial thrombosis.
- Arterial thromboembolism affecting the cerebral circulation results in either transient ischaemic attacks (TIAs) or in severe cases, cerebral infarction (stroke).
- Investigation of TIAs is necessary and prophylaxis using aspirin (or another antiplatelet agent) or warfarin is often beneficial, depending on the pathophysiology.
- If the source of embolism is from the heart, prophylaxis against TIA or stroke may be considered using warfarin.

Thrombosis is the development of a 'thrombus' consisting of platelets, fibrin, red cells and white cells in the arterial or venous circulation. If part of this thrombus in the venous circulation breaks off and enters the right heart, it may be lodged in the pulmonary arterial circulation, causing pulmonary embolism (PE). In the left-sided circulation, an embolus may result in peripheral arterial occlusion, either in the lower limbs or in the cerebral circulation (where it may cause thromboembolic stroke). Since the pathophysiology of each of these conditions differs, they will be discussed separately under the headings venous thromboembolism and arterial thromboembolism.

VENOUS THROMBOEMBOLISM

Epidemiology

Venous thromboembolism is common, with an incidence of 2–5%. PE is now the commonest cause of maternal death, and deep vein thrombosis may result in not only PE but also subsequent morbidity as a result of the postphlebitic limb. Thromboembolism appears to increase in prevalence over the age of 50 years, and the diagnosis is more often missed in this age group.

Aetiology

Venous thromboembolism occurs primarily due to a combination of stagnation of blood flow and hypercoagulability. Vascular injury is also a recognized causative factor but is not necessary for the development of venous thrombosis. In venous thromboembolism, the thrombus is different in structure from that in arterial thromboembolism. In the former, platelets seem to be uniformly distributed through a mesh of fibrin and other blood cell components, whereas in arterial thrombo-embolism the white platelet 'head' is more prominent and it appears to play a much more important initiatory role in thrombus.

Sluggishness of blood flow may be related to bed rest, surgery or reduced cardiac output (e.g. in heart failure). Factors increasing the risk of hypercoagulability include surgery, pregnancy, oestrogen administration, malignancy, myocardial infarction and several acquired or inherited disorders of coagulation (e.g. antithrombin III deficiency, protein C deficiency, resistance to activated protein C, or primary antiphospholipid syndrome).

Protein C deficiency is inherited by an autosomal dominant transmission. Such patients at increased risk not only of venous thromboembolism but also of warfarin skin necrosis. This occurs because protein C (and its closely related co-factor, protein 5) are vitamin K-dependent antithrombotic factors that can be further suppressed by the administration of warfarin. Thrombosis in the small vessels of the skin may occur if large loading (induction) doses of warfarin are given to such patients when the suppression of the antithrombotic effects of these factors occurs before the antithrombotic effects of blockade of vitamin K-dependent clotting factor (II, VII, IX and X) production has occurred. Although the prevalence of protein C deficiency is 0.2%, only one subject in 70 (i.e. 0.0003%) will be symptomatic, and the condition accounts for around 4% of patients presenting with thromboembolic disease before the age of 45 years.

Protein S deficiency is probably even rarer than protein C deficiency but the familial form, inherited in an autosomal dominant fashion, is a high-risk state, accounting for possibly 5–8% of cases of the thromboembolism in patients less than 45 years old.

The presence of another, additional clotting defect may be a trigger factor for problems in patients with deficiency of one of these factors. One of these conditions is activated protein C deficiency. This results from the presence of factor V Leiden, a point mutation in the factor V gene, which causes the activated factor V molecule to be resistant to activation by activated protein C (APC). This defect may have a prevalence of 9% in the general population, and higher in patients with thromboembolic disease, and may in itself be of little consequence until there is another risk factor, such as immobility or use of the contraceptive pill. In these circumstances, the combination of risks may be responsible for the increased predisposition to thromboembolism in a high proportion of such affected individuals.

Antithrombin III deficiency is a rare autosomal dominantly inherited abnormality associated with a reduced plasma concentration of this protein. The defect may not result in clinical problems until pregnancy, or until patients enter their fourth decade, when venous and (to a lesser extent) arterial thrombosis becomes more common. Nevertheless, it has been estimated to be responsible for between 2% and 5% of thromboembolism occurring before the 45th year of life.

Lupus anticoagulant (an antibody against phospholipid) is so named because it increases the clotting time in blood when measured by some standard cloning tests. Patients affected are more prone to thromboembolism. This factor is found in 10% of patients with systemic lupus erythematosus (SLE) where it is associated with a threefold increase in thromboembolic risk; it is also found in the primary antiphospholipid syndrome (PAPS), where it may signify an increased risk of venous and arterial thrombosis and of recurrent miscarriage.

Oestrogens increase the circulating concentrations of clotting factors I, II, VII, VIII, IX and X and reduce fibrinolytic activity. They also depress the concentrations of antithrombin III, which is protective against thrombosis. This effect is dose related, and venous thrombosis was more often seen with the high (50 microgram) oestrogen-containing contraceptive pill than with the present lower-dose preparations. Venous thromboembolism is also commoner in malignancy (the risk may be up to fivefold greater). Although first described in association with carcinoma of the pancreas, all solid tumours seem to be associated with this problem. This may be related to the expression of tissue factor or factor X activators, but several other mechanisms may also be responsible.

The increased risk of venous thromboembolism in surgery is related in part to stagnation of venous blood in the calves during the operation, but also to tissue trauma, since it appears to be more common in operations that involve marked tissue damage, such as orthopaedic surgery. This may in turn be related to release of tissue thromboplastin and to reduced fibrinolytic activity. The most important risk factors associated with clinical thromboembolism after surgery are age and obesity.

Clinical manifestations

In 90% of patients, deep vein thrombosis occurs in the veins of the lower limbs and pelvis. In up to half of cases this may not result in local symptoms or signs, and the onset of PE may be the first evidence of the presence of venous thromboembolism. In other cases patients classically present with pain involving the calf or thigh associated with swelling, redness of the overlying skin and increased warmth. In a large deep venous thrombosis that prevents venous return the leg may become discoloured and oedematous. Massive venous thrombus can occasionally result in gangrene, although this occurs very rarely now that effective drug therapies are available.

PE may occur in the absence of clinical signs of venous thrombosis. It may be very difficult to diagnose because of the non-specificity of symptoms and signs. Clinical diagnosis is often made because of the presence of associated risk factors. Obstruction with a large embolus of a major pulmonary artery may result in acute massive PE, presenting with sudden shortness of breath and dull central chest pain, together with marked haemodynamic disturbance (e.g. severe hypotension and right ventricular failure). It may increase the risk of unconsciousness and the patient may die of acute circulatory failure unless rapidly treated.

Acute submassive pulmonary embolus occurs when less than 50% of the pulmonary circulation is occluded by embolus, and the embolus normally lodges in a more distal branch of the pulmonary artery. It may result in some shortness of breath, but if the lung normally supplied by that branch of the pulmonary artery becomes necrotic, pulmonary infarction results with pleuritic pain and haemoptysis (coughing up blood), and there may be a pleural 'rub' (a sound like Velcro being torn apart when the patient breathes in) as a result of inflammation of the lung. Patients may, rarely, develop recurrent thromboembolism. This may not result in immediate symptoms or signs but the patient may present with increasing breathlessness and signs of pulmonary hypertension (right ventricular hypertrophy) and, if untreated, progressive respiratory failure.

Investigations

Although several conditions may mimic deep vein thrombus (e.g. Baker's cyst, a rupture of the posterior aspect of the synovial capsule of the knee), deep vein thrombosis is the commonest cause of pain, swelling and tenderness of the leg. The clinical diagnosis of venous thrombosis is relatively unreliable, and venography is the most specific diagnostic test. This involves injection of radiopaque contrast medium, normally into a vein on the top of the foot, and subsequent radiography of the venous system. Ultrasound is a non-invasive alternative that does not involve exposure to ionizing radiation or potentially allergenic contrast media. It is now the initial investigation of choice in clinically suspected DVT, although it is less sensitive for below-knee and isolated pelvic DVT, Magnetic resonance imaging (MRI) is also non-invasive and avoids radiation exposure. Particularly when used with direct thrombus imaging (by detecting methaemoglobin in the clot; MRI DTI), it is sensitive and specific, even with below knee and isolated pelvic DVT. However, it is not yet widely clincally available and ultrasound remains the primary initial investigation.

The diagnosis of PE is most often made using one of two techniques: pulmonary arteriography or ventilation–perfusion scanning. Pulmonary arteriography is the most specific test. This requires catheterization of the right side of the heart and an injection of contrast medium into the pulmonary artery. Adequate facilities and experienced personnel are therefore required and it is now generally reserved for those situations where massive or submassive PE is suspected but non-invasive tests have given indeterminate results.

Ventilation–perfusion scanning involves the injection of a radiolabelled substance into the vein and measurement using a scintillation counter of the perfusion via the pulmonary circulation. This, is often combined with a ventilation scan in which radiolabelled gas, normally xenon, is inhaled by the patient. PE classically results in an area of under- or non-perfusion of a part of the lung that, nevertheless, because the airways are patent, ventilates normally. This pattern is called ventilation–perfusion mismatch, and is a specific sign of PE.

Computed tomography angiography (CT angiography) using helical or spiral CT (sCT) is now being increasingly used in some centres, and has a high accuracy rate. Although subsegmental emboli can be missed, visulization of smaller arterial branches, and therefore detection of small emboli, may improve with the availability of multidetector scanners. Not only does sCT enable direct visualization of emboli, but visualization of the lung parenchyma and mediastinum may help in the differential diagnosis in non-embolic cases. Magnetic resonance imaging is also being developed for the diagnosis of PE and early results are promising.

Other findings do occur in PE, such a changes in the chest radiograph, the commonest of which is a raised right hemidiaphragm as a result of loss of lung volume (PE more commonly affects the right than the left lung). Hypoxia is also seen, and this is worse the larger the pulmonary embolus. The electrocardiogram may show signs of right ventricular strain. The echocardiogram may show right ventricular overload and dysfunction in massive PE. However, all these changes are relatively non-specific and do not obviate the need for the specific tests mentioned earlier.

Treatment

The aim of treatment of venous thrombosis is to allow normal circulation in the limbs and, wherever possible, to prevent damage to the valves of the veins, thus reducing the risk of the swollen postphlebitic limb. Second, it is important to try to prevent associated PE and also recurrence of either venous thrombosis or PE in the risk period after the initial episode.

In acute massive PE the initial priority is to correct the circulatory defect that has caused haemodynamic upset and, in these circumstances, rapid removal of the obstruction using thrombolytic drugs or surgical removal of the embolus may be necessary. In acute submassive PE, the goal of treatment is to prevent further episodes, particularly of the more serious acute massive PE. In both deep vein thrombosis and PE, a search must be made for underlying risk factors, such as carcinoma, which may occur in up to 10% of patients, and particularly in those with repeated episodes of venous thromboembolism.

The treatment of venous thromboembolism consists of the use of anticoagulants and, in severe cases, thrombolytic drugs. Anticoagulant therapy involves the use of immediate-acting agents (particularly heparin), and oral anticoagulants, the commonest of which is warfarin. Not only do these treat the acute event, but they also prevent recurrence and may be necessary for some time after the initial event, depending on the persistence of risk factors for recurrent thromboembolism.

Heparins

Conventional or unfractionated heparin (UFH) is a heterogeneous mixture of large mucopolysaccharide molecules ranging widely in molecular weight between 3000 and 30 000, with immediate anticoagulant properties. It acts by increasing the rate of the interaction of thrombin with antithrombin III by a factor of 1000. It thus prevents the production of fibrin (factor I) from fibrinogen. Heparin also has effects on the inhibition of production of activated clotting factors IX, X, XI and XII; and these effects occur at concentrations lower than its effects on thrombin.

Unlike UFH, low molecular weight heparins (LMWHs) contain polysaccharide chains ranging in molecular weight between 4000 and 6000. Whereas UFH produces its anticoagulant effect by inhibiting both thrombin and factor Xa, LMWHs predominantly inactivate only factor Xa. In addition, unlike UFH, they inactivate platelet bound factor Xa and resist inhibition by platelet factor 4, which is released during coagulation.

Because unfractionated and LMWHs all consist of high molecular weight molecules that are highly ionized (heparin is the strongest organic acid found naturally in the body) they are not absorbed via the gastrointestinal tract and must be given by intravenous infusion or deep subcutaneous (never intramuscular) injection. Unfractionated heparin is highly protein bound, and it appears to be restricted to the intravascular space with a consequently low volume of distribution. It does not cross the placenta and does not appear in breast milk. Its pharmacokinetics are complex but it appears to have a dose-dependent increase in half-life. The half-life is normally about 60 minutes, but is shorter in patients with PE. It is removed from the body by metabolism, possibly in the reticuloendothelial cells of the liver, and by renal excretion. The latter seems to be more important after high doses of the compound. LMWHs have a number of potentially desirable pharmacokinetics features compared with UFH. They are predominantly excreted renally and have longer and more predictable half-lives than UFH and so have more predictable dose response than UFH. They can therefore be given once or, at the most, twice daily in a fixed dose (sometimes based on the patient's body weight) without the need for laboratory monitoring.

The major adverse effect of all heparins is haemorrhage, which is commoner in patients with severe heart or liver disease, renal disease, general debility and in women aged over 60 years. The risk of haemorrhage is increased in those with prolonged clotting times and in those given heparin by intermittent intravenous bolus rather than by continuous intravenous administration. UFH is monitored by derivatives of the activated partial thromboplastin time, for example the kaolin–cephalin clotting time (KCCT); in those patients with a KCCT three times greater than control there is an eightfold increase in the risk of haemorrhage. The therapeutic range for the KCCT during UFH therapy therefore appears to be between 1.5 and 2.5 times the control values. Rapid reversal of the effect of heparin can be achieved using protamine sulphate, but this is rarely necessary because of the short duration of action of heparin. LMWs may produce fewer haemorrhagic complications, and monitoring of effect is not routinely required.

Heparins, particularly UFH, may also cause thrombocytopenia (low platelet count). This may occur in two forms. The first occurs 3–5 days after treatment and does not normally result in complications. The second type of thrombocytopenia occurs after about 6 days of treatment and often results in much more profound decreases in platelet count and an increased risk of thromboembolism. LMWHs are thought to be less likely to cause thrombocytopenia, but this complication has been reported, including in individuals who had previously developed thrombocytopenia after UFH.

Heparin-induced osteoporosis is rare but may occur when the drug is used during pregnancy, and may be dose related. The exact mechanism is unknown. Other adverse effects of heparin are alopecia, urticaria and anaphylaxis, but these are also rare.

It has been shown that there is a non-linear relationship between the dose of UFH infused and the KCCT. This means that disproportionate adjustments in dose are required depending on the KCCT if under-dosing or over-dosing is to be avoided (Table 21.1). Since the half-life of UFH is 1 hour it would take 5 hours (five half-lives of the drug) to reach a steady state. A loading dose is therefore administered to reduce the time to achieve adequate anticoagulation. UFH in full dose can also be given by repeated subcutaneous injection, and in these circumstances the calcium salt appears to be less painful than the sodium salt. Opinions differ as to whether the subcutaneous or intravenous route is preferable. The subcutaneous route may take longer to reach effective plasma heparin concentrations but avoids the need for infusion devices. Heparin is normally used

Table 21.1 Guidelines to control unfractionated heparin (UFH) treatment (modified from Fennerty et al 1986)

Loading dose

5000 IU over 5 minutes

Infusion

Start at 1400 IU/h (e.g. 8400 IU in 100 ml of normal saline over 6 hours). Check after 6 hours. Adjust dose according to ratio of the KCCT to the control value using the values below

KCCT ratio	Infusion rate change
> 7.0	Discontinue for 30 min to 1 h and reduce by > 500 IU/h
> 5.0	Reduce by 500 IU/h
4.1–5.0	Reduce by 300 IU/h
3.1–4.0	Reduce by 100 IU/h
2.6–3.0	Reduce by 50 IU/h
1.5–2.5	No change
1.2–1.4	Increase by 200 U/h
< 1.2	Increase by 400 U/h

After each dose change, wait 10 hours before next KCCT estimation unless KCCT > 5, when more frequent (e.g. 4-hourly) estimation is advisable Developed using Diogen (Bell and Alton); local validation may be necessary

in the immediate stages of venous thrombosis and PE until the effects of warfarin become apparent. In the past it has been continued for 7–10 days, but recent evidence indicates that 3–5 days of therapy may be sufficient in many instances. This shorter treatment may also reduce the risk of the rare but potentially very serious complications of severe heparin-induced thrombocytopenia, which normally occurs after the sixth day. LMWHs are used for similar lengths of time, but are normally given subcutaneously without a loading dose, and without routine monitoring. They are more expensive than UFH, but the increased efficacy and convenience of administration may well make them cost-effective in treatment and prevention in certain situations, for example out-patient treatment.

Heparinoids

Danaparoid

Danaparoid is a heparinoid that is licensed for prophylaxis of deep vein thrombosis in patients undergoing general or orthopaedic surgery. It is a mixture of low molecular weight sulphated glycosaminoglycuronans, heparan sulphate, dermatan sulphate and a small amount of chondroitin sulphate. It acts by inhibiting factor Xa and like LMWHs is given by subcutaneous injection. Providing there is no evidence of cross-reactivity, it also has a role in the treatment of individuals who develop thrombocytopenia in association with heparin therapy, when it is given intravenously, and monitoring of anti-Xa activity is only required in those at high risk of bleeding (e.g. renal insufficiency).

Hirudins

Lepirudin

Lepirudin, a recombinant hirudin, is licensed for anticoagulation in patients with type II (immune) heparin-induced thrombocytopenia (HIT) who require parenteral antithrombotic treatment. The dose of lepirudin is adjusted according to the activated partial thromboplastin time (APTT).

Oral anticoagulants

Although not the only coumarin anticoagulant available, warfarin is by far the most widely used drug in this group because of its potency, duration of action and more reliable bioavailability. Acenocoumarol (nicoumalone) has a much shorter duration of action and phenindione may be associated with a higher incidence of non-haemorrhagic adverse effects. When given by mouth, warfarin is completely and rapidly absorbed, although food decreases the rate (but not the extent) of absorption. It is extremely highly plasma protein bound (99%) and therefore has a small volume of distribution (7–14 l). It consists of an equal mixture of two enantiomers, (R)- and (S)-warfarin. They have different anticoagulant potencies and routes of metabolism. Both enantiomers act by inducing a functional deficiency of vitamin K and thereby prevent the normal carboxylation of the glutamic acid residues of the amino-terminal ends of clotting factors II, VII, IX and X. This renders the clotting factors unable to cross-link with calcium and thereby bind to phospholipid-containing membranes. Warfarin prevents the reduction of vitamin K epoxide to vitamin K by epoxide reductase. (S)-warfarin appears to be atleast five times more potent in this regard than (R)-warfarin. Since warfarin does not have any effect on already carboxylated clotting factors, the delay in onset of the anticoagulant effect of warfarin is dependent on the rate of clearance of the fully carboxylated factors already synthesized. In this regard the half-life of removal of factor VII is approximately 6 hours, that of factor IX 24 hours, factor X 36 hours and factor II 50 hours.

The effect of warfarin is monitored using the one-stage prothrombin time, for example the international normalized ratio (INR). This test is sensitive chiefly to factors VII, II and X (and to a lesser extent factor V, which is not a vitamin K-dependent clotting factor).

However, factor VII, to which the INR is sensitive, is the most important factor in the extrinsic pathway of clotting. The optimum therapeutic range for the INR differs for different clinical indications since the lowest INR consistent with therapeutic efficacy is the best in reducing the risk of haemorrhage. Examples of therapeutic ranges recommended for certain indications are given in Table 21.2.

Warfarin is metabolized by the liver via the cytochrome P450 system. Only very small amounts of the drug appear unchanged in the urine. The average clearance is 4.5 l/day, and the half-life ranges from 20 to 60 hours (mean 40 hours). It thus takes approximately 1 week (around five half-lives) for the steady state to be reached after warfarin has been administered. The enantiomers of warfarin are metabolized stereo-specifically, (R)- warfarin being mainly reduced at the acetyl side-chain into secondary warfarin alcohols while (S)-warfarin is predominantly metabolized at the coumarin ring to hydroxywarfarin. The clearance of

Table 21.2   Recommended target international normalized ratios (INRs)for different conditions and grade of recommendation (British Association for Haematology 1998).

Indication	Target INR	Grade of recommendation
Pulmonary embolus	2.5	A
Proximal deep vein thrombosis	2.5	A
Calf vein thrombus	2.5	A
Recurrence of venous thromboembolism when no longer on warfarin therapy	2.5	A
Recurrence of venous thromboembolism while on warfarin therapy	3.5	C
Symptomatic inherited thrombophilia	2.5	C
Antiphospholipid syndrome	3.5	B
Non-rheumatic atrial fibrillation	2.5	A
Atrial fibrillation due to rheumatic heart disease, congenital heart disease, thyrotoxicosis	2.5	C
Cardioversion	2.5	B
Mural thrombus	2.5	B
Cardiomyopathy	2.5	C
Mechanical prosthetic heart valve	3.5	B
Bioprosthetic valve	Not indicated	A
Ischaemic stroke without atrial fibrillation	Not indicated	A
Retinal vessel occlusion	Not indicated	C
Peripheral arterial thrombosis and grafts	Not indicated	A
Coronary artery thrombosis	Not indicated	A
Coronary artery graft thrombosis	Not indicated	A
Coronary angioplasty and stents	Not indicated	A

INR, international normalized ratio.
A, at least one randomized controlled trial (RCT); B, well conducted clinical trials but no RCT; C, expert opinion but no studies.

warfarin may be reduced in liver disease as well as during administration of a variety of drugs known to inhibit either the (S) or (R), or both, enantiomers. These are shown in Table 21.3. Renal function is thought to have little effect on the pharmacokinetics of, or anticoagulant response to, warfarin.

The major adverse effect of warfarin is haemorrhage, which often occurs at a predisposing abnormality such as an ulcer or tumour. The risk of bleeding is increased by excessive anticoagulation, although this may not need to be present for severe haemorrhage to occur. Close monitoring of the degree of anticoagulation of warfarin is therefore important, and guidelines for reversal of excessive anticoagulation are shown in Table 21.4. It is also important to reduce the duration of therapy of the drug to the minimum effective period in order to reduce the period of risk.

Skin reactions to warfarin may also occur but are rare. The most serious skin reaction is warfarin-induced skin necrosis, which may occur over areas of adipose tissue such as the breasts, buttocks or thighs, especially in women, and which is related to relative deficiency of protein C or S. This is important because these deficiencies result in an increased risk of thrombosis and therefore warfarin may more often be used in such subjects. Preventing excessive anticoagulation in the initial stages of induction of therapy may reduce the severity of the reaction. A scheme which helps to achieve this aim is shown in Table 21.5.

Warfarin may also be teratogenic, producing in some instances a condition called chondrodysplasia punctata. This is associated with 'punched-out' lesions at sites of ossification, particularly of the long bones but also of the facial bones, and may be associated with absence of the spleen. Although it has been associated predominantly with warfarin anticoagulation during the first trimester of pregnancy, other abnormalities, including cranial nerve palsies, hydrocephalus and microcephaly, have been reported at later stages of pregnancy if the child is exposed.

Although other oral anticoagulants are available, in the vast majority of cases these have not been shown to have any clear benefits over warfarin. They may be used occasionally where a patient does not tolerate warfarin. The necessary duration of anticoagulation in venous thrombosis and pulmonary embolus is still uncertain.

On the basis of the available evidence, therapy may be required for approximately 6 months after the first deep vein thrombosis or pulmonary embolus. It may be possible to reduce the duration of therapy in patients who have had a postoperative episode since it is likely that the risk factor has been reversed (unless immobility continues). In patients with a second episode, therapy may be required for even longer, and in patients with more than two episodes life-long treatment may be necessary in order to reduce the risk of recurrence.

Fibrinolytic drugs

Thrombolytic therapy is used in life-threatening acute massive pulmonary embolus. It has been used in deep vein thrombosis, particularly in those patients where a large amount of clot exists and venous valvular damage is likely. However, fibrinolytic drugs are potentially more dangerous than anticoagulant drugs, and evidence is not available in situations other than acute massive embolism to show a sustained benefit from their use.

Streptokinase was the first agent available in this class. It was produced from streptococci, and is a large protein that binds to and activates plasminogen, thus encouraging the breakdown of formed fibrin to fibrinogen degradation products. It also acts on the circulating fibrinogen to produce a degree of systemic anticoagulation. Since it is a large protein molecule, it cannot be administered orally and has to be given by intravenous infusion. The half-life of removal from the body is 30 minutes. It is cleared chiefly by the reticuloendothelial system in the liver.

Its major adverse effect is to increase the risk of haemorrhage but it may also be antigenic and produce an anaphylactic reaction. It may also cause hypotension during infusion, and in some patients, particularly those who have been administered the drug within the previous 12 months, a relative resistance to the drug may occur. Thrombolytic therapy is contraindicated in patients who have had major surgery or with active bleeding sites in the gastrointestinal or genitourinary tract, those who have a history of stroke, renal or liver disease, and those with hypertension. It should also be avoided during pregnancy or during the postpartum period.

Tissue plasminogen activator (rt-PA) or alteplase was developed using recombinant DNA technology. Although this agent is much more expensive, it can be used in those situations where streptokinase may be less effective because of development of antibodies, for example within 1 year of previous streptokinase use, or where allergy to streptokinase has previously occurred. Because it produces a lesser degree of systemic anticoagulation (it is more active against plasminogen associated with the clot), immediate use of heparin subsequently is necessary to prevent recurrence of thrombosis. Alteplase is now generally given.

Reteplase, and more recently tenecteplase, are also fibrin-specific agents, and so heparin is required to prevent rebound thrombosis. They have a similar efficacy to alteplase and are also more expensive than streptokinase. They are presently only licensed for acute myocardial infarction (see section on arterial thromboembolism, below). In this clinical situation, reteplase is administered as an intravenous bolus, followed by a second bolus 30 minutes later (double bolus), and tenecteplase is given as a single intravenous

Table 21.3   Some clinically important drug interactions with warfarin

Interacting drug	Effect of interaction on anticoagulant effect	Probable mechanism(s)
Colestyramine Colestipol	Reduced anticoagulant effect	Impaired absorption and increased elimination of warfarin. N.B. Long-term treatment may cause impaired vitamin K absorption and enhance anticoagulant effect
Barbiturates Carbamazepine Griseofulvin Phenytoin (see also below) Primidone Rifampicin Rifabutin St John's wort	Reduced anticoagulant effect	Induction of warfarin metabolism
Amiodarone Azapropazone Chloramphenicol Cimetidine Ciprofloxacin Clarithromycin Dextropopoxyphene Erythromycin Fluconazole Itraconazole Ketoconazole Mefenamic acid Metronidazole Miconazole Norfloxacin Ofloxacin Phenylbutazone Sulfinpyrazone Sulphonamides (e.g. in co-trimoxazole)	Increased anticoagulant effect	Inhibition of warfarin metabolism
Anabolic steroids Bezafibrate Clofibrate Danazol D-thyroxine Gemfibrozil L-thyroxine Phenytoin (see also above) Salicylates/aspirin (high-dose) Stanozolol Tamoxifen	Increased anticoagulant effect	Pharmacodynamic potentiation of anticoagulant effect
NSAIDs (including aspirin at all doses) Clopidogrel Ticlopidine	Increased risk of bleeding	Additive effects on coagulation and haemostasis
Oral contraceptives, oestrogens and progestogens	Reduced anticoagulant effect	Pharmacodynamic antagonism of anticoagulant effect
Vitamin K (e.g. in some enteral feeds)		

Table 21.4 Recommendations for management of bleeding and excessive anticoagulation in patients receiving warfarin (British Society for Haematology 1998)

Cause	Recommendation
3.0<INR<6.0 (target INR 2.5) 4.0<INR<6.0 (target INR 3.5)	1. Reduce warfarin dose or stop 2. Restart warfarin when INR<5.0
6.0<INR<8.0, no bleeding or minor bleeding	1. Stop warfarin 2. Restart when INR<5.0
INR>8.0, no bleeding or minor bleeding	1. Stop warfarin 2. Restart warfarin when INR<5.0 3. If other risk factors for bleeding give 0.5–2.5 mg of vitamin K (oral)
Major bleeding	1. Stop warfarin 2. Give prothrombin complex concentrate 50 units/kg or FFP 15 ml/kg 3. Give 5 mg of vitamin (oral or i.v.)

INR, international normalized ratio; FFP, fresh frozen plasma.

Table 21.5 Suggested warfarin induction schedule (modified from Fennerty et al 1984)

Day	INR	Warfarin dose (mg)
First	<1.4	10
Second	<1.8	10
	1.8	1
	>1.8	0.5
Third	<2.0	10
	2.0–2.1	5
	2.2–2.3	4.5
	2.4–2.5	4
	2.6–2.7	3.5
	2.8–2.9	3
	3.0–3.1	2.5
	3.2–3.3	2
	3.4	1.5
	3.5	1
	3.6–4.0	0.5
	>4.0	0 (Predicted maintenance dose)
Fourth	<1.4	>8
	1.4	8
	1.5	7.5
	1.6–1.7	7
	1.8	6.5
	1.9	6
	2.0–2.1	5.5
	2.2–2.3	5
	2.4–2.6	4.5
	2.7–3.0	4
	3.1–3.5	3.5
	3.6–4.0	3
	4.1–4.5	Miss out next day's dose then give 2 mg
	>4.5	Miss out 2 d doses then give 1 mg

INR, international normalized ratio.

bolus. They therefore have the advantage of convenience of administration compared with alteplase.

Patient care

The patient on oral anticoagulants should be given full information on what to do in case of problems and what circumstances and drugs to avoid. An anticoagulant card with previous INR values and doses should also be provided. The patient should be told of the colour code for the different strengths of warfarin tablet and should be told to carry their treatment card at all times. The likely duration of anticoagulant therapy should be made clear to the patient to avoid unnecessary and potentially dangerous prolongation of treatment. Patients who have received a fibrinolytic agent should also carry a card identifying the drug given and the date of administration.

ARTERIAL THROMBOEMBOLISM

Epidemiology

Acute myocardial infarction is the commonest cause of acute arterial thrombosis. Stroke is commonly caused by atherothromboembolism from the great vessels or embolism arising from the heart (approximately 80% of strokes). The annual incidence of stroke in the developed world is approximately 1 per 2000 of the population, and the incidence is likely to increase as the population ages. Peripheral arterial occlusive thrombosis is normally associated with atherothromboembolism but is rare, even in patients with increased risk of thromboembolism (e.g. atrial fibrillation).

Aetiology

Arterial thromboembolism is normally associated with vascular injury and hypercoagulability. Vascular injury is most often due to atheroma. Although the exact mechanism is not clear, it is thought that platelet aggregation may be induced by the sheer stresses caused by stenosis of an atherosclerotic vessel. This thrombotic material may embolize to cause occlusion further downstream. Hypercoagulability is also a risk factor. It may be associated with increased plasma fibrinogen levels and an increase in circulating cellular components (e.g. polycythaemia or thrombocythaemia). As mentioned earlier, the thrombus formed in the artery contains a much larger proportion of platelets, possibly reflecting the fact that other blood components that are not as readily adherent may be dissipated by the higher flow rates in the arterial circulation.

Oestrogens, by the mechanisms described earlier, are likely to increase the risk of arterial as well as venous thrombosis. Hyperlipidaemia may also increase the risk of hypercoagulability as well as enhancing thrombotic risk through its role in the progression of atheroma and vascular injury.

Clinical manifestations

Arterial thromboembolism affecting the cerebral circulation results in either transient ischaemic attacks (TIAs) or, in severe cases, cerebral infarction (one form of stroke). A transient ischaemic attack is defined as symptoms of acute ischaemia of the brain lasting for less than 24 hours with complete recovery. The distinction between a transient ischaemic attack and a stroke is therefore one of degree. It may involve weakness of the limbs or cause disturbance of vision. If the vertebrobasilar territory is affected, nausea, vomiting and dizziness may be the most prominent features. In stroke, features are similar but persist for longer than 24 hours. Clinical findings, however, vary markedly, and it may be difficult on clinical grounds to separate cerebral infarction from the even more serious cause of stroke, cerebral haemorrhage, although patients with haemorrhage more often have severe headache and coma, and less often have a preceding history of transient ischaemic attacks.

Arterial thromboembolism affecting a limb (normally a lower limb) most often presents as a sudden onset of pain in the limb associated with loss of peripheral pulses and coldness of the affected limb.

Investigations

The diagnosis of a transient ischaemic attack is a clinical one since, by definition, no permanent damage to the brain substance is caused by these episodes. The investigations therefore help to identify risk factors for transient ischaemia and will include investigations of factors known to increase blood viscosity or hypercoagulability, estimation of serum glucose and lipid levels, investigation of the carotid vessels (normally by Doppler ultrasound) and a search for any cardiac sources of emboli (echocardiography). Evidence of arterial disease elsewhere increases the suspicion of transient ischaemic episodes.

The diagnosis of cerebral infarction includes the investigations previously mentioned for transient ischaemic attacks but computed axial tomography (CT scanning) is the investigation of choice. In cerebral infarction, areas of low density occur within a day or two of the episode. In cerebral haemorrhage, an area of high density occurs, often immediately after the episode.

Thromboembolism in a peripheral artery may be detected by Doppler ultrasound, but angiography is the definitive modality for investigation of the site and extent of blockage and the response to treatment.

Treatment

Transient ischaemic attacks resolve spontaneously, and major aspects of their management include risk factor modification and prophylaxis (see aspirin, below). In patients with cerebral infarction aspirin in a dose of 300 mg should be administered as soon as possible after the diagnosis is established. Intravenous alteplase, if administered within 3 hours of onset of ischaemic stroke, has been shown to be beneficial but is associated with increased risk of intracerebral bleeding. Several neuroprotective agents have been investigated for treatment of ischaemic stroke but none have been shown to be effective. Anticoagulants may increase the risk of conversion of infarction of brain substance to haemorrhage and are contraindicated. Maintenance of adequate nutrition and the prevention and treatment of aspiration pneumonia, deep vein thrombosis, pressure sores and constipation are important. Risk factors for recurrent cerebral infarction such as hypertension, diabetes and hyperlipidemia should be treated. Stopping smoking, avoiding excessive alcohol consumption and exercise are also important.

Anticoagulant therapy is effective in prophylaxis against cardiothromboembolic TIA or stroke (e.g. in patients with atrial fibrillation) but is not normally instituted until at least 2 weeks after the event. If the source of emboli is from the great vessels, then prophylaxis with aspirin or other antiplatelet agent is more likely to be of benefit and is also likely to be safer than warfarin therapy (see below).

Aspirin (acetylsalicylic acid)

Aspirin is a potent inhibitor of the enzyme cyclo-oxygenase, which catalyses the production of prostaglandins. It reduces the production of thromboxane A_2 in the platelet, an effect that lasts for the life of the platelet. It also prevents the production of the anti-aggregatory prostaglandin epoprostenol (prostacyclin) in the endothelial lining of the blood vessel, but there is still debate as to what is the optimal dose for aspirin to achieve the maximum ratio of inhibition of thromboxane versus epoprostenol production.

Aspirin is well absorbed after oral administration. It is rapidly metabolized by esterases in the blood and liver to salicylic acid and other metabolites that are excreted in the urine. In the doses used in prophylaxis against thromboembolism, aspirin is largely metabolized by the liver, but in overdose, urinary excretion of salicylate becomes a limiting factor in drug elimination.

The major adverse effect of aspirin is gastrointestinal irritation and bleeding. This problem is much more common with higher doses of aspirin (600 mg or more) that were once used in the prevention of arterial thromboembolism but are less common with the doses (150–300 mg) now recommended. There is evidence that concomitant use of ulcer-healing drugs (e.g. misoprostol, H_2 receptor antagonists or omeprazole) can reduce the risk of non-steroidal anti-inflammatory drug (NSAID) induced peptic ulceration in patients susceptible to the problem, but haemorrhagic risk may not be significantly reduced. Not is there evidence that buffered or enteric-coated preparations are safer in this respect. However, the vast majority of patients tolerate low dose aspirin well, and it is normally given as a single oral dose of soluble aspirin. Aspirin may also, rarely, induce asthma, particularly in patients with coexisting reversible airways obstruction. Other patients have a form of aspirin hypersensitivity that may result in urticaria and/or angio-oedema. In this situation there may be cross-reactivity with other NSAIDs.

Clopidogrel

Clopidogrel is a pro-drug that is metabolized in part to an active thiol derivative. The latter inhibits platelet aggregation by rapidly and irreversibly inhibiting the binding of adenosine diphosphate (ADP) to its platelet receptor, thus preventing the ADP-mediated activation of the glycoprotein IIb/IIIa receptor for the life of the platelet. It is orally active and is given once daily for the reduction of atherosclerotic events in those with pre-existing atherosclerotic disease. In this respect, it may be a useful alternative to aspirin in aspirin allergic subjects, but haemorrhage occurs with the same frequency as aspirin, and thrombocytopenia (sometimes severe) may be commoner than with aspirin therapy.

Dipyridamole

Dipyridamole is used by mouth as an adjunct to oral anticoagulation for prophylaxis of thromboembolism associated with prosthetic heart valves. Modified-release preparations are licensed for secondary prevention of ischaemic stroke and transient ischaemic attacks (see treatment of stroke). It is a phosphodiesterase inhibitor and thus elevates concentrations of cyclic AMP. It may also block the uptake of adenosine by erythrocytes and other cells. Adverse effects include gastrointestinal problems, flushing and hypotension.

Ticlopidine

Ticlopidine reduces platelet aggregation by inhibiting ADP-dependent binding of fibrinogen to the platelet membrane. It is orally active and is licensed for reduction of risk of first and recurrent stroke in those with previous cerebral ischaemic events. It may also be used to reduce the risk of major ischaemic events in patients with intermittent claudication. Ticlopidine is also used (in combination with aspirin) for the prevention of subacute stent occlusion after intracoronary stenting. However, because of a significant incidence of serious haematological side-effects (2.4% incidence of neutropenia, 0.8% incidence of severe neutropenia and thrombocytopenia, sometimes associated with paradoxical thrombosis), a clinician in hospital should carry out the initiation of therapy, and frequent haematological monitoring is required for the first 3 months. The risks and benefits of ticlopidine versus aspirin should be carefully considered, and the benefit/risk ratio for ticlopidine is greater in patients for whom aspirin is not suitable. In many countries clopidogrel is preferred to ticlopidine because of its favourable adverse effect profile.

Glycoprotein IIb/IIIa inhibitors

Glycoprotein IIb/IIIa inhibitors prevent platelet aggregation by blocking the binding of fibrinogen to receptors on platelets. Abciximab is a monoclonal antibody which binds to accidents, particularly coronary glycoprotein IIb/IIIa receptors and to other related sites; it is licensed as an adjunct to heparin and aspirin for the prevention of ischaemic complications in high-risk patients undergoing percutaneous transluminal coronary intervention. Abciximab should be used once only.

Eptifibatide and tirofiban also inhibit glycoprotein IIb/IIIa receptors; they are licensed for use with heparin and aspirin to prevent early myocardial infarction in patients with unstable angina or non-Q-wave myocardial infarction. Abciximab, eptifibatide and tirofiban should be used by specialists only.

Patient care

Aspirin is normally well tolerated at the doses used for stroke prevention (150 to 300 mg). However, it should not be given to patients with gastrointestinal ulceration. Since it may induce bronchospasm in susceptible individuals, it should be used cautiously in such circumstances. It is best tolerated if taken once daily as soluble aspirin after food.

CASE STUDIES

Case 21.1

A patient receiving warfarin to prevent deep vein thrombosis and previously well controlled comes to the clinic with an INR of 12, despite having the same dose of drug. There is no evidence of bleeding.

Question

What should be done?

Answer

The patient should be given phytomenadione (vitamin K) 500 micrograms by *slow* intravenous injection. This should return the INR to the therapeutic range by 24 h without causing warfarin resistance subsequently. A search for clinical conditions or drugs which might cause warfarin sensitivity should also be made. Measurement of plasma warfarin concentration may help in difficult cases.

Case 21.2

A patient receiving heparin for 10 days for extensive venous thromboembolism develops aterial thrombosis.

Question

What would you suspect in this situation and what should be done?

Answer

The rare but serious heparin-induced thrombocytopenia may be responsible. The platelet count should be measured urgently and heparin discontinued immediately. Florinotytic therapy has been used successfully in cases of occlusive thrombosis, and surgery has also been necessary. The CSM recommends monitoring the platelet count regularly in patients given heparin for more than 5 days.

Case 21.3

A patient who is admitted with suspected myocardial intarction says that he had a myocardial intarction 6 months earlier and was treated with a drug to 'dissolve the clot in the coronary artery'.

Question

What relevance may this have to his management on this occasion?

Answer

The patient has received a thrombolytic, possibly streptokinase, within the last yeer. He should be asked if he was given a card with the identity of the therapy to carry with him. If the prior treatment was with streptokinase, consideration should be given to the use of tPA as an alternative agent because of the relative resistance to streptokinase which may last up to 12 months after prior treatment.

Case 21.4

Question

What should a 64-year-old male patient be asked before starting aspirin therapy following an acute myocardial Intarction?

Answer

The patient should be asked if he has had aspirin before and, if so, whether he toferated it. Aspirin is contraindicated in patients with gastrointestinal ulceration. It may induce bronchospasm or angio-oedema in susceptible individuals and caution should be exercised in these circumstances. Gastric irritation is minimized by taking the dose after food.

Case 21.5

A 56-year-old woman on warfarin therapy for atrial fibrillation with mitral stenosis appears to become resistant to warfarin after previously good control on 5 mg daily and her INR does not rise above 1.4 even when her warfarin dose is increased to 20 mg daily.

Question

What can be done to find the cause of the resistance?

Answer

The patient should be asked about any new medications which might have been introduced recently. Some proprietary medicines may contain vitamin K which could cause resistance. One cause of apparent resistance to warfarin is poor compliance and this should therefore be considered. Supervised administration of the dose and/or measurement of plasma warfarin concentration may be of value if the latter is suspected.

REFERENCES

British Society for Haematology 1998 Guidelines on anticoagulant therapy, 3rd edn. British Journal of Haematology 101: 374–387

Fennerty A G, Dolben J, Thomas P et al 1984 Flexible induction dosage regimen for warfarin and prediction of maintenance dose. British Medical Journal 288: 1268–1270

Fennerty A G, Renowden S, Scolding N et al 1986 Guidelines for the control of heparin treatment. British Medical Journal 292: 579–580

FURTHER READING

Hardman S M C, Cowie M R 1999 Anticoagulation in heart disease. Brish Medical Journal 318: 238–243

National Institute for Clinical Excellence 2000 Technology appraisal guidance no. 12, September 2000. Guidance on glycoprotein IIb/IIIa inhibitors for acute coronary syndromes. National Institute for Clinical Excellence, London

Shetty H G M, Backhouse G, Bentley D P et al 1992 Effective reversal of warfarin-induced excessive anticoagulation with low dose vitamin K. Thrombosis and Haemostasis 67: 13–15

Dyslipidaemia 22

R. Walker

KEY POINTS

- Elevated concentrations of total cholesterol (TC) and low-density lipoprotein (LDL-C) increase the risk of coronary heart disease (CHD), while high-density lipoprotein (HDL-C) confers protection.
- Two-thirds of the UK population have a serum TC above the desirable level of 5 mmol/l.
- Dyslipidaemia may be secondary to disorders such as diabetes mellitus, hypothyroidism, chronic renal failure, nephrotic syndrome, obesity, high alcohol intake and some drugs.
- Androgens, β-blockers, ciclosporin, oral contraceptives, diuretics, glucocorticoids and vitamin A derivatives can have an adverse effect on the lipid profile.
- The four main classes of lipid lowering agents are: statins, fibrates, resins and nicotinic acid derivatives.
- Statins are generally the drugs of choice in the treatment of primary prevention and secondary prevention of CHD.
- The aim of treatment in primary and secondary prevention includes the lowering of TC to either less than 5 mmol/l or a reduction of TC by 20% to 25%, whichever results in the lowest level. The equivalent target for LDL-C is 3 mmol/l or a reduction of 30%, whichever results in the lowest level.

Elevated serum concentrations of total cholesterol (TC) and low-density lipoprotein cholesterol (LDL-C) appear to increase the risk of an individual developing coronary heart disease (CHD). However, high-density lipoprotein (HDL-C) confers protection against coronary heart disease, with the risk reducing as HDL-C increases. It is therefore appropriate to use the term dyslipidaemia, which encompasses hypercholesterolaemia and hypolipoproteinaemia, particularly when considering the individual at risk of coronary heart disease because of a high TC and low HDL-C (TC:HDL-C ratio).

Epidemiology

Lipid and lipoprotein concentrations vary among different populations, with countries consuming a Western type of diet generally having higher TC and LDL-C levels than those where regular consumption of saturated fat is low.

The ideal serum lipid profile is actually unknown and probably varies between different populations, but for practical purposes the values presented in Table 22.1 represent the target profile in the UK. A relationship between TC and coronary heart disease is well established in Western populations at concentrations above 5 mmol/l (and LDL-C > 3 mmol/l). Unfortunately more than 68% of the population have a TC above 5 mmol/l and this is viewed as a contributory risk factor to the development of coronary heart disease, which accounts for one in four deaths in the UK. A reduction in the mean level of TC in the population will reduce the development of coronary atherosclerosis and the prevalence of coronary heart disease. However, such a population strategy will be expensive to implement and must run in parallel with programmes that identify individuals with dyslipidaemia and/or other risk factors who are at high risk of coronary heart disease.

There is increasing evidence that reductions of TC and LDL-C below 5 mmol/l and 3 mmol/l, respectively, lower the incidence of coronary heart disease. In fact, there is little evidence of a level below which a further reduction of TC or LDL-C is not associated with a lower risk of coronary heart disease.

Population studies (Table 22.2) have shown that TC increases with age in men and women after the age of 20, with men having higher levels between the ages of 25 and 54. The rate of rise slows in men after 45 and appears to decline after 75 years, presumably because men with hypercholesterolaemia have died from coronary heart disease. In women, TC continues to rise up to the age of 74 years. Beyond the age of 54 the mean TC in women exceeds that of men of a similar age. It should, however,

Table 22.1 Ideal serum lipid profile

Total cholesterol (TC)	< 5.0 mmol/l
LDL cholesterol (LDL-C)	< 3.0 mmol/l
Triglycerides	< 2.3 mmol/l
HDL cholesterol (HDL-C)	> 0.9 mmol/l

Table 22.2 Mean concentrations of TC and HDL-C and ratios of TC to HDL-C in a stratified random sample of 10 569 volunteers of whom 294 were taking lipid lowering drugs (adapted from Primatesta & Poulter 2000)

	Age 16–24	Age 25–34	Age 35–44	Age 45–54	Age 55–64	Age 65–74	Age > 75	All ages
Men	(n = 423)	(n = 912)	(n = 967)	(n = 964)	(n = 724)	(n = 621)	(n = 390)	(n = 5001)
TC (mmol/l)	4.37	5.11	5.52	5.76	5.80	5.75	5.54	5.47
HDL-C (mmol/l)	1.30	1.27	1.29	1.27	1.27	1.25	1.33	1.28
Ratio	3.55	4.31	4.64	4.89	4.92	4.96	4.51	4.61
Women	(n = 450)	(n = 967)	(n = 1071)	(n = 1092)	(n = 804)	(n = 636)	(n = 548)	(n = 5568)
TC (mmol/l)	4.56	4.92	5.22	5.67	6.16	6.43	6.33	5.59
HDL-C (mmol/l)	1.53	1.52	1.54	1.58	1.57	1.52	1.62	1.55
Ratio	3.20	3.42	3.60	3.87	4.22	4.54	4.17	3.84

be remembered that HDL-C levels of less than 0.9 mmol/l are associated with increased coronary mortality regardless of TC (Goldbourt et al 1997).

Lipid transport and lipoprotein metabolism

The major lipids in plasma (cholesterol, triglycerides and phospholipids) are transported in the form of lipoproteins. There are six main classes of lipoproteins: chylomicrons, chylomicron remnants, very low-density lipoproteins (VLDL-C), intermediate-density lipoproteins (IDL-C), low-density lipoproteins (LDL-C) and high-density lipoproteins (HDL-C).

The protein components of lipoproteins are known as apoproteins, of which apoproteins A-I, E, C and B are perhaps the most important. Apoprotein B exists in two forms: B-48, which is present in chylomicrons and associated with the transport of ingested lipids; and B-100, which is found in endogenously secreted VLDL-C and associated with the transport of lipids from the liver (Fig. 22.1).

When dietary cholesterol and triglycerides are absorbed from the intestine they are transported in the intestinal lymphatics as chylomicrons, which pass through blood capillaries in adipose tissue and skeletal muscle where the enzyme lipoprotein lipase is located, bound to the endothelium. Lipoprotein lipase is activated by apoprotein C-II (a component of apoprotein C) on the surface of the chylomicron. The lipase catalyses the breakdown of the triglyceride in the chylomicron to free fatty acid and glycerol, which then enter adipose tissue and muscle. The cholesterol-rich chylomicron remnant is

taken up by receptors on hepatocyte membranes, and in this way dietary cholesterol is delivered to the liver and cleared from the circulation.

VLDL-C is formed in the liver, transports triglycerides and contains some cholesterol. The triglyceride content of VLDL-C is removed by lipoprotein lipase in a manner analogous to that described for chylomicrons above, and forms IDL-C particles. IDL-C particles acquire cholesterol esters from HDL-C under the influence of the enzyme lecithin-cholesterol acyltransferase (LCAT). The IDL-C may be transported to the liver or be further hydrolysed and modified to lose triglyceride and apoprotein E1 and become an LDL-C particle. LDL-C is the major cholesterol-carrying particle in plasma.

LDL-C provides cholesterol, an essential component of cell membranes and a precursor of steroid hormones, to those cells that require it. LDL-C is also probably the main lipoprotein involved in atherogenesis. For reasons that are not totally clear, but probably related to minor trauma, anoxaemia or hypertension, the arterial endothelium becomes permeable to lipoproteins. Monocytes migrate through the permeable endothelium and engulf the lipoproteins. This results in the formation of lipid-laden macrophages that have a principal role in the development of atherosclerosis. The aim of treatment in hyperlipidaemia is often to reduce concentrations of LDL-C (and consequently atherogenesis) and thus reduce TC at the same time.

While VLDL-C and LDL-C are considered the 'bad' lipoproteins, HDL-C is often considered to be the 'good' antiatherogenic lipoprotein. HDL-C transports cholesterol from peripheral tissues to the liver and plays a major role in maintaining cholesterol homeostasis in the body. It is therefore considered desirable to maintain

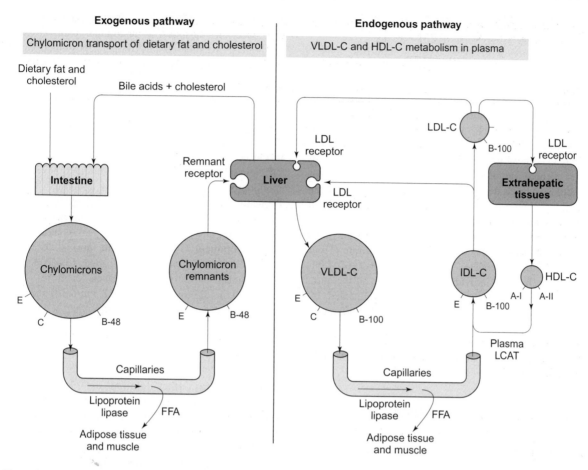

Figure 22.1   Schematic representation of lipoprotein metabolism in plasma. Dietary cholesterol and fat are transported in the exogenous pathway. Cholesterol produced in the liver is transported in the endogenous pathway.

levels of the protective HDL-C. Drugs that reduce HDL-C levels have an undesirable effect on lipid metabolism. It is now clear that there are at least two subfractions of HDL-C, HDL$_2$ and HDL$_3$, of which probably only HDL$_2$ protects against atheroma formation.

The role of hypertriglyceridaemia as an independent risk factor for coronary heart disease is unclear because triglyceride levels are confounded by an association with low HDL-C, hypertension, diabetes and obesity, and a synergistic effect with LDL-C and/or low HDL-C.

Aetiology

Primary dyslipidaemia

Up to 60% of the variability in serum fasting lipids may be genetically determined although expression is often influenced by interaction with environmental factors. The common familial (genetic) disorders can be classified as:

- the primary hypercholesterolaemias such as familial hypercholesterolaemia in which cholesterol is raised
- the primary mixed (combined) hyperlipidaemias in which both cholesterol and triglycerides are raised
- the primary hypertriglyceridaemias such as type III hyperlipoproteinaemia, familial lipoprotein lipase deficiency and familial Apo C-II deficiency.

Familial hypercholesterolaemia

Heterozygous familial hypercholesterolaemia is a common inherited metabolic disease and affects approximately 1 in 500 of the population. Familial hypercholesterolaemia is caused by a range of mutations in the LDL receptor gene that varies from family to family. Given the key role of LDL receptors in the catabolism of LDL-C, patients with familial hypercholesterolaemia may have serum levels of LDL-C two to three times higher than the general population from birth. It is important to identify and treat these individuals from birth, otherwise they will be exposed to high concentrations of LDL-C and will suffer the consequences.

In patients with heterozygous familial hypercholesterolaemia it has been estimated that coronary heart disease occurs about 20 years earlier than in the general population with some individuals, particularly men, dying from atherosclerotic heart disease often before the age of 40 years. The adult heterozygote typically exhibits the signs of cholesterol deposition such as corneal arcus (crescentic deposition of lipids in the cornea), tendon xanthomas (yellow papules or nodules of lipids deposited in tendons) and xanthelasma (yellow plaques or nodules of lipids deposited on eyelids) in their third decade.

In contrast to the heterozygous form, homozygous familial hypercholesterolaemia is extremely rare (1 per million) and associated with an absence of LDL receptors. In these individuals involvement of the aorta is evident by puberty and usually accompanied by cutaneous and tendon xanthomas. Myocardial infarction has been reported in homozygous children as early as 1.5–3 years of age. Until the 1980s, sudden death from acute coronary insufficiency before the age of 20 years was normal.

Familial combined hyperlipidaemia

Familial combined hyperlipidaemia has an incidence of 1 in 200 and is associated with excessive synthesis of VLDL. It is associated with an increased risk of atherosclerosis and occurs in approximately 15% of patients who present with coronary heart disease below the age of 60 years.

Familial type III hyperlipoproteinaemia

Familial type III hyperlipoproteinaemia has an incidence of 1 in 5000. It is characterized by the accumulation of chylomicron and VLDL remnants that fail to get cleared at a normal rate by hepatic receptors due to the presence of less active polymorphic forms of apoprotein E. Triglycerides and TC are both elevated and accompanied by corneal arcus, xanthelasma, tuberoeruptive xanthomas (groups of flat or yellowish raised nodules on the skin over joints, especially the elbows and knees) and palmar striae (yellow raised streaks across the palms of the hand). The disorder predisposes to premature atherosclerosis.

Familial lipoprotein lipase deficiency

Familial lipoprotein lipase deficiency is characterized by marked hypertriglyceridaemia and chylomicronaemia, and usually presents in childhood. It has an incidence of 1 per million and is due to a deficiency of the extrahepatic enzyme lipoprotein lipase, which results in a failure of lipolysis and the accumulation of

chylomicrons in plasma. The affected patient presents with recurrent episodes of abdominal pain, eruptive xanthomas, lipaemia retinalis (retinal deposition of lipid) and enlarged spleen. This disorder is not associated with an increased susceptibility to atherosclerosis; the major complication is acute pancreatitis.

Familial apolipoprotein C-II deficiency

In the heterozygous state, familial apolipoprotein C-II deficiency is associated with reduced levels of apolipoprotein C-II, the activator of lipoprotein lipase. Typically levels of apolipoprotein C-II are 50–80% of normal. This level of activity can maintain normal lipid levels. In the rare homozygous state there is an absence of apolipoprotein C-II, and despite normal levels of lipoprotein lipase it cannot be activated. Consequently, homozygotes have triglyceride levels of from 15 to above 100 mmol/l (normal range < 2.3 mmol/l) and may develop acute pancreatitis. Premature atherosclerosis is unusual but has been described.

Lipoprotein(a)

There are many other familial disorders of lipid metabolism in addition to those mentioned above but most are rare. However, a raised level of lipoprotein(a) (Lp(a)) is emerging as a major genetically inherited determinant of coronary heart disease. Lp(a) was first described more than 40 years ago. It is found in the serum of virtually everyone in a wide concentration range (0.01–2 g/l) with up to 70% of the variation in serum concentration being genetically determined. The concentration of Lp(a) is not normally distributed and the contribution of inheritance to circulating Lp(a) levels is more pronounced than for any other lipoprotein or apoprotein. A parental history of early onset coronary heart disease is associated with raised concentrations, and these appear to play a role in both atherogenesis and thrombosis. Lp(a) is structurally and functionally similar to plasminogen, and may competitively bind to fibrin and impair fibrinolysis (Atsumi et al 1998). Concentrations of Lp(a) above 0.3 g/l occur in about 20% of Caucasians and increase the risk of coronary atherosclerosis twofold, and this may increase to fivefold if LDL-C concentrations are also raised. However, the role of serum levels of Lp(a) in the clinical assessment of coronary heart disease risk remain unclear.

Secondary dyslipidaemia

Dyslipidaemias that occur secondary to a number of disorders (Table 22.3), dietary indiscretion or as a side-effect of drug therapy (Table 22.4) account for up to 40% of all dyslipidaemias. Fortunately, the lipid abnormalities in secondary dyslipidaemia can often be

Table 22.3 Example of disorders known to adversely affect the lipid profile

Type 1 diabetes
Type 2 diabetes
Hypothyroidism
Pregnancy
Inappropriate diet
Alcohol abuse
Chronic renal failure
Nephrotic syndrome
Renal transplantation
Cardiac transplantation
Hepatocellular disease
Cholestasis
Myeloma

Table 22.4 Example of drugs known to adversely affect the lipid profile

Androgens
β-blockers
Ciclosporin
Diuretics Thiazide Loop
Glucocorticoids
Oral contraceptives
Progestogens
Vitamin A derivatives

two notable exceptions to the rule with this example: nicotinic acid and fenofibrate. Both drugs reduce triglyceride levels but nicotinic acid increases urate levels while fenofibrate reduces them by an independent uricosuric effect.

Many of the disease states associated with secondary dyslipidaemia are listed in Table 22.3. The impact and severity of the lipid disorder will depend on the individual's genetic or nutritional predisposition to hyperlipidaemia. Some of the more common disorders that cause secondary dyslipidaemia include the following:

Diabetes mellitus

Premature atherosclerotic disease is the main cause of reduced life expectancy in patients with diabetes. The atherosclerotic disease is often widespread and complications such as plaque rupture and thrombotic occlusion occur more often and at a younger age (Donnelly et al 2000, Campbell 2001). The incidence of coronary heart disease is up to four times higher among diabetic patients.

Type 1 diabetes. In patients with type 1 diabetes HDL-C may appear high, but for reasons which are unclear it does not impart the same degree of protection against coronary heart disease as in those without diabetes. It is therefore not appropriate to use coronary risk prediction charts that utilize the TC:HDL-C ratio in patients with type 1 diabetes.

Type 2 diabetes. Patients with type 2 diabetes typically have increased triglycerides and decreased HDL-C. Levels of TC may be similar to those found in non-diabetic individuals but the patient with type 2 diabetes often has increased levels of highly atherogenic small dense LDL particles (Feher & Elkeles 1999). Individuals with type 2 diabetes but no coronary heart disease are thought to have the same coronary heart disease risk as patients without diabetes who have survived a myocardial infarction. Treatment with a statin was normally recommended if LDL-C was raised, and a fibrate recommended if LDL-C was normal but triglycerides were raised. The results of the recent Heart Protection Study (2002) suggest statins reduce vascular events regardless of cholesterol level.

Hypothyroidism

Abnormalities of serum lipid and lipoprotein levels are common in patients with untreated hypothyroidism. It is an important cause of secondary dyslipidaemia that can also lead to combined hyperlipidaemia or, less commonly, severe hypertriglyceridaemia in susceptible individuals. However, once adequate thyroid replacement has been instituted the dyslipidaemia should resolve.

corrected if the underlying disorder is treated, effective dietary advice implemented or the offending drug withdrawn.

On occasions a disorder may be associated with dyslipidaemia, but not the cause of it. For example, hyperuricaemia (gout) and hypertriglyceridaemia coexist in approximately 50% of men. In this particular example, neither is the cause of the other and treatment of one does not resolve the other. There are, however,

Chronic renal failure

Dyslipidaemia is frequently seen in patients with renal failure in the predialysis phase, during haemodialysis or when undergoing chronic ambulatory peritoneal dialysis. The hypertriglyceridaemia that most commonly occurs is associated with reduced lipoprotein lipase activity and often persists despite starting chronic maintenance renal dialysis.

Nephrotic syndrome

In patients with the nephrotic syndrome, dyslipidaemia appears to be caused by an increased production of apolipoprotein B-100 and associated LDL-C. In turn, the increased production is related to the extent of proteinuria (which depletes plasma of apolipoproteins) and the serum albumin level. The necessary use of glucocorticoids in patients with the nephrotic syndrome may exacerbate underlying lipoprotein abnormality.

Obesity

Chronic, excessive intake of calories leads to increased concentrations of triglycerides and reduced HDL-C. Obesity per se can exacerbate any underlying primary dyslipidaemia.

Alcohol

In the heavy drinker the high calorie content of beer and wine may be a cause of obesity with its associated adverse effect on the lipid profile. In addition, alcohol increases hepatic triglyceride synthesis, which in turn produces hypertriglyceridaemia.

Light to moderate drinkers (1–2 units/day) have a lower incidence of coronary heart disease and associated mortality than those who do not drink. This protective effect is probably due to an increase in HDL-C, and appears independent of the type of alcohol.

Drugs

A number of drugs can adversely affect serum lipid and lipoprotein concentrations (see Table 22.4). In particular, much attention has been given to the adverse effects of diuretic and β-blocker antihypertensive drugs on lipoprotein metabolism, but the clinical significance of these effects is unclear.

Antihypertensive agents. Hypertension is a major risk factor for atherosclerosis, and the beneficial effects of lowering blood pressure are well recognized. It is, however, a concern that treatment of patients with hypertension has reduced the incidence of cerebrovascular accidents and renal failure but had no major impact in reducing the incidence of coronary heart disease. It has been suggested that many of the antihypertensive agents used have an adverse effect on lipids and lipoproteins that override any beneficial reduction of blood pressure.

Diuretics. Thiazide and loop diuretics increase VLDL-C and LDL-C by mechanisms that are not completely understood. Whether these adverse effects are dose-dependent is also unclear. Use of a thiazide for less than 1 year has been reported to increase TC by up to 7% with no change in HDL-C. However, there is evidence that the short-term changes in lipids do not occur with the low doses in current use. Studies of 3–5 years' duration have found no effect on TC.

β-blockers. The effects of β-blockers on lipoprotein metabolism are reflected in an increase in serum triglyceride concentrations, a decrease in HDL-C, there is no discernible effect on LDL-C. β-blockers with intrinsic sympathomimetic activity appear to have little or no effect on VLDL-C or HDL-C. Pindolol has intrinsic sympathomimetic activity but is rarely used as an antihypertensive agent since it may exacerbate angina. Acebutolol and oxprenolol have half the intrinsic sypathomimetic activity of pindolol and may be useful if a β-blocker has to be used in a patient susceptible to altered lipoprotein metabolism. Alternatively, the combined α and β blocking effect of labetalol may be of use since it would appear to have a negligible effect on the lipid profile.

Overall, the need to use a diuretic or a β-blocker must be balanced against patient considerations. A patient in heart failure should receive a diuretic if indicated regardless of the lipid profile. Similarly, in patients who have had a myocardial infarction and have no signs of cardiac failure, the beneficial protective effect of a β-blocker will usually outweigh any benefit of drug withdrawal.

If an antihypertensive agent is required that is without adverse effects on lipoproteins, many studies would suggest that angiotensin-converting enzyme (ACE) inhibitors such as lisinopril, angiotensin II receptor antagonists such as valsartan, α adrenoceptor blockers such as doxazosin or calcium channel blockers such as amlodipine could be used.

Oral contraceptives. Oral contraceptives containing an oestrogen and a progestogen provide the most effective contraceptive preparations for general use and have been well studied with respect to their harmful effects.

Oestrogens and progestogens both possess mineralocorticoid and glucocorticoid properties that predispose to hypertension and diabetes mellitus, respectively. However, the effects of the two hormones on lipoproteins are different. Oestrogens cause a slight increase in hepatic production of VLDL-C and HDL-C, and reduce serum LDL-C levels. In contrast, progestogens increase LDL-C and reduce serum HDL-C and VLDL-C.

The specific effect of the oestrogen or progestogen varies with the actual dose and chemical entity used. Ethinylestradiol at a dose of 30–35 micrograms or less would appear to create few problems with lipid metabolism, while norethisterone is one of the more favourable progestogens even though it may cause a pronounced decrease in HDL-C concentrations.

Corticosteroids. The effect of glucocorticosteroid administration on lipid levels has been studied in patients treated with steroids for asthma, rheumatoid arthritis and connective tissue disorders. Administration of glucocorticosteroids, for example prednisolone, has been shown to increase TC and triglycerides by elevating LDL-C and, less consistently, VLDL-C. The changes are generally more pronounced in women. Alternate-day therapy with glucocorticosteroids has been suggested to reduce the adverse effect on lipoprotein levels in some patients.

Ciclosporin. Ciclosporin is primarily used to prevent tissue rejection in recipients of renal, hepatic and cardiac transplants. Its use has been associated with increased LDL-C levels, hypertension and glucose intolerance. These adverse effects are often exacerbated by the concurrent administration of glucocorticosteroids. Without doubt the combined use of ciclosporin and glucocorticosteroid contributes to the adverse lipid profile seen in transplant patients. Unfortunately, the administration of a lipid-lowering drug to patients treated with ciclosporin increases the incidence of myositis and rhabdomyolysis (dissolution of muscle associated with excretion of myoglobin in the urine) and its use is therefore contraindicated in such patients.

Hepatic microsomal enzyme inducers. Drugs such as carbamazepine, phenytoin, phenobarbital, rifampicin and griseofulvin, which increase hepatic microsomal enzyme activity, can also increase serum HDL-C. The administration of these drugs may also give rise to a slight increase in LDL-C and VLDL-C. The overall effect is one of a favourable increase in the TC:HDL-C ratio. It is interesting to note that patients treated for epilepsy have been reported to have a decreased incidence of coronary heart disease.

Risk assessment

Primary prevention

In patients with no evidence of coronary heart disease the revised Sheffield table (Wallis et al 2000) offers a pragmatic way forward (Table 22.5) although others may prefer the Joint British Societies Coronary Risk Prediction Chart found in the British National Formulary.

The Sheffield table identifies patients who should have their lipid levels measured and those who would benefit from treatment. Its use overcomes the need to measure lipid concentrations in everybody. The tables takes as the treatment threshold a risk of developing coronary heart disease of 3% per year and indicates when a given risk level (for example at least 30% over 10 years) has been crossed. While the table is useful, it also has limitations. For example, it does not allow quantification of risk and gives no guidance on how to manage familial lipid disorders or dyslipidaemias in ethnic minorities. The revised table uses ratios of TC:HDL-C and identifies two levels of coronary heart disease risk (15% and 30% over 10 years), and attempts to quantify the influence of family history of premature coronary heart disease and left ventricular hypertrophy on ECG. In determining the level of risk, hypertension is considered to be present or absent and an average HDL-C is assumed if not measured.

When assessing an individual's risk of coronary heart disease the possibility of familial dyslipidaemia should not be overlooked. This is important not only for the management of the individual, but also for the possible treatment of other members of the family. Criteria that should raise suspicion of a familial dyslipidaemia are presented in Table 22.6.

Secondary prevention

Patients with coronary heart disease and levels of TC > 5 mmol/l and LDL-C > 3 mmol/l are the ones most likely to benefit from treatment with lipid lowering agents. Typical of individuals who fall into this category are patients with a history of angina, myocardial infarction, coronary artery bypass graft, coronary angioplasty or cardiac transplantation.

Since few trials have included individuals aged over 75 years, several guidelines advocate this as the cut-off point beyond which treatment should not be initiated. However, it is difficult to sustain such an approach, particularly in secondary prevention, and factors such as coexisting disease and life expectancy should be taken into account.

As in the situation with primary prevention outlined above, if an individual is to receive a lipid lowering agent as part of a secondary prevention strategy, the possibility of a familial dyslipidaemia and the need to assess other family members must not be overlooked.

Treatment

Lipid profile

When a decision has been made to determine an individual's lipid profile a random serum TC and HDL-C will often suffice. If a subsequent decision is

Table 22.5 Sheffield table for primary prevention of cardiovascular disease (adapted from Wallis et al 2000) showing TC:HDL-C ratios conferring estimated risk of coronary heart disease events of 15% and 30% over 10 years

Instructions
- Choose table for men or women
- **Hypertension** means SBP ≥140 or DBP ≥90 or on antihypertensive treatment
- Identify correct column for hypertension, smoking, and diabetes
- Identify row showing age
- Read off TC:HDL-C ratios at intersection of column and row. If there is an entry,

measure TC:HDL-C ratio. If no entry, lipids need not be measured unless familiar hyperlipidaemia suspected
- If HDL-C ratio confers CHD risk of 15%, consider treatment of **mild hypertension** (SBP 140–159 or DBP 90–99) and with **aspirin**
- If TC:HDL-C ratio confers CHD risk of 30%, consider **statin** if ≥ 5.0 mmol/l
- Decisions on statin at CHD risk between 15% and 30% depend on local policy

TC:HDL-C ratio

Hypertension	Yes		No		Yes		No		Yes		No		Yes		No	
Smoking	Yes		Yes		Yes		Yes		No		No		No		No	
Diabetes	Yes		Yes		No		No		Yes		Yes		No		No	
CHD risk	15%	30%	15%	30%	15%	30%	15%	30%	15%	30%	15%	30%	15%	30%	15%	30%
Men (age)																
70	2.0	3.0	2.0	3.6	2.1	3.8	2.4	4.4	2.5	4.6	2.9	5.3	3.1	5.6	3.7	6.7
68	2.0	3.2	2.1	3.8	2.2	4.1	2.6	4.7	2.7	4.8	3.0	5.6	3.3	6.0	3.9	7.1
66	2.0	3.4	2.2	4.0	2.4	4.3	2.7	5.0	2.8	5.2	3.2	5.9	3.5	6.3	4.1	7.6
64	2.0	3.6	2.4	4.3	2.5	4.6	2.9	5.3	3.0	5.5	3.5	6.3	3.7	6.8	4.4	8.1
62	2.1	3.8	2.5	4.6	2.7	4.9	3.1	5.6	3.2	5.9	3.7	6.7	3.9	7.2	4.7	8.6
60	2.2	4.1	2.7	4.9	2.9	5.2	3.3	6.0	3.4	6.3	3.9	7.2	4.2	7.7	5.0	9.2
58	2.4	4.4	2.9	5.3	3.1	5.6	3.5	6.5	3.7	6.7	4.2	7.7	4.5	8.3	5.4	9.9
56	2.6	4.7	3.1	5.7	3.3	6.0	3.8	7.0	4.0	7.2	4.6	8.3	4.9	8.9	5.8	10.6
54	2.8	5.1	3.3	6.1	3.6	6.5	4.1	7.5	4.3	7.8	4.9	9.0	5.2	9.6	6.3	–
52	3.0	5.5	3.6	6.6	3.9	7.0	4.4	8.1	4.6	8.4	5.3	9.7	5.7	10.4	6.8	–
50	3.3	6.0	3.9	7.1	4.2	7.6	4.8	8.8	5.0	9.1	5.7	10.5	6.1	–	7.3	–
48	3.6	6.6	4.3	7.8	4.5	8.3	5.2	9.6	5.4	9.9	6.3	–	6.7	–	8.0	–
46	3.9	7.1	4.6	8.5	5.0	9.1	5.7	10.4	5.9	10.8	6.8	–	7.3	–	8.7	–
44	4.3	7.6	5.1	9.3	5.4	9.9	6.3	–	6.5	–	7.5	–	8.0	–	9.6	–
42	4.7	8.6	5.6	10.2	6.0	10.9	6.9	–	7.2	–	8.2	–	8.8	–	10.5	–
40	2.0	9.5	6.2	–	6.6	–	7.6	–	7.9	–	9.1	–	9.7	–		
38	2.0	10.5	6.9	–	7.3	–	8.5	–	8.8	–	10.1	–	10.8	–		
36	2.0	–	7.7	–	8.2	–	9.5	–	9.8	–						
34	2.0	–	8.6	–	9.2	–	10.6	–								
32	2.1	–	9.8	–	10.5	–										
30	9.4	–														
28	10.8	–														

Table 22.5 continued

Women (age) — TC:HDL-C ratio

Hypertension	Yes		No		Yes		Yes		No		No		Yes		No	
Smoking	Yes		Yes		No		Yes		No		Yes		No		No	
Diabetes	Yes		Yes		Yes		No		Yes		No		No		No	
CHD risk	15%	30%	15%	30%	15%	30%	15%	30%	15%	30%	15%	30%	15%	30%	15%	30%
70	2.3	4.1	2.7	4.9	3.3	6.1	3.8	7.0	4.0	7.2	4.6	8.3	5.6	10.2	6.7	–
68	2.3	4.2	2.7	5.0	3.4	6.1	3.9	7.0	4.0	7.3	4.6	8.4	5.7	–	6.8	–
66	2.3	4.2	2.8	5.1	3.4	6.2	3.9	7.1	4.1	7.4	4.7	8.5	5.7	–	6.9	–
64	2.4	4.9	2.8	5.2	3.5	6.4	4.0	7.3	4.2	7.6	4.8	8.7	5.9	–	7.0	–
62	2.4	4.4	2.9	5.3	3.6	6.5	4.1	7.5	4.3	7.8	4.9	9.0	6.0	–	7.2	–
60	2.5	4.6	3.0	5.5	3.7	6.7	4.2	7.7	4.4	8.1	5.1	9.3	6.2	–	7.4	–
58	2.6	4.8	3.1	5.7	3.8	7.0	4.4	8.0	4.6	8.4	5.3	9.6	6.5	–	7.8	–
56	2.7	5.0	3.3	6.0	4.0	7.4	4.6	8.4	4.8	8.8	5.5	10.1	6.8	–	8.1	–
54	2.9	5.3	3.5	6.3	4.3	7.8	4.9	8.9	5.1	9.3	5.8	–	7.2	–	8.6	–
52	3.1	5.6	3.7	6.8	4.5	8.3	5.2	9.5	5.4	9.9	6.2	–	7.7	–	9.2	–
50	3.3	6.1	4.0	7.3	4.9	9.0	5.6	–	5.9	–	6.7	–	8.3	–	9.9	–
48	3.6	6.6	4.3	7.9	5.3	9.8	6.1	–	6.4	–	7.3	–	9.0	–		
46	4.0	7.3	4.8	8.8	5.9	–	6.8	–	7.1	–	8.1	–	10.0	–		
44	4.5	8.2	5.4	9.8	6.6	–	7.6	–	7.9	–	9.1	–				
42	5.1	9.4	6.1	–	7.5	–	8.6	–	9.0	–	10.3	–				
40	5.9	–	7.1	–	8.7	–	10.0	–								
38	7.0	–	8.4	–												
36	8.5	–	10.2	–												

- **Do not use for secondary prevention:** patients with MI, angina, PVD, non-haemorrhagic stroke. TIA, or diabetes with microvascular complications have high CHD risk. Treat mild hypertension: treat with aspirin; and treat with statin if serum cholesterol ≥ 5.0 mmol/l
- **Treat hypertension above mild range** (average ≥ 160 or ≥ 100)
- **Treat mild hypertension** (140–159 or 90–99) with **target organ damage** (LVH, proteinuria, renal impairment) or with **diabetes** (type 1 or 2)
- Consider drug treatment only **after** 6 months of appropriate advice on smoking, diet and repeated BP measurements

- Use **average** of repeated TC:HDL-C measurements. If HDL-C not available, assume 1.2 mmol/l
- Those with TC:HDL-C ratio ≥ 8.0 may have **familial hyperlipidaemia**
- The table **underestimates** CHD risk in
  - LVH on ECG (risk doubled – add 20 years to age)
  - family history of premature CHD (add 6 years)
  - familial hyperlipidaemia
  - British Asians

Table 22.6   Criteria that raise suspicion of familial dyslipidaemia

Family history of dyslipidaemia, or coronary heart disease
  • in first degree female relative less than 65 years old
  • in first degree male relative less than 55 years old

Xanthelasma or corneal arcus under the age of 50

Tendon xanthomata + TC > 7.5 mmol/l at any age

made to commence treatment and monitor outcome a more detailed profile that includes triglycerides is required.

Serum concentrations of triglycerides increase after the ingestion of a meal, and therefore patients must fast for 12–15 hours before they can be measured. Patients must also be seated for at least 5 minutes prior to drawing a blood sample. Cholesterol levels are little affected by food intake, and this is therefore not a consideration if only TC is to be measured. However, it is important that whatever is being measured reflects a steady state value. For example, during periods of weight loss, lipid concentrations decline as they do following a myocardial infarction. In the case of the latter, samples drawn within 24 hours of infarct onset will reflect the preinfarction state. In general, measurement should be deferred for 2 weeks after a minor illness and for 3 months after a myocardial infarction, serious illness or pregnancy.

Once the TC, HDL-C and triglyceride values are known it is usual to calculate the value for LDL-C using the Friedewald equation:

$$LDL\text{-}C = (TC - HDL\text{-}C) - (0.45 \times triglyceride) \text{ mmol/l}$$

The Friedewald formula is not valid if the serum triglyceride concentration > 4.5 mmol/l.

Lifestyle

Before a decision is made to start treatment with a lipid lowering agent other risk factors must also be tackled as appropriate, such as smoking, obesity, high alcohol intake, lack of exercise, whilst underlying disorders should be treated where present, for example diabetes mellitus, hypertension. Issues around body weight, diet and exercise will be briefly covered below.

Body weight

The overweight patient is at increased risk of atherosclerotic disease and typically has elevated levels of serum triglycerides, raised LDL-C and a low HDL-C. This adverse lipid profile is often compounded by the presence of hypertension and raised blood glucose. A reduction in body weight will generally improve the lipid profile and reduce overall cardiovascular risk.

It is useful to classify the extent to which an individual is overweight by calculating their body mass index (BMI). The BMI in all but the most muscular individual gives a clinical measure of adiposity:

$$BMI \ (kg/m^2) = \frac{weight \ (kg)}{height^2 \ (m)}$$

where

BMI ≤ 18.5	underweight
BMI = 18.6–24.9	ideal
BMI = 25–29.9	overweight (low health risk)
BMI = 30–40	obese (moderate health risk)
BMI > 40	obese (high health risk)

Diet

Diet modification should always be encouraged in a patient with dyslipidaemia but is rarely successful alone in bringing about a significant improvement in the lipid profile. Randomized controlled trials of dietary fat reduction or modification have shown variable results on cardiovascular morbidity and mortality (Hooper et al 2001). In pragmatic, community based studies, reductions in TC of only 3–6% have been observed. The overall picture is that patients with dyslipidaemia should receive dietary advice and a small number of those who adhere to the advice will experience a substantial fall in TC.

There is a common misconception that a healthy diet is one that is low in cholesterol. However, it is the saturated fat content that is important, although many components of a healthy diet are not related to fat content. For example, the low incidence of coronary heart disease in those who consume a Mediterranean diet suggests an increased intake of fruit and vegetables is also important. The typical Meditterranean diet has an abundance of plant food (fruit, vegetables, breads, cereals, potatoes, beans, nuts, and seeds) minimally processed, seasonally fresh, and locally grown; fresh fruit as the typical daily dessert, with sweets containing concentrated sugars or honey consumed a few times per week; olive oil as the principal source of fat; dairy products (principally cheese and yoghurt) consumed daily in low to moderate amounts; zero to four eggs consumed weekly; and red meat consumed in low to moderate amounts. This diet is low in saturated fat (< 8% of energy) and varies in total fat content from < 25% to > 35% of energy.

Stanol esters and plant sterols

The availability of margarines and other foods enriched with plant sterols or stanol esters increases the likelihood that LDL-C can be reduced by dietary change. Both stanol esters and plant sterols inhibit cholesterol absorption from the gastrointestinal tract and reduce LDL-C by an average of 10%. However, as with other dietary changes the reduction seen varies between individuals and is probably dependent on the amount and frequency of sterol intake and the intial cholesterol level. The phytosterols appear less effective in individuals already on a low fat diet.

Antioxidants

Antioxidants occur naturally in fruit and vegetables and are important components of a healthy diet. Their consumption is thought to be beneficial in reducing the formation of atherogenic, oxidized LDL-C. Primary and secondary prevention trials with antioxidant vitamin supplements, however, have not been encouraging. Neither vitamin E nor beta carotene supplements would appear to reduce the risk of coronary heart disease but likewise have not been shown to be harmful.

Salt

Dietary salt (sodium) has an adverse effect on blood pressure and therefore a potential impact on coronary heart disease and stroke. As part of dietary advice the average adult intake of sodium should be reduced from approximately 150 mmol (9 g) to 100 mmol (6 g) of salt. This intake can be reduced by consumming fewer processed foods, avoiding many ready meals and not adding salt at the table.

Exercise

Moderate amounts of aerobic exercise (brisk walking, jogging, swimming, cycling) on a regular basis have a desirable effect on the lipid profile of an individual. These beneficial effects have been demonstrated within 2 months in middle-aged men exercising for 30 minutes three times a week. Current advice for adults who are not routinely active is to undertake 30 minutes of moderate intensity activity on at least 5 days of the week. For active individuals, additional aerobic exercise of vigorous intensity is recommended for 20–30 minutes three times a week.

Overall, comprehensive dietary and lifestyle changes (stopping smoking, stress management training and moderate exercise) can bring about regression of coronary atherosclerosis. Unfortunately many find it difficult to attain or sustain the necessary changes. In others, dietary and lifestyle changes alone will never be adequate or will not bring about the necessary improvement in lipid profile quickly enough. As a consequence the use of lipid lowering drugs is widespread.

Drugs

Before starting lipid lowering therapy, dietary and lifestyle changes should ideally be tried for 3–6 months. If this does not achieve the required beneficial effect on the lipid profile then drug therapy may be started but involves a long-term commitment to treatment and appropriate dietary and lifestyle adjustments. In an individual requiring treatment for secondary prevention a delay of up to 6 months in starting treatment may not be appropriate.

Primary prevention

It cannot be overemphasized that dyslipidaemia should not be treated in isolation and must be embarked upon with clear goals. In patients without evidence of arterial disease treatment must be considered if their risk of coronary heart disease is 30% or more over 10 years (Department of Health 2000). Treatment should include:

- a statin to lower TC to either less than 5 mmol/l or reduce TC by 20–25%, whichever results in the lowest level (equivalent figures for LDL-C are 3 mmol/l or a reduction of 30%, whichever results in the lowest level)
- advice to stop smoking
- personalized information on modifiable risk factors including physical activity, diet, alcohol intake, weight and diabetes
- advice and treatment to achieve blood pressure below 140/85 mmHg
- tight control of blood pressure and glucose in those with diabetes

A summary of the screening and management of dyslipidaemia in an individual with no evidence of coronary heart disease but with a 10 year risk of >30% is presented in Figure 22.2.

Secondary prevention

In individuals with diagnosed coronary heart disease or other occlusive arterial disease, treatment (Department of Health 2000) should include:

- a statin to lower TC to either less than 5 mmol/l or reduce TC by 20–25%, whichever results in the lowest level (equivalent figures for LDC-C are 3 mmol/l or a reduction of 30%, whichever results in the lowest level)
- advice to stop smoking
- personalized information on modifiable risk factors including physical activity, diet, alcohol intake, weight and diabetes
- advice and treatment to achieve blood pressure below 140/87 mmHg

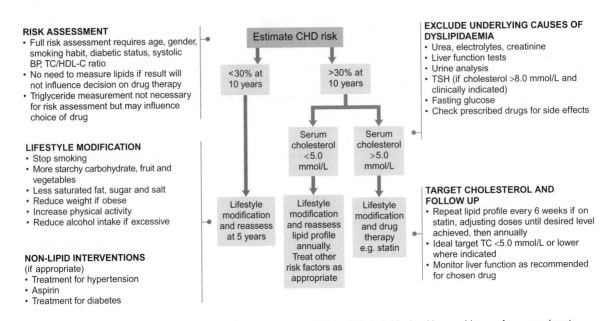

RISK ASSESSMENT
- Full risk assessment requires age, gender, smoking habit, diabetic status, systolic BP, TC/HDL-C ratio
- No need to measure lipids if result will not influence decision on drug therapy
- Triglyceride measurement not necessary for risk assessment but may influence choice of drug

LIFESTYLE MODIFICATION
- Stop smoking
- More starchy carbohydrate, fruit and vegetables
- Less saturated fat, sugar and salt
- Reduce weight if obese
- Increase physical activity
- Reduce alcohol intake if excessive

NON-LIPID INTERVENTIONS
(if appropriate)
- Treatment for hypertension
- Aspirin
- Treatment for diabetes

Estimate CHD risk

<30% at 10 years

>30% at 10 years

Serum cholesterol <5.0 mmol/L

Serum cholesterol >5.0 mmol/L

Lifestyle modification and reassess at 5 years

Lifestyle modification and reassess lipid profile annually. Treat other risk factors as appropriate

Lifestyle modification and drug therapy e.g. statin

EXCLUDE UNDERLYING CAUSES OF DYSLIPIDAEMIA
- Urea, electrolytes, creatinine
- Liver function tests
- Urine analysis
- TSH (if cholesterol >8.0 mmol/L and clinically indicated)
- Fasting glucose
- Check prescribed drugs for side effects

TARGET CHOLESTEROL AND FOLLOW UP
- Repeat lipid profile every 6 weeks if on statin, adjusting doses until desired level achieved, then annually
- Ideal target TC <5.0 mmol/L or lower where indicated
- Monitor liver function as recommended for chosen drug

Figure 22.2 Typical screening and management algorithm for dyslipidaemia in individuals with no evidence of coronary heart disease (CHD) but with a 10 year risk of CHD > 30% (adapted from SIGN 1999).

- tight control of blood pressure and glucose in those with diabetes
- low dose aspirin (75 mg daily)
- ACE inhibitors for those with left ventricular dysfunction
- β-blocker for those who have had a myocardial infarction
- Warfarin or aspirin for those over 60 years who have atrial fibrillation.

Lipid lowering therapy

There are four main classes of lipid-lowering agents available:

- HMG-CoA reductase inhibitors
- fibrates
- anion exchange resins
- nicotinic acid and derivatives.

Agents such as soluble fibre and fish oils have also been used to reduce lipid levels. A number of new agents are under investigation for their beneficial effect in the management of dyslipidaemia (Table 22.7).

The choice of lipid lowering agent depends on the underlying dyslipidaemia, the response required and patient acceptability. The various groups of drugs available have different mechanisms of action and variable efficacy depending on the lipid profile of an individual. Table 22.8 demonstrates the comparable effectiveness of the different groups in improving the

lipid profile. However, this table must be interpreted with caution as not all members of each group will bring about the changes quoted. The statins are currently the drugs of choice in the majority of patients with dyslipidaemia.

Statins

The discovery of a class of drugs, the statins, that selectively inhibit 3-hydroxy-3-methylglutaryl-CoA reductase (HMG-CoA reductase) was a significant advance in the treatment of dyslipidaemia. Their primary site of action is the liver and by inhibiting HMG-CoA reductase, the formation of mevalonic acid, the rate-limiting step in the biosynthesis of cholesterol, is inhibited. This results in a reduction in intracellular levels of cholesterol, an increase in LDL receptors on cell surfaces, enhanced receptor-mediated catabolism and clearance of LDL-C from the circulation. LDL-C production is also reduced by inhibition of the hepatic synthesis of VLDL-C, the precursor of LDL-C. The overall effect is a reduction in TC, LDL-C, VLDL-C and triglycerides with an increase in HDL-C. The reduction in LDL-C occurs in a dose-dependent manner, with a lesser and dose-independent effect on VLDL-C and triglycerides. While the effect of statins on the lipid profile contributes to their beneficial outcome in reducing morbidity and mortality from coronary heart disease, other mechanisms known as pleiotropic effects (Takemoto & Liao 2001) may also play a part. These mechanisms include plaque stabilization, inhibition of

Table 22.7 Examples of drug groups under development to treat dyslipidaemia

Drug group	Mechanism
Acyl-coenzyme A: cholesterol acyltransferase (ACAT) inhibitors	ACAT is responsible for esterifying excess intracellular cholesterol. Inhibition of ACAT prevents transport of cholesterol into the arterial wall and thereby prevents atheroma developing. Lowers VLDL-C and triglycerides Example: avasimibe
Bile acid sequestrants	Related to first generation resins but improved patient tolerance. Sequester bile acids and prevent reabsorption. Reduce LDL-C while HDL-C and triglycerides may increase or remain unchanged Example: colesevelam
Cholesterol absorption inhibitors	Inhibit absorption of cholesterol from diet and bile. Reduce LDL-C, increase HDL-C, no effect on triglycerides. Mechanism similar to plant sterols found in lipid lowering spreads but more potent Example: ezetimibe
Cholesteryl ester transfer protein (CETP) inhibitors	CETP is responsible for the transfer of cholesteryl ester from HDL-C to the atherogenic LDL-C and VLDL-C
Lipoprotein lipase (LPL) activity enhancers	LPL is responsible for VLDL-C catabolism with subsequent loss of triglycerides and increase in HDL-C. Protects against atherosclerosis Example: NO-1886
Microsomal triglyceride transfer protein (MTP) inhibitors	Inhibit absorption of lipid and reduce hepatic secretion of lipoproteins thereby reducing atherosclerotic plaque formation
Peroxisome proliferator – activated receptor (PPAR) activators	PPAR-α and -γ regulate the expression of genes involved in lipid metabolism and inhibit atherosclerotic plaque rupture. They reduce entry of cholesterol into cells, lower LDL-C and triglycerides, and increase HDL-C Example: GW-501516
Squalene synthase inhibitors	Inhibition of squalene synthase up-regulates LDL receptor activity and enhances removal of LDL-C Example: BMS-188494

Table 22.8 Examples of reported change in lipid profile at optimal dose of single drug

Drug group	TC (%)	Triglycerides (%)	LDL-C	HDL-C
Anion exchange resin	↓15–30%	↑5–30%	↓15–30%	↑ 3–8%
Fibrate	↓10–20%	↓30–50%	↓20–25%	↑10–25%
HMG-CoA reductase inhibitor	↓20–45%	↓10–45%	↓25–60%	↑2–15%
Nicotinic acid and derivatives	↓15–30%	↓20–60%	↑15–40%	↑10–20%
Fish oils	↑or ↓	↓10–60%	↑ or ↓	↑ 5–10%

thrombus formation, reduced plasma viscosity and anti-inflammatory and antioxidant activity.

Simvastatin was the first member of the group to be marketed in the UK and it was followed by pravastatin, fluvastatin, atorvastatin. The indications and relative efficacy of these four statins in reducing TC and LDL-C are shown in Table 22.9. The efficacy of statins has been demonstrated in four landmark, randomized placebo-controlled trials (Table 22.10). Statins are currently the lipid lowering agents of choice in both primary and

Table 22.9 Comparison of selected statins

Drug	Indications	Dose	Mean reduction in TC	Mean reduction in LDL-C
Atorvastatin	Primary hypercholesterolaemia	10 mg	28%	38%
	Familial hypercholesterolaemia	20 mg	35%	46%
	Mixed hyperlipidaemia	40 mg	40%	51%
	Raise HDL-C levels and lower LDL-C:HDL-C and	40 mg twice daily	42%	54%
	TC: HDL-C ratios	80 mg once daily	46%	61%
Fluvastatin	Primary hypercholesterolaemia	20 mg	13%	17%
	Mixed hyperlipidaemia	40 mg	19%	23%
	Slow progression of atherosclerosis in primary	40 mg twice daily		
	hypercholesterolaemia and coronary heart disease	80 mg once daily	25%	34%
Pravastatin	Primary hypercholesterolaemia	10 mg	13%	19%
	Prevention of coronary heart disease in	20 mg	18%	24%
	hypercholesterolaemia	40 mg	24%	34%
	Hypercholesterolaemia and coronary heart disease			
	Slow progression and reduce incidence of cardiac events in patients with previous MI or unstable angina where TC > 4.8 mmol/l, LDL-C > 3.2 mmol/l to reduce: risk of death, recurrent MI, need for revascularization procedures, number of days of hospitalization, and risk of stroke			
Simvastatin	Primary hypercholesterolaemia	10 mg	21%	28%
	Heterozygous and homozygous familial	20 mg	26%	35%
	hypercholesterolaemia	40 mg	30%	41%
	Mixed hyperlipidaemia	80 mg	37%	48%
	Lowering LDL-C:HDL-C ratio and TC: HDL-C by raising HDL-C coronary heart disease (TC ≥ 5.5 mmol/l) to reduce: risk of death, non-fatal MI, need for myocardial revascularization and to slow progression of coronary heart disease			

secondary prevention of coronary heart disease associated with dyslipidaemia.

There is much debate around which should be the statin of choice. Perhaps more important is the need to identify patients who need treatment and ensure they receive an appropriate, effective dose of a statin. It has been shown that less than a third of patients with a history of coronary heart disease or stroke receive lipid lowering treatment and of these only 1 in 8 achieves target levels of TC < 5 mmol/l or LDL-C < 3 mmol/l (Primatesta & Poulter 2000).

All the statins require the presence of LDL receptors for their optimum clinical effect, and consequently they are less effective in patients with heterozygous familial hypercholesterolaemia because of the reduced number of LDL receptors. However, even in the homozygous patient with no LDL receptors they can bring about some reduction of serum cholesterol although the mechanism is unclear.

Adverse effects.   Many side-effects appear mild and transient. The commonest include gastrointestinal symptoms, altered liver function tests and muscle aches. Less common are elevation of transaminase levels in excess of three times the upper limit of normal. Should this occur treatment must be discontinued. Myopathy (unexplained muscle soreness or weakness) leading to myoglobulinuria secondary to rhabdomyolysis is also a rare but serious adverse effect. Other less common side-effects include hepatitis, peripheral neuropathy, rash, headache, insomnia, nightmares, vivid dreams and difficulty concentrating.

The statins are a heterogenous group metabolized by different pathways. Simvastatin and atorvastatin are metabolized by the cytochrome P450 3A4 (CYP 3A4) enzyme system, Fluvastatin is metabolized by CYP 2C9, and pravastatin is not metabolized by cytochrome P450 enzymes.

Simvastatin and atorvastatin do not alter the activity of CYP 3A4 themselves, but their serum levels are increased by known inhibitors of CYP 3A4. For example, grapefruit juice contains one or more components that inhibit CYP 3A4. Ingestion of one glassful (250 ml) a day

Table 22.10 Outcome of key statin trials

Trial	Patients (% males)	Initial cholesterol (mmol/l) TC	LDL-C	Treatment	Reduction in cholesterol (%) TC	LDL-C	Outcome
Secondary prevention							
CARE[a]	4159 with previous MI (86%)	< 6.2	3–4.5	Pravastatin 40 mg/day or placebo for 5 years	– 20%	– 28%	24% relative reduction in risk of non-fatal MI or death from coronary heart disease (from 13.2% to 10.2%)
LIPID[a]	9014 with a history of MI or unstable angina (83%)	4–7		Pravastatin 40 mg daily or placebo for 6.1 years	– 18%	– 25%	24% relative reduction in death from coronary heart disease (from 8.3% to 6.4%). Reduction in the incidence of serious cardiovascular events and overall mortality
4S[a]	4444 with previous MI or angina (81%)	5.5–8		Simvastatin 20 mg daily (increased to 40 mg/daily in 37% patients) or placebo for 5.4 years	– 25%	– 35%	42% relative reduction in risk of death from coronary heart disease (from 8.5% to 5.0%). 34% relative reduction in risk of major coronary event (from 28% to 19%)
Primary prevention							
WOSCOPS[a]	6595 men with no history of MI (100%)	> 6.5	4.5–6	Pravastatin 40 mg daily or placebo for 4.9 years	– 20%	– 26%	31% relative reduction in risk of non-fatal MI or death from coronary heart disease (from 7.9% to 5.5%)

[a] See references for full details of each study.

will have little effect, but consumption of over 1 litre a day significantly increases the level of the statin and the risk of developing myopathy.

All the statins have the potential to cause muscle myopathy, particularly when serum levels are increased or when co-administered with agents such as fibrates that are themselves capable of causing myopathy. Examples of drug interactions involving statins are presented in Table 22.11.

Fibrates

Members of this group include bezafibrate, ciprofibrate, fenofibrate and gemfibrozil. They are thought to act by binding to peroxisome proliferator-activated receptor alpha (PPAR-α) on hepatocytes. This then leads to changes in the expression of genes involved in lipoprotein metabolism. Consequently, fibrates reduce triglyceride and, to a lesser extent, LDL-C levels while increasing HDL-C. In addition to their effects on serum lipids and lipoproteins, the fibrates may also have a beneficial effect on the fibrinolytic and clotting mechanisms. Fibrates take 2–5 days to have a

measurable effect on VLDL-C, with their optimum effect present after 4 weeks.

Adverse effects. Overall, the side-effects of fibrates are mild and vary between members of the group. Their apparent propensity to increase the cholesterol saturation index of bile renders them unsuitable for patients with gallbladder disease. Gastrointestinal symptoms such as nausea, diarrhoea and abdominal pain are common but transient, and often resolve after a few days of treatment. Myositis has been described, and is associated with muscle pain, unusual tiredness or weakness. The mechanism is unclear but it is thought they may have a direct toxic action on muscle cells in susceptible individuals (Ucar et al 2000).

Fibrates have been implicated in a number of drug interactions (Table 22.12), of which two in particular are potentially serious. Fibrates are known to significantly increase the effect of anticoagulants, while concurrent use with a statin is associated with an increased risk of myositis and, rarely, rhabdomyolysis. Concurrent use of cerivastatin and gemfibrozil was noted to cause rhabdomyolysis and this led to the withdrawal of cerivastatin from clinical use in 2001.

Table 22.11   Examples of drug interactions involving statins

Drug group	Interacting drug	Atorvastatin	Fluvastatin	Simvastatin	Pravastatin	Comment
Statins	**Antivirals eg**					
	Amprenavir	✓	✓	✓	✓	Protease inhibitors increase
	Indinavir	✓	–	✓	–	risk of myopathy
	Ciclosporin	✓	✓	✓	–	Increased risk of myopathy
	Digoxin	✓	x	✓	x	Increased level of digoxin
	Erythromycin	✓	–	✓	x	Increased risk of myopathy
	Clarithromycin	✓	–	✓	x	Increased risk of myopathy
	Fibrates	✓	✓	✓	–	Increased risk of myopathy
	Grapefruit juice	–	–	✓	x	Increased levels of statin
	Imidazoles and triazoles eg					
	Itraconazole	✓	–	✓	x	Increased risk of myopathy
	Ketaconazole	✓	–	✓	x	Increased risk of myopathy
	Nefazodone	–	–	✓	x	Increased risk of myopathy
	Nicotinic acid	✓	✓	✓	–	Increased risk of myopathy
	Norethisterone and ethinylestradiol oral contraceptives	✓	–	–	x	Increased levels of norethisterone and ethinylostradiol
	Phenytoin	✓	–	–	x	Increase and decrease of phenytoin levels reported
	Resins	✓	✓	✓	✓	Reduced levels of statin with concurrent administration
	Rifampicin	–	✓	–	x	Reduced levels of statin
	Warfarin	✓	–	✓	x	Anticoagulant effect enhanced

✓ interaction likely; – use combination with caution; x interaction unlikely.

There appears little to differentiate members of the group with regard to their effect on the lipid profile. In addition to their effect on lipids, they have all been reported to produce an improvement in glucose tolerance, although bezafibrate probably has the most marked effect. In the patient with elevated triglycerides and gout only fenofibrate has been reported to have a sustained uricosuric effect on chronic administration. Fibrates appear to be of particular benefit in patients with type 2 diabetes if triglyceride levels remain greater than 2.3 mmol/l

Anion exchange resins

Anion exchange resins are also known as ion exchange resins or bile acid sequestrants. The two members of this group in current use are colestyramine and colestipol. Both were formerly considered first-line agents in the management of patients with hypercholesterolaemia but now have limited use. They reduce TC levels but either have no effect on, or show a slight increase in, triglyceride levels. As a consequence they are unsuitable for use in patients with elevated triglyceride levels.

Following oral administration, neither colestyramine nor colestipol is absorbed from the gut. They bind bile acids in the intestine, prevent their reabsorption and produce an insoluble complex that is excreted in the faeces. The depletion of bile acids results in an increase in hepatic synthesis of bile acids from cholesterol. The depletion of hepatic cholesterol increases LDL receptor activity in the liver and this removes LDL-C from the blood. Both colestyramine and colestipol also increase hepatic VLDL-C synthesis and thereby increase serum triglycerides in some patients.

Colestyramine and colestipol can reduce TC levels within 24–48 hours, and thereafter continue to gradually reduce levels for up to 1 year. The starting dose of colestyramine is one 4 g sachet twice a day. Over a 3–4 week period the dose should normally be built up to 12–24 g daily taken in water or a suitable liquid as a single dose, or up to four divided doses each day. Occasionally 36 g a day may be required although the

Table 22.12 Examples of drug interactions involving resins and fibrates

Drug group	Interacting drug	Comment
Resins (colestyramine/colestipol)		All medication should be taken 1 h before or 4–6 h after colestyramine/colestipol to avoid reduced absorption caused by binding in the gut
	Acarbose	Hypoglycaemia enhanced by colestyramine
	Digoxin	Absorption reduced
	Diuretics	Absorption reduced
	Levothyroxine (thyroxine)	Absorption reduced
	Mycophenolate mofetil	Absorption reduced
	Paracetamol	Absorption reduced
	Phenylbutazone	Absorption reduced
	Raloxifene	Absorption reduced
	Valproate	Absorption reduced
	Statins	Absorption reduced by up to 50%
	Vancomycin	Effect of oral vancomycin antagonized by colestyramine
	Warfarin	Increased anticoagulant effect due to depletion of vitamin K or reduced anticoagulant effect due to binding or warfaring in gut
Fibrates	Antidiabetic agents	Improvement in glucose tolerance
	Ciclosporin	Increased risk of renal impairment
	Resin	Reduced bioavailability of fibrate if taken concomitantly
	Statin	Increased risk of myopathy
	Warfarin	Increased anticoagulant effect

benefits of increasing the dose above 16 g a day are offset by gastrointestinal disturbances and poor patient adherence. Colestipol is also available in granular form and mixed with an appropriate liquid at a dose of 5 g once or twice daily. This dose can be increased every 1–2 months to a maximum of 30 g in a single or twice daily regimen.

Adverse effects.   Side-effects with the resins are more likely to occur with high doses and in patients aged over 60 years. Bloating, flatulence, heartburn and constipation are common complaints. Constipation is the major subjective side-effect, and although usually mild and transient it may be severe.

Colestyramine and colestipol are known to interact with many drugs (see Table 22.12), primarily by interfering with absorption. Consequently, medication should be taken 1–2 hours before or 4–6 hours after the resin. For patients on multiple-drug therapy, resins are clearly not the best choice.

Nicotinic acid and derivatives

Nicotinic acid in pharmacological doses (1.5–6 g) lowers both serum LDL-C and VLDL-C levels and increases HDL-C.

The major mechanism of action for nicotinic acid appears to be the ability to reduce the release of VLDL-C, which in turn leads to decreased levels of IDL-C and LDL-C. In addition, it reduces the release of free fatty acids from adipose tissue into the general circulation and consequently reduces the available substrate for triglyceride synthesis. The mechanism by which nicotinic acid increases HDL-C is not known although a decrease in HDL-C catabolism has been reported. Nicotinic acid has also been shown to reduce levels of Lp(a).

Acipimox is structurally related to nicotinic acid, has similar beneficial effects on the lipid profile and a better side-effect profile but appears to be less potent.

Adverse effects.   Despite the established long-term safety of nicotinic acid it is of limited use in practice because of its side-effects. These are very common and unpleasant and include troublesome flushing of the skin, headache, postural hypotension, diarrhoea, exacerbation of peptic ulcers, hepatic dysfunction, gout and increase blood glucose levels. While acipimox shares many of these side-effects, though to a lesser extent, it does not have an adverse effect on blood glucose nor does it share the property of exacerbating peptic ulcers.

Fish oils

Fish oil preparations rich in ω-3 fatty acids have been shown to markedly reduce serum triglyceride levels by decreasing VLDL-C synthesis. As a consequence LDL-C levels are reduced and there is also a beneficial rise in HDL-C. However, the effect is inconsistent. Significant increases in LDL-C have also been reported to accompany the use of fish oils. On current evidence routine use cannot be recommended.

Soluble fibre

Preparations containing soluble fibre, such as ispaghula husk, have been shown to reduce lipid levels. The fibre is thought to bind bile acids in the gut and increase the conversion of cholesterol to bile acids in the liver. However, its role in the management of dyslipidaemia is unclear because it is much less effective than statins in reducing TC and LDL-C.

Patient care

Diet

The management of dyslipidaemia should always include lifestyle changes once underlying causes have been eliminated. Dietary advice (Table 22.13) is the cornerstone of management and should be supported by advice to stop smoking, undertake regular exercise and moderate alcohol intake. Patients should be encouraged to increase their intake of complex carbohydrates, fruit

and vegetables, and oily fish. Soluble fibre found in lentils, beans, peas and oats may also have some beneficial effect in reducing cholesterol.

Drugs

Statins

In patients receiving an HMG-CoA reductase inhibitor, a once-daily regimen involving an evening dose is often preferred. Several of the HMG-CoA reductase inhibitors are claimed to be more effective when given as a single dose in the evening compared to a similar dose administered in the morning. This has been attributed to the fact that cholesterol biosynthesis reaches peak activity at night. However, atorvastatin may be taken in the morning or evening with similar efficacy. A reduction in TC and LDL-C is usually seen with all HMG-CoA reductase inhibitors within 2 weeks, with a maximum response occurring by week 4 and maintained thereafter during continued therapy.

Anion exchange resins

Palatability is often a major problem with patients needing to be well motivated and prepared for the problems they may encounter.

Table 22.13   Examples of dietary modifications to lower cholesterol intake

	Avoid/decrease	Preferred alternative
Meat	Fatty cuts of meat, ham, pork, bacon, duck, liver, kidney, sausages, Scotch eggs, meat pies, pastries	Chicken and turkey without skin Lean cuts of meat Fish
Dairy produce	Whole milk, cream Full fat yoghurt Hard cheese, cream cheese, processed cheese Egg yolks	Skimmed or semi-skimmed milk Low fat yoghurt Low fat cheeses, cottage cheese Egg white
Fats	Butter, dripping, lard, suet, margarine, ghee, coconut oil	All fats should be limited Unsaturated vegetable oils and spreads made from corn, sunflower, soya, olive and rapeseed oils
Nuts	Coconut, peanuts	Intake should be limited Walnuts, almonds, hazelnuts
Fish	Fish roe, caviar, potted fish, fried fish Shellfish in excess	Fresh, frozen or smoked fish Oily fish such as mackeret, salmon, herrings, kippers and sardines to be consumed at least twice weekly
Fruit/vegetables	–	Aim for five portions per day
Cakes, biscuits, sweets	Cakes, biscuits, pastries, crisps, sweets, chocolate	Fruit

Both colestyramine and colestipol are available in an orange flavour and/or as a low-sugar (aspartame-containing) powder. Colestipol is without taste and is odourless. Each sachet of colestyramine or colestipol should be added to at least 120 ml of liquid and stirred vigorously to avoid the powder clumping. The powder does not dissolve but disperses in the chosen liquid, which may be water, fruit juice, skimmed milk or non-carbonated beverage. Both may also be taken in soups, with cereals, and with pulpy fruits with high moisture content, such as apple sauce.

All patients receiving colestipol or colestyramine must be aware that any concurrent medication must be taken 1–2 hours before or 4–6 hours after the anion exchange resin. Gemfibrozil can be administered with colestipol if the two drugs are administered 2 hours apart.

Other lipid-lowering agents

To achieve optimum effect, patients taking a fibrate should be advised to take their medication 30 minutes before a meal.

The adverse effect profile of nicotinic acid has been discussed above. For those patients who find the flushing particularly troublesome, a single dose of aspirin 75 mg, taken some 30 minutes before the nicotinic acid, has been shown to give relief from the prostaglandin-mediated flushing. Extended-release dosage forms of nicotinic acid have also been shown to reduce the incidence of flushing and pruritus.

Case 22.1

Mr D. F. is a 43-year-old man who has been relatively fit and well for the past 20 years during which he has rarely visited his GP. Two weeks ago he was admitted to hospital having suffered a myocardial infarction. On questioning it was revealed that his brother had died in a road traffic accident at the age of 19 and his father had died from coronary heart disease aged 54 years.

Examination of Mr D. F. revealed a corneal arcus and tendon xanthomas. Blood drawn within 2 h of the onset of the myocardial infarction revealed TC 7.8 mmol/l, HDL-C 0.9 mmol/l and triglycerides 2.3 mmol/l.

Questions

1. Calculate the concentration of DF's LDL-C and comment on the findings.
2. What is the likely diagnosis and treatment for DF on discharge?
3. DF wants to know why he was not identified as being at high risk of CHD before he suffered his myocardial infarction?

Answers

1. The value for LDL-C can be calculated from the Friedewald formula where:

$$\text{LDL-C} = (\text{TC} - \text{HDL-C}) - (0.45 \times \text{triglycerides})$$
mmol/l
$$= (7.8 - 0.9) - (0.45 \times 2.3)$$
$$= 5.9 \text{ mmol/l}$$

The ideal value of LDL-C is <3 mmol/l.

2. Mr D. F. has the signs and family history of classic heterozygous familial hypercholesterolaemia, most likely due to a genetic defect in the LDL receptor on hepatocytes. His level of LDL-C is high and action is required to reduce it. Appropriate lifestyle advice is necessary but a statin will be required to achieve the desired outcome. Typically a high dose of simvastatin (80 mg day) will have to be used.

3. Unfortunately Mr D. F.'s father probably died of heart disease at a time when the practice of detecting affected families and screening first degree relatives was not widespread. The early, unrelated death of his brother and Mr D. F.'s previous good health would not have given an opportunity to identify any underlying familial disorder.

From population data it is known, for example, that the prevalence of heterozygous familial hypercholesterolaemia is about 1 in 500. Consequently 120 000 cases would be expected in the UK. However, only 15 000 cases are known and screening programmes to track cases in affected families are now in place. A family history of elevated TC or death from coronary heart disease before the age of 55 in a first degree male relative, as in the case of Mr D. F., is an important sign that should highlight the potential risk to other family members.

Case 22.2

Mr P. T. is a 50-year-old man with a blood pressure of 140/85 mmHg and type 2 diabetes, but no history of coronary heart disease. He smokes 10 cigarettes a day. On a routine clinic visit he is found to have a TC of 6.4 mmol/l, HDL-C 0.8 mmol/l and triglycerides 2 mmol/l.

Questions

1. Is PT at high risk of CHD?
2. What advice and/or treatment would be appropriate?

Answers

1. Mr P. T. has a TC:HDL-C ratio of 8 which far exceeds the ratio of 6.1 (from the Sheffield table) and indicates his risk of coronary heart disease is > 30% over 10 years. Treatment, probably with a statin to reduce TC:HDL ratio, is indicated.

2. The incidence of coronary heart disease is up to four-fold greater in diabetic patients. Mr P. T. needs to achieve meticulous control of his blood glucose and reduce his blood pressure to less than 130/80 mmHg. Stopping smoking would be an extremely beneficial lifestyle intervention he could make. The use of nicotine replacement therapy or bupropion may be considered as treatment options to assist this.

A range of other lifestyle interventions should be considered including diet, exercise and reduction in both body weight and excess alcohol consumption if appropriate.

Case 22.3

Mr E. C. is a 48-year-old executive for a large multinational company who works long hours and frequently has to travel abroad. He has a family history of coronary heart disease and 9 months ago he attended a coronary screening clinic for a health check. At the clinic he was found to have a normal blood pressure but a blood screen revealed a TC of 6.7 mmol/l and triglycerides of 11.8 mmol/l. When he revisited the clinic 4 weeks later after trying to follow dietary advice a fasting blood sample revealed a TC of 5 mmol/l and triglycerides of 2.7 mmol/l. Liver function tests were normal. He is a non-smoker and claims never to drink more than 10 units of alcohol per week.

After repeated requests to revisit the clinic he eventually turned up stating he had been away from home for 6 months on a series of business trips. He was trying to keep to a low fat diet and his blood profile revealed TC 5.7 mmol/l, triglycerides 4.3 mmol/l, HDL-C 0.8 mmol/l and LDL-C 3 mmol/l.

Questions

1. Is Mr E. C. at high risk of coronary heart disease?
2. Is Mr E. C. a candidate for lipid lowering therapy?
3. Should the children of Mr E. C. be screened for dyslipidaemia?

Answers

1. Mr E.C. has a TC:HDL-C ratio of 7.1. If the Sheffield tables were used they would indicate he does not have a 10 year risk of coronary heart disease > 30%, is not at high risk of coronary heart disease and does not require lipid lowering treatment. However, the tables underestimate the risk of coronary heart disease in those with familial hyperlipidaemia or a history of premature coronary heart disease.

   Mr E. C. would appear to have a mixed lipaemia although it is difficult to interpret non-fasting triglycerides because of the influence of food intake. The low HDL-C suggests he is overweight and/or has a non-ideal lifestyle. Exclusion of diabetes, high alcohol intake, liver and renal impairment are necessary. The possibility of impaired glucose tolerance should not be overlooked and a glucose tolerance test should be performed.

2. Given the elevated triglycerides and TC, Mr E. C. is certainly a candidate for lifestyle advice. The use of a statin may be considered if the lifestyle changes do not bring about the necessary improvements in the lipid profile. However, the dyslipidaemia may be secondary to obesity, alcoholism, diabetes or hypothyroidism. If any of these disorders are present the appropriate treatment may correct the underlying dyslipidaemia.

3. The family history of coronary heart disease is important but is only significant if the age of onset in a parent or sibling was under 55 years of age for an affected male or under 65 years for an affected female. A rare familial disorder, e.g.

familial dysbetalipoproteinaemia, may be the causative factor. If this was confirmed his children should be screened after puberty as the offending gene may not express itself in the younger child.

Mr E. C. was subsequently found to have diabetes and the appropriate treatment corrected his lipid profile. However, even in this scenario where a patient is diagnosed with type 2 diabetes, it is important to consider advising children about lifestyle issues and the need to control weight throughout life.

Case 22.4

Mrs S. A. is a 49-year-old woman who visits her doctor complaining of menopausal symptoms including hot flushes, night sweats and irritability. She is concerned about her risk of coronary heart disease because both her husband and mother have angina. Her mother developed angina at the age of 68 and 5 years later was diagnosed with breast cancer. In general Mrs S. A. does not like taking medicines and would much prefer exercise to hormone replacement therapy (HRT).

Question

Is Mrs S. A. at risk of coronary heart disease and what advice would you give her about the relative benefits of exercise and HRT?

Answer

Coronary heart disease is a leading cause of mortality among women in developed countries and has often been overlooked because the focus of attention has been its impact on men at a younger age.

From the limited evidence available it would appear Mrs S. A. is not at high risk of coronary heart disease. There is unlikely to be a familial disorder given the age of onset of coronary heart disease in her mother, although it would also be necessary to clarify if her father developed coronary heart disease before the age of 55 years to exclude this. Clearly there is no genetic link with her husband although their lifestyle should be explored, e.g. are they smokers, do they have a high fat diet and/or undertake little exercise, etc.?

There is clear evidence that women who are physically active have lower coronary heart disease rates. Moreover, vigorous activity is not necessary to achieve these lower coronary heart disease rates, with walking at a light to moderate intensity sufficient to lower coronary heart disease risk. In fact, time spent walking is probably more important than pace. Several workers have shown an inverse association between physical activity and coronary heart disease risk among women who are overweight, smoke or have elevated cholesterol levels. Recent guidelines recommend moderate intensity physical activity for at least 30 minutes most days (i.e. 2.5 h per week) to decrease coronary heart disease risk. Even in women who walk at least 1 h per week coronary heart disease rates have been shown to be half those of women who do not undertake regular exercise.

It is known that the protective effect of endogenous oestrogens on the female cardiovascular system are lost after the menopause, and the risk of coronary heart disease rises thereafter to levels seen in men. The oral administration of an oestrogen as a component of hormone replacement therapy (HRT) to postmenopausal women decreases LDL-C, increases HDL-C and offers protection against the development of coronary heart disease. However, HRT should not be offered routinely to postmenopausal women solely to reduce the risk of coronary heart disease, or for secondary prevention in those with coronary heart disease. It should also not be prescribed in women with a family history of breast cancer.

Overall there is little evidence to compare the relative benefits of HRT and exercise. HRT would probably help control Mrs S. A.'s vasomotor symptoms, but given her family history of breast cancer the use of HRT would not be advised.

REFERENCES

Atsumi T, Khamashta M A, Andujar C et al 1998 Elevated plasma lipoprotein(a) level and its association with impaired fibrinolysis in patients with antiphospholipid syndrome. Journal of Rheumatology 25(1): 69–73

Campbell I W 2001 Type 2 diabetes: 'the silent killer'. Pract Diab Int 18: 187–191

Clarke R, Frost C, Collins R et al 1997 Dietary lipids and blood cholesterol: a quantitative meta-analysis of metabolic ward studies. British Medical Journal 314: 112–117

Department of Health 2000 National service framework for coronary heart disease. HMSO, London

Donnelly R, Emslie-Smith A M, Gardner I D et al 2000 Vascular complications of diabetes. British Medical Journal 320: 1062–1066

Feher M D, Elkeles R S 1999 Lipid modification and coronary heart disease in type 2 diabetes: different from the general population? Heart 81: 10–11

Goldbourt U, Yaari S, Medalie J H 1997 Isolated low HDL cholesterol as a risk factor for coronary heart disease mortality: a 21 year follow-up of 8000 men. Arteriosclerosis, Thrombosis, and Vascular Biology 17: 107–113

Heart Protection Study 2002 MRC/BHF Heart Protection Study of cholesterol lowering with simvastatin in 20 536 high-risk individuals: a randomised placebo-controlled trial. Lancet 360: 7–22

Hooper L, Summerbell C D, Higgins P T et al 2001 Dietary fat intake and prevention of cardiovascular disease: systematic review. British Medical Journal 322: 757–763

Long-term Intervention with Pravastatin in Ischaemic Disease (LIPID) Study Group 1998 Prevention of cardiovascular events and death with pravastatin in patients with coronary heart disease and a broad range of initial cholesterol levels. New England Journal of Medicine 339: 1349–1357

Primatesta P, Poulter N R 2000 Lipid concentrations and the use of lipid lowering drugs: evidence from a national cross sectional survey. British Medical Journal 321: 1322–1325

Sacks F M, Pfeffer M A, Moye L A et al for the Cholesterol and Recurrent Events (CARE) Trial Investigators 1996 The effect of pravastatin on coronary events after myocardial infarction in patients with average cholesterol levels. New England Journal of Medicine 335: 1001–1009

Scandinavian Simvastatin Survival Study Group 1994 Randomised trial of cholesterol lowering in 4444 patients with coronary heart disease: the Scandinavian Simvastatin Survival Study (4S). Lancet 344: 1383–1389

Scottish Intercollegiate Guidelines Network (SIGN) 1999 Lipids and the primary prevention of coronary heart disease: a national clinical guideline. SIGN publication number 40. SIGN, Edinburgh

Shepherd J, Cobbe S M, Ford I et al for the West of Scotland Coronary Prevention Study (WOSCOPS) Group 1995 Prevention of coronary heart disease with pravastatin in men with hypercholesterolemia. New England Journal of Medicine 33: 1301–1307

Takemoto M, Liao J K 2001 Pleiotropic effects of 3-hydroxy-3-methylglutaryl coenzyme a reductase inhibitors. Arteriosclerosis, Thrombosis and Vascular Biology 21: 1712–1719

Ucar M, Mjorndal T, Dahlqvist R 2000 HMG-CoA reductase inhibitors and myotoxicity. Drug Safety 22: 441–457

Wallis E J, Ramsay L E, Haq I U et al 2000 Coronary and cardiovascular risk estimation for primary prevention: validation of a new Sheffield table in the 1995 Scottish health survey population. British Medical Journal 320: 671–676

Asthma 23

K. P. Gibbs   M. Small

KEY POINTS

- Asthma is a common and chronic inflammatory condition of the airways whose cause is not completely understood.
- Common symptoms are caused by hyperresponsive airways, and include coughing, wheezing, chest tightness and shortness of breath.
- The only reliable, simple and objective way to diagnose asthma is to demonstrate airflow limitation.
- Asthma mortality is about 1500 per year in the UK and costs in the region of £2000 million per year in health and other costs.
- Asthma triggers should be avoided or controlled.
- Pharmacological therapy should involve early anti-inflammatory treatment in all but the mildest asthmatics.
- Optimum treatment involves the lowest doses of therapy that provide good symptom control with minimal or no side-effects, and the best drug delivery device is one that the patient can use correctly.
- Poor compliance and poor inhaler technique should be considered when asthma control proves difficult.
- Patients must be educated to take an active role in their disease management, be given individualized self-management plans and be regularly supervised by the health care team.

Asthma literally means 'panting'. It is a broad term used to refer to a disorder of the respiratory system that leads to episodic difficulty in breathing. A lack of knowledge of the exact defect, which causes the airways to be hyperreactive to various stimuli, has led to an imprecise definition. In fact the definition is actually a description of the clinical symptoms. The British Thoracic Society defines asthma as a common and chronic inflammatory condition of the airways. In susceptible individuals this inflammation causes symptoms which are usually associated with widespread but variable airflow obstruction that is often reversible, either spontaneously or with treatment, and causes an associated increase in airway responsiveness to a variety of stimuli.

Epidemiology

The exact prevalence of asthma remains uncertain because of the differing ways in which airway restriction is reported, diagnostic uncertainty (especially for children under 2 years) and the overlap with other conditions such as chronic obstructive airways disease. It has been estimated that about 4% of the British and American populations have asthma. The National Asthma Campaign estimates that there are over 3.4 million people with asthma in the UK (National Asthma Campaign 1999). Mortality from asthma is estimated at approximately 0.4 per 100 000 and is currently estimated at about 1500 per annum in the UK. However, it has been estimated that around 80% of deaths from asthma may be preventable (Harrison 1999). Most deaths occur outside hospital, and the most common reason for death is thought to be inadequate assessment of the severity of airway obstruction by the patient and/or clinician and inadequate therapy of an acute attack.

The probability of children having asthma-like symptoms is estimated to be between 5% and 12%, with a higher occurrence in boys than girls and in children whose parents have an allergic disorder. Between 30% and 70% of children will become symptom-free by adulthood. However, individuals who develop asthma at an early age do have a poorer prognosis.

The prevalence of asthma actually appears to be rising despite advances in therapy. However, there is some doubt about this due to the differing criteria for the diagnosis of asthma used in different studies. Asthma is considered to be one of the consequences of Western civilization, and appears to be related to a number of environmental factors. Air pollution resulting from industrial sources and transport may be interacting with smoking, dietary and other factors to increase the incidence of this debilitating problem.

Aetiology

The specific abnormality underlying asthma is hyper-reactivity of the lungs to one or more stimuli. This can also occur in certain patients with chronic bronchitis and allergic rhinitis but usually to a lesser extent. There are a number of possible trigger factors (Table 23.1).

One of the most common trigger factors is the allergen found in the faeces of the house dust mite, which is

Table 23.1 Examples of trigger factors that may cause asthma

Trigger	Examples
Allergens	Pollens, moulds, house dust mite, animals (dander, saliva and urine)
Industrial chemicals	Manufacture of, for example isocyanate-containing paints, epoxy resins, aluminium, hair sprays, penicillins and cimetidine
Drugs	Aspirin, ibuprofen and other prostaglandin synthetase inhibitors, β-adrenoceptor blockers
Foods	A rare cause but examples include nuts, fish, seafood, dairy products, food colouring, especially tartrazine, benzoic acid and sodium metabisulphite
Other industrial triggers	Wood or grain dust, colophony in solder, cotton dust, grain weevils and mites; also environmental pollutants such as cigarette such as cigarette smoke and sulphur dioxide
Miscellaneous	Cold air, exercise, hyperventilation, viral respiratory tract infections, emotion or stress

almost universally present in bedding, carpets and soft furnishing. Pollen from grass (prevalent in June and July) can lead to seasonal asthma. The role of occupation in the development of asthma has become apparent with increased industrialization. There are many causes of occupational asthma, and bronchial reactivity may persist for years after exposure to the trigger factor. Food allergy usually results in gastrointestinal disturbances and eczema rather than asthma. Drug-induced asthma can be severe, and the most common causes are β-blocker drugs and prostaglandin synthetase inhibitors. The administration of β adrenoceptor blockers to a patient, even in the form of eye drops, can cause $β_2$ receptor blockade and consequent bronchoconstriction. Selective β adrenoceptor blockers are thought to pose slightly less risk, but as these lose their selectivity at higher doses it is generally recommended that this group of drugs is avoided altogether in asthma patients. Aspirin and related non-steroidal anti-inflammatory drugs can cause severe bronchoconstriction in susceptible individuals. Aspirin inhibits the enzyme cyclo-oxygenase, which normally converts arachidonic acid to prostaglandins. When this pathway is blocked an alternative reaction predominates, leading to an increase in production of bronchoconstrictor leukotrienes. Approximately 5% of the adult asthma population is sensitive to aspirin.

It is generally thought that emotional disturbances cannot cause asthma but it is well known that they can provoke or worsen bronchoconstriction and may affect the effectiveness of bronchodilators used to treat asthma.

Pathophysiology

The discovery of the antibody IgE led to the description of 'extrinsic' or allergic asthma, and non-IgE-mediated 'intrinsic' asthma, also known as asthma of unknown origin. However, these definitions are considered to be of secondary importance to the classification of asthma according to the frequency and severity of symptoms. Extrinsic asthma is common in children, associated with a genetic predisposition, and is precipitated by known allergens. Intrinsic asthma tends to develop in adulthood, and symptoms are triggered by non-allergenic factors such as a viral infection, irritants which cause epithelial damage and mucosal inflammation, emotional upset which mediates excess parasympathetic input or exercise which causes water and heat loss from the airways, triggering mediator release from mast cells.

Mast cells, eosinophils, epithelial cells, macrophages and activated T lymphocytes are all key features of the inflammatory process of asthma (Fig. 23.1). These cells act on the airways to cause inflammation, either directly or through neural mechanisms.

Airway inflammation can be acute, subacute or chronic in character:

- *Acute*: early recruitment of cells to the airway.
- *Subacute*: resident and recruited cells are activated to cause a more persistent pattern of inflammation.
- *Chronic*: cell damage is persistent and subject to ongoing repair, permanent change in the airway may occur with airway remodelling.

These cell-derived mediators, therefore, play an important role in causing the main features of asthma: marked hypertrophy and hyperplasia of bronchial smooth muscle, mucus gland hypertrophy leading to excessive mucus production and airway plugging, airway oedema, acute bronchoconstriction and impaired mucociliary clearance.

Mast cell components are released as a result of an IgE-antibody-mediated reaction on the surface of the cell. Histamine and other mediators of inflammation are released from mast cells, for example leukotrienes, prostaglandins, bradykinin, adenosine, prostaglandin-generating factor of anaphylaxis, as well as various chemotactic agents that attract eosinophils and neutrophils. These mediators have a number of

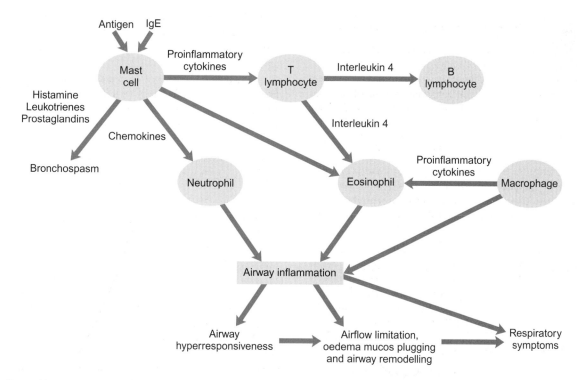

Figure 23.1 Cellular mechanisms involved in airway inflammation.

activities. For example, histamine triggers rapid bronchoconstriction whereas leukotrienes (LTs) such as LTC_4, LTD_4 and LTE_4 constrict at a slower rate. The chemotactic agents cause a slower reaction characterized by the infiltration of macrophages into the lumen of the airways. Macrophages release prostaglandins, thromboxane and platelet-activating factor (PAF). PAF appears to sustain bronchial hyperreactivity and cause respiratory capillaries to leak plasma, which increases mucosal oedema. It also facilitates the accumulation of eosinophils within the airways, a characteristic pathological feature of asthma. Eosinophils release various inflammatory mediators such as LTC_4 and PAF. Epithelial damage results, and thick viscous mucus is produced that causes further deterioration in lung function.

Mucus production is normally a defence mechanism, but in asthma patients there is an increase in the size of bronchial glands and goblet cells that produce mucus. Mucus transport is dependent on its viscosity. If it is very thick it plugs the airways, which also become blocked with epithelial and inflammatory cell debris. Mucociliary clearance is also decreased due to inflammation of epithelial cells. The epithelial cell damage can be severe, which in turn can increase access of various irritants to the cholinergic receptors. This can

result in further bronchoconstriction mediated by the parasympathetic nervous system.

Clinical manifestations

Asthma can present in a number of ways. It may manifest as a persistent cough. Most commonly it is described as recurrent episodes of difficulty in breathing (dyspnoea) associated with wheezing (a high-pitched noise due to turbulent airflow through a narrowed airway). Diagnosis is usually made from the clinical history from the patient or patient's representative confirmed by demonstration of reversible airflow obstruction, with repeated measures of lung function. The history of an asthma patient often includes the presence of atopy and allergic rhinitis in the close family. Symptoms of asthma are often intermittent, and the frequency and severity of an episode can vary from individual to individual. Between periods of wheezing and breathlessness patients may feel quite well. Tightness of the chest, shortness of breath and abnormal lung function tests that improve by 15% with administration of suitable treatment confirm the diagnosis of asthma. However, the absence of an improvement in ventilation cannot rule out asthma, and in younger children it is sometimes very difficult to perform lung function tests.

Acute severe asthma is a dangerous condition that requires hospitalization and immediate emergency treatment. It occurs when bronchospasm has progressed to a state where the patient is breathless at rest and has a degree of cardiac stress. This is usually progressive and can build up over a number of hours or even days. The breathlessness with a peak flow rate < 100 litre per minute, is so severe that the patient cannot talk or lie down. Expiration is particularly difficult and prolonged as air is trapped beneath mucosal inflammation. The pulse rate can give an indication of severity. Severe acute asthma can increase the pulse rate to more than 110 beats per minute. It is common to see hyperexpansion of the thoracic cavity and lowering of the diaphragm, which means that accessory respiratory muscles are required to try to inflate the chest. Breathing can become rapid (> 30 breaths/min) and shallow, leading to low arterial oxygen tension (Pa_{O_2}) with the patient becoming fatigued, cyanosed, confused and lethargic. The arterial carbon dioxide tension (Pa_{CO_2}) is usually low in acute asthma. If it is high it should respond quickly to emergency therapy. Hypercapnia (high Pa_{CO_2} level) that does not diminish is a more severe problem, and indicates progression towards respiratory failure.

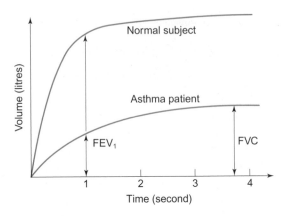

Figure 23.2 Typical lung spirometry in normal subjects and asthma patients. FEV_1/FVC is an index of airways obstruction. A decrease in FEV_1/FVC indicates obstruction.

Investigations

The function of the lungs can be measured to help diagnose and monitor various respiratory diseases. A series of routine tests has been developed to assess asthma as well as other respiratory disease such as chronic obstructive pulmonary disease (COPD). The most useful test for abnormalities in airway function is the forced expiratory volume (FEV). This is measured by means of lung function assessment apparatus such as a spirometer. The patient inhales as deeply as possible and then exhales forcefully and completely into a mouthpiece connected to a spirometer. The FEV_1 is a measure of the forced expiratory volume in the first second of exhalation. Another volume that is commonly measured is the forced vital capacity (FVC). This is an assessment of the maximum volume of air exhaled with maximum effort after maximum inspiration. The FEV_1 is usually expressed as a percentage of the total volume of air exhaled, and is reported as the FEV_1/FVC ratio. This ratio is a useful and highly reproducible measure of the capabilities of the lungs. Normal individuals can exhale at least 75% of their total capacity in 1 second. Any reduction indicates a deterioration in lung performance (Fig. 23.2).

The peak flow meter is a useful means of self-assessment for the patient. It gives slightly less reproducible results than the spirometer but has the advantage that the patient can do regular tests at home with the hand-held meter. The peak flow meter measures peak expiratory flow rate (PEFR). This is the maximum flow rate that can be forced during expiration. The PEFR can be used to assess the improvement or deterioration in the disease as well as the effectiveness of treatment. For all three measurements (FEV_1, FVC and PEFR) there are normal values with which the patient's results can be compared. However, these 'normal' values vary with age, race, gender, height and weight. The measurement of FEV_1, FVC or PEFR does not detect early deterioration of lung function such as bronchospasm and mucus plugging in the smaller airways.

Confirming the diagnosis of asthma is usually made by the response to a bronchodilator. The PEFR is measured before and after the administration of a bronchodilator. The diagnosis is confirmed if the PEFR improves by more than 15% with the bronchodilator. However, individuals may not have airflow obstruction at the time of the test so the absence of an improvement does not rule out asthma. In this situation peak flow readings can be done at home with repeated pre- and post-bronchodilator readings taken at various times of the day.

Treatment

Since asthma involves inflammation and bronchoconstriction, treatment should be directed towards reducing inflammation and increasing bronchodilatation. Restoration of normal airways function and prevention of severe acute attacks are the main goals of treatment. Anti-inflammatory drugs should be given to all patients with all but the mildest of symptoms. Other measures, such as avoidance of

Table 23.2	Common therapeutic problems in asthma

- Asthma is under-diagnosed, especially in the elderly

- Failing to avoid or reduce the effect of allergens

- Lack of patient knowledge about the condition and its management

- When to start anti-inflammatory therapy

- Taking anti-inflammatory therapy on an 'as required' basis rather than regularly as no short-term benefit is felt by the patient

- Patients or health professionals missing the signs of rapidly deteriorating asthma control

- Incorrect technique in the use of inhalers and drug delivery devices

- Little published evidence to guide the best management of asthma in children under 12 years, particularly the under 2-year-old age group

recognized trigger factors, may also contribute to the control of this disease. The lowest, effective dose of drugs should be given to minimize short-term and long-term side-effects. However, it should always be remembered that asthma is a potentially life-threatening illness and is often under-treated. Common therapeutic problems encountered in the management of asthma are outlined in Table 23.2.

Chronic asthma

The pharmacological management of asthma depends upon the frequency and severity of a patient's symptoms. Infrequent attacks can be managed by treating each attack when it occurs, but with more frequent attacks preventive therapy needs to be used.

The preferred route of administration of the agents used in the management of asthma is by inhalation. This allows the drugs to be delivered directly to the airways in smaller doses and with fewer side-effects than if systemic or parenteral routes were used. Inhaled bronchodilators also have a faster onset of action than when administered systemically and give better protection from bronchoconstriction.

Treatment of chronic asthma is usually given in a stepwise progression, as outlined in Figure 23.3, according to the severity of the patient's asthma symptoms. At each stage the patient's inhaler technique should be assessed. If necessary the type of inhalation device used should be changed to improve patient compliance. These national management guidelines will be updated in late 2002.

β adrenoceptor agonist bronchodilators

β adrenoceptor agonists are the mainstay of the management of asthma. Selective β_2 agonists such as salbutamol and terbutaline have now replaced the older, non-selective agents such as adrenaline (epinephrine), isoprenaline and orciprenaline. The selective agents have fewer β_1-mediated side-effects, particularly cardiotoxicity. However, β_2 receptors are also present in myocardial tissue. Therefore, cardiovascular stimulation resulting in tachycardia and palpitations is still the main dose-limiting toxicity with these agents. The degree of selectivity varies with the agent, dose, route and duration of therapy.

An inhaled β_2 agonist is the first-line agent in the management of asthma. These are used as required by the patient for the symptomatic relief of breathlessness and wheezing, for example salbutamol 200 micrograms when required. This may be the only treatment necessary for those with infrequent symptoms.

β_2 agonists should be initiated 'when required' for the relief of symptoms. There is no advantage to regular administration and there may be some potential clinical disadvantages (Walters & Walters 2000).

Inhaled anti-inflammatory agents

Regular anti-inflammatory treatment must be given to patients who require an inhaled bronchodilator regularly. The agents used include corticosteroids and cromones (Table 23.3). The threshold frequency of β_2 agonist use, which prompts the start of this 'preventer' therapy, has not been fully established. A review of current evidence has concluded that the threshold should be the use of β_2 agonists at an average of two or three times daily (North of England Evidence Based Guideline Development Project 1995).

At present, inhaled corticosteroids are the initial drugs of choice (British Thoracic Society 1997). Beclometasone or budesonide are used at doses of 100–400 micrograms twice daily. Higher doses are used if symptoms persist. The dose of inhaled corticosteroid should be reduced, if possible, once symptoms and peak expiratory flow rates have improved.

If a patient's asthma cannot be controlled by the above dose of inhaled corticosteroid and the inhaler technique and compliance are adequate, the dose can be increased to a maximum of 1.5–2 mg a day. Adrenal suppression may occur at these maximum doses so patients should carry a steroid warning card. Oropharyngeal side-effects such as candidiasis are also more common at the higher doses of steroids (Table 23.4) but can be minimized if patients use a large-volume spacer device and rinse the mouth with water after inhalation.

Inhaled sodium cromoglicate and nedocromil sodium could be used instead of corticosteroids in those who

- Avoidance of provoking factors where possible
- Patient's involvement and education
- Selection of best inhaler device
- Treatment stepped up as necessary to achieve good control
- Treatment stepped down if control of asthma good

Notes

- **Patients should start treatment at the step most appropriate to the initial severity. A rescue course of prednisolone may be needed at any time and at any step. The aim is to achieve early control of the condition and then to reduce treatment.**
- **Until growth is complete any child requiring beclomethasone or budesonide > 800 micrograms daily or fluticasone > 500 micrograms daily should be referred to a paediatrician with an interest in asthma**

Prescribe a peak flow meter and monitor response to treatment

Stepping down:

Review treatment every three to six months. If control is achieved a stepwise reduction in treatment may be possible. In patients whose treatment was recently started at step 4 or 5 or included steroid tablets for gaining control of asthma this reduction may take place after a short interval. In other patients with chronic asthma a three to six month period of stability should be shown before slow stepwise reduction is undertaken.

Step 5:

Addition of regular steroid tablets

Inhaled short acting β agonists as required with inhaled beclomethasone or budesonide 800–2000 micrograms daily or fluticasone 400–1000 micrograms daily via a large volume spacer and one or more of the long acting bronchodilators
plus
regular prednisolone tablets in a single daily dose.

Step 4:

High dose inhaled steroids and regular bronchodilators

Inhaled short acting β agonists as required with inhaled beclomethasone or budesonide 800–2000 micrograms daily or fluticasone 400–1000 micrograms daily via a large volume spacer
plus
a sequential therapeutic trial of one or more of
- inhaled long acting β agonists
- sustained release theophylline
- inhaled ipratropium or oxitropium
- long acting β agonist tablets
- high dose inhaled bronchodilators
- cromoglycate or nedocromil.

Step 3:

High dose inhaled steroids or low dose inhaled steroids plus long-acting inhaled β agonist bronchodilator

Inhaled short acting β agonists as required
plus either
beclomethasone or budesonide increased to 800–2000 micrograms daily or fluticasone 400–1000 micrograms daily via a large volume spacer
or
beclomethasone or budesonide 100–400 micrograms twice daily or fluticasone 50–200 micrograms twice daily plus salmeterol 50 micrograms twice daily.
In a very small number of patients who experience side effects with high dose inhaled steroids, either the long acting inhaled β agonist option is used or a sustained release theophylline may be added to step 2 medication. Cromoglycate or nedocromil may also be tried.

Step 2:

Regular inhaled anti-inflammatory agents

Inhaled short acting β agonists as required
plus
beclomethasone or budesonide 100–400 micrograms twice daily or fluticasone 50–200 micrograms twice daily.
Alternatively, use cromo-glycate or nedocromil sodium, but if control is not achieved start inhaled steroids.

Step 1:

Occasional use of relief bronchodilators

Inhaled short acting β agonists "as required" for symptom relief are acceptable. If they are needed more than once daily move to step 2. Before altering a treatment step ensure that the patient is having the treatment and has a good inhaler technique.
Address any fears.

Outcome of steps 4–5: best possible results

- Least possible symptoms
- Least possible need for relieving bronchodilators
- Least possible limitations of activity
- Least possible variation in PEF
- Best PEF
- Least adverse effects from medicine

Outcome of steps 1–3: control of asthma

- Minimal (ideally no) chronic symptoms, including nocternal symptoms
- Minimal (infrequent) exacerbations
- Minimal need for relieving bronchodilators
- No limitations on activities including exercise
- Circadian variation on peak expiratory flow (PEF) < 20%
- PEF ≥ 80% of predicted or best
- Minimal (or no) adverse effects from medicine

Figure 23.3 Guidelines for the management of chronic asthma in adults and children (reproduced by permission of the BMJ Publishing Group, from British Thoracic Society, 1997).

Table 23.3 Drugs used for the prophylaxis of asthma

Drug/route		Total daily dosage range
Beclometasone diproprionate		
Inhaled	Adult	Standard dose: 300–800 micrograms in 2–4 divided doses
		High dose: 1000–2000 micrograms in 2–4 divided doses
	Child	100–400 micrograms in 2–4 divided doses
Beclometasone diproprionate CFC-free (Qvar® brand)[a]		
Inhaled	Adult	Standard dose: 100–400 micrograms in 2 divided doses
		High dose: 400–800 micrograms in 2 divided doses
Budesonide		
Inhaled	Adult	Standard dose: 200–800 micrograms daily in up to 2 divided doses
		High dose: 800–1600 micrograms daily in 2 divided doses
	Child	100–800 micrograms daily in 2 divided doses
Nebulized	Adult	2–4 mg in 2 divided doses
	3–12 years	1–2 mg in 2 divided doses
Fluticasone		
Inhaled	Adult	Standard dose: 200–500 micrograms in 2 divided doses
		High dose: 1000–2000 micrograms in 2 divided doses
	Child	100–200 micrograms in 2 divided doses
Sodium cromoglicate		
Inhaled	Adult and child	Maintenance dose: 40 mg in 4 divided doses. Increased to 60–80 mg in severe cases or periods of risk
Nedocromil sodium		
Inhaled	Adult	8–16 mg in 2–4 divided doses

[a] Owing to the bioavailability differences in non-CFC steroid inhalers, dosing is quoted for the individual brand.

suffer unacceptable side-effects with corticosteroids and may be effective at controlling symptoms in mild to moderate asthma but are less effective in severe asthma. A systematic review of studies involving children has shown that there is little benefit of sodium cromoglicate in maintenance therapy (Tasche et al 2000), although it may be of help in preventing exercise-induced asthma

Additional bronchodilators

Additional bronchodilators may be required if the above therapy does not adequately control symptoms (Tables 23.5 and 23.6).

Inhaled anticholinergic agents

These block muscarinic receptors in bronchial smooth muscle and can be added to the treatment regimen. Ipratropium bromide 80 micrograms four times daily or oxitropium 200 micrograms twice daily are available. They have slower onsets of action than β_2 agonists but last longer. The anticholinergics may be especially helpful in the elderly where asthma may be complicated by a degree of obstructive airways disease.

Oral bronchodilators

Either β_2 agonists or theophylline can also be added for additional symptom control. Slow-release forms should be used; these are especially useful in a single night-time dose if nocturnal symptoms are troublesome although twice daily dosing is more usual. Oral bronchodilators may also become necessary in patients who are unable to use inhaler therapy effectively.

Theophylline should be started at a dose of 3 mg/kg/day in adults and increased after 7 days to 6 mg/kg/day (children 13 mg/kg/day).

Theophylline has a narrow therapeutic index, and its hepatic metabolism varies greatly between individuals. Theophylline clearance is affected by a variety of factors, including disease states and concurrent drug therapy. The dose used should therefore take into account these factors, which are outlined in Table 23.7. Serum levels may be taken after 3–4 days at the higher dose and it has been normal practice to adjust the dose to keep the serum level within a therapeutic window of 10–20 mg/l. However, some patients show a good clinical response with levels less than 10 mg/l while others tolerate levels in excess of 20 mg/l. The patient should be monitored for the emergence of serious toxic effects such as tachycardia and persistent vomiting. Only modified-release preparations should be used, and once stabilized on a particular product the patient should not be changed to another theophylline preparation, as there are large differences in serum profiles with the different preparations. Normal-release theophylline preparations

Table 23.4 Adverse reactions associated with drugs used in the management of asthma

β₂ agonists
- By inhalation: adverse drug reactions are uncommon
- More commonly (mainly by nebulization, orally or parenterally): fine tremor (usually the hands), nervous tension, headache, peripheral vasodilatation, tachycardia. The adverse reactions often diminish as tolerance develops with continued administration
- With high doses: hypokalaemia, aggravation of angina

Inhaled corticosteroids
- Hoarseness, oral or pharyngeal candidiasis
- Adrenal suppression may occur with high doses, for example beclometasone diproprionate above 1500 micrograms daily

Oral corticosteroids
- Prolonged use of these results in exaggeration of some of the normal physiological effects of steroids
- Mineralocorticoid effects include: hypertension, potassium loss, muscle weakness, and sodium and water retention. These effects are most notable with fludrocortisone, are significant with hydrocortisone, occur only slightly with prednisolone and methylprednisolone and are negligible with dexamethasone and betamethasone
- Glucocorticoid effects include: precipitation of diabetes, osteoporosis, development of a paranoic state, depression, euphoria, peptic ulceration, immunosuppression, Cushing's syndrome (moon face, striae and acne), growth suppression in children, worsening of infection: skin thinning, striae atrophicae, increased hair growth, perioral dermatitis and acne
- Adrenal suppression occurs with high doses and/or prolonged treatment. Steroid therapy must be gradually withdrawn in these patients to avoid precipitating an adrenal crisis of hypotension, weight loss, arthralgia and sometimes, death

Ipratropium bromide
- Occasionally: dry mouth
- Rarely: systemic anticholinergic effects such as urinary retention and constipation

Methotrexate
- Myelosuppression, mucositis and, rarely, pneumonitis

Nedocromil sodium
- Mild and transient nausea, coughing, transient bronchospasm, throat irritation, headache and a bitter taste

Oxitropium
- Dry mouth, local irritation of the throat and nose may occur
- Occasionally: nausea
- Rarely: systemic anticholinergic effects, e.g. blurring of vision, hesitancy of micturition. These are more likely in the elderly

Sodium cromoglicate
- Coughing, transient bronchospasm and throat irritation due to inhalation of the powder

Theophylline
- Although about 5% of the population experience minor adverse effects: nausea, diarrhoea, nervousness and headache, increasing the serum concentration results in more serious effects. The following is a guide to the serum levels at which the adverse reactions usually occur:
  – Above 20 mg/l: persistent vomiting, insomnia, gastrointestinal bleeding, cardiac arrhythmias
  – Above 35 mg/l: hyperglycaemia, hypotension, more serious cardiac arrhythmias, convulsions, permanent brain damage and death
- Individual patients may suffer these effects at serum levels other than those quoted, for example convulsions have occurred in patients at 25 mg/l.

Leukotriene receptor antagonists
- Abdominal pain, headache, diarrhoea, dizziness, upper respiratory tract infections
- Rarely: acute hepatitis (associated with zafirlukast), Churg–Strauss syndrome.

Table 23.5 Comparison of inhaled bronchodilators

Drug	Onset of action (min)	Peak action (min)	Duration of action (h)
Ipratropium	3–10	60–120	4–6
Oxitropium	5–10	60–120	7.5–12
Salbutamol	5–15	60[a]	4–6
Salmeterol	14[a]	150[a]	12[a]
Terbutaline	5–30	60–120	3–6

[a] Approximate or median value

should not be used because of their rapid absorption and highly variable clearance, giving short and unpredictable durations of action.

High-dose β₂ agonists

These are only considered if conventional doses do not achieve adequate symptom control. Nebulized drugs such as salbutamol 2.5–5 mg per dose are given. Multiple actuations of a metered-dose inhaler into a large volume spacer can be used instead of a nebulizer.

Terbutaline has been given by subcutaneous infusion in the treatment of 'brittle' asthma, where there is an unpredictable and rapid onset of airway narrowing, causing sudden onset of acute, severe life-threatening asthma.

Table 23.6 Daily dosage range for some bronchodilators

Drug/route	Age	Total daily dosage range
Aminophylline		
Intravenous Injection		5 mg/kg as a single dose
Intravenous infusion	Adult	500 micrograms/kg/h
	6 months–12 years	1 mg/kg/h
	12–18 years	500 micrograms/kg/h
Oral	Adult	225–900 mg (modified release) in 1–2 divided doses
	Child	10–12 mg/kg (modified release) in 2 divided doses
Formoterol (eformoterol)		
Inhaled	Adult	24–48 micrograms in 2 divided doses
Ipratropium bromide		
Inhaled	Adult	60–3200 micrograms in 3–4 divided doses
	Child	20–120 micrograms in 3–4 divided doses
Nebulized	Adult	100–2000 micrograms in up to 4 divided doses
	3–14 years	100–1500 micrograms in up to 3 divided doses
Oxitropium		
Inhaled		400–600 micrograms in 2–3 divided doses
Salbutamol		
Inhaled		100–800 micrograms in 3–4 divided doses
Nebulized	Adult	2.5–10 mg as a single dose, with a maximum of 40 mg daily in up to 4 divided doses
	Child	2.5–5 mg as a single dose
Intravenous injection	Adult	250 micrograms, repeated if necessary
Intravenous infusion	Adult	3–20 microgram per minute
Subcutaneous or Intramuscular injection	Adult	500 micrograms repeated every 4 h if necessary
Oral	Adult	6–16 mg in 3–4 divided doses
	< 2 years	400 micrograms/kg in 4 divided doses
	2–6 years	3–8 mg in 3–4 divided doses
	6–12 years	6–8 mg in 3–4 divided doses
Salmeterol		
Inhaled		100–200 micrograms in 1–2 divided doses
Terbutaline		
Inhaled		250–4000 micrograms in 4 divided doses
Nebulized	Adult	10–40 mg in 2–4 divided doses
	< 3 years	4–8 mg in 2–4 divided doses
	3–6 years	6–12 mg in 2–4 divided doses
	6–8 years	8–16 mg in 2–4 divided doses
	> 8 years	10–20 mg in 2–4 divided doses
Intravenous, subcutaneous or intramuscular injection	Adult	250–2000 micrograms in up to 4 divided doses
	Child	10 micrograms/kg up to a maximum of 300 micrograms
Intravenous infusion	Adult	1.5–5 micrograms/min for up to 8–10 h
Theophylline		
Oral	Adult	250–1000 mg (modified release) in 1–2 divided doses
	2–7 years	12 mg/kg (modified release) in 1–2 divided doses
	8–12 years	10 mg/kg (modified release) in 1–2 divided doses

Table 23.7 Factors affecting theophylline clearance

Decreased clearance	Increased clearance
Congestive cardiac failure Cor pulmonale Chronic obstructive pulmonary disease Viral pneumonia Acute pulmonary oedema Cirrhosis	
Premature and term babies Elderly Obesity	Children of 1–12 years Cigarette smoking
High-carbohydrate, low-protein diet	High-protein, low-carbohydrate diet Barbecued meat
Cimetidine Erythromycin Oral contraceptives Ciprofloxacin Propranolol	Carbamazepine Phenobarbital Phenytoin Sulfinpyrazone

Oral corticosteroids

Oral corticosteroids should only be used if symptom control cannot be achieved with maximum doses of inhaled bronchodilators and steroids. The dose should be given as a single morning dose to minimize adrenal suppression. Alternate day dosing produces fewer side-effects but is less effective in controlling asthma.

Short courses of high-dose oral steroids, 30–60 mg, can be safely used during exacerbations of asthma.

Steroid-sparing agents

Some agents are being investigated in patients who are dependent on systemic steroids in an attempt to reduce the steroid dose. Methotrexate, ciclosporin and gold have been tried with varying success. All have potentially toxic side-effects and need to be closely monitored.

Long-acting β adrenoreceptor agonist bronchodilators

Long-acting inhaled β_2 agonists (salmeterol and formoterol (eformoterol)) are available. These should be used in conjunction with conventional β_2 agonists, rather than as replacements, as the latter have faster onsets of action. When low-dose inhaled steroids fail to control asthma symptoms adequately, then long-acting β_2 agonists can be added instead of increasing the steroid dose. These agents may also have a place in controlling nocturnal and early morning symptoms instead of oral theophyllines and in the management of aspirin/non-steroidal-induced asthma. In all instances they should be discontinued if no benefit is gained from their use.

Leukotriene antagonists

Two types of oral drugs have been developed with the goal of attenuating the effects of leukotrienes in asthma: the leukotriene receptor blockers and the leukotriene synthesis inhibitors, for example 5-lipo-oxygenase inhibitors. Early clinical trial results suggest that both groups could be beneficial, especially in mild to moderate asthma when used alone or in combination with β_2 agonists, for exercise- or aspirin-induced asthma or in patients with poor compliance with inhaled drugs because of poor inhaler technique; however, their role remains to be defined, particularly in severe asthma.

Acute severe asthma

The management of acute asthma depends on the severity of the attack and its response to treatment, as well as an appreciation of the patient's past history and present treatment. If an acute attack becomes persistent and difficult to treat it is known as acute severe asthma.

The aims of treatment are to prevent any deterioration in the patient's condition and hasten recovery.

Prevention of an acute attack

The ideal way of treating an acute attack is to educate patients to recognize when their condition is deteriorating so that they can initiate treatment to prevent the attack becoming severe. This can be achieved with an individualized self-management plan (discussed later in the chapter).

The doses of inhaled β_2 agonist and inhaled corticosteroid should be increased and a short course of oral steroids commenced at a dose of 40–60 mg every morning for 1 week.

If the condition deteriorates further, hospital admission may become necessary. Ideally this should be a self-referral from the patient, responding to criteria drawn up by the doctor, such as the PEFR falling to 100–150 litres per minute. The education of patients and their relatives in the management of acute attacks should always stress the prompt initiation of further treatment and early referral.

Immediate management of acute severe asthma

The immediate treatment of acute severe asthma should take place in the patient's home, during the ambulance journey or immediately on admission to hospital. One suggested treatment protocol is outlined in Figure 23.4.

Recognition and assessment in hospital

Features of acute severe asthma
- Peak expiratory flow (PEF) ≤ 50% of predicted or best
- Can't complete sentences in one breath
- Respirations ≥ 25 breaths/min
- Pulse > 110 beats/min

Life threatening features
- PEF < 33% of predicted or best
- Silent chest, cyanosis, or feeble respiratory effort
- Bradycaria or hypotension
- Exhaustion, confusion, or coma

If Sao_2 < 92% or a patient has any life threatening features, measure arterial blood gases.

Blood gas markers of a very severe, life threatening attack:
- Normal (5–6 kPa, 36–45 mm Hg) or high $Paco_2$
- Severe hypoxia: Pao_2 < 8 kPa (60 mm Hg) irrespective of treatment with oxygen
- A low pH (or high H^+)

No other investigations are needed for immediate management

Caution
Patients with severe or life threatening attacks may not be distressed and may not have all these abnormalities. The presence of any should alert the doctor

1 Immediate treatment
- Oxygen 40–60% (CO_2 retention is not usually aggravated by oxygen therapy in asthma)
- Salbutamol 5 mg or terbutaline 10 mg via an oxygen driven nebulizer
- Prednisolone tablets 30–60 mg or intravenous hydrocortisone 200 mg or both if very ill
- No sedatives of any kind
- Chest radiograph to exclude pneumothorax

Peak expiratory flow in normal adults

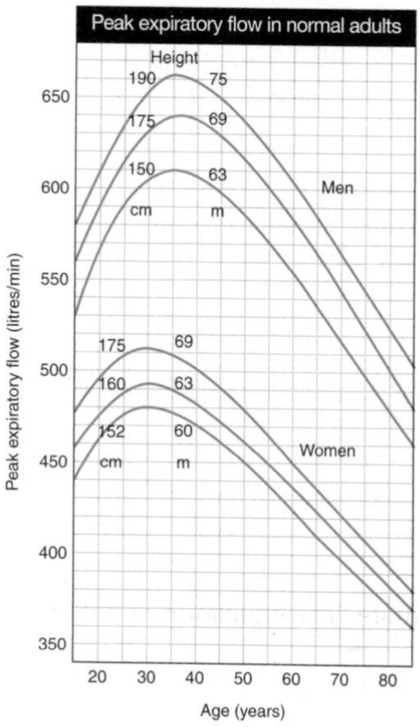

From: Gregg I, Nunn AJ, BMJ 1989; 298; 1068–70

IF LIFE THREATENING FEATURES ARE PRESENT:
- Add ipratropium 0.5 mg to the nebulized β agonist
- Give intravenous aminophylline 250 mg over 20 minutes or salbutamol or terbutaline 250 micrograms over 10 minutes.
  Do not give bolus aminophylline to patients already taking oral theophyllines

2 Subsequent management
IF PATIENT IS IMPROVING CONTINUE:
- 40–60% oxygen
- Prednisolone 30–60 mg daily or intravenous hydrocortisone 200 mg 6 hourly
- Nebulized β agonist 4 hourly

IF THE PATIENT IS NOT IMPROVING AFTER 15–30 MINUTES
- Continue oxygen and steroids
- Give nebulized β agonist more frequently, up to every 15–30 minutes
- Add ipratropium 0.5 mg to nebulizer and repeat 6 hourly until patient is improving

IF PATIENT IS STILL NOT IMPROVING GIVE:
- Aminophylline infusion (small patient 750 mg/24 hours, large patient 1500 mg/24 hours); monitor blood concentrations if it is continued for over 24 hours
- Salbutamol or terbutaline infusion as and alternative to aminophylline

3 Monitoring treatment
- Repeat measurement of PEF 15–30 minutes after starting treatment
- Oximetry: maintain Sao_2 > 92%
- Repeat blood gas measurements

- initial Pao_2 < 8 kPa (60 mmHg) unless sebsequent Sao_2 > 92%
- Pao_2 normal or raised
- patient deteriorates
- Chart PEF before and after giving nebulized or inhaled β agonists and at least 4 times daily throughout hospital stay

Transfer patient to the intensive care unit accompanied by a doctor prepared to intubate if there is:
- Deteriorating PEF, worsening or persisting hypoxia, or hypercapnia
- Exhaustion, feeble respirations, confusion or drowsiness
- Coma or repiratory arrest

4 When discharged from hospital, patients should have:
- Been on discharge medication for 24 hours and *have had inhaler technique checked and recorded*
- PEF > 75% of predicted or best and PEF diurnal variability < 25% *unless discharge is agreed with respiratory physician*
- Treatment with oral and *inhaled steroids* in addition to bronchodilators
- Own PEF meter and *written self management plan*
- GP follow up arranged *within 1 week*
- Follow up appointment in respiratory clinic *within 4 weeks*

Also
- Determine reason(s) for exacerbation and admission
- Send details of admission, discharge and potential best PEF to GP.

Figure 23.4 Guideline for the management of acute severe asthma in adults (reproduced by permission of the BMJ Publishing Group from British Thoracic Society 1997).

Oxygen is administered in a high concentration, at high flow rates, whenever possible. A nebulized β_2 agonist is administered, which should give prompt bronchodilatation lasting 4–6 hours.

Nebulizers are used in preference to conventional inhalers because they permit a high dose (10–20 times the dose of a metered dose inhaler) and they require no coordination on the part of the patient between inspiration and actuation, which is helpful in those distressed or for those who panic. Patients undergoing an acute attack often have an inspiratory rate too low to use a metered-dose inhaler effectively. If a nebulizer is not immediately available, multiple actuations of a metered-dose inhaler into a large volume spacing device is an acceptable alternative. Salbutamol at doses of 2–5 mg (20–50 puffs, given five puffs at a time in the spacer) is used.

Corticosteroids are also given in the acute attack. Oral prednisolone 0.6 mg/kg (commonly 40–60 mg) is the first-line choice with intravenous hydrocortisone 3–4 mg/kg (commonly 200 mg) if the patient cannot take oral medication. This reduces and prevents the inflammation that causes oedema and hypersecretion of mucus and hence helps to relieve the resultant smooth muscle spasm. The clinical response to both oral and parenteral steroids has an onset at 1–2 hours with a peak effect at 6–8 hours.

If life-threatening features are present, such as cyanosis, bradycardia, confusion, exhaustion or unconsciousness, intravenous bronchodilators can be used. Intravenous aminophylline can be given with a bolus dose of 250 mg over 30 minutes. A β_2 agonist such as salbutamol 200 micrograms over 10 minutes is often preferred if the patient is already taking an oral theophylline. Potential adverse effects of intravenous β_2 agonists include cardiovascular effects such as tremor and tachycardia and metabolic effects such as hypokalaemia.

Antibiotics are only indicated where there is evidence of a bacterial infection.

Subsequent management of acute severe asthma

The subsequent management depends on the patient's clinical response. All patients should be monitored throughout their treatment with objective measures of their PEFRs before and after bronchodilator treatment and with continual monitoring of their arterial blood gas concentrations to ensure adequate oxygen is being given. Initially, β_2 agonists are given every 4 hours, and the corticosteroids given orally every morning or every 6 hours if intravenous treatment is required, for example in very severe asthma or if the patient is vomiting.

If the response to the initial treatment is good, treatment is tailed off gradually. Intravenous steroids are discontinued, oral and inhaled steroids started if indicated, and the nebulized β_2 agonist is reduced in frequency to 6-hourly. As improvement continues, an inhaled β_2 agonist is substituted for the nebulized form and the oral corticosteroids stopped or reduced to a maintenance dose if clinically necessary.

If the patient's condition has not responded to the initial treatment within 15–30 minutes, nebulized ipratropium bromide 500 micrograms may be given together with each β_2 agonist dose. The addition of the anticholinergic often gives a response that is greater than that of the two agents used alone. Intravenous aminophylline or intravenous β_2 agonist is then added if progress is still unsatisfactory. Both drugs may be used earlier if life-threatening signs such as cyanosis, bradycardia or exhaustion are seen. The choice between intravenous aminophylline and β_2 agonist depends on concurrent therapy and side-effect profiles.

The dose of intravenous aminophylline used must also take into account recent theophylline therapy in addition to other factors (Table 23.8). Serious toxicity can occur with parenteral aminophylline, and patients must be carefully monitored for nausea and vomiting, the most common early signs of toxicity. If the aminophylline infusion is continued for more than 24 hours, the serum theophylline level may be measured to maintain the serum theophylline level in the optimum range of 10–20 mg/l.

Further deterioration in the condition may require assisted mechanical ventilation on an intensive care unit. Regular monitoring of arterial blood gases and oxygen saturation are performed to help detect any deterioration in condition.

As the patient responds to treatment, infusions can be stopped and other treatment changed or tailed off as described above. Throughout the treatment programme, potential drug interactions should be anticipated and managed appropriately (Table 23.9).

Table 23.8 Intravenous aminophylline dosing in acute severe asthma

	Aminophylline dose	Patient characteristics
Loading dose	5 mg/kg over 20–30 min	Adults and children
	3 mg/kg over 10–15 min	Previous theophylline therapy
Maintenance dose	0.5 mg/kg/h	Non-smoking adults
	0.7 mg/kg/h	Children under 12 and smokers
	0.2 mg/kg/h	Cardiac failure, liver impairment, pneumonia

Table 23.9   Common interactions with drugs used in the management of asthma

Drug	Interacting drug	Probable mechanism and clinical result
β$_2$ agonists	Corticosteroids	Increased risk of hypokalaemia with high-dose corticosteroids
	Theophylline	Increased risk of hypokalaemia with high-dose β$_2$ agonists
	β adrenoreceptor antagonists	Antagonism of bronchodilator effect. More marked with non-selective antagonists
Corticosteroids	Antidiabetic agents	Corticosteroids have hyperglycaemic activity
	Antihypertensive	Antagonism of hypotensive effect
	β$_2$ agonists	Increased risk of hypokalaemia with high doses
	Carbamazepine	Reduced steroid effect due to increased metabolism
	Phenobarbital	
	Phenytoin	
	Primidone	
	Rifampicin	
	Diuretics	Excessive potassium loss possible
	Oestrogens and oral contraceptives	Enhanced steroid effects, possibly due to reduced steroid metabolism
	Salicylates	Enhanced salicylate elimination
Theophylline	β adrenoreceptor antagonists	Inhibition of theophylline metabolism resulting in increased plasma levels
	Cimetidine	
	Ciprofloxacin	
	Erythromycin	
	Oral contraceptives	
	Verapamil	
	Barbiturates	Induction of theophylline metabolism resulting in decreased plasma levels
	Carbamazepine	
	Phenytoin	
	Smoking	
	Rifampicin	
	High-dose β$_2$ agonists	Increased risk of hypokalaemia
	Lithium carbonate	Theophylline enhances the renal clearance of lithium thus reducing serum lithium concentrations
	Thyroxine (starting thyroxine while on theophylline)	Increased theophylline elimination

All patients should have their inhaler technique checked, and any observed deficiencies should be corrected before discharge. A self-management plan should be drawn up and discussed with each patient.

Patient care

The correct use of drugs and the education of patients are the cornerstones of the management of asthma. There are three main steps in the education of the asthmatic patient:

1. The patient should have an understanding of the action of each of the medicines they use.
2. The appropriate choice of inhalation device(s) should be made and the patient educated to use them correctly.
3. An individualized self-management plan should be developed for each patient.

All members of the health care team should give education and support for the asthmatic patient at regular intervals. The need for each patient to understand their asthma and its management must be balanced against the

Table 23.10	Ladder of asthma knowledge
Step 1	Patient/carer *understands* what relief medication does, side-effects which may occur, aims of treatment, what is happening to them and their chest. Education material is made available
Step 2	Patient/carer *accepts and agrees* about use of medication, importance of preventers and recognition of symptoms
Step 3	Patient/carer *knows* how to monitor PEF and symptoms, when to increase dose of inhaled steroids and contact GP practice
Step 4	Patient/carer *confident* to manage own medication, increasing and decreasing using PEF or symptom monitoring, start oral steroids and attend GP practice at that point

PEF, peak expiratory flow.

dangers of overwhelming the patient with information, particularly with a newly diagnosed patient. To try to overcome this a 'ladder of asthma knowledge' has been proposed whereby patients are counselled in a gradual manner, each session adding to the previous one in content and reinforcing existing knowledge (Scottish Intercollegiate Guidelines Network 1998). This is outlined in Table 23.10.

Patient knowledge of asthma treatment

Increasing the knowledge of patients about their asthma therapy is a necessary component of asthma management. However, education alone has not been shown to have a beneficial effect on morbidity. Education programmes must, therefore, also look at modifying a patient's behaviour and attitude to asthma. A European survey has highlighted the further and continued need for asthma education. For example, 35% of patients were unaware that inflammation in the airways is the underlying cause of asthma and 20% of asthamatics believed that β_2-agonists were the most effective means of reducing inflammation (Rabe et al 2000). Counselling should lead to increased patient confidence in the ability to self-manage asthma, decrease hospital admission rates and emergency visits by general practitioners, increase compliance and improve quality of life.

Specific counselling on drug therapy should concentrate on three areas: drugs used to relieve symptoms, drugs used to prevent asthma attacks and those drugs which are given only as reserve treatment for severe attacks.

Choice of inhalation device

The choice of a suitable inhalation device is vital in asthma management. The incorrect use of inhalers will lead to suboptimal treatment. This has been demonstrated to occur in up to 75% of patients using metered-dose inhalers. Several factors need to be considered when choosing the appropriate device, including the patient's age, severity of disease, manual dexterity, coordination and personal preference. The range of different devices available for the drugs commonly used in asthma is illustrated in Table 23.11.

Metered-dose aerosol inhalers

The pressurized, metered-dose inhaler (MDI), illustrated in Figure 23.5, is the most widely prescribed inhalation device. It contains a suspension of active drug, with a typical particle size of 2–5 μm, in a liquefied propellant. Operation of the device releases a metered dose of the drug with a droplet size of 35–45 μm. The increased droplet size is due to the propellant, which evaporates when expelled from the inhaler. A transition from the older chlorofluorocarbon (CFC) propellants to newer hydrofluoroalkanes, which do not damage the ozone layer, has taken place.

MDIs have the advantage of being multidose, small and widely available for most of the drugs used for asthma management. Their main disadvantage is that correct use requires a good technique, mainly coordinating the beginning of inspiration with the actuation of the inhaler. Even when this is done correctly, MDIs only deliver about 10% of drug to the airways with 80% deposited in the oropharynx. Other disadvantages include irritation in the pharynx and bronchi, which

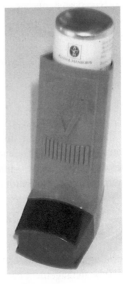

Figure 23.5 Pressurized, metered dose inhaler. (Photograph by Roger Gale.)

Table 23.11 Inhalation devices and spacer devices available

Drug	Inhaler device type						
	Metered-dose inhaler	Breath-actuated metered-dose inhaler	Single-dose dry powder	Multiple-dose dry powder	Nebulizer	Large-volume spacer for MDI	Small volume spacer for MDI
Salbutamol	✓	✓	✓	✓	✓	✓	✓
Terbutaline	✓			✓	✓	✓	✓
Salmeterol	✓	✓		✓		✓	✓
Formoterol (eformoterol)	✓		✓				
Beclometasone	✓	✓	✓	✓		✓	✓
Budesonide	✓			✓	✓	✓	✓
Fluticasone	✓			✓		✓	✓
Ipratropium	✓	✓		✓	✓	✓	✓
Oxitropium	✓	✓				✓	✓
Cromoglicate	✓		✓		✓	✓	✓
Nedocromil	✓						✓

inhibits further inspiration; this is caused by the cold propellant. Corticosteroids administered by MDIs can cause dysphonia and oral candidiasis. This candidiasis can be minimized either by advising patients to gargle with water after using the inhaler and to expel the water from the mouth afterwards, or by using a spacer device.

Younger children in particular find MDIs difficult to use and find the addition of a spacer device (see below) makes this easier and allows inhalation over several breaths.

The correct technique for using metered-dose inhalers is as follows:

1. MDIs have a mouthpiece dust-cap which has to be removed before use. Often patients do not remove this.
2. The MDI must be vigorously shaken. This distributes the drug particles uniformly throughout the propellant. The MDI must be held upright.
3. The patient should breathe out gently, but not fully.
4. The tongue should be placed on the floor of the mouth and the inhaler placed between the lips, which are then closed round the mouthpiece.
5. The patient should now start to breathe in slowly and deeply through the mouth.
6. The canister is pressed to release the dose while the patient continues to breathe in. This synchronization

of inspiration and actuation, so that there is a supporting stream of air to carry the drug to the lungs, is probably the most common failure in those with bad inhalation technique. Asthmatics very short of breath (for example during a severe attack) find this particularly difficult.

7. The breath is held for at least 10 seconds. This allows the drug particles reaching the periphery of the lung to settle under gravity. Using this technique, about 15% of a dose may reach the lungs. Exhalation should be through the nose.
8. If a second dose is called for, at least 1 minute should elapse before repeating the inhalation procedure. During actuation, the temperature of the MDI actuator stem and valve drops, and should theoretically be allowed to warm up. In practice, however, this may not be very important.

Studies indicate that personal tuition improves inhaler technique. Other methods of instruction include videos, package inserts and information leaflets or booklets provided by the National Asthma Campaign and the pharmaceutical industry.

The scoring of inhalation technique has been advocated using checklists (Table 23.12), which can be kept as a permanent record by any of the health care professionals.

Table 23.12 MDI technique score chart
1. Shake vigorously
2. Remove cap
3. Hold upright
4. Breathe out gently, not fully
5. Start breathing in slowly and deeply
6. Actuate during inspiration
7. Continue slow inhalation
8. No aerosol loss is visible
9. Hold breath 10 seconds
10. Next dose after 1 minute
Score 1 for each correct step undertaken
This gives a score out of 10 that can be used to monitor a patient's performance and highlight any problem areas.

Metered-dose inhaler with a spacer extension

Extension devices allow greater evaporation of the propellant, so reducing particle size and velocity. This also reduces oropharyngeal deposition and potentially increases lung deposition. Oral candidiasis and dysphonia (impaired voice) from inhaled corticosteroids may be reduced by using these devices. Spacers are useful for people who have poor coordination between inspiration and actuation. Several types are available. In younger children these offer advantages over MDIs alone with respect to compliance. Recommendations have been published regarding device choice (British Thoracic Society 1997, National Institute for Clinical Excellence 2000) (see Table 23.13).

Small volume spacer devices are available, either as an integral part of the design of some MDIs, as illustrated in Figure 23.6, or as an addition. Some coordination between inspiration and inhalation is required. The small volume has been shown to be superior to conventional MDIs in increasing the FEV_1 in children and has been used to try to compensate for poor inhalation technique in adults. These are also more convenient to carry around than the larger spacers.

Large-volume (750 ml) spacers are available, and are more efficient than the smaller spacers. The Volumatic (Fig. 23.7) and the Nebuhaler are two such devices. These have one-way inhalation valves that allow several inhalations of one dose from the spacer's chamber. No coordination is required between actuation of the MDI and inhalation. This type of spacer has been shown to produce greater bronchodilatation than either a conventional MDI or a nebulizer. A large-volume spacer has been used instead of a nebulizer to deliver high doses of a β_2 agonist in acute severe asthma attacks. The disadvantage of these devices is their large size, which

renders them less portable. Spacers should be washed regularly in warm, soapy water and left to drip dry without rinsing (Pierart et al 1999). Cloths should not be used for drying as this affects the antistatic coating of the spacer. Smaller versions or fitted facemasks are available for young children.

Breath-actuated metered-dose inhalers

These are MDIs that are actuated automatically by inspiratory flow rates of about 22–36 l/min. One type is illustrated in Figure 23.8. This is easily managed by adults and children and eliminates the need for the correct coordination of inspiration and actuation.

Dry powder inhalers

Several types of breath-operated dry powder inhalers are available. These are freon propellant free and are designed to be easier to use than conventional MDIs. They are useful for those who have difficulty coordinating an MDI and can be used by children as young as 4 years old. Table 23.13 gives the current recommendations for device choice in children (British Thoracic Society 1997, National Institute for Clinical Excellence 2000).

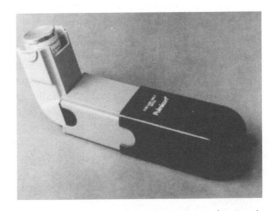

Figure 23.6 Spacer extension as integral part of metered-dose inhaler.

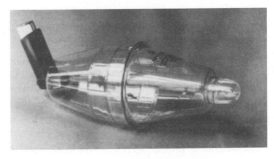

Figure 23.7 Large-volume spacer (Volumatic).

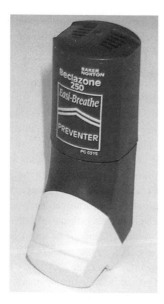

Figure 23.8 Breath-actuated metered-dose inhaler. (Photograph by Roger Gale.)

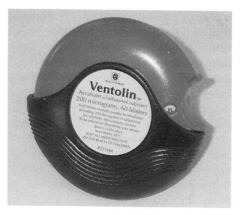

Figure 23.9 Multiple-dose dry powder inhaler. (Photograph by Roger Gale.)

Dry powder inhalers are available as either single-dose, or multiple-dose devices (Fig. 23.9). Single-dose devices pierce or break a gelatin capsule to release the contents and must be regularly cleaned to avoid powder clogging the device. Multiple-dose devices are preferred by many patients since they avoid having to reload for each dose.

Nebulizers

A nebulizer produces an aerosol by blowing air or oxygen through a solution to produce droplets of 5 μm or less in size. Nebulizers require little coordination from the patient as any drug is inhaled through a facemask or mouthpiece using normal tidal breathing. Only about 13% of the dose used is deposited in the lungs, but because the doses used are higher than those used in other aerosol devices, patients will receive 10–20 times the dose received from an MDI.

Nebulizers are therefore useful in patients who are unable to use conventional inhalers, for example children under 2 years old, patients with severe attacks of asthma unable to produce sufficient inspiratory effort and those lacking the coordination to use other inhalers. Nebulized bronchodilators can be used in acute severe asthma attacks, often avoiding the need for intravenous drugs, and in conjunction with prophylactic agents in the treatment of chronic asthma unresponsive to or poorly controlled by conventional treatment.

Most of the β_2 agonists, as well as ipratropium bromide, beclometasone, budesonide and sodium cromoglicate, are available for nebulization. The majority of these preparations are made up in isotonic 0.9% sodium chloride and are available in preservative-free, unit dose presentations. The use of solutions that are either hypertonic or hypotonic, particularly after dilution with water, or contain a preservative such as benzalkonium chloride or EDTA, has been associated with bronchoconstriction.

The safe and correct use of nebulizers requires careful counselling, especially if they are to be used in the home. The following points are critical for the correct use of a nebulizer:

1. Nebulizers should only be driven by compressed air or by oxygen at flow rates of at least 5–6 l/min to ensure that droplets of the correct size are produced.

Table 23.13	Inhaler device choice for children aged under 5 years				
Age group	1st choice device	2nd choice device	3rd choice device	Breath-actuated	Dry-powder
0–2 years	MDI + spacer + face mask	MDI + spacer	Nebulizer (rarely needed)	Avoid	Avoid
3–5 years	MDI + spacer	MDI + spacer + face mask	Nebulizer (rarely needed)	Not proven	Possible use for β_2 agonist but not recommended for corticosteroids

2. For all drugs a minimum volume of 3–4 ml should be nebulized, using 0.9% sodium chloride as a diluent if necessary. This volume is required to reduce the amount of drug that is unavoidably left in a 'dead-space' fluid volume of about 1 ml at the end of nebulization. The side of the nebulizer should be repeatedly tapped during use to ensure that no fluid builds up on the sides of the nebulizer chamber.

3. Most nebulizer chambers are disposable but will last 3–4 months when used by a patient at home. The chamber must be emptied after use and each day the chamber should be rinsed in hot water and dried by blowing air through the device. Several centres advocate that once a week the chamber should be sterilized using 0.02% hypochlorite to prevent bacterial contamination. The chamber is thoroughly rinsed to remove all traces of hypochlorite and then dried.

4. The nebulizer should be serviced at least once a year.

5. Each patient should be given a self-management plan for the correct use of his/her nebulizer. If the nebulizer is only for use in severe attacks, the patient should be advised to use it only when the peak flow reading falls below a specified amount and not to exceed a maximum dose, e.g. 5 mg of salbutamol. Patients must be informed that they should contact their doctor if the nebulizer fails to give the expected relief or the relief lasts for less than 4 hours.

There are disadvantages with the use of nebulizers. There may be over-reliance on the nebulizer by the patient which can result in a delay in seeking medical advice, while the high doses of bronchodilators used increase the incidence of side-effects.

Self-management plans

Every asthmatic should be considered for an individualized self-management plan. These plans are a means of giving patients more confidence by involving them in the management of their own asthma. The patient should then be able to deal with any fluctuation in their condition and know when to seek medical advice. Supervised patient self-management has been shown to improve patient knowledge, concordance and quality of life and reduce asthma-related incidents such as days off work (Gibson et al 1999), whereas information-only education has shown no effect on health outcomes (Gibson et al 2000).

Key elements of a self-management plan include being able to monitor symptoms, peak flow measurements, drug usage and knowing how to deal with fluctuations in severity of asthma according to written guidance. Symptom diaries, treatment/management guidance cards and peak flow reading diary cards are available from the National Asthma Campaign and from some of the pharmaceutical companies who manufacture asthma products.

A self-management plan would also include details of when to increase the dose of an inhaled steroid, when to take a short course of oral corticosteroids and when to use a nebulizer, how to monitor the effects of the nebulized dose and when to self-refer to a general practitioner or local hospital (Table 23.14).

Table 23.14 Example of part of a self-management plan

Peak flow	Symptoms	Action
> 85% of normal best value	Intermittent or few symptoms	When required, β_2 agonist for symptom relief Continue regular inhaler corticosteroid, consider reducing the dosage
70–85% of best	Waking at night 'Cold' symptoms	Double dose of inhaled corticosteroid
50–70% of best	Increasing breathlessness β_2 agonist required every 2–3 h	Start oral corticosteroid course Contact a doctor
<50% of best	Severe attack Poor response to β_2 agonist	Call emergency doctor or ambulance urgently

CASE STUDIES

Case 23.1

Mrs. M. L., a 48-year-old, recently diagnosed asthmatic patient, came into her community pharmacy looking extremely anxious and gasping for breath. She could only say a couple of words before becoming breathless again. An asthma attack was suspected.

Mrs M. L. was taken to hospital. On arrival she was given 60% oxygen 30 mg oral prednisolone and nebulized salbutamol 5 mg 4-hourly initially. Her symptoms resolved quickly and she was discharged 24 hours later. She was given the remainder of a 1 week course of prednisolone tablets 30 mg daily, an emergency supply of prednisolone tablets in the event of a further attack and a peak flow meter. She was also advised to continue to use her beclometasone MDI inhaler 400 micrograms twice a day and salbutamol MDI when required.

Questions

1. How should Mrs M. L. be managed immediately on her arrival at the pharmacy?
2. She asks if she can prevent this from happening again. What would you advise?

Answers

1. Mrs M. L. is suffering an acute asthma attack. The common symptoms of acutely deteriorating asthma control are (British Thoracic Society 1997):

   - peak expiratory flow $\leq$ 50% of the patient's predicted or best value
   - cannot complete sentences in one breath
   - respiratory rate $\geq$ 25 breaths per minute
   - pulse rate $\geq$ 110 beats per minute.

   She should initially be reassured. Her normal bronchodilator medication should then be found or an emergency supply made to her immediately. She should then be helped to administer this, preferably via a spacer. She should take two puffs, repeated 10–20 times. If oxygen is available this should be administered at 60% or more. An ambulance should be called if this is her first acute attack, if she does not respond to the medication, or if her condition deteriorates (Respiratory Disease Task Force 2000).
2. The education of asthmatic patients should involve the entire health care team and has been shown to have a positive effect on outcomes (Self & Nahata 1997). Mrs M. L. will probably have been given a follow-up appointment but all health care professionals can reinforce the key messages of self-management of asthma. Discussion with Mrs M. L. should cover:
   - The role of inflammation in the aetiology of asthma. This will enable greater understanding of the role of preventer therapy.
   - The differences between her 'preventer' and 'reliever' therapy. Patients continue to use more bronchodilator than preventer therapy (Rabe et al 2000).
   - Inhaler technique. It has been estimated that up to 75% of patients using a MDI have suboptimal inhaler technique. Careful analysis of Mrs M. L.'s technique may give some

clues to poor asthma management. The choice of device should be carefully tailored to a patient's manual dexterity, coordination, age, disease severity and personal preference. Mrs M. L. may benefit from instruction with her technique or a recommendation may be made for an alternative and more appropriate device.
   - Potential side-effects of her medication and how to minimize them, for example rinsing the mouth out with water after using a steroid inhaler to reduce the risk of oral candidiasis.
   - A review of her current medication to watch for any drugs which could trigger or exacerbate an asthma attack, such as β-blockers; a small proportion of asthmatics are sensitive to aspirin and other non-steroidal anti-inflammatory drugs.
   - How to identify trigger factors and reduce their effect.
   - How to use a peak flow meter.
   - How to recognize deteriorating asthma symptoms. A peak flow of < 70–80% of 'best' or symptoms at night are indicative of deteriorating asthma. The point at which to start the emergency steroid course should be discussed with the respiratory clinic or GP.
   - When to call for help.

However, it is important not to overwhelm any patient with too much information at once. Education can be built on, with the important basics covered first and then expanded upon at subsequent visits.

Case 23.2

Mrs S. J. is a 32-year-old housewife who has had asthma since the age of 5 years. She is a non-smoker, drinks occasional alcohol and has a pet cat. Her current medication is:

- beclometasone MDI 500 micrograms twice a day
- salbutamol MDI 200 micrograms when required.

Mrs S. J. visits her general practitioner (GP) as she has been feeling increasingly short of breath over the past few weeks.

Mrs S. J. was prescribed zafirlukast 20 mg twice a day in addition to her existing medication and also given a course of amoxicillin 250 mg three times a day for a week, as her GP suspected she might have a slight infection. She continued with her new medication with no further problems.

Two months later she was admitted to hospital experiencing flu-like symptoms, abdominal pain and loss of appetite. On examination Mrs S. J. appeared to be jaundiced.

Liver function tests were as follows:

Bilirubin:	44 μmol/l	(normal range: < 17 μmol/l)
Alanine transaminase (ALT):	200 IU/l	(normal range: 0–35 units/l)
Aspartate transaminase (AST):	150 IU/l	(normal range: 0–35 units/l)

Questions

1. What treatment should be considered by Mrs S. J.'s GP?

2. What is Mrs S. J.'s diagnosis on admission to hospital and what is the likely cause?
3. What treatment would you recommend initially?
4. After 7 days Mrs S. J.'s condition improved. What treatment would you now recommend?

....

Answers

1. As Mrs S. J.'s asthma seems uncontrolled with an inhaled corticosteroid and occasional use of a short acting β_2 stimulant, her GP could consider prescribing a leukotriene receptor antagonist. These drugs reduce airway oedema and smooth muscle constriction in patients with asthma by preventing stimulation of type 1 cysteinyl leukotriene receptors. This is beneficial in asthma, as cysteinyl leukotrienes are highly potent mediators of inflammation, causing mucus hypersecretion, constriction of bronchial smooth muscle and migration of inflammatory cells (Lipworth 1999). Her GP could prescribe either zafirlukast 20 mg twice a day or montelukast 10 mg at night.

   An alternative treatment option would be to prescribe a long acting β_2-stimulant by inhalation, such as salmeterol or formoterol (eformoterol). These drugs are given twice a day in addition to existing corticosteroid therapy. Long acting β_2-stimulants are particularly useful for patients with nocturnal symptoms, but should not be used to relieve an acute attack.

2. Mrs S. J. is showing signs of acute hepatitis as she appears jaundiced with a raised bilirubin level and has raised ALT and AST levels. Alanine transaminase is specific to the liver, while aspartate transaminase is also found in the lungs and muscle. Both substances are released in vast quantities if hepatocytes are injured, although the ALT level is usually higher than the AST level.

   Zafirlukast is likely to have caused the liver damage in Mrs S. J. as it had been recently started. Asymptomatic increases of two to three times the normal upper limit for serum liver enzyme levels were seen in 60 out of 4058 patients taking zafirlukast during pre-marketing trials but no severe hepatotoxicity was noted. Rare cases of severe hepatitis while taking zafirlukast have also been identified.

   The way in which zafirlukast causes hepatocellular damage is currently unknown, although it is postulated that it may be an immunological mechanism because the effect is idiosyncratic and hepatic eosinophils have been present in the most severe cases documented in the literature. Zafirlukast has been observed to potentially cause Churg–Strauss syndrome, an immunologic adverse reaction causing systemic vasculitis with eosinophilia and asthma. Another theory is that the cytochrome P450 pathway responsible for the metabolism of zafirlukast may also produce hepatotoxic metabolites in some patients (Reinus et al 2000).

3. Zafirlukast treatment was immediately stopped and Mrs S. J. was prescribed 60 mg of prednisolone each morning. She was also prescribed salbutamol 5 mg via the nebulizer four times a day as needed.

4. Mrs S. J.'s salbutamol nebules were discontinued and it was advised that her dose of prednisolone should be slowly reduced over the next few weeks. She was also started on a salmeterol inhaler 50 micrograms (2 puffs) twice a day to help to control her asthma. Her GP was asked to monitor her liver function tests carefully and after 3 months they returned to normal. Mrs S. J.'s asthma was still not

adequately controlled and so her GP decided to add montelukast to her existing treatment. Her liver function tests were monitored closely over the next 3 months, but remained normal. This indicates that although montelukast and zafirlukast seem to have the same mode of action, they do not seem to produce the same adverse effects.

Hepatotoxicity due to zafirlukast is an idiosyncratic reaction that is extremely rare. It is not possible to predict if a patient may suffer liver damage if treated with zafirlukast, but health professionals should be aware of this adverse reaction.

Case 23.3

Miss Z. T., a 39-year-old severe asthmatic, was admitted to hospital for the third time in 2 months with acute severe asthma. After admission these drugs were started:

- intravenous hydrocortisone 100 mg three times a day
- salbutamol 5 mg every 2 hours via a nebulizer
- ipratropium 500 micrograms four times a day via a nebulizer
- 750 mg aminophylline as an intravenous infusion over 24 hours
- Intravenous co-amoxiclav 1.2 g three times a day.

On day 2, the aminophylline infusion and the hydrocortisone were stopped. The consultant respiratory physician reviewed her current medication and in addition to her regular fluticasone and salmeterol inhalers he suggested she receive theophylline modified release tablets 250 mg twice a day and oral prednisolone 30 mg each morning.

Miss Z. T. continued to need regular salbutamol via the nebulizer over the next 2 days and so the doctor suggested a continuous subcutaneous infusion of 6 mg of terbutaline over 24 hours instead.

....

Questions

1. What advice would you give to the nurses and doctors looking after this patient about how to administer and monitor the terbutaline infusion?
2. What legal considerations should be taken in to account with your recommendations?

....

Answers

1. Terbutaline is available as terbutaline sulphate 500 micrograms/ml ampoules and also as terbutaline sulphate Respules® 2.5 mg/ml. To give a continuous subcutaneous infusion over 24 hours requires a syringe driver. Miss Z. T. will probably continue on this treatment when she goes home if it is successful and so the syringe driver needs to be as small and discreet as possible. Syringe drivers holding 10 ml syringes are generally used in such patients, as they are small and can be easily hidden under clothing. The solution for infusion over 24 hours therefore needs to be in a maximum volume of 10 ml. The product available for injection has a concentration of 500 micrograms/ml and so Miss Z. T. would require 12 ml to give a dose of 6 mg. An alternative is to use the Respules® that contain a sterile solution of terbutaline sulphate that is more concentrated

than the injection. This patient would require 2.4 ml of terbutaline sulphate from the Respules®, which could then be made up to 10 ml with 0.9% sodium chloride for injection. The infusion should then be run at a rate of 0.4 ml per hour.

While she is receiving terbutaline infusion Miss Z. T.'s potassium level should be carefully monitored owing to the risk of hypokalaemia. This risk is greater in severe asthma due to hypoxia and the concomitant use of theophylline and corticosteroids. She may experience a fine tremor, usually of the hands, while receiving terbutaline infusion but this would probably be no worse than the tremor experienced after receiving salbutamol via the nebulizer and she may already be used to this. The nurse looking after Miss Z. T. should also be reminded to check the infusion site for any signs of irritation during the infusion.

2. Terbutaline prescribed as a continuous subcutaneous infusion over 24 hours is unlicensed. It is therefore important that the consultant is aware of this and it is documented that he takes full responsibility for the prescription. Although unlicensed, this route is used for brittle asthmatics when other treatments fail. The usual starting dose is 6 mg over 24 hours, which can be increased to 8–12 mg over 24 hours if necessary. This is greater than the maximum dose recommended in the British National Formulary (BNF) for intravenous infusion. It should be noted, however, that salbutamol given via a nebulizer is commonly given in doses higher than the maximum licensed dose of 5 mg four times a day.

The use of terbutaline nebulizer Respules® for subcutaneous infusion is also unlicensed. It is therefore important that the hospital pharmacist also obtains a disclaimer signed by the consultant specifying that the prescriber accepts the responsibility for the use of the product. The use of the Respules® is seen as enhancing patient care, as Miss Z. T.'s quality of life is reduced due to her brittle asthma and multiple admissions to hospital. If she is to continue with the portable syringe driver at home it needs to be discreet and easily hidden to prevent embarrassment. The use of the higher concentration Respules® allows longer duration infusions and consequently fewer syringe changes per day, increasing the acceptance of this therapy.

REFERENCES

British Thoracic Society, National Asthma Campaign, Royal College of Physicians of London 1997 The British guidelines on asthma management: 1995 review and position statement. Thorax 52(Suppl. 1): S1–S21

Gibson P G, Coughlan J, Wilson A J et al 1999 Self management, education and regular practitioner review for adults with asthma. Cochrane Collaboration, Cochrane Library. Issue 2. Update Software, Oxford

Gibson P G Coughlan J, Wilson A L et al 2000 Limited (information only) patient education programs for adults with asthma. Cochrane Collaboration. Cochrane Database of Systematic Reviews. Update Software, Oxford

Greg I, Nunn A J 1989 New regression equations for predicting peak expiratory flow in adults. British Medical Journal 298: 1068–1070

Harrison B 1999 Acute severe asthma in adults. Medicine 27: 64–68

Lipworth B J 1999 Leukotriene-receptor antagonists. Lancet 153: 57–62

National Asthma Campaign 1999 National Asthma Audit 1999/2000. National Asthma Campaign, London

National Institute for Clinical Excellence (NICE) 2000 Guidance on the use of inhaler systems (devices) in children under 5 years with chronic asthma. Technology Appraisal Guidance, no. 20: NICE, London
http://www.nice.org.uk

North of England Evidence Based Guideline Development Project 1995 Evidence based clinical practice guideline: the primary care management of asthma in adults.
http://www.bmj.com/asthma/ast01.htm

Pierart F, Wildhaber J H, Vrancken I et al 1999 Washing plastic spacer in household detergent reduces electrostatic charge and greatly improves delivery. European Respiratory Journal 13: 673–678

Rabe K F, Vermeire P A, Soriano J B et al 2000 Clinical management of asthma in 1999: the asthma insights and reality in europe (AIRE) study. European Respiratory Journal 16: 802–807

Reinus J F, Persky S, Burkiewicz J S et al 2000 Severe liver injury after treatment with the leukotriene receptor antagonist zafirlukast. Annals of Internal Medicine 133: 964–968

Respiratory Disease Task Force 2000 Practice guidance on the care of people with asthma and chronic obstructive pulmonary disease. Royal Pharmaceutical Society of Great Britain, London

Scottish Intercollegiate Guidelines Network (SIGN) 1998 Primary care management of asthma. SIGN publication no. 33. SIGN, Edinburgh
http://www.sign.ac.uk

Self T H, Nahata M C 1997 Improving outcomes in asthma: role of pharmacy. Annals of Pharmacotherapy 31: 495–497

Tasche M J A, Uijen J H J M, Bernsen R M D et al 2000 Inhaled disodium cromoglycate (DSCG) as maintenance therapy in children with asthma: a systematic review. Thorax 55: 913–920

Walters E H, Walters J 2000 Inhaled short acting beta-2 agonist use in asthma: regular vs as needed treatment. Cochrane Review. In: Cochrane Library, issue 4. Update Software, Oxford

FURTHER READING

Beasley R, Miles J 1999 Diagnosis and management of adult asthma. Medicine 27: 58–64

Lazio G 1999 Pulmonary function tests in practice. Medicine 27: 20–26

Le Souëf P 1999 Asthma in children. Medicine 27: 54–57

Scottish Intercollegiate Guidelines Network (SIGN) 1999 Emergency management of acute asthma. SIGN publication no. 38 SIGN, Edinburgh
http://www.sign.ac.uk

Scottish Intercollegiate Guidelines Network (SIGN) 1996 Hospital in-patient management of acute asthma attacks. SIGN publication no. 6 SIGN, Edinburgh
http://www.sign.ac.uk

Chronic obstructive pulmonary disease

24

K. P. Gibbs   M. Small

KEY POINTS

- Chronic obstructive pulmonary disease (COPD) is the most prevalent manifestation of obstructive lung disease and mainly comprises chronic bronchitis and emphysema.
- Tobacco smoking is the most important risk factor for the development of COPD. Stopping smoking can help to slow disease progression and should be the primary focus of COPD management.
- Bronchodilators and corticosteroids can be used in some patients for symptom relief, to reverse airflow restriction and control inflammation.
- Drug administration via a nebulizer may not be a cost-effective way of improving symptoms in patients with severe disease.
- Influenza vaccine should be given to COPD patients every year.
- Prophylactic antibiotics have no place in the management of COPD. Antibiotic therapy is vital if a patient develops purulent sputum.
- Cor pulmonale can develop. The use of domiciliary oxygen therapy for 15 hours a day reduces the associated mortality.
- Patients should undergo non-pharmacological pulmonary rehabilitation, such as breathing exercises.

Chronic obstructive pulmonary disease (COPD) is a general term that covers a variety of other disease labels, including chronic obstructive airways disease (COAD), chronic obstructive lung disease (COLD), chronic bronchitis and emphysema.

COPD is defined as a chronic, slowly progressive disorder characterized by airflow obstruction, which does not change markedly over several months.

Chronic bronchitis is clinically diagnosed after determination of the symptoms. The epidemiological definition is a chronic or recurrent cough with sputum production on most days for at least 3 months of the year during at least 2 consecutive years, in the absence of other diseases recognized to cause sputum production. This does not necessarily mean the patient has airflow obstruction. Emphysema is defined as an abnormal permanent enlargement of the air spaces distal to the terminal bronchioles, accompanied by destruction of their walls and without obvious fibrosis. This change in the anatomy of the lungs results in a deterioration of gas exchange and impaired ventilation.

Epidemiology

COPD is a major cause of morbidity and mortality in all industrialized countries and is the largest single cause of lost working days in the UK. COPD causes about 30 000 deaths each year in the UK and is accountable for more than 12% of all hospital admissions. The burden of COPD on an average UK health care system exceeds that of asthma (Table 24.1)

Respiratory diseases including chronic bronchitis are more common in areas of high atmospheric pollution and in people with dusty occupations such as foundry workers and coal miners. Areas of northern England and Scotland that are highly industrialized show the highest incidence of COPD.

Aetiology

Chronic obstructive pulmonary disease is largely preventable as cigarette smoking is the most important and dominant risk factor in its development; non-smokers rarely develop COPD. The incidence of COPD in non-smokers has been estimated at 5% or less; the contribution of passive inhalation of tobacco smoke to this incidence is unknown. The greater the exposure to tobacco, the higher the risk of developing COPD, although only about 15% of smokers appear to be

Table 24.1   Annual health service workload due to chronic respiratory disease in an average UK health district of 250 000 people (COPD guidelines group 1997)

	Hospital admissions	In-patient bed days	GP consultations
COPD	680	9600	14 200
Asthma	410	1800	11 900

susceptible and go on to develop COPD. Tobacco exposure can be calculated in 'pack-years':

$$\text{Total pack years} = \frac{\text{(number of cigarettes smoked per day)}}{20} \times \text{number of years of smoking}$$

A person who has smoked 1–20 pack years has an approximately 10% risk of developing mild COPD and 4% risk of severe COPD. If this figure was 61 pack-years, those probabilities rise to 24% and 7%, respectively (COPD Guidelines Group 1997).

Other risk factors, outlined in Table 24.2, may be important such as working in dusty environments and genetic factors such as α_1-antitrypsin deficiency (Senior & Anthonisen 1998, MacNee 1999).

Chronic bronchitis

Chronic bronchitis is associated with cigarette smoking and air pollution. Normally cilia and mucus in the bronchi protect against inhaled irritants, which are trapped and expectorated. Persistent irritation such as that caused by cigarette smoke causes an exaggeration in the response of these protective mechanisms. Hypersecretion of mucus results from hypertrophy and proliferation of mucus-producing glands. Cigarette smoke also inhibits mucociliary clearance, which causes a further build-up of mucus in the lungs. Irritation from smoke leads to inflammation of the small bronchioles (bronchiolitis) and alveoli (alveolitis). As a result,

macrophages and neutrophils infiltrate the epithelium and trigger a degree of epithelial destruction. This, together with a proliferation of mucus-producing cells, leads to plugging of smaller bronchioles and alveoli with mucus and particulate matter.

There are a number of other risk factors for the development of bronchitis. It is known that not all smokers with a similar smoking history develop the same degree of pulmonary impairment.

An additional risk factor is the natural ageing process of the lungs. Males are currently more at risk of developing chronic bronchitis, but as the number of women who smoke increases, the incidence of chronic bronchitis in females will also rise. Occupational exposure to chemical fumes and dust are established risk factors for chronic airflow obstruction and increased mortality from COPD. The major risk factors are shown in Table 24.2.

Emphysema

Emphysema has a different aetiology to chronic bronchitis but is often found to coexist with it. Emphysema results from a gradually progressive loss of elastic tissue within the lungs due to an imbalance between proteolytic enzymes and protective factors. Macrophages and neutrophils release lysosomal enzymes such as elastase that are capable of destroying connective tissue in the lungs. Under normal circumstances a protective factor called α_1-antitrypsin,

Table 24.2 Risk factors for the development of COPD

Risk factor	Comment
Smoking	Risk increases with increasing consumption but large individual variation in susceptibility
Age	Increasing age results in ventilatory impairment; however, this is most likely to be due to cumulative smoking
Gender	Male gender was previously thought to be a higher risk factor but this may be due to a higher incidence of tobacco smoking in men. Women have greater airway reactivity and experience faster declines in FEV_1 so may be at more risk than men
Occupation	The development of COPD has been implicated with occupations such as coal and gold mining, cement, cotton, grain handling and farming
Genetic factors	α_1-antitrypsin deficiency is the strongest single risk factor but other genetic disorders involving tissue necrosis factor and epoxide hydrolase may also be risk factors
Air pollution	Death rates are higher in urban areas than in rural areas
Socioeconomic status	More common in individuals of low socioeconomic status
Airway hyper-responsiveness and allergy	Smokers show increased levels of IgE and eosinophils and airway hyper-responsiveness

also known as α_1-protease inhibitor, inhibits proteolytic enzymes and so prevents damage. A deficiency of α_1-antitrypsin is known to predispose to emphysema. Measurement of α_1-antitrypsin is sometimes useful in younger patients since it may indicate those who are predisposed to emphysema caused by smoking. Cigarette smoke has been shown to inactivate this protein. Its production is determined by the protease inhibitor gene (M). One in 2500 individuals are homozygous for the recessive (Z) gene, which causes low blood levels of α_1-antitrypsin (10–15% of normal levels) and can result in early emphysema. Heterozygous individuals with the MZ gene also have an established risk of emphysema, which is increased by smoking. It is thought that women may have protection conferred by oestrogen, which stimulates the synthesis of protease inhibitors such as α_1-antitrypsin.

Pathophysiology

Bronchitis

There are two pathological processes underlying the development of chronic bronchitis. The first is a hypersecretory disorder characterized by expectoration with increasing susceptibility to respiratory infections. The second is an obstructive disorder that results from smooth muscle constriction and may or may not be associated with emphysema. Bronchoconstriction is not apparent in all patients, but where it does occur it adds further to deterioration in ventilation.

Hypersecretion of thick and viscous mucus results from proliferation of the mucus-secreting glands and goblet cells in the bronchial epithelium. Excessive mucus production is not thought to contribute significantly to airway obstruction although it does cause distension of the alveoli and loss of their gas exchange function. Pus and infected mucus accumulate, leading to recurrent or chronic viral and bacterial infections. The primary pathogen is usually viral but bacterial infection often follows. Common bacterial pathogens include *Streptococcus pneumoniae*, *Moraxella catarrhalis* and *Haemophilus influenzae*. Ulceration occurs where there is a focal point for infection and/or inflammation. Normal columnar epithelium may be replaced by squamous epithelium.

In addition, thickening of the bronchiole and alveolar walls results from chronic inflammation and oedema. This leads to blockage and obstruction of the airways. Alveolar distension and destruction results in distortion of the blood vessels that are closely associated with the alveoli. This causes a rise in the blood pressure in the pulmonary circulation. Reduction in gas diffusion across the alveolar epithelium leads to a low partial pressure of oxygen in the blood vessels (hypoxaemia) due to an imbalance between ventilation and perfusion. By a mechanism that is not clearly established, chronic vasoconstriction results and causes a further increase in blood pressure and further compromises gas diffusion from air spaces into the bloodstream. The chronic low oxygen levels lead to polycythaemia (increase in number of erythrocytes), which makes the blood more viscous. In advanced disease, this persistent hypoxaemia develops along with pathological changes in the pulmonary circulation. Sustained pulmonary hypertension results in a thickening of the walls of the pulmonary arterioles, with associated pulmonary remodelling and an increase in right ventricular pressure within the heart. The consequence of continued high right ventricular pressure is eventual right ventricular hypertrophy, dilatation and progressive right ventricular failure (cor pulmonale). Pulmonary oedema develops as a result of physiological changes subsequent to the hypoxaemia and hypercapnia, such as activation of the rennin–angiotensin system, salt and water retention and a reduction in renal blood flow.

Bronchiectasis is a pathological change in the lungs where the bronchi become permanently dilated. It is common after early attacks of acute bronchitis during which mucus both plugs and stretches the bronchial walls. In severe infections the bronchioles and alveoli can become permanently damaged and do not return to their normal size and shape. The loss of muscle tone and loss of cilia can contribute to COPD because mucus has a tendency to accumulate in the dilated bronchi.

Emphysema

Emphysema is a term used to describe progressive destructive enlargement of the respiratory bronchioles, alveolar duct and alveolar sac. Adjacent alveoli can become indistinguishable from each other, with two main consequences. The first is loss of available gas exchange surfaces, which leads to an increase in dead space and impaired gas exchange. The second consequence is the loss of elastic recoil in the small airways (vital for maintaining the force of expiration), which leads to a tendency for them to collapse, particularly during expiration. Increased thoracic gas volume and hyperinflation of the lungs results.

There are two main types of emphysema. Centrilobular emphysema involves the destruction of respiratory bronchioles, alveolar ducts and alveoli. This type of emphysema is especially common in the upper lobes of the lungs of cigarette smokers and coal miners. Panacinar emphysema is associated with α_1-antitrypsin deficiency, but in this case the alveoli are also affected. As described above, macrophages and neutrophils release the proteolytic enzyme elastase, which is normally inhibited by α_1-antitrypsin. Evidence suggests that macrophages and neutrophils release a greater amount of elastase in response to smoke in smokers than in non-smokers. Elastase breaks down elastin, which is an integral protein of the alveoli. In addition to destruction, matrix repair may be inhibited, particularly among those who smoke cigarettes. In emphysema, destruction of the alveoli also results in the loss of the capillary network essential for adequate perfusion. The decrease in lung perfusion along with loss of ventilation capacity due to loss of elastic recoil means that, unlike bronchitis, the ventilation/perfusion ratio is normally maintained. The patient with emphysema, therefore, experiences greater dyspnoea than a bronchitic but is better able to preserve gas exchange, as the respiratory centres are more responsive to lack of oxygen in the tissues (hypoxia). As a result, pure emphysema does not tend to lead to cor pulmonale or polycythaemia at such an early stage as bronchitis.

Clinical manifestations

Diagnosis

The diagnosis of COPD can only be made with certainty after objective measurement of airways obstruction with spirometric tests, and after exclusion of other possible diagnoses such as asthma. A diagnosis requires:

- a history of chronic progressive symptoms (cough, and/or wheeze, and/or breathlessness)
- objective evidence of airways obstruction, ideally by spirometric testing, that does not return to normal with treatment (COPD Guidelines Group 1997).

A study of the criteria commonly used to diagnose COPD from a patient's history has shown three factors to be of particular value in confirming the diagnosis (Strauss et al 2000):

- a self-reported history of chronic obstructive airways disease
- smoking in excess of 40 pack years
- age greater than 45 years; age less than 45 years virtually rules out a COPD diagnosis.

COPD is a progressive disorder, which passes through a potentially asymptomatic mild phase, before the moderate phase and then severe disease. The main signs and symptoms of each stage are summarized in Table 24.3.

Clinical features

The traditional description of COPD symptoms, particularly in severe disease, depends on whether bronchitis or emphysema predominates. Chronic bronchitic patients exhibit excess mucus production and a degree of bronchospasm resulting in wheeze and dyspnoea. Hypoxia and hypercapnia (high levels of carbon dioxide in the tissues) are common. This type of patient has a productive cough, is often overweight and finds physical exertion difficult due to dyspnoea. The bronchitic patient is sometimes referred to as a 'blue bloater'. This term is used because of the tendency of the patient to retain carbon dioxide caused by a decreased responsiveness of the respiratory centre to prolonged hypoxaemia that leads to cyanosis, and also the tendency for peripheral oedema to occur. Bronchitic patients lose the ability to increase the rate and depth of ventilation in response to persistent hypoxaemia. The reason for this is not clear, but decreased ventilatory drive may result from abnormal peripheral or central respiratory receptors. In severe disease the chest diameter is often increased, giving the classical barrel chest. As obstruction worsens, hypoxaemia increases, leading to pulmonary hypertension. Right ventricular strain leads to

Table 24.3   Classification and diagnosis of COPD (COPD Guidelines Group 1997)

COPD classification	Clinical state	Results of investigations
Mild	Smoker's cough, but little or no breathlessness. No abnormal signs	FEV_1: 60–79% predicted FEV_1/ VC mildly reduced
Moderate	Breathlessness (± wheeze) on exertion, cough (± sputum) and some abnormal signs	FEV_1: 40–59% predicted Reduced T_{LCO} Some patients are hypoxaemic but not hypercapnic
Severe	Breathlessness on any exertion. Wheeze, cough prominent. Clinical overinflation usual, plus cyanosis, peripheral oedema and polycythaemia in some	FEV_1 < 40% predicted with marked hyperinflation T_{LCO} variable but often low Hypoxaemia usual and hypercapnia in some

FEV_1, forced expiratory volume produced in the first second of expiration; VC, vital capacity; T_{LCO}, diffusing capacity for carbon monoxide or gas transfer factor.

right ventricular failure, which is characterized by jugular venous distension, hepatomegaly and peripheral oedema, all of which are consequences of an increase in systemic venous blood pressure. Recurrent lower respiratory tract infections can be severe and debilitating. Signs of infection include an increase in the volume of thick and viscous sputum, which is yellow or green in colour and may contain bacterial pathogens, squamous epithelial cells, alveolar macrophages and saliva, but pyrexia may not be present.

The clinical features of emphysema are different from those of bronchitis. A patient with emphysema will experience increasing dyspnoea even at rest, but often there is minimal cough and the sputum produced is scanty and mucoid. Cough is usually more of a problem after dyspnoea is apparent. The patient will breathe rapidly (tachypnoea) because the respiratory centres are responsive to mild hypoxaemia, and will have a flushed appearance. Typically a patient with emphysema will be thin and have pursed lips in an effort to compensate for a lack of elastic recoil and exhale a larger volume of air. Such a patient will tend to use the accessory muscles of the chest and neck to assist in the work of breathing. Hypoxaemia is not a problem until the disease has progressed. Pulmonary hypertension is usually mild and cor pulmonale is uncommon until the terminal stages of the disease.

Generally, bronchial infections tend to be less common in emphysema. The patient with emphysema is sometimes referred to as a 'pink puffer' because he or she hyperventilates to compensate for hypoxia by breathing in short puffs. As a result the patient appears pink with little carbon dioxide retention and little evidence of oedema. Eventually the patient is unable to obtain enough oxygen in spite of rapid breathing.

The bronchitic 'blue bloater' and emphysemic 'pink puffer' represent two ends of the COPD spectrum. In reality the underlying pathophysiology may well be a mixture, and the resulting signs and symptoms will be somewhere between the two extremes described.

Two specific problems are common in patients with COPD:

- sleep apnoea syndrome
- acute respiratory failure.

The sleep apnoea syndrome is a respiratory disorder characterized by frequent or prolonged pauses in breathing during sleep. It leads to a deterioration in arterial blood gases and a decrease in the saturation of haemoglobin with oxygen. Hypoxaemia is often accompanied by pulmonary hypertension and cardiac arrhythmias, which may lead to premature cardiac failure.

Acute respiratory failure is said to have occurred if the Po_2 suddenly drops and there is an increase in Pco_2 that decreases the pH to 7.3 or less. The most common cause is an acute exacerbation of chronic bronchitis with an increase in volume and viscosity of sputum. This further impairs ventilation and causes more severe hypoxaemia and hypercapnia. The clinical signs and symptoms of acute respiratory failure include restlessness, confusion, tachycardia, cyanosis, sweating, hypotension and eventual unconsciousness.

Investigations

Lung function tests are used to determine the severity of the respiratory disease and can also indicate response to treatment. A spirometer is used to measure lung volumes and flow rates. The main measurement made is the forced expiratory volume in the first second of exhalation (FEV_1), as this is reproducible, objective and shown to give the best predictive estimates of future mortality. Other tests can be performed, such as:

- vital capacity (VC): the volume of air inhaled and exhaled during maximal ventilation
- forced vital capacity (FVC): the volume of air inhaled and exhaled during a forced maximal expiration after full inspiration
- residual volume (RV): the volume of air left in the lungs after maximal exhalation
- carbon monoxide transfer factor (T_{LCO}): diffusing capacity or gas transfer factor for carbon monoxide.

Vital capacity decreases in bronchitis and emphysema. Residual volume increases in both cases but tends to be higher in patients with emphysema due to air being trapped distal to the terminal bronchioles. Total lung capacity is often normal in patients with bronchitis, but is usually increased in emphysema, again due to air being trapped. Other respiratory function tests that are carried out are the same as those for asthma. In patients with COPD there are reductions in FEV_1, FVC and the FEV_1/FVC ratio. The best guide to the progression of COPD is how the FEV_1 changes over time. Smoking increases the normal deterioration over time, from about 30 ml per year to about 45 ml per year. The major criticism of measuring FEV_1 and FVC is that they detect changes only in airways greater than 2 mm in diameter. As airways less than 2 mm in diameter contribute only 10–20% of normal resistance to airflow, there is usually severe obstruction and extensive damage to the lungs by the time the lung function tests (FEV_1 and FVC) detect abnormalities.

Arterial blood gases can be measured at rest and after exercise and are useful to determine the severity of disease and response to treatment. However, they are not considered to be useful in assessing disease progression. In a chronic bronchitic there is usually a low partial pressure of oxygen (Po_2, reference range 12–16 kPa) and an elevated partial pressure of carbon dioxide (P_{CO_2}, reference range 4.6–6.0 kPa). Haemoglobin level (reference range 13.5–18 g/dl for an adult male) and haematocrit (reference range 40–80%) can increase due to polycythaemia secondary to chronic hypoxaemia. Emphysema usually leads to a higher P_{O_2} than is seen in patients with bronchitis and normal values for P_{CO_2} until later stages of the disease.

In both bronchitis and emphysema the oxygen and carbon dioxide partial pressure changes progress slowly over a period of years. The pH of blood stays near normal (pH 7.35–7.45) in chronic disease because the kidneys compensate for the acidity caused by retention of carbon dioxide by retaining bicarbonate ions (reference range 22–28 mmol/l). In acute respiratory failure (e.g. due to pneumonia) where P_{CO_2} rises rapidly there may be a temporary acidosis until the kidneys can compensate, which may take more than 24 hours. Acid/base defects can be corrected by mechanical ventilation to reverse carbon dioxide accumulation.

Chest radiographs reveal differences between the two disease states. A patient with emphysema will have a flattened diaphragm with a loss of peripheral vascular markings and the appearance of bullae. These are indicative of extensive trapping of air. A bronchitic patient will have increased bronchovascular markings and may also have cardiomegaly (increased cardiac size due to right ventricular failure) with prominent pulmonary arteries.

patients with severe COPD and hypoxaemia, long-term oxygen therapy is the only treatment known to improve the prognosis.

The aims of treatment for patients with COPD are shown in Table 24.4 and the common therapeutic problems associated with COPD in Table 24.5. Drug treatment itself can only relieve symptoms; it does not modify the underlying pathology. Most patients with COPD are considered to have irreversible obstruction, in contrast to asthmatics, but a significant number do seem to respond to bronchodilators. Treatment options at each stage of COPD are outlined in Figure 24.1.

Smoking

Smoking is the most important factor in the development of obstructive airways disease. Every smoker with chronic airflow obstruction must be advised to stop smoking.

Individually targeted advice may prove to be more successful in persuading individuals to give up, especially in those motivated to do so.

Smokers who have a strong physical type of dependence will benefit from agents such as nicotine chewing gum or patches. The nicotine absorbed reduces the effects associated with cigarette smoking such as irritability, sleep disturbances, fatigue, headache and increased appetite.

Treatment

The clinical progress of COPD depends on whether bronchitis or emphysema predominates. Bronchitic patients will experience an increasing frequency of exacerbations of acute dyspnoea triggered by excess mucus production and obstruction. There is a progressive decline in lung function with complications such as cor pulmonale, hypercapnia and polycythaemia. Eventually cardiorespiratory failure with hypercapnia will occur, which may be severe, unresponsive to treatment and result in death. Emphysema patients will become progressively dyspnoeic without exacerbations triggered by increased sputum production. Eventually cor pulmonale will develop very rapidly, usually in the late stages of the disease, and lead to intractable hypercapnia and respiratory arrest.

Drug treatment together with other measures such as physiotherapy and artificial ventilation have not been shown to improve the natural progression of COPD. Quality of life and symptoms will, however, improve with suitable treatment and it is likely that the correct management of the patient will lead to a reduction in hospital admissions and may prevent premature death. In

Table 24.4 Treatment aims for patients with COPD

- Lessen airflow limitation
- Prevent and treat secondary medical complications such as hypoxaemia and infections
- Decrease respiratory symptoms and improve quality of life

Table 24.5 Common therapeutic problems associated with COPD

- Failure of patient to stop smoking
- Inadequate inhaler technique leading to sub-therapeutic dosing.
- Poor concordance with treatment regimen
- Failure to assess corticosteroid reversibility before prescribing inhaled corticosteroids
- Prescribing antibiotics inappropriately in an acute exacerbation of COPD
- Failure to properly assess a patient for home nebulizer therapy
- Failure to ensure compliance with 15 hours a day of home oxygen therapy

The COPD escalator

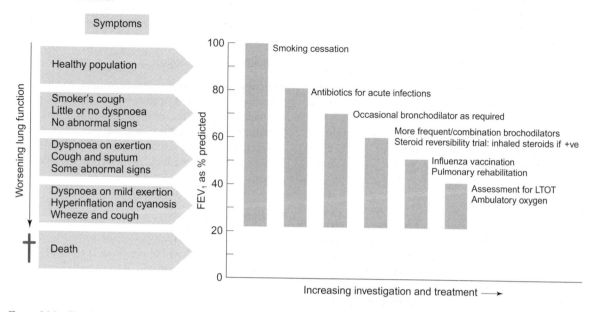

Figure 24.1 The COPD escalator (COPD Guidelines Group 1997; with the kind permission of the publishers).

Antibiotics and vaccines

Prophylactic antibiotics have no place in the management of COPD. Antibiotic therapy is, however, vital if a patient develops purulent sputum. It patients frequently develop acute infective exacerbations of bronchitis they should be given a supply of antibiotics to keep at home and start on the first sign of an exacerbation.

Initial routine sputum cultures are unhelpful in these patients as they are unreliable in identifying the pathogenic organisms.

The normal pathogens involved are *Streptococcus pneumoniae*, *Haemophilus influenzae* or *Moraxella catarrhalis*. The usual antibiotics of choice are co-amoxiclav, amoxicillin, erythromycin or doxycycline. If the infection follows influenza, *Staphylococcus aureus* may be present, and an anti-staphylococcal agent such as flucloxacillin should be added to the regimen. If the infection is considered atypical in presentation or if the purulent sputum is still present after 1 week of treatment, then sputum cultures should be taken to try to identify the pathogenic organisms.

Prophylactic immunization

The benefit of immunization in preventing acute infective exacerbations has not yet been demonstrated in all patient groups. A single dose of pneumococcal vaccine has been shown to prevent infection in the elderly, and could be offered to those with chronic airflow obstruction. There have, however, been no specific studies investigating the value of pneumococcal vaccination for patients with COPD to date and so it is not routinely recommended. Influenza vaccine should be given annually to patients with COPD, and this has been shown to reduce clinical infection rates in the general elderly population by about 70%. The prevalent strains of influenza change so the vaccine composition is, correspondingly, altered annually.

Bronchodilators

Bronchodilators in COPD are used to reverse airflow limitation. As the degree of limitation varies widely, their effectiveness should be assessed in each patient using respiratory function tests and by assessing any subjective improvement reported by the patient. Patients may report an improvement in exercise tolerance or relief of symptoms such as wheeze and cough. The use of diary cards to document daily symptoms may help.

Inhaled β_2 adrenoceptor agonists

Selective β_2 agonists should be tried initially since they provide rapid relief and have a low incidence of side-effects. Inhaled treatment is as efficacious as oral agents and is therefore preferred, having fewer side-effects. The low doses of inhaled β_2 agonists used in asthma, such as 200 micrograms of salbutamol, may not be high enough for COPD; higher doses (400–800 micrograms) may be

403

required 6-hourly. This dosing may result in an increased incidence of side-effects. Short-acting β_2 agonists should ideally be used when required for symptom relief. Used before exercise they can improve exercise tolerance. Regular dosing may be necessary in some patients and preferred by others. Poor patient response to bronchodilators may be due to poor inhalation technique and this should always be assessed and the inhaler device changed if necessary.

Long-acting β_2 agonists have no defined place in COPD treatment and should only be used after demonstrated benefit.

Anticholinergic drugs

In COPD patients, parasympathetic (vagal) airway muscle tone is the major reversible component. Inhaled anticholinergic drugs reverse this vagal tone and have a significant bronchodilator effect, especially in the elderly. The drugs of choice are the quaternary atropine derivatives ipratropium bromide and oxitropium, which when inhaled give local effects with little systemic absorption. The inhaled anticholinergics have a slower onset of bronchodilatation than the β_2 agonists. Higher doses of anticholinergics may be required than are used in patients with asthma, for example 80–120 micrograms of ipratropium bromide used 6-hourly.

Trial evidence shows short-term bronchodilatation and relief of symptoms using these agents but there is little evidence of any beneficial long-term effects on prognosis (Kerstjens 1999).

Patients vary in their response to β_2 agonists and anticholinergics. Combination therapy may produce additive bronchodilatation, but responses must always be properly assessed.

Theophyllines

Theophyllines are weak bronchodilators and are said to have additional physiological effects in COPD. These effects, such as improved right ventricular function and diaphragmatic function, have not been established as clinical benefits. The use of theophylline should only be considered in moderate to severe disease if other treatments have failed to improve symptoms. Whenever theophylline is tried in the management of COPD, an initial therapeutic trial of several weeks should be carried out. If subjective and objective measures of lung function show an improvement, then theophylline can be continued as maintenance therapy. Persistent nocturnal symptoms such as cough or wheeze may be helped by the night-time use of long-acting theophylline.

Care must be taken when prescribing theophylline. The clearance of theophylline is affected by many factors, including cigarette smoking, viral pneumonia, heart failure, and concurrent drug treatment (see Chapter 23).

The side-effects of theophylline occur at variable serum concentrations in most people, and may even occur at therapeutic concentrations in some.

Nebulized bronchodilators

Although most patients will benefit from standard dose bronchodilators, a few with severe disease will require the higher doses that only a nebulizer can deliver. Nebulizer therapy should only be prescribed after a patient has been assessed as outlined in Table 24.6. Dosage regimens should be tailored to individual patients needs.

Corticosteroids

A therapeutic trial of corticosteroids should be tried in patients with COPD whose condition is clinically stable and who are already on maximal bronchodilator therapy. It is difficult to predict which patients will benefit from steroid therapy. Patients should be given oral steroids (for example, 30 mg of prednisolone every morning) for 2 weeks. Lung function tests should be performed together with patient records of peak flow measurements, exercise tolerance and a diary of symptom frequency and severity. Maintenance steroids should be prescribed subsequently if both subjective and objective measurements are improved, for example a 20–25% increase in lung function tests.

If a patient benefits from the trial of steroids, inhaled steroids should ideally be used as maintenance treatment although only about 50% of patients who respond to oral

---

Table 24.6 Assessment of a patient for nebulized therapy at home

- Assess hand-held inhaler technique to ensure current inhaler choice is optimal for that patient
- Assessment by specialist to confirm diagnosis and review current treatment options
- Trial treatment with an oral steroid, if not already done
- Trial of high dose bronchodilator (e.g. 400 micrograms salbutamol and 160 micrograms ipratropium bromide four times a day), to assess effectiveness
- Formal trial of a home nebulizer (e.g. 2.5–5 mg salbutamol or 250–500 micrograms ipratropium bromide, singly or together)
- Patient to monitor the best of three peak expiratory flow rate measurements twice a day, morning and evening, before treatment and for a minimum of 1 week on each treatment – average peak flow should be calculated from at least five days recordings
- Monitor patient's treatment response over a period of at least 2 weeks
- Subjective and objective assessment of benefit from inhaler by patient and doctor

steroids also respond to inhaled steroids. For the transition from oral to inhaled therapy, the oral steroids should be gradually tailed off and inhaled treatment started. For example, beclometasone 200–500 micrograms should be given twice daily initially, increased to 1500 micrograms when oral therapy has been stopped. At high inhaled doses (above 1500–2000 micrograms of beclometasone), side-effects such as adrenal suppression are possible. The longer-term effect of this therapy on the rate of decline of lung function has been questioned (Vestbo et al 1999) and further study is required to define the exact place of corticosteroid therapy in COPD.

Ideally, only if maximal inhaled doses fail to control symptoms should oral steroids be used. These must be used in the smallest dose possible to minimize long-term adverse effects and should be used in conjunction with inhaled steroids.

Treatment for dyspnoea

Some patients with COPD, particularly those with emphysema, have severe breathlessness that does not respond to the conventional treatment. Such patients may benefit from low-dose opioids. Methadone and diamorphine have been used, but any opioid can be tried. These reduce the respiratory drive and perception of dyspnoea and will reduce oxygen consumption at rest and on exercise. This therapy requires close monitoring of arterial blood gases and should not be used if hypercapnia exists.

Acute exacerbations of COPD

Acute exacerbations of airflow limitation can occur in any patient with COPD. These exacerbations can be spontaneous but are often precipitated by infection and lead to respiratory failure with hypoxaemia and retention of carbon dioxide. Many patients can be managed at home but some will require admission to hospital.

Bronchodilators

Bronchodilatation is required using a β_2 agonist given by nebulization, for example salbutamol 2.5 mg, 4–6 hourly, and if necessary intravenously. The addition of a nebulized anticholinergic agent may be beneficial, depending on the clinical condition of the patient. Antibiotics and high-dose steroids may also be required if the patient does not respond to bronchodilator therapy.

Antibiotics

Antibiotics have only been shown to be effective if two or more of the following three factors are present:

1. increased breathlessness
2. increased sputum volume
3. development of purulent sputum.

Antibiotics are also given to all patients with acute on chronic respiratory failure.

The choice of antibiotic should be dependent on local policy, sensitivity patterns and any previous treatments. Amoxicillin or oxytetracycline are generally suitable as first-line agents, with a broad-spectrum cephalosporin or a macrolide reserved for more severe exacerbations.

Other treatment

If intravenous aminophylline is considered, the loading dose and maintenance dose required should be carefully chosen as these depend on various factors (see Chapter 23).

Oxygen therapy is necessary to improve hypoxia. In patients with a hypoxic drive, the administration of high concentration oxygen will cause a fall in ventilation, carbon dioxide retention and respiratory acidosis. A maximum concentration of 24% oxygen is therefore used.

Corticosteroids are rarely needed for patients with acute exacerbations managed in community settings. For these patients, and for those admitted to hospital, criteria have been suggested for starting corticosteroids:

- the patient is already taking oral corticosteroids
- there is a previously documented reponse to oral corticosteroids
- the airflow obstruction fails to respond to an increase in bronchodilator dosage
- this is the first presentation of airflow obstruction.

In either case oral steroids, such as prednisolone 30 mg every morning, are given for 7–14 days, then stopped after the acute episode.

During an acute attack, pyrexia, hyperventilation and the excessive work of breathing can result in an inability to eat or drink and thus lead to dehydration. Intravenous hydration is usually given, and any inspired gases administered are humidified. Care must be taken to avoid fluid retention, especially if pulmonary oedema is present.

Chest physiotherapy is employed to mobilize secretions, promote expectoration and expand collapsed lung segments.

A respiratory stimulant (analeptic) can be tried in patients with acute respiratory failure, carbon dioxide retention and depressed ventilation. These are non-specific central nervous system stimulants. The drug of choice is doxapram, which stimulates the respiratory and vasomotor centres in the medulla. Doxapram increases the depth of breathing and may slightly increase the rate of breathing. Arterial oxygenation is usually not improved because of the increased work of breathing induced by doxapram. This agent has a narrow therapeutic index, and side-effects such as arrhythmias, vasoconstriction, dizziness and convulsions. Doxapram is used as a continuous infusion at a rate of 1–4 mg per minute. The patient's arterial blood gases and blood pH must be monitored during treatment to allow correct dosage adjustment. Doxapram may be harmful if used when the Pa_{CO_2} is normal or low, and should be used with care in patients with epilepsy, hypertension, coronary artery disease or those taking monoamine-oxidase inhibitors.

Doxapram will generally tide a patient over until the underlying cause is determined and controlled. If the patient's condition still does not improve, assisted ventilation may be considered.

Treatment of cor pulmonale

COPD is responsible for over 90% of cases of cor pulmonale. Treatment of cor pulmonale is symptomatic and involves managing the underlying airways obstruction, hypoxaemia and any pulmonary oedema that develops. Peripheral oedema is managed by using thiazide or loop diuretics. Plasma aldosterone concentrations are often raised in chronic hypoxaemia and hypercapnia, and the patient with resistant oedema may benefit from spironolactone. Alternatively an angiotensin-converting enzyme inhibitor may be tried. Oxygen is used to treat hypoxaemia, and this should also promote a diuresis.

Domiciliary oxygen therapy

The use of oxygen should be regarded as a drug therapy. The aim of therapy is to improve oxygen delivery to the cells, increase alveolar oxygen tension and decrease the work of breathing to maintain a given Pa_{O_2}. Domiciliary oxygen therapy can be given in two ways:

Intermittent administration. Intermittent administration is used to increase mobility and capacity for exercise and to ease discomfort. Intermittent administration is of most benefit in patients with emphysema.

Continuous long-term oxygen therapy (LTOT). LTOT for at least 15 hours per day has been shown to improve survival in patients with severe, irreversible airflow obstruction, hypoxaemia and peripheral oedema (Medical Research Council Working Party 1981). The prescribing of LTOT must be according to Department of Health guidelines (Table 24.7). One of the aims of treatment is to achieve a Pa_{O_2} of at least 8 kPa without causing a rise in Pa_{CO_2} of more than 1 kPa, achieved by adjusting the oxygen flow rate. Before selecting patients for LTOT, each individual must also be assessed with respect to age, quality of life and smoking habits. Patients who smoke are a fire risk if they use LTOT.

Moreover, the carbon monoxide present in tobacco smoke binds to haemoglobin and forms carboxy-haemoglobin, which decreases the amount of oxygen that can be transported by the blood and will partially or completely negate the beneficial effects of LTOT.

Oxygen can be prescribed as oxygen cylinders but 15 hours per day at 2 l/minute requires 10 'F' size (1340 litre) cylinders a week. A more convenient system is to use a concentrator, which converts ambient air to 90% oxygen using a molecular sieve. The concentrator is sited in a well-ventilated area in the home with plastic tubing to terminals in rooms such as the living room and bedroom. Tubing from the terminals delivers oxygen to the patient, who wears a mask or uses the more convenient nasal prongs. This tubing should be long enough to allow some mobility.

Patient care

Pulmonary rehabilitation

Patients should participate in a coordinated programme of non-pharmacological treatment with support from all members of the health care team. This should include: advice and support on stopping smoking; nutritional assessment; aerobic exercise training to increase capacity and endurance for exercise; breathing retraining, for example diaphragmatic and pursed lips breathing to improve the ventilatory pattern and improve gas exchange; and psychological support because COPD patients often have decreased capacity to participate in social and recreational activities and can become anxious, depressed or fatigued. Pulmonary rehabilitation programmes that include at least 4 weeks' exercise training have been shown to improve dyspnoea and the patient's COPD control. These benefits were greater than those seen with bronchodilators. However, the long-term effect of these programmes has yet to be

---

Table 24.7 Department of Health guidelines for prescribing long-term oxygen

1. Absolute indication: COPD with Pa_{O_2} < 7.3 kPa, Pa_{CO_2} > 6.0 kPa, FEV_1 < 1.5 l, FVC < 2.0 l and oedema

   Measurements should be made with stable disease on at least two occasions, 3 weeks apart, with all reversible factors, e.g. reversible airways disease, fully treated

2. Relative indication: as in (1) with hypoxaemia but without hypercapnia or oedema

3. Palliative use: in other severe hypoxaemic lung disease

4. Palliation of chronic respiratory failure

established (Lacasse et al 1996), although personalized education to COPD patients about their condition has been shown to reduce their need for health services (Tougaard et al 1992).

Stopping smoking

Government advertising has alerted smokers to the health hazards involved with smoking. To give up smoking, which has been described as a form of drug addiction, requires self-motivation. The reported success rates of different anti-smoking methods have varied from 10% to 30%. Members of the health care team can educate smokers about the dangers and actively encourage and motivate those who want to give up.

Use of inhaled therapy

For those patients with obstructive airways disease with a degree of reversibility, the correct use of inhaled therapy is a vital part of overall management.

Medication counselling needs to highlight the modes of action of the bronchodilators, particularly the more rapid onset of the β_2 agonists to relieve breathlessness rather than the slower-acting anticholinergics. If inhaled steroids are prescribed, the importance of regular administration must be stressed.

The incorrect use of any inhaler will lead to sub-therapeutic dosing. The correct use of inhalers is, therefore, as vital in the management of obstructive airways disease patients as it is for patients with asthma

(see Chapter 23). The advantages and disadvantages of each type of inhaler device are summarized in Table 24.8.

Home nebulizer therapy

Patients who are prescribed nebulizer therapy for use at home should be counselled appropriately (Table 24.9).

Domiciliary oxygen therapy

Studies have shown that only about 50% of patients on LTOT comply with the requirement for 15 hours of treatment a day. Counselling will be required to persuade the patient to comply with this minimum figure. Emphasis must be given to the improvement in quality of life gained from treatment rather than the idea of being continually 'tied' to the oxygen supply.

The long-term, chronic nature of COPD may leave a patient with a fear of exercise as this will cause dyspnoea (breathlessness). Thus the patient with COPD may decide not to undertake any exercise. Mobility should be encouraged but is limited by the need to use domiciliary bottled oxygen or oxygen concentrators. Portable oxygen cylinders can be used to increase exercise tolerance during walking. If an oxygen concentrator is used, limited mobility can be gained by installing at least two terminals for the unit (usually in the living room and bedroom) with long tubing between the terminal and nasal prongs.

Portable cryogenic liquid oxygen units are also available. These are refilled from a larger reservoir system kept in the patient's home.

Table 24.8 **Comparison of inhaler devices**

Inhaler type	Compact	Hand–lung coordination required	Easy to use	Reduces oropharynx deposition
MDI	+	+	–	–
MDI + small spacer	+	±	±	+
MDI + large spacer	–	–	±	+
Breath-actuated MDI	+	–	+	–
Dry powder	+	–	±	–
Breath-actuated dry powder	+	–	+	–
Nebulizer	–	–	±	–

MDI, metered-dose inhaler; +, feature present; ±, feature present for some patients; –, feature absent.

Table 24.9   Practical points on using home nebulizers (British Thoracic Society 1997)

Equipment and administration

- Gas source should be from a home compressor or from a compressed air cylinder
- Oxygen should be used as the driving gas for asthma patients and air for COPD patients
- A gas flow rate of 6–8 l/min is usually used to nebulize 50% of the particles to 2–5 μm in diameter to aid deposition into the small airways
- If a nebulizer only leaves around 0.5 ml fluid after nebulization (residual volume) then the nebulizer should be initially filled with 2–2.5 ml. If the nebulizer has a greater residual volume, then 2–4.5 ml should be used initially
- β_2 agonists and ipratropium nebulizer solutions can be mixed together

Ten minutes should be sufficient for nebulization (antibiotics and steroids may take longer)

Patient counselling

- Patients should be advised at what point in their treatment they should call for medical help
- Use a mask for babies and young children with coordination difficulties, and for acutely ill patients when holding a nebulizer is tiring
- Use a mouthpiece for nebulized steroids, nebulized antibiotics (with a filter), and for anticholinergic drugs in patients with glaucoma
- Drugs should only be put into the nebulizer immediately before use
- Disposable nebulizer chambers should last for up to 3 months.
- The nebulizer chamber should be emptied after each use, and washed at least once a day in warm water with a little detergent

CASE STUDIES

Case 24.1

Mr L. P. is a 65-year-old ex-ship builder who has smoked 20 cigarettes a day for the past 40 years. He has had a chronic cough for the past 6 years, often producing grey sputum. He is overweight and occasionally becomes breathless.

Mr L. P. was admitted to hospital with increasing breathlessness, wheeze and a productive cough. His sputum was thick and green and he had a temperature of 39°C. His present medication includes:

- **salbutamol + ipratropium combined inhaler 2 puffs four times a day**
- **beclometasone inhaler 500 micrograms twice a day**
- **Aminophylline slow release tablets 225 mg twice a day.**

Questions

1. What is the probable diagnosis for this patient, and what factors lead to this answer?
2. Does this patient require antibiotic therapy? If so what would you recommend and why?
3. What other measures could be used to prevent further exacerbations?

Answers

1. Mr L. P. has acute-on-chronic bronchitis because his sputum has turned from grey to green; he has increased breathlessness, a productive cough and a raised temperature. The features of chronic bronchitis include the presence of a chronic cough, the production of grey sputum and occasional breathlessness. Other features of Mr L. P. that are characteristic of chronic bronchitis are that he smokes and is overweight. Smoking is one of the most important risk factors for the development of chronic bronchitis. The degree of risk depends on the cumulative dose or the number of pack-years. Mr L. P. has been smoking 20 cigarettes a day for 40 years, which is equivalent to 40 pack years.

2. Mr L. P. requires antibiotics because he has increased breathlessness and has developed green sputum. The most likely bacterial causes are *Haemophilus influenzae*, *Streptococcus pneumoniae* or *Moraxella catarrhalis*. Sometimes infection can be caused by *Chlamydia pneumoniae*. Acute bronchitis may also be caused by a viral infection, which would not be treated with antibiotics.

   The antibiotic of choice will depend on local guidelines but needs to cover the above organisms. A suitable first-line agent would be amoxicillin or erythromycin. Amoxicillin does not cover all *Haemophilus influenzae* infections and so co-amoxiclav may be a good alternative, especially if β-lactamase organisms are present. Erythromycin is usually kept for patients allergic to penicillin. It has a high incidence of gastrointestinal side-effects and so newer macrolides such as clarithromycin or azithromycin may be preferred. Ciprofloxacin is a particularly effective treatment for pneumococcal infections but should be kept as a second-line agent.

   Another factor to be considered is the extent to which the antibiotic penetrates the sputum. Commonly the amount of penetration reduces as COAD tissue damage progresses. β-lactam antibiotics such as amoxicillin only reach sputum concentrations of approximately 5–20% of those in serum. Erythromycin usually reaches a concentration sufficient to treat streptococcal infections, but higher concentrations may sometimes be needed to treat *Haemophilus influenzae* infections. In order to obtain sufficient concentrations of antibiotics in the sputum, intravenous therapy may be required in patients with severe exacerbations or those unable to take medication orally.

3. Immunization with pneumococcal and influenza vaccines may prevent acute infective exacerbations of bronchitis, particularly in the elderly. However, there have been no specific studies into the value of pneumococcal vaccine in patients with COPD to date, and so it is not routinely recommended.

The risk of persistent or repeated infections is high, particularly in patients with bronchiectasis. These patients may sometimes be given prophylactic antibiotics daily to prevent acute infections. Antibiotics may be given in rotation so as not to become resistant to one particular drug. The antibiotics chosen will depend on local policies and local bacteriological sensitivity data.

COPD patients may also be given a supply of antibiotics to keep at home. Patients are told to start taking the antibiotics at the onset of an infection, to prevent treatment delay.

Case 24.2

Mr A. G. is a 56-year-old mechanic with chronic emphysema. He has had two admissions to hospital in the past year due to chest infections. Mr A. G. enters your community pharmacy and asks for advice on the best way to give up smoking. He usually smokes 20 cigarettes a day and has been doing so for the past 40 years.

Questions

1. Why is it important for Mr A. G. to give up smoking?
2. What smoking cessation products are currently available both over the counter and on prescription?
3. What benefits and problems are associated with the various products available?

Answers

1. It is very important for Mr A. G. to give up smoking, as it is a major risk factor for chronic obstructive pulmonary disease (COPD). Smoking is the single greatest cause of preventable illness and early death in the UK and each year causes over 120 000 deaths. Stopping smoking is the single most important way of affecting a patient's outcome at all stages of COPD. Mr A. G. should be told that stopping smoking will not prevent the onset of heart disease but that it will 'reduce the odds' for him personally. Stopping smoking now will not have an immediate effect: a reduction in COPD mortality is not seen until about 10 years or more after cessation of smoking. Giving up smoking will slow down the gradual decline in FEV_1 that is seen in smokers, and the onset of disability from COPD may be postponed by 10–15 years.

Motivation from the patient is the key to giving up smoking. Nicotine replacement will help about 15% of smokers who are motivated to give up, but the relapse rate is about 50% at 1 year. Smokers need both initial advice from all health care professionals and also follow-up support. For example, especially in the early stages, symptoms such as coughing increase after the cigarettes are stopped. The patient must be closely supported to avoid a return to the habit.

2. There are several types of nicotine replacement therapy available to the patient, including gum, patches, nasal spray, inhaler, lozenges and sublingual tablets. Also available on prescription is the drug amfebutamone (bupropion).

British Thoracic Society guidelines recommend that health professionals should ask about smoking at every opportunity, advise all smokers to stop, assist cessation by advising on nicotine replacement therapy and refer patients to a specialist smoking cessation service if necessary (Raw et al 1999, COPD Guidelines Group 1997).

Nicotine replacement therapy (NRT) approximately doubles smoking cessation rates compared with controls (either placebo or no nicotine replacement therapy), irrespective of the intensity of adjunctive therapy. There is little research comparing the relative effectiveness of nicotine replacement therapy products, but all seem to have similar success rates. Choice of product should be made on the number of cigarettes smoked (irrespective of the nicotine content), the smoker's personal preference and tolerance to side-effects. Certain products may be better suited to certain individuals, meaning that the patient is more likely to stick to the cessation programme. Sublingual tablets are the only NRT product to be licensed for use during pregnancy. Other NRT products may reasonably be used during pregnancy though, providing the fetal nicotine exposure is kept lower than if the mother continued to smoke (Israel 1999).

Nicotine patches

These are considered to be most suitable for people who smoke regularly through the day. The 24-hour patch that is worn overnight is considered to be better for people who crave nicotine first thing in the morning, whereas the 16-hour patch may be better for people who experience vivid dreams when using the 24-hour patch. The main side-effect is skin irritation and so patches may not be the ideal form of NRT for people with skin problems or allergies to adhesive tape.

Nicotine gum

It is very important to chew correctly when using nicotine gum. It is advised that the gum should be chewed slowly until the taste becomes strong and then allowed to rest between the cheek and teeth to allow absorption. When the taste has faded the gum should be chewed again. Nicotine gum is therefore not a good choice for people with dentures or other vulnerable dental work.

Nicotine inhaler

This method of NRT may be particularly useful for people who miss the physical act of smoking. Its main side-effect is local irritation to the throat and mouth, so it should be used with caution in patients with asthma.

Nicotine nasal spray

This is most useful for people who smoke 20 or more cigarettes per day. Nasal and sinus irritations are common side-effects and so it is not recommended for people with nasal or sinus conditions, allergies or asthma.

Nicotine sublingual tablets

These tablets dissolve under the tongue and so may be useful for people with dentures who have difficulty using nicotine gum. This is a particularly discreet form of NRT.

Amfebutamone (bupropion)

Originally used as an antidepressant, this drug has been licensed for use in smoking cessation. It is thought to work first because depression and anxiety are symptoms of nicotine withdrawal and second because it may increase the levels of the central neurotransmitters dopamine, serotonin and noradrenaline (norepinephrine) which seem to be depleted by smoking. Treatment should be started while the patient is still smoking and a target stop date set during the second week. Treatment should then be continued for 7–9 weeks, initially at a dose of 150 mg daily for 6 days, increasing to 150 mg twice a day thereafter.

Clinical trials have compared amfebutamone with placebo, a nicotine patch and a combination of both. It was found that the use of amfebutamone alone resulted in significantly higher long-term rates of smoking cessation than the use of either a nicotine patch alone or placebo. Combining amfebutamone with a nicotine patch produced even more successful results, although they were not statistically significant.

Amfebutamone should not be used in patients with a current or previous seizure disorder or in patients with bulimia, anorexia nervosa, bipolar disorder or severe hepatic cirrhosis. Amfebutamone inhibits cytochrome P450 enzymes and so may inhibit the metabolism of other drugs. The main side-effects experienced include dry mouth, insomnia, headache, dizziness, rash and taste disorders.

Other methods

Other non-nicotine methods of cessation include hypnosis, acupuncture, clonidine and lobeline although most have little evidence of efficacy other than a placebo effect. Clonidine is not recommended as first-line treatment due to the high incidence of side-effects and lobeline is now not recommended due to inadequate evidence of efficacy.

Mr A. G. should, therefore, be offered accurate information on all available smoking cessation therapies so that he can decide on the best method for him personally.

Case 24.3

Mr G. M., a 50-year-old farmer, and has suffered with 'a touch of asthma' for 10 years for which he uses a salbutamol metered dose inhaler as necessary. He currently smokes 25 cigarettes a day and has done so for 35 years. He has been noticing a progressive increase in his coughing over the past 5 years, which his salbutamol no longer seems able to control. He now becomes breathless walking to nearby shops and is regularly coughing up sputum. He has only now visited his GP, not having wanted to bother her before.

His GP diagnoses moderate chronic obstructive pulmonary disease (COPD). As he seems to be failing to respond to inhaled bronchodilators, she refers him to the local hospital for a corticosteroid reversibility test.

Questions

1. What are the main differences between asthma and COPD?
2. What is a corticosteroid reversibility test, when should one be preformed, and how are the results interpreted?

3. If corticosteroids are beneficial, what formulation should be prescribed?
4. How can the usefulness of bronchodilators be assessed in COPD patients?

Answers

1. Both asthma and COPD may present with similar symptoms. Both have been associated with cough, breathlessness and wheezing. COPD patients are breathless and wheezy mainly on exertion and do not have the nocturnal attacks of wheezing or breathlessness at rest that are seen in asthmatic patients. Asthmatics generally only cough occasionally whereas the cough of COPD patients tends to be persistent. Sputum production is regular in COPD but occassional in asthma.

2. Corticosteroid reversibility tests should be performed in all COPD patients with moderate or severe disease and in those with mild disease who are using inhaled bronchodilators more than once a day. A course of oral prednisolone 30 mg every morning for 2 weeks is taken. The spirometric test FEV_1 is performed before and at the end of the steroid course. Alternatively an inhaled steroid such as beclometasone 500 micrograms twice a day can be taken for 6 weeks.

   A rise in FEV_1 that is greater than 200 ml and 15% more than the pre-test level is accepted as a significant response. This is generally seen in about 10–20% of COPD patients and indicates that steroid therapy is worthwhile.

3. Patients who show an objective response to corticosteroids should be prescribed inhaled steroids as first choice therapy. Patients can be managed on inhaled steroids according to the same criteria for dosage adjustment as asthma patients. The equivalent of up to beclometasone 1000 micrograms per day can be used. Oral steroids may confer some extra benefit over inhaled steroids in the short term but there is no evidence for a longer-term benefit. One factor that must be taken into account when assessing the risks of steroids is that patients with COPD are generally at higher risk of osteoporosis, mainly due to their age, inactivity and tobacco intake.

4. Reversibility tests to bronchodilators should be performed at all stages of COPD. The objectives of these tests are:

   - to detect those patients whose FEV_1 increases substantially and are thus really asthmatic
   - to establish the post-bronchodilator FEV_1 which is the best predictor of long-term prognosis.

   The test should measure the FEV_1:

   - before and 15 minutes after 2.5–5 mg nebulized salbutamol
   - before and 30 minutes after 500 micrograms nebulized ipratropium bromide
   - before and 30 minutes after both salbutamol and ipratropium bromide in combination.

   Reversibility is said to have occurred if there is an increase in FEV_1 that is both greater than 200 ml and if there is a 15% increase over the pre-bronchodilator value that is greater than the natural variability of the FEV_1 (Quanjer 1993).

REFERENCES

British Thoracic Society 1997 Current best practice for nebuliser treatment. Thorax 52(Suppl.2): S1–S106

COPD Guidelines Group of the Standards of Care Committee of the British Thoracic Society 1997 British Thoracic Society guidelines for the management of chronic obstructive pulmonary disease. Thorax 52(Suppl.1): S1–S28

Israel M 1999 Smoking cessation. Pharm J 262: 226–228

Kerstjens H A M 1999 Clinical evidence: stable chronic obstructive pulmonary disease. British Medical Journal 319: 495–500

Lacasse Y, Wong E, Guyatt G H et al 1996 Meta-analysis of respiratory rehabilitation in chronic obstructive pulmonary disease. Lancet 348: 1115–1119

MacNee W 1999 Chronic obstructive pulmonary disease: causes and pathology. Medicine 27: 68–72

Medical Research Council Working Party, 1981 Long-term domiciliary oxygen therapy in chronic hypoxic cor pulmonale complicating chronic bronchitis and emphysema Lancet 1(8222): 681–686

Quanjer P H 1993 Standardized lung function testing: official statement of the European Respiratory Society. European Respiratory Journal 6(Suppl. 16): 5–40

Raw M, McNeill A, West R 1999 Smoking cessation: evidence based recommendations for the healthcare system. British Medical Journal 318: 182–185

Senior R M, Anthonisen N 1998 Chronic obstructive pulmonary disease. American Journal of Respiratory and Critical Care Medicine 157: S139–S147

Strauss E S, McAlister F A, Sackett D L et al 2000 The accuracy of patient history, wheezing, and laryngeal measurements in diagnosing obstructive airways disease. Journal of the American Medical Association 283: 1853–1857

Tougaard L, Krone T, Sorknaes A et al 1992 The PASTMA Group. Economic benefits of teaching patients with chronic obstructive pulmonary disease about their illness. Lancet 339: 1517–1520

Vestbo J, Sorensen T, Lange P et al 1999 Long-term effect of inhaled budesonide in mild and moderate chronic obstructive pulmonary disease: a randomised controlled trial. 353: 1819–1823

Drug-induced lung disease

25

N. P. Keaney

KEY POINTS

- The signs and symptoms of drug-induced lung disease may not be easily, distinguished from those of a naturally occurring illness.
- Antibiotics, particularly penicillins; are the drugs most often responsible for allergic bronchospasm.
- Aspirin and other non-steroidal anti-inflammatory drugs (NSAIDs) precipitate asthma via altered mediator synthesis. Individuals with this type of sensitivity can cross-react to tartrazine (E102).
- In asthmatics the hypersensitivity of the airways has paradoxically resulted in bronchoconstriction to a number of inhaled drugs, (e.g. sodium cromoglicate, beclometasone), due to excipients causing non-specific stimulation of bronchial mucosal irritant receptors.
- Cholinoceptor agonists such as pilocarpine eye drops can produce bronchoconstriction by a direct effect on bronchial smooth muscle.
- Angiotensin-converting enzyme (ACE) inhibitors (e.g. captopril, lisinopril) also inhibit proteases that inactivate kinins and other vasoactive peptides. ACE inhibitor induced cough has been ascribed to sensitization of non-myelinated nerve fibres in the airways by kinins.
- In patients with asthma, drugs with β adrenoreceptor blocking properties must be avoided even if applied topically (e.g. timolol eye drops).
- NSAIDs have been widely implicated as causative agents in hypersensitivity pneumonitis.
- Drug-induced pulmonary fibrosis is more reliably diagnosed than other parenchymal reactions, particularly with cytotoxic drugs such as bleomycin, busulfan, chlorambucil, cyclophosphamide and melphalan.
- The unique pharmacokinetic profile of amiodarone and its principal desethyl metabolite predisposes to chronic pneumonitis with fibrosis.

An adverse drug reaction (ADR) can involve the lung in a variety of ways, and the clinical presentation is mainly determined by the site of the damage. Thus the airways may be principally involved, as in an allergic reaction to penicillin; or the parenchyma of the lung may be the sole site of a chronic fibrotic reaction. The symptoms and signs of an ADR may not, therefore, be easily distinguished from those of a naturally occurring illness. Likewise, the changes in pulmonary function, as measured by spirometry or by the carbon monoxide transfer factor, and the radiological abnormalities seen on a chest radiograph are usually non-specific. A high index of suspicion is required if an ADR is to be diagnosed and, although respiratory toxicity is a recognized problem with drugs such as methotrexate, it can be very difficult to establish a cause and effect relationship without re-exposing the patient to one or more suspected drugs. Because of many uncertainties this is not a technique that is regularly used to confirm a suspected pulmonary ADR; for example, a chronic reaction may have so disabled a patient that the risk:benefit ratio is unfavourable or provocation of an asthma attack may cause a life-threatening situation. The role of all members of the health care team in the surveillance of ADRs is developing with the impact of clinical governance. For example, the monitoring of disease modifying anti-rheumatic drugs (DMARDs) by pharmacists is perceived as valuable by patients who are anxious to receive more information about the potential toxicity of their therapy.

Other dilemmas of drug rechallenge relate to the size and duration of dosage to ensure, on the one hand, that an ADR is identifiable and, on the other, that only a safe reaction occurs. In some circumstances rechallenge may not be necessary either because the ADR is merely an aspect of the therapeutic effect of a suspected drug, or an alternative is readily available, or because of previous reports of a similar ADR to the drug. ADRs are typically classified into those that are predictable on the basis of the known pharmacological action of the drug, and these are usually dose-related (augmented; type A). Those that are non-dose-related have been described as idiosyncratic in nature (bizarre; type B). Allergic (anaphylactic) reactions are defined as bizarre (type B), although in the airways some apparently allergic reactions – i.e. asthmatic reactions – may be due to a recognized non-allergic mechanism (Table 25.1). For most ADRs, however, the underlying mechanism is poorly understood, and the classification into type A and B reactions cannot be easily applied. For example, some pulmonary reactions to cytotoxic drugs, although unpredictable in any particular patient, in essence may be a direct consequence of some as yet unidentified action of the drug. It is convenient, therefore, to discuss induced lung disease on the basis of the respiratory structure affected and giving rise to the clinical syndrome characteristic for that site. Thus the bronchi and small airways, the parenchyma of the lung, the pulmonary circulation and the pleural space will be treated separately as far as possible. All the ADRs described below are infrequent or rare phenomena (except for cough with ACE inhibitors), and the descriptions of incidence, whether explicit or implied, should be read with that in mind.

Bronchi and small airways

Airflow obstruction

Local anaphylaxis in airways causes asthma due to the release of preformed and newly synthesized mediators and involves IgE and mast cells in immediate reactions and polymorph neutrophils, eosinophils, lymphocytes and platelets in late and sustained reactions. It is helpful to consider the various ways in which drugs may interact with the above processes as they modify the physiological control of the calibre of the airways (see Table 25.1).

Drugs as antigens

Antibiotics are the drugs most often responsible for allergic reactions. These reactions vary in severity, and acute asthma may be accompanied by systemic anaphylaxis or merely local cutaneous reactions with erythema. For penicillins, the group most commonly involved, there is almost always a history of uneventful exposure to a previous course of treatment. Fatal reactions seem to occur in patients with a recognized allergic predisposition such as asthma or a previous ADR to a penicillin. Sensitivity to penicillin is sometimes due to persisting impurities such as a

polyvalent penicilloyl antigen, and is sometimes due to the β-lactam itself. Identification of penicillin sensitivity by patch or prick skin testing is not reliable, and intradermal testing has been associated with fatality. As penicillin allergy may not be attributable to the β-lactam ring itself, it can be appreciated that cross-reactivity with another group of β-lactam antibiotics, the cephalosporins, is not an inevitable consequence of allergy to penicillin.

Direct release of mediators

Histamine can be released from mast cells by a number of drugs. This phenomenon is readily demonstrated by intradermal injection of morphine or quaternary ammonium compounds such as tubocurarine; also, in the clinical context, marked bronchoconstriction has been reported after intravenous injection of muscle relaxants. This latter group of drugs is used in conjunction with intravenous anaesthetic agents, which themselves can cause anaphylaxis. The combination of thiopental and suxamethonium was commonly implicated in anaesthetic ADRs affecting the airways. Individual patients often cross-react with other induction agents and relaxants, which means that an allergic process is unlikely. Direct release of mediators is probable with this combination of drugs and is clearly the mechanism for the high incidence of anaphylactoid reactions with the former intravenous anaesthetic agent Althesin (a combination of two steroids solubilized with polyoxyethylated castor oil, Cremophor EL). This surface-active agent effected disruption of the membrane of mast cells, with release of granules and mediators ensuing. The cytotoxic agents the Taxols are also formulated with Cremophor EL, and even with a slower rate of infusion there have been anaphylactoid reactions.

Table 25.1 Mechanisms whereby bronchospasm may occur as an adverse drug reaction

Site of reaction	Mechanism	Drug
Interaction with IgE	Drug as antigen	Penicillin, dextrans
Direct release of mediators	Displacement of histamine	Iodinated contrast media, quaternary amines
Altered mediator synthesis	Cyclo-oxygenase inhibition	Aspirin, NSAIDs
Reflex bronchoconstriction	Non-specific irritation	Dry powder propellant metabisulphite
Direct effect on smooth muscle	Agonist	Pilocarpine
Inhibit hydrolysis of mediator	Inhibition of enzyme	Neostigmine ACE inhibitor (cough)
Antagonism at β adrenoreceptors	Mast cell sensitization (?)	Timolol, propafenone
Agonists at β adrenoreceptors	Tolerance (genetic polymorphism)	Isoprenaline, fenoterol, salmeterol (?)

Iodinated intravenous radiological contrast media have been systematically studied, and in one survey the incidence of anaphylaxis was 1 in 14 000, accompanied in 12% of cases by severe bronchospasm. Individuals who are thought to be sensitive to contrast media can be tested with small intravenous doses. Pretreatment with an H_1 antagonist such as chlorphenamine (chlorpheniramine) may only be prophylactic in two-thirds of susceptible patients. Other drugs for which direct mediator release has been invoked include hydrocortisone sodium succinate, methylprednisolone and N-acetylcysteine. Using the phosphate salt of hydrocortisone, however, avoids this problem. Benzalkonium, which is incorporated as a preservative in a number of preparations, probably acts in the same way and, because of reports of bronchospasm, has been removed from solutions for administration by nebulization (e.g. ipratropium).

Altered mediator synthesis

Aspirin and other non-steroidal anti-inflammatory drugs (NSAIDs) can precipitate asthma in sensitive individuals. These attacks develop about half an hour after ingestion and are frequently accompanied by flushing and rhinorrhoea. Cross-sensitivity between aspirin and the many differently structured NSAID molecules argues against an allergic mechanism. One theory suggests that their common action as inhibitors of cyclo-oxygenase and prostaglandin synthesis creates an imbalance between bronchodilator and bronchoconstrictor prostanoids and leukotrienes, respectively, with both series deriving from the same precursor, arachidonic acid. Some individuals with this type of sensitivity to aspirin cross-react to the food colourant tartrazine (E102). About 10% of asthmatics have been estimated to be affected. A syndrome of late-onset asthma, nasal polyposis and intermittent attacks of rhinorrhoea, angio-oedema or urticaria has been reported. Extrinsic asthmatics are also susceptible. The severity of an attack is variable, but even mild asthmatics have been known to suffer a fatal reaction. A genetic predisposition may be relevant to familial clustering of cases but the expression of the abnormality is variable with challenge results positive in those unaware of any history and negative in a significant proportion of those reporting previous aspirin sensitivity. Interestingly, a refractory period occurs for 2–5 days after a reaction to aspirin or an NSAID during which rechallenge does not precipitate asthma. This phenomenon has been used to desensitize patients who must take the drug regularly to maintain the refractory state. Analgesia in this group of patients can be safely provided by the use of codeine or dihydrocodeine; paracetamol is without hazard for all but a very few. Evidence is emerging that novel cyclo-oxygenase (COX)-2 inhibitors may be used safely.

Reflex bronchoconstriction

The modern management of bronchial asthma utilizes the inhaled route of administration. In view of the hyperreactivity of the airways in asthmatics it should not be surprising that with a number of inhaled drugs bronchoconstriction may be brought about by a vagal reflex due to a non-specific stimulation of bronchial mucosal irritant receptors. This is especially problematic with dry powders. As an example of the need to overcome this side-effect the dry powder, sodium cromoglicate, administered via an inhaler, was formerly marketed as a combination formulation with isoprenaline, a bronchodilator with a rapid onset of action.

Wheeze following inhalation of beclometasone dipropionate is well recognized and may be of some concern if an allergic reaction is responsible. In one study the abnormal reaction could be prevented by prior inhalation of cromoglicate, suggesting that an allergic basis was possible. However, the patients had a similar response to a placebo inhaler containing propellant alone which suggested that a non-specific irritant action was the cause. A dry powder formulation of beclometasone (with lactose as a filler) or use of a multidose budesonide inhaler (with no filler) could be regarded as safe alternatives in this situation. The prior use of a bronchodilator would, of course, prevent this particular adverse drug reaction.

Paradoxical bronchoconstrictor reactions to inhaled ipratropium have been reported with the nebulizer solution and, as mentioned above, the preservative benzalkonium was implicated. However, the major factor in this adverse response was undoubtedly the hypotonicity of the solution. Unit-dose vials with an isotonic preservative-free sterile formulation have more or less eliminated this ADR. Sporadic reports are now likely to be due to non-specific irritation and involve metered-dose inhalers.

Direct effect on smooth muscle

Cholinoceptor agonists such as carbachol, pilocarpine (eye drops) and methacholine (bronchial challenge testing) have all been identified as causative agents that can aggravate asthma or produce unexpectedly severe bronchoconstriction.

Inhibition of mediator hydrolysis

Anticholinesterases such as neostigmine are used after general anaesthesia to reverse the effects of competitive muscle antagonists. Because of the risks of bradycardia and bronchospasm the muscarinic antagonist atropine is given simultaneously. Use of the novel antimuscarinic drug glycopyrronium failed to prevent such bronchospasm.

Angiotensin-converting enzyme (ACE) inhibitors such as captopril and lisinopril also inhibit other proteases such as those that inactivate bradykinin and other vasoactive peptides. The incidence of cough with this group of drugs has been reported to vary from 0.2 to 3%. This adverse effect has been ascribed to sensitization of non-myelinated nerve fibres in the airways by excess kinins. Modulation of the response can be effected by prostaglandins, for example the NSAID sulindac has been shown to prevent the induction of cough due to ACE inhibitors. There is conflicting evidence as to whether ACE inhibitors affect bronchial hyperreactivity, however, it is clear cough is very much more frequent as an ADR.

Antagonism at β adrenoceptors

Non-selective β-blockers given orally block the β adrenoceptors in the heart, peripheral vasculature, bronchi, pancreas and liver, etc. There may be some argument for using a selective β agonist such as atenolol, metoprolol or bisoprolol in a patient with reversible airflow obstruction due to chronic bronchitis and without asthma. In this situation one might expect the inhaled $β_2$ agonist would need to be administered in a large dose to overcome the bronchial $β_2$ blockade that occurs to some extent even with 'selective' $β_2$ blockers. The issue is not simply one of agonist/antagonist interaction as pharmacokinetic considerations must be borne in mind. The inhaled route of administration results in selective distribution of supramaximal doses of bronchodilator to the airways. The effect is most likely to be inhibited by a competitive β receptor antagonist towards the end of the expected duration of action, when the concentration of agonist will have declined substantially – i.e. after 3–4 hours. While it would appear appropriate to use a β agonist more frequently or to change to the anticholinergic agent ipratropium, the solution is really to avoid the use of oral β-blockers in susceptible patients. This recommendation is consistent with advice from the Committee on the Safety of Medicines. Nowadays there are many alternatives to β-blockers that can be used in the treatment of disorders such as hypertension and angina.

In asthmatic subjects there is an added risk to the use of a β-blocker, namely that acute severe bronchospasm may be precipitated. This can occur even with the low systemic concentrations achieved following topical application of timolol eye drops. The mechanism of this ADR is uncertain. It is unlikely to be due to simple antagonism of the bronchodilator activity of circulating adrenaline (epinephrine) or neurally released nor-adrenaline (norepinephrine). It may possibly relate to their effect on mast cells that are stablized in vitro by β agonists at physiological concentrations and it is of interest that pretreatment of asthmatic subjects with cromoglicate, which stabilizes mast cells, protects from bronchoconstriction induced by propranolol. One must be aware that some drugs may have β-blocking properties and can exacerbate asthma even though this may not be obvious at first sight. Examples of such agents include xamoterol, which was marketed for use in mild cardiac failure, and propafenone, a class IC antiarrhythmic drug.

Agonists at β adrenoceptors

The suggestion has been made in the past, and resurrected recently, that regular use of bronchodilators may result in a deterioration in the control of asthma. High doses of isoprenaline were implicated as the principal factor in the epidemic of sudden death from asthma that was recorded in a number of countries in the 1960s. This concern has been made all the more relevant by more recent epidemiological findings from New Zealand that attributed an increase in asthmatic mortality to self-treatment with nebulized high-dose β agonists. With isoprenaline it seemed likely that inadequate education of patients about the use of prophylactic and emergency steroid therapy was combined with an over-reliance on high doses of a non-selective β agonist bronchodilator. Similar arguments have been presented for the data from New Zealand, where fenoterol was the standard nebulized bronchodilator therapy for severe asthma.

Tolerance may develop in a proportion of patients who abuse high-dose inhaled isoprenaline. The indirect evidence is based on an increase in the duration of action seen in those who revert to using the drug appropriately. Experiments designed to test tolerance to high-dose salbutamol by establishing successive dose–response curves before, during and after chronic dosing with oral or inhaled β agonists have not consistently demonstrated tolerance either in asthmatic patients or volunteers. One possible explanation for the variation in these experiments is the recent finding of genetic polymorphism of β adrenoreceptors. People with one genotype show a propensity to develop functional tolerance. The discussion about the safety of β agonists has been further developed by evidence that regular bronchodilator therapy might itself result in a deterioration of asthma control even when prophylactic inhaled steroid therapy is constant. This concern has been related to the long acting β agonists salmeterol and formoterol that have a duration of bronchodilator action of up to 12 hours – i.e. they provide virtually constant stimulation of β adrenoceptors when taken twice daily. However, it is clear that combining either salmeterol with beclometasone or fluticasone or formoterol with budesonide improves the control of asthma as judged by lung function, exacerbation rate, symptoms and health-related quality of life. Many guidelines for the management of asthma recommend that an informed, motivated, self-monitoring patient using anti-inflammatory prophylactic therapy should use bronchodilators as required for symptomatic relief. For more symptomatic patients a long-acting bronchodilator should be added.

Lung parenchyma

Adverse drug reactions affecting the lung parenchyma can be broadly classified into acute and chronic reactions, reflecting hypersensitivity and fibrosis, respectively, as the predominant mechanisms of toxic response. Subacute reactions, intermediate between acute and chronic in their onset, also occur. Although there is little understanding of the processes underlying the aetiology and pathogenesis of these ADRs, certain clinical patterns are identifiable and the radiological manifestations have been clarified over the last 10 years by the introduction of high resolution computed tomography (HRCT). A 'ground glass' appearance on HRCT is indicative of alveolitis and usually predicts steroid responsiveness.

Hypersensitivity pneumonitis

In general, these acute reactions are of an allergic nature, have a dramatic clinical presentation, and demand urgent diagnosis and withdrawal of the offending agent. With early treatment the affected individual has an excellent chance of a complete recovery, particularly when methotrexate is used intermittently as a DMARD. However, when most patients develop a cough with breathlessness and wheezing, many probable causes are considered before this symptom complex is attributed to an ADR. Eosinophilia on a blood count is characteristic of allergy and a patchy bilateral infiltrate distributed peripherally on the chest radiograph should lead to a review of recent drug therapy. Such a presentation in an individual whose lungs have previously been normal and in whom infection has been excluded can be confidently identified as an ADR if the history reveals ingestion of a candidate drug. A diagnosis will usually be made on the grounds of high clinical suspicion, but further investigations will include pulmonary function testing with spirometry and measurement of the transfer factor for carbon monoxide. However, these results will merely show the type of defect and will not be diagnostic for an ADR. In recent years the technique of bronchoscopic bronchoalveolar lavage has been applied to these cases. It has proved possible to identify an increase in the cellular yield (pleocytosis) in hypersensitivity pneumonitis with eosinophilia and/or lymphocytosis in the fluid obtained. With more sophisticated facilities the pattern of various lymphocytic subtypes can be assessed

or an in vitro analysis of the transformation of lavaged lymphocytes can be performed and the effects of challenge with the suspected drug studied. Pleural effusions sometimes feature, and eosinophilia may be found in the pleural fluid or on pleural biopsy. The rapid onset of the symptoms will usually ensure the speedy withdrawal of the offending drug (usually by the patient), and it seems likely that many minor reactions are never reported. The probability of complete recovery is excellent, and the rate of improvement will be accelerated by systemic corticosteroid therapy. Drug-induced hypersensitivity pneumonitis is not a sufficiently frequent occurrence for trials of treatment to be compared. It seems logical to use a corticosteroid with a view to suppressing the inflammatory reaction and so prevent chronic inflammation that could progress to pulmonary fibrosis, a permanent injury.

Non-steroidal anti-inflammatory drugs (NSAIDs)

NSAIDs such as indometacin, azapropazone, diclofenac and ibuprofen are prominent among the drugs that are recognized as causing hypersensitivity pneumonitis. The NSAIDs are a group of drugs with a high risk of various ADRs, making it very important that they are prescribed for positive indications and that their continued use is kept under review. Experience with the novel COX-2 selective inhibitors is insufficient to be able to quantify this risk.

Gold

Parenteral gold (aurothiomalate) when used in the treatment of rheumatoid arthritis has also been found to cause acute breathlessness with bilateral 'alveolar' infiltrates on the chest radiograph. The symptoms can follow the second to the fifth or sixth injection. There is approximately a 50% chance of complete resolution if the gold treatment is discontinued. A genetic predisposition to this ADR is probable.

Sulfasalazine

Sulfasalazine is now widely used in the management of patients with rheumatoid arthritis. It too has been implicated as a cause of pulmonary eosinophilia although the majority of reports have related to its use in inflammatory bowel disease. The reaction is mostly related to the sulphonamide rather than the 5-aminosalicylate moiety (mesalazine).

Other drugs

Many other drugs have featured in sporadic reports of drug-induced pulmonary eosinophilia, especially antibiotics. Nitrofurantoin causes both acute pneumonitis (90% of cases) and, rarely, chronic pulmonary fibrosis. Nitrofurantoin is of particular interest as it resembles paraquat in its capacity to undergo cyclical reduction and oxidation. The reoxidation liberates a free electron and generates toxic O_2-radicals and reactive nitrofurantoin molecules that may act as a hapten. The acute reaction usually occurs after 4 weeks or so of continuous treatment although even more rapid reactions have been observed.

With cytotoxic drugs, acute reactions are uncommon. Methotrexate is implicated most often, but this reflects its higher usage compared with procarbazine, mitomycin, bleomycin or azathioprine, all of which have been associated with the development of a corticosteroid-responsive eosinophilic pneumonitis. Re-exposure to the offending drug is not recommended.

Pulmonary fibrosis

Drug-induced pulmonary fibrosis is an ADR that is somewhat more reliably diagnosed than other parenchymal reactions, particularly with cytotoxic drugs. For such drugs the cumulative dose, the patient's age, renal dysfunction, previous radiotherapy, oxygen administration and concurrent cytotoxic therapy have been implicated as predisposing factors. The antiarrhythmic agent amiodarone has also been frequently implicated as a cause of pulmonary fibrosis

Bleomycin

Bleomycin was found to cause pulmonary damage during early animal experiments. Nevertheless it was introduced into clinical practice and the predictability of this reaction led to its experimental use for research into mechanisms of toxicity. The high ambient oxygen tension in the lung facilitates the generation of superoxide radicals by bleomycin, and this effect also accounts for the risks of oxygen therapy mentioned above. A relationship between the cumulative dose of bleomycin and its toxicity becomes evident when more than 450 mg has been administered – below this dose toxicity occurs in 3–5% of patients, whereas at 450–550 mg and over 550 mg, incidences of 13% and 17%, respectively, have been observed (1 mg = 550 000 IU).

The clinical onset of the chronic pneumonitis/pulmonary fibrosis syndrome is usually insidious, with symptoms of malaise, dry cough, fever and breathlessness developing and progressing over a period of several weeks or months. The chest radiograph is usually abnormal with basal infiltrates initially and widespread infiltrates in more severely affected patients. HRCT is a more sensitive method of detecting pulmonary abnormalities. Pulmonary function testing may be abnormal in asymptomatic individuals with no radiological changes, yielding presumed prevalences of toxicity of 33% and 71% in two surveys. However, some of the effects attributed to bleomycin were minor and unlikely to be clinically deleterious, for example a 10% reduction in gas transfer occurred after the first dose of bleomycin in one study but did not decrease further.

The course of the pulmonary damage caused by bleomycin is variable. With mild disease the radiological changes may resolve over a period of 6–12 months if the drug is withdrawn, and symptoms may disappear. High-dose corticosteroid therapy in more severely affected patients has led to improvement. Mortality from bleomycin-induced pulmonary fibrosis ranges from 1% to 2% in large series to 10% in patients receiving 550 mg (550 000 IU). Despite this profile of toxicity, bleomycin is widely used in a variety of malignant tumours as it is often curative.

Busulfan

Pulmonary parenchymal damage caused by other cytotoxic drugs is regularly observed and reported in the literature. The alkylating agent busulfan has a low risk estimated at 4%, but autopsy studies have found a much higher incidence of abnormalities (46%) that had not been clinically evident during life. Chlorambucil, cyclophosphamide and melphalan are the subjects of sporadic reports of fibrotic ADRs involving the lung. In one bizarre incident, a pharmacist treated himself with melphalan because myelomatosis had been mentioned in a differential diagnosis. He died from progressive pulmonary fibrosis and did not have any disorder requiring cytotoxic therapy.

Carmustine

The nitrosoureas, especially carmustine, seem to be capable of causing a syndrome of delayed pulmonary fibrosis. Carmustine was usually used alone in primary cerebral malignant tumours, which rarely involve the lung. The attribution of a pulmonary ADR to this drug can therefore be made much more clearly and confidently in this circumstance than, for example, when multiple cytotoxic drugs are used for an intrathoracic tumour that is subsequently irradiated. For carmustine, high dosage is correlated with the early development of pulmonary fibrosis but the incidence of this ADR increases as survivors are followed up. In one series of 31 children treated with carmustine only 17 were cured of their tumour. Of these survivors, six died from pulmonary fibrosis (two within 3 years of treatment) and six of the remaining eight patients who could be traced were found to have evidence of severe fibrotic damage to the lungs with an active fibrotic process recognized up to 17 years after treatment.

Amiodarone

The antiarrhythmic drug amiodarone has an unusual pharmacokinetic profile due to its high lipid solubility. The parent drug and its principal desethyl metabolite have exceptionally low rates of elimination ($t_{1/2} > 45$–60 days) from huge volumes of distribution (5000 litres), resulting in concentrations in the lung 1000 times greater than in serum. This accumulation favours a direct toxic effect, and daily doses in excess of 400 mg for more than 2 months result in pulmonary toxicity in 6% of patients. A mortality rate of 10–20% is expected. Chronic pneumonitis with fibrosis is the usual toxic manifestation, and this can be readily diagnosed on transbronchial biopsy performed via a bronchoscope. Foamy alveolar macrophages seen on light microscopy contain dense lamellar cytoplasmic inclusions on electron microscopy, which are a consequence of pulmonary accumulation of phospholipid with amiodarone and desethylamiodarone and are seen even in the absence of clinical evidence of pneumonitis or fibrosis.

Up to 25% of patients with amiodarone-induced pulmonary damage may have 'organizing pneumonia', a steroid-responsive condition with characteristic histological features. This type of reaction is thought to have an immunological basis, and treatment with prednisolone is recommended for all patients in case some areas of pneumonitis are of this nature. This treatment should be continued for some months after withdrawal of amiodarone, because of its prolonged elimination half-life.

Amiodarone is heavily iodinated and increases the density of tissues, for example pulmonary opacities seen on HRCT can be ascribed to the toxicity of this drug from the radiological appearances. Oxygen therapy, for example during general anaesthesia, may aggravate pulmonary toxicity and in some instances precipitate respiratory failure in patients with subclinical amiodarone toxicity.

Pulmonary vasculature

Venous thromboembolism (VTE)

In the early 1960s there were many reports of venous thrombosis in association with the use of oral contraceptive agents. The sporadic reports were followed by many systematic surveys both retrospective and prospective that established a risk of venous thromboembolism (VTE) five to six times greater in women taking the contraceptive pill. Further studies related the risk to the dose of oestrogen, and despite a general dose reduction a small risk persists. In a prospective study of 17 000 married women aged between 25 and 39 years, 105 episodes of VTE occurred, the incidence (events per 1000 woman-years) being 0.43 in users and 0.06 in non-users of oral contraceptives. Of the certain or probable diagnoses, 71 were in postoperative patients and confined to current users of oral contraceptives. Further analysis suggests, however, that the risk of pregnancy and its associated incidence of VTE is such that a combined oral contraceptive should not be discontinued preoperatively. The use of a progestogen-only pill would undoubtedly carry less risk.

The implications of oestrogen in hormone replacement therapy (HRT) have been extensively examined in three recent studies, each of which has shown a two- to fourfold risk of thromboembolism with oestrogen only as well as with oestrogen/progestogen combinations. HRT is a purely preventive therapy, and so the risk/benefit relationships should be assessed, bearing in mind that in an older population of women factors such as gross obesity, previous venous thrombosis and/or a family history of venous thrombosis must be taken into account.

Pulmonary hypertension

About 30 years ago a small epidemic of pulmonary hypertension was identified, particularly in Switzerland. The problem seemed to be confined to countries where the appetite suppressant aminorex fumarate was marketed. The evidence for this ADR was circumstantial as no animal model was found that reproduced the syndrome. Withdrawal of the drug brought the epidemic to an end. Now sporadic cases associated with other anorectic drugs such as amfetamines, fenfluramine and, most recently, dexfenfluramine have been reported. Pulmonary hypertension, once initiated, usually progresses to a clinical syndrome characterized by increasing breathlessness, right-sided cardiac failure and sudden death. Pulmonary hypertension also follows severe or recurrent pulmonary thromboembolism, and is therefore linked with oestrogen therapy and the oral contraceptive. Intravenous drug abusers inject particulate matter, for example from crushed tablets, impaction of which in pulmonary arterioles may give rise to a clinical presentation typical of pulmonary embolism. Progression to severe pulmonary hypertension does occur, and corn starch, talc and microcrystalline cellulose have each been found in the lung on histological examination.

Eosinophilia/myalgia with L-tryptophan

In 1989 a new syndrome occurred typified by pain in muscles and a rash with cough and breathlessness being common. There was marked eosinophilia of peripheral blood, but even in the most breathless patients the chest radiograph looked surprisingly normal. Pulmonary hypertension was often found and was the cause of the respiratory distress. Treatment with an anti-inflammatory high-dose corticosteroid was rapidly beneficial.

The majority of patients were taking L-tryptophan as a 'health food' supplement, but subsequently cases were described from psychiatric clinics where L-tryptophan was prescribed for a depressive illness. The causative factor of this eosinophilia/myalgia syndrome is obscure. It is intriguing that such an adverse reaction should appear to be due to a naturally occurring amino acid. An individual producer of L-tryptophan was linked epidemiologically to many cases in the USA, and it has been suggested that an impurity, 1,1'-ethylene (bis)tryptophan, arising from the manufacturing process was the cause. While this may seem now only of historical interest, its relevance relates to a need for continued vigilance with over-the-counter medication.

Pulmonary vasculitis

Drug-induced pulmonary vasculitis is caused by an immune mechanism, for example, due to the presence of intravascular immune complexes formed when excess antigen (drug or metabolite) and antibody combine and are deposited on the vascular endothelium. The complement system is then activated, and the sequential changes set up an inflammatory reaction. The result is a vasculitis that produces different clinical manifestations, the pattern of which depends on the size and site of the blood vessels targeted by the immune complexes and on the persistence of the cellular response. Our understanding of these and other parenchymal reactions is limited by the absence of suitable animal models and the paucity of adequate histological evidence in most patients, so that many cases of pulmonary vasculitis will be overlooked.

Pulmonary vasculitis is frequently a capillaritis and the conventional diagnostic appearances associated with an arteritis will be absent. The involvement of capillaries weakens them and as they are largely unsupported by connective tissue, bleeding into the alveolar walls and alveoli occurs. If this diffuse alveolar haemorrhage is associated with glomerulonephritis and is of idiopathic aetiology it is called Goodpasture's syndrome. The diagnostic marker is a circulating antibody against the glomerular basement membrane (anti-GBM). Anti-GBM is not detected in drug-induced diffuse alveolar haemorrhage (with or without glomerulonephritis) due to penicillamine, aminoglutethimide, nitrofurantoin, amphotericin and cocaine smoking.

Pulmonary oedema

Non-cardiogenic pulmonary oedema or adult respiratory distress syndrome (ARDS) occurs as a consequence of increased pulmonary alveolar capillary permeability. Classically the air spaces in the lung become filled with a proteinaceous fluid. This ADR can be mistaken for left ventricular failure, from which it differs by having a normal cardiac size on chest X-ray (and a normal pulmonary venous 'wedge' pressure). Breathlessness and hypoxaemia may progress to respiratory failure. In 1880 Osler described pulmonary oedema as a complication of heroin abuse, and it still occurs in addicts. This particular ADR occurs with both intravenously and orally administered opiates. It has been reported after overdose of dextropropoxyphene and codeine and even with naloxone (although this drug is only likely to be given to patients who have already taken an opiate). Other drugs known to cause non-cardiogenic pulmonary oedema are listed in Table 25.2.

Pleural reactions

Pleural reactions, either effusions or fibrosis, may be associated with various parenchymal adverse drug reactions or may be an isolated finding. Bromocriptine,

Table 25.2 Drugs causing non-cardiogenic pulmonary oedema

Adrenaline (epinephrine)
Amitriptyline[a]
Antilymphocytic globulin
Aspirin
Codeine[a]
Dextropropoxyphene[a]
Diamorphine (heroin)
Hydrochlorothiazide
Indometacin
Interleukin-2
Methadone
Mono-octanoin
Ritodrine
Salbutamol
Terbutaline

[a]Adverse drug reaction described with overdose.

like methysergide, is an ergot derivative and, while both have been found to cause pulmonary fibrosis, an unusual feature of this ADR has been the presence of pleural effusions and/or pleural thickening. It is tempting to relate the reaction to an effect involving 5-hydroxy-tryptamine (5-HT) receptors, although which subtype is involved is unclear. Other drugs associated with pleural effusion are listed in Table 25.3, and at least six subgroups can be identified.

Table 25.3 Examples of drugs associated with pleural effusion and/or thickening

Drug	Association
Amiodarone	Parenchymal reaction
Cytotoxics	
Methotrexate	Pleuritic pain
Dantrolene	Eosinophilia
Nitrofurantoin	
L-Tryptophan	
Interleukin-2	
Bromocriptine	5-HT receptors (?)
Methysergide	
Pergolide	
Oesophageal sclerosants	Direct toxicity
Procainamide	Drug-induced systemic lupus erythematosus

FURTHER READING

Allen I, Cooper D Jun (eds) 1990 Clinics in Chest Medicine 11(1)

Camus Ph, Gibson G J 2002 Adverse pulmonary effects of drugs and radiation. In: Gibson J, Sterk P, Geddes D, Costabel U, Corrin B (eds) Respiratory medicine. Saunders, London

Foucher P, Biour M, Blayac J P et al 1997 Drugs that may injure the respiratory system. European Respiratory Journal 10: 265–279. Updated on the Internet: http://www.pneumotox.com

Keaney N P 1998 Respiratory disorders. In: Davies D M, Ferner R E, De Glanville (eds) Davies's textbook of adverse drug reactions. Oxford University Press, Oxford

White D A, Matthy R 1986 Drug induced pulmonary disease. American Review of Respiratory Diseases 133: 321–340, 488–505

Insomnia and anxiety 26

C. H. Ashton

KEY POINTS

- Hypnotic and anxiolytic drugs do not cure insomnia or anxiety but can provide useful short-term symptomatic treatment.
- Before starting symptomatic medication, the primary cause of insomnia or anxiety should be investigated and treated appropriately where possible.
- Hypnotic and anxiolytic drugs should only be used short term (2–3 weeks); long-term regular use leads to tolerance, dependence and other adverse effects.
- Long-term benzodiazepine users should be offered advice on withdrawal.
- If benzodiazepines are indicated, the smallest effective dose should be used. Start with small doses, increasing if necessary. Use half adult dose in elderly.
- Sleep hygiene, counselling and psychological methods are more appropriate than hypnotics as long-term treatment for patients with insomnia.
- Antidepressant drugs and psychological methods are more appropriate than anxiolytics in long-term treatment for anxiety disorders.
- Newer non-benzodiazepine hypnotics (such as zopiclone and zolpidem) have similar pharmacological and adverse effects to benzodiazepines, offer few advantages, and are more expensive.

Definitions and epidemiology

Insomnia and anxiety are among the commonest symptoms seen in general practice. Each can arise from a number of causes and often, though not always, they occur together. Insomnia refers to difficulty in falling asleep or staying asleep, or to lack of refreshment from sleep. Complaints of poor sleep increase with increasing age and are twice as common in women as in men (Morgan & Clarke 1997). Thus by the age of 50 years a quarter of the population are dissatisfied with their sleep, the proportion rising to 30–40% (two-thirds of them women) among individuals over 65 years.

Anxiety, a feeling of apprehension or fear, combined with symptoms of increased sympathetic activity, is a normal response to stress. A clinical problem may arise if the anxiety becomes severe or persistent, and interferes with everyday performance. Clinical subtypes of anxiety include panic disorder, agoraphobia, other phobias and generalized anxiety. The prevalence of such syndromes in the general population is about 10–20%, and there is a high rate of co-morbidity with depressive disorders (Judd et al 1998). The overall female to male ratio is nearly 2:1. The age of onset of most anxiety disorders is in young adulthood (twenties and thirties), although the maximum prevalence of generalized anxiety and agoraphobia-panic in the general population is in the 50–64 year age group.

Pathophysiology

Anxiety and insomnia reflect disturbances of arousal and/or sleep systems in the brain. These systems are functionally interrelated, and their activity determines the degree and type of alertness during wakefulness and the depth and quality of sleep.

Arousal systems

Arousal is maintained by at least three interconnected systems: a general arousal system, an 'emotional' arousal system and an endocrine/autonomic arousal system (Fig. 26.1). The general arousal system, mediated by the brainstem reticular formation, thalamic nuclei and basal forebrain bundle, serves to link the cerebral cortex with incoming sensory stimuli and provides a tonic influence on cortical reactivity or alertness. Excessive activity in this system, due to internal or external stresses, can lead to a state of hyperarousal as seen in anxiety and insomnia. Emotional aspects of arousal, such as fear and anxiety, are contributed by the limbic system which also serves to focus attention on selected aspects of the environment. There is evidence that increased activity in certain limbic pathways is associated with anxiety and panic attacks.

These arousal systems activate somatic responses to arousal, such as increased muscle tone, increased sympathetic activity, and increased output of anterior and posterior pituitary hormones. Inappropriate increases in autonomic activity are often associated with anxiety states; the resulting symptoms (palpitations, sweating, tremor, etc.) may initiate a vicious circle which increases the anxiety.

423

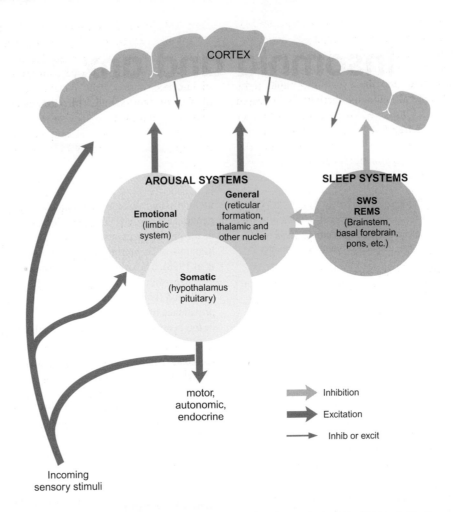

Figure 26.1 Diagram of arousal and sleep systems. Arousal systems receive environmental and internal stimuli, cause cortical activation, and mediate motor, autonomic and endocrine responses to arousal. Reciprocally connected sleep systems generate slow-wave sleep (SWS) and rapid eye movement sleep (REMS). Either system can be excited or inhibited by cognitive activity generated in the cortex.

Several neurotransmitters have been particularly implicated in arousal systems. Acetylcholine is the main transmitter maintaining general arousal, but there is evidence that heightened emotional arousal is particularly associated with increased noradrenergic and serotonergic activity. Drugs which antagonize such activity have anxiolytic effects. In addition, the inhibitory neurotransmitter γ-aminobutyric acid (GABA) exerts an inhibitory control on other transmitter pathways, and increased GABA activity may have a protective effect against excessive stress reactions. Many drugs which increase GABA activity are potent anxiolytics.

Sleep systems

At the other end of the arousal spectrum, the phenomenon of sleep is actively induced and maintained by neural mechanisms in several brain areas, including the lower brainstem, pons and parts of the limbic system. These mechanisms have reciprocal inhibitory connections with arousal systems, so that activation of sleep systems at the same time inhibits waking, and vice versa (see Fig. 26.1). Normal sleep includes two distinct levels of consciousness, orthodox sleep and paradoxical sleep, which are promoted from separate neural centres.

Orthodox sleep normally takes up about 75% of sleeping time. It is somewhat arbitrarily divided into four stages (1–4) which merge into each other, forming a continuum of decreasing cortical and behavioural arousal. Stages 3 and 4 are associated with increasing amounts of high-voltage δ slow waves (1–3 Hz) shown on the electroencephalograph (EEG). These latter stages represent the deepest level of sleep and are also termed slow-wave sleep (SWS).

Paradoxical sleep (rapid eye movement sleep, REMS) normally takes up about 25% of sleeping time and has quite different characteristics. The EEG shows unsynchronized fast activity similar to that found in the alert conscious state, and the eyes show rapid jerky movements. Peripheral autonomic activity is increased during REMS, and there is an increased output of catecholamines and free fatty acids. Vivid dreams and nightmares most often occur in REMS, although brief frightening dreams (hypnagogic hallucinations) can occur in orthodox sleep, especially at the transition between sleeping and waking. Figure 26.2 shows the normal distribution of sleep stages during the night: stage 4 sleep occurs mostly in the first few hours, while REMS is most prominent towards the morning. Brief awakenings during the night are normal. Both SWS and REMS are thought to be essential for brain function and both show a rebound after a period of deprivation, usually at the expense of lighter (stage 1 and 2) sleep which appears to be expendable.

Aetiology and clinical manifestations

Insomnia

Insomnia may be caused by any factor which increases activity in arousal systems or decreases activity in sleep systems. Many causes act on both systems. Increased sensory stimulation activates arousal systems, resulting in difficulty in falling asleep. Common causes include pain or discomfort and external stimuli such as noise, bright lights and extremes of temperature. Anxiety may also delay sleep onset as a result of increased emotional arousal.

Drugs are an important cause of insomnia. Difficulty in falling asleep may result directly from the action of stimulants, including caffeine, theophylline, sympathomimetic amines and some antidepressants.

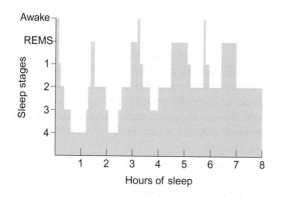

Figure 26.2 Diagram of normal sleep stages in young adults. (From Horne 1988.)

Drug withdrawal after chronic use of central nervous system depressants, including hypnotics, anxiolytics and alcohol, commonly cause rebound insomnia with delayed or interrupted sleep, increased REMS and nightmares. With rapidly metabolized drugs, such as alcohol or short-acting benzodiazepines, this rebound may occur in the latter part of the night, resulting in early waking. Certain drugs, including neuroleptics, tricyclic antidepressants and propranolol, may occasionally cause nightmares.

Difficulty in staying asleep is characteristic of depression. Patients typically complain of early waking, but sleep records show frequent awakenings, early onset of REMS, and reduced SWS. Alteration of sleep stages, increased dreaming and nightmares may also occur in schizophrenia, while recurring nightmares are a feature of post-traumatic stress disorder. Interference with circadian rhythms, as in shift work or rapid travel across time zones, can cause difficulty in falling asleep or early waking.

Frequent arousals from sleep are associated with myoclonus, 'restless legs syndrome', muscle cramps, bruxism (tooth-grinding), head banging and sleep apnoea syndromes. Reversal of the sleep pattern, with a tendency to poor nocturnal sleep but a need for daytime naps, is common in the elderly, in whom it may be associated with cerebrovascular disease or dementia.

Anxiety

Anxiety is commonly precipitated by stress, but vulnerability to stress appears to be linked to genetic factors such as trait anxiety, and many patients presenting for the first time with anxiety symptoms have a long history of high anxiety levels going back to childhood. Anxiety may also be induced by central stimulant drugs (caffeine, amphetamines), withdrawal from chronic use of central nervous system depressant drugs (alcohol, hypnotics, anxiolytics) and metabolic disturbances (hyperventilation, hypoglycaemia, thyrotoxicosis). It may form part of a depressive disorder and may occur in temporal lobe lesions and in rare hormone-secreting tumours such as phaeochromocytoma or carcinoid.

Apart from the psychological symptoms of apprehension and fear, somatic symptoms may be prominent in anxiety and include palpitations, chest pain, shortness of breath, dizziness, dysphagia, gastrointestinal disturbances, loss of libido, headaches and tremor. Panic attacks are experienced as storms of increased autonomic activity combined with a fear of imminent death or loss of control. If panics become associated with a particular environment, commonly a crowded place with no easy escape route, the patient may actively avoid similar situations and eventually become agoraphobic.

Investigations, differential diagnosis

Many patients complaining of insomnia overestimate their sleep requirements. Although most people sleep for 7–8 hours daily, some healthy subjects require as little as 3 hours of sleep, and sleep requirements decline with age. Such 'physiological insomnia' does not usually cause daytime fatigue, although the elderly may take daytime naps. If insomnia is causing distress, primary causes such as pain, drugs which disturb sleep, psychiatric disturbance including anxiety and depression, and organic causes such as sleep apnoea should be identified and treated before hypnotic therapy is prescribed. There is growing concern that daytime sleepiness resulting from insomnia increases the risk of industrial, traffic and other accidents (Balter & Uhlenuth 1992).

In patients presenting with symptoms and clinical signs of anxiety, it is important to exclude organic causes such as thyrotoxicosis, excessive use of stimulant drugs such as caffeine, and the possibility of alcoholism or withdrawal effects from benzodiazepines. However, unnecessary investigations should be avoided if possible. Extensive gastroenterological, cardiological and neurological tests may increase anxiety by reinforcing the patient's fear of serious underlying physical disease.

Treatment

Hypnotic drugs

Hypnotic drugs provide only symptomatic treatment for insomnia. Although often efficacious in the short term, they do little to alter the underlying cause which should be sought and treated where possible. Simple explanation of sleep requirements, attention to sleep hygiene, reduction in caffeine or alcohol intake, and the use of analgesics where indicated may obviate the need for hypnotics (Lader 1992). Behavioural techniques are sometimes helpful. Nevertheless, about 20 million prescriptions for hypnotics are issued each year in the UK, and these drugs can improve the quality of life if used rationally.

The ideal hypnotic would gently suppress all arousal systems while simultaneously stimulating the systems for deep and satisfying sleep. It would allow a natural return of normal sleep patterns and would be suitable for long-term use. Unfortunately, no such hypnotic exists; all presently available hypnotics are general central nervous system depressants which inhibit both arousal and sleep mechanisms. Thus they do not induce normal sleep and often have adverse effects including daytime sedation ('hangover') and rebound insomnia on withdrawal. They are unsuitable for long-term use because of the development of tolerance and dependence.

Benzodiazepines

By far the most commonly prescribed hypnotics are the benzodiazepines. A number of different benzodiazepines are available (Table 26.1). These drugs differ considerably in potency (equivalent dosage) and in rate of elimination but only slightly in clinical effects. All benzodiazepines have sedative/hypnotic, anxiolytic, amnesic, muscular relaxant and anticonvulsant actions with minor differences in the relative potency of these effects.

Pharmacokinetics. Most benzodiazepines marketed as hypnotics are well absorbed and rapidly penetrate the brain, producing hypnotic effects within half an hour after oral administration. Rates of elimination, however, vary, with elimination half-lives of from 6 to 100 hours (see Table 26.1). The drugs undergo hepatic metabolism via oxidation or conjugation, and some form pharmacologically active metabolites with even longer elimination half-lives. Oxidation of benzodiazepines is decreased in the elderly, in patients with hepatic impairment and in the presence of some drugs including alcohol.

Pharmacokinetic characteristics are important in selecting a hypnotic drug. A rapid onset of action combined with a medium duration of action (elimination half-life about 6–8 hours) is usually desirable. Too short a duration of action may lead to, or fail to control, early morning waking, while a long duration of action (nitrazepam) may produce residual effects the next day and may lead to cumulation if the drug is used regularly. However, frequency of use and dosage are important. For example, diazepam (5–10 mg) produces few residual effects when used occasionally, despite its slow elimination, although chronic use impairs daytime performance. Large doses of short-acting drugs may produce hangover effects, while small doses of longer-acting drugs may cause little or no hangover.

Effects on sleep. A major site of the hypnotic action of benzodiazepines is the brainstem reticular formation which, as mentioned above, is of central importance in arousal. The reticular formation is extremely sensitive to depression by benzodiazepines which decrease both spontaneous activity and responses to afferent stimuli. Similar depression of limbic arousal systems adds to hypnotic efficacy in patients with insomnia due to anxiety. However, active sleep mechanisms are also suppressed, and this effect leads to disruption of the normal sleep pattern.

Benzodiazepines are effective hypnotics: they hasten sleep onset; decrease nocturnal awakenings; increase total sleeping time; and often impart a sense of deep, refreshing sleep. However, they produce changes in the relative proportion of different sleep stages. Stage 2 (light

Table 26.1   Profile of some hypnotic drugs

Drug	Site of action	Elimination half-life (h)	Recommended hypnotic dose (mg)[a]
Benzodiazepines	GABA-BZ receptor		
Diazepam[b]		20–100 (36–200)[c]	5–10
Loprazolam		6–12	1
Lormetazepam		10–12	0.5–1.5
Nitrazepam		15–38	5–10
Temazepam		8–15	10–20
Non-benzodiazepines	GABA-BZ receptor		
Zaleplon		1	5–10
Zolpidem		2	10
Zopiclone		5–6	7.5
Chloral hydrate		(8)	500–1000
Clomethiazole		4	192–384
Antihistamines	Histamine (H_1) receptor		
Promethazine		17–34	25–50

BZ, benzodiazepine.
[a] Doses are recommended adult doses based on the *British National Formulary* (March 2001) and are approximately equivalent in hypnotic potency. Dosage should be reduced in the elderly.
[b] Diazepam, though classed as an anxiolytic drug, has useful hypnotic properties when administered as a single dose.
[c] Half-life of pharmacologically active metabolite shown in parentheses.

sleep) is prolonged and mainly accounts for the increased sleeping time. By contrast, the duration of SWS may be considerably reduced. REMS is also decreased (Fig. 26.3); the latency to the first REMS episode is prolonged and dreaming is diminished. This abnormal sleep profile probably arises because of the unselective depression of both arousal and sleep mechanisms. The suppression of REMS may be an important factor in determining rebound effects on drug withdrawal (see below).

Mechanism of action. Most of the effects of benzodiazepines result from their interaction with specific binding sites associated with postsynaptic $GABA_A$ receptors in the brain. All benzodiazepines bind to these sites although with varying degrees of affinity.

$GABA_A$ receptors are multimolecular complexes that control a chloride ion channel and contain specific binding sites for GABA, benzodiazepines and several other drugs, including non-benzodiazepine hypnotics and some convulsant drugs (Fig. 26.4).

The various effects of benzodiazepines (hypnotic, anxiolytic, anticonvulsant) probably result from GABA potentiation in specific brain sites, and some actions may result from secondary effects on other neurotransmitter systems. For example, a reduction in serotonergic activity may underlie the anxiolytic effects. In addition, different subtypes of benzodiazepine-binding sites may mediate more selective drug effects (Haefely 1990).

Adverse effects of hypnotic use

Tolerance. Tolerance to the hypnotic effects of benzodiazepines develops rapidly. Sleep latency, stage 2 sleep, SWS, REMS, dreaming and intrasleep awakenings all tend to return to pre-treatment levels after a few weeks of regular use. Nevertheless, poor sleepers may report continued efficacy, and the drugs are often used long term because of difficulties in withdrawal.

Rebound insomnia. Rebound insomnia, in which sleep is poorer than before drug treatment, is common on withdrawal of benzodiazepines. Sleep latency is prolonged; intrasleep wakenings become more frequent; and REMS duration and intensity is increased, with vivid dreams or nightmares which may add to frequent awakenings. These symptoms are most marked when the drugs have been taken in high doses or for long periods but can occur after only a week of low-dose administration. They are conspicuous with moderately rapidly eliminated benzodiazepines (temazepam, lorazepam) and may last for many weeks. With slowly eliminated benzodiazepines (diazepam), SWS and REMS may remain depressed for some weeks and then slowly return to the baseline, sometimes without a rebound effect. Tolerance and rebound effects are probably a reflection of down-

A Slow wave sleep

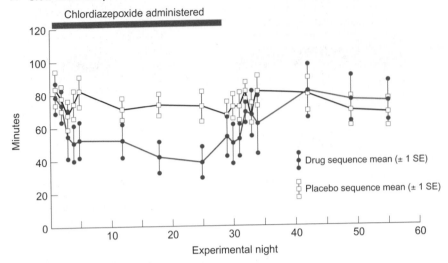

B Rapid eye movement sleep

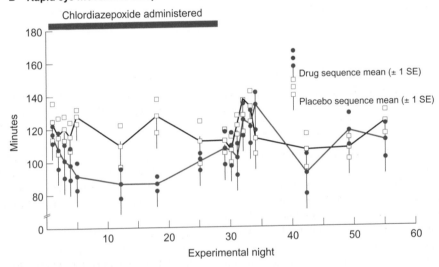

Figure 26.3 Effect of chlordiazepoxide on **A** total slow-wave sleep (SWS) and **B** total rapid eye movement sleep (REMS). Open symbols and dotted lines are placebo; filled symbols and solid line are chlordiazepoxide. Upper trace effect on SWS ($n = 9$). Lower trace, effects on total REMS time ($n = 9$). (From Hartmann 1976.)

regulation of GABA–benzodiazepine receptors, a homeostatic response to regular drug use. They encourage continued hypnotic usage and contribute to the development of drug dependence (see later section on benzodiazepines).

Oversedation, hangover effects. Many benzodiazepines used as hypnotics can give rise to a subjective 'hangover', and after most of them, even those with short elimination half-lives, psychomotor performance and memory may be impaired on the following day. Oversedation is most likely with slowly eliminated benzodiazepines, especially if used chronically, and is most marked in the elderly in whom drowsiness, incoordination and ataxia, leading to falls and fractures,

and acute confusional states may result even from small doses. Paradoxical excitement may occur occasionally.

Some benzodiazepines in hypnotic doses may decrease alveolar ventilation and depress the respiratory response to hypercapnia, increasing the risk of cerebral hypoxia, especially in the elderly and in patients with chronic respiratory disease.

Drug interactions. Benzodiazepines have additive effects with other central nervous system depressants. Combinations of benzodiazepines with alcohol, other hypnotics, sedative tricyclic antidepressants, antihistamines or opioids can cause marked sedation and may lead to accidents or severe respiratory depression.

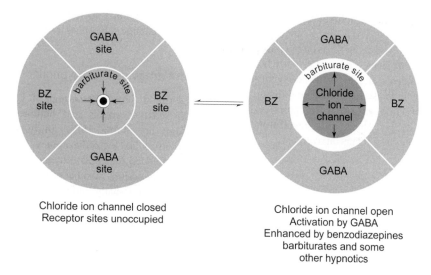

Figure 26.4 Schematic cross-sectional diagram of the GABA-benzodiazepine (BZ) receptor complex. On the left, the diagram shows the inactive state of the receptor, with the chloride ion channel closed and receptor sites unoccupied. Activation of the receptor by GABA, benzodiazepines, barbiturates and some other hypnotics (diagram on right) opens the chloride channel, causing hyperpolarization (inhibition) of the neurone.

Pregnancy and lactation. The regular use of benzodiazepines is contraindicated in pregnancy since the drugs are concentrated in fetal tissues where hepatic metabolism is minimal. They can cause neonatal depression, hypotonia and feeding difficulties if given in late pregnancy, and infants exposed in utero to regular hypnotic maternal doses may develop withdrawal symptoms 2–3 weeks after birth (irritability, crying, muscle twitches). They also enter breast milk, and long-acting benzodiazepines are contraindicated during lactation, although short- to medium-acting benzo-diazepines appear to be safe.

Zopiclone

Zopiclone a cyclopyrrolone, is a non-benzodiazepine that nevertheless binds to benzodiazepine receptors. It has hypnotic effects similar to benzodiazepines and carries the same potential for adverse effects including dependence and abstinence effects on withdrawal. Psychiatric reactions, including hallucinations and behavioural disturbances, have been reported to occur shortly after the first dose. This drug appears to have no particular advantages over benzodiazepines, although it may cause less alteration of sleep stages.

Zolpidem

Zolpidem is an imidazopyridine that binds preferentially to one benzodiazepine receptor subtype (ω-1; benzodiazepine-1) thought to mediate hypnotic effects. It is an effective hypnotic with only weak anticonvulsant

and myorelaxant properties. (In contrast, benzodiazepines bind to three known subtypes and zopiclone to two.) Because of its short elimination half-life (2 hours) hangover effects are rare, but rebound effects may occur in the later part of the night, causing early morning waking and daytime anxiety. With high doses, brief psychotic episodes, tolerance and withdrawal effects have been reported. Both zopiclone and zolpidem are more expensive than other hypnotics.

Zaleplon

Zaleplon is a pyrazolopyrimidine which, like zolpidem, binds selectively to the ω-1 benzodiazepine receptor. It is an effective hypnotic at a dose of 5–10 mg, has a very short elimination half-life (1 hour), and appears to cause minimal residual effects on psychomotor or cognitive function after 5 hours. No tolerance to the hypnotic action or withdrawal effects such as rebound insomnia were observed after 4 weeks treatment in 615 patients with primary insomnia (Elie et al 1999) and the drug appears suitable for use in the elderly (Hedner et al 2000). The recommended maximal duration of treatment is 2 weeks, and the drug may have abuse potential when used in doses of 25 mg or more. Zaleplon has only recently been introduced and its therapeutic use awaits full evaluation.

Chloral derivatives (chloral hydrate, triclofos, dichloralphenazone)

Chloral derivatives still have some use as hypnotics in general practice. They are all metabolized to

429

trichlorethanol, which has an elimination half-life of 8 hours (see Table 26.1). These drugs are moderately effective as hypnotics, and their effects on sleep are similar to those of benzodiazepines. They can produce hangover effects, drug dependence and an abstinence syndrome on withdrawal and may cause gastrointestinal disturbance. The mechanism of action (on $GABA_A$ receptors) is similar to that of benzodiazepines, but respiratory and cardiovascular depression occurs on overdose.

Clomethiazole

Clomethiazole has hypnotic and anticonvulsant properties and a mode of action on $GABA_A$ receptors similar to that of benzodiazepines. It is fairly rapidly eliminated (half-life 4 hours; see Table 26.1) and produces little respiratory depression at therapeutic doses. For these reasons it has been advocated for use in the elderly and is sometimes used in alcohol and narcotic detoxification. However, it has a low therapeutic index, produces a profound respiratory depression in overdose, and carries an appreciable risk of dependence, especially in combination with alcohol.

Promethazine

Promethazine is one of the few drugs with useful hypnotic properties which does not act on GABA-benzodiazepine receptors. It is a sedative antihistamine with antagonistic effects on H_1 receptors in the brain. Promethazine is related to the phenothiazines, and has additional slight neuroleptic and anticholinergic effects. In suitable dosage (see Table 26.1), promethazine has mild to moderate hypnotic efficacy, but the onset of action is slow (1.5–3 hours) and it is only slowly eliminated (elimination half-life 12 hours). Hangover effects are common, and it occasionally produces excitement rather than sedation. Nevertheless, promethazine is sometimes of value in paediatric practice and in cases where other hypnotics are contraindicated. Other sedative antihistamines with similar effects include diphenhydramine and chlorphenamine (chlorpheniramine).

Other drugs used as hypnotics

Prescribing data suggest that tricyclic antidepressants with sedative effects and neuroleptic drugs in low dosage are being increasingly used as hypnotic alternatives to benzodiazepines. Such drugs are not recommended for general hypnotic use since they have potentially serious adverse effects. Alcohol is used as a 'nightcap' by many individuals, often with the tacit approval of their doctors. Alcohol (which also acts on $GABA_A$ receptors) may indeed help to induce sleep but may lead to late-night restlessness, and excessive use of alcohol is a common cause of insomnia.

Rational drug treatment of insomnia

A hypnotic drug may be indicated for insomnia when it is severe, disabling, unresponsive to other measures or likely to be temporary. In choosing an appropriate agent, individual variables relating to the patient and to the drug need to be considered (Table 26.2).

Patient care

Type of insomnia

The duration of insomnia is important in deciding on a hypnotic regimen. Transient insomnia may be caused by changes of routine such as overnight travel, change in time zone, alteration of shift work or temporary admission to hospital. In these circumstances a hypnotic with a rapid onset and medium duration of action and few residual effects could be used on one or two occasions.

Short-term insomnia may result from temporary environmental stress. In this case a hypnotic may

Table 26.2 Drug treatment in insomnia

Type of insomnia	Choice of drugs	Administration
Transient insomnia	Benzodiazepine (temazepam, diazepam)	Once or twice only
Short-term insomnia	Benzodiazepine (medium duration of action)	1–2 weeks only, or intermittent
Chronic insomnia	1. Treat primary cause (education, sleep hygiene, pain relief, psychiatric treatment) 2. Benzodiazepine (medium duration of action) 3. Zopiclone 4. Sedative antihistamine	2–3 weeks maximum; preferably intermittent; lowest effective dose

occasionally be indicated, but should be prescribed in low dosage for 1 or 2 weeks only, preferably intermittently on alternate nights or one night in three.

Chronic insomnia presents a much greater therapeutic problem. It is usually secondary to other conditions (organic or psychiatric) at which treatment should initially be aimed. In selected cases a hypnotic may be helpful but it is recommended that such drugs should be prescribed at the minimal effective dosage and administered intermittently (one night in three) or temporarily (not more than 2 or 3 weeks). Occasionally it is necessary to repeat short, intermittent courses at intervals of a few months.

The elderly

The elderly are especially vulnerable both to insomnia and to adverse effects from hypnotic drugs. They may have reduced metabolism of some drugs and may be at risk of cumulative effects. They are also more susceptible than younger people to central nervous system depression including cognitive impairment and ataxia (which may lead to falls and fractures). They are sensitive to respiratory depression, prone to sleep apnoea and other sleep disorders, and are more likely to have 'sociological', psychiatric and somatic illnesses which both disturb sleep and may be aggravated by hypnotics. For some of these elderly patients, hypnotics can improve the quality of life but the dosage should be adjusted (usually half the recommended adult dose) and hypnotics with long elimination half-lives should be avoided. A considerable number of elderly patients give a history of regular hypnotic use going back for 20 or 30 years. In some of these patients, gradual reduction of hypnotic dosage or even withdrawal may be indicated (see below).

The young

Hypnotics are generally contraindicated for children. Where sedation is required, sedative antihistamines are usually recommended. However, a single dose of a benzodiazepine (with appropriate dosage reduction) may be more effective.

Pregnancy and lactation

Regular use of slowly eliminated hypnotics are contraindicated. If hypnotics are required, intermittent doses of relatively rapidly eliminated hypnotics may be used and have been shown to be safe during breastfeeding.

Disease states

Hypnotics are contraindicated in patients with acute pulmonary insufficiency, significant respiratory depression, obstructive sleep apnoea or severe hepatic impairment. In patients with chronic pain or terminal conditions suitable analgesics including non-steroidal anti-inflammatory agents or opiates, sometimes combined with neuroleptics, usually provide satisfactory sedation. In such patients the possibility of drug dependence becomes a less important issue and regular use of hypnotics with a medium duration of action should not be denied if they provide symptomatic relief of insomnia.

Choice of drug

There is little difference in hypnotic efficacy between most of the available agents. The main factors to consider in the rational choice of a hypnotic regimen are duration of action and the risk of adverse effects, especially oversedation and the development of tolerance and dependence. Cost may be a factor with new drugs.

Rate of elimination

In general, very short-acting drugs such as zolpidem should be avoided as they tend to cause late-night insomnia and daytime anxiety (the place of zaleplon has not yet been fully assessed). Regular use of slowly eliminated drugs should also be avoided because of the increased risk of oversedation and hangover effects. Drugs with a medium elimination half-life (6–8 hours) appear to have the most suitable profile for hypnotic use. These may include temazepam and loprazolam, which are the drugs of first choice in most situations where hypnotics are indicated. Zopiclone is a reasonable second choice. A sedative antihistamine such as promethazine is a safe third choice and it is useful in children although it may produce daytime drowsiness.

Dosage

The minimum effective dosage should always be used as there is considerable individual variation in response and susceptibility to oversedation. It is best to start with a small dose which may be increased if necessary. Dosage should, in general, be halved in the elderly and caution exercised in the presence of respiratory or hepatic disease.

Duration and timing of administration

In order to prevent the development of tolerance and dependence, the maximum duration of treatment should be limited to 2 or 3 weeks and treatment should, where possible, be intermittent (one night in two or three). Dosage should be tapered slowly if hypnotics have been taken regularly for more than a few weeks. Doses should be taken 20 minutes before retiring in order to allow dissolution in the stomach and absorption to commence before the patient lies down in bed.

Anxiolytic drugs

As with insomnia, drugs provide only symptomatic treatment for anxiety. They may temporarily help a patient to cope with an otherwise overwhelming stress and can provide a short-term cover which allows time for more specific treatments to take effect, but they do not cure the underlying disorder. Most anxiety states are more effectively treated in the long term by non-pharmacological interventions including counselling, psychotherapy, behavioural and cognitive methods, relaxation, and anxiety management training. Essentially, all these methods involve a learning process which enables the patient to develop improved stress-coping techniques. However, these methods are time consuming, labour intensive and costly.

The ideal anxiolytic drug would selectively damp down excess activity in limbic (emotional) and somatic arousal systems, without inhibiting learning processes or producing undue sedation. The onset of action would be rapid and the drugs would be suitable for long-term use. No available drug meets all these requirements. The 'classic' anxiolytics, such as the benzodiazepines, have a rapid onset of action but impair cognitive processes and have undesirable long-term effects. Antidepressants are effective in some types of anxiety but have a delayed onset of action, are potentially toxic, and may be difficult to withdraw. Some of the somatic manifestations of anxiety can be alleviated by β adrenoreceptor antagonists, but these drugs have little effect on subjective symptoms. Some drugs used in anxiety disorders are shown in Table 26.3.

Table 26.3   Profile of some drugs used in anxiety disorders

Drug	Elimination half-life (h)	Approximate anxiolytic dosage[a]
Benzodiazepines		
Chlordiazepoxide	5–30 (36–200)[b]	15–30 mg three times daily
Diazepam	20–100 (36–200)	2–5 mg three times daily
Lorazepam	10–18	1 mg three times daily
Oxazepam	4–15	10–30 mg three times daily
Buspirone	2–11	5–10 mg three times daily
β adrenoceptor antagonist		
Propranolol	2–4	40 mg twice daily
Tricyclic antidepressants		
Amitriptyline	10–25 (13–93)	75–150 mg daily
Clomipramine	16–20	10–100 mg daily
Dosulepin (dothiepin)	14–40	75–150 mg daily
Imipramine	4–18 (12–61)	50–100 mg daily
Selective serotonin reuptake inhibitors		
Fluoxetine	2–3 days (7–15 days)	20 mg daily
Fluvoxamine	15	100 mg daily
Paroxetine	20	20 mg daily
Sertraline	26 (36)	50 mg daily
Citalopram	33	10–20 mg daily
Monoamine oxidase inhibitors		
Moclobemide	1–4	300–600 mg daily
Phenelzine	1[c]	15 mg three time daily

[a] Doses based on *British National Formulary* (March 2001), but requirements vary and dosage may need individual titration. Starting doses should be less. Dosage should be reduced in the elderly.
[b] Half-life of pharmacologically active metabolite shown in parentheses.
[c] Causes irreversible enzyme inhibition; effects last for 2 weeks after cessation of treatment.
Moclobemide is a short-acting reversible monoamine oxidase inhibitor.

Benzodiazepines

Benzodiazepines are still the most commonly prescribed drugs for anxiety. About 7.5 million prescriptions for benzodiazepines classed as anxiolytics are issued each year in the UK, and many anxious patients are also prescribed hypnotics.

Benzodiazepines have potent anxiolytic effects which are exerted at low doses that produce minimal sedation. A major advantage in acute situations is the rapid onset of action that occurs within an hour of the first effective dose. Many clinical trials have shown short-term efficacy in patients with anxiety disorders. Anxiolytic effects have also been reported in normal volunteers with high trait anxiety and in patients with anticipatory anxiety before surgery. However, in subjects with low trait anxiety and in non-stressful conditions benzodiazepines may paradoxically increase anxiety and impair psychomotor performance.

The major site of anxiolytic action is the limbic system (see above). This effect is mediated by a primary action at $GABA_A$ receptors, resulting in enhancement of inhibitory GABA activity (see Fig. 26.2). Secondary suppression of noradrenergic and/or serotonergic pathways may be of particular importance in relation to anxiolytic effects.

Adverse effects of anxiolytic use

Tolerance. Tolerance to the anxiolytic effects of benzodiazepines seems to develop more slowly than to the hypnotic effects. In clinical use, most patients reporting initial drowsiness find that it wears off in a few days while the anxiolytic effect remains for some weeks. However, benzodiazepines are usually no longer effective in the treatment of anxiety after 1–4 months of regular use (Drug and Therapeutics Bulletin 1980).

Psychomotor impairment. Although oversedation is not usually a problem in anxious patients, there is evidence that long-term use of benzodiazepines results in psychomotor impairment and has adverse effects on memory. Many patients on long-term benzodiazepines complain of poor memory, and incidents of shoplifting have been attributed to memory lapses caused by benzodiazepine use. In elderly patients the amnesic effects may falsely suggest the development of dementia. There is some evidence that benzodiazepines also inhibit the learning of alternative stress-coping strategies, such as behavioural treatments for agoraphobia. Additive effects with other central nervous system depressants including alcohol occur, as with hypnotic use of benzodiazepines, and may contribute to traffic and other accidents.

Disinhibition, paradoxical effects. Occasionally, benzodiazepines produce paradoxical stimulant effects. These effects are most marked in anxious subjects and include excitement, increased anxiety, irritability and outbursts of rage. Violent behaviour, including baby battering, have sometimes been attributed to disinhibition by benzodiazepines of behaviour normally suppressed by social restraints, fear or anxiety. Increased daytime anxiety can occur with rapidly eliminated benzodiazepines, such as lorazepam, and is probably a withdrawal effect.

Affective reactions. Chronic use of benzodiazepines can aggravate depression and provoke suicide in depressed patients, and can cause depression in patients with no previous history of depressive disorder (Committee on Safety of Medicines 1988). Aggravation of depression is a particular risk in anxious patients who often have mixed anxiety/depression. Some patients on long-term benzodiazepines complain of 'emotional anaesthesia' with inability to experience either pleasure or distress. However, in some patients, benzodiazepines induce euphoria, and they are increasingly used as drugs of abuse when taken in high doses or self-administered intravenously.

Dependence. The greatest drawback of chronic benzodiazepine use is the development of drug dependence. It is now generally agreed that the regular use of therapeutic doses of benzodiazepines as hypnotics or anxiolytics for more than a few weeks can give rise to dependence, with withdrawal symptoms on cessation of drug use in over 40% of patients. It is estimated that there are about 1 million long-term benzodiazepine users in the UK, and many of these are likely to be dependent. People with anxious or 'passive-dependent' personalities seem to be most vulnerable to dependence and withdrawal symptoms. Such individuals make up a large proportion of anxious patients in psychiatric practice, are often described as suffering from 'chronic anxiety', and are the type of patient for whom benzodiazepines are most likely to be prescribed. Such patients often continue to take benzodiazepines for many years because attempts at dosage reduction or drug withdrawal result in abstinence symptoms which they are unable to tolerate. Nevertheless, these patients continue to suffer from anxiety symptoms despite continued benzodiazepine use, possibly because they have become tolerant to the anxiolytic effects and may also suffer from other adverse effects of long-term benzodiazepine use such as depression or psychomotor impairment (Ashton 1987).

Abuse. In the last decade there has been a growing problem with benzodiazepine abuse. Some patients escalate their prescribed dosage and may obtain prescriptions from several doctors. These tend to be anxious patients with 'passive-dependent' personalities who may have a history of alcohol misuse; they often combine large doses of benzodiazepines with excessive alcohol consumption. In addition, a high proportion (30–90%) of illicit recreational drug abusers also use benzodiazepines, and some take them as euphoriants in their own right. Recreational use of most benzodiazepines has been reported in various countries; in the UK, temazepam is most commonly abused. Exceedingly large doses (over 1 g) may be taken and sometimes injected intravenously (Strang et al 1993). Benzodiazepines became easily available due to widespread prescribing which favoured their entrance into the illicit drug scene. Abusers become dependent and suffer the same adverse effects and withdrawal symptoms as prescribed dose users.

Benzodiazepine withdrawal. Many patients on long-term benzodiazepines seek help with drug withdrawal. Clinical experience shows that withdrawal is feasible in most patients if carried out with care. Abrupt withdrawal in dependent subjects is dangerous, and can induce acute anxiety, psychosis or convulsions. However, gradual withdrawal, coupled where necessary with counselling or psychological treatments, can be successful in the majority of patients (Ashton 1994). The duration of withdrawal should be tailored to individual needs, and may last many months. Dosage decrements may be of the order of 1–2 mg of diazepam per month. Even with slow dosage reduction, a variety of withdrawal symptoms may be experienced, including increased anxiety, insomnia, hypersensitivity to sensory stimuli, perceptual distortions, paraesthesiae, muscle twitching, depression and many others. These may last for many weeks, though diminishing in intensity, but occasionally the withdrawal syndrome is protracted for a year or more. Temporary use of other drugs, particularly sedative tricyclic antidepressants, may be indicated during the withdrawal period. The eventual outcome does not appear to be influenced by dosage, type of benzodiazepine, duration of use, personality disorder, psychiatric history, age, severity of withdrawal symptoms or rate of withdrawal (Ashton 1987). Hence benzodiazepine withdrawal is worth attempting in patients who are motivated to stop, and most patients report that they feel better after withdrawal than when they were taking the benzodiazepine. Community pharmacists may be ideally suited to advise doctors and patients on the management of benzodiazepine withdrawal.

Choice of benzodiazepine in anxiety

Despite the drawbacks of chronic use, benzodiazepines can be valuable in the short-term management of anxiety because of their anxiolytic efficacy and rapid onset of action. The choice of an appropriate benzodiazepine, as with hypnotics, depends largely on pharmacokinetic characteristics. Potent benzodiazepines such as lorazepam (see Table 26.3) have been widely used for anxiety disorders but are probably inappropriate. Lorazepam is moderately rapidly eliminated and needs to be taken several times daily. Declining blood concentrations may lead to inter-dose anxiety as the anxiolytic effect of each tablet wears off. The high potency of lorazepam (approximately 10 times that of diazepam), and the fact that it is available only in 1 and 2.5 mg tablet strengths, has often led to excessive dosage. Such doses lead to adverse effects, a high probability of dependence and difficulties in withdrawal. A slowly eliminated benzodiazepine such as diazepam is more appropriate in most cases. Diazepam has a rapid onset of action, and its slow elimination ensures a steady blood concentration. It should be prescribed in the minimal effective dosage to avoid cumulative effects, and it can also be used as a hypnotic, thus avoiding the need for a separate hypnotic drug. However, as with hypnotics, the anxiolytic use of benzodiazepines should generally be limited to short-term (2 weeks) or intermittent use. Parenteral administration of lorazepam or diazepam may occasionally be indicated for severely agitated psychiatric patients.

Buspirone

Buspirone has a structure and mode of action completely different from that of the benzodiazepines. It has mixed agonist/antagonist actions at serotonergic receptors that are thought to be involved in anxiety. In clinical trials it appears to have anxiolytic effects comparable with those of benzodiazepines, but it is without sedative/hypnotic, anticonvulsant or muscle relaxant effects. A major disadvantage is that anxiolytic effects are delayed for up to 3 weeks, and in some patients buspirone produces dysphoria and may actually increase anxiety. Furthermore, it does not usually alleviate anxiety associated with benzodiazepine withdrawal. Buspirone does not appear to produce dependence or a withdrawal syndrome, although most clinical studies have been of limited duration, and the drug is recommended for short-term use only. Its place in the treatment of anxiety is doubtful at present.

Antidepressant drugs

A number of tricyclic and other antidepressants have additional sedative or anxiolytic effects (see Table 26.3). They appear to be as effective as benzodiazepines in generalized anxiety and superior in panic disorder and agoraphobia. They are also of value in depressive states associated with anxiety and in anxiety/depression associated with benzodiazepine withdrawal. Selective serotonin reuptake inhibitors (SSRIs) and monoamine oxidase inhibitors (MAOIs) are also effective in phobic states and panic disorders. A disadvantage of all these drugs is their slow onset of action which may be delayed for 2–4 weeks and they may initially exacerbate anxiety symptoms. For this reason it is advisable to start with small doses. The mode of action of these drugs is thought to be an initial increase in central serotonergic and noradrenergic activity, which may cause further anxiety, followed by a down-regulation of adrenergic and serotonergic receptors, accounting for the delayed anxiolytic effect. Nevertheless, the sedative effect of some tricyclic antidepressants may be a separate action and is often manifested early in the treatment. A second disadvantage of antidepressants is that some are toxic in overdose and have many adverse effects including anticholinergic actions, cardiovascular actions, especially in the elderly, drug interactions, and interactions with certain foods (see Chapter 27). They are, however, more suitable for long-term use than benzodiazepines, and can be continued for several months. They are often effective in low to moderate doses and do not cause cognitive impairment. Some patients have difficulty in stopping these drugs because of withdrawal symptoms, which include rebound excessive cholinergic activity and increased anxiety or depression. Withdrawal should therefore be carried out gradually.

β adrenoreceptor blockers

Some somatic symptoms of anxiety such as palpitations and tremor are due to excessive sympathetic activity acting on peripheral β adrenoreceptors. These symptoms can be alleviated by β adrenoreceptor blockers such as propranolol. These drugs, when used in small doses which do not induce hypotension, can be of value in acutely stressful situations or panic attacks where physical symptoms dominate the picture, although they have little effect on subjective symptoms. If used regularly, withdrawal should be gradual to prevent rebound tachycardia and return of palpitations.

Antipsychotic drugs

Some antipsychotic drugs such as chlorpromazine and haloperidol have sedative and anxiolytic effects and may, on occasion, be of short-term use in severe anxiety disorders associated with panic. They have a rapid onset of action (within 1 hour) but should be used in minimal dosage and only short-term since they carry a risk of inducing dyskinesias and other adverse effects. Anxious patients may have withdrawal problems after regular use. The growing tendency to prescribe these drugs as alternatives to benzodiazepines is to be deprecated.

Rational use of drugs in anxiety

It is clear that drugs do not provide a long-term solution for anxiety. In acute anxiety states, often precipitated by stress, short-term benzodiazepines may help to cope with the immediate situation as they have high efficacy and a rapid onset of action (Table 26.4). Diazepam, prescribed in hypnotic or anxiolytic doses, depending on the circumstances, is probably the drug of choice. A single dose may be sufficient, and it should not be continued regularly for more than 1 or 2 weeks. It can be given intermittently and intermittent courses can be repeated if necessary. Potent, short-acting benzodiazepines such as alprazolam and lorazepam should be avoided. Benzodiazepines are not recommended in bereavement because their amnesic actions may interfere with subsequent readjustment (Tyrer 1989). The aims and limitations of benzodiazepine treatment for anxiety, and the risk of drug dependence should be explained to patients.

If longer-term treatment is required in generalized anxiety, anxiety/depression or phobic states, sedative tricyclic antidepressants or SSRIs are preferred. These drugs are efficacious, can be used for several months, and do not interfere with non-pharmacological treatments. However, their therapeutic effects may be delayed for 2 or 3 weeks and they can initially exacerbate anxiety. For this reason it is best to start with small doses which can be gradually increased. MAOIs are effective in panic and phobic disorders. β adrenoreceptor blockers are effective in controlling somatic symptoms such as palpitations and tremor, and have a role for patients in whom such symptoms are prominent.

The most effective long-term treatment of anxiety is by psychological methods, which can include self-help groups, counselling, behavioural and cognitive techniques, anxiety management training and psychotherapy. These measures all take time to be effective: the main role of drugs is to alleviate symptoms during the learning process involved.

Common therapeutic problems in the management of insomnia and anxiety are summarized in Table 26.5.

Table 26.4   Drug treatment in anxiety[a]

Drug	Efficacy	Onset of therapeutic effect	Risk of withdrawal symptoms	Administration
Benzodiazepines	++	Immediate	++	Single dose, intermittent (2 weeks)
Buspirone	+	Delayed (2–4 weeks)	–	Short term (4 weeks)
β adrenoreceptor blockers	+ (some patients)	Immediate	+	Medium term (weeks to months)
Tricyclic antidepressants	++ (hypnotic effect earlier)	Delayed (2–4 weeks)	+	Medium to long term (3–12 months)
SSRIs	++	Delayed (2–4 weeks) (least with fluoxetine)	+ (3–12 months) (most with paroxetine)	Medium to long term
MAOIs (selected patients)	++	Delayed (3–6 weeks)	+ (3–12 months)	Medium to long term

[a] Wherever possible, psychological treatments are preferred (counselling, anxiety management training, cognitive and behaviour therapy, psychotherapy).

CASE STUDIES

Case 26.1

A 40-year-old nursing sister consulted a psychiatrist for help in withdrawing from lorazepam which she had taken regularly in a dose of 1 mg three times a day for 10 years. She had tried on several occasions to stop the lorazepam but had been unsuccessful because of the appearance of anxiety and insomnia. The psychiatrist advised a schedule of dosage reduction, cutting her daily lorazepam intake by half a 1 mg tablet each week, but the patient was unable to continue the withdrawal because of increasing daytime anxiety and severe insomnia which interfered with her work. In order to help her sleep, the psychiatrist prescribed zopiclone 7.5 mg nightly, soon increased to 15 mg at night. The nursing sister remarked that the zopiclone was remarkably effective in alleviating all her withdrawal symptoms. It was so effective that she began to take it during the day as well as at night and was soon consuming half a zopiclone tablet six times daily as well as the nightly dose. At this point the psychiatrist consulted a pharmacologist for further information about zopiclone.

Question

What advice did the psychiatrist receive from the pharmacologist? Outline a better course of action that could have been taken to help this patient.

Answer

Zopiclone has similar pharmacological actions to benzodiazepines and acts on GABA/BZ receptors. The psychiatrist had merely substituted dependence on zopiclone for the original dependence on lorazepam.

A better course of action would have been to change the patient gradually from lorazepam to an equivalent dosage of diazepam (25–30 mg) and to withdraw this very slowly at the approximate rate of 1 mg every 1–2 weeks. Diazepam has a longer half-life than lorazepam and the available tablet strengths allow small dosage decrements which are not possible with lorazepam or zopiclone. Gradual withdrawal over a period of months is tolerable to most patients, and can be combined if necessary with anxiety management techniques. Psychological health improves after withdrawal in most long-term benzodiazepine users.

Diazepam was prescribed for this patient instead of zopiclone and she subsequently became drug-free with normal sleep and disappearance of her daytime anxiety. She was able to continue her duties as a nursing sister.

Case 26.2

A 20-year-old man, known to have schizophrenia, was acutely admitted to a psychiatric ward in a highly agitated and disturbed state. He was panicking because of 'voices' threatening to kill him. He was aggressive and violent towards the hospital staff whom he feared were in league with the voices. He was eventually sedated by an intramuscular injection of lorazepam which was repeated 6 hours and 12 hours later, and he was also given haloperidol by mouth. He remained in hospital for 4 weeks, during which time his condition was controlled with oral haloperidol and lorazepam. On discharge, he was taking haloperidol 10 mg and lorazepam 6 mg daily. His general practitioner continued with the same drug regimen but

Table 26.5 Common therapeutic problems in the management of insomnia and anxiety

Problem	Prevalence	Contributing factors	Management
Benzodiazepine overdose	Occurs in ~ 40% of all self-poisoning incidents 1512 deaths due to benzodiazepines were reported in the UK 1980–89 ($^2/_3$ benzodiazepines alone); temazepam was reported to be the most toxic (11.9 deaths/million prescriptions)	Benzodiazepine often taken with other drugs including antidepressants, paracetamol, alcohol and opiates Benzodiazepines plus opiates are responsible for 100 deaths per year in Glasgow alone	Flumazenil (a competitive antagonist at benzodiazepine receptors) may be administered cautiously.[a] This will reverse benzodiazepine actions and may reveal the extent to which other drugs are contributing to the patient's condition. However, in benzodiazepine-dependent patients, flumazenil may precipitate withdrawal reactions
Insomnia treated with zopiclone during or after benzodiazepine withdrawal	Many patients are prescribed zopiclone as an alternative hypnotic, since it is not a benzodiazepine, and is thought to have a different action	Patients often report that zopiclone alleviates benzodiazepine withdrawal symptoms, but tend to escalate dosage and take it during the day as well as at night	Zopiclone (and zolpidem) act on benzodiazepine receptors[b] and cause dependence in the same way. These drugs have also been abused in escalating doses. They should not be prescribed as a substitute for benzodiazepines
Patients wishing to withdraw from lorazepam or other potent, relatively short-acting benzodiazepines	Many UK patients are still being prescribed relatively large doses of lorazepam (e.g. >7.5mg daily).	Lorazepam is 10 times more potent than diazepam but is available in only 1 mg or 2.5 mg formulations, which makes it difficult to reduce dosage gradually	If benzodiazepine withdrawal is indicated, it is usually advisable to switch to diazepam. The substitution should be carried out stepwise, replacing one dose of lorazepam at a time with the equivalent dose of diazepam. Withdrawal can then be carried out gradually at the rate of 1–2 mg diazepam every 2–4 weeks
Patients taking a combination of a benzodiazepine and an antidepressant drug	Many patients on long-term benzodiazepines are also taking a prescribed antidepressant	An antidepressant may have been prescribed for depression caused by chronic benzodiazepine use, or for patients with anxiety/depression, although this is not recommended (CSM 1988)	Gradual withdrawal from the benzodiazepine may be indicated. In this case, the patient should continue on the antidepressant drug until benzodiazepine withdrawal is complete and probably for a month or more afterwards. The advisability of continuing or slowly withdrawing the antidepressant can then be considered
Patients attending pharmacies for several months to obtain repeat prescriptions for benzodiazepines	An estimated 1 million patients in the UK are taking prescribed benzodiazepines regularly for over a year (often for many years)	A considerable proportion of these patients are likely to be dependent and to be at risk of adverse effects, especially if elderly	The pharmacist may wish to contact the community pharmacist service who may approach the prescriber and suggest methods of withdrawal and help in supervision of withdrawal
Benzodiazepine abuse	Well over 100 000 people abuse illicitly obtained benzodiazepines in the UK	Illicit benzodiazepine abuse is common among polydrug users, alcoholics, and psychiatric patients. Some of these inject benzodiazepines and are at risk of HIV and hepatitis as well as local consequences of injection	The source of most illicitly obtained benzodiazepines is stolen prescriptions. Reduction in benzodiazepine prescribing would help to alleviate this problem

[a] Flumazenil is short-acting; repeated administration may be required if a long-acting benzodiazepine has been taken in overdose.
[b] See Table 26.1

noticed that the patient seemed drowsy and depressed over the next few months although the voices did not reappear.

Question

What would have been a better procedure for the hospital to follow?

Answer

Although lorazepam is helpful in controlling acute severe agitated states, it is not indicated for long-term use. Lorazepam dosage should have been gradually withdrawn while the patient was in hospital. It is not helpful long-term in schizophrenia and discharging the patient still taking lorazepam opened the way to long-term use and the risk of adverse effects including depression. In addition, benzodiazepines have additive effects with other sedative drugs and would have added to drowsiness and depression which can be caused by haloperidol.

Case 26.3

An widow aged 70, living alone, had taken nitrazepam, 10 mg at night, to help her sleep since her husband's death 3

years previously. At first this prescription had seemed efficacious but for the past year she had noticed increasing insomnia. She would get up and wander at night, sometimes turning on the gas cooker and leaving it burning. During the day she was confused and forgetful and would frequently fall asleep. She often forgot her keys and locked herself out of the house. She was involved in a road traffic accident after driving through a red traffic light. Her daughter consulted a doctor, wondering if her mother was developing Alzheimer's disease.

Question

Other than age-related dementia, what could have caused the patient's altered behaviour? Suggest a suitable course of action for the doctor to take.

Answer

Benzodiazepines, especially slowly eliminated hypnotics such as nitrazepam, can cause confusional states suggesting dementia in the elderly. The doctor advised gradual dosage reduction and withdrawal of the nitrazepam over 3 months, using an oral suspension (2.5 mg/ml). After withdrawal, the patient slept better and her memory and cognitive functions returned. She also went through a normal grieving period which she had not experienced after her husband's death.

REFERENCES

Ashton H 1987 Benzodiazepine withdrawal: outcome in 50 patients. British Journal of Addiction 83: 665–671

Ashton H 1994 The treatment of benzodiazepine dependence. Addiction 89: 1535–1541

Balter M B, Uhlenuth E H 1992 New epidemiological findings about insomnia and its treatment. Journal of Clinical Psychiatry 53: 34–42

Committee on Safety of Medicines 1988 Benzodiazepines, dependence and withdrawal symptoms. Current Problems 21: 1–2

Drug and Therapeutics Bulletin 1980 The CRM on benzodiazepines. Drug and Therapeutics Bulletin 17: 76

Elie R, Eckart R, Farr I et al 1999 Sleep latency is shortened during 4 weeks of treatment with zaleplon, a novel nonbenzodiazepine hypnotic. Journal of Clinical Psychiatry 60(8): 536–544

Haefely W 1990 Benzodiazepine receptor and ligands: structural and functional differences. In: Hindmarch I, Beaumont G, Brandon S et al (eds) Benzodiazepines: current concepts. Wiley, Chichester, pp. 1–18

Hartmann E 1976 Long term administration of psychotropic drugs: effects on human sleep. In: Williams R L, Karacan I

Pharmacology of sleep. Willey, New York, pp. 211–224

Hedner J, Yaeche R, Emilien G et al 2000 Zaleplon shortens subjective sleep latency and improves subjective sleep quality in elderly patients with insomnia. International Journal of Geriatric Psychiatry 15: 704–712

Horne J 1988 Why we sleep. Oxford University Press, Oxford

Judd L L, Kessler R C, Paulus M P et al 1998 Comorbidity as a fundamental feature of generalised anxiety disorders: results from the national comorbidity study (NCS). Acta Psychiatrica Scandinavica 98(Suppl. 393): 6–11

Lader M (ed) 1992 The medical management of insomnia in general practice. Royal Society of Medicine, London

Morgan K, Clarke D 1997 Longitudinal trends in late-life insomnia: implications for prescribing. Age Ageing 26: 179–184

Strang J, Seivewright N, Farrell M 1993 Oral and intravenous abuse of benzodiazepines. In: Hallstrom C (ed) Benzodiazepine dependence. Oxford University Press, Oxford, pp. 128–142

Tyrer P 1989 Choice of treatment in anxiety. In: Tyrer P (ed) The psychopharmacology of anxiety. Oxford University Press, Oxford, pp. 255–281

FURTHER READING

Ashton H 1992 Brain function and psychotropic drugs. Oxford University Press, Oxford

Ashton H 1994 Guidelines for the rational use of benzodiazepines. When and what to use. Drugs 48: 25–40

Ashton H 1995 Protracted withdrawal from benzodiazepines: the post-withdrawal syndrome. Psychiatric Annals 25: 174–179

Ashton H 1995 Toxicity and adverse consequences of benzodiazepines use. Psychiatric Annals 25: 158–165

Ashton C H, Young A H 1999 SSRIs, drug withdrawal and abuse: problem or treatment. In: Stanford S C (ed) Selective serotonin reuptake inhibitors (SSRIs) R G Landes, Austin, Texas, pp. 65–80

Gale C, Oakley-Browne M 2000 Extracts from 'Clinical Evidence': anxiety disorder. British Medical Journal 321: 1204–1207

Affective disorders **27**

P. Pratt

The central feature of an affective disorder is an alteration in mood. The most common presentation is that of a low mood or depression. Less commonly the mood may become high or elated, as in mania.

Depression

The term 'depression' can in itself be misleading. Everyone in the normal course of daily life will experience alterations in mood. Depressed mood in this context does not represent a disorder or illness; in fact, lowered mood as a response to the ups and downs of living is considered normal and termed sadness or unhappiness. Sometimes clinical depression may present in a mild form, so it is important to differentiate this from normal unhappiness.

Mania

If the mood becomes elated or irritable this may be a symptom of mania. The term 'mania' is used to describe severe cases, frequently associated with psychotic symptoms. Hypomania describes a less severe form of the disorder. In clinical practice this distinction is often blurred, with hypomania being seen as patients develop, or recover from mania.

Bipolar and unipolar disorders

If a patient develops one or more manic episodes the condition may be termed a bipolar disorder. Although it may be accompanied by depressive episodes, the existence of repeated manic episodes alone is sufficient to be termed a bipolar disorder. The term 'manic–depressive' is a somewhat outdated way of describing a bipolar disorder. The term 'unipolar' is used to describe single episodes of depression.

Epidemiology

Differences in diagnosis, particularly of depression, make it difficult to estimate the true incidence of affective disorders. The lifetime risk of developing a bipolar disorder is said to be about 1% (0.5–1.5%). While the incidence is reported by some to be the same for both men and women, other studies suggest the disorder may be slightly more common in women.

By comparison, the overall incidence of depression is much higher and there does appear to be a significant difference between the sexes. Studies from America and Europe, using standard assessment tools, found a lifetime prevalence of between 16% and 17%, with a 6-month prevalence of about 6%. Higher rates are consistently found in women, with reports suggesting that women are twice as likely as men to suffer depression. The differences between the sexes have been explained by the fact that women are more likely to express their feelings of depression to a doctor whereas in many cases men may present as alcoholics.

Although depression can occur at any age, including infancy, it is estimated that the average age of onset of depression is in the late 20s. Some earlier studies found the incidence and prevalence of depression in women peaking at the age of 35–45 years. In bipolar disorder an earlier age of onset is suggested, perhaps in late adolescence.

Aetiology

Like most psychiatric disorders, the causes of affective disorders are unknown. Despite this uncertainty, several factors can be identified which may have a role in their development. There appears to be general agreement that a genetic predisposition exists, with major life events able to precipitate an episode. These may bring about some of the biochemical changes often described in depressed patients.

Genetic causes

The incidence of affective disorder in first-degree relatives of someone with severe depression may be about 20%, which is almost three times the risk for relatives in control groups. Comparisons of the risk of affective disorder in the children of both parents with an affective disorder show a four times greater risk, and the risk is doubled in children with one parent with an affective disorder.

Social, environmental and genetic factors could all account for the findings of higher familial rates of affective disorders. Studies looking at twins have found fairly strong evidence for a genetic factor.

Evidence of a genetic link has been found in studies of children from parents with affective disorder who were adopted by healthy parents. A higher incidence of affective disorder was found in the biological parents of adopted children with affective disorder than in the adoptive parents.

Environmental factors

Although environmental stresses can often be identified prior to an episode of mania or depression, a causal relationship between a major event in someone's life and the development of an affective disorder has not been firmly established. It may be that life events described as 'threatening' are more likely to be associated with depression.

The lack of prospective studies makes it difficult to interpret data linking early life events, such as loss of a parent, to the development of an affective disorder. The fact that specific environmental stresses have not been identified should not lead to the conclusion that the environment or lifestyle is irrelevant to the course or development of affective disorders. Employment and the existence of a close and confiding relationship have been noted to offer some protection.

Biochemical factors

In its simplistic form the biochemical theory of depression postulates a deficiency of neurotransmitter amines in certain areas of the brain. This theory has been developed to suggest receptor sensitivity changes may be important.

The hypothesis in affective disorders focuses on an involvement of the neurotransmitters noradrenaline (norepinephrine), 5-hydroxytryptamine (5-HT) and dopamine. This arose out of the findings that both the monoamine-oxidase inhibitors (MAOIs) and the tricyclic antidepressants appeared to increase neurotransmitter amines (particularly noradrenaline (norepinephrine)) at important sites in the brain. When it was found that reserpine, previously used as an antihypertensive, caused both a depletion of neurotransmitter and also induced depression, this was taken as an apparent confirmation of the theory.

By looking at the metabolites of noradrenaline (norepinephrine) and 5-HT some investigators have suggested different types of depression may exist. It has been found that some depressed patients appear to have reduced cerebral concentrations of 5-hydroxyindolacetic acid (5-HIAA) (the metabolite of 5-HT) whereas others appear to have reduced levels of methoxyhydroxyphenylglycerol (MHPG), a metabolite of noradrenaline (norepinephrine). Although much less attention has been paid to dopaminergic activity, some studies have found reduced activity in depressed patients, and an overactivity has been postulated in mania.

The concept of noradrenergic (norepinephrinergic) and serotonergic forms of depression has not gained widespread support, and there is little justification in measuring noradrenaline (norepinephrine) or serotonin metabolites in routine practice.

Endocrine factors

Some endocrine disorders such as hypothyroidism and Cushing's syndrome have been associated with changes in mood. Apart from disorders occurring premenstrually or following childbirth, there appears little direct evidence to link endocrine changes with affective disorders.

Some investigators have found that a proportion of depressed people have increased cortisol levels. This finding has been used as the basis for the dexamethasone suppression test in depression.

Physical illness and side-effects of medication

Disorders of mood, particularly depression, have been associated with several types of medication and a number of physical illnesses (Table 27.1).

Table 27.1 Drugs and physical illnesses implicated in disorders of mood

Drugs

Analgesics	Antipsychotics
Antidepressants	Benzodiazepines
Antihypertensives	Antiparkinsonism agents
Anticonvulsants	Steroids
Opiate withdrawal	
Amfetamine withdrawal	
Benzodiazepine withdrawal	

Physical illness

Viral illness	Thyroid disease
Carcinoma	Addison's disease
Neurological disorders	Systemic lupus
Diabetes	erythematosus
	Pernicious anaemia

An individual's ideas may become grandiose, and they may develop fantastic projects which lead nowhere and inevitably are left incomplete and disjointed. Clothing is usually flamboyant, and if makeup is worn it is usually excessive and involves bright colours.

Severity

The severity of the disorder may vary from mild through moderate to severe. In most circumstances, mild forms of the disorders are unlikely to come to the attention of specialist services, but many cases of mild to moderate depression will be seen by the primary health care team.

If left untreated, it is important to remember that affective disorders carry a risk of mortality. As well as suicidal attempts by someone who is depressed, the lack of self-care and physical exhaustion resulting from mania may be life-threatening.

Clinical manifestations

Depression

A low mood is the central feature of depression. This is often accompanied by a loss of interest or pleasure in normally enjoyable activities. Thinking is pessimistic and in some cases suicidal. A depressed person may complain they have little or no energy. In severe cases, psychotic symptoms such as hallucination or delusion may be present.

Anxiety or agitation frequently accompany the disorder, and the so-called biological features of sleep disturbances, weight loss and loss of appetite are often present. Depressed people typically complain of somatic symptoms, particularly gastric problems, and non-specific aches are common.

Normal sexual drive is reduced, and some people may lose interest in sex altogether. In some cases the biological features are reversed and excessive eating and sleeping may occur. In contrast to agitation, psychomotor retardation may be a presenting feature.

Bipolar disorder

At least one episode of mania must have occurred for a diagnosis of bipolar disorder to be made; depression may also occur, but it is not essential for this diagnosis to be made.

In mania the mood is elated or irritable and the accompanying overactivity is usually unproductive. Disinhibition may result in excessive spending sprees or inappropriate sexual activity. Manic people may describe their thoughts as racing, with ideas rapidly changing from one topic to another. Speech may be very rapid with frequent punning and rhyming.

Investigations

There are no universally accepted tests which will confirm the presence of an affective disorder.

Various rating scales have been developed that may help demonstrate the severity of depressive disorder or distinguish a predominantly anxious patient from a depressed patient.

As discussed earlier, biochemical tests have not been particularly helpful in determining the treatment plan or management of affective disorders. The dexamethasone suppression test is still used by some clinicians as an aid to diagnosis, but it must be considered as having limited value in practice.

The American Psychiatric Association has developed a precise system of diagnosis, based on the description of symptoms in the Diagnostic and Statistical Manual of Mental Disorders, now in its fourth edition (DSM IV). Within the UK, mental and behavioural disorders are commonly classified using the International Classification of Diseases, ICD 10 (WHO 1992).

A systematic approach to the diagnosis of affective disorders is particularly helpful when considering the effectiveness of medication; most new clinical trials for antidepressants or neuroleptics will require a DSM diagnosis as an entry criterion.

From a practical clinical point of view it is uncommon for clinicians to treat affective disorders against such rigid diagnostic criteria, but recording target symptoms may be useful in evaluating the response to treatment. In routine clinical practice antidepressant medication should be considered when four or more of the signs and symptoms listed in Table 27.2 are present in a patient with persistent low mood or loss of interest or pleasure.

Rating scales

Various rating scales have been developed which may help in the assessment of the severity of the disorder. Two of the more common ones used in practice are the Beck depression inventory and the Hamilton depression rating scale.

Beck depression inventory

This is a self-reporting scale looking at 21 depressive symptoms. The subject is asked to read a series of statements and mark on a scale of 1 to 4 how severe the symptoms are. The higher the score the more severely depressed a person may be.

Hamilton depression rating scale

This rating scale is used by a health care professional at the end of an interview to rate the severity of the depression.

Dexamethasone suppression test

This test involves the administration of 1 mg of dexamethasone at 11 p.m., which is said to coincide with the low point of cortisol secretion. It would be expected that normally dexamethasone would suppress the secretion of cortisol for about 24 hours. Blood samples are taken the following day, at 8 a.m., 4 p.m. and 11 p.m. If it is found that plasma cortisol levels are elevated between 9 and 24 hours after the administration of dexamethasone, then this is taken as a positive result (i.e. dexamethasone has failed to suppress normal cortisol secretion).

It is important to note that this test is not specific to depression, and other disorders may account for an apparent positive result. Similarly, there may be a high proportion of depressed people who show a negative result with the test.

Table 27.2 Signs and symptoms of depression

Fatigue or loss of energy
Disturbed sleep
Inappropriate guilt
Poor concentration
Thought of death or suicide
Disturbed appetite
Agitation or slowing of speech

Diagnostic and statistical manual of mental disorders

The majority of modern drug trials demonstrating the benefit of antidepressant treatment will use the DSM criteria for the diagnosis of affective disorder (Tables 27.3 and 27.4).

Table 27.3 DSM IV diagnostic criteria for a major depressive episode (American Psychiatric Association 1994)

A. Five (or more) of the following symptoms have been present during the same 2-week period and represent a change from previous functioning; at least one of the symptoms is either (1) depressed mood or (2) loss of interest or pleasure:

1. Depressed mood most of the day, nearly every day, as indicated by either subjective report (e.g. feels sad or empty) or observation made by others (e.g. appears tearful).
2. Markedly diminished pleasure or interest in all or almost all activities, most of the day, nearly every day (as indicated by either subjective account or observation made by others).
3. Significant weight loss when not dieting or weight gain (e.g. a change of more than 5% of bodyweight within a month), or increase or decrease in appetite nearly every day.
4. Insomnia or hypersomnia nearly every day.
5. Psychomotor retardation or agitation nearly every day (observable by others, not merely subjective feeling of being slowed down or restless).
6. Fatigue or loss of energy nearly every day.
7. Feelings of worthlessness or excessive or inappropriate guilt (which may be delusional) nearly every day. (Not merely self-reproach or guilt about being sick.)
8. Diminished ability to think or concentrate or indecisiveness, nearly every day (either by subjective account or as observed by others).
9. Recurrent thought of death (not just fear of dying), recurrent suicidal ideation, without a specific plan, or a suicide attempt or a specific plan for committing suicide.

B. The symptoms do not meet criteria for mixed episode.

C. The symptoms caused clinically significant distress or impairment in social, occupational or other important areas of functioning.

D. The symptoms are not due to the direct physiological effect of a substance (e.g. a drug of abuse, a medication) or a general medical condition (e.g. hypothyroidism).

E. The symptoms are not better accounted for by bereavement, i.e. after the loss of a loved one, the symptoms persist for longer than 2 months or are characterized by marked functional impairment, morbid preoccupation with worthlessness, suicidal ideation, psychotic symptoms or psychomotor retardation.

Table 27.4   DSM IV diagnostic criterion for a manic episode (American Psychiatric Association 1994)

A. A distinct period of abnormality and persistently elevated, expansive, or irritable mood lasting at least 1 week (or any duration if hospitalization is necessary).

B. During the period of mood disturbances, three (or more) of the following symptoms have persisted (four if only the mood is irritable) and have been present to a significant degree:
   1. Inflated self-esteem or grandiosity.
   2. Decreased need for sleep (e.g. feels rested after only 3 hours of sleep).
   3. More talkative than usual or pressure to keep talking.
   4. Flight of ideas or subjective experience that thoughts are racing.
   5. Distractibility (i.e. attention too easily drawn to unimportant or irrelevant external stimuli).
   6. Increase in goal-directed activity (either socially, at work or school, or sexually) or psychomotor agitation.
   7. Excessive involvement in pleasurable activities which have a high potential for painful consequences (e.g. engaging in unrestrained buying sprees, sexual indiscretions, or foolish business investments).

C. The symptoms do not meet the criteria for a mixed episode.

D. The mood disturbance is sufficiently severe to cause marked impairment in occupational functioning or in usual social activities or relationships with others, or to necessitate hospitalization to prevent harm to others or self, or there are psychotic features.

E. The symptoms are not due to the direct physiological effects of a substance (e.g. a drug of abuse, a medication or other treatment) or a general medical condition (e.g. hyperthyroidism).

Treatment

The aim of treatment is to prevent harm and to relieve distress or to be prophylactic. It is important to differentiate symptoms of the disorder from the premorbid personality. With the exception of valproate semisodium, the drugs which are used to control the symptoms of mania are not specifically antimanic. They are also used in schizophrenia and other disorders; therefore the diagnosis will primarily influence the way in which these drugs are used rather than the choice of drug per se.

In the treatment of depression all the antidepressants are generally considered to be equally effective. There is no convincing evidence from clinical trials that any one drug is faster acting or any better or any worse than any other in relieving the symptoms of depression. Limited evidence suggests that severely depressed patients may be more likely to respond to antidepressants affecting

more than one neurotransmitter system, but the existence of a particular biochemical subtype of depression has not been established. Overall the major difference between agents is in their side-effect profile and toxicity in overdose. There can also be significant variations in the costs of different agents.

Treatment of depression

In moderate and severe depression, antidepressant medication should be considered the mainstay of treatment. In milder depressive states non-drug strategies may be considered preferable to drug treatment.

Sometimes a view is expressed that non-drug treatments and antidepressant medication are somehow mutually exclusive. In moderate to severe depression this is wrong: just as antidepressants should never be seen as the sole answer to a depression, the use of non-drug strategies should not be used as the reason for withholding treatment with antidepressant drugs.

Drug treatment

Despite the many new antidepressants available today, the therapeutic effectiveness of these agents has changed little since the discovery of the antidepressant properties of imipramine over 30 years ago.

Given an accurate diagnosis of moderate to severe depression, the majority of antidepressants currently available can be considered to be effective in up to 80% of patients. They must be taken in adequate doses for some 4–6 weeks (up to 12 weeks in some patients) in order to produce a full response, and treatment should be continued for 6 months at a full therapeutic dose before attempting withdrawal.

Unless the patient is experiencing severe problems, withdrawal of antidepressants should always be undertaken gradually. Following abrupt discontinuation patients may experience gastrointestinal symptoms, together with headache, giddiness, sweating, shaking and insomnia. In addition, extrapyramidal reactions may be associated with abrupt withdrawal of the selective serotonin re-uptake inhibitors (SSRI) antidepressants, for example like paroxetine. Following successful treatment antidepressants should be gradually reduced over a period of 4 weeks. This should be extended in patients experiencing problems, or where medication has been given for extended periods.

Generally, the long half-life of fluoxetine enables the drug to be stopped without the need for tapering from the standard antidepressant dose of 20 mg. Patients taking monoamine-oxidase inhibitors may experience psychomotor agitation following discontinuation.

Overall, antidepressants are not generally considered to be 'addictive' as there is no substantial evidence to support the existence of a physical dependency on antidepressants. However, some patients do report that they are dependant on their antidepressants and are unable to stop taking them.

As discussed earlier, there is no strong evidence for the existence of a particular biochemical subtype of depression. However, for unknown reasons certain patients do respond better to particular antidepressants. This has led to the widely held view that previous response to treatment is a strong indication to use that particular drug in the treatment of a future episode.

As well as previous response, the other important considerations to take into account when selecting an antidepressant are side-effects, contraindications, toxicity in overdose, patient preference and clinician familiarity.

Generally speaking, the older drugs have a poorer side-effect (Barbui et al 2001) and toxicity profile than the more recently introduced agents. Traditionally the antidepressant drugs are categorized by their chemical structure (e.g. tricyclic) or their predominant pharmacological action (e.g. MAOI or selective serotonin (5-HT) re-uptake inhibitor (SSRI).

Tricyclic antidepressants. A greater understanding of the pharmacology of antidepressants has lent much support to the biochemical theory of depression.

Although substantial data on the pharmacological effects of the tricyclic antidepressants exist, it is still not clear how the drugs relieve the symptoms of depression. Originally it was thought that the primary effect of the drugs was related to their ability to block the re-uptake of noradrenaline (norepinephrine) and/or 5-HT following their release and action as neurotransmitters. As this effect occurs some weeks before the antidepressant response, clearly this is not the whole story.

Following chronic administration, further biochemical changes take place, particularly with pre- and post-synaptic receptor sensitivity. Reduction of pre-synaptic α_2 receptor sensitivity occurs, and this increases the production of noradrenaline (norepinephrine). Other effects which may be relevant include an increase in α_1 and β_1 receptor sensitivity. It is now felt that these receptor changes in the cerebral cortex and hippocampus may be more related to the antidepressant response than simple re-uptake inhibition.

There are at least 12 tricyclic antidepressants in current clinical use. although the basic chemical structures of these compounds are similar there are differences between them. All the tricyclic antidepressants block the re-uptake of noradrenaline (norepinephrine) and 5-HT to a greater or lesser degree.

Imipramine. This is probably the most well established antidepressant. Its antidepressant effect was demonstrated over 30 years ago, and its is still widely prescribed today. Although less sedating than some other tricyclic drugs, some patients may still experience problems. As well as cardiovascular problems, significant antimuscarinic effects such as dry mouth, blurred vision and constipation occur.

For an effective antidepressant response it is important that the drug is given in full therapeutic doses; the British National Formulary advises that doses should be gradually increased to at least 150 mg daily and higher in some cases (up to 300 mg). Some patients, particularly the elderly, will not require such high doses, but even so they may still be unable to tolerate adequate doses.

Tolerance may develop to some of the unpleasant side-effects, and this may be facilitated by starting with a lower dose of the drug and gradually increasing the dose over a week.

In addition to the unpleasant side-effect profile, imipramine is toxic following overdose. Bearing in mind that the drug is used to treat a disorder which involves suicide, this relative lack of safety is an important disadvantage.

Imipramine is metabolized by demethylation to an active metabolite, desipramine. Both the parent drug and its metabolite have long half-lives (9–20 hours and 10–35 hours, respectively) that permit single daily dosing. Unfortunately the drug is only available in 10 mg or 25 mg tablets, and some patients do not like taking large numbers of tablets at once.

Amitriptyline. Another well-established and widely prescribed antidepressant, it has a similar poor side-effect and toxicity profile to imipramine, but is more sedative. Additional sedative properties are sometimes considered an advantage in selected patients.

Like imipramine, the drug and its active metabolite (nortriptyline) have long half-lives (9–46 hours and 18–56 hours). The dose range is similar to imipramine. Slow-release versions of amitriptyline exist, but apart from the convenience of swallowing fewer tablets they offer little advantage over conventional tablets.

Amoxapine. Unlike many of the other recently introduced antidepressants, amoxapine does not appear to have a significantly improved side-effect or toxicity profile.

Like other drugs in this class it is an effective antidepressant. Although some data have suggested the drug may have a particularly rapid onset of action, this does not appear to have been confirmed.

In standard doses, amoxapine may be less cardiotoxic than some other tricyclics but its effects following overdose are particularly severe, with renal failure and a high rate of seizures making management more difficult.

Another difference between amoxapine and the rest of the group is its dopamine-blocking effect. At first sight an antidepressant drug with inherent antipsychotic effects would appear to be useful, but in practice this is unlikely, and the potential for antidopaminergic side-effects is a significant disadvantage.

Clomipramine. This was one of the first antidepressants found to be a potent 5-HT re-uptake inhibitor. Some clinicians believe this drug is more effective than other antidepressants, but little evidence exists to support this anecdotal view. In addition to its antidepressant effect the drug has also been found to be of value in obsessional states.

Data from a fatal toxicity index (Cassidy & Henry 1987) show clomipramine to have a lower than expected toxicity per million prescriptions. This may be accounted for by the high rate of prescribing in non-depressive states, rather than any specific effect of the drug.

Dosulepin (dothiepin). Although produced over 20 years ago, this continues to be a widely prescribed antidepressant in the UK. Originally the drug was considered an improvement over amitriptyline and imipramine due to its improved side-effect profile. However, since the introduction of many of the newer antidepressants, further improvements in the side-effect profile of antidepressants have been made.

Doxepin. Doxepin has similar effects and side-effects to the traditional tricyclics. Limited evidence suggests that doxepin may have fewer cardiac effects on patients pre-existing cardiac disease than other traditional tricyclics. However, direct comparisons do not exist and a newer agent should be considered as an alternative to doxepin in patients with cardiac disease.

Lofepramine. Although desipramine is a metabolite of lofepramine, the latter should not be considered purely as a pro-drug. Important differences exist between lofepramine and the other traditional tricyclics.

Antimuscarinic effects occur with lofepramine, but these are less severe than with other tricyclics. Despite being metabolized to desipramine, lofepramine is significantly safer than the traditional agents, following overdose.

Lofepramine does not have a significant sedative effect, which may be an advantage in some patients, but in others the lack of sedation may be seen as a disadvantage. Some patients may complain of an alerting effect from lofepramine, particularly if the majority of the dose is given at bedtime.

Despite a few reports of hepatic problems, given the favourable side-effect profile and low toxicity in overdose, lofepramine may be considered as a first line treatment in the pharmacological management of depression.

Nortriptyline. Nortriptyline is the major metabolite of amitriptyline, but appears to have little effect on blood pressure. Plasma levels seem to show an inverted 'U' relationship with antidepressant effect. Patients respond best to intermediate levels of the drug, but higher or lower levels may be associated with a poorer response. Apart from these differences, nortriptyline shares many of the properties of the traditional tricyclic antidepressants.

Trimipramine. This is a particularly sedative tricyclic antidepressant with little difference from the rest of the traditional tricyclics.

Monoamine-oxidase inhibitors. Two types of MAOI are available: the traditional ones, which are both non-selective and irreversible, and moclobemide, which is a selective reversible inhibitor of monoamine-oxidase type A (RIMA)

In practice the traditional MAOIs are used much less than the tricyclic antidepressants. Some clinicians believe that the MAOIs are less effective than other antidepressants in moderate to severe depression. This is probably based on some of the original work that showed the MAOIs to be little different from placebos. Certainly the drugs do have anxiolytic properties, and if used in adequate doses are effective antidepressants. Some workers have suggested that MAOIs may be more effective in atypical depression or mild depression with a significant anxiety component. Due to the potential for drug and food interactions, MAOIs should be reserved for use when first-line antidepressant treatments have failed.

The potential for traditional MAOIs to interact with other drugs and tyramine-containing foods has been well known since the 1960s. It is important that patients are made aware of the advice printed on the MAOI warning card and follow the dietary restrictions. Occasionally other foods are added to this list of banned foods. For the majority of patients it is unhelpful to extend this list, which only compounds the difficulty for the depressed patients to construct a suitable diet.

An understanding of the mechanism of the interaction between foods and the MAOIs added weight to the biochemical hypothesis of depression. Although the effect of these drugs on monoamines is well understood, it is still not clear exactly how the MAOIs exert their antidepressant effect.

MAOIs inhibit the enzymes responsible for the oxidation of noradrenaline (norepinephrine), 5-HT and other biogenic amines. Two forms of monoamine-oxidase have been found to exist, MAO-A and MAO-B. The traditional MAOIs are all non-selective, and inhibit both forms of the enzyme.

Inhibition of MAO-A is thought to be responsible for the antidepressant effects. It is also responsible for metabolizing tyramine and producing the cheese interaction. Moclobemide is an antidepressant that acts as a reversible inhibitor of MAO-A. As tyramine is metabolized by both forms of the enzyme, if tyramine-containing foods are consumed, tyramine is metabolized by MAO-B enzymes as well as being able to reverse the inhibition of MAO-A. Unless very large quantities of tyramine are ingested, this appears to prevent the typical hypertensive reaction seen with conventional MAOIs and tyramine-containing foods.

Selegiline is a selective MAO-B inhibitor that does not seem to produce this interaction with foods, but neither does it appear to have a significant antidepressant effect.

Generally speaking, the traditional MAOIs and moclobemide have little anticholinergic effect; even so, some patients do experience dry mouth, constipation and urinary retention. In contrast to the hypertension which follows an interaction of tyramine-rich foods and the traditional MAOIs, these drugs are liable to cause postural hypotension as a side-effect. This side-effect may be particularly noticeable with phenelzine and may prevent adequate dosages being achieved.

Traditional MAOIs.

Tranylcypromine. Tranylcypromine has a structure that closely resembles amfetamine. It has a significant stimulant effect, and is more likely to give rise to dependence because of this. Unlike the other MAOIs it does not irreversibly inhibit monoamine-oxidase, which is said to recover some 5 days after withdrawal of the drug. Even so, the precautions associated with the MAOIs must still be continued for 2 weeks after discontinuing the drug.

Due to the amfetamine-like alerting effect of tranylcypromine the last dose should not be given after about 3 p.m. Some clinicians believe that the onset of action of this drug may be somewhat faster than the other MAOIs. However, the risk of interaction is also said to be greater with tranylcypromine than with other MAOIs.

Phenelzine. Unlike tranylcypromine, phenelzine belongs to the hydrazine group of MAOIs. The distinction is important as the hydrazines have been associated with hepatocellular jaundice. Although hydrazine MAOIs such as phenelzine should be avoided in patients with hepatic impairment, jaundice is rarely seen with their use in practice.

In most patients, phenelzine is neither sedative nor stimulant, and may be considered as an alternative to tranylcypromine, when its amfetamine-like effects are undesirable. As with other antidepressants it is important that phenelzine is prescribed in an adequate dosage (at least 1 mg/kg bodyweight).

Isocarboxazid. This is the least potent of the MAOIs, and may be considered if side-effects from the other agents are particularly troublesome.

Reversible inhibitors of monoamine-oxidase.

Moclobemide. Although an effective antidepressant, with less propensity for interactions with tyramine rich foods, caution should still be exercised as other drug interactions do occur. It is difficult to know the place of this agent in the treatment of depression as the drug does not appear to be as well established as the traditional MAOIs in atypical depression or depression unresponsive to other treatments. It cannot be assumed that moclobemide should replace the traditional MAOIs solely on the basis of the reduced propensity for interaction with certain foods.

Specific serotonin re-uptake inhibitors (SSRIs).

In an attempt to reduce some of the problems associated with the tricyclic antidepressants, a series of agents which are specific to 5-HT have been developed, the so-called selective (or specific) serotonin re-uptake inhibitors (SSRIs).

As a group these drugs appear to be no more, but also no less, effective than the tricyclics. Generally speaking, they have less troublesome side-effects and are significantly less toxic following overdose than the traditional antidepressants.

All the SSRIs currently available have different chemical structures, but they all have a specific effect which inhibits serotonin re-uptake. The SSRIs have similar side-effect profiles, but there are differences in the intensity of different side-effects. As with the antidepressants in general, there are differences between the individual agents which may be important for some patients (Edwards & Anderson 1999).

The degree of specificity for serotonin re-uptake differs between the SSRIs, but this does not correlate with clinical efficacy. If given in adequate doses for an adequate period of time, all the drugs in this class appear equally effective.

Prior to the availability of generic forms, these drugs were considerably more expensive than the traditional tricyclic agents. This led to considerable debate over the use of these agents. Several meta-analyses attempted to determine whether or not this class of drugs represented any overall benefit over the traditional tricyclic agents. (Song F et al 1993, Anderson & Tomenson 1995, Hotopf et al 1996). The only definitive conclusion that was drawn was that the SSRIs were neither more nor less effective than traditional tricyclics. They may be better tolerated than tricyclics as measured by fewer drop-outs from clinical trials, but the significance of this for clinical practice is unclear.

Many clinicians now consider the SSRIs as first-line treatment, particularly in primary care. This may be due to a combination of factors, including lack of toxicity in overdose, tolerability and simplicity of dosage. However, the impact of promotion by the pharmaceutical industry must not be overlooked. Data on fluoxetine indicate that a maximum response is achieved at 20 mg with little benefit to be gained by increasing the dose further. As large numbers of patients are given subtherapeutic doses of antidepressants, this simple dose regimen does appear to offer a practical advantage.

Fluvoxamine. This was the first SSRI available in the UK. Although patients experience few antimuscarinic side-effects, other problems related to serotonergic enhancement such as nausea, headache and nervousness have been reported.

Fluoxetine. The main difference between fluoxetine and the other SSRIs is the long half-lives of both the parent drug and its primary active metabolite, desmethylfluoxetine. In the initial stages of treatment some patients may experience a greater feeling of nervousness with fluoxetine than with the other SSRIs, but in most cases tolerance to this develops.

The long half-life of fluoxetine and its major metabolite is a problem if severe side-effects develop or the prescriber wishes to change to an MAOI. It will take 5 weeks to clear fluoxetine, and in some patients this delay may make management difficult.

Paroxetine. Although all the SSRIs have been reported to cause extrapyramidal-type movements, paroxetine appears to be more commonly implicated. The problem may be particularly severe following abrupt discontinuation of high doses.

Sertraline. Like the other SSRIs, sertraline is an effective antidepressant. Although doses of up to 200 mg have been used, doses of 150 mg and above should not be given for longer than 8 weeks.

Citalopram. The efficacy and side-effect profile of citalopram appear similar to the other agents, but like sertraline the reduced propensity for interactions with drugs metabolized by the cyctochrome P4502D6 isoenzyme has been suggested as a theoretical advantage.

Lithium. Lithium does have antidepressant properties, but will be discussed in more detail in the antimanic section.

Other drugs.

Maprotiline. Although maprotiline has slightly fewer antimuscarinic side-effects than the tricyclics, it also has many of the cardiovascular problems associated with these drugs. It induces seizures to a greater extent than the other antidepressants, particularly at higher doses.

Trazodone. In vitro the drug appears to operate as a mixed serotonin agonist/antagonist, but clinically it is thought to operate as a serotonin agonist. Trazodone is much safer than the tricyclics following overdose but causes pronounced sedative and hypotensive effects in some patients. Priapism has also been noted as a rare but distressing side-effect. This is probably due to its potent α receptor blocking properties.

Nefazodone. Structurally related to trazodone, nefazodone acts as a weak 5-HT and noradrenergic (norepinephrinergic) re-uptake inhibitor and a selective 5-HT_2 antagonist. The overall effect is to facilitate 5-HT_{1A} neurotransmission without up-regulating 5-HT_2 receptors (an effect thought to be related to increased violence or suicide early in treatment).

In practice the main difference between nefazodone and other antidepressants appears to be the lack of sexual dysfunction associated with this agent. Although nefazodone has few antimuscarinic or cardiac side-effects, 5-HT-related problems such as nausea and headache still occur.

Mianserin. Mianserin was one of the first antidepressants to have a significantly improved toxicity profile following overdose. Like many of the newer drugs, it has fewer antimuscarinic side-effects than the traditional tricyclics. One drawback in using mianserin is the need for monthly blood counts during the first 3 months of treatment, due to a high reported incidence of blood dyscrasias, particularly in the elderly. These blood tests should not be considered a substitute for the routine clinical monitoring of the patient.

Venlafaxine. Venlafaxine represents the first in a new class of antidepressants, the serotonin–noradrenaline (serotonin–norepinephrine) re-uptake inhibitors (SNRIs). These antidepressants were developed in an attempt to improve efficacy over the standard agents. As the name suggests, they prevent the re-uptake of both serotonin and noradrenaline (norepinephrine) (like the tricyclic antidepressants), but without the antimuscarinic, cardiac or toxic effects of the older drugs. Although venlafaxine shares many of the benefits of the other newer antidepressants, such as lack of antimuscarinic side-effects and safety in overdose, the suggestions of increased speed of response or benefit in treatment resistance remain to be confirmed.

As well as a similar side-effect profile to the SSRIs, at higher doses venlafaxine is also associated with a rise in blood pressure. Changing to the slow release formulation may reduce some of the gastrointestinal problems associated with the conventional release product.

Reboxetine. A specific noradrenergic (norepinephrinergic) re-uptake inhibitor. Response rates appear similar to other antidepressants. This casts further doubt on the existence of particular subtypes of depression likely to respond to particular antidepressants. Patients experiencing problems with serotonergic related side-effects may benefit from a switch to reboxetine.

Mirtazapine. Mirtazapine enhances both noradrenergic (norepinephrinergic) and 5HT_1 serotonergic transmission. Specific 5HT_1 neurotransmission is achieved as the drug also acts as a 5HT_2 and 5HT_3 antagonist. This preferential effect on noradrenaline (norepinephrine) and serotonin has led to the drug being referred to as a noradrenergic (norepinephrinergic) and specific serotonergic antidepressant (NaSSA). Despite the novel pharmacology, mirtazapine appears little different from other antidepressants in terms of efficacy.

Other treatments.

Electroconvulsive therapy. Electroconvulsive therapy (ECT) would only be considered after referral to a psychiatrist. Although it is said to have a faster onset of action, its effects are fairly short lived, and antidepressants are normally required to prevent relapse. Although the treatment itself is considered safe, there are risks from the anaesthetic agent, and some patients suffer short-term memory loss following treatment.

Non-drug treatments. In addition to drug treatment, most patients will need help and support to cope with depression. As well as this type of therapy, other forms of psychotherapy are available from specialist services. For mild forms of depression non-drug strategies are often considered as first-line treatment.

St John's wort (Hypericum perforatum). Extracts of hypericum are effective in the short term management of mild or moderately severe depression (Linde & Mulrow 2001). Hypericum may induce the metabolism of other drugs, which may lead to toxicity on discontinuation. There is currently insufficient evidence to support the use of this product in severe depression.

Choice of antidepressant. There is no robust evidence to guide the clinican's choice of antidepressant. As no antidepressant has been found to be any more effective than any other, the choice will be determined by other factors. In some areas, cost has become a major factor in choice. In general the newer drugs appear to have a better side-effect profile and are less toxic following overdose. Recent experiences with some new antidepressants now withdrawn due to severe and unexpected side-effects quite rightly serve as a caution against significant changes in traditional prescribing habits based on limited data.

There is substantial experience of using drugs such as lofepramine and fluoxetine, which may lead to their use as first-line treatments. All the modern antidepressants appear better tolerated than the traditional tricyclics but the margin of benefit is reported to be small. However, the continued prescribing of antidepressants (particularly common with tricyclics) in subtherapeutic doses remains a major issue, particularly within primary care.

In an attempt to curtail the use of the newer, more expensive drugs, suggestions have been made to reserve these drugs for patients intolerant of the older less expensive drugs, or in those considered to be at high suicidal risk. In clinical practice the identification of suicidality is difficult, and all patients with severe depression should be considered at risk of self-harm. A more enlightened view would be to concentrate on areas such as non-compliance as a way of preserving health care resources. The issue of simplicity of dose should not be underestimated.

As long as there are no contraindications, then previous response to a particular drug is considered the strongest indication for use. Standard texts such as the British National Formulary suggest that patients who are agitated or anxious may respond to antidepressants with sedating side-effects, and those who are withdrawn or apathetic to the less sedating ones. In practice, antidepressants, both sedating and nonsedating, appear to be helpful in anxiety (Rickels et al 1993).

In the absence of previous treatment and obvious contraindications, where sedation is not required, then lofepramine or one of the well-established SSRIs could be considered as first-line treatment. If the patient requires additional sedative effects, then trazodone may be more appropriate. Although still based on largely anecdotal evidence, some clinicians advocate the use of venlafaxine, or tricyclic antidepressants in severely depressed hospitalized patients (Spigset & Martensson 1999).

Treatment of mania

Valproate semisodium is the only available drug which is a specific antimanic agent. In addition the neuroleptics, lithium and benzodiazepine sedatives all have a place in the management of mania. In most cases neuroleptics or valproate semisodium are the treatments of choice in the acute stages. Benzodiazepines, either alone or in combination, may also be effective. Lithium is the drug of choice for long-term use to prevent recurrence or relapse. In time further evidence may establish the place of sodium valproate along with carbamazepine as alternatives. When used prophylactically these agents are commonly referred to as mood stabilizers.

Valproate semisodium

This is a 1:1 molar combination of sodium valproate and valproic acid. Following administration, valproate ion is released and subsequently absorbed. The therapeutic differences between sodium valproate and valproate semisodium have not been established. However, the latter is the only form of valproate licensed for the acute treatment of mania. The mechanism of action in mania is unclear but may be related to increased levels of γ-aminobutyric acid (GABA). The antimanic effects of valproate are seen within 3 days, but the full benefit of treatment may not be apparent for up to 3 weeks. Dosage should be rapidly titrated up to between 1000 mg and 2000 mg per day. Routine plasma levels are not necessary, but levels above 50 micrograms/ml and below 100 micrograms/ml are reported to be associated with optimal response.

Although the risks of liver damage are greater in young children, liver function tests should be performed prior to initiation of therapy and periodically thereafter in all patients. In addition the patient must be instructed to report any problems, such as unexplained bruising, that may indicate abnormalities in coagulation.

Neuroleptics

All these drugs share a common effect of blocking dopamine D_2 post-synaptic receptors. There is little evidence supporting the use of any one neuroleptic over any other, but in practice haloperidol, chlorpromazine or zuclopenthixol (Acuphase) tend to be used most frequently. Their effect may become apparent within several days of initiatng treatment. Droperidol, another commonly used neuroleptic, was discontinued in the UK in 2001.

In most circumstances, haloperidol is probably the neuroleptic of choice as it is free from many of the cardiovascular problems of chlorpromazine. As haloperidol is less sedating than chlorpromazine it may occasionally be necessary to control severe behaviour disturbances with additional sedatives such as lorazepam, either orally or by injection. Neuroleptics may also be required in combination with valproate semisodium if significant psychotic symptoms exist.

Zuclopenthixol acetate (Acuphase) is formulated as a long-acting injection (up to 3 days) and may be appropriate as an alternative to repeated attempts to control disturbed behaviour with other injections.

Dosage and duration of treatment are important when treating acute mania. The dose of neuroleptic should be reduced as the patient improves, and in most cases the neuroleptic can be stopped as the patient becomes euthymic.

As the parenteral forms of the atypical neuroleptics become widely available, they offer therapeutic benefits in the acute management of mania.

Lithium

Although lithium is effective in the acute management of mania, other treatments are generally preferred. This is due to the delay in response and variability of fluid intake which may compromise the safe use of lithium. In the acute situation lithium make take up to 10–14 days to exert an effect. Higher plasma levels are also required (around 1.2 mmol/l).

Neuroleptics or valproate semisodium, either alone or in combination, along with benzodiazepines should be considered the first-line treatment in the acute phase of mania.

Following an acute episode lithium remains the primary consideration for prophylaxis (Baldessarini & Tondo 2000). Generally speaking, continuation therapy with a prophylactic mood stabilizer should be considered in all bipolar patients who have had two or more acute episodes within 2–4 years. It may also be reasonable to consider prophylaxis in any patient following a severe manic episode. As treatment is long term, the cooperation of the patient is essential, and so a thorough explanation of the risks and benefits of the treatment is vital.

Before lithium treatment is initiated, an assessment of the patient's physical state is essential. Thyroid, renal and cardiac function should all be within normal limits, but it is still possible to use lithium, with caution, in patients with mild to moderate renal failure or cardiovascular impairment. Thyroid deficiency should be corrected before lithium treatment is commenced.

Plasma levels. There is a narrow therapeutic window for lithium plasma levels. Levels above 1.2 mmol/l are considered to be toxic and levels below 0.4 mmol/l are not considered to be effective. If lithium plasma levels are kept in the range 0.5–0.8 mmol/l, then lithium is usually well tolerated with minimal side-effects.

The range of 0.5–0.8 mmol/l is appropriate for prophylaxis, but if lithium is used to control the acute phase, levels may need to be around 1.0 mmol/l.

In order to accurately interpret lithium levels it is important that the correct schedule is followed. In order to establish consistent results the 12-hour standard serum lithium protocol has been devised. This means that lithium levels should be taken in the morning as near as possible to 12 hours after the last dose of lithium.

As the absorption and bioavailability of lithium may vary from brand to brand, it is important that patients do not inadvertently change brands or dosage forms without levels being checked.

Even though lithium has a narrow therapeutic range and is particularly toxic in overdose, it is still well tolerated by most people if the blood levels are kept at the lower end of the therapeutic range. The most common side-effects reported by patients are tremor, thirst, polyuria, weight gain and lethargy. As well as complaints of side-effects, some patients may not like taking prophylactic mood stabilizers as they like the slight 'highs' in their illness. There is a significant risk of relapse if lithium is suddenly discontinued.

Patients taking a prophylactic mood stabilizer may occasionally stop taking their medication when they feel they no longer need it, or want to see if they can overcome the disorder without the need for drugs. Patients commonly have several trials on a mood stabilizer before they accept the fact that they will need it long term and that they frequently relapse when they no longer take the drug.

Carbamazepine

Carbamazepine has been shown to be both antidepressant and antimanic, but its main use is as an alternative to lithium in the prophylaxis of bipolar disorders. In most patients a daily dose of 600 mg or above is required.

Mood stabilizer combinations

In patients who cannot be controlled on a single mood stabilizer, consideration should be given to combining treatments. Although not entirely without risks, all of the above drugs have been used in various combinations in resistant cases. (Freeman & Stoll 1998).

Patient care

In the acute phase of an affective disorder a patient will have little or no insight into his or her condition. This often makes it difficult to prescribe medication following an informed discussion on the risks and benefits of treatment. Depressed patients may say they are not worth treating; most manic patients will find it impossible to engage in meaningful dialogue, or they may insist they do not need medication and consistently refuse treatment. Thus in the initial stages of treatment some patients are treated against their will. As people respond to treatment it is crucial that the benefits as well as the risks of treatment are explained. This may need to be repeated and backed up by written information. Engaging the patient and including them in the choice of treatment not only supports their basic human rights but is also likely to lead to a better therapeutic outcome. This is particularly important with long-term prophylactic mood stabilizers where a patient may feel well for many months (apart from the side-effects of medication!).

Patients with an affective disorder may have a low attention span and will often forget what they have been told about medication. They may repeatedly seek

Table 27.5	Some important drug interactions (consult specialist texts for a comprehensive review)	
Antidepressant	Interacting drug	Effect
Tricyclics	Adrenaline (epinephrine) (and other directly acting sympathomimetics)	Greatly enhances effect. Dangerous
	Alcohol	Enhanced sedation
	Antiarrhythmics	Risk of ventricular arrhythmias
	Anticonvulsants	Lowered seizure threshold and possible lowered tricyclic levels
	MAOIs	Severe hypertension
	Fluoxetine	Increased tricyclic plasma levels
SSRIs	Anticoagulants	Enhanced effects
	MAOIs	Dangerous
	Lithium	Possible serotonin syndrome
MAOIs	Alcohol, fermented beverages, tyramine rich foods	Hypertensive crisis
	Antihypertensives	Increased effect
	Anticonvulsants	Lowered seizure threshold
	Levodopa	Hypertensive crisis
	Sympathomimetics	Hypertensive crisis
Neuroleptics	Anaesthetic agents	Hypotension
	Anticonvulsants	Lowered seizure threshold
	Antiarrhythmics	Risk of ventricular arrhythmias
	Astemizole and terfenadine	Risk of ventricular arrhythmias
Lithium	Non-steroidal anti-inflammatory drugs (NSAIDs)	Enhanced lithium plasma levels
	SSRIs	Possible serotonin syndrome
Diuretics	Enhanced lithium plasma levels particularly with thiazides	
	Angiotensin-converting enzyme (ACE) inhibitors	Enhanced lithium plasma levels
	Sumatriptan	Possible central nervous system toxicity
St John's wort	Induces cytochrome P450 enzymes particularly 1A2, 2C9, and 3A4	
	Indinavir	Reduced plasma concentration (avoid)
	Warfarin	Reduced anticoagulant effect (avoid)
	SSRIs	Increased serotonergic effect (avoid)
	Carbamazepine (and other anticonvulsants)	Reduced plasma concentrations (avoid)
	Digoxin	Reduced plasma concentration (avoid)
	Oestrogens and progestogens	Reduced contraceptive effect (avoid)
	Theophylline	Reduced plasma concentration (avoid)
	Ciclosporin	Reduced plasma concentration (avoid)

information and reassurance, even after someone has already fully discussed the effects of medication with them.

Many people are understandably frightened by the idea of taking medication that will affect their mind. Taking an antidepressant is frequently considered a sign of weakness by the patient as well as their family and friends. This often leads patients to try and deal with their depression without medication. This may be fine for the milder forms of the disorder, but could have life-threatening consequences for those with severe depression or mania. The use of patient information leaflets and the involvement of the family or close friends may help patients to understand the risks and benefits of their treatment. Patients should always be offered the opportunity of discussing their medication with a specialist pharmacist involved in their care.

Many of the drugs used in the treatment of affective disorders have the potential to interact with other drugs that have been prescribed or purchased. Some of these are summarized in Table 27.5.

Common therapeutic problems in the management of affective disorder are outlined in Table 27.6.

CASE STUDIES

Case 27.1

Mrs G. S. is a 24-year-old woman who presents to her general practitioner with a 2-month history of difficulty in getting to sleep. She has lost interest in most things but does get up and dresses every day. She complains of little energy and spends most of the day sitting in the front room with the television on.

She has a 3-month-old child, and feels guilty because she finds it hard to care for the baby. Mrs G. S.'s parents-in-law are staying with the family to help out with the baby.

Question

What diagnosis is likely to be given to Mrs G. S. and what are the important factors to take into account when advising on treatment?

Answer

Mrs G. S. has a puerperal depressive disorder of moderate severity. She feels guilty at not being able to look after her child.

It should be established that Mrs G. S. is not a high suicidal risk, and the health visitor and other professionals must be consulted to establish that the baby is not at risk. Even though

Table 27.6   Common therapeutic problems in the management of affective disorder

Problem	Possible solution
Antidepressants	
Treatment failure (30–40% of patients will not respond to first antidepressant)	Ensure adequate dose and duration of treatment
	Check compliance – engage the patient – develop therapeutic relationship
	Reassess response against target symptoms
	Reconfirm diagnosis; identify compounding factors, e.g. high levels of alcohol consumption
Risk of self-harm	Prescribe/dispense limited quantities. Involve family or carer in supervising medication. Avoid traditional tricyclics in unsupervised situations
Withdrawal reactions	Ensure gradual withdrawal
Relapse on discontinuation	Consider long-term treatment
Intolerance	Consider changing to a different class
Antimanic agents	
Treatment failure	Ensure adequate dose, check plasma levels. Consider drug combinations
Toxicity adverse effects	Determine dose by clinical response, guided by plasma levels
	Ensure patient is well informed and able to recognize impending toxicity and adverse effects of treatment
Weight gain	Dietary advice; consider alternative pharmacotherapy
Lithium levels	Ensure plasma levels are 12 hours post-dose, taken in the morning. Regular monitoring is important

the patient may not be breastfeeding, it is still important that mother and child are not separated. Regular professional contact and assessment of Mrs G. S. should be maintained.

In terms of efficacy, none of the antidepressants is likely to be any more effective than any other in puerperal depression, and so the choice of treatment will be determined by other factors.

Although the patient finds it difficult to get off to sleep she still spends most of the day sitting around feeling tired and sleepy. A sedative antidepressant may help sleep initially, but sedative side-effects during the day would be a problem. The effects of medication should be explained, particularly the likely side-effects, lack of dependence potential and the duration of treatment.

During the first 1–2 weeks of treatment with an antidepressant, the patient will notice an improvement in her sleep pattern. Lofepramine 70 mg initially twice daily or fluoxetine 20 mg daily would be suitable choices because of their low side-effect profile and absence of sedation.

Case 27.2

Mr P. D. is a 70-year-old man with a longstanding history of bipolar disorder. He was admitted to an acute psychiatric ward, with a 3-day history of increasing irritability. He had been brought into hospital by the police, who had been contacted by a neighbour, because he had been standing in the window exposing himself.

Mr P. D. said he felt 'fine, fine all the time' and 'never been better'. He wanted to go home as he had important business to deal with, and insisted he was within his rights to go home. He would not discuss this but said everyone would soon find out.

Mr P. D.'s speech was very rapid, and it was sometimes difficult to understand what he was saying. He was dressed in a very untidy fashion and had obviously not taken care of his personal hygiene for some time.

On his last admission 18 months ago he was treated with haloperidol.

Question

What treatment is appropriate for Mr P. D.?

Answer

Mr P. D.'s symptoms of mania need to be brought under control. Haloperidol would be a suitable choice, in view of his previous response. A medication review should be carried out, which would confirm the circumstances of the response to haloperidol during his previous admission.

When Mr P. D.'s manic symptoms are controlled, lithium treatment should be discussed with him. This should include the provision of written information and the opportunity for contact in the future. Renal, thyroid and cardiac function should be assessed, and if within normal limits, lithium carbonate 400 mg at night may be prescribed.

One week later a 12-hour standard serum lithium level should be performed and the dose of lithium adjusted to achieve 12-hour levels between 0.4 and 0.8 mmol/l.

Mr P. D. should be monitored closely for side-effects, as the combination of neuroleptic and lithium may increase the severity of drug-induced rigidity and tremor. The side-effects and signs of impending toxicity from lithium should be explained to Mr P. D. He should be warned of the possibility of interaction with drugs he may obtain from doctors or pharmacists in the future.

Case 27.3

Mr A. F. is a 40-year-old salesman who was admitted following an overdose attempt with 20 paracetamol tablets. He felt that everything in his life had gone wrong and there was no point in going on.

Question

What course of action would you advise?

Answer

It is important to use an antidepressant with a low side-effect profile and a good safety profile following overdose in this patient. One of the SSRIs would be a suitable choice for Mr A. F. He should be told that he is being prescribed a drug that will relieve the symptoms of his depression. While pointing out the benefits of antidepressant treatment, the common side-effects should be discussed. Mr A. F. should be told how long it will take his antidepressant medication to work and that this type of medication is normally prescribed for at least 6 months.

Mr A. F. should be reassured that his antidepressant is not addictive and is not related to tranquillizers such as Valium. As his symptoms improve he should be offered the opportunity of discussing any concerns about his medication.

Case 27.4

Mr O. S. is a 49-year-old unemployed gentleman. He was admitted to a psychiatric unit at the request of his general practitioner, who had prescribed fluoxetine 20 mg daily 2 weeks earlier. On admission he was noted to be withdrawn, lacking motivation and just gave 'yes' or 'no' in response to questioning. He reported no interests in his life, and it was noted that he had attempted to harm himself in the past.

One month after admission there was no significant improvement in his symptoms.

Question

What treatment options are appropriate for Mr O. S.?

Answer

Before considering a change in treatment, it must be confirmed that Mr O. S. has regularly taken his fluoxetine. Plasma levels are not generally available, or particularly helpful. Scrutiny of the medicine charts, discussion with nursing staff and the patient will enable a reasonable judgment to be formed. A dose increase could be considered if the patient had shown a limited response to fluoxetine. In this case, the patient had received no apparent benefit and a change in treatment was warranted.

An in-depth review of his previous medication should be undertaken. This should include discussion with the patient about any previous antidepressant treatment he had found to be particularly effective, or troublesome.

This review revealed that Mr O. S. had received several different antidepressants over the past 20 years. Two years ago he was treated with venlafaxine S/R 75 mg daily. The medical records confirmed Mr O. S.'s view that this medication had helped him in the past, but on further questioning he stated that he had not taken medication for long after discharge from hospital as he did not want to get 'hooked' on it.

The importance of long-term treatment and the proposed treatment plan should be discussed with Mr O. S. Fluoxetine should be discontinued and venlafaxine started 1 week later.

Case 27.5

Ms Y. S. is a 28-year-old student with a history of bipolar disorder. She was admitted to an acute psychiatric unit at the request of her key worker. She had recently become increasingly elated and her partner was very concerned about the increased credit card bills she was incurring.

On the ward she attempted to develop sexual relationships with several young male patients.

Question

Describe the treatment options available for Ms Y. S.

Answer

There is insufficient information to determine whether or not Ms Y. S. was being treated with a prophylactic mood stabilizer. It is important to determine if the current episode was related to inadequate prophylactic treatment.

The current episode of hypomania must be treated. She is currently at risk though her promiscuity and the excessive use of her credit card. Both behaviours are likely to affect her ability to maintain a relationship with her partner.

Initially treatment with valproate semisodium should be considered. A neuroleptic such as haloperidol could be considered, but as she had no psychotic symptoms, valproate is the preferred option. An assessment of liver function, prothrombin rate and full blood count should be performed prior to initiating therapy.

The patient should be informed of the important adverse effects of therapy. In particular she should be advised to report any unexplained bruising and to avoid the use of salicylates. Treatment should be commenced at 250 mg three times daily and increased in accordance with response and tolerability. Benzodiazepines may also be considered as a short-term adjunct if additional sedation is required.

Following resolution of the acute episode, long-term prophylaxis must be considered. In this case Ms Y. S. had previously been treated with lithium, but had refused to continue as this had caused significant weight gain.

In view of the patient's refusal to consider lithium, prophylactic options are carbamazepine or valproate semisodium (valproate semisodium is not licensed for prophylactic use in the UK). Little hard evidence currently exists to guide the choice. It is important to take the patient's view into account.

As the patient had no significant depressive episode during the course of her illness she should be encouraged to consider prophylactic treatment with valproate, albeit currently not licensed for this indication.

Case 27.6

Ms A. B. is a 55-year-old unemployed lady with a longstanding history of depression. She has been treated with numerous antidepressants over the years and is currently under the care of the community mental health team.

The only treatment that appears to have had any effect on her depressive episodes has been dosulepin (dothiepin). She has taken several overdoses in the past and her psychiatrist is reluctant to prescribe this drug.

Question

What measures could be taken to enable Ms A. B. to be treated effectively.

Answer

Ms A. B. does not have treatment resistant depression. She has been succesfully treated with dosulepin (dothiepin) in the past, but impulsively takes an overdose as a way of dealing with difficult circumstances.

Non-drug strategies by the mental health team should be directed at enabling Ms A. B. to find alternative ways of dealing with these difficulties.

Despite the obvious risk of fatality, dosulepin (dothiepin) remains the treatment of choice for Ms A. B. due to her previous response to this drug and her lack of response to other antidepressants. Practical measures of controlling the quantities of medication should be introduced. These include gaining the agreement, where possible, of the local community pharmacist to dispense dosulepin (dothiepin) every 2 or 3 days. Alternatively, medication could be supplied as part of the regular contact between Ms A. B. and the community team.

Communication between all those involved in the care of Ms A. B. is crucial. When individualizing the supply of medication in this way all those involved must be alert to the possibility that the system of supply may break down. In this case an apparently routine prescription for 1 month's supply of medication may have fatal consequences.

REFERENCES

American Psychiatric Association 1994 Diagnostic and statistical manual of mental disorders, 4th edn. American Psychiatric Association, Washington, DC

Anderson I M, Tomenson B M 1995 Treatment discontinuation with selective serotonin re- uptake inhibitors compared with tricyclic antidepressants: a meta-analysis. British Medical Journal 310: 1433–1438

Baldessarini R J, Tondo L 2000 Does lithium treatment still work? Evidence of stable responses over three decades. Archives of General Psychiatry 57(2): 187–908

Barbui C, Hotopf M, Freemantle N et al 2001 Selective serotonin re-uptake inhibitors versus tricyclic and heterocyclic antidepressants: comparison of drug adherence. Cochrane Review. Cochrane Library, issue 2. Update Software, Oxford

British National Formulary, no. 41 2001 British Medical Association and Royal Pharmaceutical Society of Great Britain, London

Cassidy S, Henry J 1987 Fatal toxicity of antidepressant drugs in overdose. British Medical Journal 295: 1021–1024

Edwards J G, Anderson I 1999 Systematic review and guide to selection of selective serotonin re-uptake inhibitors. Drugs 57(4): 507–533

Freeman M O, Stoll A L 1998 Mood stabilizer combinations: a review of safety and efficacy. American Journal of Psychiatry 155(1): 12–21

Hotopf M, Lewis G, Normand C 1996 Are SSRIs a cost effective alternative to tricyclics? British Journal of Psychiatry 168: 404–409

Linde K, Mulrow C D 2001 St John's wort for depression. Cochrane Review. Cochrane Library, issue 2. Update Software, Oxford

Rickels K, Downing R, Schweizer E et al 1993 Antidepressants for treatment of generalized anxiety disorder. Archives of General Psychiatry 50: 884–895

Song F, Freemantle N, Sheldon T A et al 1993 Selective serotonin re-uptake inhibitors: a meta analysis of efficacy and acceptability. British Medical Journal 306: 683–687

Spigset O, Martensson B 1999 Fortnightly review: drug treatment of depression. British Medical Journal 318(7192): 1188–1191

World Health Organization 1992 Tenth revision of the international classification of diseases and related health problems (ICD-10). WHO, Geneva

FURTHER READING

Anderson I M, Nutt D J, Deakin J F 2000 Evidence-based guidelines for treating depressive disorders with antidepressants: a revision of the 1993 British Association for Psychopharmacology guidelines. British Association for Psychopharmacology. Journal of Psychopharmacology 14(1): 3–20

De Jonghe F, Swinkels J 1997 Selective serotonin re-uptake inhibitors: relevance of differences in their pharmacological and clinical profiles. CNS Drugs 7(6): 452–467

Gelder M, Gath D, Mayou R et al (eds) 1996 Oxford textbook of psychiatry, 4th edn. Oxford Medical Publications, Oxford

Kent J M 2000 SnaRIs, NaSSAs, and NaRIs: new agents for the treatment of depression. Lancet 355(9207): 911–918

Licht R W 1998 Drug treatment of mania: a critical review. Acta Psychiatrica Scandinavica 97(6): 387–397

Moller H J, Volz H P 1996 Drug treatment of depression in the 1990s. Drugs 52(5): 625–638

Peet M, Pratt J P 1993 Lithium: current status in psychiatric disorders. Drugs 46: 7–17

Taylor D, Duncan D 1997 Doses of carbamazepine and valproate in bipolar affective disorder. Psychiatric Bulletin 21: 221–223

Schizophrenia 28

D. Branford

KEY POINTS

- Schizophrenia is a complex illness which varies greatly in presentation.
- Positive symptoms such as hallucinations, delusions and thought disorder, which commonly occur in the acute phase of the illness, usually respond to antipsychotic drug therapy.
- Negative symptoms such as apathy, social withdrawal and lack of drive, which occur commonly in the chronic phase of the illness are more resistant to drug treatment.
- The term 'atypical' is used to describe those antipsychotic drugs that do not cause extrapyramidal side-effects.
- Typical antipsychotic drugs are often associated with anticholinergic, sedative and cardiovascular side-effects in addition to extrapyramidal side-effects.
- Long-term treatment with typical antipsychotic drugs is associated with the development of tardive dyskinesia.
- Most typical antipsychotic drugs have similar efficacy for the treatment of schizophrenia.
- Clozapine has a broader spectrum of activity than traditional antipsychotic drugs with some efficacy for treatment-resistant schizophrenia and negative symptoms.

The concept of schizophrenia can be difficult to understand. People who do not suffer from schizophrenia can have little idea of what the experience of hallucinations and delusions is like. The presentation of schizophrenia can be extremely varied, with a great range of possible symptoms. There are also many misconceptions about the condition of schizophrenia that have led to prejudice against sufferers of the illness. Schizophrenics are commonly thought to have low intelligence and to be dangerous. In fact only a minority of patients show violent behaviour, with social withdrawal being a more common picture. Up to 10% of people with schizophrenia commit suicide.

Classification

Since the late 19th century there have been frequent attempts to define the illness we now call schizophrenia.

Kraepelin, in the late 1890s, coined the term 'dementia praecox' (early madness) to describe an illness where there was a deterioration of the personality at a young age. Kraepelin also coined the terms 'catatonic' (where motor symptoms are prevalent and changes in activity vary), 'hebephrenic' (silly, childish behaviour, affective symptoms and thought disorder prominent), and 'paranoid' (clinical picture dominated by paranoid delusions). A few years later a Swiss psychiatrist called Bleuler introduced the term 'schizophrenia', derived from the Greek words *skhizo* (to split) and *phren* (mind), meaning the split between the emotions and the intellect.

Schneider (1957) attempted to make diagnosis more reliable by identifying symptoms of first rank importance, but in recent years, two systems of classification have become more widely used. These are the *Diagnostic and Statistical Manual of Mental Disorders,* fourth edition (DSM IV) (American Psychiatric Association) and the *International Classification of Diseases,* 10th edition (ICD 10) (World Health Organization).

Symptoms of schizophrenia

Symptoms common in acute psychotic illness

To establish a definite diagnosis of schizophrenia it is important to follow the diagnostic criteria in either DSM IV or ICD 10, but symptoms which commonly occur in the acute phase of a psychotic illness include the following:

- awkward social behaviour, appearing preoccupied, perplexed and withdrawn, or showing unexpected changes in behaviour
- initial vagueness in speech which can progress to disorders of the stream of thought or poverty of thought
- abnormality of mood such as anxiety, depression, irritability or euphoria
- auditory hallucinations, the most common of which are referred to as 'voices'; such voices can give commands to patients, or may discuss the person in the third person, or comment on their action

- delusions of which those relating to control of thoughts are the most diagnostic, for example patients feel that thoughts are being inserted into or withdrawn from their mind
- lack of insight into the illness.

These symptoms are commonly called positive symptoms.

Factors affecting diagnosis and prognosis

There is a reluctance to classify people as suffering schizophrenia on the basis of one psychotic illness, but there are a number of features which lead one to predict whether an acute illness will become chronic.

These features include:

- age of onset, which, typically for schizophrenia, is late teenage to age 30 years
- reports of childhood which indicate not mixing or a rather shy and withdrawn personality
- a poor work record
- a desire for social isolation
- being single and not seeming to have sexual relationships
- a gradual onset of the illness and deterioration from previous level of functioning
- grossly disorganized behaviour.

Treatment

There is a wide range of antipsychotic drugs available for the treatment of a psychotic illness. Although most antipsychotic drugs are equally effective in the treatment of psychotic symptoms some individuals respond better to one drug than another.

There is some controversy over how long people should remain on an antipsychotic drug following first acute illness. Some would argue that, if the prognosis is poor, long-term therapy should be advocated. Others would want to see a second illness before advocating long-term therapy.

Symptoms common in chronic schizophrenia

Between 60% and 80% of patients who suffer from an acute psychotic illness will suffer further illness and become chronically affected. For these patients the diagnosis of schizophrenia can be applied.

As schizophrenia progresses, there may be periods of relapse with acute symptoms but the underlying trend is towards symptoms of lack of drive, social withdrawal and emotional apathy. Such symptoms are sometimes called negative symptoms and respond poorly to most antipsychotic drugs.

Causes of schizophrenia

Although the cause of schizophrenia remains unknown, there are many theories and models.

Vulnerability model

The vulnerability model postulates that the persistent characteristic of schizophrenia is not the schizophrenic episode itself but the vulnerability to the development of such episodes of the disorder. The episodes of the illness are time limited but the vulnerability remains, awaiting the trigger of some stress. Such vulnerability can depend on premorbid personality, social network or the environment. Manipulation and avoidance of such stress can abort a potential schizophrenic episode.

Developmental model

The developmental model postulates that there are critical periods in the development of neuronal cells which, if adversely affected, may result in schizophrenia. Two such critical periods are postulated to occur when migrant neural cells do not reach their goal in fetal development and when supernumerary neural cells slough off at adolescence. This model is supported by neuroimaging studies which show structural brain abnormalities in patients with schizophrenia.

Ecological model

The ecological model postulates that external factors involving social, cultural and physical forces in the environment, such as population density, individual space, socio–economic status and racial status, influence the development of the disorder. The evidence in support of such a model remains weak.

Genetic model

There is undoubtably a genetic component to schizophrenia with a higher incidence in the siblings of schizophrenics. However, even in monozygotic twins there are many cases where only one sibling has developed schizophrenia.

Transmitter abnormality model

The suggestion that schizophrenia is caused primarily by an abnormality of dopamine receptors and, in particular, D_2 receptors, has largely emerged from research into the effect of antipsychotic drugs Such a theory is increasingly being questioned.

Other factors involved in schizophrenia

Numerous other factors have been implicated in the development and cause of schizophrenia. These include migration, socio-economic factors, perinatal insult, infections, season of birth, viruses, toxins and family environment.

In reality all of these factors may influence both the development and progression of schizophrenia Social familial and biological factors may lead to premorbid vulnerability and subsequently influence both the acute psychosis and the progression to chronic states. What is then likely is that the illness will feed back to influence social, familial and biological factors, thus leading to future vulnerability.

Drug treatment in schizophrenia

Mode of action of antipsychotic drugs

Although the cause of schizophrenia remains an enigma, an understanding of the mode of action of antipsychotic drugs has led to the dopamine theory of schizophrenia. This theory postulates that the symptoms experienced in schizophrenia are caused by an alteration to the level of dopamine activity in the brain. It is based on knowledge that dopamine receptor antagonists are often effective antipsychotics while drugs which increase dopamine activity, such as amphetamine, can either induce psychosis or exacerbate a schizophrenic illness.

At least six dopamine receptors exist in the brain, with much recent activity being focused on the D_2 receptor as being responsible for antipsychotic drug action. Drugs such as pimozide which claim to have a more specific effect on D_2 receptors have less effect on blood pressure and a low risk of anticholinergic side-effects but do not appear superior in antipsychotic effect when compared to other agents.

Research into the mode of action of clozapine has caused a change of attention to the mesolimbic system in the brain and to different receptors. Clozapine does not chronically alter striatal D_2 receptors but does appear to affect striatal D_1 receptors. It also appears to have more effect on the limbic system and on serotonin ($5-HT_2$) receptors, which may explain its reduced risk of extrapyramidal symptoms. The term 'atypical' is used to categorize those antipsychotic drugs that, like clozapine, rarely produce extrapyramidal side-effects.

Rationale and mode of use of drugs

Although a variety of social and psychological therapies are helpful in the treatment of schizophrenia, drugs form the essential cornerstone. The aim of all therapies is to minimize the level of handicap and achieve the best level of mental functioning. Drugs do not cure schizophrenia. At the same time, benefits have to be balanced against side-effects and the need to suppress particular symptoms. For example, if the person has a delusion that he or she is responsible for famine in Africa, but this does not in any way influence the person's behaviour or mood, there would be little point in increasing antipsychotic drug therapy. If, on the other hand, this delusion led to great distress, or violent or dangerous behaviour, then an increase in antipsychotic drugs may be indicated.

It is now accepted that antipsychotic drugs can control or modify symptoms such as hallucinations and delusions that are evident in the acute episode of illness. Except for clozapine and the other atypicals, there is little evidence for antipsychotic drugs being of value in the treatment of the negative symptoms, although the matter remains controversial. Antipsychotic drugs increase the length of time between breakdowns and shorten the length of the acute episode in most patients.

Drug selection and dose

Concerns about side-effect profiles and toxicity of typical antipsychotic drugs has led to calls for the 'atypical' drugs to be prescribed more widely and as first choice (Taylor et al 2001, NICE 2002). This view is supported by evidence from clinical trials which demonstrate that atypicals are better tolerated at normal clinical doses than typicals (Tran et al 1997). In addition patients are put at less risk of developing tardive dyskinesia (Beasley et al 1999). However, this view is not supported by either the Royal College of Psychiatrists (1999) or the NHS Centre for Reviews and Dissemination (1999). The Royal College of Psychiatrists' guidelines recommend low doses of typical antipsychotic drugs for first line use although the definition of low dose remains unclear. The NHS Centre for Reviews and Dissemination reviewed atypicals and could not advocate first line use of atypicals and this was supported by Geddes et al (2000). They concluded that there was no clear evidence that atypical antipsychotic drugs were either more effective or better tolerated than conventional antipsychotics.

Other factors that have influenced drug selection or dose are:

- the withdrawal of some antipsychotic drugs from routine clinical practice and changes to the product licences of others
- guidelines warning about the use of high doses of antipsychotic drugs (Thompson 1994)
- a move away from routine use of antipsychotic drugs for emergency tranquillization to the short-term use of benzodiazepines such as lorazepan and diazepam

- changes to dose ranges advocated by some pharmaceutical companies (e.g. haloperidol maximum dose was reduced from 120 mg to 30 mg daily).

There will be further changes in practice with the introduction of both intramuscular and depot formulations of the atypical antipsychotic drugs.

Another factor that has influenced prescribing practice in schizophrenia in recent years has been agreement over the role of clozapine. Clozapine is an atypical antipsychotic drug that has demonstrated a greater efficacy than other antipsychotics. Unfortunately, it is associated with a 1–2% incidence of neutropenia which makes routine monitoring of blood mandatory. Clozapine is now established as the drug of choice in treatment-resistant schizophrenia.

Despite all these changes, many of the issues relevant to drug selection and dose remain. These are:

- Side effects
  - for the older, typical drugs, side-effects such as hypotension, extrapyramidal symptoms and anticholinergic effects are key factors in the choice of drug
  - for the newer atypical drugs side-effects, such as weight gain (Taylor & McAskill 2000), affects adherence in many patients
  - sedation remains a factor for all antipsychotic drugs.
- Selection should not be based on chemical group alone since individual response to a particular drug or dose may be more important.
- Polypharmacy remains a matter of concern. Reasons why polypharmacy occurs include:
  - poor response to standard drug treatments
  - unrealistic expectations about the speed of action and the extent of treatment control
  - prescribers feeling inhibited about exceeding the licensed dose and resorting to prescribing two or more antipsychotic drugs to achieve control, particularly in the acute situation. Increasingly, though, prescribers are being encouraged to use clozapine at an earlier stage for patients who do not fully respond to treatment
  - once control has been achieved there may be reluctance to reduce doses for fear of the re-emergence of symptoms
  - confusion arising between the perceived need in the ward situation for sedation and the antipsychotic effects. The sedating side-effects of antipsychotic drugs may be evident within hours; they are rapid in onset but may begin to wear off after 2–3 weeks. The antipsychotic effects on thought disorder, hallucinations and delusions may take some weeks to appear, although if there has been no response within 2–3 weeks a change of antipsychotic or change of dose may be indicated.

The consensus view is that very high doses of antipsychotic drugs are not beneficial in improving either the speed or the overall level of response in acute psychosis.

The antipsychotic drugs in use are listed in Table 28.1, along with some of their common adverse effects. A treatment algorithm for schizophreniia is presented in Figure 28.1.

Maintenance dosages

Once control of symptoms is achieved, the issue of maintenance dosages then comes to the fore. In particular, concerns about tardive dyskinesia have led to a series of new approaches to maintenance therapy. The aim of maintenance therapy should be to maintain the patient in a state of remission, but at the same time achieve the best possible level of functioning.

A review of the literature up to 1980 found that there was no difference in outcome in patients maintained on doses of antipsychotic drugs above the equivalent of 310 mg of chlorpromazine per day, compared with those on doses below that level, and to date no evidence has emerged to refute that. Patients may also remain stable on reducing doses. Three strategies that have been tried to maintain remission and reduce antipsychotic drug intake are described below.

Drug holidays. These are no longer advocated as patients become clinically disadvantaged without any reduction in risk of tardive dyskinesia.

Low-dose regimens. Trials using low-dose regimens of flupentixol decanoate and fluphenazine decanoate have produced unclear results, but indications are that with careful patient selection and good supervision some patients can remain in remission on low doses.

Brief intermittent treatment. Such treatments rely on patient recognition of prodromal symptoms and rapid access to drug therapy. Although some studies have demonstrated encouraging results others have found such an approach to be associated with a higher rate of both psychotic and dysphoric symptoms.

Neuroleptic equivalence

Although antipsychotic drugs vary in potency, studies on relative dopamine receptor binding have led to the concept of chlorpromazine equivalents as a useful method of transferring dosage from one product to another. Concern has been expressed about the variation between sources for such values, in particular about the quoted chlorpromazine equivalents of the butyrophenones and the conversion of depot doses to oral (Table 28.2). Likewise, there is no agreement on the equivalent doses of the atypicals.

Table 28.1 Neuroleptics/antipsychotics and common therapeutic problems associated with them

Drug group	Drug	Comment
Butyrophenones	Haloperidol	Extrapyramidal side-effects of Parkinsonian rigidity, dystonia, akathisia Tardive dyskinesia with long term use Drug most associated with neuroleptic malignant syndrome Sedation Hormonal effects Available as depot formulation
	Benperidol	As haloperidol Claimed to reduce sexual drive
Phenothiazines piperidines	Thioridazine	Marked anticholinergic side-effects of dry mouth, blurred vision and constipation High incidence of QT abnormalities on ECG has resulted in limitations to licence Postural hypotension and falls in the elderly Low incidence of extrapyramidal side-effects
	Pericyazine	Side-effects similar to thioridazine
	Pipotiazine	As thioridazine but only available as depot formulation
aliphatic	Chlorpromazine	As haloperidol but in addition postural hypotension, low body temperature, rashes and photosensitivity Increased sedation Jaundice
	Promazine	As chlorpromazine but low potency Considered by some to have weak antipsychotic effect
	Levomepromazine (methotrimeprazine)	Very sedative Mostly used in terminal illness
piperazine	Trifluoperazine	As chlorpromazine but greater incidence of extrapyramidal side-effects and lower incidence of anticholinergic effects Some antiemetic properties
	Fluphenazine	As trifluoperazine but also available as depot formulation
	Perphenazine	As trifluoperazine
	Prochlorperazine	Useful antinauseant but implicated in falls in the elderly
Thioxanthines	Flupentixol	Similar to fluphenazine but also available as depot formulation
	Zuclopenthixol	Similar to chlorpromazine but also available as depot formulation
Diphenylbutylpiperidines	Pimozide	As haloperidol but concerns about cardiac effects at high dose
Benzamides	Sulpiride	Lower incidence of extrapyramidal effects Few anticholinergic effects Claim of efficacy against negative symptoms
	Amisulpride	As sulpiride
Dibenoxazepine tricyclics	Loxapine	High incidence of extrapyramidal side-effects Few anticholinergic effects
	Clozapine	Drug of choice for resistant schizophrenia Low incidence of extrapyramidal side-effects or tardive dyskinesia Neutropenia in 1–2% of cases Enhanced efficacy against both positive and negative symptoms Sedation, dribbling, drooling, weight gain
Thienobenzodiazepines	Olanzapine	Similar to clozapine but no efficacy against treatment resistance
	Quetiapine	Similar to clozapine but no efficacy against treatment resistance
	Zotepine	Similar to clozapine but no proven efficacy against treatment resistance Higher rate of drug induced seizures
Serotonin–dopamine antagonists	Risperidone	As olanzapine but extrapyramidal side-effects at higher doses
	Ziprasidone	As risperidone

STEP 1 – FIRST EPISODE

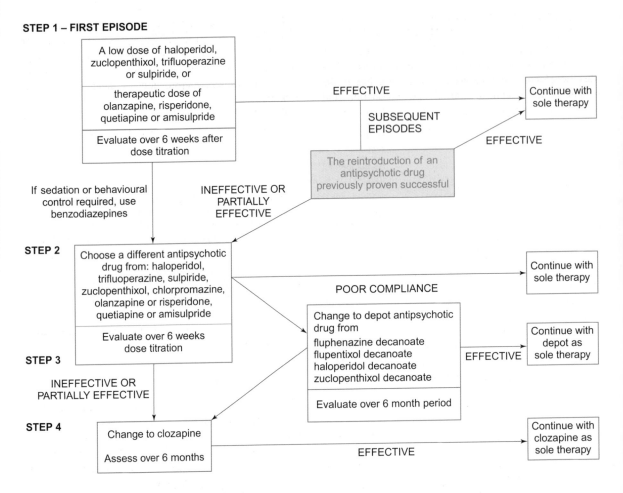

Figure 28.1   Treatment algorithm for schizophrenia.

Long-acting formulation of antipsychotic drugs

Most long-acting (depot) formulations are synthesized by esterification of the hydroxyl group of the antipsychotic drug to a long-chain fatty acid such as decanoic acid. The esters which are more lipophilic and soluble are dissolved in an oily vehicle such as sesame oil or a vegetable oil (viscoleo). Once the drug is injected into muscle it is slowly released from the oil vehicle. Active drug becomes available following hydrolysis for distribution to the site of the action.

Although the ideal long-acting antipsychotic formulation should release the drug at a constant rate so that plasma level variations are kept to a minimum, all the available products produce significant variations (Table 28.3). This can result in increased side-effects at the time of peak plasma concentrations and increased patient irritability towards the end of the period, as plasma concentrations decline. The long-acting risperidone involves a novel microsphere formulation new to clinical practice.

Table 28.2   Neuroleptic equivalent of antipsychotic drugs to 100 mg chlorpromazine (from Foster 1989)

Drug	Usual dose (mg) equivalent to 100 mg of chlorpromazine	Variations in quoted dosage (mg) equivalent to 100 mg of chlorpromazine
Oral antipsychotics		
Promazine	200	100–250
Thioridazine	100	50–120
Trifluoperazine	5	3.5–7.5
Haloperidol	2	1.5–5
Sulpiride	200	–
Depot antipsychotics administered every 2 weeks (all administered as the decanoate)		
Zuclopenthixol	200	80–200
Flupentixol	40	16–40
Fluphenazine	25	10–25
Haloperidol	20	–

In addition to the principles of drug choice and dosage selection that apply to oral drugs, with depot therapy there is also a need to consider the future habitation of the patient. If the patient is to live an independent lifestyle, depot formulations are indicated, but if the person is to remain in staffed accommodation and receive other medicines via routine administration by nurses, the use of depot formulations may not be logical.

Advantages and disadvantages of long-acting formulations of antipsychotic drugs

Non-compliance with oral medicines is a major problem in patients with psychiatric illnesses and the administration of depot formulations guarantees drug delivery. It has been argued that, although depot injections are expensive, they have economic advantages because they reduce hospital admissions, improve drug bioavailability by avoiding the deactivating processes which occur in the gut and liver and result in more consistent plasma levels of drug.

Depot formulations have the disadvantages of reduced flexibility of dosage, the painful nature of administration and high incidence of both extrapyramidal side-effects and weight gain.

Anticholinergic drugs

Anticholinergic drugs are prescribed to counter the extrapyramidal side-effects of typical antipsychotics, and at one time were routinely prescribed. It is generally accepted that, with the possible exception of the first few weeks of treatment with antipsychotic drugs known to have a high incidence of extrapyramidal side-effects, anticholinergic drugs should only be prescribed when a need has been shown. A number of studies have looked at the discontinuation of anticholinergic agents and reported re-emergence of the symptoms. One such study reported up to 62% of patients being affected. Between 25% and 30% of patients will have a continuing need for anticholinergic drugs.

The anticholinergic drugs are not without problems, having their own range of side-effects, including dry mouth, constipation and blurred vision. Trihexyphenidyl (benzhexol), in particular, is renowned for its euphoric effects and withdrawal problems can include cholinergic rebound.

One of the benefits of the atypical antipsychotic drugs is the reduced need for co-prescription of anticholinergic drugs.

Interactions involving antipsychotic drugs

There are claimed to be many interactions involving antipsychotic drugs but few appear to be clinically significant. Propranolol increases the plasma concentration of chlorpromazine, and carbamazepine accelerates the metabolism of haloperidol and olanzapine. When tricyclics are administered with phenothiazines increased antimuscarinic effects can occur and most antipsychotic drugs increase the sedative effect of alcohol.

Adverse effects of antipsychotic drugs

There are a large number of adverse effects associated with antipsychotic drugs. Some of these effects such as sedation, antilibido effect and weight gain, may be considered to be of value with particular patients, but the susceptibility to such adverse effects is often a major factor in determining drug choice.

The major groups of side-effects are described below.

Sedation. Although sedation is greatest with chlorpromazine, it is primarily related to dosage with most other antipsychotics. Products claiming to be less sedating can often only substantiate such claims for low doses.

Anticholinergic side-effects. Side-effects such as dry mouth, constipation and blurred vision are particularly associated with piperidine phenothiazines.

Extrapyramidal side-effects. Side-effects such as akathisia, dystonia and parkinsonian effects are

Table 28.3	Comparison of depot antipsychotics (from Jann et al 1985)			
Drug	Ester	Oily vehicle	Time to peak (days)	Half-life (days)
Haloperidol	Decanoate	Sesame	3–9	21
Flupentixol	Decanoate	Viscoleo	7	17
Zuclopenthixol	Decanoate	Viscoleo	4–7	19
Fluphenazine	Decanoate	Sesame	0.3–1.5	6–9
Pipotiazine	Palmitate	Sesame	10–15	15

associated with typical antipsychotic drugs, and occur frequently, particularly with depot antipsychotics, piperazine phenothiazines and butyrophenones. These side-effects are reversible by using anticholinergic drugs or by dosage reduction. The common extrapyramidal effects include:

- *Akathisia*, motor restlessness, which primarily presents as restlessness. This causes patients to pace up and down, constantly shift their leg position or tap their feet.
- *Dystonia* is the result of sustained muscle contraction. It can present as grimacing and facial distortion, neck twisting and laboured breathing. Occasionally the patient may have an oculogyric crisis in which, after a few moments of fixed staring, the eyeballs move upwards and then sideways, remaining in that position. In addition to these eye movements, the mouth is usually wide open, the tongue protruding and the head tilting backwards.
- *Parkinson-like side-effects*, which usually present as tremor, rigidity and poverty of facial expression. Drooling and excessive salivation are also common. A shuffling gait may be seen and the patient may show signs of fatigue when performing repetitive motor activities.

Hormonal effects. These are primarily influenced by the effect on prolactin. This may result in galactorrhoea, missed menstrual periods and loss of libido.

Postural hypotension and photosensitivity. These are particularly associated with the aliphatic phenothiazines.

Tardive dyskinesla. Classically the syndrome of tardive dyskinesia affects the tongue, facial and neck muscles but will often also affect the extremities. It is usual to find abnormalities of posture and movements of the fingers in addition to the oral–lingual–masticatory movements.

Epidemiological studies support the association between the prescribing of antipsychotic drugs and the development of tardive dyskinesia. Other factors which also appear to be associated are: the duration of exposure to antipsychotic drugs; the co-prescribing of anticholinergic drugs; the co-prescribing of lithium; advanced age; prior experience of acute extrapyramidal symptoms; and brain damage. Many other factors have been postulated to be associated with tardive dyskinesia such as depot formulations of antipsychotic drugs, dosage of antipsychotic drug, and antipsychotic drugs with high anticholinergic activity, but such associations remain unproven.

Although the mechanism by which tardive dyskinesia arises is unclear, the leading hypothesis is that after prolonged blockade of dopamine receptors a paradoxical increase in the functional activity of dopamine in the basal ganglia occurs. This altered functional state is thought to come about through a phenomenon of disuse supersensitivity of dopamine receptors. The primary clinical evidence to support such a theory is that tardive dyskinesia is late in onset after prolonged exposure to antipsychotic drugs, has a tendency to worsen upon abrupt discontinuation of the antipsychotic drug and that in terms of response to drugs presents as the opposite of Parkinson's disease; a disease postulated to be caused by a deficiency of dopamine in the caudate nucleus of the brain.

The attempts to treat tardive dyskinesia have been many and varied, but they include dopamine-depleting agents such as reserpine and tetrabenazine, dopamine-blocking agents such as antipsychotic drugs, blockers of catecholamine synthesis such as methyldopa, cholinergic agents such as choline and lecithin, GABA antagonists such as sodium valproate and baclofen and the provision of drug holidays. Such strategies are rarely successful. Most strategies currently involve a gradual withdrawal of the typical antipsychotic drug, if at all possible, or maintenance of the lowest dosage or the use of an atypical antipsychotic drug.

CASE STUDIES

Case 28.1

Wayne is a 19-year-old man. His childhood was unremarkable and by the age of 16 he was achieving well at school. There were some reports of him engaging in strange behaviours during childhood but generally these did not give rise for concern. Aged 17 he became involved with the illicit drug culture and increasingly lost interest in his studies. His parents became concerned as he appeared to undergo a change of personality, communicating with them very little. He eventually dropped out of school and took various short-term jobs. He moved into a flat and seemed to live a twilight existence involving illicit drugs and all night raves. Police were called to his flat following a disturbance. They found Wayne living in squalor. He was surrounded by pieces of paper containing incomprehensible messages and was incoherent. He sat with a fixed stare appearing quite inaccessible. He kept laughing and responding to imaginary people. He was very resistant to hospital admission requiring to be admitted under a section of the Mental Health Act 1983. On the ward he has remained quiet but appears to be in conversation with people who are not there.

....

Questions

1. Outline the drug(s) of choice for Wayne and the rationale for selection.
2. What factors would influence the likely prognosis?
3. Outline the drug(s) of choice if there is the need for rapid tranquillization.

Answers

1. The first need is to ascertain whether the patient's behaviour results from abuse of illicit substances or the onset of a schizophrenic illness. If the former, he would be expected to recover within a few days with little or no drug treatment. If, however, this is the first presentation of a schizophrenic illness, the symptoms are likely to persist, and it would be appropriate to prescribe an antipsychotic drug. The choice of antipsychotic drug for first illness psychosis remains a matter of controversy. The alternatives are either a low dose of a typical antipsychotic drug (such as haloperidol, 3–5 mg twice daily) or an atypical such as risperidone or olanzapine. Advocates of prescribing low doses of typicals maintain that at such doses the risk of extrapyramidal side-effects is small and the efficacy maintained. Advocates of the atypicals maintain that the risk of extrapyramidal side-effects, even at low doses of typicals, remains a problem and is likely to have a negative impact on the patient's attitude to future drug treatment.

2. A number of factors in Wayne's history indicate a poor prognosis:
   - there has been a deterioration in function
   - his age, which is typical for a first breakdown
   - his poor work record
   - grossly disorganized behaviour
   - a number of positive symptoms such as hallucinations.

3. If Wayne's symptoms became such that there was a need for rapid tranquillization a decision would have to be made about whether to use antipsychotic drugs or benzodiazepines. In the past, sedative antipsychotic drugs such as chlorpromazine, haloperidol or zuclopenthixol were favoured, but increasing concern of sudden death has resulted in a move to use benzodiazepines such as lorazepam or diazepam in such situations.

Case 28.2

Brian has recently been admitted to hospital for the third time this year, the pattern for the last two admissions being the same. His positive symptoms responded rapidly on both previous admissions. On the first admission he suffered severe extrapyramidal side-effects with 300 mg daily of chlorpromazine and was stabilized and discharged on sulpiride 400 mg twice daily and procyclidine 5 mg twice daily. He almost immediately stopped taking the sulpiride, claiming not to be ill. During his second admission he was successfully treated with olanzapine 10 mg daily but again stopped the medicine as soon as he was discharged.

Questions

1. Was Brian's drug treatment appropriate?
2. What strategies could be adopted to maintain Brian in treatment?

Answers

1. Yes, Brian's treatment was appropriate. Except for the initial treatment with a large dose of chlorpromazine in a drug-naive patient, the treatment was according to agreed guidelines. The initial choice of a low dose typical antipsychotic was followed by a second choice of an atypical because the patient still suffered extrapyramidal side-effects.

2. Brian has no insight into his illness or the need for continuing treatment. This could be for a number of reasons:
   - it is part of the illness, and his failure to gain insight is symptomatic of incomplete recovery
   - he lacks a supportive environment to ensure that he takes medicines
   - he is suffering from side-effects that deter him from taking the medicines.

In most cases the use of a depot antipsychotic injection would be the easiest way to ensure compliance, although if Brian is determined to avoid drug treatment this strategy is unlikely to be successful. In his case the history of severe extrapyramidal side-effects would also need to be taken into account as most of the depot antipsychotic drugs are associated with a high incidence of such side-effects.

Case 28.3

Justin, aged 25, has a 3-year history of schizophrenia with many admissions to hospital. Throughout the period of his illness he has received a range of different oral antipsychotic drugs including chlorpromazine, haloperidol, sulpiride, risperidone and olanzapine, as well as the depot antipsychotic drugs haloperidol and zuclopenthixol. For most of this time he has had a fixed belief that he is involved in a complex battle involving the devil, Jesus Christ and many other cosmic beings with whom he communicates. When he is ill these beings torment him while at other times he quite enjoys his involvement with them as they make him feel special. He currently receives zuclopenthixol 500 mg by intramuscular injection every week, olanzapine 10 mg at night, carbamazepine 200 mg three times daily, haloperidol 10 mg four times daily, and procyclidine 10 mg three times daily. He has remained on the ward for the last 4 months with no sign of improvement. The team wish to consider clozapine for Justin.

Questions

1. Comment on the current drug therapy Justin is receiving.
2. What action is required before Justin can receive clozapine?

Answers

1. Although it is not uncommon for polypharmacy to occur when there has been poor response, the practice is frowned upon. Additional medicines are often added in a crisis or in the hope of achieving a greater degree of response. As in this case, the strategy is often unsuccessful. The particular issues of note with this patient's drug regimen are:
   - the combination of a typical and an atypical antipsychotic drug reduces the potential benefit of using a drug with a low incidence of extrapyramidal side-effects because the patient still suffers extrapyramidal side-effects, requires procyclidine, and is at risk of developing tardive dyskinesia

- the very large total dose he is receiving from the combination of antipsychotic drugs.
- the dose of anticholinergic drug (procyclidine) is high and likely to result in its own side-effects
- the need for such frequent dosing of the intramuscular depot might not be necessary – administration at 2-week intervals would normally be appropriate – there is little evidence to support the value of carbamazepine, either for schizophrenia or as an adjunctive treatment.

2. The preparation for treatment with clozapine involves a number of steps. These include:
   - registration with the clozapine monitoring scheme

- background blood tests to ensure that the patient is not already suffering from neutropenia or other blood disorder
- stopping the depot antipsychotic drug – this would usually occur some weeks before starting clozapine
- stopping carbamazepine as this interacts with clozapine
- slowly reducing haloperidol
- gradually stopping procyclidine.

Ideally one would want to have removed all other treatments and prescribe clozapine alone but sometimes the final step of withdrawing other medicines may occur during the initiation phase with clozapine.

REFERENCES

Beasley C M, Dellva M A, Tamura R N et al 1999 Randomised double-blind comparison of the incidence of tardive dyskinesia in patients with schizophrenia during long term treatment with olanzapine or haloperidol. British Journal of Psychiatry 174: 23–30

Foster P 1989 Neuroleptic equivalence. Pharmaceutical Journal 243: 431–432

Geddes J, Freemantle N, Harrison P et al 2000 Atypical antipsychotics in the treatment of schizophrenia: systematic overview and meta-regression analysis. British Medical Journal 321: 1371–1376

Jann M W, Ereshefsky L, Saklad S R 1985 Clinical pharmacokinetics of the depot antipsychotics. Clinical Pharmacokinetics 10(4): 315–333

National Institute for Clinical Excellence (NICE) 2002 Technology Appraisal Guidance No 43. Guidance on the use of newer (atypical) antipsychotic drugs for the treatment of schizophrenia. NICE, London

NHS Centre for Reviews and Dissemination 1999 Drug treatment in schizophrenia. Effective Healthcare Bulletin 5, no. 6. Latimer Trend and Co., Plymouth

Royal College of Psychiatrists 1999 The management of schizophrenia. Part 1: Pharmacological treatments. Royal College of Psychiatrists, London

Taylor D M, McAskill R 2000 Atypical antipsychotics and weight gain: a systematic review. Acta Psychiatrica Scandinavica 101: 416–432

Taylor D M, McConnell H, McConnell D et al 2001 The Maudsley 2001 prescribing guidelines, 6th edn. Martin Dunitz, London

Thompson C 1994 The use of high dose antipsychotic medication. British Journal of Psychiatry 164: 448–458

Tran P V, Dellva M A, Tollefson G D et al 1997 Extrapyramidal symptoms and tolerability of olanzapine versus haloperidol in the acute treatment of schizophrenia. Journal of Clinical Psychiatry 58: 205–211

FURTHER READING

Gilbody S M, Bagnall A M, Duggan L et al 2000 Risperidone versus other atypical antipsychotic medication for schizophrenia. Cochrane Library, Issue 4. Update Software, Oxford

Scottish Intercollegiate Guidelines Network 1998 Psychosocial interventions in the management of schizophrenia. Guideline 30. Updated at www.sign.ac.uk/guidelines

Johnstone E C, Humphreys M S, Lang F H et al (eds) 1999 Schizophrenia: concepts and clinical management. Cambridge University Press, Cambridge, p 271

Epilepsy 29

S. Dhillon   J. W. Sander

KEY POINTS

- An epileptic seizure is a transient paroxysm of uncontrolled discharges of neurones causing an event which is discernible by the person experiencing the seizure and/or an observer.
- The incidence of epileptic seizures has been estimated at between 20 and 70 cases per 100 000 of the population.
- About 70–80% of all those who develop epilepsy will become seizure-free on treatment and about 50% will successfully withdraw their medication.
- Generalized seizures result in impairment of consciousness from the onset; they include tonic–clonic convulsions, absence attacks and myoclonic seizures.
- Partial seizures include simple partial seizures, complex partial seizures and secondarily generalized seizures.
- Treatment of epilepsy is usually for at least 3 years and, depending on circumstances, sometimes for life.
- Treatment aims to control seizures using one drug.

An epileptic seizure is a transient paroxysm of uncontrolled discharges of neurones causing an event that is discernible by the person experiencing the seizure and/or by an observer. The tendency to have recurrent attacks is known as epilepsy – by definition a single attack does not constitute epilepsy. Epileptic seizures or attacks are a symptom of many different diseases, and the term 'epilepsy' is loosely applied to a number of conditions that have in common only a tendency to have recurrent epileptic attacks. A patient with epilepsy will show recurrent epileptic seizures that occur unexpectedly and stop spontaneously.

Epidemiology

There are problems in establishing precise epidemiological statistics for a heterogeneous condition such as epilepsy. Unlike most ailments, epilepsy is episodic; between seizures patients may be perfectly normal and have normal investigations. Thus, the diagnosis is essentially clinical, relying heavily on eyewitness descriptions of the attacks. In addition, there are a number of other conditions in which consciousness may be transiently impaired and which may be confused with epilepsy. Another problem area is that of case identification. Sometimes the patient may be unaware of the nature of the attacks and so may not seek medical help. Patients with milder epilepsy may also not be receiving ongoing medical care and so may be missed in epidemiological surveys. Furthermore, since there is some degree of stigma attached to epilepsy, patients may sometimes be reluctant to admit their condition.

Incidence and prevalence

Epileptic seizures are common. The incidence (number of new cases per given population per year) has been estimated at between 20 and 70 cases per 100 000 persons, and the cumulative incidence (the risk of having the condition at some point in life) at 2–5%. The incidence is higher in the first two decades of life but falls over the next few decades, only to increase again in late life, owing mainly to cerebrovascular diseases. Most studies of the prevalence of active epilepsy (the number of cases in the population at any given time) have estimated figures between 4 and 8 per 1000, and a rate of 5/1000 is commonly quoted.

Prognosis

Up to 5% of people will suffer at least one seizure in their lifetime. However, the prevalence of active epilepsy is much lower and most patients who develop seizures have a very good prognosis. About 70–80% of all people developing epilepsy will eventually become seizure-free, and about half will successfully withdraw their medication. Once a substantial period of remission has been achieved, the risk of further seizures is greatly reduced. A minority of patients (20–30%) will develop chronic epilepsy, and in such cases, treatment is more difficult. Patients with symptomatic epilepsy, more than one seizure type, associated mental retardation or neurological or psychiatric disorders are more likely to have a poor outcome. Of chronic patients, fewer than 5% will be unable to live in the community or will depend on others for their day-to-day needs. Most patients are entirely normal between seizures but a small minority of patients with severe epilepsy may suffer physical and intellectual deterioration.

Mortality

There is an increased mortality in people with epilepsy, especially among younger patients and those with severe epilepsy. Most studies have given overall standardized mortality ratios between two and three times higher than that of the general population. Common causes of death in people with epilepsy include accidents (e.g. drowning, head injury, road traffic accidents), status epilepticus, tumours, cerebrovascular disease, pneumonia and suicide. Sudden unexpected death, an entity which remains unexplained, is common in chronic epilepsy, particularly among the young who have convulsive forms of epilepsy.

Aetiology

Epileptic seizures are produced by abnormal discharges of neurones that may be caused by any pathological process which affects the brain. The idiopathic epilepsies are those in which there is a clear genetic component, and they probably account for a third of all new cases of epilepsy. In a significant proportion of cases, however, no cause can be determined, and these are known as the cryptogenic epilepsies. Possible explanations for cryptogenic epilepsy include as yet unexplained metabolic or biochemical abnormalities and microscopic lesions in the brain resulting from brain malformation or trauma during birth or other injury. The term 'symptomatic epilepsy' indicates that a probable cause has been identified.

The likely aetiology of epilepsy depends upon the age of the patient and the type of seizure. The commonest causes in young infants are hypoxia or birth asphyxia, intracranial trauma during birth, metabolic disturbances, congenital malformations of the brain or infection. In young children and adolescents, idiopathic seizures account for the majority of the epilepsies, although trauma and infection also play a role. In this age group, particularly in children aged between 6 months and 5 years, seizures may occur in association with febrile illness. These are usually short, generalized tonic–clonic convulsions that occur during the early phase of a febrile disease. They must be distinguished from seizures that are triggered by central nervous system infections which produce fever, for example meningitis or encephalitis. Unless febrile seizures are prolonged, focal, recurrent or there is a background of neurological handicap, the prognosis is excellent, and it is unlikely that the child will develop epilepsy.

The range of causes of adult onset epilepsy is very wide. Both idiopathic epilepsy and epilepsy due to birth trauma may also begin in early adulthood. Other important causes are head injury, alcohol abuse, cortical dysplasias, brain tumours and cerebrovascular diseases. Brain tumours are responsible for the development of epilepsy in up to a third of patients between the ages of 30 and 50 years. Over the age of 50 years, cerebrovascular disease is the commonest cause of epilepsy, and may be present in up to half of patients.

Pathophysiology

Epilepsy differs from most neurological conditions as it has no pathognomonic lesion. A variety of different electrical or chemical stimuli can easily give rise to a seizure in any normal brain. The hallmark of epilepsy is a rather rhythmic and repetitive hypersynchronous discharge of neurones, either localized in an area of the cerebral cortex or generalized throughout the cortex, which can be observed on an electroencephalogram (EEG).

Neurones are interconnected in a complex network in which each individual neurone is linked through synapses with hundreds of others. A small electrical current is discharged by neurones to release neurotransmitters at synaptic levels to permit communication with each other. Neurotransmitters fall into two basic categories: inhibitory or excitatory. Therefore, a neurone discharging can either excite or inhibit neurones connected to it. An excited neurone will activate the next neurone whereas an inhibited neurone will not. In this manner, information is conveyed, transmitted and processed throughout the central nervous system.

A normal neurone discharges repetitively at a low baseline frequency, and it is the integrated electrical activity generated by the neurones of the superficial layers of the cortex that is recorded in a normal EEG. If neurones are damaged, injured or suffer a chemical or metabolic insult, a change in the discharge pattern may develop. In the case of epilepsy, regular low-frequency discharges are replaced by bursts of high-frequency discharges usually followed by periods of inactivity. A single neurone discharging in an abnormal manner usually has no clinical significance. It is only when a whole population of neurones discharge synchronously in an abnormal way that an epileptic seizure may be triggered. This abnormal discharge may remain localized or it may spread to adjacent areas, recruiting more neurones as it expands. It may also generalize throughout the brain via cortical and subcortical routes, including collosal and thalamocortical pathways. The area from which the abnormal discharge originates is known as the epileptic focus. An EEG recording carried out during one of these abnormal discharges may show a variety of atypical signs, depending on which area of the brain is involved, its progression and how the discharging areas project to the superficial cortex.

Clinical manifestations

The clinical manifestation of a seizure will depend on the location of the focus and the pathways involved in its spread. An international seizure classification scheme based on the clinical features of seizures combined with EEG data is widely used to describe seizures. It divides seizures into two main groups according to the area of the brain in which the abnormal discharge originates. If it involves initial activation of both hemispheres of the brain simultaneously, the seizures are termed 'generalized'. If a discharge starts in a localized area of the brain, they are termed 'partial' or 'focal' seizures.

Generalized seizures

Generalized seizures result in impairment of consciousness from the onset. There are various types of generalized seizures, including the following.

Tonic–clonic convulsions.   Often called 'grand mal' attacks, these are the commonest of all epileptic seizures. Without warning, the patient suddenly goes stiff, falls and convulses, with laboured breathing and salivation. Cyanosis, incontinence and tongue biting may occur. The convulsion ceases after a few minutes and may often be followed by a period of drowsiness, confusion, headache and sleep.

Absence attacks.   Also known as 'petit mal', these are a much rarer form of generalized seizure. They happen almost exclusively in childhood and early adolescence. The child goes blank and stares; fluttering of the eyelids and flopping of the head may occur. The attacks last only a few seconds and often go unrecognized even by the child having them.

Myoclonic seizures.   These are abrupt, very brief involuntary shock-like jerks, which may involve the whole body, or the arms or the head. They usually happen in the morning, shortly after waking. They may sometimes cause the person to fall, but recovery is immediate. It should be noted that there are forms of non-epileptic myoclonic jerks that occur in a variety of other nerve diseases and may also occur in healthy people, particularly when they are just going off to sleep.

Atonic seizures.   These comprise a sudden loss of muscle tone causing the person to collapse to the ground. Recovery afterwards is quick. They are rare, accounting for less than 1% of the epileptic seizures seen in the general population, but much commoner in patients with severe epilepsy starting in infancy.

Partial seizures

Simple partial seizures.   In these seizures the discharge remains localized and consciousness is fully preserved. Simple partial attacks on their own are rare

and they usually progress to the other forms of partial seizure. What actually happens during a simple partial seizure depends on the area of the discharge and may vary widely from patient to patient but will always be stereotyped in one patient. Localized jerking of a limb or the face, stiffness or twitching of one part of the body, numbness or abnormal sensations are examples of what may occur during a simple partial seizure. If the seizure progresses with impairment of consciousness, it is termed a complex partial seizure. If it develops further and a convulsive seizure occurs, it is then called a partial seizure with secondary generalization. In attacks which progress, the early part of the seizure, in which consciousness is preserved, may manifest as a sensation or abnormal feeling, and is called the 'aura'.

Complex partial seizures.   The patient may present with altered or 'automatic' behaviour: plucking his or her clothes, fiddling with various objects and acting in a confused manner. Lipsmacking or chewing movements, grimacing, undressing, performing aimless activities, and wandering around in a drunken fashion may occur on their own or in different combinations during complex partial seizures. Most of these seizures originate in the frontal or temporal lobes of the brain and can sometimes progress to secondarily generalized seizures.

Secondarily generalized seizures.   These are partial seizures, either simple or complex, in which the discharge spreads to the entire brain. The patient may have a warning, but this is not always the case. The spread of the discharge can occur so quickly that no feature of the localized onset is apparent to the patient or an observer, and only an EEG can demonstrate the partial nature of the seizure. The involvement of the entire brain leads to a convulsive attack with the same characteristics as a generalized tonic–clonic convulsion.

Diagnosis

Diagnosing epilepsy can be difficult as it is first necessary to demonstrate a tendency to recurrent epileptic seizures. The one feature that distinguishes epilepsy from all other conditions is its unpredictability and transient nature. The diagnosis of epilepsy is clinical and depends on a reliable account of what happened during the attacks, if possible both from the patient and from an eyewitness, but some investigations may help, and the EEG is usually one of them. However, these investigations cannot conclusively confirm or refute the diagnosis of epilepsy.

There are other conditions that may cause impairment or loss of consciousness and which can be misdiagnosed as epilepsy; these include syncope, breath-holding attacks, transient ischaemic attacks, psychogenic attacks, etc. In addition, patients may present with acute epileptic seizures as a result of other problems such as drug intake, metabolic dysfunction, infection, head trauma or flashing lights (photosensitive seizures). These conditions have to be clearly ruled out before a diagnosis of epilepsy is made. Epilepsy must only be diagnosed when seizures occur spontaneously and are recurrent. The diagnosis must be accurate since the label 'suffering with epilepsy' carries a social stigma that has tremendous implications for the patient.

The EEG is often the only examination required, and it aims to record abnormal neuronal discharges. However, EEGs have limitations that should be clearly understood. Up to 5% of people without epilepsy may have non-specific abnormalities in their EEG recording, while up to 40% of people with epilepsy may have a normal EEG recording between seizures. Therefore the diagnosis of epilepsy should be strongly supported by a bona fide history of epileptic attacks. Nevertheless, the EEG is invaluable in classifying seizures.

The chance of recording the discharges of an actual seizure during a routine EEG, which usually takes 20–30 minutes, is slight, and because of this, ambulatory EEG monitoring and EEG video-telemetry are sometimes required. Ambulatory EEG allows recording in day-to-day circumstances using a small cassette recorder. EEG video-telemetry is useful in the assessment of difficult cases, particularly if surgery is considered. The patient is usually admitted to hospital and remains under continuous monitoring. This is only helpful in a very few cases, and it is best suited for patients who have frequent seizures. Neuroimaging with magnetic resonance imaging (MRI) is the most valuable investigation when structural abnormalities such as stroke, tumour, congenital abnormalities or hydrochephalus are suspected.

Treatment

During seizures

Convulsive seizures may look frightening, but the patient is not in pain, will usually have no recollection of the event afterwards and is usually not seriously injured. Emergency treatment is seldom necessary. Patients should, however, be made as comfortable as possible, preferably lying down (ease to the floor if sitting), cushioning the head and loosening any tight clothing or neckwear. During seizures, patients should not be moved unless they are in a dangerous place, for example in a road, by a fire or hot radiator, at the top of stairs or by the edge of water. No attempt should be made to open the patient's mouth or force anything between the teeth. This usually results in damage, and broken teeth may be inhaled, causing secondary lung damage. When the seizure stops, patients should be turned over into the recovery position, and the airway checked for any blockage.

Partial attacks are usually less dramatic. During automatisms, patients may behave in a confused fashion and should generally be left undisturbed. Gentle restraint may be necessary if the automatism leads to dangerous wandering. Attempts at firm restraint, however, may increase agitation and confusion. No drinks should be given after an attack, nor should extra antiepileptic drugs (AEDs) be administered. It is commonly felt that seizures may be life-threatening, but this is seldom the case. After a seizure, it is important to stay with the patient and offer reassurance until the confused period has completely subsided and the patient has recovered fully.

If a seizure persists for more than 10 minutes, if a series of seizures occur, or if the seizure is particularly severe, then intravenous or rectal administration of 10–20 mg diazepam for adults, with lower doses being used in children, is advisable.

Long-term treatment

In most cases, epilepsy can only be treated by long-term regular drug therapy. The objective of therapy is to suppress epileptic discharges and prevent the development of epileptic seizures. In the majority of cases, full seizure control can be obtained, and in other patients drugs may reduce the frequency or severity of seizures.

Initiating treatment with an AED is a major event in the life of a patient, and the diagnosis should be unequivocal. Treatment options must be considered with careful evaluation of all relevant factors, including the number and frequency of attacks, the presence of precipitating factors such as alcohol, drugs or flashing lights, and the presence of other medical conditions (Feely 1999). Single seizures do not require treatment unless they are associated with a progressive brain disorder or there is a clearly abnormal EEG. If there are long intervals between seizures (over 2 years) there is a case for not starting treatment. If there are more than two attacks that are clearly associated with a precipitating factor, fever or alcohol for instance, then treatment may not be necessary.

Therapy is long term, usually for at least 3 years, and, depending on circumstances, sometimes for life. A full explanation of all the implications must be given to the patient. The patient must be involved in all stages of the treatment plan. It is vital that the patient understands the implications of treatment and agrees with the treatment goals. Empowerment of patients to be actively involved in the decision-making process will ensure good adherence and is essential for effective clinical management. Antiepileptic treatment will fail unless the patient fully understands the importance of regular therapy and the objectives of treatment. Poor compliance is still a major factor which results in hospital admissions and poor seizure control and leads to the clinical use of multiple antiepileptic drugs.

General principles of treatment

Therapy aims to control seizures using one drug, with the lowest possible dose that cause the fewest side-effects possible. The established AEDs, carbamazepine, ethosuximide, phenytoin and sodium valproate, form the mainstay of treatment. Acetazolamide, clobazam, clonazepam, phenobarbital and primidone are also occasionally used in the treatment of epilepsy. More recently, in the last decade new drugs such as gabapentin, lamotrigine, levetiracetam, oxcarbazepine, topiramate, tiagabine and vigabatrin have been introduced, and felbamate and zonisamide may be launched in the near future. The choice of drugs depends largely on the seizure type, and so correct diagnosis and classification are essential. Table 29.1 lists the main indications for the more commonly used AEDs currently available, and Table 29.2 summarizes the clinical use of the newer AEDs.

Initiation of therapy in newly diagnosed patients

The first-line AED most suitable for the patient's seizure type should be introduced slowly, starting with a small dose, as too rapid an introduction may induce side-effects that will lose the patient's confidence. For most drugs, this gradual introduction will produce a therapeutic effect just as fast as a rapid introduction, and the patient should be reassured about this.

Maintenance dosage

There is no single optimum dose of any AED that suits all patients. The required dose varies from patient to patient, and from drug to drug. Drugs should be introduced slowly and then increased incrementally to an initial maintenance dosage. Seizure control should then be assessed, and the dose of the drug changed if necessary. For most AEDs, dosage increments are constant over a wide range. However, more care is needed with phenytoin as the serum level–dose relationship is not linear, and small dose changes may result in considerable serum level changes. Generic prescribing for epilepsy remains controversial. Most specialists would prefer patients to remain on the same brand of medication, and this is also preferred by the majority of patients. This is obviously important in those patients where the dosage has been carefully titrated to achieve optimal control.

Altering drug regimens

If the maximal tolerated dose of a drug does not control seizures, or if side-effects develop, the first drug can be substituted with another first-line AED. To do this, the second drug should be added gradually to the first. Once a good dose of the new drug is established, the first drug should then slowly be withdrawn. The withdrawal of individual AEDs should be carried out in a slow stepwise fashion to avoid the precipitation of withdrawal seizures (e.g. over 2–3 months). This risk is particularly great with barbiturates (phenobarbital and primidone) and benzodiazepines (clobazam and clonazepam). If a drug needs to be withdrawn rapidly – for example if there are life-threatening side-effects – then diazepam or another benzodiazepine can be used to cover the withdrawal phase.

Examples of withdrawal regimes are given below:

- Carbamazepine
  a. 100–200 mg every 2 weeks (as part of a drug change)
  b. 100–200 mg every 4 weeks (total withdrawal)

- Phenobarbital
  a. 15–30 mg every 2 weeks (as part of a drug change)
  b. 15–30 mg every 4 weeks (total withdrawal)

- Phenytoin
  a. 50 mg every 2 weeks (as part of a drug change)
  b. 50 mg every 4 weeks (total withdrawal)

- Sodium valproate
  a. 200–400 mg every 2 weeks (as part of a drug change)
  b. 200–400 mg every 4 weeks (total withdrawal)

Table 29.1 Antiepileptic drugs for different seizure types

Seizure type	First-line treatment	Second-line treatment
Partial seizures		
Simple partial	Carbamazepine	Vigabatrin
Complex partial	Phenytoin	Clobazam
Secondarily generalized	Valproate	Phenobarbital
	Lamotrigine	Acetazolamide
		Gabapentin
		Topiramate
Generalized seizures		
Tonic–clonic	Valproate	Vigabatrin
Tonic	Carbamazepine	Clobazam
Clonic	Phenytoin	Phenobarbital
	Lamotrigine	
Absence	Ethosuximide	Clonazepam
	Valproate	Lamotrigine
		Acetazolamide
Atypical absences	Valproate	Phenobarbital
Atonic	Clonazepam	Lamotrigine
	Clobazam	Carbamazepine
		Phenytoin
		Acetazolamide
Myoclonic	Valproate	Phenobarbital
	Clonazepam	Acetazolamide

The frequency of monitoring varies: stabilized patients may routinely have serum levels checked only once or twice a year. TDM may be used more often in some patients, for one or more of the above indications. A number of the newer antiepileptic drugs do not require TDM. However, since most are used as adjuvant therapy it is useful to establish baseline levels of existing drugs before the new agent is introduced. Clinical effects should be monitored and TDM, where appropriate, carried out at 6–12 months.

Antiepileptic drug developments

The older, more established AEDs were developed in animal models. Potential AEDs were administered to the animal to test the drug's ability to raise seizure threshold or prevent spread of seizure discharge. Models include maximal electroshock and the subcutaneous pentylenetetrazole models (Solomon 2000). AEDs were then identified as exerting their pharmacologic effect by modulating sodium and calcium channels, increasing GABA concentrations, altering serotonin neurotransmission or reducing glutamate-mediated excitation by NMDA (N-methyl D-aspartate) and AMPA (alpha-amino-3-hydroxy-5-methyl-4-isoxazole propionic acid) receptors (Fig. 29.1).

Established therapeutic drugs such as phenytoin, phenobarbital, sodium valproate, carbamazepine, ethosuximide, clonazepam and diazepam, though effective, have poor side-effect profiles, many interactions and difficult pharmacokinetics. Over the past 10–15 years, there has been renewed interest in the development of new AEDs with a better understanding of excitatory and inhibitory pathways in the brain.

The new drugs that have been developed are vigabatrin, lamotrigine, gabapentin, tiagabine, topiramate, felbamate, oxcarbazepine and zonisamide. Unlike most of the older agents, vigabatrin, lamotrigine, gabapentin, tiagabine and zonisamide are devoid of significant enzyme inhibiting or inducing properties. Although tiagabine is extensively metabolized by cyctochrome P450, it does not influence the pharmacokinetics of conventional AEDs, theophylline, warfarin, digoxin or oral contraceptives (Mengel et al 1995). Topiramate and oxcarbazepine, however, induce cytochrome P450 CYP3A4 which is responsible for the metabolism of oral contraceptives (Sabers & Gram 2000).

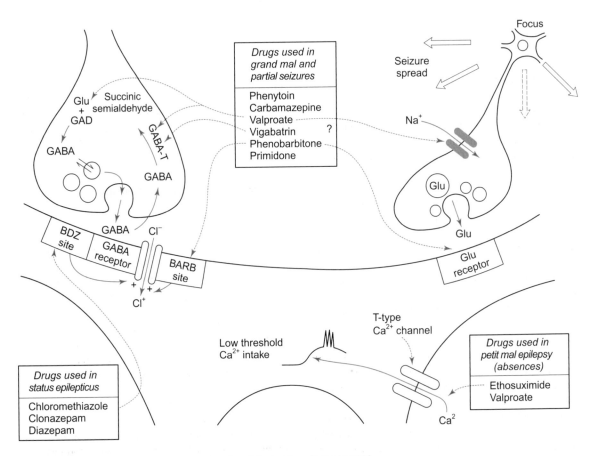

Fig. 29.1 Action of epileptic drugs on receptor sites. Adapted from Solomon 2000.

Table 29.3 Commonly used starting and maintenance doses of antiepileptic drugs for adults

AED	Starting dose (mg)	Average maintenance (total mg/day)	Doses/day
Acetazolamide	250	500–1500	2
Carbamazepine	100	600–2400	2–4 (retard 2)
Clobazam	10	10–30	1–2
Clonazepam	0.5	0.5–3	1–2
Ethosuximide	250	500–1500	1–2
Gabapentin	300	900–1200	3
Lamotrigine	50*	100–500[a]	2
Levetiracetam	1000	2000–3000	2
Oxcarbazepine	300	900–1800	2–3
Phenobarbital	60	60–180	1
Phenytoin	200–300	200–400	1–2
Valproate	500	2000–2500	1–2
Vigabatrin	500	2000–4000	1–2

[a] Reduce by 50% if on valproate.

Antiepileptic drug profiles

The maintenance doses for the more widely used AEDs are given in Table 29.3, while their pharmacokinetic profile is presented in Table 29.4. Drug interactions are summarized in Table 29.5, and common side-effects in Table 29.6.

Acetazolamide. Acetazolamide is occasionally used as an AED. It can be prescribed as a second-line drug for most types of seizures, but particularly for partial seizures, absence seizures and myoclonic seizures. Its intermittent use in catamenial seizures has also been suggested. Acetazolamide has only limited use as long-term therapy because of the development of tolerance in the majority of patients. Side-effects include skin rashes, weight loss, paraesthesia, drowsiness and depression. Routine TDM is not available for this drug.

Carbamazepine. Carbamazepine is a drug of first choice in tonic–clonic and partial seizures, and may be of benefit in all other seizure types except generalized absence seizures and myoclonic seizures. Tolerance to its beneficial effect does not usually develop. Adverse events may occur in up to a third of patients treated with carbamazepine but only about 5% will necessitate drug withdrawal, usually due to skin rash, gastrointestinal disturbances or hyponatraemia. Dose-related adverse reactions including ataxia, dizziness, blurred vision and diplopia are common. Serious adverse events including hepatic failure and bone marrow depression are extremely uncommon. Carbamazepine shows autoinduction, – i.e. induces its own metabolism as well as inducing the metabolism of other drugs. It should therefore be introduced at low dosage and the dose optimized over a period of a month. The target serum concentration therapeutic range is 4–12 micrograms/ml. In addition, a number of clinically important pharmacokinetic interactions may occur, and caution should be exercised when co-medication is instituted (see Table 29.5). For patients requiring higher doses, the slow-release preparation of carbamazepine has distinct advantages, allowing twice daily ingestion and avoiding high peak serum concentrations. A 'chewtab' formulation is also available, and pharmacokinetic studies have shown that it performs well even if inadvertently swallowed whole. Carbamazepine retard offers paediatric patients in particular a dosage form that reduces fluctuations in the peak-to-trough serum levels and hence allows a twice daily regimen. The latter can assist compliance.

Clobazam. Clobazam is a 1,5-benzodiazepine that is said to be less sedative than 1,4-benzodiazepine drugs such as clonazepam and diazepam. Although the

Table 29.4 Pharmacokinetic data summary

Drug	Absorption				Elimination		
	F(%)	T_{peak} (h)	V_d (L/kg)	Protein binding (% bound)	$T_{1/2}$ (h)	Renal excretion (%)	Active metabolite
Carbamazepine	75–85	1–5 (chronic dose)	0.8–1.6	70–78	24–45 (single), 8–24 (chronic)	< 1	Yes
Diazepam	90	1–2	1–2	96	20–95	2	Yes
Clonazepam	80–90	1–2	2.1–4.3	80–90	19–40	2	–
Gabapentin	51–59	2–3	57.7L	0	5–7	100	No
Lamotrigine	100	2–3	0.92–1.22	55	24–35 (induces its own metabolism)	< 10	No
Ethosuximide	90–95	3–7	0.6–0.9	0	20–60	10–20	No
Phenobarbital	95–100	1–3	0.6	40–50	50–144	20–40	No
Phenytoin	85–95	4–7	0.5–0.7	90–95	9–40 (non-linear kinetics)	< 5	No
Primidone	90–100	1–3	0.4–1.1	20–30	3–19	40	Yes
Sodium valproate	100	0.5–1.0	0.1–0.5	88–92	7–17	< 5	No
Vigabatrin	60–80	2	0.6–1.0	0	5–7	100	No

development of tolerance is common, clobazam is used as an adjunctive therapy for patients with partial or generalized seizures who have proved unresponsive to other antiepileptic medication. Its intermittent use in catamenial epilepsy has also been suggested. Clobazam may produce less sedation than other benzodiazepines, but otherwise its adverse effects are similar, including dizziness, behavioural disturbances and dry mouth. Withdrawal may be difficult.

Clonazepam. Clonazepam, a 1,4-benzodiazepine, is a drug of choice for myoclonic seizures and a second-line drug for generalized tonic–clonic seizures, absences, and as adjunctive therapy for partial seizures, but, as with clobazam, effectiveness often wears off with time as tolerance develops. Parenteral clonazepam is useful in status epilepticus. It has an adverse effect profile similar to that of clobazam, but may be more sedating.

Diazepam. Diazepam is used mainly in the treatment of status epilepticus, intravenously or in the acute management of febrile convulsions as a rectal solution. Absorption from suppositories or following intramuscular injection is slow and erratic. The rectal

solution may also be useful in status epilepticus if it is not possible to give the drug intravenously.

Ethosuximide. Ethosuximide is a drug of first choice for generalized absence seizures, and has no useful effect against any other seizure type. Tolerance does not seem to be a problem. The most commonly encountered adverse effects are gastrointestinal symptoms, which occur frequently at the beginning of therapy. Behaviour disorders, anorexia, fatigue, sleep disturbances and headaches may also occur. The therapeutic range commonly quoted is 40–100 micrograms/ml but some patients may require higher concentrations, sometimes as high as 150 micrograms/ml. The absorption of ethosuximide is complete, the bioavailability of the syrup and capsule formulations being equivalent. Increase in daily dose may lead to disproportionately higher increases in average plasma concentrations, therefore careful monitoring is indicated at high doses.

Gabapentin. Gabapentin is a second-line treatment of partial seizures although its main use currently is for the treatment of neuropathic pain. The optimal dose remains

Table 29.5 Drug interactions

Drug affected	Effect on plasma level	Drug implicated	Possible mechanism
Carbamazepine	Increase	Sodium valproate Cimetidine Dextropropoxyphene, propoxyphene Erythromycin Isoniazid Troleandomycin Danazol	Enzyme inhibition
	Decrease	Phenytoin Phenobarbital	Enzyme induction
Phenytoin	Increase	Sodium valproate Chloramphenicol Isoniazid Disulfiram Fluconazole Flu vaccine	Enzyme inhibition
		Amiodarone Fluoxetine	Mechanism unclear
	Decrease	Phenobarbital Rifampicin Carbamazepine	Enzyme induction
		Furosemide (frusemide)	Decreased responsiveness of renal tubules
		Acetazolamide	Increased osteomalacia
Sodium valproate	Increase	Salicylates	Displacement from protein binding sites and possible enzyme inhibition
	Decrease	Potential enzyme inducers	Enzyme induction
Phenobarbital	Increase	Sodium valproate	Enzyme inhibition
	Decrease	Bifampicin	Enzyme induction
Lamotrigine	Increase	Sodium valproate	Enzyme inhibition
	Decrease	Phenytoin, carbamazepine	Enzyme induction
Topiramate	Decrease	Phenytoin, carbamazepine	Enzyme induction
Ethosuximide	Increase	Sodium valproate	Enzyme inhibition
	Decrease	Carbamazepine	Enzyme induction

to be established: the maximum recommended dose is currently 3600 mg/day, but the efficacy of higher doses is presently being investigated in clinical trials. In view of its pharmacokinetic profile, a three times daily dosage must be used. To date, no clinical significant interactions of gabapentin with other AEDs or other drugs have been reported. The most frequently reported side-effects are drowsiness, dizziness, diplopia, ataxia and headache. No idiosyncratic side-effects have been reported so far.

Lamotrigine. Lamotrigine may be used as a first-line drug in patients with partial seizures, with or without secondary generalization, and in tonic–clonic convulsions. The recommended starting dose is 50 mg when used as monotherapy, and 25 mg when used as an add-on therapy; the latter dose is given on alternate days in patients receiving concomitant sodium valproate and daily in patients receiving other AEDs, with a maximum recommended dose of 400 mg/day in two divided doses. It should be slowly titrated as too rapid titration may be associated with an increased incidence of skin rash. Lamotrigine does not seem to interact with other concomitantly administered antiepileptic drugs. However, hepatic enzyme inducers increase the metabolism of lamotrigine, reducing its half-life. Therefore, higher doses of lamotrigine need to be administered if it is used in conjunction with enzyme inducer drugs such as phenytoin and carbamazepine. Inhibitors of hepatic enzymes such as sodium valproate block the metabolism of lamotrigine and reduced doses of lamotrigine need to be used if both drugs are given in combination. Headaches, drowsiness, ataxia

Table 29.6   Side-effect profile of anticonvulsants

Drug	Dose related (predictable)	Non-dose related (idiosyncratic)
Carbamazepine	Diplopia, drowsiness, headache, nausea, orofacial dyskinesia, arrhythmias	Photosensitivity, Stevens–Johnson syndrome, agranulocytosis, aplastic anaemia, hepatotoxicity
Sodium valproate	Dyspepsia, nausea, vomiting, hair loss, anorexia, drowsiness	Acute pancreatitis, aplastic anaemia, thrombocytopenia, hepatotoxicity
Phenytoin	Ataxia, nystagmus, drowsiness, gingival hyperplasia, hirsutism, diplopia, asterixis, orofacial dyskinesia, folate deficiency	Blood dyscrasias, rash, Dupuytren's contracture, hepatotoxicity
Phenobarbital	Fatigue, listlessness, depression, poor memory, impotence, hypocalcaemia, osteomalacia, folate deficiency	Macropapular rash, exfoliation, hepatotoxicity
Ethosuximide	Nausea, vomiting, drowsinesss, headache, lethargy	Rash, erythema multiforme, Stevens–Johnson syndrome
Clonazepam	Fatigue, drowsiness, ataxia	Rash, thrombocytopenia
Lamotrigine	Headaches, drowsiness, diplopia, ataxia	Liver failure, disseminated intravascular coagulation
Gabapentin	Drowsiness, diplopia, ataxia, headache	Not reported
Topiramate	Dizziness, drowsiness, nervousness, fatigue, weight loss	Not reported
Vigabatrin	Drowsiness, dizziness, weight gain	Behavioural disturbances, severe psychosis

and diplopia, usually transient, are the most commonly reported acute adverse effects, particularly during dose escalation. A skin rash is the commonest idiosyncratic side-effect of this drug, and affects up to 3% of patients. There have been a few reports of fatalities due to disseminated intravascular coagulation and fulminant liver failure associated with the use of lamotrigine, but these rare events have to be seen in the context of more than 100 000 patients exposed to the drug.

Levetiracetam. Levetiracetam is a recently marketed AED that is indicated for the treatment of refractory partial epilepsy. Placebo controlled trials in refractory partial epilepsy have shown a 50% seizure reduction in up to 40% of patients. In these trials 8% became seizure-free compared to none on placebo. The usual dose is between 1500 and 3000 mg a day. It is usually started at 500 mg a day and the dose is titrated upwards in incremental steps of 500 mg every 1 or 2 weeks. It is well tolerated and the most frequent central nervous system adverse events are dizziness, asthenia and somnolence. No idiosyncratic adverse events have yet been reported.

Oxcarbazepine. Oxcarbazepine is an analogue of carbamazepine. It is an inactive pro-drug that is converted in the liver to the active 10-hydroxy metabolite and bypasses the 10,11-epoxide, the primary metabolite of carbamazepine. The usual dose is between 900 and 2400 mg/day. The spectrum of efficacy and side-effects is broadly comparable to carbamazepine. The principal advantage of oxcarbazepine over carbamazepine is the lack of induction of hepatic enzymes, with the consequence that there is no autoinduction of the metabolism of the drug and fewer pharmacokinetic interactions. In addition, two-thirds of patients who are allergic to carbamazepine can tolerate oxcarbazepine.

Phenobarbital. Phenobarbital, a barbiturate, is a second-line drug for the treatment of tonic–clonic, tonic and partial seizures. It may also be used in other seizure types. Its antiepileptic efficacy is similar to that of phenytoin or carbamazepine. Adverse effects on cognitive function, the propensity to produce tolerance and the risk of serious seizure exacerbation on withdrawal make it an unattractive option, and it should be used only as a last resort. In addition to cognitive effects, barbiturates may cause skin rashes, ataxia, folate deficiency, osteomalacia, behavioural disturbances (particularly in children) and an increased risk of connective tissue disorders such as Dupuytren's contracture and frozen shoulder. Phenobarbital is a potent enzyme inducer and is implicated in several clinically important drug interactions (see Table 29.5) The normal adult serum target range of 15–40 micrograms/ml should be interpreted with caution due to development of tolerance to some of the pharmacological effects as well as to the antiepileptic action. Decreased elimination is expected in patients with impaired renal or hepatic function. Once a day dosage is usually adequate in most adults because of the long half-life. However, as the steady state is not reached for 2–3 weeks the administration of a loading dose is recommended. Routine monitoring is not necessary on initiating therapy as the dose can be adequately titrated according to the clinical response. However, monitoring is indicated if patients do not respond or exhibit toxicity.

Primidone. Primidone is principally metabolized to phenobarbital in vivo and has similar effects and a more severe side-effect profile than phenobarbital. There is nothing to recommend primidone as an AED over phenobarbital.

Phenytoin. Phenytoin is a drug of first choice for tonic–clonic, tonic and partial seizures, and a second-line drug for atonic seizures and atypical absences. It is not effective in typical generalized absences and myoclonic seizures. Tolerance to its antiepileptic action does not usually occur. Phenytoin has non-linear kinetics and a low therapeutic index, and in some patients frequent drug serum level measurements may be necessary. Drug interactions (see Table 29.5) are common as phenytoin metabolism is very susceptible to inhibition by other drugs, while it may enhance the metabolism of others. Caution should be exercised when other medication is introduced or withdrawn. Adverse events may occur in up to a half of patients treated with phenytoin, but only about 10% will necessitate drug withdrawal, most commonly due to skin rash. Dose-related adverse reactions including nystagmus, ataxia and lethargy are common. Cosmetic effects such as gum hypertrophy, hirsutism and acne are well recognized adverse effects, and should be taken into account when prescribing for children and young women. Chronic adverse effects include folate deficiency, osteomalacia, Dupuytren's contractures and cerebellar atrophy. Serious idiosyncratic adverse events, including hepatic failure and bone marrow depression, are extremely uncommon. Most patients require dosages from 250 to 400 mg daily. The drug shows slow and fast metabolism, hence slow metabolizers may require doses of 100–200 mg/day and fast metabolizers doses of 400–600 mg/day. The target serum range for phenytoin is 10–20 micrograms/ml (although a number of patients are controlled outside the range). Once patients achieve levels within the target range the majority require once a day dosage. Phenytoin is available in capsule, tablet, suspension and injection form. It is usually prescribed orally although it may be given intravenously. Oral preparations of phenytoin may present differences in bioavailability. Patients stabilized on one formulation should continue to receive the same formulation. Care is required when changing from the elixir to the capsule or tablet formulation due to the different bioavailability. Intravenous phenytoin should be administered with caution and at a rate not exceeding 50 mg/min. Intravenous phenytoin may be indicated when patients are on a nil by mouth regimen or require the drug for status epilepticus. Phenytoin ready mixed parenteral formulation should not be added to intravenous fluids due to a risk of acid precipitation. The drug should never be given intramuscularly.

Sodium valproate. Sodium valproate is a drug of first choice for the treatment of generalized absence seizures, myoclonic seizures and generalized tonic–clonic seizures, especially if these occur as part of the syndrome of primary generalized epilepsy. Tolerance to its antiepileptic action does not usually occur. Drug interactions with other antiepileptic drugs may be problematic. Phenobarbital levels increase with co-medication with valproate, and a combination of these two drugs may result in severe sedation. Sodium valproate may also inhibit the metabolism of lamotrigine, phenytoin and carbamazepine. Enzyme-inducing drugs enhance the metabolism of sodium valproate, so caution should be exercised when other AEDs are introduced or withdrawn. Up to a third of patients may experience adverse effects, but fewer than 5% will require the drug to be stopped. Adverse effects include anorexia, nausea, diarrhoea, weight gain, alopecia, skin rash and thrombocytopenia. Confusion, stupor, tremor and hyperammonaemia are usually dose related. Serious adverse events including fatal pancreatic and hepatic failure are extremely uncommon. In children under 2 years, on other AEDs and with pre-existing neurological deficit, the risk of this is 1/500. In adults on valproate monotherapy the risk is 1/37 000. The usual therapeutic range quoted is 50–100 micrograms/ml; however, because of the lack of a good correlation between total valproate concentrations and effect, serum level monitoring of the drug has limited use. TDM should only be performed in cases of suspected toxicity, deterioration in seizure control, to check compliance or to monitor drug interactions. Routine monitoring of this drug is not necessary.

Tiagabine. Tiagabine is a new drug with mild to moderate efficacy in seizure control. It is used as a second-line drug in partial seizures with or without secondary generalization. Results from controlled trials have shown that up to one-third of patients on tiagabine achieve a 50% reduction in seizure frequency, although complete remission from seizures is an infrequent occurrence. The usual dose is between 30 and 45 mg a day, and it is normally started at 10 mg day in two divided doses, with incremental steps of 5 mg every 2 weeks. The commonest adverse events are on the central nervous system and consist of sedation, tremor, headache, mental slowing, tiredness and dizziness. Confusion, irritability and depression may occur. Increases in seizure frequency and episodes of non-convulsive status have also been reported. So far, no life-threatening idiosyncratic reactions have been reported. Use in pregnancy is not recommended although no teratogenicity has been reported in humans.

Topiramate. Topiramate is chemically unrelated to other AEDs and is used as a second-line drug for patients with partial seizures. Usual doses are between 200 and 600 mg/day. It has to be titrated slowly, and the recommended starting dose is 25 mg once daily, titrating upwards in 25 mg/day increments every 2 weeks up to 200 mg/day in two divided doses. After that the dose should be increased by 50 mg every 2 weeks until seizure control is achieved or side-effects develop. It has no clinical significant interaction with other AEDs, although hepatic enzyme inducers accelerate its metabolism and topiramate doses need to be adjusted downwards if patients are coming off carbamazepine or phenytoin. Side-effects of topiramate include dizziness, drowsiness, nervousness, impaired concentration, paraesthesias, nephrolithiasis and fatigue. Patients starting topiramate should increase their fluid intake to reduce the risk of kidney stones. Weight loss is seen in up to 30% of patients.

Vigabatrin. Vigabatrin, a suicide inhibitor of γ-aminobutyrate (GABA) transaminase, in view of its safety profile, is a last resort drug for partial seizures. Vigabatrin may also be useful in West's syndrome, particularly if associated with tuberous sclerosis. Vigabatrin does not interact with other drugs apart from decreasing phenytoin levels, probably by blocking its absorption. The commonest adverse events associated with vigabatrin are behavioural disturbances ranging from agitation and confusion to frank psychosis and visual field defects. Other known adverse effects include drowsiness, headaches, ataxia, weight gain, depression and tremor. Careful monitoring for side-effects, particularly ophthalmological, on initiation of therapy is essential. Routine TDM is not available for this drug.

New antiepileptic drugs

A number of antiepileptic drugs are under development, and the following section provides a summary profile on two of those.

Felbamate. Felbamate may be used as a drug of last resort in patients with intractable epilepsy. Its mechanism of action is unknown. The usual dose is between 1200 and 3600 mg/day. Felbamate exhibits significant pharmacokinetic interactions with phenytoin, carbamazepine and valproic acid. Side-effects of felbamate include diplopia, insomnia, dizziness, headache, ataxia, anorexia, nausea and vomiting. A major use-limiting problem is its potential to cause aplastic anaemia and liver failure, affecting as many as 1 in 4000 patients exposed to the drug. Hence, it seems prudent to limit its use to specialist centres and severe intractable cases.

Table 29.7 Common therapeutic problems in epilepsy

Problem	Comment
Hepatic enzyme induction	Enzyme induction occurs with carbamazepine, phenytoin, phenobarbital, primidone and topiramate. Interactions occur with a large number of drugs including oral contraceptives
Use of progesterone-only contraceptives with enzyme-inducing AED	Best avoided. If no acceptable alternative, patient should take at least double usual dose of progesterone-only pill
Use of combined oral contraceptive with enzyme-inducing AED	Preparations containing 50 micrograms of oestrogen should be used
Continuation of AED during pregnancy	Ideally review before attempting pregnancy to determine if reducing or discontinuing treatment is possible
Use of phenytoin as monotherapy	Less frequently considered first line monotherapy due to poor side-effect profile, narrow therapeutic index and saturation pharmacokinetics
Prescribing of branded AEDs	Debate continues about whether significant differences exist between generic and branded AEDs

AED, antiepileptic drug

Zonisamide. Zonisamide is an antiepileptic drug that is effective as add-on treatment for refractory partial seizures and refractory myoclonic seizures. Clinical trials suggest that about 50% of patients with refractory partial seizures will experience a reduction of 50% or more in seizures after the introduction of zonisamide. The common side-effects of zonisamide include sedation, fatigue weight loss and kidney stones.

Table 29.7 lists some common therapeutic problems in epilepsy.

CASE STUDIES

Case 29.1

J. B. is a 31-year-old woman with a history of early morning myoclonic jerks starting at the age of 16. When she was 18 years old she had her first generalized tonic–clonic convulsive seizure. A diagnosis of juvenile myoclonic epilepsy was made and she was started on sodium valproate 1200 mg a day which controlled her seizures.

At the age of 21 the patient had a healthy baby and experienced no problems with epilepsy control. Aged 22, she had her second pregnancy and delivered a healthy baby girl. Three weeks after delivery early morning myoclonic seizures returned. The dose of sodium valproate was increased to 1500 mg to control jerks. However, 6 months later she experienced a recurrence of her convulsive attacks with no clear precipitating factor. Sodium valproate was increased to 2000 mg a day. Early morning myoclonic seizures crept back and she had further convulsive seizures. Lamotrigine was started at 200 mg daily. She has been completely seizure-free for the last 2 years and is now driving again.

J. B. wants to discuss her medication with you and would like to stop treatment. She has no plans to increase her family.

Question

What advice would you give J. B.?

Answer

J. B. should be advised to continue on medication. She has juvenile myoclonic epilepsy, which tends to recur when medication is withdrawn. The patient has no intention of having further children and therefore pregnancy need not be a consideration in the choice of her continued drug therapy. She is generally well and hence it would be sensible to advise her to continue with the present regimen, as sodium valproate and lamotrigine have a synergistic effect in juvenile myoclonic epilepsy. If, however, she wants to reduce medication, then a slow decrease of valproate with optimization of treatment with lamotrigine should be considered.

Case 29.2

O. B. is a 44-year-old man who suffers from partial epilepsy. An MRI scan shows a choroid cyst on the right

temporal lobe, bilateral hippocampal sclerosis and cerebral atrophy. Seizures take the form of complex partial attacks and at night secondary generalizations occur. He has had trials of treatment with every single drug in the book and almost every combination.

Six months ago, he was taking 225 mg of topiramate (could not tolerate more), 400 mg of phenytoin and 10 mg of clobazam each day. At this point levetiracetam was added and titrated up to 2000 mg a day. This led to a significant improvement in seizure control. Indeed, seizures have almost completely been abolished and he is only having occasional nocturnal events. He is, however, complaining of drowsiness and periods of unsteadiness.

Question

What treatment advice is appropriate for this patient?

Answer

Mr. O. B. needs his drug regimen optimizing. The decision should be made to reduce either the dose of topiramate or that of phenytoin. The consensus view is that phenytoin should probably be reduced first. However, this patient had a bad experience in the past when an attempt was made to discontinue phenytoin, at which time he had a significant increase in seizure frequency. It would therefore be more appropriate to discontinue topiramate in Mr. O. B.

This was done and his improvement has been maintained.

Case 29.3

V. P. is a 33-year-old patient who started to have complex partial seizures with a clear temporal lobe element at about the age of 8. Occasionally she would have secondary generalized seizures. Her epilepsy was thought to be cryptogenic but 6 years ago she was referred to a hospital clinic. A high resolution MRI scan showed that she had a right temporal lobe abnormality. This was thought to be amenable to surgery. The patient, however, declined any consideration of a surgical approach.

When initially seen at the clinic, V. P. was taking 600 mg of carbamazepine and 750 mg of primidone. Treatment with carbamazepine was optimized and an attempt was made to discontinue primidone but her seizure frequency increased. Clobazam was added to her treatment and she became seizure-free. Primidone was restarted, increasing at a rate of 125 mg every 8 weeks. Over the last 2 years she has remained seizure-free on 20 mg clobazam and 1800 mg carbamazepine controlled release.

Question

Would you now consider reducing this patient to monotherapy with carbamazepine?

Answer

In view of the long-standing epilepsy in this patient and the clear-cut aetiology, there must be a reluctance to advise any change in treatment. Although tolerance to clobazam may develop, this is not always the case. V. P. would probably be better off on therapy with carbamazepine and clobazam. Of course, if her seizures recurred, the question of surgery should be reconsidered.

Case 29.4

J. O. is a 59-year-old patient who has suffered with seizures since the age of 14. No putative aetiology has been identified. A recent high resolution MRI scan did not show any structural abnormality apart from mild cerebral atrophy. J. O. is currently taking 1600 mg of carbamazepine controlled release and 2000 mg of sodium valproate each day.

A trial of treatment with gabapentin was attempted, and doses of up to 3600 mg were used. This had no impact on the frequency of the patient's complex partial seizures and, if anything, he felt unsteady and drowsy on this dose. The decision was made to replace gabapentin with other medication. Of the antiepileptic drugs available, he has not had trials of treatment with tiagabine, oxcarbazepine or levetiracetam. On discussing options with the patient, the decision was made to try levetiracetam.

Questions

1. Should gabapentin be discontinued before levetiracetam is started?
2. Should consideration be given to the withdrawal of sodium valproate or carbamazepine at this stage?

Answers

1. Levetiracetam should be started concomitantly with the discontinuation of gabapentin. Gabapentin should be reduced in 600 mg decremental steps at the same time that levetiracetam is titrated upwards. This should be done at incremental steps of 500 mg every week.
2. If J. O. derives benefit from the trial of treatment with levetiracetam, then it would be appropriate to consider withdrawing either sodium valproate or carbamazepine.

Case 29.5

D. G. is a 22-year-old student studying maths at university. He was involved in a road traffic accident and admitted to hospital with a fractured neck of femur and head injuries. The clinician starts carbamazepine following a number of complex partial seizures. Four weeks after dischage D. G. develops a severe upper respiratory chest infection. His GP prescribes ciprofloxacin. Three days later the patient has ataxia, blurred vision and is very drowsy.

Questions

1. How should carbamazepine therapy be initiated?
2. Comment on the patient's deterioration following initiation of carbamazepine.

Answers

1. Carbamazepine is an enzyme inducer and induces its own metabolism. The drug should be started slowly and the dose titrated over 3–4 weeks. A suitable dose schedule would be 100 mg twice daily increasing to 200 mg after 2 weeks and then to 300 mg twice daily. Serum drug levels should be taken to monitor therapy.
2. Ciprofloxacin is not a good choice since it causes hepatic enzyme inhibition. The patient shows signs of carbamazepine toxicity and this could be explained by raised serum carbamazepine levels. The antibiotic also causes a reduction in seizure threshold and hence should be avoided in patients with epilepsy

Case 29.6

E. M. is a 75-year-old retired schoolteacher who lives in a residential home and has long-standing epilepsy. Her current medication includes phenytoin, phenobarbital and sodium valproate. She routinely has sub-therapeutic levels of all three drugs. One evening she is found unconscious in her bedroom and in her bathroom an empty bottle of phenytoin capsules is discovered. She is taken to hospital in an ambulance and on arrival an urgent request for blood levels of the anticonvulsants is made. Serum levels are available the same day and show a toxic level of phenytoin of 65 mg/l (normal therapaeutic range 10–20 mg/l).

Question

How long will it take for the toxic levels of phenytoin to fall within the therapeutic range?

Answer

Phenytoin shows non-linear pharmacokinetic handling. It is difficult to work out how long it will take for levels to fall within the normal therapeutic range. Hence daily monitoring of serum levels is advisable. If the hepatic enzymes are fully saturated with phenytoin then at maximum metabolic capacity approximately 10 mg/l of the drug will be eliminated. Initially the drug will redistribute into plasma, hence for the first 2–3 days serum phenytoin levels will fall slowly. It is usual for the levels to take up to 6–7 days to fall within the therapeutic range. Therapy will then need to be reviewed.

REFERENCES

Feely M 1999 Drug treatment of epilepsy. British Medical Journal 318: 106–109

Marson A G, Kadir Z A, Hutton J L, Chadwick D W 1997 The new antiepileptic drugs: a systematic review of their efficacy and tolerability. Epilepsia 38: 859–80.

Mengel H, Jansen J A, Sommerville K et al 1995 Tiagabine: evaluation of the risk of interaction with theophylline, warfarin, digoxin, cimetidine, oral contraceptives, triazolam or ethanol.

Epilepsia 36 S(3): 12

Sabers A, Gram L 2000 Newer anticonvulsants: comparative review of drug interactions and adverse effects. Drugs 60: 23–33

Shorvon S, Stefan H 1997 Overview of the safety of newer antiepileptic drugs. Epilepsia 38 (S1): S45–51

Solomon L M 2000 Mechanisms of action of anticonvulsant agents. Neurology 55 (S1): S32–S40

FURTHER READING

Duncan J S, Shorvon S D, Fish D R (eds) 1995 Clinical epilepsy. Churchill Livingstone, Edinburgh

Sander J W A S, Shorvon S D 1996 The epidemiology of the epilepsies. Journal of Neurology, Neurosurgery and Psychiatry

61: 433–443

Marson A G, Kadir Z A, Hutton J L et al 1997 The new antiepileptic drugs: a systematic review of their efficacy and tolerability. Epilepsia 38: 859–880.

Parkinson's disease 30

D. J. Burn

KEY POINTS

- Parkinson's disease is the second most common neurodegenerative disease, affecting 1% of the population over the age of 65.
- Parkinson's disease is characterized by bradykinesia, rest tremor, rigidity and, later in the disease course, postural instability.
- Neuronal loss in the brainstem (substantia nigra) leads to a profound dopamine deficiency in the striatum. This provides the rationale for dopaminergic replacement therapies.
- Parkinson's disease is not always easy to diagnose. The diagnosis is clinically-based. Error rates of ~ 25% have been reported in clinicopathological studies.
- Depression is common in Parkinson's disease. It is the major determinant of quality of life and is often missed. The depression of Parkinson's disease can be readily treated.
- Levodopa, coupled with a dopa-decarboxylase inhibitor, remains the most potent oral drug available for the treatment of Parkinson's disease. There is debate as to whether levodopa should be deferred in biologically young patients, in an attempt to delay the onset of motor complications.
- Several other drug treatments are available for the management of Parkinson's disease. When given as adjunctive therapy to levodopa, the primary aim of these agents is to smooth out motor fluctuations.
- End of dose deterioration and the on–off phenomenon are motor complications synonymous with the use of levodopa, usually for a number of years. Despite advances in oral pharmacotherapy for Parkinson's disease, the on–off phenomenon, in particular, remains difficult to treat effectively.
- Surgical treatments of Parkinson's disease show promise, but require further evaluation.
- Advanced Parkinson's disease is difficult to manage, particularly neuropsychiatric problems. Reduction of dopaminergic therapy may be the best compromise.
- Next to levodopa, the introduction of Parkinson's disease nurse specialists has been the most important advance in the management of Parkinson's disease.

Parkinson's disease is the most common cause of parkinsonism and is the second most common neurodegenerative disease, after Alzheimer's disease. Although descriptions of the condition appeared before the 19th century, it was James Parkinson's eloquent account in 1817 that fully documented the clinical features of the illness now bearing his name. The identification of dopamine deficiency in the brains of people with Parkinson's disease and the subsequent introduction of replacement therapy with levodopa represents a considerable (and still unparalleled) success story in the treatment of neurodegenerative illness in general. There remain, however, a number of significant management problems in Parkinson's disease, particularly in the advanced stages of the condition.

Epidemiology

Parkinson's disease affects 1% of the population over 65 years of age, rising to 2% over the age of 80. One in 20 patients are, however, diagnosed before their 40th year. It is estimated that 110 000 people have Parkinson's disease in the UK. The condition is found worldwide, although it may be less common in China and West Africa. Most epidemiological studies have indicated a small male to female predominance.

Other causes of parkinsonism include the neurodegenerative conditions multiple system atrophy and progressive supranuclear palsy. Prevalences for these conditions are 4.3 and 5.0 per 100 000, respectively. Drug-induced parkinsonism is a common form of so-called 'symptomatic' parkinsonism. It affects 10–15% of individuals exposed to dopamine receptor blocking agents (including neuroleptics and some labyrinthine sedatives).

Aetiology

Both genetic and environmental factors have been implicated as a cause of Parkinson's disease. While initially opinions were polarized, it now seems probable that in the majority of cases there is an admixture of influences, with environmental factors precipitating the onset of Parkinson's disease in a genetically susceptible individual.

Environmental factors became pre-eminent in the 1980s, when drug addicts attempting to manufacture heroin accidently produced a toxin called MPTP (1-methyl-4-phenyl-1,2,3,6-tetrahydropyridine). Ingestion or inhalation of MPTP rapidly produced a severe parkinsonian state, indistinguishable from advanced Parkinson's disease. MPTP is a relatively simple compound, and is not too dissimilar from paraquat. More recently, the demonstration that chronic systemic pesticide exposure can reproduce the clinical and pathological features of Parkinson's disease in rotenone-treated rats has generated considerable interest.

In a small number of patients, genetic factors are dominant. The discovery of a mutation in the gene coding for a synaptic protein called α-synuclein has provided tremendous impetus to research. Such mutations have been described in fewer than 10 families worldwide. Nevertheless, because α-synuclein is a major component of the pathological hallmark of Parkinson's disease, the Lewy body (see below), the challenge now is to discover how a mutation in this protein in a tiny minority can relate to the formation of Lewy bodies in the vast majority.

Pathophysiology

The characteristic pathological features of Parkinson's disease are neuronal loss in pigmented brainstem nuclei, together with the presence of eosinophilic inclusion bodies, called Lewy bodies, in surviving cells. The pars compacta of the substantia nigra in the midbrain is particularly affected. Dopaminergic neurones within this nucleus project to the striatum, which is therefore deprived of the neurotransmitter dopamine.

In Parkinson's disease there is a loss of over 80% of nigral neurones before symptoms appear. There is controversy over the duration of this preclinical period, but current evidence favours a relatively short latency, of the order of 5 years.

Dopaminergic neurones are not the only cells to die within the brainstem, and a host of other nuclei and neurotransmitter systems are involved. For example, cholinergic neurones within the pedunculopontine nucleus degenerate, providing potential clinicopathological correlates with postural instability, swallowing difficulty (dysphagia) and sleep disturbance (REM sleep behavioural disturbance). The involvement of this nucleus in Parkinson's disease may account for why dopaminergic therapy is relatively ineffective in treating these particular clinical problems. Within the striatum, changes occur within γ-aminobutyric acid-positive neurones, as a consequence of nigrostriatal dopaminergic deficiency and also non-physiological dopaminergic replacement. These changes are thought to play a key role in mediating the development of involuntary movements (dyskinesias) which develop after a number of years of levodopa treatment. The loss of noradrenergic and serotonergic neurones within the locus coeruleus and the raphé nucleus, respectively, may provide a pathophysiological basis for depression, which is common in Parkinson's disease.

Clinical features

Bradykinesia is a *sine qua non* for parkinsonism in general. If a person does not have slowness of movement, they cannot have either parkinsonism or Parkinson's disease. Rest tremor, extrapyramidal rigidity (so-called 'lead pipe' and/or 'cog-wheel') and postural instability comprise the remaining classical tetrad of clinical features for Parkinson's disease. Asymmetry of signs at disease onset is very common. The rest tremor is a rhythmic movement with a frequency of 4–6 Hz (cycles per second), typically noticed with the patient at rest. It is sometimes described as 'pill-rolling' in nature, from the movement of the thumb across the fingers. However, 15–20% of patients do not develop a tremor. Postural instability is a late feature of Parkinson's disease, and comprises an impairment of righting reflexes with a tendency to fall. There may be a flexed truncal posture and loss of arm swing when walking. There is reduced blink frequency and facial expression, which, together with rather reduced volume (hypophonic) and monotonous speech, may lead to significant difficulties in communication. The patient may drool and have greasy skin (seborrhoea). Writing becomes small (micrographia) and barely legible.

Autonomic dysfunction may occur in Parkinson's disease. Urogenital difficulties, with erectile dysfunction in males and urinary urgency in both sexes, are commonly encountered. Frank incontinence is, however, rare. Constipation is invariable and is multifactorial in origin. Falling blood pressure on standing (postural hypotension) may contribute to falls later in the disease course. Neuropsychiatric disturbances affect approximately 40% of people with Parkinson's disease and are a major determinant of both carer stress and nursing home placement. Depression can be a very early feature, and may precede the onset, of Parkinson's disease. Recent studies have demonstrated that depression, above any other factor, is the most significant determinant of quality of life in the person with Parkinson's disease, yet it is generally underdiagnosed. The occurrence of dementia in Parkinson's disease is related to the age of onset of the illness, as well as the disease duration. The cognitive impairment may be accompanied by hallucinations (often visual), paranoid ideation and frank confusion.

Differential diagnosis

It is important to remember that, while Parkinson's disease is a common form of parkinsonism, there are numerous other degenerative and symptomatic causes. Furthermore, 'all that shakes is not Parkinson's disease'. Table 30.1 gives a differential diagnosis for causes of parkinsonism. These are separated into degenerative and symptomatic categories. The list is not exhaustive and excludes, for instance, rare parkinsonian manifestations in uncommon diseases. A detailed description of these different causes of parkinsonism is beyond the scope of this chapter, but a few points should be highlighted. Essential tremor is not included in Table 30.1, as this common condition does not cause bradykinesia. Nevertheless, it may be very difficult to differentiate from tremor-dominant Parkinson's disease. A positive family history and good response to alcohol may provide vital clues towards the diagnosis of essential tremor.

Several clinical and clinicopathological series have confirmed our fallibility in not making a correct diagnosis of Parkinson's disease. If clinical criteria, such as those produced by the UK Parkinson's Disease Brain Bank, are not applied, then the error rate (false-negative diagnosis) may be as high as 25–30% (Hughes et al 1992, Meara et al 1999). These criteria are listed in Table 30.2. Degenerative conditions commonly masquerading as Parkinson's disease are progressive supranuclear palsy, multiple system atrophy and Alzheimer's disease.

Perhaps the most important differential diagnosis to consider when a patient presents with parkinsonism is whether their symptoms and signs may be drug-induced. This is because drug-induced parkinsonism (DIP) is potentially reversible upon cessation of the offending agent. Reports linking DIP with the neuroleptic chlorpromazine were first published in the 1950s. Since then, numerous other agents have been associated with DIP. Many of these are widely recognized, although others are not (Table 30.3). Compound antidepressants may contain neuroleptic drugs (trifluoperazine in Motival, for example) and are not always recognized as

potential culprits. Repeat prescription of vestibular sedatives and antiemetics (particularly prochlorperazine and cinnarizine) is another commonly encountered cause of DIP. The pathogenesis of DIP is unlikely to be only due to dopamine receptor blockade. If this were the case the incidence and severity of DIP should correlate with the drug dosage and length of exposure, and this is not clearly observed.

DIP is more common in the elderly and in women. The clinical features of DIP can be indistinguishable from Parkinson's disease, although the signs in DIP are more likely to be bilateral at the onset. Withdrawal of the offending agent will lead to improvement and resolution of symptoms and signs in approximately 80% of patients within 8 weeks of discontinuation. DIP may, however, take up to 18 months to fully resolve in some cases. Furthermore, in other patients the parkinsonism may improve after stopping the drug, only to then deteriorate. In this situation, the drug may have unmasked previously latent Parkinson's disease. This contention is supported by the findings of one recent study, which noted an increased risk of Parkinson's disease in subjects who had experienced a previous reversible episode of DIP.

Investigations

The diagnosis of Parkinson's disease is a clinical one, and should be based, preferably, upon validated criteria. In young onset or clinically atypical Parkinson's disease, a number of investigations may be appropriate. These include copper studies and DNA testing to exclude Wilson's disease and Huntington's disease, respectively. Brain imaging by computed tomography (CT) or magnetic resonance imaging (MRI) may be appropriate to exclude hydrocephalus, cerebrovascular disease or

Table 30.1 The differential diagnosis of parkinsonism

Degenerative causes	Symptomatic causes
Parkinson's disease	Dopamine receptor blocking agents
Progressive supranuclear palsy (Steele–Richardson–Olszewski syndrome)	Cerebrovascular disease
	Hydrocephalus (especially so-called 'normal pressure' hydrocephalus)
Multiple system atrophy	Toxic (e.g. manganese, carbon monoxide, carbon disulphide, hydrocarbon, MPTP exposure)
Alzheimer's disease	
Corticobasal ganglionic degeneration	Post-encephalitic parkinsonism
	Wilson's disease
	Young-onset Huntington's disease (Westphal variant)
	Dementia pugilistica ('punch drunk' syndrome)

Table 30.2   Clinical criteria for the diagnosis of Parkinson's disease (from Hughes et al 1992)

Step 1 Diagnosis of parkinsonian syndrome

The patient has bradykinesia, plus one or more of the following:

a) classic rest tremor

b) muscular rigidity

c) postural instability, without other explanation

Step 2 Exclusion criteria for Parkinson's disease

a) history of repeated strokes	i) supranuclear gaze palsy
b) history of repeated head injury	j) cerebellar signs
c) history of definite encephalitis	k) early severe autonomic involvement
d) oculogyric crises	l) early severe dementia
e) dopamine receptor blocking agent exposure at onset of symptoms	m) extensor plantar
f) more than one affected relative	n) cerebral tumour or hydrocephalus on CT
g) sustained remission	o) negative response to large doses of levodopa
h) strictly unilateral features after 3 years	p) MPTP exposure

Step 3 Supportive prospective positive criteria for Parkinson's disease (three or more required for diagnosis of definite Parkinson's disease)

a) unilateral onset	e) an excellent (> 70%) response to levodopa
b) rest tremor present	f) a sustained (> 5 years) response to levodopa
c) progressive disorder	g) severe levodopa-induced dyskinesias
d) progressive persistent asymmetry	h) clinical course > 10 years

Table 30.3   Non-neuroleptic drugs associated with drug-induced parkinsonism

Tetrabenazine
Calcium-channel blockers (e.g. cinnarizine)
Amiodarone
Lithium[a]
Phenelzine[b]
Amphotericin B[c]
5-Fluorouracil[b]
Vincristine-Adriamycin[b]
Pethidine[b]

[a] Lithium causes postural tremor. Reports of parkinsonism occurring with lithium have usually been in the context of prior exposure to neuroleptics.
[b] Only single case reports of drug-induced parkinsonism with these drugs.
[c] One case report of drug-induced parkinsonism in a child after bone marrow transplantation and a second in association with cytosine arabinoside therapy.

basal ganglia abnormalities suggestive of an underlying metabolic cause.

The differentiation of Parkinson's disease from multiple system atrophy and progressive supranuclear palsy is a not uncommon clinical problem and may be very difficult, particularly in the early disease stages. Anal sphincter electromyography, tilt table testing for orthostatic hypotension and eye movement recordings may all be of some help, although they are rarely diagnostic in their own right.

Treatment

A general approach

When treatment becomes necessary, it is impossible to generalize about which drug should be commenced. All currently available drugs for Parkinson's disease are symptomatic, since no agent has yet been shown, beyond reasonable doubt, to have disease modifying or neuroprotective properties.

A number of factors, including age, severity and type of disease (tremor-dominant versus bradykinesia-dominant) and co-morbidity, need to be taken into account. In 1967 Cotzias and co-workers described the efficacy and tolerability of levodopa in Parkinson's disease patients, when the drug was started in low doses and gradually increased thereafter. Unfortunately, despite dramatic initial benefits, the limitations of levodopa treatment were quickly realized, and a phenomenon termed the 'long-term levodopa syndrome' was recognized in the USA. This syndrome comprises premature wearing-off of the antiparkinsonian effects of levodopa, and response fluctuations. The wearing-off effect is the time before a patient is due their next dose of medication, during which they become increasingly bradykinetic. Response fluctuations can include dramatic swings between gross involuntary movements (dyskinesias) and a frozen, immobile state. The rapid and sudden switching between the dyskinetic state and profound akinesia is also termed the 'on–off' phenomenon. These problems emerge at a rate of approximately 10% per year, so that by 10 years into their illness all Parkinson's disease patients can expect to be experiencing such unpredictable responses. Notably, however, levodopa-induced dyskinesias and fluctuations develop earlier in younger Parkinson's disease patients than in older patients. On–off episodes may be extremely disabling, and remain a major therapeutic challenge in the management of Parkinson's disease.

Current trends have therefore shifted towards either late administration of levodopa (provided that alternative treatments can give adequate symptomatic control) or the use of combination therapies, in an effort to reduce the longer-term problems associated with levodopa. The evidence that such strategies benefit the patient beyond 5 years into their disease course is weak, however, and this remains an area of debate (Montastruc et al 1999, Weiner 1999).

Drug treatment

Levodopa preparations

Immediate-release levodopa. Irrespective of the debate regarding early or late levodopa therapy, there is no doubt that levodopa remains the most effective oral symptomatic treatment for Parkinson's disease. It is administered with a peripheral dopa-decarboxylase inhibitor: carbidopa plus levodopa = co-careldopa (Sinemet) and benserazide plus levodopa = co-beneldopa (Madopar). The decarboxylase inhibitor blocks the peripheral conversion of levodopa to dopamine and thereby allows a lower dose of levodopa to be administered. Levodopa readily crosses the blood–brain barrier, where it is converted by endogenous aromatic amino acid decarboxylase to dopamine, and then stored in surviving nigrostriatal nerve terminals.

Immediate-release levodopa is usually commenced in a dose of 50 mg per day, increasing every 3–4 days until a dose of 50 mg three times daily is reached. The patient should be instructed in the early stage of the illness to take the drug with food to minimize nausea. Paradoxically, in more advanced Parkinson's disease it may be beneficial to take levodopa 30 minutes or so before food, since dietary protein can critically interfere with the absorption of the drug at this time.

If there is little or no response to 50 mg three times daily, the unit dose may be doubled to 100 mg. Should the patient's levodopa dose escalate to 600 mg per day with no significant response, the diagnosis of Parkinson's disease should be reviewed. Levodopa, commenced in the above way, is usually well tolerated. Nausea, vomiting and orthostatic hypotension are the most commonly encountered side-effects. These adverse events may be circumvented by increasing the levodopa dose even more slowly, or co-prescribing domperidone 10 or 20 mg three times daily. Later in the illness, and in common with all antiparkinsonian drugs, levodopa may cause vivid dreams, nightmares, or even a toxic confusional state.

Clinically relevant drug interactions with levodopa include hypertensive crises with monoamine-oxidase type A inhibitors. Levodopa should therefore be avoided for at least 2 weeks after stopping the inhibitor. Levodopa can also enhance the hypotensive effects of antihypertensive agents and may antagonize the action of antipsychotics. The absorption of levodopa may be reduced by concomitant administration of oral iron preparations.

Controlled-release levodopa. Both Sinemet and Madopar are available as controlled release (CR) preparations. The nomenclature for Sinemet CR is confusing, as the drug is marketed as Sinemet CR (carbidopa/levodopa 50/200) and also as Half Sinemet CR (carbidopa/levodopa 25/100). Trying to prescribe Half Sinemet CR unambiguously can be difficult. If the instruction is misinterpreted and a tablet of Sinemet CR is halved, the slow-release mechanism is disrupted.

Levodopa in CR preparations has a bioavailability of 60–70%, which is less than the 90–100% obtained from immediate release formulations. CR preparations have response duration of 2–4 hours, compared with 1–3 hours for immediate release.

Two large studies in early Parkinson's disease over 5 years have not shown any benefit for CR use over immediate release levodopa in terms of dyskinesias and response fluctuation frequency (Dupont et al 1996, Block et al 1997). However, CR preparations may be of help in simplifying drug regimens, in relieving nocturnal akinesia, and in co-prescribing with immediate release levodopa during the day to relieve end-of-dose deterioration.

Two commonly encountered problems with CR preparations are, first, changing the patient from all immediate release to all CR levodopa. This is poorly tolerated, as CR levodopa has a longer latency than immediate release levodopa to turn the patient 'on' (typically 60–90 versus 30–50 minutes), and the patient's perception is that the quality of their 'on' period is poorer. Second, CR preparations should not be prescribed more than four times a day, as the levodopa may accumulate, causing unpredictable motor fluctuations.

Dopamine agonists

In theory, dopamine agonists, which stimulate dopamine receptors both post- and presynaptically, would seem to be a very attractive therapeutic option in Parkinson's disease, since they may bypass the degenerating nigrostriatal dopaminergic neurones. Unfortunately, experience to date with the oral agents available has usually shown them to be less potent than levodopa and less well tolerated. One drug in this class, apomorphine, is available in a parenteral form. It is particularly potent, and is described in detail below (page 490).

Dopamine agonists differ in their affinity for a number of receptors, including the dopamine receptor family. It is not known whether these differences are clinically significant. Cabergoline is a relatively new ergot dopamine agonist with a much longer plasma half-life than other agents in this class of 63–68 hours. This means that once daily dosing is possible. Prolonged and non-pulsatile stimulation of dopamine receptors may, theoretically, be less likely to cause dyskinesias. Ropinirole and pramipexole are non-ergot derivatives.

Four double-blind, randomized and controlled studies of up to 5 years' duration have compared the use of a dopamine agonist (cabergoline, ropinirole, pramipexole and pergolide) with levodopa in the treatment of early Parkinson's disease (Rinne et al 1999, Rascol et al 2000, Parkinson's Study Group 2000, Oertel 2000). Although the studies differed in a number of ways (for instance, levodopa supplementation was not permitted in the pergolide study), the results provide a consistent message, that the use of dopamine agonists in early Parkinson's disease is associated with a lower incidence of dyskinesias when compared with levodopa. Supplementary levodopa was, however, required in a significant number of patients in the cabergoline (65% of patients initially randomized to cabergoline), ropinirole (66% of patients initially randomized to ropinirole) and pramipexole (53% of patients initially randomized to pramipexole) studies, suggesting that only a subgroup of patients derive adequate benefit from agonist monotherapy alone. Further clinical follow-up will hopefully address the issue of what happens to patients receiving agonist monotherapy when they finally require levodopa. Notably, will the dyskinesia rate rapidly increase and catch up with other patients previously exposed to levodopa, or will it remain at a lower frequency?

All the agonists may be used as add-on therapy to levodopa in the later stages of the disease, when motor control has become suboptimal. This may necessitate a concomitant reduction in levodopa dosage to avoid excessive dopaminergic side-effects.

There have been very few comparative studies performed between the dopamine agonists, so it is not possible to be definitive as to which drug should be recommended. In practice, it is often worth changing from one agonist to another if side-effects are a problem, since there is variability in a given patient's tolerance to the different drugs.

The principal side-effects of the dopamine agonists are nausea and vomiting, postural hypotension, hallucinations and confusion, and exacerbation of dyskinesias. Ergot derivatives run the risk of causing pleuropulmonary fibrosis. This occurs in 2–6% of patients on long-term bromocriptine treatment. Annual monitoring with chest X-ray and erythrocyte sedimentation rate (ESR) has been suggested for patients taking ergot derivative agonists, although the utility and cost-effectiveness of this recommendation have not been established. There is also an increased risk of toxicity when erythromycin is co-prescribed with an agonist.

Both ropinirole and pramipexole have recently been implicated in causing 'sleep attacks', with sudden onset of drowsiness, leading to driving accidents in some cases. The term 'sleep attack' is almost certainly a misnomer, however, as patients do have warning of impending sleepiness, although they may subsequently be amnesic for up to several minutes while in this state. Excessive sleepiness attributable to antiparkinsonian drugs is not a new phenomenon, and has previously been reported with levodopa. It is essential to advise patients taking all antiparkinsonian agents, and especially ropinirole and pramipexole, that they may be prone to excessive drowsiness. This may be compounded by the use of other sedative drugs and alcohol.

Catechol-O-methyl transferase inhibitors

Inhibitors of the enzyme catechol-O-methyl transferase (COMT) represent a recent and novel addition to the range of therapies available for Parkinson's disease. Unfortunately, use of the first agent in this class, tolcapone, was suspended in the EU because of fears over hepatotoxicity. Entacapone is still available and studies have not shown derangement of liver function with this drug.

COMT itself is a ubiquitous enzyme, found in gut, liver, kidney and brain among other sites. In theory, COMT inhibition may occur both centrally (where the degradation of dopamine to homovanillic acid is inhibited) and peripherally (where conversion of levodopa to the inert 3-*O*-methyldopa is inhibited) to benefit the patient with Parkinson's disease. In practice, both tolcapone and entacapone act primarily as peripheral COMT inhibitors.

Three large and one small double-blind, placebo controlled studies in fluctuating Parkinson's disease have confirmed efficacy for entacapone in decreasing 'off' time, and permitting a concomitant reduction in levodopa dose (Ruottinen & Rinne 1996, Parkinson's Study Group 1997, Rinne et al 1998, Sagar et al 2000). A 20% reduction in 'off' time is reported, translating into nearly 1.5 hours less immobility per day. This reduction tends to occur towards the end of the day, a time when many Parkinson's disease patients are at their worst in terms of motor function.

When entacapone is prescribed, a 200 mg dose is used with each dose of levodopa administered, up to a frequency of 10 doses per day. Because of increased dyskinesias, an overall reduction of 10–30% in the daily dose of levodopa may be anticipated. Entacapone can be employed with any other antiparkinsonian drug (although caution may be needed with apomorphine).

The optimal way to use entacapone is unknown. A patient experiencing end-of-dose deterioration, or generally underdosed, would seem to be the ideal candidate. However, there are no comparative studies of entacapone versus dopamine agonists available to provide guidance as to which class of drug is best to use, and when. Trials are underway to assess the potential benefits of combined treatment with levodopa and COMT inhibitors in de novo Parkinson's disease patients. These studies will address whether this combined treatment is associated with a lower incidence of motor complications.

Other than exacerbation of dyskinesias, COMT inhibitors may also cause diarrhoea (the mechanism for this is unknown), abdominal pain, and a dryness of the mouth. Urine discolouration is reported in approximately 8% of patients.

It is best to avoid non-selective monoamine-oxidase inhibitors or a daily dose of selegiline in excess of 10 mg when using entacapone. In addition, the co-prescription of venlafaxine and other noradrenaline (norepinephrine) re-uptake inhibitors is best avoided. Entacapone may potentiate the action of apomorphine. Patients taking iron preparations should be advised to separate this medication and entacapone by at least 2 hours.

Selegiline

Selegiline is a selective, irreversible inhibitor of monoamine-oxidase type B. Inhibition of this enzyme slows the breakdown of dopamine in the striatum. Selegiline may also have an anti-apoptotic effect (apoptosis is a form of programmed cell death thought to be important in several neurodegenerative conditions including Parkinson's disease). Whether or not the drug has a neuroprotective effect by this or some other means remains controversial.

A single daily dose of 5 mg or 10 mg of selegiline is prescribed. Higher doses are associated with only minimal additional inhibition of monoamine-oxidase. Following the publication of the UK Parkinson's Disease Research Group study in 1995, where excess mortality in a group of patients taking selegiline was demonstrated, prescription of the drug in the UK (but not in the USA) dropped by nearly 50%. This study drew much criticism, both in its design and also in the analysis of the data. Nevertheless, a subsequent observational study from the UK General Practice Research Database also suggested a small excess mortality in patients taking selegiline.

The reason for the possible excess mortality is uncertain. It has, however, been suggested that the drug may be best avoided in patients with falls, confusion and postural hypotension. The use of selegiline in younger patients with early Parkinson's disease, as a means of deferring levodopa treatment, still has its advocates. Selegiline can cause hallucinations and confusion, particularly in moderate to advanced disease. The withdrawal of selegiline may then be associated with significant deterioration in motor function. Selegiline should probably not be co-prescribed with selective serotonin re-uptake inhibitors, since a serotonin syndrome, including hypertension and neuropsychiatric features, has been reported in a small minority of cases.

Amantadine

Amantadine was introduced as an antiparkinsonian treatment in the late 1960s. It has a number of possible modes of action, including facilitation of presynaptic dopamine release, blocking dopamine re-uptake, an anticholinergic effect, and also as a *N*-methyl-D-aspartate (NMDA) receptor antagonist. Initially employed in the early stages of treatment, where its effects are mild and relatively short-lived, interest has focused more recently upon the use of amantadine as an antidyskinetic agent in advanced disease (Verhagen-Metman et al 1999).

Daily doses of 100–300 mg amantadine may be used (some recommend even higher doses for improved antidyskinetic effect) although side-effects become much more frequent at higher doses. These include a toxic confusional state, peripheral oedema and livedo reticularis (a persistent patchy reddish-blue mottling of the legs, and occasionally the arms). There may be significant 'rebound' worsening of parkinsonism when amantadine is withdrawn. The mechanism for this is unknown.

Anticholinergic drugs

The availability of anticholinergic drugs such as trihexyphenidyl (benzhexol) and orphenadrine predated the introduction of levodopa by nearly 90 years. Anticholinergic drugs have a moderate effect in reducing tremor but do not have any significant benefit upon bradykinesia.

The use of these agents has fallen because of troublesome side-effects, including constipation, urinary retention, cognitive impairment and toxic confusional states. In selected younger patients an anticholinergic drug may still be helpful, but close monitoring is advised.

Tricyclic antidepressants have anticholinergic properties, normally regarded as a disadvantage in the treatment of depression. These drugs are generally longer acting than other anticholinergic agents and may have a potential benefit in Parkinson's disease, both for their anticholinergic effects and also their effect in inhibiting monoamine re-uptake at adrenergic nerve endings. A low dose of a tricyclic antidepressant (e.g. amitriptyline 10–25 mg) at night is sometimes useful in alleviating nocturnal akinesia, improving sleep, and improving performance early in the morning.

Apomorphine

Apomorphine is a specialized, but almost certainly underused, drug in the treatment of Parkinson's disease (Poewe & Wenning 2000). It is the most potent dopamine agonist available, and is administered either by bolus subcutaneous injection or by continuous subcutaneous infusion. The drug is acidic, and is generally difficult to administer in a stable form which does not lead to irritation of skin or mucosal surfaces. Alternative methods of administration, including transdermal and intranasal routes, are being evaluated.

The drug produces a reliable 'on' effect with short latency of action. A single bolus lasts for up to 60 minutes, depending upon the dose given. Continuous subcutaneous apomorphine may significantly improve dyskinesias in advanced Parkinson's disease, as well as lessening akinesia and rigidity (Colzi et al 1998). This may allow oral antiparkinsonian medications to be reduced.

Apomorphine causes profound nausea, vomiting and orthostatic hypotension. These problems are counteracted by pre-dosing for 2–3 days with 20 mg three times daily domperidone. Neuropsychiatric disturbance (probably at a lower frequency than with oral agonists) and skin reactions (including nodule formation), are other potential side-effects. Apomorphine, in conjunction with levodopa, may cause a Coomb's positive haemolytic anaemia, which is reversible. It is recommended that patients be screened before beginning treatment and at 6-monthly intervals thereafter. Establishing a patient on apomorphine is greatly helped by the supervision of a nurse specialist, if available.

Surgery

There has been renewed interest in the use of neurosurgical techniques for the treatment of Parkinson's disease. This has resulted not only from recognition of the shortcomings of medical treatment currently available, but also from an improved understanding of basal ganglia circuitry and better neuroimaging methods. A detailed consideration of this topic is beyond the scope of this chapter (see Further reading section). Table 30.4 summarizes techniques currently being employed and evaluated. The functional effects of lesioning (-otomy), and the use of deep brain stimulation, are similar, in that the high frequency used in stimulation is believed to act by 'blocking' neurones. Deep brain stimulation has the advantage of being reversible, but is costly, and programming of the stimulator may be very time-consuming.

Table 30.4   A summary of anatomical targets for the treatment of Parkinson's disease

Target	Bradykinesia	Tremor	Dyskinesia	Comments
Thalamus	–	+++	–	Bilateral thalamotomy is not recommended because of a high incidence of bulbar dysfunction
Globus pallidus	++	++	+++	10–15% incidence of persistent adverse events with unilateral pallidotomy; no reliable data of bilateral procedures
Subthalamic nucleus	+++	+++	++	Weight gain, contralateral dyskinesia, involuntary eyelid closure and speech disturbance reported

+ to +++ refers to the relative efficacy of the procedure for the clinical feature; – refers no benefit for the procedure for the clinical feature.
For each of the three targets listed, both ablation and stimulation procedures have been evaluated.

The subthalamic nucleus target appears to hold great promise, but the number of published patient-years experience with this surgical approach is very limited. A forthcoming multicentre UK study of surgery targeted to this structure versus optimal medical therapy should clarify the potential benefits to be gained from a subthalamic target.

Surgery may also play a role in so-called neurorestorative treatments. Such approaches include stem cell and fetal cell transplantation, and also xenotransplantation (use of tissue from another species, for example the pig). To date, there have been conflicting results regarding the efficacy of fetal cell transplants. These differences may well reflect transplantation technique, the nature of the tissue being implanted, whether immunosuppression is prescribed, and how patients are selected and assessed. Despite the seemingly negative results from a recent double-blind US study of embryonic cell implantation (Freed et al 2001), other groups will be reporting their findings in the near future. This should, hopefully, provide clarification of these complex medical and ethical issues.

Patient care

After diagnosis, the provision of an explanation of the condition, education and support are essential. If available, a Parkinson's disease nurse specialist is invaluable at this early stage. The Parkinson's Disease Society produces an excellent range of literature to help the newly diagnosed patient come to terms with the condition. In accordance with advice given by the society itself, patients who drive are advised to inform their insurance company and also the Driver and Vehicle Licensing Agency.

A doctor will record impairments in the clinic, while the patient is more concerned with their disability and handicap. Thus, a patient can be noted to have seemingly marked impairments and yet may not complain about significant disability. The converse may also be true. Not all patients, therefore, require immediate treatment.

Furthermore, concomitant depression may distort the patient's perception of their disability, leading to inappropriate prescribing of antiparkinsonian therapy. In this situation, the use of an antidepressant may be more helpful. There is no good evidence base for which antidepressant should be used, and both the tricyclic agents and selective serotonin re-uptake inhibitors have their advocates.

Accurate compliance with the timing of therapy may be particularly important in patients who are beginning to develop long-term treatment complications. It can be helpful for patients to keep diary cards when they begin to experience problems with either bradykinesia or dyskinesia, so that these symptoms can be related to drug and food intake. Careful changes in timing of drug therapy or meals may initially be sufficient to reduce variation in performance. Some patients experience troublesome early morning bradykinesia. It may then be beneficial to prescribe an initial dose of a rapidly acting agent, such as dispersible oral co-beneldopa, to take on first wakening so that the patient can then get up and dress. A combination of levodopa with dopamine agonists, which are more slow acting, may be useful in the patient with motor fluctuations. A combination of levodopa and a COMT inhibitor may be more appropriate in a patient with end-of-dose deterioration (or 'wearing-off' effects).

Other factors that need to be considered in patients with Parkinson's disease are the benefits of adequate sleep and rest at night, which may be made more difficult if they have urinary frequency or problems with nocturnal bradykinesia. Judicious use of hypnotic therapy may be appropriate, while a tricyclic antidepressant may offer the dual benefit of sedation with anticholinergic effect. Low friction sheets to assist turning and encouragement of mobility through physiotherapy may also be helpful. The treatment of the patient with severe disease remains one of the greatest challenges in the management of Parkinson's disease. On–off fluctuations may be refractory to oral dopaminergic therapies. Sudden freezing episodes compound failing postural stability, leading to increasing falls and injuries. In select patients, the use of apomorphine, either as a bolus injection or as a continuous subcutaneous infusion, may be very helpful in this situation. When cognitive impairment is problematic the use of conventional antipsychotic medication is inappropriate because such drugs can precipitate a catastrophic worsening of parkinsonism. Behavioural disturbances require discussion with carers and, if possible, with the patient him- or herself. A graded withdrawal of antiparkinsonian drugs is often indicated, aiming to simplify the regimen to levodopa monotherapy. In rare cases it may be necessary to reduce the dose, or even completely withdraw levodopa therapy in order to control aggressive, sexually demanding or psychotic features.

The role of cholinesterase inhibitors in the treatment of the neuropsychiatric features of Parkinson's disease is currently being evaluated. Such drugs offer the prospect of improving psychotic features and attentional problems without immobilizing the patient.

Patients' relatives also need emotional and social support through what can be a very demanding period. The loss of physical mobility, together with a personality change, can be very difficult for relatives to cope with. The involvement of occupational therapists and social workers in this situation is important.

Other coexisting medical complications that may need attention include disorders of gut motility, which present as constipation or difficulty with swallowing, disturbances of micturition, sometimes presenting as nocturia, and postural hypotension.

Constipation can be managed in the usual way with bulking agents, and, if necessary, stimulant laxatives and stool-softening agents.

The management of postural hypotension includes assessment of the patient's autonomic function in order to establish whether this is primarily drug related or associated with autonomic neuropathy. If the patient is dizzy on standing, simple measures such as advice on rising slowly may be adequate. The use of elastic stockings, to reduce pooling of the blood in the lower limbs, is sometimes helpful. Pharmacological approaches include the use of fludrocortisone or occasionally midodrine (a selective α_1 adrenergic agonist). It is also important to consider what other therapies the patient is receiving that might contribute to such symptoms (e.g. diuretics), and to stop these if possible.

The presence of reduced dexterity in virtually all people with Parkinson's disease means that thought needs to be given to the way in which medication is dispensed and stored. If the patient is taking a complex regimen of drugs, or has early cognitive problems, the use of pre-packaged therapies may improve compliance.

Table 30.5 lists some common therapeutic problems encountered in the management of people with Parkinson's disease.

CASE STUDIES

Case 30.1

A 70-year-old man, Mr X., was diagnosed as having mild Parkinson's disease 6 months ago. This did not require any treatment. He returns with his wife stating that he is 'terrible' and cannot do what he wants to do. Examination continues to confirm only mild motor impairment.

Questions

1. What additional problem would one consider in this gentleman's case?
2. What therapeutic strategy (if any) would you consider?

Answers

1. Given the disparity between Mr. X.'s reported disability and the observed impairment, coexisting depression must be a possibility. This is a major, and often unrecognized, determinant of quality of life in Parkinson's disease. Talking to his wife might clarify the issue, supported by the administration to the patient of a validated depression questionnaire (e.g. the hospital anxiety and depression scale or 15 item geriatric depression scale).
2. A simple explanation and/or referral to a Parkinson's disease nurse specialist may suffice. Alternatively, it might be necessary to prescribe an antidepressant. A selective serotonin re-uptake inhibitor (e.g. paroxetine 20 mg daily) would be a reasonable choice for Mr X.

Table 30.5   Common therapeutic problems in Parkinson's disease

Problem	Cause	Possible solution
Early-onset dyskinesias in young Parkinson's disease patients	Exposure to levodopa? Biological factors?	Delay introduction of levodopa (e.g. use a dopamine agonist)
One dose of levodopa does not last to the next ('wearing off')	Advancing disease (pre- and post-synaptic changes)	More frequent doses of levodopa; COMT inhibitor or dopamine agonist
Pain and immobility during the night	Evening dose of levodopa not lasting long enough	Use of slow-release levodopa or dopamine agonist
Freezing episodes and/or unpredictable motor fluctuations	Advancing disease (pre- and post-synaptic changes)	Apomorphine (Surgery?)
Mismatch between patient's symptoms and signs	Underlying depression?	Antidepressant
Confusion and hallucinations with preserved cognition	Toxic (drug-related) psychosis	Review and reduce antiparkinsonian therapy
Confusion and hallucinations with impaired cognition	Underlying brain pathology ± drug effects	Reduce and simplify antiparkinsonian drugs as far as possible. Support team. (Cholinesterase inhibitor?)

Case 30.2

A 53-year-old lady, Mrs Y., is referred by her GP because of suspected Parkinson's disease. This is bilateral and tremor-dominant. She has a long history of dyspepsia and reflux. Her father may have had Parkinson's disease, and she is worried that she has the same disease.

Questions

1. Which question might give additional diagnostic help in this lady's social history?
2. What features should one look for in the drug history?

Answers

1. A history of tremor that is alcohol-responsive, coupled with a possible positive family history, should always raise the possibility of essential tremor as the correct diagnosis, rather than Parkinson's disease. In fact, Mrs Y.'s tremor was not alcohol-responsive, and she had bradykinesia on neurological examination.
2. Given this patient's history of reflux and dyspepsia, the use of dopamine receptor blocking agents, such as metoclopramide, might be relevant. Mrs Y. had been taking this drug for nearly 12 months. Drug-induced parkinsonism was therefore suspected, and when reviewed 3 months after stopping the metoclopramide, her symptoms and signs had resolved.

Case 30.3

Mr Z. has a 6-year history of Parkinson's disease. He is 75 years old. His motor symptoms are well controlled on a combination of one tablet of co-careldopa (25/100), three times a day and selegiline 10 mg daily. His wife comes to clinic with him and reports that he has recently been confused at night. Furthermore, he has been hallucinating, seeing gnomes at the bottom of the garden. She is very frightened.

Question

What should be done?

Answer

The problem here is to what extent the features of Mr Z.'s psychosis relate to his drugs, or to the underlying disease process. Dementia associated with Parkinson's disease is more common in the older patient with longstanding disease.

A mini-mental state examination to assess cognitive function in more detail would be appropriate. Intercurrent infection should also be excluded.

Selegiline is best avoided in cases like this and should be discontinued. This may lead to an improvement in Mr Z.'s psychotic features, without any other action being necessary. The use of an antipsychotic agent in Mr Z. is absolutely contraindicated, as it will only serve to worsen his Parkinson's disease.

REFERENCES

Block G, Liss C, Reines S et al 1997 Comparison of immediate-release and controlled-release carbidopa/levodopa in Parkinson's disease. European Neurology 37: 23–27

Colzi A, Turner K, Lees A J 1998 Continuous subcutaneous waking day apomorphine in the long term treatment of levodopa induced interdose dyskinesia in Parkinson's disease. Journal of Neurology, Neurosurgery and Psychiatry 64: 573–576

Dupont E, Andersen A, Boas J et al 1996 Sustained-release Madopar HBS compared with standard Madopar in the long-term treatment of de novo parkinsonian patients. Acta Neurologica Scandinavica 93: 14–20

Freed C R, Greene P E, Breeze R E et al 2001 Transplantation of embryonic dopamine neurons for severe Parkinson's disease. New England Journal of Medicine 344: 710–719

Hughes A J, Daniel S E, Kilford L et al 1992 Accuracy of clinical diagnosis of idiopathic Parkinson's disease: a clinico-pathological study of 100 cases. Journal of Neurology, Neurosurgery and Psychiatry 55: 181–184

Meara J, Bhowmick B K, Hobson P 1999 Accuracy of diagnosis in patients with presumed Parkinson's disease. Age and Ageing 28: 99–102

Montastruc J L, Rascol O, Senard J M 1999 Treatment of Parkinson's disease should begin with a dopamine agonist. Movement Disorders 14: 725–730

Oertel W H 2000 Pergolide vs levodopa (PELMOPET). Movement Disorders 15: 4

Parkinson's Study Group 1997 Entacapone improves motor fluctuations in levodopa-treated Parkinson's disease patients. Annals of Neurology 42: 747–755

Parkinson's Study Group 2000 Pramipexole vs levodopa as initial treatment for Parkinson's disease. Journal of the American Medical Association 284: 1931–1938

Poewe W, Wenning G K 2000 Apomorphine: an underutilized therapy for Parkinson's disease. Movement Disorders 15: 789–794

Rascol O, Brooks D J, Korczyn A D et al 2000 A five-year study of the incidence of dyskinesias in patients with early Parkinson's disease who were treated with ropinirole or levodopa. New England Journal of Medicine 342: 1484–1491

Rinne U K, Larsen J P, Siden A et al 1998 Entacapone enhances the response to levodopa in parkinsonian patients with motor fluctuations. Neurology 51: 1309–1314

Rinne U K, Bracco F, Chouza C et al 1999 Early treatment of Parkinson's disease with cabergoline delays the onset of motor complications: results of a double-blind levodopa controlled trial. European Journal of Neurology 6(Suppl. 5): S17–S23

Ruottinen H M, Rinne U K 1996 Entacapone prolongs levodopa response in a one month double blind study in parkinsonian patients with levodopa related fluctuations. Journal of Neurology, Neurosurgery and Psychiatry 60: 36–40

Sagar H, Brooks D J, UK-Irish Entacapone Study Group 2000 The UK-Irish double-blind study of entacapone in Parkinson's disease. Movement Disorders 15: 135

Verhagen-Metman L, Del Dotto P, LePoole K et al 1999 Amantadine for levodopa-induced dyskinesias. Archives of Neurology 56: 1383–1386

Weiner W J 1999 The initial treatment of Parkinson's disease should begin with levodopa. Movement Disorders 14: 716–724

FURTHER READING

Allain H, Schuck S, Mauduit N 2000 Depression in Parkinson's disease. British Medical Journal 320: 1287–1288

Bhatia K, Brooks D J, Burn D J et al 1998 Guidelines for the management of Parkinson's disease. Hospital Medicine 59: 469–480

Friedman J H, Factor S A 2000 Atypical antipsychotics in the treatment of drug-induced psychosis in Parkinson's disease. Movement Disorders 15: 201–211

Lang A E, Lozano A M 1998 Parkinson's disease: II. New England Journal of Medicine 339: 1130–1143

Krack P, Hamel W, Mehdorn H M et al 1999 Surgical treatment of Parkinson's disease. Current Opinion in Neurology 12: 417–425

Quinn N P 1997 Parkinson's disease: clinical features. In: Quinn N P (ed) Parkinsonism. London: Baillière Tindall, vol. 6:1, pp. 1–13

Thomas S, MacMahon D, Henry S, on behalf of the Parkinson's Disease Society UK. Primary Care Task Force 1999 Moving and shaping – the future: commissioning services for people with Parkinson's disease. Parkinson's Disease Society, London

Pain 31

S. Woolfrey   D. Kapur

KEY POINTS

- Pain is multifactorial.
- Single modality treatment may not be appropriate for pain.
- The World Health Organization (WHO) analgesic ladder forms the basis of the use of analgesic drugs, although the step of weak opioids may sometimes be omitted and strong opioids used earlier.
- The pain arising from malignancy may change. The prescribed drug should be appropriate for the type or intensity of the pain and should be reviewed regularly.
- Many pains do not respond to opioids, particularly that arising from nerve damage or psychogenic pain. Adjuvant drugs should be considered.
- Patients taking long-acting opioids should have 'escape' doses of fast-acting opioid for breakthrough and incident pain.
- Patients taking opioids should initially be co-prescribed antiemetics and during chronic use, laxatives.

The International Association for the Study of Pain has defined pain as 'an unpleasant sensory and emotional experience associated with actual or potential tissue damage, or described in terms of such damage'.

Acute pain may be viewed as a symptom of a disease process and has a biological function by allowing the patient to avoid or minimize injury. Chronic pain, on the other hand, may be described more as a disease than a symptom.

Aetiology and neurophysiology

Neuroanatomy of pain transmission

The majority of tissues and organs are innervated by special sensory receptors (nociceptors) connected to primary afferent nerve fibres of different diameters. Small myelinated, Aδ fibres and unmyelinated C fibres are believed to be responsible for the transmission of painful stimuli. These afferent primary fibres terminate in the dorsal horn of the spinal grey matter.

Pain transmission onward is far more complex and understood less well. The most important parts of this process are the wide dynamic range cells that project to the thalamus and beyond in the spinothalamic tract. Modulation or inhibition also occurs at the level of the spinal cord. This process can be activated by stress or certain analgesic drugs such as morphine. When the pain modulation system is active, noxious stimuli produce less activity in the pain transmission pathway. The description of this process is the most significant contribution of the gate theory of pain. Conversely, certain factors can lead to an increased sensitivity to noxious stimuli. The most important of these is pain itself and it is clear that painful stimuli can lead to further pain from relatively trivial insults. This occurs through neurochemical and even anatomical changes within the central nervous system that have been termed 'central sensitization'.

Neurotransmitters and pain

Various neurotransmitters found in the dorsal horn of the spinal cord may be involved in pain modulation. These include amino acids such as glutamate and γ-aminobutyric acid (GABA), monoamines such as noradrenaline (norepinephrine) and 5-hydroxytryptamine (5-HT) and certain peptide molecules, of which the opioid peptides are the most important. Opioid receptors are found in both the central nervous system (CNS) and the periphery; in the CNS they are found in high concentrations in the limbic system, the brainstem and the spinal cord. The natural ligands (molecules that bind to the receptor) for opioid receptors are a group of neuropeptides known as endorphins. Opioid analgesics mimic the actions of these natural ligands and exert their effect through the μ, δ and, to a lesser extent, the κ receptors. These receptors mediate the analgesic effect of morphine-like drugs.

Assessment of pain

Evaluation of pain should include a careful description of the pain and an assessment of its consequences. There should be a full history, psychosocial assessment, medication history and assessment of previous pain problems, paying attention to factors that influence the pain. Where necessary, diagnostic tests should be organized. These may include radiography, various imaging techniques, and diagnostic and prognostic nerve blocks.

Pain is a subjective phenomenon, and quantitative assessment is difficult. The most commonly used instruments are visual analogue and verbal rating scales. Visual analogue scales are lines 10 cm long with the extremes at each end labelled usually 'no pain at all' and 'worst pain imaginable' respectively. The patient is required to mark the severity of the pain between the two extremes of the scale. Verbal rating scales use adjectival descriptors such as 'none', 'mild', 'moderate' and 'excruciating'. More elaborate questionnaires such as the McGill pain questionnaire help to describe other aspects of the pain, and pain diaries record the influence of activity and medication on pain.

Management

Acute pain results from noxious stimulation, such as injury. It can be managed by analgesic drugs and is often self-limiting.

Chronic pain can be defined as pain which has lasted for 6 months or more. Treatment must be comprehensive, and may involve pain clinics, hospices and a multidisciplinary approach that manages medical and behavioural aspects. Initial treatment should be directed at the underlying disease process with surgery or antitumour therapy. Pain can be modulated by means other than drugs, for example stimulation-produced analgesia such as transcutaneous electrical nerve stimulation (TENS), acupuncture and massage, or invasive procedures such as neurosurgery or neurolytic nerve blocks. Non-medical treatment, for example physical therapy and various psychological techniques such as cognitive techniques, relaxation training or hypnosis, may also form part of a management programme.

The analgesic ladder

The analgesic ladder forms the basis of many approaches to the use of analgesic drugs. There are essentially three steps: non-opioid analgesics, weak opioids and strong opioids. The analgesic efficacy of non-opioids such as non-steroidal anti-inflammatory drugs (NSAIDs), aspirin and paracetamol is limited by side-effects and ceiling effects (i.e. beyond a certain dose, no further pharmacological effect is seen). Beyond the non-opioids, there are a number of drugs in the mild opioid group such as codeine and dextropropoxyphene which are of some value clinically. There may be some virtue in combining a mild opioid with a non-opioid drug although many commercial preparations contain inadequate quantities of both components and are no more effective than a non-opioid alone. Strong opioids, of which morphine is the standard, have no ceiling effect, and therefore increased dosage gives increased analgesia. The relative potencies of the major opioids are summarized in Table 31.1.

Adjuvant medication

In some types of pain such as the pain of cancer or nerve pain, the addition of non-analgesic drugs to analgesic therapy can enhance pain relief. A list of such adjuvant drugs is given in Table 31.2. It should be remembered that some drugs, for example tricyclic antidepressants, have intrinsic analgesic activity, perhaps related to their ability to affect 5-HT and noradrenergic neuro-transmission.

Special techniques

Patient-controlled analgesia (PCA)

Patient-controlled analgesia (PCA) is a system in which the patient titrates the dose of opioid to suit individual analgesic requirements. The drug is contained in a system (usually a syringe attached to either an electronic or non-electronic pump) that delivers a pre-set dose when activated by the patient depressing a button. A lock-out period, during which the machine is programmed not to respond, ensures that a second dose is not delivered before the previous one has had an effect. Some devices allow an additional background infusion of drug to be delivered continuously. A maximum dose facility ensures that the machine does not deliver more than a pre-set dose over a given time.

Table 31.1 Relative potencies of opioid drugs	
Drug	Potency (morphine = 1)
Codeine	0.1
Dihydrocodeine	0.1
Tramadol	0.2
Pethidine	0.1
Morphine	1
Diamorphine	2.5
Hydromorphone	7
Methadone	2–10 (with repeat dosing)
Fentanyl (transdermal)	150

Table 31.2 Adjuvant drugs used in the treatment of pain

Drug class	Type of pain	Example
Anticonvulsants	Neuropathic pain Migraine Cluster headache	Carbamazepine Sodium valproate Gabapentin Lamotrigine
Antidepressants	Neuropathic pain Musculoskeletal pain	Amitryptyline Imipramine Venlafaxine
i.v. anaesthetic agents	Neuropathic pain Burn pain Cancer pain	Ketamine
Skeletal muscle relaxants	Muscle spasm Spasticity	Baclofen Dantrolene Botulinum toxin (type A)
Steroids	Raised intracranial pressure Nerve compression	Dexamethasone Prednisolone
Antibiotics	Infection	As indicated by culture and sensitivity
Antispasmodics	Colic Smooth muscle spasm	Hyoscine butylbromide Loperamide
Hormones/hormonal analogues	Malignant bone pain Spinal stenosis Intestinal obstruction	Calcitonin (salmon) (salcatonin) Octreotide
Bisphosphonates	Bone pain (secondary to either malignancy or osteoporosis).	Disodium pamidronate (i.v. in malignancy) Alendronic acid

PCA is a useful technique for the management of pain after surgery. The system is convenient and enjoys a high degree of patient acceptability. The traditional intermittent intramuscular injection of opioids can be effective but is less versatile than titrated intravenous administration. The subcutaneous route is subject to most of the problems associated with intramuscular administration, but may be useful for pain relief in children as it avoids multiple injections if a short catheter is left in place. Opioid use via any route is associated with nausea and antiemetics should be prescribed routinely. Administration of compound preparations containing both opioids and antiemetics is not recommended as few preparations contain drugs with similar pharmacokinetic profiles and accumulation (usually of the antiemetic) may occur.

Neural blockade

Local anaesthetic drugs injected close to a sensory nerve or plexus will block the conduction of pain impulses and provide excellent analgesia. Agents in common use are lidocaine (lignocaine), prilocaine and bupivacaine. Some are given with adrenaline (epinephrine) to reduce systemic toxicity and increase the duration of action.

Local anaesthetics can be applied directly to wounds or by local infiltration to produce postoperative analgesia, but will not normally block pain arising from deep internal organs. Local anaesthetic techniques are particularly useful in day-stay surgery and in children. Continuous infusions via a catheter will permit prolonged analgesia. More permanent nerve blockade for the control of cancer pain is best achieved by using a neurolytic agent such as absolute alcohol or phenol.

Epidural analgesia

Epidural injections may be effective in relieving pain arising from non-malignant and malignant disease. They are very effective in postoperative and labour pain. Various combinations of local anaesthetics, opioids or steroids can be introduced into the epidural space near to the level of the pain.

Epidural local anaesthetics

Long-acting local anaesthetic drugs such as bupivacaine are most effective in relieving pain after major surgery. They work by blocking nerves in the spinal canal serving both superficial and deep tissues, and thus analgesia can be obtained in deep internal organs. Sensory nerves will be blocked and also sympathetic nerves that maintain smooth muscle tone in blood vessels. As a result, vasodilatation can occur, which may result in significant hypotension. Epidural catheters allow continuous infusions and long-term therapy by this route. Adverse effects may include muscle weakness in the area supplied by the nerve and, rarely, infection and haematomas.

Epidural opioids

Effective analgesia can be obtained by adding small doses of opioids to the epidural space, because there are opioid receptors in the spinal cord. They can be given with and without long-acting local anaesthetic drugs. However, severe respiratory depression, nausea and vomiting, urinary retention and pruritus can occur after their use. Life-threatening respiratory depression can occur when additional opioids are given by other routes to patients already receiving epidural opioids, and this practice should be actively discouraged. The respiratory depression encountered soon after administration (due to intravascular absorption) is relatively common and is simple to detect and treat. However, respiratory depression can occur many hours after opioid administration, particularly with the most commonly used drug, morphine, probably because of its lower lipophilicity, compared with fentanyl and diamorphine. Fentanyl is a drug with much greater stability than diamorphine, and it can be used with bupivacaine in a terminally sterilized formulation with potential risk management benefits. Respiratory depression can still occur.

Stimulation-produced analgesia

TENS and acupuncture

TENS (transcutaneous electrical nerve stimulation) machines are portable battery-powered devices that generate a small current to electrodes applied to the skin. The electrodes are placed at the painful site or close to the course of the peripheral nerve innervating the painful area, and the current is increased until paraesthesiae are felt at the site of the pain.

The current stimulates the large, rapidly conducting (Aβ) fibres which close the gating mechanism in the dorsal horn cells, and this inhibits the small, slowly conducting fibres (Aδ and C). TENS may also exert an additional effect by stimulating endogenous opioids.

Acupuncture also works in a similar fashion, although additional factors may be involved. Stimulation-produced analgesia can be used for trauma, postoperative pain, labour pain and various chronic pains. TENS, in particular, offers the patient a simple, non-invasive, self-controlled method of pain relief with few adverse effects.

Analgesic drugs

Non-steroidal anti-inflammatory drugs (NSAIDs)

NSAIDs produce their effect through cyclo-oxygenase inhibition, and are used widely to relieve pain, with or without inflammation, in people with acute and chronic musculoskeletal disorders. In single doses, NSAIDs have analgesic activity comparable to that of paracetamol (Cashman 1996). In regular higher dosages they have both a long analgesic and an anti-inflammatory effect, which makes them particularly useful for the treatment of continuous or regular pain associated with inflammation. They have been shown to be suitable for the relief of pain in dysmenorrhoea, toothache and some headaches, and to treat the pain caused by secondary bone tumours, many of which produce lysis of bone and release of prostaglandins.

Clinical considerations

Differences in anti-inflammatory activity between NSAIDs are small, but there is considerable variation in individual patient response as well as the incidence and type of side-effects. About 60% of patients will respond to any NSAID. Of the remaining patients, those who do not respond to one NSAID may well respond to another. An analgesic effect should normally be seen within a week, whereas an anti-inflammatory effect may not be achieved, or be assessable clinically, for up to 3 weeks.

The potential benefits of treatment with an NSAID must be weighed against the risks. NSAIDs are contraindicated in patients with known active peptic ulceration and should be used with caution in the elderly and in those with renal impairment or asthma.

COX-2 specific drugs

Cyclo-oxygenase exists in two forms: cyclo-oxygenase-1 (COX-1) and cyclo-oxygenase-2 (COX-2). COX-1 is a constitutive enzyme that exists under normal conditions in a variety of tissues where it catalyses the formation of essential prostaglandins. It does not have a role in nociception or inflammation. COX-2 is an inducible enzyme that appears in damaged tissues shortly after injury and leads to the formation of inflammatory prostaglandins within these tissues. COX-2 specific NSAIDs should, theoretically, inhibit the formation of inflammatory prostaglandins without affecting the activity of COX-1 in areas such as the gut. A number of studies have examined the safety of these drugs and shown that the use of COX-2 specific drugs is associated with reduced risks of gastrointestinal side-effects when compared with non-selective drugs

Weak opioids

Drugs of this type are prescribed frequently by primary care physicians, either alone or in combination with other analgesics, for a wide variety of painful disorders. There are three major drugs in this group: codeine, dihydrocodeine and dextropropoxyphene. They are recommended by the World Health Organization for pain that is not responsive to non-opioid analgesics. Despite this recommendation, there are almost no modern data to show that these drugs are of any benefit in the relief of chronic pain, and it may be of more benefit to go straight to prescribing strong opioids.

Codeine

Codeine is suggested as the first choice drug in this group. It is structurally similar to morphine and about 10% is demethylated to form morphine, and the analgesic effect may be due to this, at least in part. It is a powerful cough suppressant as well as being very constipating. In combination with aspirin-like drugs the analgesic effects are usually additive, but the variability in response is considerable. A degree of genetic polymorphism occurs within the population such that the hepatic microsomal enzyme CYP2D6 that is responsible for the conversion of codeine to morphine does not catalyze this conversion in approximately 8% of the population. Codeine's duration of analgesic action is about 3 hours.

Dihydrocodeine

Dihydrocodeine is only available in a few countries and is chemically related to codeine. It has similar properties to codeine when used at the same dosage and is slightly more potent. It has a shorter duration of action than codeine, and this makes its value in the management of chronic pain extremely limited.

Dextropropoxyphene

Dextropropoxyphene is prescribed either alone or in combination with other analgesics such as aspirin and paracetamol. There are few hard data on its therapeutic value, and at least one major review has concluded that the analgesic efficacy of this drug is less than aspirin and barely more than placebo. At best, dextropropoxyphene has failed to show any superiority over paracetamol (Li Wan Po & Zhang 1997). At worst it is a dangerous drug which has the potential for steadily developing toxicity. Patients with hepatic dysfunction and poor renal function are particularly at risk. It is associated with problems in overdosage, notably a non-naloxone-reversible depression of the cardiac conducting system. Dextropropoxyphene interacts unpredictably with a number of drugs, including carbamazepine and warfarin.

Strong opioids

Morphine

Morphine is the standard strong opioid analgesic. It is available as oral, rectal and injectable formulations and has a duration of effect of about 4 hours. There is no ceiling effect when the dose is increased. A general protocol for morphine use is to obtain rapid control of acute pain with an intravenous dose of 2–5 mg titrated against relief of the patient's pain. For control of chronic pain or pain arising from malignancy, an oral regimen is appropriate using a quick-release formulation of morphine. A suitable starting dose is 5–10 mg every 4 hours, and the patient should be advised to take the same dose as often as is necessary for breakthrough pain. It may be necessary to double the dose every 24 hours until pain relief is achieved, although a slower dose escalation will often suffice. After control is achieved it is appropriate to change to an oral sustained-release preparation, which offers twice-daily dosing. Maximum daily doses of up to 1 or 2 g of morphine can be achieved if necessary, but few patients require more than about 200 mg daily. Morphine is metabolized in the liver, and one metabolite, morphine 6-glucuronide, is pharmacologically active; this should be taken into consideration in patients who have renal failure.

Other strong opioids

Opioids such as pethidine and dextromoramide offer little advantage over morphine in that they are generally milder in action with a relatively short duration of action (2 hours). Dipipanone is only available in a preparation which contains an antiemetic (cyclizine), and increasing doses lead to sedation and the risk of developing a tardive dyskinesia with long-term use. Methadone has a long elimination half-life of 15–25 hours, and accumulation may occur in the early stages of use. It has a low side-effect profile with long-term use, and some patients who experience serious adverse effects with morphine may tolerate methadone.

Hydromorphone and oxycodone are synthetic opioids that have been used for many years in North America and more recently in Europe. They are available in both standard and sustained-release preparations. Some patients appear to tolerate hydromorphone or oxycodone better than morphine but there is no evidence to suggest which patients achieve the best effect with either of these drugs and morphine should remain the first-line treatment.

Fentanyl is now available as a sustained-release transdermal patch for long-term use. The patch is designed to release the drug continuously for 3 days. When starting the drug, existing analgesic therapy should be continued for the first 12 hours until therapeutic levels are achieved, and a short-acting opioid should be available for breakthrough pain. Patches are replaced every 72 hours.

Clinical considerations

As a general rule, strong opioids work best against visceral pain or pain arising from a somatic cause. They work moderately against sympathetically maintained pain, and poorly against neurogenic or psychogenic pain. Their use is almost universally accepted in cancer pain but many patients with chronic non-cancer pain can find considerable relief with potent opioids and barriers to their use in this setting appear to be based more on ignorance and political fashions than clinical evidence (Portenoy 1990, McQuay 1997).

Agonist–antagonist and partial agonists

Most of the drugs in this category are either competitive antagonists at the μ receptor, that is to say they can bind to this site but exert no action; or they exert only limited actions, that is to say they are partial agonists. Those that are antagonist at the μ receptor can provoke a withdrawal syndrome in patients receiving concomitant agonist opioids such as morphine. These properties make it difficult to use these agents in the control of chronic pain, and the process of conversion from one group of drugs to another can be complex.

Pentazocine. Pentazocine is a benzomorphan derivative that is an agonist and at the same time a very weak antagonist at the μ receptor. This drug became popular in the 1960s, when it was thought that it would have little or no abuse potential. This is now known to be untrue, although its abuse potential is less than that of the conventional agonists such as morphine. It produces an analgesia that is clearly different from morphine and is probably due to agonist actions at the κ receptor. There are no detailed studies of its use in chronic pain, but its short duration of action (about 3 hours) and the high incidence of psychomimetic side-effects make it a totally unsuitable drug for such use.

Buprenorphine. This drug is a semi-synthetic, highly lipophilic opioid that is a partial agonist. It undergoes extensive metabolism when administered orally, and to avoid this effect it is given sublingually. It has high receptor affinity and, through this property, a duration of action of 6 hours.

A long duration of action and high bioavailability would suggest a role for buprenorphine in the management of chronic pain. However, it is difficult to find any controlled studies in the literature and the high incidence of adverse effects seems the likely reason. The incidence of nausea and vomiting appears to be substantially higher than with morphine, though respiratory depression and constipation are less. Patients who can tolerate this drug appear to experience long-lasting effective analgesia.

Tramadol

Tramadol is a centrally acting analgesic that has opioid agonist activity and also has potent monoamine re-uptake properties similar to many antidepressants. Indeed, tramadol appears to have intrinsic antidepressant activity. It is not as powerful as morphine and its value in the management of acute pain is limited by an unfavourably high risk of nausea and vomiting. Its place in the treatment of chronic pain has not been established, but it may be an acceptable alternative to the weak opioids (Sunshine 1994). Its monoaminergic activity seems to be valuable in the management of neuropathic pain.

Adverse effects of opioids

The adverse effects of opioids are nearly all dose related, and tolerance develops to the majority with long-term use.

Respiratory depression. Respiratory depression is potentially dangerous in patients with impaired respiratory function, but tolerance is said to develop rapidly with chronic dosing. It can be reversed by naloxone.

Sedation. Sedation is usually mild and self-limiting. Smaller doses, given more frequently, may counteract the problem. Rarely, amfetamine or methylphenidate has been used to counteract this effect.

Nausea and vomiting. Antiemetics should be co-prescribed routinely with opioids for the first 10 days. Choice of antiemetic will depend upon the cause, and a single drug will be sufficient in two-thirds of patients. Where nausea is persistent, additional causes should be sought and prescribing reviewed. If another antiemetic is used it should have a different mode of action.

Constipation. Opioids reduce intestinal secretions and peristalsis, causing a dry stool and a hypotonic colon. When opioids are used on a long-term basis most patients need a stool softener and a laxative on a routine basis. Suitable routine laxatives include docusate sodium, co-danthramer and co-danthrusate. Dosage should be titrated to give a comfortable stool. High-fibre diets and bulking agents do not work very well in preventing constipation in patients on opioids.

Tolerance. Chronic drug treatment with opioids often causes tolerance to the analgesic effect. When this occurs the dosage should be increased or, alternatively, another opioid can be substituted, since cross-tolerance is not usually complete. Addiction is very rare when opioids are prescribed for pain relief.

Smooth muscle spasm. Morphine causes spasm of the sphincter of Oddi in the biliary tract and may cause biliary colic, as well as urinary sphincter spasm and retention of urine. Thus, in biliary or renal colic, it is preferable to use another opioid without these effects. Pethidine is believed to be the most effective in these circumstances.

Non-opioid analgesics

The pharmacological actions and use of the conventional non-opioids such as paracetamol, aspirin and NSAIDs are well known and will not be discussed further here.

Nefopam is a drug which is chemically related to orphenadrine and diphenhydramine. It is not an opioid, anti-inflammatory drug or antihistamine. The mechanism of analgesic action is unknown. As a non-opioid, it is free from problems of habituation and respiratory depression. The drug has a very high number of dose-related effects in clinical use. These may be linked to the anticholinergic actions of the drug. Nefopam may be useful in asthmatic patients and in those who are intolerant of NSAIDs.

Adjuvant analgesics

To be an analgesic, a drug must relieve pain in animal models of pain and must give demonstrable and reliable pain relief in patients. Drugs such as the opioids and the NSAIDs clearly are analgesics. The evidence is less clear for the drugs in this section, and traditional methods would not classify them as analgesics. However, all appear to have given some benefit in the control of chronic pain.

Anticonvulsants

The usefulness of this group of drugs has been established for the treatment of neuropathic pain (McQuay et al 1995). Conditions which may respond to anticonvulsants include trigeminal neuralgia, glossopharyngeal neuralgia, various neuropathies, lancinating pain arising from conditions such as postherpetic neuralgia and multiple sclerosis and similar pains that may follow amputation or surgery. Several classes of drugs show anticonvulsant activity. These can

be broadly classed as sodium channel blockers (carbamazepine, phenytoin), glutamate inhibitors (lamotrigine, gabapentin), GABA potentiators (sodium valproate, tiagabine) or drugs showing a mixture of these effects (topiramate). Failure to respond to one particular drug does not indicate that anticonvulsants as a broad class will be ineffective. A drug with a different mechanism of action or combination therapy could be considered.

Anticonvulsants are surprisingly effective in the prophylaxis of migraine and cluster headache. Their mode of action is unclear but both of these conditions are associated with abnormal excitability of certain groups of neurones and the neuronal depression caused by anticonvulsants is probably important.

Antidepressants

Persistent chronic pain is frequently accompanied by anxiety and depression. Thus it is not surprising that the use of antidepressants and other psychoactive drugs are part of standard pain management. There is evidence that some of these drugs have analgesic properties that are independent of their psychotropic effects.

The tricyclic antidepressants (TCAs) are frequently used for the treatment of chronic pain conditions, with and without anticonvulsants, and there is a substantial body of literature about their analgesic action (McQuay et al 1996).

The biochemical activity of the TCAs suggests that their main effect will be on serotonergic and noradrenergic neurones. The TCAs inhibit the re-uptake of the monoamines 5-HT and/or noradrenaline (norepinephrine) at neurones in the brain and spinal cord. Through a rather complex mechanism, this causes an initial fall in the release of these transmitters followed by a sustained rise in the concentration of neurotransmitter at synapses in the pain neural pathways. This rise usually takes 2–3 weeks to develop. Since pain is a common presenting complaint of depression it seems reasonable to assume that some relief of pain will be associated with the reversal of depression. TCAs are effective analgesics in headache, facial pain, low back pain, arthritis, denervation pain and, to a lesser degree, cancer.

Clinical use of antidepressants in chronic pain

Various TCAs have been utilized (usually methylated tricyclics), with or without phenothiazines and anticonvulsants. Drug doses have varied considerably, but most are low, of the order of 25–75 mg/day. Evidence tends to support the use of higher doses (greater than 75 mg/day) for somatic and neuropathic pain. Where depression is prominent, a full antidepressant dose schedule should be employed and in the case of amitryptyline, a target dose of 150–250 mg/day would usually be appropriate.

TCAs have a wide range of adverse effects, and these may cause a marked reduction in patient adherence. Newer antidepressant drugs have generally been disappointing from the analgesic perspective. However, much of the research has looked at the selective serotonin re-uptake inhibitors (SSRIs). Recent work suggests that both noradrenergic and serotonergic transmission needs to be enhanced for an analgesic effect to be seen. The serotonin/noradrenaline (norepinephrine) re-uptake inhibitor venlafaxine has effects on both monoamines and does appear to posses analgesic activity at higher dose ranges (150 mg/day and above). A number of antidepressant compounds do not act via monoamine re-uptake inhibition and do not appear to possess intrinsic analgesic activity. Examples are trazodone and mirtazapine. They are effective antidepressants and may have a place in the treatment of coexisting depression but analgesia should be tackled separately.

Ketamine

Ketamine is an intravenous anaesthetic agent with a variety of actions within the central nervous system. Many of its effects are related to its activity at central glutamate receptors although it also has actions at certain voltage-gated ion channels and opioid receptors. Low doses of ketamine (0.1–0.3 mg/kg/hr via the intravenous route) can produce profound analgesia, even in situations where opioids have been ineffective such as neuropathic pain. Despite its variable oral availability, oral administration of ketamine can be surprisingly effective (Mercadante 1996). Its usefulness is limited by troublesome psychotropic side-effects although the simultaneous administration of benzodiazepines or antipsychotics can reduce these problems.

Neuroleptics

Phenothiazines, with the exception of levomepromazine (methotrimeprazine), have no effect in the treatment of pain. A dose of 15 mg of levomepromazine (methotrimeprazine) has an analgesic activity equivalent to 10 mg of intramuscular morphine. Levomepromazine (methotrimeprazine) also has profound hypnotic, anxiolytic and antiemetic effects which make it a useful drug in the palliative care setting.

Anxiolytics

Benzodiazepines may be used for pain relief in conditions associated with acute muscle spasm and are sometimes prescribed to reduce the anxiety and muscle tension associated with chronic pain conditions. Many authorities believe that they reduce pain tolerance and there is good evidence that they can reduce the effectiveness of opioid analgesics although the mechanism is unclear. Clonazepam has been used in the management of neurogenic pain but some of the more modern anticonvulsants have clearer evidence of efficacy. Diazepam can be used to control painful spasticity due to acute or spinal cord injury but sedation may be troublesome, and baclofen (see below) is probably a more suitable choice.

Antihistamines

These agents were introduced into the management of chronic pain because of their sedative muscle relaxant properties. These actions are non-specific, and it is not clear whether the clinical effect is mediated centrally or peripherally. Most clinical studies have been carried out with hydroxyzine, which has shown benefit in acute pain, tension headache and cancer pain.

There is evidence that analgesic combinations of antihistamines, NSAIDs and opioids may yield greater analgesia than that provided by each drug alone.

Skeletal muscle relaxants

Drugs described in this section are used for the relief of muscle spasm or spasticity. It is axiomatic that the underlying cause of the spasticity and any aggravating factors such as pressure sores or infections should be treated. This group of drugs will usually help spasticity, but this may be at the cost of decreased muscle tone elsewhere, which may lead to a decrease in the mobility of the patient and thus make matters worse.

The drug of first choice is probably baclofen, which has a peripheral site of action, working directly on the skeletal muscle. Baclofen is a derivative of the inhibitory neurotransmitter GABA and appears to be an agonist at the $GABA_B$ receptor. It is alleged that it is most effective for the treatment of spasticity caused by multiple sclerosis or other diseases of the spinal cord, especially traumatic lesions. There are reports of its use in trigeminal neuralgia and a number of painful conditions, including postherpetic neuralgia.

Dantrolene is an alternative that is effective orally and which may have fewer (but potentially more serious) adverse effects. Its effect is due to a direct effect on skeletal muscle and takes several weeks to develop.

The α_2-adrenergic agonist tizanidine has potent muscle relaxant activity and is an alternative to baclofen. It may also have some direct analgesic effects.

Botulinum toxin

The bacterium *Clostridium botulinum* produces a potent toxin that interferes directly with neuromuscular transmission. Purified preparations of the type A toxin produce long-lasting relaxation of skeletal muscle. The effect often lasts in excess of 3 months and avoids the systemic side-effects of agents such as baclofen. Great care must be taken in administering this drug as spread may occur to adjacent muscle groups producing excessive weakness. Overdosage, with systemic absorbtion, may lead to generalized muscle weakness and even respiratory failure.

Clonidine

The α-adrenergic agonist clonidine has been shown to produce analgesia, and there is evidence that both morphine and clonidine produce a dose-dependent inhibition of spinal nociceptive transmission that is mediated through different receptors for each drug. This may explain why clonidine has been shown to work synergistically with morphine when given intrathecally or epidurally. Clonidine also appears to work when given by other routes or even topically, but may cause severe hypotension by any route.

Cannabinoids

Cannabis has been used as an analgesic for hundreds of years. Despite the historical record, problems concerning the legal status of cannabis in most countries has hindered scientific investigation of its analgesic properties. The active ingredient in preparations made from the hemp plant *Cannabis sativa* is δ-9 tetrahydrocannabinol. This compound has analgesic activity in animal models of experimental pain as well as in the clinical situation (Hirst et al 1998). Overall analgesic activity appears relatively weak and it has not proved possible to separate the analgesic activity from the potent psychotropic effects characteristic of these drugs. There may be a clearer analgesic effect in neuropathic pain but the evidence for this remains anecdotal.

Treatment of selected pain syndromes

Herpetic and postherpetic neuralgia

The pain associated with *Herpes zoster* infection is severe, continuous and often described as burning and lancinating. Antiviral therapy such as aciclovir initiated at the first sign of the rash can reduce the duration of the pain, particularly postherpetic pain, which follows the disappearance of the rash. Analgesics such as NSAIDs provide some benefit. TCAs such as amitriptyline are the mainstay of treatment, commencing with a dose of 50 mg at night and increasing to 150 mg if required. They may be combined with anticonvulsants if the response is poor or incomplete. Carbamazepine is historically the most important drug of this group but modern anticonvulsant drugs (see above) have also proved useful and may be better tolerated. Recent work has suggested that direct injection of long-acting steroid preparations into the spinal fluid may help refractory cases but this remains to be confirmed.

Trigeminal neuralgia

Trigeminal neuralgia presents as abrupt, intense bursts of severe, lancinating pain, provoked by touching sensitive trigger areas on one side of the face. The disorder may spontaneously remit for periods of several weeks or months. Anticonvulsants have been used successfully. If drug therapy is ineffective, surgical techniques such as decompression of the nucleus of the fifth cranial nerve, glycerol injection or gangliolysis can be of great benefit. If surgery becomes necessary, anticonvulsants should be withdrawn gradually afterwards.

Peripheral nerve injury and neuropathy

Damage to, or entrapment of, nerves can cause pain, unpleasant sensations and paraesthesiae. Tricyclics and anticonvulsants have been used with some success to reduce neuropathic pain. A neuroma occurs when damaged or severed nerve fibres sprout new small fibres in an attempt to regenerate. Pain develops several weeks after the nerve injury, and is often due to the neuroma growing into scar tissue, causing pain as it is stretched or mobilized. Treatment of neuroma is very difficult and few treatments are successful. Options include surgery and injections of steroid and local anaesthetic agents.

Sympathetically maintained pain

Causalgia and reflex sympathetic dystrophy are names for an important group of painful conditions that may follow trauma or damage to nerves and which are associated with overactivity of the sympathetic nervous system. Treatment is directed at blocking sympathetic overactivity, reducing pain and instituting aggressive physiotherapy to facilitate a return to normal function. Sympathetic blockade can be achieved by blocking appropriate nerves using local anaesthetics, or by injecting a dose of an α-adrenergic blocking agent such as phentolamine, which may give sufficient pain relief to permit the institution of regular physiotherapy and for recovery to take place. Other drugs that have been used successfully include oral corticosteroids, other α-adrenergic agonists and blockers and calcium channel blocking drugs (Kingery 1997).

Musculoskeletal (myofascial) pain

Myofascial pain is that arising from muscles and is associated with stiffness and neuralgic symptoms such as tingling and paraesthesiae. It may occur spontaneously or following trauma, such as whiplash injury. Myofascial pain syndrome is also known as myositis, fibrositis, myalgia and myofascitis. Acute muscle injury can be treated by first aid with the application of a cooling spray or ice to reduce inflammation and spasm, followed by passive stretching of the muscle to restore its full range of motion. Injection therapy is used to disrupt sensitive muscle trigger points, and may involve injecting local anaesthetic or saline. Local injections of botulinum toxin have also been shown to be effective where muscle spasm is prolonged and severe. TENS and acupuncture have an important role to play in reducing pain and muscle spasm. Treatment of chronic myofascial syndromes should always include a programme of physical therapy.

Postamputation and phantom limb pain

The majority of amputees suffer significant stump or phantom limb pain for at least a few weeks each year. Pain will be present immediately postoperatively in the stump. This may be caused by muscle spasm, nerve injury and sensitivity of the wound and surrounding skin. As the wound heals, the pain should subside. If it does not, the reason may be vascular insufficiency or infection. Pain occurring some number of years after amputation may be caused by changes in the structure of the bones or skin in the stump, or ischaemia. For instance, reduction in the thickness of overlying tissue with age may expose nerve endings to increased stimuli.

TCAs may be helpful for stump pain. Standard analgesics can be given, and surgery may be necessary to restore the vascular supply or reduce trauma to nerve endings.

Phantom pain is a referred pain which produces a burning or throbbing sensation, felt in the absent limb. Cramping sensations are caused by muscular spasm in the stump. The patient with phantom limb pain is often anxious, depressed and frightened, all of which exacerbate the pain. Analgesic drugs alone are generally not adequate for phantom pain, but TCAs and anticonvulsants are useful adjuvants. Other therapy which can be effective includes TENS and sympathetic blockade (Sherman 1980). These patients frequently require management at specialist pain centres.

Postoperative pain

The majority of patients suffer postoperative pain. The site and nature of surgery influence the severity of pain, although individual variations among patients do not allow the amount of pain to be predicted according to the type of operation.

Apart from the obvious benefit of relieving suffering, pain relief is desirable for a number of physiological reasons after surgery or any form of major tissue injury. For example, poor-quality analgesia reduces lung function, increases heart rate and blood pressure, and magnifies the stress response to surgery (Kehlet 1994). The use of intermittent and patient-controlled intermittent intravenous injections of opioids has been described earlier. However, opioids themselves may delay recovery and are associated with adverse events in the postoperative period (Kehlet et al 1996). It is now common to treat postoperative pain with combinations of opioids and local anaesthetic blocks or infiltrations. In addition, NSAIDs can be used as adjuvants to opioids. Agents such as diclofenac and ketorolac are used frequently, but care must be taken because in situations where there is a possibility of renal stress, such as blood loss, the normal protective effect of prostaglandins on the kidney will be lost and renal failure may result. There is no evidence to support the use of either NSAIDs or local anaesthetic techniques pre-emptively, although there is some theoretical and clinical evidence that opioids given prior to surgery may be more effective than when given postoperatively.

Headache

Tension headaches are caused by muscle contraction over the neck and scalp. They respond well to TENS and methylated TCA drugs given as a single dose at night. Propranolol and minor tranquilizers have also been used. NSAIDs may be indicated if the headache is associated with cervical spondylosis or neck injury.

Migraine

Most migraine attacks respond to simple analgesics such as aspirin or paracetamol. Soluble forms are best, as gut motility is reduced during a migraine attack and absorption of oral medication may be delayed. Migraine treatment has altered markedly in recent years with the advent of the triptan drugs such as sumatriptan, zolmitriptan and naratriptan (Ferrari 1998, Goadsby & Olesen 1996). These are $5-HT_{1B/D}$ agonists that will often abort an attack, especially when given by the subcutaneous route. Their vasoconstrictor activity precludes their use in patients with angina or cerebrovascular disease but their side-effects are less serious than the ergot derivatives they have replaced.

Prophylactic drug treatment of migraine includes β-adrenergic blockers, anticonvulsants and tricyclic antidepressants. Chronic treatment is undesirable.

Cluster headache

Cluster headache is a disabling condition characterized by severe unilateral head pain occurring in clusters of attacks varying from minutes to hours. It shares some pathological features with migraine and treatment is similar although recent high resolution magnetic resonance imaging studies have shown specific anatomical differences in the brains of people with cluster headache. Triptans are effective in acute attacks, as is inhalation of 100% oxygen. Prophylaxis is similar to that of migraine.

Dysmenorrhoea

Dysmenorrhoea is a common cause of pelvic pain. It can be helped by the prescription of oral contraceptives, since pain is absent in anovulatory cycles. NSAIDs are effective because of their action on cyclo-oxygenase inhibition. Dysmenorrhoea due to endometriosis may require therapy with androgenic drugs such as danazol or regulators of the gonadotrophins such as norethisterone.

Burn pain

Patients with burns may require a series of painful procedures such as physiotherapy, debridement or skin grafting. Premedication with a strong opioid before the procedure coupled with intravenous opioids and the use of entonox (premixed 50% nitrous oxide and 50% oxygen) may be necessary to control the pain. Regular, time-contingent opioids such as morphine or methadone may be useful to prevent the pain induced by movement or touch in the burn area. The anaesthetic drug ketamine (see above) has potent analgesic activity when used in sub-hypnotic doses. It has a short duration of action and may be used to reduce the pain of dressing changes or other forms of incident pain. Even with low doses, a significant proportion of patients will experience side-effects of dysphoria or hallucinations. These can be treated with benzodiazepines or antipsychotic compounds such as haloperidol.

Pain of malignancy

The pain associated with cancer may arise from many different sources, and has the characteristics of both acute and chronic pain. It should be emphasized that the sources of the pain may change and continual assessment on a regular basis is required. Although this chapter is concerned only with the management of pain, care of the patient with a terminal illness requires management of all aspects of the patient. Cancer occurs more frequently in the elderly, who have a larger proportion of painful ailments than the general population. Pain may be arising from these sources too, and these require treatment at the same time. Pain can be treated both with drugs and other techniques such as radiotherapy and nerve blocks. Drug treatment is based on the analgesic ladder together with the use of adjuvant analgesics. When considering non-opioid analgesics, the NSAIDs have a special role, especially in bone metastases. Some clinicians progress from non-opioid to strong opioid drugs such as morphine, omitting the middle step of the analgesic ladder. It can be argued that the middle step of the current analgesic ladder, weak opioids, be eliminated and that another step added when strong opioids are not working. This last step would be the use of neurolytic or neurosurgical procedures to overcome pain that is non-opioid responsive.

However, strong opioids are the mainstay for the treatment of cancer pain, and virtually every form of cancer pain will respond to some degree.

Opioid use in cancer pain

Morphine is the standard opioid in standard or sustained-release oral form. If morphine is not tolerated, hydromorphone or methadone, both with relatively long half-lives, may be considered. Optimal dosage is determined on an individual basis for each patient by titration against the pain. Patients on long-term sustained-release opioids should have additional oral doses of rapidly acting opioid to act as an 'escape' medicine for incident or breakthrough pain. Pain arising from malignancy may change and, as with pain arising from any source, the cause and the treatment must be subject to regular review.

Where the oral route is not available, non-oral routes of administration such as buccal, rectal, transdermal, inhaled or injection should be used. Injection means subcutaneous, intravenous or via epidural or spinal catheter. Implanted pumps and syringe drivers may be used to provide analgesia in cases where conventional opioid delivery is ineffective. The proportion of patients who need invasive forms of drug delivery is small and is confined to those who are persistently troubled with unacceptable adverse effects. Such patients can achieve pain relief with lower doses of opioid and have few problems with side-effects. Long-term maintenance of indwelling lines and catheters requires training for patient, physicians and nursing teams, but excellent long-term results are possible. Morphine, oxycodone and hydromorphone are suitable for use. In the UK diamorphine is also suitable and readily available. Diamorphine has the advantage of being very soluble, so a high dose may be given in a small volume, which reduces the frequency of changes of syringes and refills necessary to provide adequate pain relief.

Use of adjuvant drugs in cancer pain

Neuropathic pain is common in cancer. As many as 40% of patients with cancer pain may have a neuropathic component. TCAs and anticonvulsants should be introduced early but where these are ineffective, ketamine has found an important role.

Levomepromazine (methotrimeprazine), a phenothiazine with analgesic activity, is a useful alternative when opioids cannot be tolerated. It causes neither constipation nor respiratory depression and has antiemetic and anxiolytic activity. It is sedative, which may be either a virtue or a problem in palliative care.

Corticosteroids are useful in managing certain aspects of acute and chronic cancer pain. They are particularly useful for raised intracranial pressure and for relieving pressure caused by tumours on the spinal cord or peripheral nerves.

Dexamethasone (16 mg/day) is the most commonly used steroid to ameliorate raised intracranial pressure in patients with brain tumours. High steroid doses given for 1 or 2 weeks do not require a reducing-dosage regimen. They also produce a feeling of well-being, increased appetite and weight gain, although the central effects are usually transient. It is axiomatic that underlying causes of pain be treated; therefore it is appropriate to use antibiotics to treat infections, radiotherapy to reduce tumour bulk or control bone pain, or surgery to achieve fracture fixation or to relieve bowel obstruction in conjunction with antispasmodics such as hyoscine butylbromide.

Pain arising from bone also responds to NSAIDs, which may be given orally or rectally. Bisphosphonates have a place in management of this problem, and new drugs in this group are being introduced into clinical practice.

Table 31.3 Common therapeutic problems in pain management

Problem	Solution	Example
Neuropathic pain	Anticonvulsants	Carbamazepine Sodium valproate Gabapentin Lamotrigine
	Antidepressants	Amitriptyline Imipramine
	i.v. anaesthetic agents	Ketamine
Malignant bone pain	Bisphosphonates	Disodium pamidronate Calcitonin (salmon) (salcatonin)
Muscle spasm/spasticity	Skeletal muscle relaxants	Baclofen Dantrolene Botulinum toxin (type A)
Raised intracranial pressure	Corticosteroids	Dexamethasone Prednisolone
Nausea with morphine	Antiemetics	Metoclopramide Domperidone
	Use an alternative route of administration	Topical Subcutaneous
Constipation	?drug therapy – opioids, antidepressants. Co-prescribe laxatives	Docusate sodium Co-danthramer
Use of antidepressants in patients with ischaemic heart disease	Use a non-cardiotoxic antidepressant	Venlafaxine
Drug interactions with carbamazepine	Use an anticonvulsant which does not affect hepatic enzymes	Gabapentin
Renal failure	Morphine accumulates – use lower dose Use a drug which is not handled renally	Fentanyl
Sedation/impaired cognition	Identify any drug-related causes and adjust dose/stop drug	

Specific cancer pain syndromes

Three types of malignant pain are briefly outlined below to indicate various therapeutic approaches.

Cancer of the pancreas. Pain is caused by infiltration of the tumour into the pancreas as well as by obstruction of the bowel and biliary tract and metastases in the liver. Patients will also experience anorexia, nausea, vomiting and diarrhoea, and are often depressed. Surgery, radiotherapy and chemotherapy may relieve pain for long periods, as does neurolytic blockade of the coeliac plexus. Opioid analgesics are useful and may be administered intravenously or epidurally either by bolus injection or continuous infusion.

Mesothelioma of the lung. Mesothelioma causes pain when the tumour penetrates surrounding tissues such as the pleura, chest wall and nerve plexuses. The analgesic ladder should be used first, and it should be remembered that any NSAID is useful because inflammation is often a component of the chest wall involvement. Adjuvants such as tricyclic antidepressants or steroids may be helpful. As the tumour progresses, nerve blocks or neurosurgery may be necessary, and invasion of the vertebrae can lead to nerve root or spinal cord compression. In the latter case, high-dose steroids such as dexamethasone may be given intravenously, but radiotherapy is also useful in reducing the size of the tumour.

Metastatic bone pain. Metastatic bone pain is usually treated with courses of chemotherapy and radiotherapy, but analgesics can be used. A prostaglandin-like substance has been isolated from bone metastases, and therefore NSAIDs and, more recently, bisphosphonates are often used in bone pain. Steroids also interfere with prostaglandin formation, and so dexamethasone has a role, especially where there is nerve root or spinal cord compression.

Some common problems in the treatment of pain are outlined in Table 31.3.

CASE STUDIES

Case 31.1

An 85-year-old man is admitted to hospital after falling down a flight of stairs and landing heavily on his right side. On admission, he is in severe pain and finds breathing and especially coughing, unbearably painful. Chest X-ray reveals that he has fractures of the fifth to eighth ribs on the right hand side.

Question

How should this patient's pain be managed and what are the risks of undertreatment?

Answer

Multiple rib fractures are potentially very serious and good analgesia can prevent potentially dangerous complications. Initial analgesia should include both potent opioids and NSAIDs (unless contraindicated). Opioids should be administered parenterally in the acute situation and patient-controlled analgesia would offer the safest means of dose titration. The chest injury may well result in damage to the underlying lung and it is essential to administer unrestricted high flow oxygen to the patient as the combination of lung injury and ventilatory suppression secondary to either pain or the effects of opioids could lead to dangerous hypoxia. TENS may also prove helpful.

Arterial oxygen saturation (and preferably arterial blood gases) should be monitored. If pain remains poorly controlled or the patient's oxygenation deteriorates, thoracic epidural analgesia using a mixture of local anaesthetic and opioid should be considered.

Failure to treat pain adequately in this situation may lead to a reduction in the patient's ability to cough and clear secretions from the chest. This can lead to respiratory failure and even death. Analgesia should be sufficient to allow regular physiotherapy in order to minimize the risk of such complications.

Case 31.2

A 45-year-old woman presents to her general practitioner with a 2-day history of back pain following a lifting injury at work. The pain is constant and aching in character with radiation into the posterior aspect of both thighs as far as the knee. Physical examination shows her to be maintaining a very rigid posture with some spasm of the large muscles of the back. Her range of movement is very poor but there are no neurological signs in the legs.

Question

Which drugs may help this lady's pain? What other advice should be given?

Answer

Acute back pain is very common and is rarely associated with serious spinal pathology. The absence of neurological signs is reassuring and indicates that early activity, possibly aided by a short course of analgesics, is the best way forward. NSAIDs, if tolerated, would be the drugs of choice. A low dose muscle relaxant such as baclofen 20–40 mg per day in divided doses might also help although it would be unwise to continue such drugs beyond 2 weeks. If NSAIDs are contraindicated, then paracetamol can be substituted and should be given every 6 hours. The role of opioids is less clear. Short term (7–14 days) use of a mild opioid such as codeine or tramadol is probably safe. Longer term use is less satisfactory as there is no clear evidence of their efficacy, and sedative side-effects may reduce the patient's capacity and motivation to remain active.

The patient should be advised to remain active and accept that some pain is likely during the recovery phase. Failure to remain active and, in particular, excessive bed rest are both associated with worse outcomes.

Case 31.3

A 50-year-old man is admitted to hospital with an acute onset of severe mid-thoracic spinal pain. He is found to be anaemic and investigations show that he has multiple myeloma with widespread bony lesions including fresh spinal fractures.

Question

Which drugs may help this man's pain? What particular hazards may occur in this condition?

Answer

This patient is extremely ill and even with aggressive chemotherapy, he is unlikely to survive more than a few months. Most of his pain will be related to the destruction of bone and the aim should be to provide pain relief via a 'central' mechanism through the use of opioids as well as reducing the rate of bone destruction and associated inflammatory responses. A potent opioid will be required and oral morphine would usually be the drug of first choice. In this situation, a combination of a sustained-release preparation together with liberal 'as required' dosing would be appropriate. The correct dose is the dose needed to produce adequate pain relief without producing excessive sedation. Inflammatory pain may be improved by the use of NSAIDs and these should be given regularly although they may be contraindicated in this condition (see below). High dose corticosteroids may achieve a similar effect and may also reduce the hypercalcaemia that is often seen in myeloma. Bone destruction and its associated pain may be reduced by the use of bisphosphonate compounds. In this case intravenous pamidronate should be given.

Renal failure is common in myeloma. This may be due to obstruction of renal tubules by myeloma proteins or the effects of some chemotherapeutic agents. If renal impairment occurs, opioids should be used with caution so as to avoid problems with accumulation. Transdermal fentanyl may be a more appropriate drug. NSAIDs can precipitate acute renal failure in the presence of reduced renal blood flow. Finally, platelet function is often poor in patients with myeloma. This can be due to direct effects of myeloma proteins on platelets, bone marrow replacement by myeloma or the effects of chemotherapy. Use of NSAIDs may be associated with increased risk of gastrointestinal haemorrage.

REFERENCES

Cashman J N 1996 The mechanisms of action of NSAIDs in analgesia. Drugs 52(Suppl. 5): 13–23

Ferrari M D 1998 Migraine. Lancet 351: 1043–1051

Goadsby P J, Olesen J 1996 Diagnosis and management of migraine. British Medical Journal 312: 1279–1283

Hirst R A, Lambert D G, Notcutt W G 1998 Pharmacology and potential therapeutic uses of cannabis. British Journal of Anaesthesia 81: 77–84

Kehlet H 1994 Postoperative pain relief: what is the issue? British Journal of Anaesthesia 72: 375–378

Kehlet H, Rung G W, Callesen T 1996 Postoperative opioid analgesia: time for a reconsideration? Journal of Clinical Anaesthesia 8: 441–445

Kingery W S 1997 A critical review of controlled clinical trials for peripheral neuropathic pain and complex regional pain syndromes. Pain 73: 123–139

Li Wan Po A, Zhang W Y 1997 Systematic overview of co-proxamol to assess analgesic effects of addition of dextropropoxyphene to paracetamol. British Medical Journal 315: 1565–1571

McQuay H J 1997 Opioid use in chronic pain. Acta Anaesthesiologica Scandinavica 41: 175–183

McQuay H, Carroll D, Jadad A R et al 1995 Anticonvulsant drugs for management of pain: a systematic review. British Medical Journal 311: 1047–1052

McQuay H J, Tramer M, Nye B A et al 1996 A systematic review of antidepressants in neuropathic pain. Pain 68: 217–227

Mercadante S 1996 Ketamine in cancer pain: an update. Palliative Medicine 10: 225–230

Portenoy R K 1990 Chronic opioid therapy in nonmalignant pain. Journal of Pain and Symptom Management 5: S46–S62

Sherman R A 1980 Published treatments of phantom limb pain. American Journal of Physical Medicine 59: 232–244

Sunshine A 1994 New clinical experience with tramadol. Drugs 47(Suppl. 1): 8–18

FURTHER READING

McQuay H, Moore R A 1998 An evidence based resource for pain relief. Oxford University Press, Oxford

Hanks G W, Justins D M 1992 Cancer pain: management. Lancet 339: 1031–1036

Twycross R G 1997 Symptom management in advanced cancer, 2nd edn. Radcliffe Medical Press, Oxford

Regnard C, Hockley J 2002 A clinical decision guide to symptom relief in palliative care. Radcliffe Medical Press, Oxford

Wall P D, Melzack R (eds) 2000 Textbook of pain, 4th edn. Churchill Livingstone, Edinburgh

Benzon H T, Raja S, Molloy R E et al (eds) 2000 Essentials of pain medicine and regional anaesthesia. Churchill Livingstone, Edinburgh

Nausea and vomiting 32

K. Teahon

It is important to differentiate vomiting from regurgitation, rumination and bulimia. Regurgitation is the return of oesophageal or gastric contents into the hypopharynx with little effort. Rumination is the passive regurgitation of recently ingested food into the mouth followed by rechewing, reswallowing or spitting out. It is not preceded by nausea and does not include the various physical phenomena associated with vomiting. Bulimia involves overeating followed by self-induced vomiting. Nausea and vomiting are symptoms. Treatment directed only at the symptoms does not deal with the underlying pathology which has to be identified and treated before symptoms will resolve.

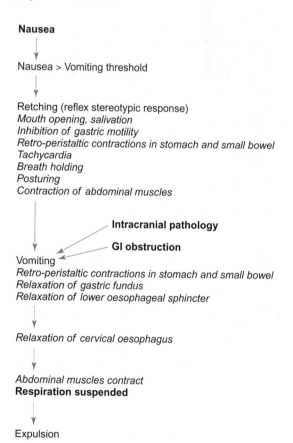

Figure 32.1 Schematic representation of nausea and vomiting.

The word nausea is derived from the Greek *nautia*, meaning sea-sickness, while vomiting is derived from the Latin *vomere*, meaning to discharge. Nausea is a subjective sensation whereas vomiting is the reflex physical act of expulsion of gastric contents.

Vomiting may or may not be preceded by nausea and involves a complex physiological process. When nausea precedes vomiting the sensation gradually increases until a certain threshold is reached when the act of vomiting is stimulated (Fig. 32.1).

Epidemiology

Enteric or systemic infection is probably the commonest cause of nausea and vomiting. The personal, social and economic impact of nausea and vomiting is significant. In Britain alone 8.5 million working days are lost because of nausea and vomiting associated with pregnancy (AGA 2000) and general practitioners write in excess of 5 million prescriptions for antiemetic drugs each year.

In hospitals nausea and vomiting occurs postoperatively (PONV) or in association with chemotherapy (CINV) or radiotherapy. It severely curtails many treatment schedules and makes treatment intolerable for some patients.

Pathophysiology (Fig. 32.2)

Complex interactions between central and peripheral pathways occur in the production of the clinical features of nausea and vomiting. The most important areas involved peripherally are the gastric mucosa and smooth muscle (the enteric brain) and the afferent pathways of the vagus and sympathetic nerves. Centrally the significant areas involved are the area postrema, the chemoreceptor trigger zone, the nucleus tractus solitarus (NTS) and the vomiting centre.

From a pharmacotherapeutic point of view the most important aspect of this complex pathophysiology is the variety of receptors involved, including dopaminergic, serotonergic, histaminergic and muscuranic receptors. In the clinical situation these become targets for various drugs directed at controlling the symptoms.

There are 10^8 neurones in the intestine (the enteric brain) and a complex interaction occurs between these, the mucosa, the smooth muscle in the intestine, the parasympathetic (vagus nerve) and sympathetic nerves and the higher centres in the spinal cord and brain to result in normal gastrointestinal peristaltic activity. The enteric brain and the vagus nerve monitor stimuli from mucosal irritation and smooth muscle stretch which may result in nausea and/or vomiting.

The area postrema in the floor of the fourth ventricle contains the chemoreceptor trigger zone (CTZ) and is a special sensory organ rich in dopaminergic, serotonergic, histaminergic and muscarinic receptors. It is located outside the blood–brain barrier and it is likely that chemicals, toxins, peptides, drugs and neurotransmitters in the cerebrospinal fluid (CSF) and bloodstream interact with this area to cause nausea and vomiting. However, the precise mechanism is not known.

The vomiting centre is situated in the dorsolateral reticular formation close to the respiratory centre and receives impulses from higher centres, visceral efferents, the eighth (auditory) nerve (the latter two through the nucleus tractus solitarus) and from the chemoreceptor trigger zone. It includes a number of brainstem nuclei required to integrate the responses of the gastrointestinal tract, pharyngeal muscles, respiratory muscles and somatic muscles to result in a vomiting episode. The vomiting centre may be stimulated in association with, or in isolation from, the nausea process.

The vomiting reflex can be elicited either directly via afferent neuronal connections, especially from the GI tract (probably dependent on the integrity of the nucleus tractus solitarus), or from humoral factors (dependent on the integrity of the area postrema).

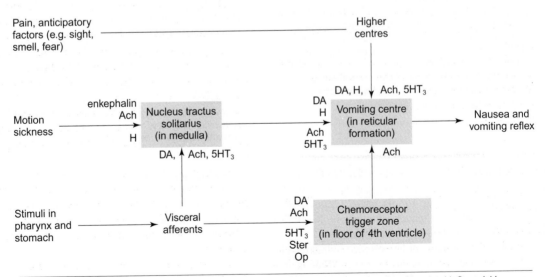

Putative receptors: Ach, acetylcholine (muscarinic); DA, dopamine; 5HT$_3$, serotonin; H, histamine; Ster, steroid; Op, opioid.

Figure 32.2 Diagrammatic representation of pathways involved in nausea and vomiting.

The sequence of muscle excitation and inhibition necessary for the act of vomiting (see Fig. 32.1) is probably controlled by a central pattern generator located in the NTS, and information from the chemoreceptor trigger zone and vagus nerve converge at this point.

The central mechanisms of nausea and vomiting include increased intracranial pressure, dilation of cerebral arteries during migraine and stimulation of the labyrinthine mechanism or of the senses of sight, smell and taste.

The peripheral mechanisms of nausea and vomiting include gastric dysrhythmias, motion sickness, delayed gastric emptying and gastric mucosal irritation (ulceration, NSAIDs). These mechanisms are all mediated through the vagal afferent neurones. The vomiting associated with distension or obstruction of the gastrointestinal tract is mediated through both the sympathetic and vagal afferent neurones.

Antiemetic drugs

Drug classes

Several classes of antiemetic drugs are available that antagonize the neurotransmitter receptors involved in the pathophysiology of nausea and vomiting. These drugs are classed according to their target receptor and some drugs affect multiple receptors. The drug classes available, their target receptors, main therapeutic indications and main side-effects are detailed in Table 32.1.

Choice of drug regimen

The choice of drug regimen for any patient involves:

- an understanding of the likely pathophysiology of the symptoms and receptors involved in an individual patient
- complementary combinations of antiemetics targeted at as many receptors as possible in the pathophysiological pathway for the particular condition
- the preferred route of administration
- the side-effects of available agents.

Management of the patient

Management of the patient with nausea and vomiting is approached in three main steps:

1. Recognize and correct any complications. This includes dehydration, hypokalaemia and metabolic alkalosis in the acute situation with symptoms of less than 4 weeks duration. Weight loss and malnutrition are features in the chronic situation when symptoms have been present for longer than 4 weeks.

2. Identify where possible the underlying cause (Table 32.2) and institute appropriate treatment. Here it is important to be aware that metabolic conditions such as hypercalcaemia, hyponatraemia and hyperthyroidism can result in vomiting and the cause will not readily be apparent from history and examination.

3. Implement therapeutic strategies to suppress or eliminate symptoms (these depend on the severity and clinical context).

Drug treatment of the most common therapeutic problems

Postoperative nausea and vomiting (PONV)

The overall incidence of postoperative nausea and vomiting (PONV) is estimated to be 25–30% (Kovac 2000). The aetiology is complex and multifactorial and includes patient, medical, surgical and anaesthetic related factors. The management approach is multimodal and involves multiple antiemetic drugs, less emetogenic anaesthesia, adequate hydration and adequate pain control.

Most hospitals will have devised management algorithms for PONV depending on the risk of occurrence (risk scores are available) and the likely severity. A good algorithm will contain a standard prophylaxis regimen and suggested rescue therapy, should prophylactic therapy fail. Many drugs have some efficacy but combination drug therapy is the best current answer. Sample algorithms are shown in Table 32.3. For minor uncomplicated or day surgery, a simple regimen containing cyclizine or prochlorperazine, administered at induction of anaesthesia, is commonly used. Rescue therapy might be the alternative of these two drugs which was not given at induction. Home rescue treatment might include rectal prochlorperazine. For major procedures, combinations of antiemetics may be used, especially if the patient has a history of PONV (see Fig. 32.3). These therapeutic strategies involve activity at dopaminergic, histaminergic and serotonergic receptors. It is of note that metoclopramide is of little or no value in the management of PONV.

Dexamethasone has been shown to be a safe and effective antiemetic after abdominal and other types of surgery (Wang et al 2000) in intravenous doses of 8–32 mg at induction. The mechanism of action is unclear but steroid receptors are thought to exist in the area postrema.

Pre-medication with opioids increases the incidence of PONV and this may be reduced by concurrent administration of either atropine or hyoscine, which are primarily used as antisecretory drugs at pre-medication.

Table 32.1a–1e   Antiemetic drug classes, target receptor, main therapeutic indications and side-effects

Drug Class	Generic name	Route of administration	Main indication in nausea and vomiting	Main side-effects	Comments
1a Target receptor: dopamine (D_2)					
Phenothiazines	Prochlorperazine	Oral, i.v., IM. rectal	PONV, GI induced emesis mild CINV	Dystonia, tardive dyskinesia in prolonged use, lower seizure threshold, hypotension	Also some muscarinic, histaminergic and serotonergic (5-HT_2) activity
	Chlorpromazine	Oral, i.v., rectal	Not often used		
	Levomepromazine (methotrimeprazine)	Oral, s.c. bolus or infusion	Terminal care		Has tranquillizing, anxiolytic and analgesic effects
Benzamides	Metoclopramide	Oral, i.v.	GI induced emesis, gastric stasis (e.g. migraine) CINV	Akathisia, dystonia, tardive dyskinesia	Blocks the inhibitory effect of DA on the cholinergic stimulation of gut smooth muscle
	Domperidone	Oral, rectal	GI induced emesis, nausea caused by dopamine agonists	Dystonia (rarely)	Penetrates brain poorly
	Cisapride		Gastric stasis (see comments)	Arrhythmias, multiple drug interactions	No longer used in UK because of adverse cardiac effects
Butyrophenones	Droperidol		PONV (see comments)	Arrhythmias	No longer used in UK because of adverse cardiac effects
	Haloperidol	Oral, i.m. i.v.	Palliative care, PONV	Dyskinesia	Acts at CTZ Long half-life (18 hours)
1b Target receptor: 5-hydroxytryptamine-3 (serotonin 5-HT_3)					
Serotonin (5-HT_3) antagonists	Ondansetron	Oral, i.v., rectal	CINV, PONV, radiotherapy	Mild headache, constipation, dizziness	
	Granisetron	Oral, i.v.			12 hourly dosing
	Tropisetron	Oral, i.v.,			See ondansetron
					See ondansetron
1c Target receptor: acetylcholine (muscarinic)					
Anticholinergics	Hyoscine (scopolamine)	t.d.	Motion sickness	Blurred vision, urinary retention, constipation	Hydrobromide salt used

Table 32.1a–1e continued

Drug Class	Generic name	Route of administration	Main indication in nausea and vomiting	Main side-effects	Comments
1d Target receptor: histamine (H₁)					
Antihistamines	Cyclizine	Oral, i.m. i.v.	PONV, motion sickness, hyperemesis gravidum	Sedation	
	Promethazine	Oral	Motion sickness, hyperemesis gravidum		Used as the teoclate salt (longer than the hydrochloride)
acting	Cinnarizine	Oral	Motion sickness		
1e Target receptor variable					
Corticosteroids	Dexamethasone	Oral, i.v.	CINV, PONV	Insomnia, mood changes	Receptor affected uncertain, but steroid receptors may exist in NTS area postrema
and	Erythromycin		Gastric stasis		Acts on motilin receptors
Alternative therapy	Acupuncture		Motion sickness		Receptor affected uncertain
Cannabinoids	Nabilone	Oral	CINV	Dysphoria, sedation, depression, hypotension	

t.d. transdermal; s.c. subcutaneous; i.v. intravenous; i.m. intramuscular, GI, gastrointestinal; CTZ, chemoreceptor trigger zone; PONV, postoperative nausea and vomiting; CINV, chemotherapy-induced nausea and vomiting; NTS, nucleus tractus solitarus

Table 32.2 Causes of nausea and vomiting
Infections (acute)
Drug use (acute)
Uncontrolled diabetes mellitus (acute)
Gastric mucosal disease (neoplasm, amyloid, eosinophilic gastroenteritis)
Motion sickness
Labyrinthitis (associated with vertigo and nystagmus)
Dietary indiscretion/over-indulgence
Migraine
Early pregnancy
Drugs (cytotoxics)
Radiotherapy
Postoperative (anaesthetic, type of surgery, length of surgery)
Diseases of gastrointestinal tract
Neurogenic (may be positional, projectile, or associated with neurologic symptoms or signs)
Gastric motility

Table 32.3   Approaches to postoperative nausea and vomiting (PONV)

For major in-patient surgery	For uncomplicated or out-patient surgery
At induction: Ondansetron 4 mg Cyclizine 50 mg Prochlorperazine 12.5 mg	**At induction:** Cyclizine 50 mg i.v. i.m. or prochlorperazine 12.5 mg i.m. plus ondansetron 4 mg i.v. if necessary (e.g. history of PONV)
Rescue if necessary: Ondansetron 4 mg Plus cyclizine 50 mg } for at least 24 hours	**Rescue if necessary:** Prochlorperazine 12.5 mg i.m. or cyclizine 50 mg i.v.
	Rescue at home after out-patient surgery: Prochlorperazine 10 mg every 5 hours, rectal

Risk scores

Prophylaxis is preferable to treatment and this can often be achieved not only by the use of antiemetic drugs but also by suitable planning. For example, not all patients undergoing surgery will experience PONV and a scoring system may be used to assess the risk of it occurring (Koivuranta et al 1997). This takes into account such factors as the patient's medical condition and the length and type of the anaesthesia and the surgery. A simple scoring system has been devised in which the score increases relative to the presence or absence of the following four factors: female gender, history of motion sickness or PONV, non-smoker and use of postoperative opioids (Apfel et al 1999).

Chemotherapy-induced nausea and vomiting (CINV)

Three different types of CINV have been identified: acute, delayed and anticipatory. Acute emesis begins within 1 or 2 hours of treatment and peaks in the first 4–6 hours. Delayed emesis occurs more than 24 hours after treatment, peaks at 48–72 hours and then subsides over 2–3 days. It is a characteristic feature of high dose cisplatin but also occurs with carboplatin, cyclophosphamide and anthracyclines. Anticipatory emesis is a conditioned response in patients who have developed significant CINV during previous cycles of therapy. Acute CINV is often associated with an increase in plasma serotonin concentrations for the most emetogenic agents, while delayed and anticipatory vomiting seem to be mediated by serotonin-independent pathways.

Management of CINV depends on the emetogenicity of the chemotherapy regimen and the use of combinations of antiemetic drugs based on their varying target receptors. Chemotherapy agents are divided into five emetogenic levels defined by expected frequency of emesis (Hesketh et al 1997) (Table 32.4). A CINV management strategy is outlined in Table 32.5.

In high level acute emesis, a single dose of 5-HT_3 antagonist given before chemotherapy is therapeutically equivalent to a multidose regimen. Oral formulations of antiemetics are often as effective as intravenous ones. In lower level acute emesis the cost of the 5-HT_3 antagonists is prohibitive and metoclopramide or prochlorperazine are commonly used and are effective. Dexamethasone is the most extensively evaluated steroid in the management of CINV. Used alone it is not sufficiently potent. However, it enhances the effect of other agents such as 5-HT_3 antagonists and metoclopramide and is particularly effective in treating delayed emesis. The best management for anticipatory emesis is the avoidance of acute and delayed emesis during previous cycles. However, when anticipatory nausea and vomiting is a problem, a low dose of a benzodiazepine such as lorazepam is often effective.

When apparently appropriate antiemesis regimens fail, consideration should be given to other disease and medication related issues (Table 32.6).

Pregnancy-associated nausea and vomiting

Pregnancy associated nausea and vomiting occurs in about 70% of women during the first trimester. Symptoms usually begin 4 weeks after the last menses and end at 12 weeks, having peaked at 9 weeks. First trimester nausea and vomiting are usually not harmful to either the fetus or the mother and need to be distinguished from hyperemesis gravidarum which is a condition of intractable vomiting complicating between 1% and 5% of pregnancies and sometimes resulting in serious fluid and electrolyte disturbance.

In first trimester nausea and vomiting, simple measures such as small frequent carbohydrate-rich meals and reassurance are sufficient to control symptoms. It is important to avoid drugs if possible. In hyperemesis gravidarum, drug therapy may be helpful in association with fluid and electrolyte replacement, rest and if necessary post-pyloric or parenteral feeding.

Table 32.4   Emetogenicity of chemotherapy drugs (Hesketh et al 1997)

Level	Agent	Dose (mg/m^2)
5	Carmustine	> 250
	Cisplatin	≥ 50
	Cyclophosphamide	*> 1500*
	Dacarbazine	
4	Carboplatin	
	Carmustine	≤ 250
	Cisplatin	< 50
	Cyclophosphamide	> 750 up to 1500
	Cytarabine	> 1000
	Doxorubicin	> 60
	Methotrexate	> 1000
	Procarbazine (oral)	
3	Cyclophosphamide	≤ 750
	Cyclophosphamide (oral)	
	Doxorubicin	20–60
	Epirubicin	≤ 90
	Idarubicin	
	Ifosfamide	
	Methotrexate	250–1000
	Mitoxantrone (mitozantrone)	< 15
2	Docetaxel	
	Etoposide	
	5-fluorouracil	< 1000
	Methotrexate	> 50 < 250
	Mitomycin	
	Paclitaxel	
1	Bleomycin	
	Busulfan	
	Chlorambucil (oral)	
	Hydroxycarbamide (hydroxyurea)	
	Methotrexate	≤ 50
	Tioguanine (oral)	
	Vinblastine	
	Vincristine	

Level 5 = > 90% of patients experience acute emesis without antiemetic drugs.
Level 4 = 60–90; level 3 = 30–60%; level 2 = 10–30%; level 1 = < 10%.

Table 32.5   Approaches to the treatment of chemotherapy induced nausea and vomiting (CINV)

Anticipatory nausea and vomiting
Lorazepam 1–2 mg oral/i.v. prior to chemotherapy

Highly emetogenic chemotherapy (Level 4/5 in Table 32.4)
Ondansetron 8 mg i.v. plus dexamethasone 8 mg i.v. pre-chemotherapy
Then:
Ondansetron 8 mg oral twice daily for up to 4 days and oral dexamethasone 4 mg four times a day for 2–3 days
Then:
Metoclopramide oral 10–20 mg four times a day if required
Continue oral dexamethasone at a dose of 4 mg daily for 5 days if delayed vomiting occurs

Moderately emetogenic chemotherapy (Level 3)
Ondansetron 8 mg i.v. plus dexamethasone 8 mg slow i.v. pre-chemotherapy
Then:
Metoclopramide oral 10–20 mg four times a day for 5 days if required
Add oral dexamethasone 4 mg daily if delayed emesis occurs

Mildly emetogenic chemotherapy (Level 2)
Metoclopramide 10 mg i.v. pre-chemotherapy. If necessary add dexamethasone 8 mg i.v. with chemotherapy
Then:
Metoclopramide oral 10–20 mg four times a day as required

Chemotherapy unlikely to cause emesis (Level 1)
Metoclopramide oral 10 mg every 4–6 hours as required

Table 32.6   Failure of apparently appropriate CINV prophylaxis regimens

Consider other causes of nausea and vomiting such as:
- Hypercalcaemia or other metabolic disturbance
- CNS metastases
- Antibiotics such as erythromycin
- GI obstruction
- Radiotherapy enteropathy

For hyperemesis gravidarum and for severe symptoms in early pregnancy there are few safety or efficacy data on which to base drug selection but there is reasonable evidence for the safety of antiemetics such as cyclizine, dimenhydrinate, metoclopramide, prochlorperazine, and promethazine, and all are likely to be effective. In resistant cases there is some suggestion that the use of corticosteroids or pyridoxine may help (Safari et al 1998). The drugs in the first group should be the treatment of choice, but steroids may offer a useful second-line therapy in patients with resistant symptoms.

Migraine

Migraine is a paroxysmal disorder with attacks of headaches, nausea, vomiting, photophobia, phonophobia and malaise. Treatment is directed at:

1. prophylaxis (avoid triggers, try β-blockers, pizotifen and in severe cases a 5-HT$_{1B/D}$ receptor agonist such as sumatriptan)
2. analgesia, including aspirin, paracetamol, opioids, NSAIDs and in severe cases a triptan
3. antiemetics.

Nausea and vomiting in migraine are commonly associated with gastric stasis which in addition to aggravating the symptoms also results in delayed or suppressed absorption of analgesics. Metoclopramide and domperidone attenuate the autonomic dysfunction and promote gastric emptying. The major adverse effect of acute dystonic crisis with metoclopramide therapy should be borne in mind, especially in young women and children.

Labyrinthitis

Labyrinthine dysfunction results in vertigo, nausea and vomiting. Episodes may last a few hours or days. Causes include labyrinth viral infections, tumours and Ménière's disease. The onset of episodes is often unpredictable and disabling. Betahistine has some prophylactic effect. The anticholinergics, antihistamines, phenothiazines or benzodiazepines can be used to suppress the vestibular system. Usually scopolamine, meclozine or diphenhydramine are sufficient, but if there is severe vomiting prochlorperazine or metoclopramide are of value.

Motion sickness

Motion sickness is a syndrome, a collection of symptoms without an identifiable cause. It is brought on by chronic repetitive movements which stimulate afferent pathways to the vestibular nuclei and lead to activation of the brainstem nuclei. Histaminergic and muscarinic pathways are involved.

The symptoms include vague epigastric discomfort, headache, cold sweating and nausea which may culminate in vomiting. This is often followed by marked fatigue which can last hours or days. Onset of symptoms may be abrupt or gradual. Anticholinergic and antihistamine drugs are equally effective but adverse effects are common and troublesome. Hence the relative duration of action and available dose form are usually the main criteria for drug selection. Hyoscine is probably the drug of choice, but frequently causes blurred vision and drowsiness, even after transdermal administration. Cinnarizine is also effective and is claimed to cause drowsiness less often. In tablet form, both are absorbed from the buccal or sublingual mucosa when chewed, which may facilitate administration, especially in children. Antihistamine drugs are also effective, including cyclizine, promethazine and dimenhydrinate. Treatment should be started before travel; for long journeys, promethazine or transdermal hyoscine may be preferred for their longer duration (24 hours and 3 days, respectively). Otherwise, repeated doses will be needed. Cyclizine should probably be avoided because of its abuse potential.

The most important adverse reaction of the useful drugs is sedation, and for anticholinergic drugs, blurred vision, urinary retention and constipation. In laboratory studies, the degree to which these effects impair performance, for example driving a car, is highly variable, but subjects who take anti-motion sickness drugs should normally be deemed unfit for such tasks. These drugs also potentiate the effects of alcohol.

It is of note that dopamine and 5-HT$_3$ antagonists are generally not effective in the treatment of motion sickness.

Many non-drug treatments have been advocated for alleviation, including wristbands, which act on acupuncture points, variously positioned pieces of coloured paper or card, as well as plant extracts such as ginger. Controlled or comparative studies have generally not incorporated any of the wide range of alternative options and, except for the effects of wrist bands, there seems to be no sound basis for their proposed effects.

Drug-associated nausea and vomiting

Drugs such as syrup of ipecacuanha which contains the alkaloids emetine and cephaeline may be used to cause vomiting in the treatment of poisoning. Common drugs which cause nausea and vomiting are opiates, dopamine agonists, theophylline, erythromycin and amino-glycosides. High dose oestrogen, as in post-coital contraception, often causes nausea and vomiting. There are no trial data but antihistamines such as cinnarizine seem to help. In the management of such symptoms consideration should be given to altering the dose and administering with food. With many drugs tolerance may develop. Tolerance to the emetic effects of opiates develops within a few days and therefore antiemetic therapy is not needed for long-term use.

Palliative care

Nausea and vomiting are common in patients with carcinomas and may be due to a variety of factors related to the site of the tumour itself, or to infection, renal failure or drugs. About one-third of patients who receive morphine will suffer from nausea and vomiting initially but tolerance develops and the effect disappears after 5–10 days. Various drugs can be used to counter the emetogenic effects of morphine such as metoclopramide, prochlorperazine, cyclizine and domperidone.

In advanced cancer, haloperidol is an effective antiemetic which can be given as a single dose at night (1.5 mg orally or subcutaneously). Levomepromazine (methotrimeprazine) is a phenothiazine which acts at dopaminergic, muscarinic, histaminergic and 5HT$_2$ receptors. It is useful in the treatment of nausea and vomiting, especially in the last few days of terminal illness. This drug also has analgesic, anxiolytic and tranquillizing activity. Its duration of action is between 12 and 24 hours which allows once daily administration, either orally or subcutaneously. It can also be given as a subcutaneous infusion.

Table 32.7 examines some common therapeutic problems in the management of nausea and vomiting.

Table 32.7 Common therapeutic problems in nausea and vomiting

Problem	Possible cause/solution
Persistent nausea and vomiting despite treatment	Is the cause correctly diagnosed? Review the antiemetic drug and the dose: if both correct, change to or add a second drug
Patient with PONV is vomiting despite correct antiemetic regimen	Check analgesia: pain may be causing nausea and vomiting or patient may be receiving maximum doses of patient controlled analgesia (PCA) which may require adjustment
Patient with bowel obstruction is passing flatus	Pro-kinetic drug is first choice antiemetic. 5-HT$_3$ antagonists may also be effective
Patient with bowel obstruction is not passing flatus	Spasmolytic drug is first choice. Pro-kinetic drugs are contraindicated. Similarly bulk forming, osmotic and stimulant laxatives are inappropriate; phosphate enemas and faecal softeners are better
A terminally ill patient receiving diamorphine is vomiting despite haloperidol	Levomepromazine (methotrimeprazine) given as a 24-hour subcutaneous infusion is very effective
A patient with renal failure is vomiting	Try a 5-HT$_3$ antagonist
A patient develops an acute dystonic reaction to metoclopramide	Give an intramuscular injection of diphenhydramine. Such extrapyramidal reactions to metoclopramide are more common in young female adults and its use is best avoided in these patients if possible

PONV, postoperative nausea and vomiting.

CASE STUDIES

Case 32.1

A 30-year-old man presents seeking a remedy for vomiting which had an acute onset, 12 hours previously.

Question

What questions should be asked to determine the nature, cause and seriousness of these symptoms?

Answer

The cause of vomiting requires eliciting where possible to allow appropriate treatment to be initiated. The following questions should be asked:

- Are there symptoms of infection, such as diarrhoea, sore throat, dysuria, photophobia, fever? (Infection is one of the commonest causes of vomiting.)
- Is there headache? (Raised intracranial pressure and meningitis can present with vomiting as an early symptom, usually without any nausea.)
- Is there abdominal pain? (Abdominal pain before vomiting usually means an organic gastrointestinal cause. Pain after vomiting may be due to muscle tenderness.)
- Has the patient started any new drugs? (Opiates, chemotherapeutic agents, digoxin, nicotine, non-steroidal anti-inflammatory drugs, oral hypoglycaemics and some antibiotics are common causes.)
- Is there vertigo? (If present, this is suggestive of labyrinthitis.)

Case 32.2

A 19-year-old girl who is 12 weeks pregnant presents to hospital with intractable nausea and vomiting which has not responded to home therapy and which has resulted in hypotension and dehydration.

Question

List, in order of importance, the therapeutic strategies.

Answer

1. Intravenous re-hydration and electrolyte replacement
2. Bed rest
3. Individually introduced antiemetics such as cyclizine, dimenhydrinate, metoclopramide, prochlorperazine or perphenazine are likely to be effective and there is little evidence to suggest that they have teratogenic effects
4. Post-pyloric feeding
5. Steroids
6. Parenteral nutrition.

Case 32.3

A 45-year-old woman presents with ovarian carcinoma for which she is due to receive a course of cancer chemotherapy.

Question

What drugs might be appropriate, when should they be given, and what advice should be given to the patient regarding monitoring of symptoms after treatment with the chemotherapy?

Answer

This woman is likely to receive repeated cycles of emetic chemotherapy and therefore should be given prophylactic antiemetics before the start of chemotherapy. The choice of drugs lies between metoclopramide combined with steroids and a benzodiazepine, and one of the 5-HT$_3$ receptor antagonists ondansetron, granisetron or tropisetron. The monitoring of emesis and nausea both within and outside hospital for up to 5 days after treatment is a useful exercise in deciding which patients may need other therapies. It is also important to remember that patients should be given appropriate doses of antiemetics as rescue therapy to cover delayed-onset nausea.

Case 32.4

A hospital with a large number of surgical specialities including major in-patient thoraco-abdominal and day care procedures wishes to update its PONV programme.

Question

What principles for a PONV programme should be taken into account?

Answer

The programme should contain a PONV risk score which can be used in pre-operation assessment and which includes the medical condition of the patient, the length and type of surgery, the length and type of anaesthesia and the postoperative recovery period. This would help decide which PONV prophylaxis therapy is appropriate. PONV rescue therapy should be devised depending on the postoperative clinical situation.

REFERENCES

AGA Technical Review 2000 American Gastroenterology Association Clinical Practice and Practice Economics Committee. Nausea and vomiting, May 2000. AGA National Office, Bethesda, Maryland

Apfel C, Laara E, Koivuranta M et al 1999 A simplified risk score for predicting post-anaesthetic nausea and vomiting. Anaesthesiology 91: 693–700

Hesketh P J, Kris M G, Grunberg S M et al 1997 Proposal for classifying the acute emetogenicity of cancer chemotherapy. Journal of Clinical Oncology 15: 103

Koivuranta M, Laara E, Snare L et al 1997 A survey of postoperative nausea and vomiting. Anaesthesia 52: 443–449

Kovac A L 2000 Prevention and treatment of postoperative nausea and vomiting. Drugs 59(2): 213–243

Safari H R, Alsulyman O M, Gherman R B et al 1998 Experience with oral methylprednisolone in the treatment of refractory hyperemesis gravidarum. American Journal of Obstetrics and Gynecology 178(5): 1054–1058

Wang J J, Ho S T, Liu H S et al 2000 Prophylactic antiemetic effect of dexamethasone in women undergoing ambulatory laparoscopic surgery. British Journal of Anaesthesia 84(4): 459–462

FURTHER READING

Anon. 1998 Managing migraine. Drugs and Therapeutic Bulletin 36(6): 41–44

Diener H C, Kaube H, Limmroth V 1998 A practical guide to management and prevention of migraine. Drugs 56(5): 811–824

Heffernan A M, Rowbotham D J 2000 Post-operative nausea and vomiting: time for balanced antiemesis. British Journal of Anaesthesia 85(5): 675–677

Morganstern D E, Hesketh P J 1999 Chemotherapy induced nausea and vomiting. In: Vokes E E, Golomb H M (eds) Oncologic Therapies. Springer Verlag, Berlin, pp. 1115–1135

Nolte M J, Berkery R, Pizzo B et al 1998 Assuring the optimal use of serotonin antagonist antiemetics: the process for development and implementation of institutional antiemetic guidelines at Memorial Sloan-Kettering Cancer Center. Journal of Clinical Oncology 16(2): 771–778

Skinner J and Skinner A 1999 Levomepromazine for nausea and vomiting in advanced cancer. Hospital Medicine 60(8): 568–570

Tramer M R, Carroll D, Campbell F A et al 2001 Cannabinoids for control of chemotherapy induced nausea and vomiting: quantitative systematic review. British Medical Journal 323: 16–21

Respiratory infections

33

S. J. Pedler   A. W. Berrington

KEY POINTS

- An oral cephalosporin gives greater bacteriological and clinical efficacy than a penicillin in the treatment of streptococcal pharyngitis.
- There is controversy about whether otitis media should be treated with antibiotics or allowed to run its course.
- Exacerbations of chronic bronchitis may be infective in origin and antibiotics are part of their treatment, although other therapeutic modalities are also important.
- *Streptococcus pneumoniae* remains the single commonest cause of community-acquired pneumonia, but increasing resistance to penicillin in this organism may lead to problems in the treatment of serious pneumococcal infections.
- Community-acquired pneumonia usually requires treatment on a best-guess basis to cover a variety of possible pathogens. Amoxicillin plus erythromycin would be a typical regimen.
- There are many potential causes for hospital-acquired (nosocomial) pneumonia and each unit where patients are at risk of this condition will have its own resident bacterial flora; this will strongly influence the choice of antibiotics for empirical therapy.
- *Pseudomonas aeruginosa* remains the most important respiratory pathogen in cystic fibrosis patients, and antibiotic treatment is often aimed specifically at this organism.

Respiratory tract infections are the commonest group of infections seen in the UK. Most are viral in origin, for which generally there is only symptomatic therapy available, but bacterial infections are a major cause of treatable respiratory illness.

The respiratory tract is divided into upper and lower parts: the upper respiratory tract comprises the sinuses, middle ear, pharynx, epiglottis and larynx, while the lower respiratory tract consists of the structures below the larynx – the bronchi, bronchioles and alveoli. Although there are anatomical and functional divisions both within and between these regions, it should be remembered that infections do not necessarily respect such boundaries. Nevertheless, it is clinically and bacteriologically convenient to retain these distinctions. Upper respiratory tract infections are described first.

Upper respiratory tract infections

Colds and flu

Viral upper respiratory tract infections causing coryzal symptoms, rhinitis, pharyngitis and laryngitis, associated with varying degrees of systemic symptoms, are extremely common. These infections are usually caused by viruses from the rhinovirus, coronavirus, parainfluenza virus, respiratory syncytial virus, influenza virus and adenovirus families. Colloquially, milder infections are usually termed 'colds', while more severe infections may be known as 'flu'. However, true influenza, that is infection with one of the influenza viruses, A, B or rarely C, can be a serious condition characterized by marked malaise and myalgia, and potentially complicated by life-threatening secondary bacterial infections such as staphylococcal pneumonia.

In general the treatment of these infections is symptomatic, consisting of rest, adequate hydration, simple analgesics and antipyretics. However, influenza A and B infections are amenable to both prevention and treatment with neuraminidase inhibitors such as zanamivir. Inhaled zanamivir is about 75% effective in preventing influenza during periods of exposure, and treatment has been shown to reduce the duration of symptoms from about 5 days to 4 (Jefferson et al 2000). However, there is controversy about whether these figures justify the costs involved, and current recommendations in the UK state that zanamivir should be reserved for patients with specific risk factors who can commence treatment within 48 hours of onset (National Institute of Clinical Excellence 2000).

Sore throat (pharyngitis)

Causative organisms. Pharyngitis is a common condition and most cases never come to medical attention, being treated with simple therapy directed at symptom relief. Many cases are not due to infection at all, but are caused by other factors such as smoking. Where infection is the cause, most cases are of viral aetiology and reflect part of the 'colds and flu' spectrum.

Epstein–Barr virus (EBV), the cause of glandular fever (infectious mononucleosis), is a less common but important cause of sore throat since it may be confused with streptococcal infection.

There is only one common bacterial cause of sore throat, *Streptococcus pyogenes*, the group A β-haemolytic streptococcus. Less frequent causes include β-haemolytic streptococci of groups C and G, *Arcanobacterium haemolyticum*, *Neisseria gonorrhoeae*, and mycoplasmas. *Corynebacterium diphtheriae*, the cause of diphtheria, is rare in the UK but should be borne in mind in travellers returning from parts of the world where diphtheria is common.

Clinical features. The presenting complaint of pharyngitis is a sore throat. Many cases are associated with fever, often mild, and the usual symptoms of the common cold. More severe cases are associated with infection due to EBV or *Strep. pyogenes* and in these patients there may be marked inflammation of the pharynx with a whitish exudate on the tonsils, plus enlarged and tender cervical lymph nodes. Previously, streptococcal infection was frequently accompanied by a macular rash and sometimes considerable systemic illness (scarlet fever). This presentation is now very uncommon for reasons that are not clear, but may be a result of the huge increase in the use of antibiotics during the past three decades.

Group A streptococcal infection has a number of potential complications. Pharyngeal infection may occasionally give rise to disseminated infection elsewhere, but this is rare. However, otitis media and/or sinusitis are frequent accompaniments. More important are the non-suppurative complications of streptococcal infection, rheumatic fever and glomerulonephritis. Discussion of these is outside the scope of this chapter but occasional cases are still seen in the UK, and rheumatic fever remains common in developing countries.

Diagnosis. In most cases of pharyngitis a bacteriological diagnosis cannot be made, and these are presumed to be viral in origin. The aim of any diagnostic procedure is to distinguish the streptococcal sore throat, which is amenable to antibiotic treatment, from viral infections, which are not. Unfortunately, the presentation of glandular fever is similar to that of streptococcal infection and it may not be possible to differentiate between the two on clinical grounds alone. Therefore if streptococcal infection is suspected a throat swab should be taken for culture. Unless the details of a particular case prompt a search for more unusual organisms, culture techniques are directed towards detecting β-haemolytic streptococci. If bacterial culture is negative and EBV infection is suspected, blood should be taken for serology. Other viruses may be diagnosed by viral culture or serology, but this does not usually contribute to management.

Treatment. Treatment of viral sore throats is directed at symptomatic relief, for example with rest, antipyretics and aspirin gargles. Antibiotic treatment of streptococcal sore throat has been shown to relieve symptoms and reduce the incidence of suppurative and non-suppurative complications (Del Mar et al 2000). If streptococcal infection is suspected, treatment may be started before the results of throat swab culture are known; alternatively it is perfectly acceptable to await culture results before starting treatment. Although many busy clinicians would commence treatment on clinical grounds alone, the problem of resistance has led to increasing pressure on prescribers to restrict empirical antibiotic use, particularly for conditions that are frequently viral, of which pharyngitis is a good example.

Antibiotics effective against *Strep. pyogenes* include penicillins, cephalosporins and macrolides. Resistance to the penicillins and cephalosporins in group A streptococci has not so far been described, although occasional strains resistant to erythromycin are seen.

Penicillins such as benzylpenicillin (penicillin G) or phenoxymethylpenicillin (penicillin V) have traditionally been regarded as the treatment of choice for streptococcal sore throat. However, there is now convincing evidence that cephalosporins are more effective both in terms of clinical response and eradication of the organism from the oropharynx. This was summarized in a large meta-analysis (Pichichero & Margolis 1991) which reviewed 19 studies in which oral cephalosporins and penicillin were compared. Although individually these studies lacked statistical power, overall the bacteriological cure rate was 92% in the cephalosporin group compared with 84% in the penicillin group ($P < 0.0001$). The corresponding clinical cure rates were 95% for the cephalosporin and 89% for penicillin ($P < 0.001$). The reason for this may be that the penicillins are hydrolysed by β-lactamase producing organisms (such as anaerobes) naturally resident in the oropharynx, whereas the cephalosporins are not.

Despite this difference, it remains controversial whether the extra expense of prescribing a cephalosporin is worth it, and the two classes should probably be viewed jointly as first-line agents. Cefalexin is the preferred cephalosporin. Among the penicillins, amoxicillin is well absorbed and is conveniently given three times daily. However, since patients with glandular fever are highly likely to develop a skin rash if prescribed ampicillin, amoxicillin or related drugs, these should not be used unless EBV infection has been confidently excluded. Even against sensitive strains, macrolides such as erythromycin are demonstrably less effective than β-lactams.

Further controversy surrounds the preferred duration of treatment. Generally, patients feel better within 2–3 days, but to prevent transmission of infection or the development of rheumatic fever not only must symptoms be relieved but the organism must also be eradicated from the pharynx. With penicillin this requires 10 days of treatment, although it may be difficult to persuade patients of the benefits of continuing for so long after clinical cure. With the cephalosporins there is evidence that shorter courses may be as effective, but this awaits definitive study.

Acute epiglottitis

Acute epiglottitis is a rapidly progressive cellulitis of the epiglottis and adjacent structures. Local swelling has the potential to cause rapid-onset airway obstruction, and for this reason the condition is a medical emergency. Previously, almost all childhood cases and a high proportion of adult cases were caused by *Haemophilus influenzae* type b (Hib). A smaller proportion were caused by other organisms such as pneumococci, streptococci, and staphylococci. With the advent of routine vaccination against Hib this disease has become uncommon.

The typical patient is a child between 2 and 4 years with fever and difficulty speaking and breathing. The patient may drool because of impaired swallowing. The diagnosis is made clinically, and the initial management is concentrated upon establishing or maintaining an airway. This takes priority over all other diagnostic and therapeutic manoeuvres. Thereafter the diagnosis may be confirmed by visualization of the cherry-red epiglottis. Microbiological confirmation may be obtained by culturing the epiglottis and the blood.

In view of the high prevalence of amoxicillin resistance among encapsulated *H. influenzae*, the treatment of choice is with a third generation cephalosporin such as cefotaxime or ceftriaxone. If a sensitive organism is recovered, high dose parenteral amoxicillin may be substituted.

Otitis media

Causative organisms. Inflammation of the middle ear (otitis media) is a common condition seen most frequently in children under 3 years of age. Most cases are due to bacteria, although viruses such as influenza virus and rhinoviruses have been implicated in a sizeable minority. *Streptococcus pneumoniae* and *H. influenzae* are the two most commonly encountered bacterial pathogens. *Moraxella catarrhalis* and *Strep. pyogenes* account for a smaller proportion of cases, perhaps 10%, and other bacteria are seen only rarely.

Clinical features. Classically, otitis media presents with ear pain, which may be severe. If the drum perforates the pain is relieved and a purulent discharge from the ear may follow. There may be a degree of hearing impairment, plus non-specific symptoms such as fever or vomiting in very young children. Complications of otitis media include mastoiditis (now rare), meningitis

and, particularly in the case of *H. influenzae* infection, septicaemia and disseminated infection. With the advent of routine vaccination against Hib these complications have become uncommon.

Diagnosis. The diagnosis of otitis media is essentially made clinically and laboratory investigations have little role to play. Unless the drum is perforated there is little sense in sending a swab of the external auditory canal, the results of which are likely to be unhelpful or misleading. For this reason a causative organism is rarely isolated and treatment has to be given empirically.

Treatment. There has been much debate about whether or not antibiotics should be used for the initial treatment of otitis media. A large meta-analysis of placebo-controlled trials demonstrated that even without antibiotics, only 15% of cases fail to resolve spontaneously within 2 days (Glasziou et al 2000). Antibiotics reduce this to about 10%, meaning that 20 children need to be treated in order to prevent one having pain that persists beyond the first 2 days. Moreover there is no conclusive evidence that antibiotics reduce the risk of complications such as deafness or mastoiditis. It is debatable whether the limited benefits of antibiotics outweigh the disadvantages of cost, side-effects and promotion of antibiotic resistance, at least in first world countries in which the incidence of complications is low.

If treatment is to be given, it should be effective against the three main bacterial pathogens, *Strep. pneumoniae*, *H. influenzae* and *Strep. pyogenes*. *Strep. pyogenes* and the pneumococcus are both sensitive to penicillin, but penicillin is much less active against *H. influenzae* so the broader spectrum agents amoxicillin or ampicillin should be used instead. These two drugs have identical antibacterial activity, but amoxicillin is recommended for oral treatment since it is better absorbed from the gastrointestinal tract (80% vs. 50%). Patients with penicillin allergy may be treated with a later generation cephalosporin (see below).

Up to 15% of *H. influenzae* strains are resistant to amoxicillin due to production of β-lactamase. This may manifest clinically as treatment failure, so if there is no response to amoxicillin an alternative agent should be chosen. Both erythromycin and the earlier oral cephalosporins such as cefalexin are insufficiently active against *H. influenzae* and should not be used. Alternatives include co-amoxiclav (a combination of amoxicillin and the β-lactamase inhibitor clavulanic acid) or one of the newer oral cephalosporins such as cefixime, which possesses high activity against *H. influenzae*. Cefuroxime axetil, while active in vitro, is poorly absorbed and often causes diarrhoea.

Acute sinusitis

Causative organisms. Normally the paranasal sinuses are sterile, and sinusitis follows damage to the mucous membrane which lines them. This usually occurs following a viral upper respiratory tract infection but is sometimes associated with the presence of dental disease. Acute sinusitis is usually caused by the same organisms which cause otitis media but occasionally other organisms such as *Staphylococcus aureus*, viridans streptococci and anaerobes may be found. Viruses are occasionally found in conjunction with the bacteria.

Clinical features. The main feature of acute sinusitis is facial pain and tenderness, often accompanied by headache and a purulent nasal discharge. Complications include frontal bone osteomyelitis, meningitis and brain abscess. The condition may become chronic with persistent low grade pain and nasal discharge, sometimes with acute exacerbations.

Diagnosis. As with otitis media this is a clinical diagnosis, and obtaining specimens for bacteriological examination is not usually practicable. In patients with chronic sinusitis therapeutic sinus washouts may yield specimens for microbiology.

Treatment. Since the causative organisms are the same as those found in otitis media, the same recommendations for treatment apply. Proximity to the mouth means that anaerobes are implicated quite frequently in acute sinusitis, particularly if associated with dental disease, and in such cases the addition of metronidazole may be worthwhile. Doxycycline has proved popular, particularly in chronic sinusitis, due to its broad spectrum of activity and once daily dosage.

Lower respiratory infections

Bronchitis

Bronchitis means inflammation of the bronchi. It is important to distinguish between acute bronchitis, which is usually infective, and chronic bronchitis, which is not primarily an infective condition. Chronic bronchitis is defined both clinically (production of sputum on most days for 3 or more consecutive months during 2 or more years), and pathologically (thickened, oedematous bronchial mucosa with mucus gland hypertrophy), and often coexists with emphysema, giving rise to an all too common syndrome known by terms such as chronic obstructive airways disease (COAD), chronic obstructive pulmonary disease (COPD), and chronic airflow limitation (CAL). The main risk factor is smoking, with repeated viral or bacterial respiratory infections and dust inhalation being important secondary factors. For the purposes of this chapter the importance of chronic bronchitis is that it renders the patient more susceptible to acute infections, and more likely to suffer respiratory compromise as a result. These 'acute exacerbations of chronic bronchitis' are a frequent cause of morbidity and admission to hospital.

Causative organisms. In otherwise healthy patients, the causes of acute bronchitis include viruses such as rhinovirus, coronavirus, adenovirus and influenza virus, and bacteria such as *Bordetella pertussis*, *Mycoplasma pneumoniae* and *Chlamydia pneumoniae*. The role of bacteria such as *Strep. pneumoniae* and *H. influenzae* is uncertain because these organisms are nasopharyngeal commensals and their isolation can be misleading.

Similarly, in patients with chronic bronchitis, examination of sputum at times other than during an exacerbation frequently yields potential pathogens, particularly *Strep. pneumoniae* and *H. influenzae*. During an acute exacerbation the same two pathogens are found, and the rate of isolation is not markedly increased. Other organisms which may be detected are *Moraxella catarrhalis*, which is becoming increasingly recognized in this condition, *Staph. aureus*, haemolytic streptococci, and Gram-negative bacilli. A considerable proportion (perhaps up to half) of acute exacerbations are associated with viral infections such as colds or influenza.

Since no single pathogen has been unequivocally associated with causing acute exacerbations of COAD, and since the two main suspect organisms are isolated at almost the same frequency during an exacerbation as in the absence of one, doubt has been cast on the role of bacterial infection in this condition. Nevertheless, antibiotics are now accepted as part of the standard treatment for exacerbations of COAD.

Clinical features. The characteristic feature of acute bronchitis is a cough productive of purulent sputum (i.e. phlegm that is yellow or green, the colour reflecting the presence of pus cells), sometimes with wheezing and breathlessness. In patients with pre-existing lung disease the lack of reserve may lead to respiratory compromise, which in turn may exacerbate, or be exacerbated by, cardiac failure. Sometimes the condition progresses into a frank bronchopneumonia (see below), although the dividing line between a severe exacerbation of COAD and bronchopneumonia is blurred.

Diagnosis. The diagnosis of acute bronchitis or an acute exacerbation of COAD is made clinically. Where possible a sputum sample should be sent for bacteriology, which will at least allow antibiotic sensitivity tests to be performed on potential pathogens. The sputum of patients who have received broad-spectrum agents such as amoxicillin or cephalosporins frequently yields organisms such as Gram-negative bacilli, staphylococci and yeasts. Care should be taken when interpreting such results as the oropharynx often becomes colonized with these organisms due to elimination of the normal upper respiratory flora, and they are not usually representative of the bronchial pathogen.

Treatment. There are two main arms of treatment, antibiotic therapy and supportive care. Supportive care consists of physiotherapy to aid expectoration of secretions, bronchodilators and sometimes corticosteroids. In severe cases a period of artificial ventilation may be required, an intervention which may become more common with the advent of non-invasive ventilation techniques.

Empirical antibiotic therapy should be directed against the main infecting organisms as described above. Amoxicillin is the drug of choice, with co-amoxiclav if β-lactamase producing strains of *H. influenzae* are confirmed or suspected. For penicillin-allergic patients, neither erythromycin nor the earlier oral cephalosporins such as cefalexin or cefradine are sufficiently active against *H. influenzae*. Cefaclor is slightly more active but is associated with a higher incidence of skin side-effects, especially in children, and the slightly greater activity does not justify the increased risk to the patient. Newer oral cephalosporins such as cefixime and cefpodoxime are much more active against *H. influenzae* while retaining activity against pneumococci. The macrolide clarithromycin is also active, and most strains are also sensitive to trimethoprim or tetracyclines. *M. catarrhalis* usually produces β-lactamase, but most strains are sensitive to co-amoxiclav and the newer oral cephalosporins.

Accordingly, the following recommendations can be made for the antibiotic treatment of acute bronchitis and exacerbations of COAD:

First line agents:

- amoxicillin
- doxycycline
- trimethoprim.

Second line agents:

- co-amoxiclav
- cefixime
- clarithromycin.

A number of other drugs are sometimes promoted for the treatment of exacerbations of COAD. Of these, azithromycin is not recommended since it is less active against *Strep. pneumoniae* than clarithromycin. The activity of ciprofloxacin against *Strep. pneumoniae* is generally felt to be insufficient to justify its use as monotherapy against pneumococcal infections. Levofloxacin does not seem to possess any microbiological advantage over ciprofloxacin, but newer quinolones (such as moxifloxacin) promising greater activity against Gram-positive organisms are likely to become widely used. There is good evidence that trimethoprim is as effective as co-trimoxazole in this condition, so trimethoprim alone is preferred due to the higher toxicity of co-trimoxazole.

Bronchiolitis

Bronchiolitis is characterized by inflammatory changes in the small bronchi and bronchioles, but not by consolidation. It is particularly recognized as a disease of infants in the first year of life, in whom a small degree of airway narrowing can have drastic effects on airflow, but the causal organisms are no less capable of infecting adults, who may act as a reservoir of infection. Most cases are caused by respiratory syncytial virus (RSV), which occurs in annual winter epidemics, but parainfluenzaviruses, rhinoviruses, adenoviruses and occasionally *Mycoplasma pneumoniae* have also been implicated.

The disease is characterized by a prodrome of fever and coryzal symptoms which progresses to wheezing, respiratory distress and hypoxia of varying degrees. Aetiological confirmation may be made by immunofluorescence and viral culture of respiratory secretions, but increasingly, diagnosis of RSV is made using rapid antigen detection tests.

The treatment of bronchiolitis is mainly supportive, consisting of oxygen, adequate hydration and ventilatory assistance if required. Severe cases of RSV disease may be treated with ribavirin, a synthetic nucleoside which is administered by nebulization for 12–18 hours on each of 3–7 successive days.

Pneumonia

Pneumonia is defined as inflammation of the lung parenchyma (i.e. of the alveoli rather than the bronchi), of infective origin and characterized by consolidation. Consolidation is a pathological process in which the alveoli are filled with a mixture of inflammatory exudate, bacteria and white blood cells, which is revealed on chest X-ray as an opaque area in the normally clear lung fields.

The range of organisms which can cause pneumonia is wide, so it is useful to apply some kind of classification system. Pneumonia may be classified clinically into lobar pneumonia, bronchopneumonia or atypical pneumonia, but this does not correlate entirely with the bacteriological cause; a better method is to classify pneumonia by place of origin, as either community-acquired pneumonia (CAP) or hospital-acquired pneumonia (HAP, sometimes known as nosocomial pneumonia).

Community-acquired pneumonia

Causative organisms. The causes of community-acquired pneumonia are summarized in Table 33.1. The commonest is *Strep. pneumoniae*, the pneumococcus. Classically this organism causes lobar pneumonia, but now it is more frequently seen as a cause of bronchopneumonia. The other major bacterial causes are

Table 33.1	Causes of community-acquired pneumonia
Organism	**Comments**
Streptococcus pneumoniae	Classically causes lobar pneumonia, bronchopneumonia now common
Haemophilus influenzae	Cause of bronchopneumonia, usually non-capsulate strains
Staphylococcus aureus	Severe pneumonia with abscess formation, typically following influenza
Klebsiella pneumoniae	Friedlander's bacillus, which causes an uncommon but severe necrotizing pneumonia
Legionella pneumophila	Particularly serogroup 1; causes Legionnaire's disease, usually acquired from aquatic environmental sources
Mycoplasma pneumoniae	Cause of acute pneumonia in young people, symptoms often overshadowed by systemic upset
Chlamydia pneumoniae	Mild but prolonged illness usually seen in older people, symptoms often overshadowed by systemic upset
Chlamydia psittaci	Causes psittacosis, a respiratory and multisystem disease acquired from infected birds
Coxiella burnetii	Causes Q fever, a respiratory and multisystem disease acquired from animals such as sheep
Viruses	Several viruses can cause pneumonia in adults, including influenza, parainfluenza, and varicella zoster viruses

non-capsulate strains of *H. influenzae*; here the usual picture is of a bronchopneumonia.

The so-called atypical pneumonias comprise a heterogeneous group of diseases which nevertheless have several clinical features in common. Aetiological agents include *Mycoplasma pneumoniae*, *Chlamydia pneumoniae*, *Chlamydia psittaci*, *Coxiella burnetii*, and viruses. *Legionella pneumophila* is the cause of Legionnaire's disease. This infection occurs mainly in

outbreaks associated with contaminated air-conditioning or water systems, but sporadic cases arise occasionally. It may be rapidly progressive with very extensive consolidation and respiratory failure.

Clinical features. The clinical presentation of lobar pneumonia is with cough, initially dry but later producing purulent or bloodstained, rust-coloured sputum, together with dyspnoea, fever and pleuritic chest pain. There is usually a markedly elevated peripheral white blood cell count, and the patient may be bacteraemic. Chest X-ray shows consolidation confined to one or more lobes (or segments of lobes) of the lungs. This classical picture is now quite rare perhaps because the early use of antibiotics modifies the natural history of the disease. Bronchopneumonia is an ill-defined entity with similar symptoms but with a chest X-ray that shows patchy consolidation, usually in the bases of both lungs. This disease is very common and is typically seen in patients with severe COAD or in those who are terminally ill.

The atypical pneumonias are characterized clinically by fever, systemic symptoms and a dry cough, radiologically by widespread patchy consolidation in both lung fields, and biochemically by abnormalities in liver enzymes and perhaps evidence of inappropriate antidiuretic hormone secretion. However, clinical features alone are not usually sufficient to make a confident bacteriological diagnosis, and this has major implications for the empirical treatment of pneumonia (see below).

Diagnosis. Sputum culture is the mainstay of diagnosis for pneumonia caused by pneumococci and *H. influenzae*. Sputum microscopy is unreliable because oropharyngeal contaminants are often indistinguishable from pathogens. In pneumococcal disease blood cultures are frequently positive, and some laboratories also perform serum and urine testing for pneumococcal antigen. *Legionella* may be cultured if appropriate media are used, but culture of mycoplasmata and chlamydia is beyond the scope of most routine diagnostic laboratories. In atypical pneumonia the cause is usually determined serologically, if at all.

The success of sputum culture is very dependent upon the quality of the specimen, which may be inadequate either because the patient is unable to expectorate or because the nature of the disease is such that sputum production is not a major feature. Techniques which have been used to overcome this problem include trans-tracheal aspiration (in which a cannula is inserted into the trachea through the cricothyroid membrane and sputum aspirated with a syringe), which is popular in the USA but has never been used widely in the UK, and open lung biopsy. However, the most commonly used procedure is bronchoscopy with bronchoalveolar lavage. Lavage fluid, being uncontaminated by mouth flora, is suitable for microscopy as well as culture.

Treatment. The treatment of choice for pneumococcal pneumonia is benzylpenicillin or amoxicillin. Erythromycin may be used in penicillin-hypersensitive patients, but resistance rates are rising. Pneumococci with reduced sensitivity to penicillin are becoming increasingly common, particularly in continental Europe and the USA, and it is likely that these organisms will be seen with increasing frequency in the UK. Reduced sensitivity to penicillin may result in treatment failures in conditions such as otitis media or meningitis, infections at sites where antibiotic penetration is reduced. Fortunately antibiotic penetration into the lungs is sufficiently good that penicillin and amoxicillin remain effective for infections caused by all but the most resistant strains (minimum inhibitory concentration > 1 microgram/ml). Such strains are often co-resistant to macrolides and other first-line agents, and may require treatment with a later generation cephalosporin or a glycopeptide.

The sensitivity of *H. influenzae* to antibiotics has been discussed above. Amoxicillin is the agent of choice, with co-amoxiclav, parenteral cefuroxime, cefixime or ciprofloxacin as alternatives.

M. pneumoniae does not possess a cell wall and is therefore not susceptible to β-lactams. A tetracycline or a macrolide are suitable alternatives. Tetracyclines are also effective against *Chlamydia pneumoniae*, *C. psittaci* and *Coxiella burnetii*, but erythromycin is probably less effective. Treatment should be continued for at least 14 days. It is increasingly recognized that quinolones are active against these organisms.

Staphylococcal pneumonia is usually treated with flucloxacillin plus another agent such as rifampicin, fusidic acid or gentamicin. MRSA (methicillin-resistant *Staph. aureus*) pneumonia is rarely seen outside hospital, and its management demands specialist microbiological advice.

Treatment recommendations for Legionnaire's disease are based on a retrospective review of the well-known Philadelphia outbreak of 1976 (Fraser et al 1977), in which two deaths occurred among the 18 patients who were given erythromycin, compared to 16 deaths in 71 patients treated with penicillin or amoxicillin. This is plausible, given that *Legionella* is an intracellular pathogen, and macrolides penetrate more efficiently than β-lactams into cells. Experimental data suggest that azithromycin is likely to be the most effective of the macrolide/azalide derivatives, but clinical evidence to confirm this is lacking. Other agents with proven clinical efficacy and good intracellular activity against *Legionella* include rifampicin and quinolones. There have been no randomized controlled clinical trials, nor are there likely to be. Current practice is that Legionnaire's disease is treated with high dose erythromycin (1 g four times daily), with the addition of rifampicin in severe cases. Some experts recommend first-line use of quinolones such as ciprofloxacin, particularly in immunocompromised patients.

All of these recommendations presuppose that the infecting organism is known before treatment is commenced. In practice, this is rarely, if ever, the case and therapy will initially be empirical or 'best-guess' in nature (Table 33.2).

Hospital-acquired (nosocomial) pneumonia

Causative organisms. There is a predominance of Gram-negative bacilli among the causative organisms of nosocomial pneumonia (Table 33.3), although it is important to remember that pneumococcal pneumonia may develop in hospitalized patients, and also that hospital water supplies have been implicated in outbreaks and sporadic cases of *Legionella* infection. Furthermore, it must be recognized that the common Gram-negative causes of nosocomial pneumonia will vary between hospitals and even between different units within the same hospital. This is especially true of ventilator-associated pneumonia, which for obvious reasons is usually acquired on intensive care units where broad-spectrum antibiotics are frequently used, and where there may be a particular 'resident flora' with an established antibiotic resistance pattern.

In immunocompromised patients the range of potential nosocomial pathogens is wider, and includes fungi such as *Candida* and *Aspergillus*. These infections may be particularly difficult to diagnose, and treatment is often commenced on suspicion alone.

Clinical features. Nosocomial pneumonia accounts for 10–15% of all hospital-acquired infections, usually presenting with sepsis and/or respiratory failure. Up to 50% of cases are acquired on intensive care units. Predisposing features include:

- stroke
- mechanical ventilation
- chronic lung disease
- recent surgery
- immunosuppression
- previous antibiotics.

Diagnosis. Sputum is the commonest specimen sent for culture but this is sometimes unhelpful as it may be contaminated by mouth flora. If the patient has received antibiotics, the normal mouth flora is often replaced by resistant organisms such as staphylococci or Gram-negative bacilli, making the interpretation of culture results difficult. For this reason bronchoscopy and bronchoalveolar lavage are often performed. Blood cultures may be positive.

Treatment. The range of organisms which may cause nosocomial pneumonia is very large and therapy

Table 33.2   Treatment of community-acquired pneumonia

Scenario	Regime	Comments
Mild to moderate pneumonia, organism unknown	Amoxicillin plus erythromycin	Erythromycin added to provide cover against atypical pathogens
Severe pneumonia, organism unknown	Cefuroxime plus erythromycin	Cefuroxime provides cover against *Staph. aureus* and coliform bacilli while retaining the pneumococcal and *Haemophilus* cover of amoxicillin
Pneumococcal disease	Penicillin or amoxicillin	Cefotaxime or vancomycin if high level penicillin-resistant
H. influenzae	Amoxicillin	Cefuroxime, co-amoxiclav or ciprofloxacin if β-lactamase producer
Staphylococcal pneumonia	High dose flucloxacillin plus second agent, e.g. rifampicin or fusidic acid	Isolation of *Staph. aureus* from sputum may reflect contamination with oropharyngeal commensals – see Table 33.6
Mycoplasma pneumoniae	Erythromycin or tetracycline	Treat for 14 days
Chlamydia spp.	Tetracycline preferred	Treat for 14 days
Legionella spp.	Erythromycin plus rifampicin	Quinolones also active

Table 33.3   Causes of hospital-acquired pneumonia

Common organisms
1. Gram-negative bacteria:
   Escherichia coli
   Klebsiella spp.
   Pseudomonas aeruginosa

2. Gram-positive bacteria:
   Streptococcus pneumoniae
   Staphylococcus aureus

Less common organisms
1. Gram-negative bacilli:
   Other 'coliforms':
      Enterobacter spp.
      Proteus spp.
      Serratia marcescens
      Citrobacter spp.
   Acinetobacter spp.
   Other *Pseudomonas* spp.
   Legionella pneumophila (and other species)

2. Anaerobic bacteria

3. Fungi:
   Candida albicans (and other species)
   Aspergillus fumigatus

4. Viruses:
   Cytomegalovirus
   Herpes simplex virus

must be correspondingly broad spectrum. The patient's underlying condition may give important clues to the infecting organism, such as the possibility of fungi in a neutropenic patient. The choice of antibiotics will be influenced by any preceding antibiotic therapy, and above all by the individual unit's experience with hospital bacteria. The combinations shown in Table 33.4 have all been used at some time and all have advantages and disadvantages. Several of the combinations include an aminoglycoside and this may not be desirable in all patients. Single agent therapy is attractive for ease of administration, and two agents, ceftazidime and meropenem, have suitably broad spectra. Unfortunately treatment failures have been recorded when ceftazidime is used alone due to the emergence of resistance while the patient is on treatment. In all cases erythromycin would be added if Legionnaire's disease was suspected and, except for the regimens containing clindamycin or meropenem, metronidazole would be required for suspected anaerobic infection.

Prevention. Since mechanical ventilation is an important predisposing factor for nosocomial pneumonia, a strategy termed selective decontamination of the digestive tract (SDD) has been proposed to try to prevent it. This technique is based on the premise that most organisms which cause ventilator-associated pneumonia initially colonize the patient's oropharynx or intestinal tract. By administering non-absorbable antibiotics such as an aminoglycoside or colistin to the gut, and applying

Table 33.4 Treatment of hospital-acquired pneumonia

Regime	Comments
Ureidopenicillin plus aminoglycoside (e.g. piperacillin plus gentamicin)	Good activity against Gram-negative bacilli such as *Ps. aeruginosa*, and pneumococci. Some strains of *E. coli*, *Klebsiella*, etc. are resistant to piperacillin. Relatively low activity against *Staph. aureus*. Poorly active against anaerobes. Some of these deficiences can be overcome by using piperacillin plus tazobactam, a b-lactamase inhibitor
Cephalosporin plus an aminoglycoside (e.g. cefuroxime or cefotaxime plus gentamicin)	Good activity against Gram-negative bacilli such as *E. coli*, *Klebsiella*, and Gram-positive organisms; relatively poor against *Ps. aeruginosa*. Poor activity against anaerobes
Clindamycin plus aminoglycoside	Good activity against Gram-positive organisms and anaerobes, but much less so against Gram-negatives. Favoured in the USA where metronidazole is unpopular for the treatment of anaerobic infections
Ciprofloxacin plus glycopeptide (vancomycin or teicoplanin)	Good activity against most Gram-negative bacilli including *Ps. aeruginosa*. Good activity against *Staph. aureus* and pneumococci but poor against anaerobes
Ceftazidime (monotherapy)	Convenient and avoids risk of aminoglycoside toxicity. Very active against Gram-negative bacilli including *Pseudomonas*, but less so against Gram-positive organisms and anaerobes
Meropenem (monotherapy)	Very broad spectrum agent but expensive

a paste containing these agents to the oropharynx, it is argued that the potential causative organisms will be eradicated and the incidence of pneumonia thereby reduced. In some centres an antifungal agent such as amphotericin B has been added, and others have added a systemic broad-spectrum agent such as cefotaxime.

The role of SDD remains extremely controversial. It has never become particularly popular in the UK, and concerns have been expressed about cost, the promotion of antibiotic resistance in Gram-negative bacilli and the establishment of conditions that favour the spread of antibiotic-resistant enterococci. A number of clinical trials have been performed and several meta-analyses published. Generally these have shown that there is indeed a reduction in pneumonia, but a reduction in mortality is much more difficult to demonstrate. One recent meta-analysis suggests that reduction in mortality requires the systemic component as well as the topical components (D'Amico et al 1998). Another demonstrates efficacy in surgical patients but not in medical patients (Nathens & Marshall 1999). While it seems likely that some SDD regimens are of benefit to some patients, these variables require more rigorous definition before SDD can be recommended.

Aspiration pneumonia

One further condition which may be seen either in hospitals or the community is aspiration pneumonia,

caused by inhalation of stomach contents contaminated by bacteria from the mouth. Risk factors include alcohol, hypnotic drugs and general anaesthesia – that is, those factors which may make a patient vomit while unconscious. Gastric acid is very destructive to lung tissue, causing severe tissue necrosis and infection often with abscess formation. Anaerobic bacteria are particularly implicated but these are often accompanied by aerobic organisms such as viridans streptococci. Treatment with metronidazole plus amoxicillin is usually adequate, or metronidazole plus cefuroxime if there are reasons to suspect a Gram-negative infection, for instance if the patient has been in hospital or previously exposed to antibiotics.

Cystic fibrosis: a special case.   Cystic fibrosis is an inherited, autosomal recessive disease which at the cellular level is due to a defect in the transport of ions in and out of cells. This leads to changes in the consistency and chemical composition of exocrine secretions, which in the lungs is manifest by the production of very sticky, tenacious mucus which is difficult to clear by mucociliary action. The production of such mucus leads to airway obstruction with resulting infection. Repeated episodes of infection lead eventually to bronchiectasis and permanent lung damage, which in turn predisposes the patient to further infection.

Infecting organisms.   In infants and young children *Staph. aureus* is the commonest pathogen. *H. influenzae* is sometimes encountered, but from the age of about 5 years onwards *Pseudomonas aeruginosa* is seen with increasing frequency until by the age of 18 most patients are chronically infected with this organism, which once present is never completely eradicated. Occasionally other Gram-negative bacteria such as *Escherichia coli* or *Stenotrophomonas maltophilia* are seen, and in some centres *Burkholderia cepacia* has been a particular problem due to its exceptional antibiotic resistance.

An important feature of those *Ps. aeruginosa* strains which infect cystic fibrosis patients is their production of large amounts of alginate, a polymer of mannuronic and glucuronic acid. This seems to be a virulence factor for the organism in that it inhibits opsonization and phagocytosis and enables the bacteria to adhere to the bronchial epithelium, thus inhibiting clearance. It does not confer additional antibiotic resistance. Strains which produce large amounts of alginate have a wet, slimy appearance on laboratory culture media and are termed 'mucoid' strains. Interestingly, other organisms such as *E. coli* may also produce alginate in these patients, a characteristic which is otherwise very rare.

Clinical features. Cystic fibrosis is characterized by persistent cough with copious sputum production. Many patients are chronically breathless. At times acute exacerbations occur in which there is fever, increased cough with purulent sputum, and increased dyspnoea. Systemic sepsis, however, is very rare. Eventually, chronic pulmonary infection leads to respiratory insufficiency, cardiac failure and death.

Treatment. This section will concentrate mainly on antibiotic therapy, but it should not be forgotten that other means of treatment, such as physiotherapy, play a vital part. The initial treatment of infection in a patient with cystic fibrosis will probably be directed against staphylococci, for which the usual anti-staphylococcal antibiotics such as flucloxacillin or erythromycin can be used. In some centres prophylaxis is given with agents such as co-trimoxazole, which may lead to the appearance of unusual resistant strains, for example thymidine-dependent *Staph. aureus*. These are strains which are dependent for growth on the nucleotide precursor thymidine, which confers resistance to co-trimoxazole by completely bypassing the biochemical sites of action of the sulphonamides and trimethoprim.

Once the patient is colonized by *Ps. aeruginosa*, treatment depends on early and vigorous therapy with antipseudomonal antibiotics. Physiotherapy between exacerbations may help to prevent some episodes of exacerbation, but the role of prophylactic antibiotics is uncertain. *Ps. aeruginosa* can be very antibiotic-resistant, but fortunately there is now a reasonable range of antipseudomonal antibiotics available; these are listed in Table 33.5. At present a β-lactam/aminoglycoside combination (such as ceftazidime plus gentamicin) is usually used. Agents such as meropenem or a quinolone are usually reserved for treatment failures or when

Table 33.5 Antipseudomonal antibiotics

Antibiotic	Comment
Ticarcillin	One of the first b-lactam agents effective against *Pseudomonas* but now considered insufficiently active. In combination with the b-lactamase inhibitor clavulanic acid, it may be active against some otherwise resistant strains
Ureidopenicillins	Piperacillin is the only one of these agents now available in the UK. It should be given in combination with an aminoglycoside, with which it is synergistic. Combination with the b-lactamase inhibitor tazobactam may render some resistant strains sensitive
Cephalosporins	Ceftazidime is the most active antipseudomonal cephalosporin and is very active against other Gram-negative bacilli. It has rather lower activity against Gram-positive bacteria. *Pseudomonas* may develop resistance during treatment
Aminoglycosides	Gentamicin and tobramycin have very similar activity; tobramycin is perhaps slightly more active. Netilmicin is less active, while amikacin may be active against some gentamicin-resistant strains
Quinolones	Ciprofloxacin can be given orally and parenterally but as with ceftazidime, resistance can develop while the patient is on treatment
Polymyxins	These peptide antibiotics are usually considered too toxic for systemic use but colistin (polymyxin E) can be given by inhalation
Carbapenems	Broad-spectrum agents with good activity against *Ps. aeruginosa*. Related species *Stenotrophomonas maltophilia* is resistant. Imipenem was the first of these agents, but CNS toxicity and its requirement for combination with the renal dipeptidase inhibitor cilastatin, are leading to its replacement by the newer agent meropenem

resistant organisms are encountered. The prolonged use of ceftazidime or ciprofloxacin alone should be avoided if possible since strains of *Ps. aeruginosa* (and some other Gram-negative bacilli) may become resistant to these agents while the patient is receiving treatment.

Interestingly, patients with cystic fibrosis have a more rapid clearance of some antibiotics than other patients. This is particularly noticeable with the aminoglycosides, and larger doses are often required to achieve satisfactory serum levels. Despite this, aminoglycoside toxicity is unusual in these patients.

Children with cystic fibrosis are admitted to hospital very frequently, sometimes for long periods of time, and it is not surprising that some develop an intense dislike of hospitals. This has encouraged the use of long-term indwelling central venous cannulae to allow administration of intravenous antibiotics at home by the parents. Ciprofloxacin can be given orally and offers the possibility of treatment for less severe exacerbations at home, perhaps after a brief time in hospital for parenteral therapy.

B. cepacia is often very difficult to treat, and strains may be resistant to all available antibiotics. Under these circumstances combination therapy is often used; there is some evidence with this organism that *in vitro* resistance does not always correlate with treatment failure in the patient.

The use of inhaled (usually nebulized) antibiotics as an adjunct to parenteral therapy has attracted some attention, both for treatment of acute exacerbations and for longer-term use in an attempt to reduce the pseudomonas load. Agents which have been administered in this way include colistin, gentamicin and other aminoglycosides, carbenicillin and ceftazidime. The best evidence that long-term administration can improve lung function comes from a large multicentre trial of nebulized tobramycin (Ramsey et al 1999) in which 520 patients were randomized to receive once daily nebulized tobramycin or placebo in on–off cycles for 24 weeks. At the end of the study patients in the treatment group had significantly better lung function, lower pseudomonal counts in their sputum, and had had fewer hospital admissions than those in the placebo group. This was at the expense of a degree of tobramycin resistance, although this did not seem to be clinically significant.

Some common therapeutic problems in respiratory infections are summarized in Table 33.6.

CASE STUDIES

Case 33.1

A 3-year-old boy complains of earache which has persisted despite 48 hours of symptomatic treatment with analgesics. Otitis media is diagnosed and oral cefaclor is prescribed. Three days later the parents return with the child stating that he is no better.

Questions

1. Why did the original treatment fail?
2. What treatment should now be given?

Answers

1. The most likely causes of otitis media are *Strep. pneumoniae*, *H. influenzae* and *Strep. pyogenes*. While cefaclor (or any of the early oral cephalosporins) would be active against the streptococci, they possess inadequate activity against *H. influenzae*, and this may have resulted in treatment failure.
2. A change to co-amoxiclav (because of the risk that the organism is a β-lactamase producer) or to cefixime would be appropriate. In patients hypersensitive to penicillins, one of the newer macrolides could be considered.

Case 33.2

An elderly man is admitted extremely unwell during December. For the past week he has been complaining of flu-like symptoms, but has deteriorated rapidly over the 24 hours before admission. Chest X-ray shows extensive consolidation with early cavitation. The patient is moved to the intensive care unit for monitoring and is commenced on i.v. amoxicillin and erythromycin.

Questions

1. Could the initial choice of antibiotics have been improved?
2. What precautions should be taken by the nursing and medical staff?
3. How could this infection have been prevented?

Answers

1. The clinical features suggest the possibility of staphylococcal pneumonia, perhaps as a consequence of influenza infection. Ninety-five percent of *Staph. aureus* strains produce b-lactamase and are resistant to amoxicillin. The erythromycin may have some activity but this would be insufficient for a severe infection such as this. Cefuroxime, or the addition of high dose flucloxacillin, would have been better choices than amoxicillin.
2. Influenza is highly infectious and can be transmitted in hospital to patients and staff. The patient should be isolated pending the results of virology investigations. In this case, tracheal secretions were positive for influenza A infection by immunofluorescence, and the virus was subsequently cultured.

Table 33.6 Common therapeutic problems

Problem	Comments
No pathogens isolated on sputum culture	Possibilities include an inadequate specimen such as saliva, non-infected or sterilized sputum, or a pathogen that cannot be cultured on routine media (e.g. *Chlamydia pneumoniae*, *Mycobacterium tuberculosis*). Pneumococci are susceptible to autolysis, and may fail to grow even from a well-taken specimen
Staphylococcus aureus isolated	*Staph. aureus* pneumonia is a severe disease with characteristic clinical features, often associated with bacteraemia. However, the organism is frequently isolated from the sputum of patients with bronchitis or bronchopneumonia. In these instances it usually reflects contamination of the specimen with oropharyngeal commensals, although some patients undoubtedly have a clinical infection which responds to antistaphylococcal antibiotics
Candida spp. isolated	Unless there are reasons to suspect a candida pneumonia (as a consequence of neutropenia, for example), the isolation of yeasts is likely to reflect oropharyngeal contamination of the specimen. Yeasts can be carried commensally in the mouth, particularly in the presence of dentures, but a search for clinical candidiasis should be made
Aspergillus spp. isolated	Invasive aspergillosis, allergic bronchopulmonary aspergillosis and aspergilloma should be considered. Alternatively the finding might reflect inconsequential oropharyngeal carriage
Penicillin-resistant pneumococci isolated	Respiratory infections caused by strains with low level resistance (MIC 0.1–1 mg/l) may be treated with penicillins. Strains with high level resistance should be treated according to their sensitivity profile, for example using a later generation cephalosporin, and the patient should be isolated
Coliforms isolated	Significance depends on the clinical context: unlikely to be responsible for community-acquired infection unless there is bronchiectasis, but may be relevant to hospital-acquired infections
Failure of a chest infection to respond to antibiotics	Consider poor compliance, inadequate dosage, viral or otherwise insensitive aetiology. β-lactams are ineffective against *Chlamydia*, *Mycoplasma* and *Legionella* infections
Sore throat, no pathogens isolated	Consider viral aetiology, particularly EBV (glandular fever) in teenagers and young adults
Persistent illness following treatment for pneumococcal pneumonia	Consider the possibility of an empyema (pus in the pleural space) – a condition which usually requires surgical drainage

3. Influenza vaccine is made available each winter to risk groups, including the elderly. The role of neuraminidase inhibitors such as zanamivir remains to be defined.

Case 33.3

A GP sends a throat swab on a 25-year-old hospital pharmacist with a sore throat, but omits to provide clinical details on the request form. A heavy growth of MRSA (methicillin-resistant *Staph. aureus*) is reported.

Questions

1. How should the patient be treated?

2. The patient is given amoxicillin, and promptly develops a rash. She has previously had penicillins without evidence of allergy. What is the diagnosis?

Answers

1. *Staph. aureus*, whether methicillin-resistant or not, may be carried commensally in the throat and is not a recognized cause of pharyngitis. The patient probably has a viral infection, and should be advised about rest and symptomatic treatment. She should be also advised on recovery to contact the infection control team at the hospital in which she works, for management of her MRSA carriage.

2. It is likely that she has infectious mononucleosis caused by Epstein–Barr virus. For reasons unknown, treatment with amoxicillin during EBV infection usually results in the development of a widespread erythematous rash. The diagnosis could be confirmed serologically.

Case 33.4

A 76-year-old man who continues to smoke despite three heart attacks, breathlessness at rest and repeated hospital admissions for exacerbations of his chronic bronchitis, says that his usually creamy sputum has turned green. On this occasion he is not so unwell that he requires admission. He says that he is allergic to penicillin, and is commenced on erythromycin.

Questions

1. What are the likely pathogens?
2. Why might the treatment fail?
3. What further questions should be asked?

Answers

1. The most likely bacterial causes of this man's acute bronchitis are *H. influenzae* and *Strep. pneumoniae*. It may even be a viral infection.
2. As well as having a high incidence of gastrointestinal side-effects, erythromycin is poorly active against *H. influenzae*, and furthermore the resistance rate among pneumococci is increasing.
3. Many patients who claim to be allergic to penicillin in fact have formed this opinion erroneously, for example because of vomiting or other non-allergic side-effect in the past. It is worth clarifying the allergy story, because it may prove possible to contradict this and use a penicillin such as amoxicillin.

REFERENCES

D'Amico R, Pifferi S, Leonetti C et al 1998 Effectiveness of antibiotic prophylaxis in critically ill adult patients: systematic review of randomised controlled trials. British Medical Journal 316: 1275–1285

Del Mar C B, Glasziou P P, Spinks A B 2000 Antibiotics for sore throat (Cochrane Review). In: The Cochrane Library, Issue 4. Update Software, Oxford

Fraser D W, Tsai T R, Orenstein W et al 1977 Legionnaire's disease, description of an epidemic of pneumonia. New England Journal of Medicine 297: 1189–1197

Glasziou P P, Hayem M, Del Mar C B 2000 Antibiotics for acute otitis media in children (Cochrane Review). In: The Cochrane Library, Issue 4. Update Software, Oxford

Jefferson T, Demicheli V, Deeks J et al 2000 Neuraminidase inhibitors for preventing and treating influenza in healthy adults (Cochrane Review). In: The Cochrane Library, Issue 4. Update Software, Oxford

Nathens A B, Marshall J C 1999 Selective decontamination of the digestive tract in surgical patients: a systematic review of the evidence. Archives of Surgery 134: 170–176

National Institute of Clinical Excellence 2000 Guidance on the use of zanamivir (Relenza) in the treatment of influenza. http://www.nice.org.uk/pdf/NiceZANAMIVIR15guidance.pdf (accessed 6 March 2002)

Pichichero M E, Margolis P A 1991 A comparison of cephalosporins and penicillins in the treatment of group A beta-hemolytic streptococcal pharyngitis: a meta-analysis supporting the concept of microbial copathogenicity. Pediatric Infectious Disease Journal 10: 275–281.

Ramsey B W, Pepe M S, Quan J M et al 1999 Intermittent administration of inhaled tobramycin in patients with cystic fibrosis. New England Journal of Medicine 340: 23–30

FURTHER READING

Cystic Fibrosis Trust 2000 Antibiotic treatment for cystic fibrosis. Report of the UK Cystic Fibrosis Trust's antibiotic group. Cystic Fibrosis Trust; London

Dedicoat M, Venkatesan P 1999 The treatment of Legionnaire's disease. Journal of Antimicrobial Chemotherapy 43: 747–752

Donowitz G R, Mandell G L 2000 Acute pneumonia. In: Mandell G L, Bennett J E, Dolin R (eds) Principles and practice of infectious diseases, 5th edn. Churchill Livingstone; New York, pp 717–742

Friedland I R 1995 Treatment of pneumococcal infections in the era of increasing penicillin resistance. Current Opinion in Infectious Diseases 8: 213–217

Reynolds H Y 2000 Chronic bronchitis and acute infectious exacerbations. In: Mandell G L, Bennett J E, Dolin R (eds) Principles and practice of infectious diseases, 5th edn. Churchill Livingstone, New York, pp 706–709

Urinary tract infections

34

A. J. Bint   A. W. Berrington

KEY POINTS

- Urinary tract infection (UTI) is one of the most common complaints seen in general practice and accounts for about one-third of hospital acquired infections.
- *Escherichia coli* is the most frequent pathogen, accounting for more than three-quarters of community acquired urinary tract infections.
- Symptoms are variable: many UTIs are asymptomatic, and some present atypically, particularly in children and the elderly.
- The concept of significant bacteriuria (at least 100 000 organisms per ml of urine) is used to distinguish between contamination and infection, but lower counts than this can cause symptoms and disease.
- Asymptomatic UTI should be treated in children and pregnant women.
- Catheter-related UTI should be treated only when the patient has systemic evidence of infection.
- Antimicrobial sensitivity patterns are changing. *E. coli* is becoming increasingly resistant to amoxicillin and trimethoprim, and evidence from other countries demonstrates its capacity to become resistant to quinolones.
- A 3-day treatment course is sufficient in uncomplicated lower UTI in women. Longer, 7–10 day courses are recommended for men, children and pregnant women.
- Antibiotic prophylaxis may be beneficial in women with recurrent UTIs and in children with structural or functional abnormalities.

The term urinary tract infection (UTI) usually refers to the presence of organisms in the urinary tract together with symptoms, and sometimes signs, of inflammation. However, it is more precise to use one of the following terms:

- *Significant bacteriuria:* defined as the presence of at least 100 000 bacteria per ml of urine. A quantitative definition such as this is needed because small numbers of bacteria are normally found in the anterior urethra and may be washed out into urine samples. Counts of fewer than 1000 bacteria per ml are normally considered to be urethral contaminants.
- *Asymptomatic bacteriuria:* significant bacteriuria in the absence of symptoms in the patient.

- *Cystitis:* a syndrome of frequency, dysuria and urgency, which usually suggests infection restricted to the lower urinary tract (i.e. the bladder and urethra).
- *Acute pyelonephritis:* an acute infection of one or both kidneys. Usually the lower urinary tract is also involved.
- *Chronic pyelonephritis:* difficult to define, chronic pyelonephritis usually refers to a particular type of pathology of the kidney, which may or may not be due to infection.
- *Relapse and reinfection:* recurrence of urinary infection may be due to either relapse or reinfection. Relapse is recurrence caused by the same organism that caused the original infection. Reinfection is recurrence caused by a different organism, and is therefore a new infection.

Epidemiology

Urinary tract infection is a problem in all age groups, although its prevalence varies markedly. In infants up to the age of 6 months UTI has a prevalence of about two cases per 1000, and is much more common in boys than in girls. In pre-school children UTI becomes more common, and the sex ratio reverses such that the prevalence of bacteriuria is 4.5% in girls and 0.5% in boys. In older children, the prevalence of bacteriuria is 1.2% among girls and 0.03% among boys. At least 8% of girls and 2% of boys will experience a UTI during childhood. In girls about two-thirds of these infections are asymptomatic. The occurrence of bacteriuria during childhood appears to lead to a higher incidence of bacteriuria in adulthood.

When women reach adulthood, the prevalence of bacteriuria rises to between 3% and 5%. Each year about a quarter of these bacteriuric women clear their infections spontaneously and are replaced by an equal number of newly infected women, who are often those with a history of previous infections. Up to 50% of adult women report that they have had a symptomatic UTI at some time. UTI is uncommon in young healthy men.

In the elderly of both sexes the prevalence of bacteriuria rises dramatically, reaching 20% among women and 10% among men. In hospitals, a major predisposing cause of UTI is urinary catheterization. With time, even with closed drainage systems and scrupulous hygiene, almost all catheters become infected.

Aetiology

In acute uncomplicated UTI acquired in the community, *Escherichia coli* is by far the commonest causative bacterium, being responsible for about 80% of infections. The remaining 20% are caused by other Gram-negative enteric bacteria such as *Klebsiella* and *Proteus* species, and by Gram-positive cocci, particularly enterococci and *Staphylococcus saprophyticus*. The latter organism is almost entirely restricted to infections in young, sexually active women.

UTI associated with underlying structural abnormalities (such as congenital anomalies, neurogenic bladder and obstructive uropathy) is often caused by more resistant organisms such as *Pseudomonas aeruginosa*, *Enterobacter* and *Serratia* species. Organisms such as these are also more commonly implicated in hospital-acquired urinary infections, including those in patients with urinary catheters.

Rare causes of urinary infection – nearly always in association with structural abnormalities or catheterization – include anaerobic bacteria and fungi. Urinary tract tuberculosis is an infrequent but important diagnosis which may be missed through lack of clinical suspicion. A number of viruses are excreted in urine (and may be detected by culture or nucleic acid detection) but symptomatic infection is confined to immunocompromised patients, particularly children following bone marrow transplantation, in whom adenoviruses and polyomaviruses such as BK virus are associated with haemorrhagic cystitis.

Pathogenesis

There are three possible routes by which organisms might reach the urinary tract: the ascending, blood-borne and lymphatic routes. There is little evidence for the last route in humans. Blood-borne spread to the kidney can occur in bacteraemic illnesses, most notably *Staphylococcus aureus* septicaemia, but by far the most frequent route is the ascending route.

In women, UTI is preceded by colonization of the perineum and periurethral area by the pathogen, which then ascends into the bladder via the urethra. That the urethra in women is shorter than that in men, and that the urethral meatus is closer to the anus, are probably important factors in explaining the preponderance of UTI in females. Furthermore, sexual intercourse appears to be important in forcing bacteria into the female bladder, and this risk is increased by the use of diaphragms and spermicides.

The organism

As stated, most UTIs are caused by *E. coli*. Although there are many serotypes of this organism, a few of these are responsible for a disproportionate number of infections. Some strains of *E. coli* possess certain virulence factors that enhance their ability to cause infection, particularly infections of the upper urinary tract. Recognized virulence factors include bacterial surface structures called P fimbriae (which mediate adherence to glycolipid receptors on renal epithelial cells), possession of the iron-scavenging aerobactin system, and increased amounts of capsular K antigen (which mediates resistance to phagocytosis).

The host

Although many bacteria can readily grow in urine, the high urea concentration and extremes of osmolality and pH inhibit growth. Other defence mechanisms include the flushing mechanism of bladder emptying, since small numbers of bacteria finding their way into the bladder are likely to be eliminated when the bladder is emptied. Moreover, the bladder mucosa, by virtue of a surface glycosaminoglycan, is intrinsically resistant to bacterial adherence. Presumably, in sufficient numbers, bacteria with strong adhesive properties can overcome this defence. Finally, when the bladder is infected, white blood cells are mobilized to the bladder surface to ingest and destroy invading bacteria. The role of humoral immunity in defence against infection of the urinary tract remains unclear.

Abnormalities of the urinary tract

Any structural abnormality leading to the obstruction of flow and urinary stasis increases the likelihood of infection. Such abnormalities include congenital anomalies of the ureter or urethra, renal stones and, in men, enlargement of the prostate. Renal stones can become infected with bacteria, particularly *Proteus* and *Klebsiella* species, and thereby become a source of 'relapsing' infection. Vesicoureteric reflux (VUR) is a condition caused by failure of physiological valves at the junction of the ureters and the bladder which allows urine to reflux towards the kidneys when the bladder contracts. It is probable that VUR plays an important role in childhood urinary tract infections that lead to chronic renal damage (scarring) and persistence of infection.

Clinical manifestations

Most UTIs are asymptomatic. Symptoms, when they do occur, are principally the result of irritation of the bladder and urethral mucosa. However, the clinical features of UTI are extremely variable and to some extent depend on the age of the patient.

Babies and infants

Infections in newborn babies and infants are often overlooked or misdiagnosed because the signs may not be referable to the urinary tract. Common but non-specific presenting symptoms include failure to thrive, vomiting, fever, diarrhoea and apathy. Furthermore, confirmation may be difficult because of problems in obtaining adequate specimens. UTI in infancy and childhood is a major risk factor for the development of renal scarring, which in turn is associated with future complications such as chronic pyelonephritis in adulthood, hypertension and renal failure. It is therefore vital to make the diagnosis early, and any child with a suspected UTI should receive urgent expert assessment.

Children

Above the age of two, children with UTI are more likely to present with some of the classical symptoms such as frequency, dysuria and haematuria. However, some children present with acute abdominal pain and vomiting, and this may be so marked as to raise suspicions of appendicitis or other intra-abdominal pathology. Again however, it is extremely important that the diagnosis of UTI is made promptly in order to pre-empt the potential long term consequences.

Adults

In adults the typical symptoms of lower UTI include frequency, dysuria, urgency and haematuria. Acute pyelonephritis (upper UTI) usually causes fever, rigors and loin pain in addition to lower tract symptoms. Systemic symptoms may vary from insignificant to extreme malaise. Importantly, untreated cystitis in adults rarely progresses to pyelonephritis, and bacteriuria does not seem to carry the adverse long-term consequences that it does in children.

In about 40% of women with dysuria, urgency and frequency the urine sample contains fewer than 100 000 bacteria per ml. These patients are said to have the urethral syndrome. Some have a true bacterial infection but with relatively low counts (100–1000 bacteria per ml). Some have urethral infection with *Chlamydia trachomatis*, *Neisseria gonorrhoeae* or mycoplasmas, any of which might give rise to symptoms indistinguishable from those of cystitis. In others no known cause can be found. However, most cases of urethral syndrome will respond to standard antibiotic regimens as used for treating confirmed UTI (Baerheim et al 1999).

Elderly patients

Although UTI is frequent in the elderly, the great majority of cases are asymptomatic, and even when present, symptoms are not diagnostic because frequency, dysuria, hesitancy and incontinence are fairly common in elderly people without infection. Furthermore there may be non-specific systemic manifestations such as confusion and falls, or alternatively the infection may be the cause of deterioration in pre-existing conditions such as diabetes mellitus or congestive cardiac failure, whose clinical features might predominate. UTI is one of the most frequent causes of admission to hospital among the elderly.

Investigation

The key to successful laboratory diagnosis of UTI lies in obtaining an uncontaminated urine sample for microscopy and culture. Contaminating bacteria can arise from skin, vaginal flora in women and penile flora in men. Patients therefore need to be instructed in how to produce a midstream urine sample (MSU). This requires careful cleansing of the perineum and external genitalia with soap and water, followed by a controlled micturition in which only the middle portion is collected, the initial and final components being voided into the toilet or bedpan. Understandably this is not always possible, and many so-called MSUs are in fact clean catch specimens in which the whole urine volume is collected into a sterile receptacle and an aliquot transferred into a specimen pot for submission to the laboratory. These are more likely to contain urethral contaminants. In very young children, stick-on bags are a useful way of obtaining a urine sample. Occasionally, in–out catheterization or even suprapubic aspiration directly from the bladder are necessary.

For general practitioners located at some distance from the laboratory, transport of specimens is a problem. Specimens must reach the laboratory within 2 hours, or should be refrigerated; otherwise any bacteria in the specimen will multiply and might give rise to a false-positive result. Methods of overcoming bacterial multiplication in urine include the addition of boric acid to the container, and the use of dip-slides, in which an agar-coated paddle is dipped into the urine and submitted directly to the laboratory for incubation.

Concerns about the relative expense and slow turn-around time of urine microscopy and culture have stimulated interest in alternative diagnostic strategies. Some advocate a policy of empirical antimicrobial treatment in the first instance, and reserve investigation only for those cases which do not respond. Others are in favour of using cheaper, more convenient screening tests, for example urine dipsticks for blood, protein, nitrites and leucocyte esterase, although there are concerns that these are reliable only when applied to fresh urine samples tested at the point of care (Jones et al 1998). Generally their negative predictive value is better than their positive predictive value, so their preferred use is as screening tests to identify those specimens which are least likely to be infected, and which therefore do not require culture. A perfectly valid alternative is just to hold the specimen up to the light: specimens which are visibly clear are very likely to be sterile (Bulloch et al 2000). There are other rapid methods available, and no shortage of data concerning their sensitivity and specificity, but the optimal strategy will always be a compromise between accuracy, speed, convenience and cost, and is likely to be different for different populations. Urine microscopy and culture remain the standard by which other investigations are measured.

Microscopy

Microscopy is the first step in the laboratory diagnosis of UTI, and is readily performed in ward side-rooms and GPs' surgeries as well as in laboratories. A drop of uncentrifuged urine is placed on a slide, covered with a coverslip and examined under a × 40 objective. Excess white cells are usually seen in the urine of patients with symptomatic UTI, and more than five per high-power field is abnormal. It should be noted that there are other methods in common use, and laboratories may report white cell counts per microlitre (cubic millimetre) of urine, or even per millilitre. It is important not to be too rigid in the interpretation of the white cell count: UTI may occur in the absence of pyuria, particularly at the extremes of age, in pregnancy and in pyelonephritis. Red blood cells may be seen, as may white cell casts, which are suggestive of pyelonephritis. As a rule of thumb, the presence of at least one bacterium per field correlates with 100 000 bacteria per ml.

Culture

Bladder urine is normally sterile, but when passed via the urethra it is inevitable that some contamination with the urethral bacterial flora will occur. This is why it is important that laboratories quantify the number of bacteria in urine specimens. In work carried out over 40 years ago Kass (1957) demonstrated that patients with UTI usually have at least 100 000 bacteria per ml, while in patients without infection the count is usually below 1000 bacteria per ml. Between these figures lies a grey area, and it should be appreciated that the MSU is not an infallible guide to the presence or absence of urinary infection. True infections may be associated with low counts, particularly when the urine is very dilute because of excessive fluid intake, or where the pathogen is slow-growing. Most genuine infections are caused by one single bacterial species; mixed cultures suggest contamination.

Treatment

Although many – perhaps most – cases would clear spontaneously given time, symptomatic UTI usually merits antibiotic treatment to eradicate both symptoms and pathogen. Asymptomatic bacteriuria may or may not need treatment depending upon the circumstances of the individual case. Bacteriuria in children and in pregnant women requires treatment because of the potential complications. On the other hand, in non-pregnant, asymptomatic bacteriuric adults without any obstructive lesion, treatment is probably unwarranted. Some common therapeutic problems are summarized in Table 34.3, later in the chapter.

Non-specific treatment

Advising patients with UTI to drink a lot of fluids is common practice on the theoretical basis that more infected urine is removed by frequent bladder emptying. This is plausible, although not evidence based. Some clinicians recommend urinary analgesics such as potassium or sodium citrate, which alkalinize the urine, but these should be used as an adjunct to antibiotics. They should not be used in conjunction with nitrofurantoin, which is active only at acidic pH.

Antimicrobial chemotherapy

The principles of antimicrobial treatment of UTI are the same as those of treating any other infection: from a group of suitable drugs chosen on the basis of efficacy, safety and cost, select the agent with the narrowest possible spectrum and administer it for the shortest possible time. In general there is no evidence that bactericidal antibiotics are superior to bacteriostatic agents in treating UTI, except perhaps in relapsing infections. Blood levels of antibiotics appear to be unimportant in the treatment of lower UTI – what matters is the concentration in the urine. However, blood levels are probably important in treating pyelonephritis, which may progress to bacteraemia. Drugs suitable for the oral treatment of cystitis include β-lactams (particularly amoxicillin, co-amoxiclav and oral cephalosporins), fluoroquinolones (such as ciprofloxacin, norfloxacin and ofloxacin), trimethoprim, and nitrofurantoin. Where intravenous administration is required, suitable agents include β-lactams such as amoxicillin and cefuroxime, quinolones such as ciprofloxacin, and aminoglycosides such as gentamicin.

In renal failure it may be difficult to achieve adequate therapeutic concentrations of some drugs in the urine, particularly nitrofurantoin and quinolones. Furthermore the use of aminoglycosides may be complicated by accumulation and toxicity. Penicillins and cephalosporins attain satisfactory concentrations and are relatively non-toxic, and are therefore the agents of choice for treating UTI in the presence of renal failure.

Uncomplicated lower UTI

Adults

Therapeutic decisions should be based on accurate, up-to-date antimicrobial susceptibility patterns. Interim data have been published from a recent European multicentre survey which examined the prevalence and antimicrobial susceptibility of community-acquired pathogens causing uncomplicated UTI in women (Kahlmeter 2000). Among the first 1163 *E. coli* isolates the resistance rates were 29.9% for amoxicillin, 15.6% for trimethoprim, 2.9% for ciprofloxacin, 2.3% for cefadroxil, 2.1% for co-amoxiclav, and 1.4% for nitrofurantoin. These figures are lower than routine laboratory data would suggest (Winstanley et al 1997), but it should be remembered that

the experience of diagnostic laboratories is likely to be biased by the over-representation of specimens from patients in whom empirical treatment has already failed. While it is important to be aware of local variations in sensitivity pattern, the preference for best-guess therapy would seem to be a choice between nitrofurantoin, an oral cephalosporin, and co-amoxiclav, with the proviso that therapy can be refined once sensitivities are available. The quinolones are best reserved for treatment failures and more difficult infections, since overuse of these important agents is likely to lead to an increase in resistance as it has already in countries such as Spain and Portugal. These recommendations are summarized in Table 34.1.

Other drugs which have been used for the treatment of UTI include co-trimoxazole, pivmecillinam, and earlier quinolones such as nalidixic acid. Co-trimoxazole is now recognized as a cause of bone marrow suppression and other haematological side-effects, and in the UK its use is greatly restricted. Furthermore, despite superior activity in vitro, there is no convincing evidence that it is clinically superior to trimethoprim alone in the treatment of UTI. Pivmecillinam is metabolized to mecillinam, a β-lactam agent with a particularly high affinity for Gram-negative penicillin binding protein 2 and a low affinity for commonly encountered β-lactamases, and which therefore has theoretical advantages in the treatment of UTI. Pivmecillinam has been extensively used for cystitis in Scandinavian countries, where it does not seem to have led to the development of resistance, and for this reason there have been calls for wider recognition of its usefulness. Finally, older quinolones such as nalidixic acid and cinoxacin were once widely used, but generally

Table 34.1 Oral antibiotics used for lower urinary tract infections

Antibiotic	Dose (adult)	Side-effects	Contraindications	Comments
Amoxicillin	250–500 mg three times a day	Nausea, diarrhoea, allergy	Penicillin hypersensitivity	High levels of resistance in *E. coli*
Co-amoxiclav	375–625 mg three times a day	*See* amoxicillin	*See* amoxicillin	Amoxicillin and clavulanic acid
Cefalexin	250–500 mg four times a day	Nausea, diarrhoea, allergy	Cephalosporin hypersensitivity, porphyria	
Trimethoprim	200 mg twice a day	Nausea, pruritus, allergy	Pregnancy, neonates, folate deficiency, porphyria	
Nitrofurantoin	50 mg four times a day	Nausea, allergy, rarely pneumonitis, pulmonary fibrosis, neuropathy	Renal failure, neonates, porphyria, G6PD deficiency	Modified release form may be given twice daily
Ciprofloxacin	250–500 mg twice a day	Rash, pruritis, tendinitis	Pregnancy, children	Reserve for difficult cases

G6PD, Glucose 6-phosphate dehydrogenase.

these agents have given ground to the more active fluorinated quinolones.

Duration of treatment. The question of duration of treatment has received much attention. Traditionally, a course of 7–10 days has been advocated, and this is still the recommendation for treating men, in whom the possibility of occult prostatitis should be borne in mind. For women though, there has been particular emphasis on the suitability of short course regimens such as 3 day or even single-dose therapy. The consensus of an international expert working group was that 3 day regimens are as effective as longer regimens in the cases of trimethoprim and quinolones, that β-lactams have been inadequately investigated on this point but are generally less effective than trimethoprim and quinolones, and that nitrofurantoin requires further study before conclusions can be drawn (Warren et al 1999). Single-dose therapy, with its advantages of cost, compliance and the minimization of side-effects, has been used successfully in many studies but in general is less effective than when the same agent is used for longer. This view may be challenged in future by the advent of newer fluoroquinolones.

In the urethral syndrome, it is worth trying a 3 day course of one of the agents mentioned above. If this fails, a 7 day course of tetracycline could be tried to deal with possible chlamydia or mycoplasma infection.

Children

In children, the risk of renal scarring is such that UTI should be diagnosed and treated promptly, even if asymptomatic. The drugs of choice include β-lactams, trimethoprim and nitrofurantoin. Quinolones are relatively contraindicated in children because of the theoretical risk of causing cartilage and joint problems. Children should be treated for 7–10 days.

Renal scarring occurs in 5–15% of children with UTI, who should be identified in order that appropriate treatment can be instituted. Unfortunately, the subgroup at high risk cannot be predicted, and for this reason many clinicians choose to investigate all children with UTI, for example using ultrasound and radioisotope scanning.

Acute pyelonephritis

Patients with pyelonephritis may be severely ill, and if so will require admission to hospital and initial treatment with a parenteral antibiotic. Suitable agents with good activity against *E. coli* and other Gram-negative bacilli include cephalosporins such as cefuroxime and ceftazidime, some penicillins such as co-amoxiclav, quinolones, and aminoglycosides such as gentamicin (Table 34.2). A first-choice agent would be parenteral cefuroxime, gentamicin or ciprofloxacin. When the patient is improving, the route of administration may be switched to oral therapy, typically using a quinolone. Conventionally, treatment is continued for 10–14 days.

Patients who are less severely ill at the outset may be treated with an oral antibiotic, and possibly with a shorter course of treatment. The safety of this approach has been proved in a study of adult women with acute uncomplicated pyelonephritis (Talan et al 2000). Among 113 patients treated with oral ciprofloxacin 500 mg twice daily for 7 days (+/– an initial intravenous dose), the cure rate was 96%.

Table 34.2 Parenteral antibiotics used for pyelonephritis

Antibiotic	Dose (adult)	Side-effects	Contraindications	Comments
Cefuroxime	750 mg three times a day	Nausea, diarrhoea, allergy	Cephalosporin hypersensitivity, porphyria	
Ceftazidime	1 g three times a day	*See* cefuroxime	*See* cefuroxime	
Co-amoxiclav	1.2 g three times a day	Nausea, diarrhoea, allergy	Penicillin hypersensitivity	
Gentamicin	80–120 mg three times a day or 5 mg/kg once daily	Nephrotoxicity, ototoxicity	Pregnancy, myasthenia gravis	Monitor levels
Ciprofloxacin	200–400 mg twice a day	Rash, pruritis, tendinitis	Pregnancy, children	
Meropenem	500 mg three times a day	Nausea, rash, convulsions		Reserve for difficult cases

In hospital-acquired pyelonephritis there is a risk that the infecting organism may be resistant to the usual first line drugs. In such cases it may be advisable to start a broad-spectrum agent such as ceftazidime, ciprofloxacin or meropenem.

Relapsing UTI

The main causes of persistent relapsing UTI are renal infection, structural abnormalities of the urinary tract and, in men, chronic prostatitis. Patients who fail on a 7–10 day course should be given a 2 week course, and if that fails a 6 week course can be considered. Structural abnormalities may need surgical correction before cure can be maintained. It is essential that prolonged courses (i.e. more than 4 weeks) are managed under bacteriological control, with monthly cultures.

Catheter-associated infections

In most large hospitals 10–15% of patients have an indwelling urinary catheter. Even with the very best catheter care, most will have infected urine after 10–14 days of catheterization, although most of these infections will be asymptomatic. Antibiotic treatment will often appear to eradicate the infecting organism, but as long as the catheter remains in place the organism, or another more resistant one, will quickly return. The principles of antibiotic therapy for catheter-associated UTI are therefore as follows:

- do not treat asymptomatic infection
- if possible, remove the catheter before treating symptomatic infection.

Although it often prompts investigation, cloudy or strong smelling urine is not per se an indication for antimicrobial therapy. In these situations, saline or antiseptic bladder washouts are often performed, but there is little evidence that they make a difference. Similarly, encrusted catheters are often changed on aesthetic grounds, but it is not known whether this reduces the likelihood of future symptoms.

Following catheter removal, bacteriuria may resolve spontaneously but more often it persists and may become symptomatic. In a study of women with catheter-associated infection, asymptomatic bacteriuria resolved spontaneously within 2 weeks in only 15 of 42 patients (Godfrey et al 1991). However, those with persistent and symptomatic bacteriuria responded well to single dose treatment.

Bacteriuria of pregnancy

The prevalence of asymptomatic bacteriuria of pregnancy is about 5%, and about a third of these women proceed to develop acute pyelonephritis, with its attendant consequences for the health of both mother and pregnancy. Furthermore, there is evidence that asymptomatic bacteriuria is associated with low birth weight, prematurity, hypertension and pre-eclampsia. For these reasons it is recommended that screening is carried out, preferably by culture of a properly taken MSU, which should be repeated if positive for confirmation.

Rigorous meta-analysis of published trials (Smaill 2000) has shown that antibiotic treatment of bacteriuria in pregnancy is effective at clearing bacteriuria, reducing the incidence of pyelonephritis and reducing the risk of preterm delivery. The drugs of choice are amoxicillin, cefalexin or nitrofurantoin depending on the sensitivity profile of the infecting organism. Co-amoxiclav is cautioned in pregnancy because of lack of clinical experience in pregnant women, as is ciprofloxacin. Trimethoprim is contraindicated because of its theoretical risk of causing neural tube defects. There are insufficient data concerning short course therapy in pregnancy, and 7 days of treatment remains the standard. Patients should be followed up for the duration of the pregnancy to confirm cure and to ensure that any reinfection is promptly addressed.

Prevention and prophylaxis

There are a number of folklore and naturopathic recommendations for the prevention of UTI. Most of these have not been put to statistical study, but at least are unlikely to cause harm.

Cranberry juice has long been thought to be beneficial in preventing UTI, and this has been studied in a number of clinical trials. In elderly women, a daily intake of 300 ml cranberry juice was associated with a halving of the risk of bacteriuria (Avorn et al 1994), but this and other studies have been criticized for methodological flaws. Currently there is no incontrovertible evidence that cranberry juice is effective at preventing UTI (Jepson et al 2000), and there have been no investigations of its use in the treatment of established infection.

In some patients, mainly women, reinfections are so frequent that long-term antimicrobial prophylaxis is indicated. If the reinfections are clearly related to sexual intercourse, then a single dose of an antibiotic after intercourse is appropriate. In other cases, long-term, low-dose prophylaxis may be beneficial. One dose of trimethoprim (100 mg) or nitrofurantoin (50 mg) at night will suffice. These drugs are unlikely to lead to the emergence of resistant bacteria.

In children, recurrence of UTI is common and the complications potentially hazardous, so many clinicians recommend antimicrobial prophylaxis following documented infection. The evidence in favour of this practice is not strong (Le Saux et al 2000), and although it has been shown to reduce the incidence of UTI, it has not been shown to reduce the incidence of renal complications. Furthermore, important variables remain to be clarified, such as when to begin prophylaxis, which agent to use, and when to stop.

Some of the common therapeutic problems are summarized in Table 34.3.

CASE STUDIES

Case 34.1

Two days after transurethral resection of the prostate, a 75-year-old man becomes unwell with rigors, fever and loin pain. Microscopy of his urine shows over 200 white cells/mm³. Blood cultures are taken and rapidly become positive, with Gram-negative bacilli seen in the Gram film.

Question

What antibiotic therapy is indicated?

Answer

The patient should be started on intravenous antibiotic therapy for presumed pyelonephritis and consequent bacteraemia. The antibiotic should cover Gram-negative organisms found in the hospital environment such as *Klebsiella* spp., *Enterobacter* spp. and *Pseudomonas* spp. Appropriate agents would be ceftazidime, ciprofloxacin or meropenem. An alternative would be an aminoglycoside such as gentamicin, provided the patient has satisfactory renal function.

Table 34.3 Common therapeutic problems

Problem	Comments
Asymptomatic infection	Asymptomatic bacteriuria should be treated where there is a risk of serious consequences (i.e. in childhood), where there is renal scarring, and in pregnancy. Otherwise treatment is not usually required
Catheter in situ, patient unwell	Systemic symptoms may result from catheter-associated UTI, and should respond to antibiotics although the catheter is likely to remain colonized. Local symptoms such as urgency are more likely to reflect urethral irritation than infection
Catheter in situ, urine cloudy or smelly	Unless the patient is systemically unwell, antibiotics are unlikely to achieve much and may give rise to resistance. Interventions of uncertain benefit include bladder washouts or a change of catheter
Penicillin allergy	Clarify 'allergy': vomiting or diarrhoea are not allergic phenomena and do not contraindicate penicillins. Penicillin-induced rash is a contraindication to amoxicillin but cephalosporins are likely to be tolerated. Penicillin-induced anaphylaxis suggests that all beta-lactams should be avoided
Symptoms of UTI but no bacteriuria	Exclude urethritis, candidiasis, etc. Otherwise likely to be urethral syndrome, which usually responds to conventional antibiotics
Bacteriuria but no pyuria	May suggest contamination. However, pyuria is not invariable in UTI, and may be absent particularly in pyelonephritis, pregnancy, neonates, the elderly, and *Proteus* infections.
Pyuria but no bacteriuria	Usually the patient has started antibiotics before taking the specimen. Rarely, a feature of unusual infections (e.g. anaerobes, tuberculosis, etc.)
Urine grows Candida	Usually reflects perineal candidiasis and contamination. True candiduria is rare, and may reflect renal candidiasis or systemic infection with candidaemia
Urine grows two or more organisms	Mixed UTI is unusual – mixed cultures are likely to reflect perineal contamination. A repeat should be sent unless this is impractical (e.g. frail elderly patients), in which case best guess treatment should be instituted if clinically indicated
Symptoms recur shortly after treatment	May represent relapse or reinfection. A repeat urine culture should be performed

UTI, urinary tract infection.

Case 34.2

A pregnant woman aged 26 years is found to have bacteriuria at her first antenatal visit. There are no white or red cells seen in her urine. Urine culture demonstrates *E. coli* at a count of more than 100 000 bacteria per ml, sensitive to trimethoprim, nitrofurantoin and cefalexin but resistant to amoxicillin. Other than a degree of urinary frequency, which she ascribes to the pregnancy itself, the patient does not complain of any urinary symptoms.

Question

Does this patient need antibiotic treatment, and if so, which drugs could be safely used?

Answer

The patient may be correct that her urinary frequency is a consequence of pregnancy. However, because of the consequences of untreated infection during pregnancy, even asymptomatic bacteriuria should be treated. A repeat urine specimen should be obtained to confirm the finding, and treatment started with either nitrofurantoin or cefalexin for 7 days. Trimethoprim should be avoided during pregnancy because of its theoretical risk of teratogenicity. Following treatment she should be reviewed throughout the pregnancy to ensure eradication of the bacteriuria, and to permit early treatment of any relapse or reinfection.

Case 34.3

A boy aged 2 is admitted to hospital with vomiting and abdominal pain. His mother reports that he was treated for urinary tract infection 6 months previously, but was not investigated further at the time. A clean catch urine sample shows over 50 white cells/mm^3, and bacteria are seen on microscopy.

Question

What action should be taken?

Answer

It seems that this child is suffering from a recurrent urinary tract infection. An intravenous antibiotic such as cefuroxime should be started, since the child will not tolerate oral antibiotics at present. If the organism proves to be sensitive to amoxicillin, the treatment could be changed accordingly. Further investigations (for example ultrasonography and radioisotope scan) should be carried out to determine any underlying cause of the infection and to look for already established renal scarring. The child may require long term prophylaxis to prevent recurrence.

Case 34.4

An elderly lady on an orthopaedic ward is catheterized because of incontinence. She is afebrile but has been confused since her hip replacement 5 days earlier, and remains on cefuroxime, which was started as prophylaxis at the time of the operation. The urine in her catheter bag is cloudy, has a high white cell count, and grows *Enterococcus faecalis* sensitive to amoxicillin but resistant to cephalosporins.

Question

How should this patient be managed?

Answer

The patient's confusion may have a number of causes, including her recent surgery, sleep disturbance, drug toxicity, deep venous thrombosis, or infection. If, following clinical examination and investigation (which should include blood cultures), her catheter-associated infection is thought to be contributing to her systemic problems, it should be treated with amoxicillin. If possible the catheter should be removed, even if this is inconvenient for the nursing staff. Unless it has another indication, the cefuroxime is achieving nothing and may be stopped.

Case 34.5

A woman aged 45 suffers from recurrent episodes of cystitis. Examination is unremarkable. On the occasions when a specimen has been sent, the urine has contained few white cells and no significant growth of organisms.

Question

How should the patient be managed?

Answer

This patient is suffering from the urethral syndrome, in which symptoms of infection are not associated with objective evidence of urinary tract infection. It may be felt necessary to investigate her to exclude causes of urethritis such as *Chlamydia trachomatis*, *Neisseria gonorrhoeae* and *Mycoplasma hominis*. Otherwise, her symptoms are likely to respond to conventional courses of antibiotics.

Case 34.6

During an admission for the investigation of long-standing confusion, an elderly man is found to have a heavy mixed growth of organisms in his urine.

Question

Should he be treated with an antibiotic, and if so, which one?

Answer

The question cannot be fully addressed using the available information, but mixed cultures are usually the result of contamination. Unless his clinical condition demands urgent antimicrobial therapy, his urine culture should be carefully repeated in the first instance with attempts to avoid contamination.

REFERENCES

Avorn J, Monane M, Gurwitz J H et al 1994 Reduction of bacteriuria and pyuria after ingestion of cranberry juice. Journal of the American Medical Association 271: 751–754

Baerheim A, Digranes A, Hunskaar S 1999 Equal symptomatic outcome after antibacterial treatment of acute lower urinary tract infection and the acute urethral syndrome in adult women. Scandinavian Journal of Primary Health Care 17: 170–173

Bulloch B, Bauscher J C, Pomerantz W J et al 2000 Can urine clarity exclude the diagnosis of urinary tract infection? Pediatrics 106 (5): E60

Godfrey K M, Lindsay E N, Ronald A R et al 1991 How long should catheter-acquired urinary tract infection in women be treated? Annals of Internal Medicine 114: 713–719

Jepson R G, Mihaljevic L, Craig J 2000 Cranberries for preventing urinary tract infections (Cochrane Review). In: The Cochrane Library, Issue 4. Update Software, Oxford

Jones C, Bennitt W, Halloran S P 1998 Evaluation of urine reagent strips. Medical Devices Directorate Evaluation Report. HMSO, London

Kahlmeter G 2000 The ECOSENS project: a prospective, multinational, multicentre epidemiological survey of the prevalence and antimicrobial susceptibility of urinary tract pathogens. Interim report. Journal of Antimicrobial Chemotherapy (Suppl. S1): 15–22

Kass E H 1957 Bacteriuria and the diagnosis of infections of the urinary tract. Archives of Internal Medicine 100: 709–714

Le Saux N, Pham B, Moher D 2000 Evaluating the benefits of antimicrobial prophylaxis to prevent urinary tract infections in children: a systematic review. Canadian Medical Association Journal 163: 523–529

Smaill F 2000 Antibiotics for asymptomatic bacteriuria in pregnancy (Cochrane Review). In: The Cochrane Library, Issue 4. Update Software, Oxford

Talan D A, Stamm W E, Hooton T M 2000 Comparison of ciprofloxacin (7 days) and trimethoprim-sulfamethoxazole (14 days) for acute uncomplicated pyelonephritis in women: a randomized trial. Journal of the American Medical Association 283: 1583–1590

Warren J W, Abrutyn E, Hebel J R et al 1999 Guidelines for antimicrobial treatment of uncomplicated acute bacterial cystitis and acute pyelonephritis in women. Clinical Infectious Diseases 29: 745–758

Winstanley T G, Limb D I, Eggington R et al 1997 A 10-year survey of the antimicrobial susceptibility of urinary tract isolates in the UK: the Microbe Base project. Journal of Antimicrobial Chemotherapy 40: 591–594

FURTHER READING

Berrington A W, Bint A J 1999 Diagnosis and management of urinary tract infection in pregnancy. Reviews in Medical Microbiology 10 (1): 27–36

Hooton T M 2000 Pathogenesis of urinary tract infections: an update. Journal of Antimicrobial Chemotherapy 46 (Suppl. S1): 1–7

Larcombe J 2000 Urinary tract infection in children. British Medical Journal 319: 1173–1175

Naber K G 2000 Treatment options for acute uncomplicated cystitis in adults. Journal of Antimicrobial Chemotherapy 46 (Suppl. S1): 23–27

Sobel J D, Kaye D 1995 Urinary tract infections. In: Mandell G L, Bennett J E, Dolin R (eds) 2000 Principles and practice of infectious diseases, 5th edn. Philadelphia, Churchill Livingstone, pp 773–805

Gastrointestinal infections 35

J. W. Gray

Gastrointestinal infections represent a major public health and clinical problem worldwide. Many species of bacteria, viruses and protozoa cause gastrointestinal infection, resulting in two main clinical syndromes. Gastroenteritis is a non-invasive infection of the small or large bowel that manifests clinically as diarrhoea and vomiting. Other infections are invasive, causing systemic illness, often with few gastrointestinal symptoms. *Helicobacter pylori*, and its association with gastritis, peptic ulceration and gastric carcinoma, is discussed in Chapter 10.

Epidemiology and aetiology

In Western countries the average person probably experiences one or two episodes of gastrointestinal infection each year. Infections are rarely severe, and the vast majority never reach medical attention. In the UK,

Campylobacter, followed by non-typhoidal *Salmonella* species, are much the commonest reported causes of bacterial gastroenteritis. Gastroenteritis due to viruses such as rotaviruses, adenoviruses and small round structured viruses is also common. Cryptosporidiosis is the most commonly reported parasitic infection.

In developing countries the incidence of gastrointestinal infection is at least twice as high, and the range of common pathogens is much wider. Infections are more often severe, and represent a major cause of mortality, especially in children. Gastrointestinal infections can be transmitted by consumption of contaminated food or water, or by direct faecal–oral spread. Airborne spread of viruses that cause gastroenteritis also occurs. The most important causes of gastrointestinal infection, and their usual modes of spread, are shown in Table 35.1.

In developed countries, the majority of gastrointestinal infections are food-borne. Farm animals are often colonized by gastrointestinal pathogens, especially *Salmonella* and *Campylobacter*. Therefore, raw foods such as poultry, meat, eggs and unpasteurized dairy products are commonly contaminated, and must be thoroughly cooked in order to kill such organisms. Raw foods also represent a potential source of cross-contamination of other foods, through hands, surfaces or utensils that have been inadequately cleaned. Food handlers who are excreting pathogens in their faeces can also contaminate food. This is most likely when diarrhoea is present, but continued excretion of pathogens during convalescence also represents a risk. Food handlers are the usual source of *Staphylococcus aureus* food poisoning, where toxin-producing strains of *Staph. aureus* carried in the nose or on skin are transferred to foods. Bacterial food poisoning is often associated with inadequate cooking and/or prolonged storage of food at ambient temperature before consumption.

Water-borne gastrointestinal infection is primarily a problem in countries without a sanitary water supply or sewerage system, although outbreaks of water-borne cryptosporidiosis occur from time to time in the UK.

Spread of pathogens such as *Shigella* or enteropathogenic *Escherichia coli* by the faecal–oral

Table 35.1   Important causes of gastrointestinal infection their modes of spread and pathogenic mechanisms

Causative agent	Chief mode(s) of spread	Pathogenic mechanisms
Bacteria		
Campylobacter	Food, especially poultry, milk	Mucosal invasion Enterotoxin
Salmonella species other than *S. typhi* and *S. paratyphi* *S. typhi* and *S. paratyphi*	Food, especially poultry, eggs, meat Food, water	Mucosal invasion Enterotoxin Systemic invasion
Shigella	Faecal–oral	Mucosal invasion

Escherichia coli
    Enteropathogenic
    Enterotoxigenic
    Enteroinvasive
    Verotoxin-producing
	
	Faecal–oral
	Faecal–oral, water
	Faecal–oral, food
	Food, especially beef
		Enterotoxin
		Mucosal adhesion
		Enterotoxin
		Mucosal invasion
		Verotoxin

Staphylococcus aureus	Food, especially meat, dairy produce	Emetic toxin
Clostridium perfringens	Food, especially meat	Enterotoxin

Bacillus cereus
    Short incubation period
    Long incubation period
	
	Food, especially rice
	Food, especially meat and vegetable dishes
		
		Emetic toxin
		Enterotoxin

Vibrio cholerae O1, O139	Water	Enterotoxin
Vibrio parahaemolyticus	Seafoods	Mucosal invasion Enterotoxin
Clostridium difficile	Uncertain – nosocomial transmission common	Cytotoxin Enterotoxin
Clostridium botulinum	Inadequately heat-treated canned/preserved foods	Neurotoxin
Protozoa *Giardia lamblia* *Cryptosporidium* *Entamoeba histolytica*	 Water Water, animal contact Food, water	 Mucosal invasion Mucosal invasion Mucosal invasion
Viruses	Food, faecal–oral, respiratory secretions	Small intestinal mucosal damage

route is favoured by overcrowding and poor standards of personal hygiene. Such infections in developed countries are commonest in children, and can cause troublesome outbreaks in paediatric wards, nurseries and residential children's homes.

Treatment with broad-spectrum antibiotics alters the bowel flora, creating conditions that favour superinfection with micro-organisms (principally *Clostridium difficile*) that can cause diarrhoea. *C. difficile* infection may be associated with any antibiotic, but clindamycin, ampicillin and the cephalosporins are most commonly implicated. *C. difficile*-associated diarrhoea is more common in patients with serious underlying disease and in the elderly. Although some sporadic cases are probably due to overgrowth of endogenous organisms, person-to-person transmission also occurs in hospitals and nursing homes, sometimes resulting in large outbreaks.

Pathophysiology

Development of symptoms after ingestion of gastrointestinal pathogens depends on two factors. First, sufficient organisms must be ingested and then survive host defence mechanisms, and second, the pathogens must possess one or more virulence mechanisms in order to cause disease.

Host factors

Healthy individuals possess a number of defence mechanisms that protect against infection by enteropathogens. Therefore, large numbers of many pathogens must be ingested for infection to ensue; for example, the infective dose for *Salmonella* is typically around 10^5 organisms. Other species, however, are better able to survive host defence mechanisms; for example, infection with *Shigella* or verotoxin-producing *E. coli* (VTEC) can result from ingestion of fewer than 100 organisms. VTEC (principally *E. coli* O157) are especially important because of the risk of a life-threatening complication, haemolytic uraemic syndrome (HUS).

Gastric acidity

Most micro-organisms are rapidly killed at normal gastric pH. Patients whose gastric pH is less acid, as for example following treatment with antacids or ulcer-healing drugs, are more susceptible to gastrointestinal infections.

Intestinal motility

It is widely held that intestinal motility helps to rid the host of enteric pathogens, and that antimotility agents are therefore potentially hazardous in patients with infective gastroenteritis. However there is little evidence for this belief.

Resident microflora

The resident microflora, largely composed of anaerobic bacteria, help to resist colonization by enteropathogens.

Immune system

Phagocytic, humoral and cell-mediated elements are important in resistance to different pathogens. Individuals with inherited or acquired immunodeficiencies are therefore susceptible to specific gastrointestinal infections, depending on which components of their immune system are affected.

Organism factors

The symptoms of gastrointestinal infection can be mediated by several different mechanisms (see Table 35.1).

Toxins

Toxins produced by gastrointestinal pathogens can be classified as enterotoxins, neurotoxins and cytotoxins. Enterotoxins act on intestinal mucosal cells to cause net loss of fluid and electrolytes. The classical enterotoxin-mediated disease is cholera, the result of infection with toxigenic serotypes of *Vibrio cholera*. Many other bacteria produce enterotoxins, including enterotoxigenic *E. coli* and *Clostridium perfringens*.

The emetic toxins of *Staph. aureus* and *Bacillus cereus* are neurotoxins that induce vomiting by an action on the central nervous system. The symptoms of botulism are mediated by a neurotoxin that blocks release of acetylcholine at nerve endings. Cytotoxins cause mucosal destruction and inflammation (see below). Verotoxins are potent cytotoxins that bind to specific receptors only expressed on the surface of certain cells, especially endothelial cells. This is believed to be central to the pathogenesis of the complications of VTEC-associated diarrhoea: destruction of the intestinal vasculature causing haemorrhagic colitis, and damage to the glomerular microvasculature leading to haemolytic uraemic syndrome.

Mucosal damage

Cytotoxins are important in mediating mucosal invasion, but other mechanisms are also involved. Enteropathogenic *E. coli* appears to cause diarrhoea by adhering to the intestinal mucosa and damaging microvilli. Organisms such as *Shigella* and enteroinvasive *E. coli* express surface proteins that facilitate mucosal invasion. Diarrhoea due to mucosal damage may be due to reduction in the absorptive surface area, or the presence of increased numbers of immature enterocytes which are secretory rather than absorptive.

Systemic invasion

The lipopolysaccharide outer membrane and possession of an antiphagocytic outer capsule are important virulence factors in invasive *Salmonella* infections.

Clinical manifestations

Many cases of gastrointestinal infection are asymptomatic or cause subclinical illness.

Gastroenteritis is the commonest syndrome of gastrointestinal infection, presenting with symptoms such as vomiting, diarrhoea and abdominal pain. The term 'dysentery' is sometimes applied to infections with *Shigella* (bacillary dysentery) and *Entamoeba histolytica* (amoebic dysentery), where severe colonic mucosal inflammation causes frequent diarrhoea with blood and pus. Table 35.2 shows the most important causes of gastroenteritis together with a brief description of the typical illness that each causes. However, the symptoms experienced by individuals infected with the same organism can differ considerably.

Gastrointestinal manifestations of infection with VTEC range from non-bloody diarrhoea to haemorrhagic colitis. In addition, VTEC are the most important cause of haemolytic uraemic syndrome (HUS), a serious complication which is most common in young children and the elderly. HUS is defined by the triad of microangiopathic haemolytic anaemia, thrombocytopenia and acute renal dysfunction. The mortality is about 5%, and up to half of survivors suffer long-term renal damage.

The clinical spectrum of infection with *C. difficile* ranges from asymptomatic carriage to life-threatening pseudomembranous colitis (so called because yellow-white plaques or membranes consisting of fibrin, mucus, leucocytes and necrotic epithelial cells are found adherent to the inflamed colonic mucosa).

Enteric fever, resulting from infection with *Salmonella typhi* or *S. paratyphi*, presents with symptoms such as headache, malaise and abdominal distension after an incubation period of 3–21 days. During the first week of the illness the temperature gradually increases but the pulse characteristically remains slow. Without treatment, during the second and third weeks the symptoms become more pronounced. Diarrhoea develops in about half of cases. Examination usually reveals splenomegaly, and a few erythematous macules (rose spots) may be found, usually on the trunk.

Table 35.2 Characteristic clinical features of various causes of gastroenteritis

Causative agent	Incubation period	Symptoms (syndrome)
Campylobacter	2–5 days	Bloody diarrhoea Abdominal pain Systemic upset
Salmonella	6–72 h	Diarrhoea and vomiting Fever; may be associated bacteraemia
Shigella	1–4 days	Diarrhoea, fever (bacillary dysentery)

Escherichia coli
  Enteropathogenic
  Enterotoxigenic
  Enteroinvasive
  Verotoxin-producing
	
	12–72 h
	1–3 days
	1–3 days
	1–3 days
		
		Infantile diarrhoea
		Traveller's diarrhoea
		Similar to *Shigella*
		Bloody diarrhoea (haemorrhagic colitis)
		Haemolytic uraemic syndrome

Staphylococcus aureus	4–8 h	Severe nausea and vomiting
Clostridium perfringens	6–24 h	Diarrhoea

Bacillus cereus
  Short incubation period
  Long Incubation period
	
	1–6 h
	6–18 h
		
		Vomiting
		Diarrhoea

Vibrio cholerae O1, O139	1–5 days	Profuse diarrhoea (cholera)
Vibrio parahaemolyticus	12–48 h	Diarrhoea, abdominal pain
Clostridium difficile	Usually occurs during/just after antibiotic therapy	Diarrhoea, pseudomembranous enterocolitis
Giardia lamblia	1–2 weeks	Watery diarrhoea
Cryptosporidium	2 days–2 weeks	Watery diarrhoea
Entamoeba histolytica	2–4 weeks	Diarrhoea with blood and mucus (amoebic dysentery) liver abscess
Viruses	1–2 days	Vomiting, diarrhoea

Serious gastrointestinal complications such as haemorrhage and perforation are commonest during the third week. Symptoms begin to subside slowly during the fourth week. In general, paratyphoid fever is less severe than typhoid fever.

Botulism typically presents with autonomic nervous system effects, including diplopia and dysphagia, followed by symmetrical descending motor paralysis. There is no sensory involvement.

Gastrointestinal infections are often followed by a period of convalescent carriage of the pathogen. This usually lasts for no more than 4–6 weeks, but can be for considerably longer, especially for *Salmonella*.

Investigations

The mainstay of investigation of diarrhoeal illness is examination of faeces. Bacterial infections are usually diagnosed by stool culture. Various selective culture media designed to suppress growth of normal faecal organisms and/or enhance the growth of a particular pathogen are used. When sending specimens to the laboratory it is important that details of the age of the patient, the clinical presentation, and recent foreign travel are provided, so that appropriate media for the likely pathogens can be selected.

Various other procedures are sometimes useful in investigating patients with suspected bacterial gastroenteritis. Blood cultures should be taken from patients with severe systemic upset. In *Staph. aureus* and *B. cereus* food poisoning the pathogen can sometimes be isolated from vomitus. In cases of food poisoning, suspect foods may also be cultured. In general, serological investigations are of little value in the diagnosis of bacterial gastroenteritis. However, demonstration of serum antibodies to *E. coli* O157 can be helpful in retrospectively determining the cause of the haemolytic uraemic syndrome. Parasitic infestations are usually detected by microscopic examination of faeces. Electron microscopy remains the only method for detecting many viruses in faeces, but it is time-consuming and not widely available. Immunological and molecular-based detection techniques for some viruses are becoming available: in particular, tests for antigens of rotaviruses and adenoviruses are now widely used.

Tests are available for detection of *C. difficile* toxin in faeces, while sigmoidoscopy may be helpful in diagnosing pseudomembranous colitis. Suspected enteric fever should be investigated by culture of urine, faeces, blood and sometimes, bone marrow. Serological tests for typhoid and paratyphoid fever are sometimes helpful, but the results must be interpreted with caution. Botulism is diagnosed by demonstration of toxin in serum.

Treatment

Many gastrointestinal infections are mild and self-limiting and never reach medical attention. Where treatment is required there are three main therapeutic considerations. Fluid and electrolyte replacement is the cornerstone of treatment of diarrhoeal disease. Most patients can be managed with oral rehydration regimens, but severely dehydrated patients require rapid volume expansion with intravenous fluids. Symptomatic treatment with antiemetics and antidiarrhoeal agents is occasionally prescribed, but the efficacy and safety of these agents in infective gastroenteritis are uncertain. Antimicrobial agents may be useful both in effecting symptomatic improvement and in eliminating faecal carriage of pathogens (and therefore reducing the risk of transmitting infection to others).

Antiemetics and antidiarrhoeal drugs are discussed in Chapters 32 and 12, respectively. This chapter focuses on the place of antibiotic therapy in gastrointestinal infections.

Antibiotic therapy

The requirement for antibiotic treatment in gastrointestinal infection depends on the causative agent, the type and severity of symptoms, and the presence of underlying disease. Antibiotics are ineffective in some forms of gastroenteritis, including bacterial intoxications and viral infections. For many other infections, such as salmonellosis and campylobacteriosis, effective agents are available, but antimicrobial therapy is often not clinically necessary. Serious infections such as enteric fever always require antibiotic therapy.

Conditions for which antibiotic therapy is not available or not usually required

The symptoms of *Staph. aureus* and short incubation period *B. cereus* food poisoning and botulism are usually caused by ingestion of preformed toxin, and therefore antibiotic therapy would not influence the illness. Pathogens such as *C. perfringens*, *Vibrio parahaemolyticus* and enteropathogenic *E. coli* usually cause a brief self-limiting illness that does not require specific treatment.

None of the presently available antiviral agents are useful in viral gastroenteritis. While most viral infections are self-limiting, chronic rotavirus diarrhoea can occur in immunocompromised patients. Immunoglobulin-containing preparations, administered orally or directly into the duodenum via a nasogastric tube, have been reported to be effective in such circumstances (Hammarstrom 1999). As well as human serum immunoglobulin, antibodies from other species (e.g.

immunized bovine colostrum) have been used. Immunotherapy of rotavirus infection remains experimental, and dosages and frequency of administration of immunoglobulin preparations cannot be recommended.

Conditions for which antimicrobial therapy should be considered

The place for antibiotics in the management of uncomplicated gastroenteritis due to organisms such as *Salmonella*, *Campylobacter* and *Shigella* is not clear-cut. Certain antibiotics are reasonably effective in reducing the duration and severity of clinical illness and in eradicating the organisms from faeces. However, many microbiologists are cautious about the widespread use of antibiotics in diarrhoeal illness because of the risk of promoting antibiotic resistance (Sack et al 1997). Another difficulty with respect to antibiotic prescribing is that it is not usually possible to determine the aetiological agent of diarrhoea on clinical grounds, and stool culture takes at least 48 hours. Patients with severe illness, especially systemic symptoms, may require antibiotic therapy before the aetiological agent has been established. In such circumstances a quinolone antibiotic such as ciprofloxacin would usually be the most appropriate empiric agent, at least in adults. Otherwise, it is reasonable to limit antibiotic use to microbiologically proven cases where there is serious underlying disease and/or continuing severe symptoms. Antibiotics may also be used to try to eliminate faecal carriage, for example in controlling outbreaks in institutions, or in food handlers who may be prevented from returning to work until they are no longer excreting gastrointestinal pathogens.

Campylobacteriosis. Erythromycin is effective in terminating faecal excretion of *Campylobacter*. Some studies have shown that treatment commenced within the first 72–96 hours of illness can also shorten the duration of clinical illness, especially in patients with severe dysenteric symptoms. The recommended dosage for adults is 250–500 mg four times a day orally for 5–7 days, and for children 30–50 mg/kg/day in four divided doses. The newer macrolide antibiotics such as azithromycin and clarithromycin are also effective, but are only recommended where the patient is unable to tolerate erythromycin. Ciprofloxacin, at a dose of 500 mg twice daily orally for adults, may also be effective in *Campylobacter* enteritis. However, whereas resistance rates to erythromycin have generally remained below 5%, resistance to ciprofloxacin has emerged rapidly, exceeding 10% in the UK and 50% in some countries (Thwaites & Frost 1997).

Salmonellosis. Most cases of *Salmonella* gastroenteritis are self-limiting, and antibiotic therapy is unnecessary. However, antimicrobial therapy of salmonellosis is routinely recommended for young infants and immunocompromised patients, who are susceptible to complicated infections. Most antibiotics, even those with good in vitro activity, are ineffective in uncomplicated *Salmonella* gastroenteritis. The fluoroquinolones, such as ciprofloxacin, can often shorten both the symptomatic period and the duration of faecal carriage. However ciprofloxacin resistance is now seen in about 2.5% of European and up to 10% of non-European *Salmonella* isolates. The recommended dose of ciprofloxacin for adults is 500 mg twice daily orally for 1 week. Fluoroquinolones are not licensed for this indication in children, although there is increasing evidence that they can safely be given to children. The recommended dose of ciprofloxacin in childhood is 7.5 mg/kg twice daily orally. Trimethoprim at a dose of 25–100 mg twice daily orally may be used in children if it is preferred not to use a quinolone.

Ciprofloxacin given orally at a dose of 500–750 mg twice daily in adults (7.5–12.5 mg/kg twice daily in children) or 200 mg i.v. twice daily in adults (5–7.5 mg/kg twice daily in children) is recommended for invasive salmonellosis. Alternative agents include ampicillin or amoxicillin, trimethoprim or chloramphenicol (see under enteric fever). However, some strains of *Salmonella* (e.g. *S. typhimurium* DT104, *S. virchow* and *S. hadar*) are commonly resistant to some or all of these agents.

Enteric fever. Fluoroquinolones are now widely regarded as the drugs of choice for typhoid and paratyphoid fevers. The clinical response is at least as rapid as with the older treatments, there is a lower relapse rate, and convalescent faecal carriage is shortened. Moreover, multidrug-resistant *S. typhi* (MDRST) that are resistant to co-trimoxazole, chloramphenicol and ampicillin now account for up to 95% of isolates in some parts of the Indian subcontinent, from where most infections seen in the UK originate (Rowe et al 1997). However, ciprofloxacin resistance is also beginning to emerge, and has recently been found in 5–10% of isolates in India and the UK. Agents that have been reported to be successful in treating infections with MDRST that are also ciprofloxacin-resistant include imipenem, meropenem, ceftriaxone and azithromycin.

Doses of ciprofloxacin are as outlined for non-typhoidal salmonellosis (see above). The usual dose of chloramphenicol is 50 mg/kg/day in four divided doses, and for ampicillin 100 mg/kg/day in four divided doses. Two weeks of antibiotic therapy is usually recommended, although shorter courses of ciprofloxacin (7–10 days) may be as effective. There is insufficient experience of using other agents to permit recommendation of dosages.

Chronic carriers of *Salmonella*. Patients may become chronic carriers after *Salmonella* infection, especially in the presence of underlying biliary tract disease. Oral ciprofloxacin 500–750 mg twice daily continued for 2–6 weeks is usually effective in eradicating carriage, and has largely superseded the use of oral amoxicillin at a dose of 3 g twice daily.

Shigellosis. *Shigella sonnei*, which accounts for most cases of shigellosis in the UK, usually causes a mild self-limiting illness. Although often not required on clinical grounds, antibiotic therapy of shigellosis is usually recommended in order to eliminate faecal carriage, and therefore prevent person-to-person transmission. In contrast to salmonellosis, a number of antibiotics are effective in shortening the duration of illness and terminating faecal carriage. These include oral trimethoprim at a dose of 200 mg twice daily in adults (25 mg twice daily for infants aged 2–5 months; 50 mg twice daily for children aged 6 months to 5 years, and 100 mg. twice daily for children aged 6–12 years), or amoxicillin 250–500 mg three times daily in adults (62.5–125 mg three times daily in children). However, resistance to these agents is increasing throughout the world. The fluoroquinolones are also highly active in shigellosis, and may now be the treatment of choice, in children as well as adults (Salam et al 1998). The dose of ciprofloxacin is 500 mg twice daily orally in adults (7.5 mg/kg twice daily in children). Antibiotic therapy is usually given for a maximum of 5 days.

Cholera. Fluid and electrolyte replacement is the key aspect of the management of cholera. However, antibiotics do shorten the duration of diarrhoea, and therefore reduce the overall fluid loss, and also rapidly terminate faecal excretion of the organism. Effective agents include tetracyclines, erythromycin, trimethoprim, ampicillin or amoxicillin, chloramphenicol and furazolidine. However, antibiotic resistance is being increasingly seen, and in particular *V. cholerae* O139 is intrinsically resistant to furazolidine and trimethoprim. Choice of antibiotics is therefore governed by knowledge of local resistance patterns. Tetracycline 250 mg four times daily, or doxycycline 100 mg once daily by mouth, is probably the most widely used therapy in adults. Ampicillin, amoxicillin or erythromycin are the generally preferred agents for children. Treatment is usually given for 3–5 days.

E. coli infections. While most infections with enteropathogenic *E. coli* can be managed conservatively, small trials suggest that trimethoprim may be effective, especially in controlling nursery or hospital outbreaks. On the basis that enteroinvasive *E. coli* are closely related to *Shigella*, and cause a similar clinical syndrome, similar therapy may be appropriate. Antibiotic therapy for enterotoxigenic *E. coli* infection is often unnecessary, but troublesome symptoms will respond to a 3–5 day course of ciprofloxacin or trimethoprim, although resistance to trimethoprim is becoming increasingly common in some areas. At least one recent study found that the risk of HUS in children with diarrhoea due to VTEC was much higher in those who received antibiotics (Wong et al 2000). On that basis it is advised in the UK that antibiotics are contraindicated in children with VTEC infection.

C. difficile infection. In antibiotic-associated diarrhoea, current antibiotic therapy should, if possible, be stopped. Although mild cases may resolve without specific therapy, treatment of all hospitalized patients with diarrhoea due to *C. difficile* is recommended, both to shorten the duration of illness, and to reduce environmental contamination (and therefore the risk of nosocomial transmission). However, treatment of asymptomatic individuals is not usually necessary. Oral metronidazole 400 mg three times daily for 10 days is the treatment of choice. Oral vancomycin is no more effective, is around 200-fold more expensive, and its use may be an important factor in the emergence and spread of vancomycin-resistant enterococci (Brar & Surawicz 2000, Wilcox 1998). Oral vancomycin 125–500 mg four times daily (there is little evidence that higher doses are more effective) should therefore be reserved for those who cannot tolerate or have not responded to metronidazole. Vancomycin is sometimes also preferred for severe potentially life-threatening cases, although evidence of greater efficacy is lacking. In patients unable to take oral medication, either drug can be administered via a nasogastric tube. Metronidazole suppositories may be used, and vancomycin has been instilled into the rectum and caecum via a tube. Intravenous therapy should be a last resort.

Recurrence of symptoms occurs in about 20% of patients treated for *C. difficile* infection. Although some recurrences are due to germination of spores that have persisted in the colon since the original infection, it is now recognized that the majority of these cases are due to reinfection, rather than relapse caused by the original strain (Wilcox 1998). Most recurrences respond to a further 10–14 day course of metronidazole or vancomycin, but a few patients experience repeated recurrences. There is no reliable means of managing these patients. Recognizing that recurrences may be due to repeated reinfections, enhanced infection control precautions may be the most important measure. Prolonged, tapered or pulsed antibiotic therapy is effective in some cases. Promising results have been obtained from trials of biotherapy to try to normalize the faecal flora, for example using the yeast *Saccharomyces boulardii*. Preliminary studies of immunotherapy with anti-*C. difficile* bovine immunoglobulin concentrates have also shown potential.

Cryptosporidiosis. Cryptosporidiosis in immunocompetent individuals is generally self-limiting. However, in immunosuppressed patients, severe diarrhoea can persist indefinitely, and can even contribute to death. Unfortunately there is no reliable antimicrobial therapy. There have been a number of reports of successful treatment of individual patients using azithromycin at a dose of 500 mg once daily (10 mg/kg once daily in children). Treatment should be continued until *Cryptosporidium* oocysts are no longer detectable in faeces (typically 2 weeks), in order to minimize the risk of relapse post-treatment. Occasionally therapy has to be continued indefinitely to prevent relapse. Most other agents (e.g. spiramycin, paromomycin and letrazuril) that have been investigated for treatment of cryptosporidiosis are unlicensed in the UK. None of these appears to be more effective than azithromycin.

Giardiasis. Metronidazole is the treatment of choice for giardiasis (Vesy & Peterson 1999). Various oral regimens are effective, for example 400 mg three times daily (children 7.5 mg/kg) for 5 days, or 2 g/day (children 500 mg to 1 g) for 3 days. Alternative treatments are tinidazole 2 g as a single dose, or mepacrine hydrochloride 100 mg (children 2 mg/kg) three times daily for 5–7 days. A single course of treatment for giardiasis has a failure rate of up to 10%. A further course of the same or another agent is often successful. Sometimes repeated relapses are due to reinfection from an asymptomatic family member. In such cases all affected family members should be treated simultaneously.

Amoebiasis. The aim of treatment in amoebiasis is to kill all vegetative amoebae and also to eradicate cysts from the bowel lumen. Metronidazole is highly active against vegetative amoebae, and is the treatment of choice for acute amoebic dysentery and amoebic liver abscess. The dose for adults is 800 mg (children 100–400 mg) three times daily for 5–10 days. In order to eradicate cysts, metronidazole therapy is followed by a 5 day course of diloxanide furoate 500 mg three times daily (20 mg/kg daily in three divided doses for children).

Asymptomatic excretors of cysts living in areas with a high prevalence of *E. histolytica* infection do not merit treatment because most individuals would quickly become reinfected. However, asymptomatic excretors of cysts in Europe or North America are usually treated with diloxanide furoate for 5–10 days, sometimes combined with metronidazole.

Patient care

Prevention of person-to-person transmission of gastrointestinal infections

People excreting gastrointestinal pathogens are potentially infectious to others. Liquid stools are particularly likely to contaminate the hands and the environment. All cases of gastrointestinal infection should be excluded from work or school at least until the patients are symptom-free. Patients should be advised on

general hygiene, and in particular on thorough handwashing and drying after visiting the toilet, and before handling food.

In most countries many gastrointestinal infections are statutorily notifiable. Following notification, the authorities will judge whether the implications for public health merit investigation of the source of infection, contact screening, or follow-up clearance stool samples from the original case.

Common therapeutic problems in the management of gastrointestinal infection are summarized in Table 35.3.

CASE STUDIES

Case 35.1

A 35-year-old man presents with a history of fever, weight loss and malaise 2 weeks after returning from undertaking voluntary work in the Indian countryside. Examination is unremarkable, except that the tip of his spleen is just palpable. His symptoms began a month before leaving India, when he also had mild diarrhoea. A stool sample at that time had shown that he had an infection, and he was treated with chloramphenicol for 5 days with no significant clinical response.

Questions

1. Which gastrointestinal infection would be at the top of the differential diagnosis?
2. What microbiological investigations might help to confirm this?
3. Give two reasons why he might not have responded to the treatment given in India.
4. Which antibiotic would be most appropriate as empirical therapy? Assuming that the diagnosis is confirmed, what is the likelihood that this antibiotic will be effective?

Answers

1. This presentation is typical of enteric fever (typhoid or paratyphoid fever). The patient's previous positive stool culture is also consistent with this diagnosis. However, it is also important to consider non-gastrointestinal infections, especially malaria, in a case such as this.
2. Enteric fever is usually diagnosed by isolation of the causative bacterium in stool or blood cultures. Culture of other specimens such as urine or bone marrow is occasionally helpful. Serology would be of limited value in this case, because it would be difficult to distinguish between continuing infection and an infection that has recently been adequately treated.
3. Chloramphenicol resistance is common in *Salmonella typhi* in the Indian subcontinent. Even if this strain had been chloramphenicol-sensitive, 5 days treatment would have been inadequate to reliably achieve a long-term cure.
4. Fluoroquinolones (usually ciprofloxacin) are generally regarded as the treatment of choice for enteric fever. Fewer than 10% of *S. typhi* are resistant to ciprofloxacin.

Table 35.3   Common therapeutic problems in the management of gastrointestinal infections

Infection	Antibiotic	Common problems	Resolution
Campylobacteriosis	Erythromycin	Not always effective, especially if commenced > 72 h after onset of symptoms	Reserve therapy for cases where symptoms are severe or worsening at time of diagnosis
	Ciprofloxacin[a]	Up to 50% of strains are resistant	Use only as a second line agent for isolates that have been shown to be sensitive
Salmonellosis	Ciprofloxacin[a]	Not always effective. Resistance is increasing	Reserve therapy for cases where symptoms are severe or worsening at time of diagnosis
Enteric fever	Ciprofloxacin[a]	Resistance is increasing	Alternative therapies must be guided by antibiotic sensitivities of the isolate
	Ampicillin or amoxicillin	Resistance to these agents now common	Ciprofloxacin[1] now generally regarded as treatment of choice
	Chloramphenicol	Higher incidence of chronic carriage and relapse than with ciprofloxacin	
	Co-trimoxazole		
Shigellosis	Trimethoprim	Resistance is increasing	Therapy should be guided by antibiotic sensitivities of the isolate. Most trimethoprim-resistant strains are ciprofloxacin-sensitive
Clostridium difficile	Metronidazole	Relapse rate up to 20%	Repeat course of treatment. Enhanced infection control precautions to prevent reinfection
	Vancomycin	Comparable efficacy to, but much more expensive than, metronidazole. Risk of promoting emergence and spread of vancomycin-resistant enterococci	Generally reserved as a second line agent, e.g. where no response to metronidazole, or occasionally for patients with severe infection
Cryptosporidiosis	Azithromycin	Not always effective. Recommended only for patients who are immunocompromised or have unusually severe or protracted symptoms	Long-term therapy may be required to control symptoms. Possible alternative agents are experimental

[a] Ciprofloxacin is not licensed for general paediatric use; it is widely used to treat gastrointestinal infections in children.

Case 35.2

A four-year-old child presents with a 4-day history of diarrhoea, which has occasionally been bloody. The child is otherwise well and is taking fluids; examination is unremarkable. The parents are anxious that she should be given an antibiotic to ensure that she recovers as soon as possible.

Questions

1. What are the possible infective causes of this child's diarrhoea?
2. Why is antibiotic therapy not appropriate?

Answers

1. Infections that invade the bowel mucosa can cause bloody diarrhoea. *Salmonella*, *Campylobacter* and verotoxin-producing *E. coli* (VTEC) are the most likely causes in developed countries.
2. Most cases of infective diarrhoea settle without antibiotic therapy. Widespread use of antibiotics to treat mild gastrointestinal tract infections would be likely to promote antibiotic resistance, thus compromising the effectiveness of antibiotics in serious infections. Moreover, antibiotic therapy in children with VTEC infection may increase the risk of them developing haemolytic uraemic syndrome. In general, antibiotic therapy should be considered only for patients whose symptoms are severe or worsening at the time when a pathogen has been cultured from a stool sample.

Case 35.3

A young woman is due to embark on a trekking holiday in Central America. There will be no access to medical services, and she has been advised to carry antibiotics that she can take if she develops diarrhoea.

Questions

1. Which two antibiotics would you recommend that she carry?
2. How would you advise her to use them?

Answers

1. The fluoroquinolones, such as ciprofloxacin, have the broadest activity against bacterial gastrointestinal

pathogens, including those associated with traveller's diarrhoea. Metronidazole is effective in common parasitic infections, such as giardiasis and amoebiasis.
2. Ciprofloxacin should be commenced at the onset of diarrhoea. Concurrent treatment with an antimotility agent, such as loperamide, is sometimes recommended. In bacterial gastroenteritis a response to ciprofloxacin would be expected within 48 hours. If there is no improvement in symptoms after 48–72 hours, metronidazole can be commenced.

Case 35.4

An 80-year-old woman on a geriatric ward develops profuse diarrhoea 5 days after commencing therapy with cefuroxime for a respiratory tract infection. *Clostridium difficile* toxin is detected in a stool sample. An increasing number of other patients on the ward have been developing *C. difficile*-associated diarrhoea during the past 6 months, which appears to have coincided with an increase in antibiotic prescribing.

Questions

1. How should this patient be managed?
2. What measures might be taken to try to reduce the number of cases of *C. difficile*-associated diarrhoea on the ward?

Answers

1. If possible, treatment with cefuroxime should be discontinued. If further antibiotic therapy for her respiratory tract infection is required, an antibiotic that is less likely to disturb the bowel flora should be prescribed. Metronidazole is the preferred treatment for infection with *C. difficile*. The patient should be isolated to reduce the risk of spread of the infection.
2. There are two elements to control of *C. difficile* in hospitals. First, strict infection control precautions and improved standards of environmental cleanliness can reduce the risk of patients being exposed to the bacterium. Second, the antibiotic policy on the ward should be reviewed with a view to both minimizing the use of antibiotics in general and, where antibiotic therapy is essential, to selecting agents that have least effect on the bowel flora.

REFERENCES

Brar H S, Surawicz C M 2000 Pseudomembranous colitis: an update. Canadian Journal of Gastroenterology 14: 51–56

Hammarstrom L 1999 Passive immunity against rotavirus in infants. Acta Paediatriatica 88(Suppl.): 127–132

Rowe B, Ward L R, Threlfall E J 1997 Multidrug-resistant *Salmonella typhi*: a worldwide epidemic. Clinical Infectious Diseases 24(Suppl. 1): S106–S109

Sack R B, Rahman M, Yunus M et al 1997 Antimicrobial resistance in organisms causing diarrheal disease. Clinical Infectious Diseases 24(Suppl. 1): S102–S105

Salam M A, Dhar U, Khan W A et al 1998 Randomised comparison of ciprofloxacin suspension and pivmecillinam for childhood shigellosis. Lancet 352: 522–527

Thwaites R T, Frost J A 1999 Drug resistance in *Campylobacter jejuni, C. coli* and *C. lari* isolated from humans in north west England and Wales, 1997. Journal of Clinical Pathology 52: 812–814

Vesy C J, Peterson W L 1999 Review article: the management of giardiasis. Alimentary Pharmacology and Therapeutics 13: 843–850

Wilcox M H 1998 Treatment of *Clostridium difficile* infection. Journal of Antimicrobial Chemotherapy 41(Suppl. C): 41–46

Wong C S, Jelacic S, Habeeb R L et al 2000 The risk of hemolytic-uremic syndrome after antibiotic treatment of *Escherichia coli* O157:H7 infections. New England Journal of Medicine 342: 1930–1936

FURTHER READING

Baird R W 1999 Gastroenteritis in adults: new aspects of diagnosis and treatment. Australian Family Physician 28: 324–328

Eliason B C, Lewan R B 1998 Gastroenteritis in children: principles of diagnosis and treatment. American Family Physician 58: 1769–1776

Gastanaduy A S, Begue R E 1999 Acute gastroenteritis. Clinical Pediatrics 38: 1–12

Goodman L, Segreti J 1999 Infectious diarrhea. Disease-A-Month 45: 268–299

Mead P S, Griffin P M 1998 *Escherichia coli* O157:H7. Lancet 352: 1207–1212

Lamont J T (ed) 1997 Gastrointestinal infections. Marcel Dekker, New York

Shanson D C 1999 Microbiology in clinical practice, 3rd edn. Arnold, London

Szajewska H, Hoekstra J H, Sandhu B 2000 Management of acute gastroenteritis in Europe and the impact of the new recommendations: a multicenter study. Working Group on Acute Diarrhoea of the European Society for Paediatric Gastroenterology, Hepatology and Nutrition. Journal of Pediatric Gastroenterology and Nutrition 30: 522–527

Infective meningitis

36

J. W. Gray

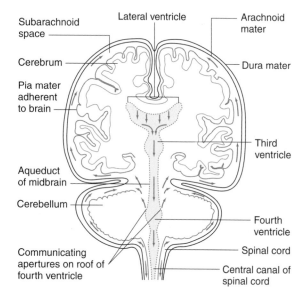

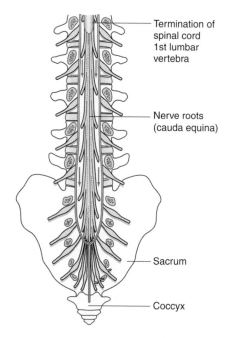

The brain and spinal cord are surrounded by three membranes, which from the outside inwards are the dura mater, the arachnoid mater and the pia mater. Between the arachnoid mater and the pia mater, in the subarachnoid space, is found the cerebrospinal fluid (CSF) (Fig. 36.1). This fluid, of which there is approximately 150 ml in a normal adult, is secreted by the choroid plexuses and vascular structures which are in the third, fourth and lateral ventricles. CSF passes from the ventricles via communicating apertures to the subarachnoid space, whence it flows over the surface of the brain and the spinal cord (see Fig. 36.1). The amount of CSF is controlled by resorption into the bloodstream by vascular structures in the subarachnoid space called the arachnoid villi. Infective meningitis is an

Figure 36.1 The meninges covering the brain and spinal cord and the flow of cerebrospinal fluid (arrowed). (Modified from Ross & Wilson (1981), by permission of Churchill Livingstone.)

inflammation of the arachnoid and pia mater associated with the presence of bacteria, viruses, fungi or protozoa in the CSF. Meningitis is one of the most emotive of infectious diseases. Even today, meningitis is associated with significant mortality and serious morbidity.

Aetiology and epidemiology

In the UK, approximately 2500 cases of bacterial meningitis are notified annually. Overall, two organisms, *Neisseria meningitidis* and *Streptococcus pneumoniae*, account for about 75% of cases. However, the pattern of bacteria causing meningitis is related to the age of the patient and the presence of underlying disease.

In the neonatal period, group B streptococci are the most common cause of bacterial meningitis. Other causes of neonatal meningitis include *Escherichia coli* and other coliform bacteria, *Listeria monocytogenes* and enterococci. In most cases infection is acquired from the maternal genital tract around the time of delivery, but transmission between patients can also occur in hospitals.

N. meningitidis is the most common cause of bacterial meningitis from infancy through to middle age, with peaks of incidence during infancy and adolescence. There are several serogroups of *N. meningitidis*, including A, B, C and the less common W135 and Y. Until recently, groups B and C accounted for 60–65% and 35–40% of infections in the UK, respectively. However, following inclusion of a vaccine against *N. meningitidis* group C (MenC) into the routine imunization programme in 1999 the incidence of infection with this serogroup has decreased markedly (Anon 2001a). There is currently no vaccine available for *N. meningitidis* serogroup B. Serogroup A predominates in Africa and the Middle East. A vaccine is available to protect travellers to these areas. *Strep. pneumoniae* is the most common cause of meningitis in adults aged over 45 years. *Haemophilus influenzae* type b (Hib) was once the major cause of bacterial meningitis in children aged 3 months to 5 years, but introduction of routine immunization in 1992 has almost eliminated Hib disease in the UK and other developed countries.

Although patients with meningococcal or Hib meningitis are potentially infectious, most cases of meningitis due to these bacteria are acquired from individuals who are asymptomatic nasopharyngeal carriers. People living in the same household as a case of meningococcal disease have a 500–1200-fold increased risk of developing infection if they do not receive chemoprophylaxis (see later). Susceptible young children who are household contacts of a case of Hib disease have a similarly increased risk of becoming infected. Epidemics of meningococcal disease sometimes occur. In developed countries these take the form of clusters of cases among people living in close proximity (for example in schools or army camps) or in a particular geographical area. In Africa, large epidemics with many thousands of cases occur, usually during the dry season.

Meningitis may occur as a complication of neurosurgery, especially in patients who have ventriculoatrial or ventriculoperitoneal shunts. Coagulase-negative staphylococci are the major causes of shunt-associated meningitis, but other bacteria are important, including coliform bacteria and *Staphylococcus aureus*. Meningitis due to *Staph. aureus* may also be secondary to trauma, or local or haematogenous spread from another infective focus. Meningitis may also be a feature of multisystem bacterial diseases such as syphilis, leptospirosis and Lyme disease. *L. monocytogenes* is an occasional cause of meningitis in immunocompromised patients.

The decline in the incidence of tuberculous meningitis in developed countries has mirrored the fall in the incidence of tuberculosis in these countries. Tuberculous meningitis may occur as part of the primary infection, or as a result of recrudescence of a previous infection.

Enteroviruses such as echoviruses and coxsackieviruses account for about 70% of cases of viral meningitis in the UK. Other agents include mumps virus, herpes viruses and human immunodeficiency viruses.

In Europe, fungal meningitis is rare in individuals without underlying disease. *Candida* species are an occasional cause of shunt meningitis. *Cryptococcus neoformans* has emerged as an important cause of meningitis in patients with the acquired immune deficiency syndrome (AIDS) and other severe defects of T cell function. In certain other areas of the world, infections with fungi such as *Coccidioides immitis* and *Histoplasma capsulatum* are endemic.

Pathophysiology

Most cases of bacterial meningitis are preceded by nasopharyngeal colonization by the causative organism. In most colonized individuals, infection will progress no further, but in susceptible individuals, local invasion occurs, leading to bacteraemia and meningeal invasion. Other routes by which micro-organisms can reach the meninges include:

- direct spread from the nasopharynx
- blood-borne spread from other foci of colonization or infection
- abnormal communications with the skin or mucous membranes, for example skull fractures, anatomical defects or a meningocele
- spread from an infected adjacent focus, for example brain abscess, tuberculoma, infected paranasal air sinus or infection of the middle ear.

Once in the subarachnoid space the infection spreads widely. The cerebral tissue is not usually directly involved although cerebral abscess may complicate some types of meningitis.

The micro-organisms that most frequently cause meningitis are capable of doing so because they have a variety of virulence factors, including mechanisms for:

- attachment to host mucosal surfaces
- evasion of phagocytosis and other host defences
- meningeal invasion
- disruption of the blood–brain barrier
- induction of pathophysiological changes in the CSF space
- secondary brain damage.

Both *H. influenzae* and *N. meningitidis* have pili that mediate attachment to specific host cell surface receptors. All common bacterial pathogens are encapsulated, which helps them resist neutrophil phagocytosis and complement-mediated bactericidal activity. Other surface structures may protect bacteria from antibody and complement-mediated bacteriolysis.

Virulence factors that facilitate access of micro-organisms into the CSF, and disruption of the blood–brain barrier, are poorly understood, but components of the cell envelope, including fimbriae and outer membrane proteins, are probably important. Inflammatory mediators such as interleukin-1, tumour necrosis factor, prostaglandins and platelet-activating factor released by the host in response to microbial components also contribute to mucosal invasion and disruption of the blood–brain barrier. Cell wall components, such as teichoic acid in Gram-positive bacteria, and lipo-oligosaccharides and lipo-polysaccharides from Gram-negative bacteria are potent inducers of the inflammatory response.

Cranial nerves may be damaged by the presence of inflammatory exudate. The local inflammatory response can cause obstruction of blood vessels and cerebral oedema, leading to impaired CSF flow, increased intracranial pressure, reduced cerebral blood flow and a risk of cerebral infarction. Brain damage may also be due to reactive oxygen species, nitric oxide and excitatory amino acids.

Clinical manifestations

Acute bacterial meningitis usually presents with sudden-onset headache, neck stiffness, photophobia, fever and vomiting. On examination, Kernig's sign may be positive. This is resistance to extension of the leg when the hip is flexed, due to meningeal irritation in the lumbar area. Where meningitis is complicated by septicaemia, there may be septic shock. The presence of a haemorrhagic skin rash is highly suggestive, but not pathognomic, of meningococcal infection. Untreated, patients with bacterial meningitis deteriorate rapidly, with development of seizures, focal cerebral signs and cranial nerve palsies. Finally, obtundation and loss of consciousness herald death.

In infants with meningitis the physical signs are usually non-specific and include fever, diarrhoea, lethargy, feeding difficulties and respiratory distress. Focal signs such as seizures or a bulging fontanelle usually only occur at a late stage.

Viral meningitis usually presents with acute onset of low-grade fever, headache, photophobia and neck stiffness. Unless they develop encephalitis, patients usually remain alert and oriented.

Although tuberculous and fungal meningitis sometimes present acutely, these infections typically have a more indolent course. The early stages of the diseases are dominated by general symptoms such as malaise, apathy and anorexia. As they progress, symptoms and signs more typical of meningitis usually appear.

Diagnosis

The definitive diagnosis of meningitis is established by detection of the causative organism and/or demonstration of biochemical changes and a cellular response in CSF. CSF is obtained by lumbar puncture, where a needle is inserted between the posterior space of the third and fourth lumbar vertebrae into the subarachnoid space. Before performing lumbar puncture the possibility of precipitating or aggravating existing brain herniation in patients with intracranial hypertension must be considered, increasingly patients are being investigated beforehand by computed tomography.

In health the CSF is a clear colourless fluid, which in the lumbar region of the spinal cord is at a pressure of 50–150 mmH$_2$O. There may be up to 5 cells/μl, the protein concentration is up to 0.4 g/l, and the glucose concentration is at least 60% of the blood glucose (usually 2.2–4.4 mmol/l). Table 36.1 shows how the cell count and biochemical measurements can be helpful in determining the type of aetiological agent in meningitis.

In bacterial meningitis, organisms may be visible in Gram stained smears of the CSF. The common causes of bacterial meningitis are easily distinguished from each other by their Gram stain appearance. Special stains, such as the Ziehl–Neelsen method, are necessary to visualize mycobacteria. However, only small numbers of mycobacteria are present in the CSF in tuberculous meningitis, and direct microscopy is often unrevealing. Although cryptococci can be visualized by Gram staining, they are often more easily seen with India ink staining, which highlights their prominent capsules.

Table 36.1 Cellular and biochemical responses in different forms of infective meningitis

Type of meningitis	Cell count	Protein (g/l)	Glucose
Bacterial	Predominantly polymorphs, 500–2000 μl (lymphocytes may predominate in early or partially treated cases)	1–3	< 50% blood glucose
Tuberculous	Predominantly lymphocytes, 100–600 μl	1–6	< 50% blood glucose
Viral	Predominantly lymphocytes, 50–500 μl	0.5–1	Usually normal
Cryptococcal	Predominantly lymphocytes, 50–1000 μl	1–3	< 50% blood glucose

Regardless of the microscopic findings, CSF should be cultured in order to try to confirm the identity of the causative organism and to facilitate further investigations such as antibiotic sensitivity testing and typing. Special cultural techniques are required for mycobacteria, fungi and viruses. Cultures of other sites are sometimes helpful. In suspected bacterial meningitis, blood for culture should always be obtained. Bacteraemia occurs in only 10% of patients with meningiciccal meningitis, but is more commonly associated with some other forms of meningitis. CSF and blood cultures may be negative in patients with meningococcal disease, especially if antibiotics have been administered prior to the cultures being taken. Cultures from sites where antibiotic penetration is less good, for example haemorrhagic skin lesions and the nasopharynx, may be helpful in such cases.

Non-culture-based methods may also be helpful in determining the aetiology of meningitis. Techniques include antigen detection and detection of microbial genomic material using molecular methods such as polymerase chain reaction (PCR). PCR is now established as a standard investigation in suspected meningococcal meningitis, and may be the only positive test in up to 50% of cases (Ragunathan et al 2000). PCR assays are also widely available for detection of *M. tuberculosis* and several viruses, including herpes simplex virus and enteroviruses. Serum antibodies to *N. meningitidis* and various viruses may be detected, but these investigations usually depend on demonstration of seroconversion between two samples collected a week or more apart, and therefore have no role in the early diagnosis of infections. Patients with tuberculous meningitis may have a positive Mantoux test.

Drug treatment

Acute bacterial meningitis is a medical emergency that requires urgent administration of antibiotics. Other considerations in some forms of meningitis include the use of adjunctive therapy such as steroids, and the administration of antibiotics to prevent secondary cases. The antimicrobial therapy of meningitis requires the attainment of adequate levels of bactericidal agents within the CSF. The principal route of entry of antibiotics into CSF is by the choroid plexus; an alternative route is via the capillaries of the central nervous system into the extracellular fluid and thence into the ventricles and subarachnoid space. The passage of antibiotics into CSF is dependent on the degree of meningeal inflammation and integrity of the blood–brain barrier, as well as following properties of the antibiotic:

- lipid solubility (the choroidal epithelium is highly impermeable to lipid-insoluble molecules)
- ionic dissociation at blood pH
- protein binding
- molecular size
- the concentration of the drug in the serum.

Antimicrobials fall into three categories according to their ability to penetrate the CSF:

- those that penetrate even when the meninges are not inflamed, for example chloramphenicol, metronidazole, isoniazid and pyrazinamide
- those that generally penetrate only when the meninges are inflamed, and used in high doses, for example most β-lactam antibiotics, the quinolones and rifampicin
- those that penetrate poorly under all circumstances, including the aminoglycosides, vancomycin and erythromycin.

Clinical urgency determines that empirical antimicrobial therapy will usually have to be prescribed before the identity of the causative organism or its antibiotic sensitivities are known. Consideration of the epidemiological features of the case, together with microscopic examination of the CSF, is often helpful in identifying the likely pathogen. However, there is a trend towards the use of broad-spectrum antimicrobial therapy to cover all likely pathogens, at least until definite microbiological information is available. For the purpose of selecting empirical antimicrobial therapy, patients with acute bacterial meningitis can be categorized into four broad groups: neonates and infants aged below 3 months; immunocompetent older infants, children and adults; immunocompromised patients; and those with CSF shunts.

Meningitis in neonates and infants aged below 3 months

The most important pathogens in neonates include group B streptococci, *E. coli* and other coliform bacteria, and *L. monocytogenes*. In many centres a third-generation cephalosporin such as cefotaxime or ceftazidime, along with amoxicillin or ampicillin, is the empiric therapy of choice for neonatal meningitis (Harvey et al 1999). Cephalosporins penetrate into CSF better than aminoglycosides, and their use in Gram-negative bacillary meningitis has contributed to a reduction in mortality to less than 10%. Other centres continue to use an aminoglycoside, such as gentamicin, together with benzyl penicillin, ampicillin or amoxicillin as empiric

therapy. This approach remains appropriate, especially in countries such as the UK where group B streptococci are by far the predominant cause of early onset neonatal meningitis. Whichever empiric regimen is used, therapy can be altered as appropriate once the pathogen has been identified. Suitable dosages are shown in Table 36.2.

In infants outside the immediate neonatal period the classical neonatal pathogens account for a decreasing number of cases of meningitis, and the common bacteria of meningitis in childhood (see below) become increasingly important. Amoxicillin or ampicillin plus cefotaxime or ceftriaxone is the recommended treatment. Therapy with amoxicillin or ampicillin and gentamicin is unsuitable for this age group because it provides inadequate cover against *H. influenzae*.

Meningitis in older infants, children and adults

Antimicrobial therapy has to cover *Strep. pneumoniae*, *N. meningitidis* and, in children aged below 5 years, *H. influenzae*. Achievable antibiotic CSF concentrations are compared with the susceptibilities of the common agents of meningitis in Table 36.3. The third-generation

Table 36.2 Suitable antibiotic regimens for treatment of acute bacterial meningitis in different age groups

Age group	First-choice antibiotic therapy	Alternative therapies
Neonates, aged ≤ 7 days	Ampicillin, 50 mg/kg twice daily or amoxicillin 25 mg/kg twice daily and cefotaxime 50 mg/kg twice daily or ceftazidime 50 mg/kg twice daily	Benzylpenicillin 50 mg twice daily and ampicillin 50 mg/kg twice daily or amoxicillin 25 mg/kg twice daily and gentamicin 2.5 mg/kg twice daily
Neonates, aged 8–28 days	Ampicillin 50 mg/kg four times daily or amoxicillin 25 mg/kg three times daily and cefotaxime 50 mg/kg three times daily or ceftazidime 50 mg/kg three times daily	Benzylpencillin 50 mg three or four times daily or ampicillin 50 mg/kg three or four times daily or amoxicillin 25 mg/kg three times daily and gentamicin 2.5 mg/kg three times daily
Infants, aged 1–3 months	Ampicillin 50 mg/kg four times daily or amoxicillin 25 mg/kg three times daily and cefotaxime 50 mg/kg three times daily or ceftriaxone 75–100 mg/kg once daily	
Infants and children aged > 3 months[a]	Cefotaxime 50 mg/kg three times daily or ceftriaxone 75–100 mg/kg once daily	Ampicillin 50 mg/kg four times daily or amoxicillin 25 mg/kg three times daily or benzylpenicillin[b] 30 mg/kg 4-hourly and chloramphenicol[c] 12.5–25 mg/kg four times daily
Adults	Cefotaxime[d] 2 g three times daily or ceftriaxone[d] 2–4 g once daily	Benzylpenicillin 2.4 g 4-hourly or ampicillin 2–3 g four times daily or amoxicillin 2 g three or four times daily and chloramphenicol[c] 12.5–25 mg/kg four times daily

[a] Calculated doses for children should not exceed maximum recommended doses for adults.
[b] Benzylpenicillin is inactive against *H. influenzae*, and should therefore not be used for children aged < 5 years.
[c] Monitoring of serum chloramphenicol levels is recommended, especially in children aged ≤ 4 years.
[d] Add ampicillin or amoxicillin to cover *L. monocytogenes* in elderly patients, or where Gram-positive bacilli seen in CSF.

Table 36.3 Achievable CSF concentrations of antibiotics in meningitis, and minimum inhibitory concentration (MIC) values for common CNS pathogens

Antibiotic	CSF: serum ratio	Peak CSF level (mg/l)	MIC$_{90}$ (mg/l) values for:		
			N. meningitidis	H. influenzae	Strep. pneumoniae
Ampicillin	1:10	10	0.02	0.25	0.05
Benzylpenicillin	1:20	1.5	0.02	1.0	0.02
Cefotaxime	1:20	10	0.01	0.06	0.25
Ceftriaxone	1:15	15	0.01	0.06	0.12
Chloramphenicol	1:2	15	1.0	1.0	2.5
Ciprofloxacin	1:5	0.6	0.004	0.015	1.0
Gentamicin	1:40	< 0.5	2.0	0.5	16
Imipenem	1:15	2.0	0.1	1.0	0.05
Meropenem	1:15	4.0	0.03	0.1	0.1
Rifampicin	1:20	1.0	0.5	1.0	2.0
Vancomycin	1:40	1.0	> 4.0	> 4.0	0.2

MIC$_{90}$, minimum concentration of antibiotic that is inhibitory for 90% of isolates; CSF, cerebrospinal fluid.

cephalosporins cefotaxime and ceftriaxone are now widely used in place of the traditional agents of choice, chloramphenicol, ampicillin, amoxicillin and penicillin (see Table 36.2). This change has stemmed from concern over the rare but potentially serious adverse effects of chloramphenicol and the emergence of resistance to penicillin, ampicillin and chloramphenicol among *Strep. pneumoniae* and *H. influenzae* in particular. Chloramphenicol resistance has also recently been reported in *N. meningitidis* (Galimand et al 1998). Cefotaxime and ceftriaxone have a broad spectrum of activity that encompasses not only the three classical causes of bacterial meningitis but also many other bacteria that are infrequent causes of meningitis. However, cephalosporins are inactive against *L. monocytogenes,* and amoxicillin or ampicillin should be added where it is possible that the patient may have listeriosis, for example in elderly patients, or where Gram-positive bacilli are seen on Gram stain. Although earlier generation cephalosporins such as cefuroxime achieve good CSF penetration and are active against the agents of meningitis in vitro, they do not effectively sterilize the CSF and should not be used to treat meningitis.

In meningitis due to *N. meningitidis* and *H. influenzae,* prompt administration of chemoprophylaxis to eliminate nasopharyngeal carriage can reduce the risk of secondary cases in close contacts of the case (see later).

Neisseria meningitidis

In view of the potentially rapid clinical progression of meningococcal disease, treatment should begin with the emergency administration of benzylpenicillin. General practitioners should give penicillin while arranging transfer of the patient to hospital. The dose is 1200 mg for adults and children aged 10 years and above, 600 mg for children aged 1–9 years, and 300 mg for children aged below 1 year. Ideally this should be given intravenously. The intramuscular route is less likely to be effective in shocked patients but can be used if venous access cannot be obtained. The only contraindication is a history of anaphylaxis to penicillin, where chloramphenicol (1.2 g for adults, 25 mg/kg for children aged < 12 years) may be given, if available.

Strains of *N. meningitidis* with reduced sensitivity to penicillin are well known and presently account for 5–10% of isolates in Europe and the USA. In general these cases respond to treatment with adequate doses of benzylpenicillin, and failure of penicillin treatment has rarely been reported. Nevertheless, cefotaxime or ceftriaxone are now widely used in preference to benzylpenicillin or chloramphenicol.

Streptococcus pneumoniae

Benzylpenicillin was once widely regarded as the treatment of choice for pneumococcal meningitis. However, pneumococci that are resistant to penicillin have now emerged across the world, and cefotaxime or ceftriaxone are now the usual preferred treatment.

Although currently only about 5% of pneumococci in the UK are penicillin-resistant, the frequency of resistance is increasing. Penicillin resistance rates of more than 50% have been reported in other countries, including Spain, Hungary and South Africa. Penicillin resistance of pneumococci is defined in terms of the minimum inhibitory concentration (MIC) of penicillin. Most strains have an MIC value of 0.1–1.0 mg/l, and are defined as having moderate resistance; strains with an MIC of 2 mg/l or more are considered highly resistant. This distinction is important because highly resistant strains are less likely to respond to treatment with β-lactam antibiotics. It is sometimes recommended that pneumococcal meningitis should be treated with vancomycin together with a cephalosporin pending the results of antibiotic susceptibility testing (Jacobs 1999). This approach would appear justified at least for patients who might have acquired their infection in a location where the incidence of penicillin resistance is high.

Strains with moderate resistance to penicillin can usually be successfully treated with cefotaxime or ceftriaxone, although treatment failures have sometimes been reported. Addition of rifampicin is sometimes recommended, but there are few data confirming this can improve the response rate. The dose of rifampicin is 600 mg twice daily in adults or 10 mg/kg (maximum 600 mg) twice daily in children. Meningitis due to fully resistant strains is usually treated with vancomycin, often in combination with a cephalosporin and/or rifampicin. Because of concern over limited CSF penetration of vancomycin, it has been suggested that trough serum levels of 15–20 mg/l should be aimed for, rather than the usual 5–10 mg/l. Alternatively vancomycin can be given intraventricularly (see later), usually in addition to systemic administration.

Chloramphenicol is a suitable alternative to penicillin for treatment of meningitis due to penicillin-sensitive strains, for example in patients who are penicillin-allergic. However, chloramphenicol is not recommended for treating penicillin-resistant pneumococcal meningitis. Although isolates may appear sensitive to chloramphenicol on routine laboratory testing, bactericidal activity is often absent, and the clinical response is usually poor. Recently, strains of *Strep. pneumoniae* that are penicillin-resistant and tolerant to both chloramphenicol and vancomycin have emerged

(Novak et al 1999). Although rare, infections with these bacteria present a major therapeutic difficulty. The carbapenem antibiotics imipenem and meropenem are active in vitro against the majority of intermediately and fully penicillin-resistant pneumococci. However, clinical experience with these agents in this setting has been variable. Imipenem is not licensed for treatment of meningitis because it can cause seizures in patients with underlying CNS disease. Moxifloxacin is a new generation quinolone antibiotic with enhanced activity against Gram-positive bacteria, including *Strep. pneumoniae,* which has shown promise in experimental pneumococcal meningitis (Schmidt et al 1998). Because of the unpredictable nature of the response to therapy of penicillin-resistant pneumococcal meningitis, patients require close observation during treatment, for example monitoring of C-reactive protein (CRP) and repeated examination of CSF during therapy.

Haemophilus influenzae

A third-generation cephalosporin such as cefotaxime or ceftriaxone is generally the treatment of choice for *H. influenzae* meningitis. These agents have superseded the traditional therapy where chloramphenicol and ampicillin or amoxicillin were used in combination until the sensitivities of the organism were known and therapy could be rationalized to a single agent.

Other bacteria

Meningitis in immunocompetent individuals is rarely due to other bacteria. The definitive treatment of such cases requires to be considered on an individual basis in the light of careful clinical and microbiological assessment.

Chemoprophylaxis

In meningococcal meningitis, spread between family members and other close contacts is well recognized, these individuals should receive chemoprophylaxis as soon as possible, preferably within 24 hours. Sometimes chemoprophylaxis may be indicated for other contacts, but the decision to offer prophylaxis beyond household contacts should only be made after obtaining expert advice (Table 36.4). Of the antibiotics conventionally used to treat meningococcal infections only ceftriaxone reliably eliminates nasopharyngeal carriage; where another antibiotic has been used for treatment, the index case also requires chemoprophylaxis. A number of antibiotics are suitable as prophylaxis (Table 36.5).

Ciprofloxacin is now widely recommended for adults because of the convenience of single dose administration, and, unlike rifampicin, it does not interact with oral contraceptives and is readily available

Table 36.4 Indications for chemoprophylaxis in contacts of cases of infection with *Neisseria meningitidis* or *Haemophilus influenzae* type b

Neisseria meningitidis

Household and other close contacts: prophylaxis usually initiated as soon as possible by clinicians caring for the case
- Persons who have slept in the same house as the patient at any time during the 7 days before the onset of symptoms
- Boy/girl friends of the case
- Unless treated with ceftriaxone (which reliably eliminates nasopharyngeal carriage), the index case should also receive antibiotic prophylaxis as soon as he or she is able to take oral medication

Healthcare workers: prophylaxis should only by initiated after consultation with hospital infection control team or public health doctor
- Individuals who have administered mouth-to-mouth resuscitation, or had some other form of prolonged close face-to-face contact with the patient

Other contacts: prophylaxis should only be initiated be a public health doctor
- Schools, nurseries, universities and other closed communities where two or more linked cases have occurred

Invasive *Haemophilus influenzae* type b infection

Household and other close contacts: prophylaxis usually initiated as soon as possible by clinicians caring for the case
- Indicated only where there is another child aged less than 4 years who has not been immunized in the same household as the index case. In such circumstances prophylaxis should be given to all household contacts aged 1 month or older, unless there are contraindications. The index case should also receive antibiotic prophylaxis as soon as he or she is able to take oral medication

Other contacts: prophylaxis very rarely necessary, and should only be initiated by a public health physician

Table 36.5 Recommended prophylactic regimens for contacts of cases of infection with *Neisseria meningitidis* or *Haemophilus influenzae* type b

Meningococcal infection	
Rifampicin (oral)	
Children aged < 1 year	5 mg/kg twice daily on 2 consecutive days
Children aged 1–12 years	10 mg/kg (max 600 mg) twice daily on 2 consecutive days
Adults[b]	600 mg twice daily on 2 consecutive days
Ciprofloxacin[a] (oral)	
Children	Obtain expert advice
Adults[b]	500 mg as a single dose
Ceftriaxone[a] (intramuscular)	
Children aged < 12 years	125 mg as a single dose
Adults[b]	250 mg as a single dose
Invasive *Haemophilus influenzae* type b infection	
Rifampicin (oral)	
Children aged 1–3 months	10 mg/kg once daily for 4 days
Children aged > 3 months	20 mg/kg once daily (max 600 mg) for 4 days
Adults[b]	600 mg once daily for 4 days

[a] Not licensed for this indication.
[b] For pregnant women, obtain expert advice.

in community pharmacies. Anaphylactoid reactions have been reported to occur in about 1:1000 individuals receiving ciprofloxacin as chemoprophylaxis. None of these reactions has been fatal; however, both the prescriber and recipient of the drug must be aware of the risk of side-effects such as facial swelling, tightness in the throat or breathing difficulty (Anon 2001 b). If the strain is confirmed as group C (or A, W135 or Y), vaccination is normally offered to contacts who were given prophylaxis. There is no need to vaccinate the patient. There is currently no vaccine that protects against group B disease, which accounts for about 70% of cases of meningococcal disease in Europe.

Chemoprophylaxis against Hib infection is usually only indicated where there is an unimmunized child in the vulnerable age-group in the household (see Table 36.4). Only rifampicin has been proved to be effective in eliminating nasopharyngeal carriage (see Table 36.5). Unimmunized household contacts aged below 4 years should also receive Hib vaccine. The index case should also receive rifampicin in order to eliminate nasopharyngeal carriage, and should be immunized, irrespective of age.

Meningitis in the immunocompromised host

The meninges are an uncommon site of infection in neutropenic patients. Possible causes of meningitis include coliform bacteria and *Pseudomonas aeruginosa*, as well as the common causes of bacterial meningitis in immunocompetent individuals. The choice of therapy is governed by the need to attain broad-spectrum coverage, using agents with good CSF penetration. Meropenem may now be the drug of choice for meningitis in this setting, although many other regimens are also appropriate.

Patients with cellular immune dysfunction are vulnerable to meningitis due to *L. monocytogenes* and *C. neoformans*. Ampicillin or amoxicillin, along with cefotaxime or ceftriaxone, is recommended as empirical antimicrobial therapy for meningitis in these patients. Definitive treatment of listeria meningitis is normally with high-dose ampicillin (3 g four times daily) or amoxicillin (2 g four times daily), with the addition of gentamicin in order to obtain a synergistic effect (Mylonakis et al 1998). The most appropriate treatment for patients who are penicillin-allergic, or in the rare circumstance of infection with a strain that is ampicillin-resistant, is uncertain, and specialist microbiological advice should be sought. Specific therapies for cryptococcal meningitis are described in detail below.

Splenectomized patients are susceptible to invasive infections with encapsulated bacteria, including *Strep. pneumoniae* and Hib. Standard therapy with either cefotaxime or ceftriaxone is appropriate.

Shunt meningitis

Shunt infections are classified according to the site of initial infection. Internal infections, where the lumen of the shunt is colonized, constitute the majority of cases. External shunt infections involve the tissues surrounding the shunt. Most internal shunt infections are caused by coagulase-negative staphylococci. *Staph. aureus* and coliforms account for most external infections. It is generally held that management of shunt infections should include shunt removal, as well as antibiotic therapy (Working Party 1995). However, recent work suggests that infections with coagulase-negative staphylococci can at least sometimes be successfully managed without shunt removal. Appropriate antimicrobial regimens are shown in Table 36.6.

Tuberculous meningitis

The outcome in tuberculous meningitis relates directly to the severity of the patient's clinical condition on commencement of therapy. A satisfactory response demands a high degree of clinical suspicion such that appropriate chemotherapy is initiated early, even if tubercle bacilli are not demonstrated on initial microscopy. Most currently used antituberculous agents achieve effective concentrations in the CSF in tuberculous meningitis. Detailed discussion of antituberculous therapy is given in Chapter 38. Adjunctive steroid therapy is of value in patients with more severe disease, particularly those who suddenly develop cerebral oedema soon after starting treatment, or who appear to be developing a spinal block. However, routine use of steroids is not recommended. They may suppress informative changes in the CSF, and interfere with antibiotic penetration by restoring the blood–brain barrier. Early neurosurgical management of hydrocephalus by means of a ventriculoperitoneal or ventriculoatrial shunt is also important in improving the prospects for neurological recovery.

Use of steroids as adjunctive therapy in the management of bacterial meningitis

In pharmacological doses, adrenal corticosteroids regulate many components of the inflammatory response and also lower CSF hydrostatic pressure. Steroids have therefore been extensively investigated in the initial management of meningitis. However, with the exception of meningitis due to *M. tuberculosis* (see above) and Hib, there is little evidence that steroids are beneficial (Coyle 1999). Indeed steroids might have an adverse effect by reducing inflammation and restoring the blood–brain barrier and consequently reducing CSF penetration of antibiotics. In Hib meningitis dexamethasone commenced early at a dose of 0.6–1.5 mg/kg/day in four divided doses for 4 days significantly reduces sensorineural hearing loss and possibly other long-term sequelae. The best protection appears to be obtained from early treatment.

Cryptococcal meningitis

The standard treatment of cryptococcal meningitis is amphotericin B (AMB), given intravenously at a dose of 0.7–1.0 mg/kg/day, together with flucytosine (FC) 100

Surgical antibiotic prophylaxis

37

J. C. Graham   S. J. Pedler

KEY POINTS

- Surgical antibiotic prophylaxis aims to reduce the rate of postoperative wound infections.
- The risk of infection depends primarily on the anatomical site of surgery; however, host and operative factors are also important.
- Prophylaxis has a definite value in operations with high infection rates, but remains questionable in low-risk surgery.
- Antibiotics chosen for prophylaxis should be active against bacteria most likely to cause significant infection.
- Optimum prophylaxis requires adequate tissue concentrations of antibiotics throughout the operation.
- Long courses of postoperative antibiotics are usually unnecessary.
- Errors in surgical antibiotic prophylaxis are not infrequent and regimens need to be audited.
- Ideally, antibiotic prophylaxis regimens should be based on the results of controlled clinical trials.

Introduction

Infection at the site of incision is a common but avoidable complication of a surgical procedure. The term surgical site infection (SSI) encompasses infections of implants, prosthetic devices and adjacent tissues involved in the operation. Such infections result in significant morbidity and the average hospital cost of SSI is over £1500 per patient. Antibiotic prophylaxis is one component of a preventative strategy that is based on good surgical technique, strict asepsis in the operating theatre and control of infection within the hospital or general practice. The decision to use antibiotics to prevent infection in an individual patient depends upon the patient's risk of surgical infection, the severity of the consequences of SSI, the effectiveness of prophylaxis in that operation and adverse consequences of prophylaxis for that patient. Administration of these agents should be monitored to ensure a quality standard is met (Dellinger et al 1994).

The goals of antibiotic prophylaxis are to:

- reduce the incidence of SSI
- use antibiotics in a manner that is supported by evidence of effectiveness
- minimize the effect on the patient's normal flora
- minimize adverse effects
- cause minimal alteration of the host defences.

Risk factors for infection

Following the initial development of antibiotics in the 1940s it was believed that these agents would be effective in reducing SSI. However, early studies suggested otherwise (Fry 1988). This was due to inconsistent timing of antibiotic administration and methodological problems as relatively clean procedures were compared with procedures where bacterial contamination was likely. This led to the stratification system outlined in Table 37.1 (Waddell & Rotstein 1994). Other factors affecting the incidence of SSI include:

- Insertion of prosthetic implants. All implants have a detrimental effect on host defences and therefore a lower bacterial inoculum is required to initiate infection when compared to tissue. Hence there is a greater risk of infection of the wound and surgical site.
- Duration of surgery. The longer the operation, the greater the risk of wound infection; this risk is additional to that of the classification of the operation.
- Co-morbidities. Based on the American Society of Anesthesiology (ASA) preoperative risk score based on the comorbidities at time of operation, a score greater than 2 (Table 37.2) is associated with an increased risk of wound infection (additional to classification of operation and duration). A risk index can be ascertained for an individual patient based on the presence of a co-morbidity (ASA score > 2) and duration of operation (> 75th percentile). As the index increases, the risk of infection rises, as it does from clean to contaminated surgery (Table 37.3).

There are a number of other risk factors that may contribute to the risk of SSI for an individual patient but

Table 37.1 Classification of surgical procedures by risk of infection

Type of procedure	Definition	Wound infection rate (%)
Clean	Atraumatic; no break in technique; gastrointestinal, genitourinary and respiratory tracts not entered	1–2
Clean-contaminated	Gastrointestinal or respiratory tract entered but without spillage; oropharynx, sterile genitourinary or biliary tract entered; minor break in technique	2–4
Contaminated	Acute inflammation; infected bile or urine; gross spillage from gastrointestinal tract	7–10
Dirty	Established infection	10–40

Table 37.2 American Society of Anesthesiology (ASA) classification of physical status

ASA score	Physical status
1	A normal healthy patient
2	A patient with mild systemic disease
3	A patient with a severe systemic disease that limits activity but is not incapacitating
4	A patient with an incapacitating systemic disease that is a constant threat to life
5	A moribund patient that is not expected to survive 24 hours with or without operation

Table 37.3 Risk index based on presence of co-morbidity and duration of operation

Risk index 0 = when neither risk factor is present

Risk index 1 = when either one of the risk factors is present

Risk index 2 = when both risk factors are present

have not been classified as well as those listed above. These include the following patient and operative factors:

Patient risk factors:

- advanced age
- malnutrition
- obesity
- concurrent infection
- diabetes mellitus
- liver impairment
- renal impairment
- immune deficiency states
- prolonged preoperative stay
- blood transfusion.

Operative risk factors:

- tissue ischaemia
- lack of haemostasis
- tissue damage, e.g. crushing by surgical instruments
- presence of necrotic tissue
- presence of foreign bodies including surgical materials.

Benefits and risk of antibiotic prophylaxis

The prophylactic use of antibiotics has important implications. It requires a risk–benefit analysis which is distinct from that used when antibiotics are given to treat active infections. On the risk side, patients without an immediate need for therapy are potentially exposed to dose-related toxicity, drug interactions and idiosyncratic toxic reactions including potentially fatal allergic responses. More generally the routine and widespread use of antibiotics in hospitals is a powerful ecological pressure in favour of bacterial antibiotic-resistance genes, threatening the therapy of real infections. The financial costs of antibiotics are a complex additional consideration. An additional problem is the colitis due to *Clostridium difficile* infection. Infection with this organism is related to antibiotic usage, especially third-generation cephalosporins. *C. difficile* infection increases morbidity and mortality and prolongs hospital stay leading to an overall increase in health care costs (estimated to be £4000 per episode).

Individual patients whose infections have been prevented will benefit, although who these patients are can never be known with certainty. At a more subtle level, other patients who perhaps did not receive antibiotics for their operations may also benefit from prevented infections in fellow patients, since an opportunity for transmission of infection from patient to patient will have been avoided.

It is important to be aware of the definitions used in wound infection studies, and caution should be used when comparing infection rates between studies, centres or surgeons. The Centers for Disease Control in the USA have published guidelines that define wound infections from both clinical and microbiological perspectives, which may allow comparison of wound infection rates (Table 37.4). Similarly, one must recognize that SSI may present following discharge from hospital; in fact, using the National Nosocomial Infection Surveillance (NNIS) data, 16% are detected through post-discharge surveillance with a further 38% requiring readmission (Gaynes et al 2001).

Table 37.4   Centers for Disease Control (CDC) definitions of surgical site (wound) infections (Horan et al 1992)

Incisional SSI

Superficial incisional SSI

BOTH:

- Infection involves only skin or subcutaneous tissue of incision
- Occurs within 30 days of operation

AND AT LEAST ONE OF THE FOLLOWING:

- Purulent drainage from the incision
- Organisms isolated from an aseptically taken culture of fluid or tissue from the superficial incision
- At least one of the following signs or symptoms:
    Pain or tenderness
    Localized swelling, redness or heat
- Diagnosis of superficial SSI by a clinician

Exclusions from definition include:

- Suture abscess (minimal inflammation and discharge confined to the points of suture penetration)
- Infected burn wound
- Incisional SSI that extends into the fascial and muscle layers (these are deep incisional SSI)

Deep incisional SSI

BOTH:

- Infection involves deep soft tissues (fascia or muscle layers)
- Occurs within 30 days of operation if no non-human-derived implantable foreign body is left in place OR within 1 year if an implant is left in place and infection is related to operative procedure

AND AT LEAST ONE OF THE FOLLOWING:

- Purulent drainage from the deep incision but not from the organ/space component of the surgical site
- A deep microbiological culture positive incision that spontaneously dehisces or is deliberately opened surgically in the presence of one or more of the following features:
    Pyrexia > 38°C
    Local pain
- Objective evidence of abscess formation or other forms of infection in the deep part of the incision
- Diagnosis of deep incisional SSI by a clinician

Organ/space SSI

BOTH:

- Infection involves any part of the anatomy (organs or spaces) opened or manipulated during the operation other than the incision
- Occurs within 30 days of operation if no non-human-derived implantable foreign body is left in place OR within 1 year if an implant is left in place and infection is related to operative procedure

AND AT LEAST ONE OF THE FOLLOWING:

- Purulent drainage from a drain placed in the organ/space
- Organisms isolated from an aseptically obtained culture of fluid or tissue from the organ/space
- Objective evidence of abscess formation or other forms of infection in the organ/space
- Diagnosis of organ/space SSI by a clinician

SSI, surgical site infection.

Pathogenesis

It is not surprising that the most frequent infectious complication of surgery is local wound infection. The epithelial surfaces of the body act as efficient boundaries between the sterile contents of the body and the bacteria-rich external world. Epithelial surfaces include not only the skin but also the conjunctiva, tympanic membranes and the mucosal surfaces of the respiratory, gastrointestinal and genitourinary tracts. Topologically the external world includes the luminal contents of these tracts. Any surgical operation will breach at least one of these surfaces and allow entry of bacteria. Whether an infection follows depends on the ability of the other defences to kill the invading bacteria. Important host mechanisms include antibodies, complement and phagocytic cells.

Organisms and sources

The identities and quantities of bacteria entering a wound are important factors in determining outcome, and to a large extent these depend on the nature of the operation (Table 37.5). In some circumstances bacteria will have already entered sterile tissues before the patient reaches hospital, as when an appendix perforates into the peritoneal cavity, or when they are introduced into soft tissues in a road traffic accident, for example. In the former event many different species of normal bowel flora, including enterococci, coliforms and anaerobes, will be involved, potentially in massive numbers. In the latter, organisms not normally associated with the human body will have entered the wound from the external environment.

Many surgical operations involve incision of the skin. This will permit the inoculation of Gram-positive skin flora, including *Staphylococcus aureus,* coagulase-negative staphylococci, and *Corynebacterium* spp. Some skin sites, the groin for example, carry both typical skin flora and gut bacteria, and this extended spectrum of organisms needs to be considered when constructing prophylaxis protocols. Skin diseases such as eczema and psoriasis, although not of infectious origin, support abnormally large populations of skin bacteria including *Staph. aureus.* Patients with these diseases, regardless of whether or not the surgical incision involves diseased skin, are at increased risk of wound infection simply because of heavy skin colonization. In all patients a vital step in prevention of wound infection is preoperative skin disinfection. This both dilutes the number of bacteria and kills many of those remaining.

The upper gastrointestinal tract supports the growth of few bacteria. The acid environment of the stomach and alkaline and bile salt content of the small bowel are inimical to the survival of most bacteria. However, gastric disease such as cancer, and drugs inhibiting acid production, can allow gastric overgrowth with coliforms. In contrast, the large bowel is heavily colonized with a wide range of bacteria. While they are contained within the lumen of the colon they have a broadly beneficial role. However, if they are released into the peritoneal cavity by disease or surgery they can cause fulminating sepsis. Elective bowel surgery is usually preceded by attempts to physically reduce bowel contents with enemas and purgatives so that there is less potential for

---

Table 37.5 Most likely pathogens in postoperative wound infections

Category of surgery	Most likely pathogen(s)
Clean	
Cardiac/vascular	Coagulase-negative staphylococci, *Staphylococcus aureus*, Gram-negative bacilli
Breast	*Staphylococcus aureus*
Orthopaedic	Coagulase-negative staphylococci, *Staph. aureus*, coliforms
Dialysis access	Coagulase-negative staphylococci, *Staph. aureus*
Neurological	Coagulase-negative staphylococci, *Staph. aureus*, coliforms
Clean-contaminated	
Burn	*Staph. aureus, Pseudomonas aeruginosa*
Head and neck	*Staph. aureus, Streptococcus* spp., anaerobes (from oral cavity)
Gastrointestinal tract	Coliforms, anaerobes (*Bacteroides fragilis*)
Urogenital tract	Coliforms, *Enterococcus* spp.
Dirty	
Ruptured viscera	Coliforms, anaerobes (*Bacteroides fragilis*)
Traumatic wound	*Staph. aureus, Streptococcus pyogenes, Clostridium* spp.

spillage during surgery. Even so, colonic and rectal surgery frequently results in significant wound contamination, making prophylaxis a prime concern. An additional worry is the effect of prophylaxis on large bowel flora. Many antibiotics can produce an overgrowth of *C. difficile,* which may progress to pseudomembranous colitis, a sometimes fatal complication.

The vagina and, in both sexes, the urethra are normally colonized with organisms drawn from large bowel flora. For the vagina this is especially so in both the prepubertal and postmenopausal age groups. In the intervening years the vaginal pH is kept acid by the action of lactobacilli, and this keeps the growth of coliforms in check. Although bladder urine is normally sterile, most urological operations are associated with disease that predisposes to infected bladder urine. Incisions of the urinary epithelium in such circumstances can permit rapid and large amounts of bacterial bloodstream invasion, with a high risk of septicaemia.

The upper respiratory tract supports large and complex communities of bacteria, which may infect both local pharyngeal and respiratory tract wounds. Aerosol transmission may result in contamination of more distant wounds. The nares can be heavily colonized by *Staph. aureus.* Measures to reduce this in renal dialysis patients have been followed by a decline in skin wound infection rates.

An important advance in surgery was the recognition that the skin and respiratory tract flora of the surgical team can cause postoperative infection. This understanding is the basis for hand disinfection, gloves, gowns and masks for operators.

As in the example of the road traffic accident, wound infections can follow contamination by organisms from the environment. Unfortunately, the source of these can occasionally be contaminated equipment in the operating theatre, for example contaminated water in a blood transfusion bag warming bath, or a surgeon's favourite shaving brush used in shaving skin prior to surgery. Characteristically such sources are only uncovered after several patients have been infected with the same unusual organism, typically a multiply antibiotic-resistant Gram-negative bacillus such as *Acinetobacter* or *Pseudomonas* spp., and can be traced to breakdowns in approved procedures such as sterilization between patients or the improper multiple use of single use only products. Disinfectants have been contaminated during preparation and have acted as sources of infection.

Although many species of bacteria may enter wounds, only a small range is commonly associated with infection. This may be partly due to poor recognition of some organisms, but it is undoubtedly true that bacteria such as *Staph. aureus* are better adapted to reproduction in human wounds and will outgrow many other species.

Consequences of infection

So far this discussion has not drawn a distinction between the consequences of wound infections at different sites. It is important to do so. Skin and superficial soft tissue infections are generally readily amenable to antibiotic therapy. However, they can impair the aesthetic quality of the surgical scar, which may be of major importance to the patient. Deeper soft tissue infections can progress to cellulitis and abscess formation, both of which can prolong hospital stay, and in some cases can be fatal. Infection of bone and joint prostheses can cause long-term disability, and may necessitate further operations. Cardiac valve infection can result in sudden and catastrophic dysfunction, or chronic ill health, again forcing additional operations. Eye infections can produce irreversible blindness. Central nervous system infections may be disastrous.

In skin and soft tissue infections the responsible organisms are usually major pathogens such as *Staph. aureus,* β-haemolytic streptococci and anaerobes. Their antibiotic susceptibilities are usually easily predictable, and to an extent they are more readily controlled than other less commonly involved organisms, such as coagulase-negative staphylococci, enterococci, *Corynebacterium* spp., *Pseudomonas* spp. and *Acinetobacter* spp., which are often multiply antibiotic-resistant.

It can be appreciated that organisms that are of little importance to a general surgeon may be of grave concern to a neurosurgeon. Hence, when considering the value of surgical antibiotic prophylaxis, an eye needs to be kept on the surgical down-side: what is the worst outcome of infection?

Choice of antibiotic regimen for prophylaxis

Antibiotic regimens consist of not only the antibiotic (or antibiotics) themselves but also the dose, route and timing of administration. The choice of a particular regimen is the product of scientific principles, practical considerations, empiricism and cost. One obvious principle is that the antibiotic should be active against organisms most likely to cause infection. Early approaches were to give antibiotics at a dose that would exceed the minimum inhibitory concentration (MIC), an in vitro measurement of the lowest concentration of a particular antibiotic required to inhibit growth of a particular organism. This parallels the approach to therapy of active infections. Apart from the presumption that such doses were required for effective prophylaxis, there was a fear that lower doses would lead to the development of antibiotic resistance. Although subinhibitory antibiotic concentrations may have enough antibacterial activity to halt the establishment of infection, most would use therapeutic doses for prophylaxis. The assumption that all organisms should be covered is now also less favoured. Several studies have shown that infections by mixed flora can be lessened or prevented by targeting just one component of the bacterial population. Although regimens may be recommended by national bodies, local treatment policies may have to be altered on the basis of local incidence of resistant bacteria. Similarly many regimens do not offer alternatives for patients with a history of anaphylaxis or urticaria immediately following penicillin therapy for whom β-lactams are contraindicated.

The timing of administration is one of the most important aspects of prophylaxis regimens. Animal studies, and latterly clinical observational studies, have shown that prophylaxis is most effective when given immediately before an operation (within 30 minutes of induction of anaesthesia), so that antibiotic activity is present for the duration of the operation and for about 4 hours afterwards (Classen et al 1992). Antibiotics given too early are associated with prophylaxis failure, presumably because of elimination of the drug before the end of wound contamination. Conversely, one study showed an increasing rate of wound infection for each hour that antibiotic administration was delayed after the start of the operation, suggesting that bacterial reproduction, once commenced, could no longer be eliminated by antibiotic regimens designed for prophylaxis. The microbiological basis for these observations is likely to be that bacterial reproduction at a logarithmic rate follows a lag phase of relatively little increase in bacterial population. The lag phase for wound infection bacteria lasts typically 3–4 hours. If bacteria inoculated into a wound can be killed or inhibited by antibiotics given early, the immune system has a relatively easier job mopping up remaining organisms. If antibiotics are given only when the growth curve has entered the logarithmic phase the chances of successful prophylaxis are reduced.

As a net result of this research, the duration of many prophylaxis regimens has been curtailed. Formerly protocols extended for several postoperative days. Now single-dose schedules are increasingly common. Greater emphasis is being placed on ensuring immediate preoperative administration. Since surgery may be delayed at short notice, sometimes between the time the patient leaves the ward and arrives at the theatre, it is sensible to take the responsibility for giving antibiotics away from ward staff and transfer it to the operating team, when prophylaxis can be given at induction of anaesthesia.

The adoption of short-course protocols obviates the need for dosage adjustment in patients with reduced ability to excrete the drug, usually due to renal failure, for it is unlikely that small numbers of doses will have significant dose-related adverse effects, and idiosyncratic reactions are dose-independent. Although the half-life of many drugs used is relatively short (1–2 hours in normal volunteers), surgical patients often have slower clearance of antibiotics from the blood. However, additional doses may be needed when there is significant blood loss (> 1500 ml) as plasma is effectively diluted by intraoperative transfusions and fluid replacement. Long operations may also need extra antibiotic doses during the operation but additional doses postoperatively do not provide an additional prophylactic benefit, therefore any decision to continue must be explicit and supported by an evidence base.

Antibiotic administration by theatre staff has practical implications for the route of administration. Ward-based prophylaxis could be given orally, if appropriate preparations exist, but this route is impractical in sedated or unconscious patients. The oral route tends to suffer from variable absorption, especially in the presence of anaesthetic pre-medication, and this also makes it unsatisfactory. However, for some oral antibiotics, for example the aminoglycosides neomycin and kanamycin, absorption is not the intention. Instead they are given preoperatively to patients planned for colorectal surgery, in order to reduce numbers of large bowel bacteria. The intravenous route is the most reliable way of ensuring effective serum levels and is the only route supported by a substantial body of evidence.

Several protocols using local application of antibiotics have been tested. These have included subcutaneous and intramuscular injection along the proposed incision line (in anaesthetized patients), application of antibiotic powder to the edges of the wound and antibiotic washouts at the end of the operation. Although some of these approaches have been effective they have generally been seen as unnecessarily complicated when compared with an intravenous bolus injection, or less frequently an intravenous infusion, of antibiotic. However, there remains a role for local antibiotic applications in specialties such as ophthalmic surgery where the addition of antibiotics to irrigation fluid is common practice. Some eye surgeons use preoperative antibiotic drops, but the value of these is debatable.

Antibiotics have also been incorporated into foreign bodies implanted at surgery, including the cement used to secure joint prosthesis. However, there has been concern that antibiotics leaching from the cement leave a surface that allows easier subsequent bacterial colonization. Some neurosurgeons advocate rinsing ventriculoperitoneal shunts in antibiotic solutions before insertion.

Once scientific principles and practical considerations have indicated a limited range of potentially useful regimens, the next step should be to compare them empirically against current best practice in the form of a randomized clinical trial. There are many pitfalls at this stage, and criteria for judging antibiotic trials are listed below:

- Trials should be prospective, blinded and randomized with control groups.
- Selection and exclusion criteria for patients should be specified.
- Regimens should be clearly specified.
- Operative practices and procedures should be standardized as much as possible. This is especially important when more than one centre is involved.
- The period of postoperative follow-up should be defined, and should be long enough to realistically detect most infections.
- Reasons for patient failure to complete the study protocol should be given – high exclusion and failure rates render a trial clinically unrealistic.
- Appropriate statistical analyses should be performed.
- Sufficient numbers of patients must be enrolled to avoid the appearance of a difference when none exists (type 1 error) or of no apparent difference when one does exist (type 2 error).

The greatest problem is recruiting a large enough number of similar patients to show a statistically meaningful difference. This is especially the case for surgical specialties with low wound infection rates, but is especially important when such infections have dire outcomes, for example meningitis in neurosurgery. Multicentre trials may be necessary to enroll large enough patient groups. Ideally, any conclusions should be applicable to similar patients undergoing treatment elsewhere, but this cannot be assumed.

An increasingly important complication in the application of clinical trial data is the risk of infection by multiply resistant bacteria, for example methicillin-resistant *Staphylococcus aureus* (MRSA). This is more likely when a patient has had a prolonged preoperative in-patient stay, increasing the chance of colonization by hospital flora. Antibiotic prophylaxis protocols that were once effective may be invalidated by such developments.

A final hurdle is calculating the cost of prophylaxis and setting this against potential savings from prevented infection. Perhaps fortunately, postoperative infections are so expensive that nearly all clinically effective prophylactic regimens are also cost effective.

Prophylaxis protocols in practice

This section describes a number of approaches to antibiotic prophylaxis in some surgical specialties. A recurrent feature in this discussion is that there is often little objective evidence to show that prophylaxis is effective in many situations, and consequently there is often wide variation in the approach to prophylaxis. Two extremes can be discerned. One approach is to cover all possible bacteria by using broad-spectrum antibiotics, the other is a minimalist approach, which concentrates on a few key pathogens, for example *Staph. aureus*. It is often not certain which approach is best.

Gastrointestinal surgery

The medical management of peptic ulcer disease has led to a reduction in gastric and duodenal surgery for complications of ulcers. However, many operations are still performed for malignancies involving the oesophagus and stomach, and these are associated with an infection rate of nearly 20%. Contributing factors to this high rate include overgrowth of the stomach and oesophagus by Gram-negative bacteria and poor patient physical condition leading to immunosuppression. Anaerobic bacteria from the mouth may also contribute to infection. Consequently, first- and second-generation cephalosporins, with or without metronidazole, have been chosen to reduce infection rates. A single preoperative dose of ciprofloxacin has been compared with a single dose of cefuroxime, and was shown to be as effective, even when the ciprofloxacin was given orally (Kogler et al 1989). Whether an oral route is useful or appropriate has been discussed earlier in the chapter.

Small bowel surgery is uncommon, but when it is necessary the luminal flora often resembles large bowel conditions both in number and species, and so broad-spectrum cover with a second-generation cephalosporin and metronidazole is appropriate.

Biliary tract surgery (open) has infection rates of about 10%. Frequent causes of postoperative infections include enterococci and Enterobacteriaceae. Aminoglycosides have been frequently used as prophylaxis, and their success, despite poor bile levels, indicates the importance of high tissue and blood antibiotic levels. Quinolones do reach high bile levels and have also been shown to give good protection against infections. Oral preparations make them useful for endoscopic manipulations of the biliary tract, but opiate premedication reduces bioavailability and so other premedications would need to be used. Antibiotic prophylaxis is not recommended for laparoscopic cholecystectomy.

Surgery for appendicitis has an overall wound infection rate of about 16% in the absence of prophylactic antibiotics. Antibiotics reduce infection rates when the appendix is gangrenous or perforated, but there is little difference between prophylaxis and no-prophylaxis groups when the appendix is normal or mildly inflamed. Unfortunately, it is difficult to predict the severity of inflammation preoperatively, and prophylaxis is recommended in all cases, especially in adults, who have higher postoperative infection rates than children. Although prophylaxis against both aerobes and anaerobes is usual, using a first- or second-generation cephalosporin and metronidazole, there is evidence that a single preoperative dose of metronidazole alone is as effective as cefuroxime/metronidazole together, even in perforated appendicitis (Soderquist-Elinder et al 1995).

Colorectal surgery requires antibiotic prophylaxis beyond all doubt. However, there are many regimens in use. Several preoperative days of antibiotics given orally, for example aminoglycosides combined with erythromycin, tetracycline and metronidazole, have been employed in order to reduce absolute bacterial numbers in the large bowel. These protocols expose the patient to antibiotics for a relatively long time, increasing the risk of unwanted effects. Newer antibiotics allow single-agent parenteral prophylaxis, for example perioperative cefoxitin or co-amoxiclav, both of which have activity against methicillin-sensitive *Staph. aureus,* Enterobacteriaceae and bowel anaerobes. Combinations of metronidazole with amoxicillin, second-generation cephalosporins such as cefuroxime, or aminoglycosides have all been used with some success. Cefuroxime and metronidazole has become a frequent combination, at least in the UK. More emphasis is now concentrated on appropriate timing of prophylaxis. Administration as the peritoneum is opened so that maximum tissue concentrations coincide with the period of maximum contamination has been advocated, with top-up doses as dictated by the length of the operation. It should also be noted that laparoscopic or non-laparoscopic hernia repair without mesh insertion does not require antibiotic prophylaxis.

Minimally invasive surgery

In the last decade, endoscopic techniques have dramatically changed approaches to general surgery. Many procedures including cholecystectomies, appendicectomies and hernia repairs, can now be performed using laparoscopes. The minimal trauma associated with endoscopic surgery has led to faster postoperative recovery. Reduced tissue damage and smaller incisions also appear to reduce wound infection rates, although such figures may be biased by exclusion from laparoscopic surgery of patients with conditions that make such surgery difficult, for example peritoneal adhesions. Surgeons performing laparoscopic surgery must therefore reassess the need for prophylaxis. It is possible that antibiotic usage is no longer justified in at least some types of operations. Good quality trials are urgently required in this area so that the full benefits of this technique can be delivered.

Cardiac surgery

The most important thoracic infectious complications of cardiac surgery are endocarditis, mediastinitis and sternal wound infection. Sternal wound infection is a consequence of about 5% of cardiac operations, and is frequently due to staphylococcal infection, both coagulase-negative staphylococci and *Staph. aureus.* Enterobacteriaceae have also been implicated in sternal infections. The severe consequences of sternal infections are sufficient incentive to use antibiotics prophylactically, and several trials of antibiotic regimens have shown them to be effective (Kreter & Woods 1992). Antibiotics are recommended for permanent pacemaker insertion, open heart surgery including coronary artery bypass grafting and prosthetic valve insertion. Cephalosporins, including cefazolin and cefuroxime, have been used to cover methicillin-sensitive staphylococci and Enterobacteriaceae. However, the increasing proportion of infections due to methicillin-resistant coagulase-negative staphylococci and *Staph. aureus* in some hospitals has reduced the effectiveness of this class of antibiotics. Consequently there has been a divergence of opinions in the approach to prophylaxis in this type of surgery, with some groups advocating broad antibiotic cover against Gram-positive organisms with glycopeptides such as teicoplanin, while others suggest using flucloxacillin, either alone or with antibiotics such as aminoglycosides which are active against Gram-negative organisms. Leg veins may be used to replace blocked coronary arteries, and incisions made to harvest veins can also become infected, although these are generally prevented by the antibiotics chosen to prevent sternal infections.

Urological surgery

The most important determinant of infectious complications of urological surgery is the presence or absence of bacteria in the urine. A level higher than 10^5 organisms/ml in a mid-stream specimen of urine is indicative of infection although lower amounts may be significant. Any bacteria in urine collected aseptically from the bladder, ureters or pelvis of the kidneys is abnormal and should be taken into account when considering prophylaxis. Common causes of infected urine are Enterobacteriaceae, especially *Escherichia coli,* and also enterococci and *Pseudomonas aeruginosa.* The last is frequent in patients who are catheterized and who have received antibiotics. Patients with abnormal structure or function of the urinary tract leading to residual urine post-voiding are also at increased risk of Gram-negative urinary tract infections. The great danger of operating on a urinary tract containing infected urine is one of bacteraemia leading to septic shock. This is especially dangerous when Gram-negative organisms are involved. Ideally, urine samples should be cultured a few days before a planned procedure so that appropriate antibiotics can be chosen. Such antibiotics should reach good blood and tissue levels, and it is an advantage if they are excreted renally. If preoperative culture is not possible, broad spectrum antibiotics likely to be effective against all Gram-negative bacteria should be used, for example aminoglycosides or quinolones, possibly in conjunction with antibiotics such as amoxicillin, which is active against enterococci. In the absence of urine culture results, antibiotics are recommended for transrectal prostate biopsy, shock-wave lithotripsy and transurethral resection of the prostate but not transurethral resection of bladder tumours.

Obstetrics and gynaecology

Most births in developed countries are unaccompanied by significant infections, which is remarkable given the high levels of faecal organisms around the perineum. This was not always the case. Puerperal sepsis was a leading cause of death in women until the need for good hygiene practices was appreciated. However, there is no indication for routine antibiotic prophylaxis for either normal vaginal deliveries or forceps deliveries unless the episiotomy or tear extends to include the rectum.

Infection rates following caesarean sections vary considerably depending on the population studied. Mothers with iron deficiency anaemia, those from poor social backgrounds and those with obstetric complications are more likely to develop infections. Some obstetricians give prophylaxis to all their caesarean section patients; others use prophylaxis selectively in high-risk patients. Antibiotics should ideally cover *Staph. aureus*, enterococci, Enterobacteriaceae and anaerobes such as *Bacteroides* spp. Single-agent drugs such as cefoxitin and co-amoxiclav, or combinations such as cefuroxime and metronidazole, have been used, although enterococci have innate resistance to cephalosporins. The baby can be protected against antibiotic exposure, if required, by withholding antibiotics until the umbilical cord has been clamped.

Gynaecological procedures are also subject to infection by the range of organisms detailed above. Infections can occur at the suture line of the vaginal cuff and extend into the tissues of the pelvis. An abdominal hysterectomy can additionally be complicated by skin incision infections. It is likely that wound infection rates are decreased by prophylaxis, and the antibiotics usually used for caesarean sections are indicated for both vaginal and abdominal hysterectomy and induced abortion.

Vascular surgery

Wound infection rates vary with body site. Surgery performed on vessels of the neck or upper limbs carries a low risk of infection, and prophylaxis is usually not necessary. Operations involving groin incisions have the highest rate of infection, and prophylaxis is indicated here

as well as with abdominal and lower limb procedures. Organisms often involved are *Staph. aureus* and Enterobacteriaceae. However, the worst complication of postoperative infection in vascular surgery is infection of the implanted graft. Once grafts are infected they are almost impossible to sterilize with antibiotic therapy, and often require removal. This may jeopardize the survival of the limb or the patient. Frequent causes of graft infections are coagulase-negative staphylococci and *Corynebacterium* spp. The antibiotic susceptibilities of these organisms are unpredictable. Other organisms such as the Enterobacteriaceae and enterococci are also likely to cause infections of grafts implanted through abdominal and groin incisions. The range of potential pathogens precludes the use of narrow-spectrum antibiotics, and many regimens have been proposed. Aminoglycosides with antistaphylococcal penicillins, several cephalosporins, and penicillins combined with β-lactamase inhibitors have all been used. The optimum duration of prophylaxis is unclear. Courses lasting for up to 14 days have been given, but 24 hours of antibiotics is probably adequate. Amputations also require prophylaxis to be given.

Neurosurgery

Any postoperative infection of the central nervous system can have devastating consequences. Avoidance of infection in neurosurgery should therefore always be a high priority. Using microbiological principles, an appropriate antibiotic would be one which is active against the most common causes of neurosurgical infection, namely *Staph. aureus,* which accounts for half of all postoperative infections, coagulase-negative staphylococci (15%), streptococci (9%) and Gram-negative rods (16%). Unfortunately this is a wide range, and, if they are all to be countered, either a single broad-spectrum antibiotic or a combination of at least two antibiotics would be required. Some surgeons use vancomycin and an aminoglycoside such as gentamicin. However, there are concerns that broad-spectrum cover may promote antibiotic multi-resistant bacteria. Additionally, both of these antibiotics penetrate the blood–brain barrier poorly. At the other extreme, narrow-spectrum cover with benzylpenicillin (again penetrates the uninflamed blood–brain barrier poorly) or rifampicin has been used with apparent success. Intermediate alternatives, predominantly cephalosporins, have been suggested in a British Society Working Party report, which also points out the need for repeated intraoperative doses during operations of more than 3 hours' duration (Infection in Neurosurgery Working Party 1994).

Similar obstacles and considerations apply to the use of antibiotics in cerebrospinal fluid shunt implantation surgery. Recent reports indicate an infection rate of about 10%, although children less than 6 months old at the time of the operation have a higher rate than older children (15.7% versus 5.6% in one report). Approximately 70% of shunt infections present within 2 months of surgery, indicating that the causative organisms are introduced into the cerebrospinal fluid at the time of operation. Half of the infections are due to coagulase-negative staphylococci. The remainder are predominantly caused by enterococci, *Staph. aureus* and Enterobacteriaceae. Less common causes are *Pseudomonas* spp. and *Candida* spp. Again there is no consensus as to appropriate regimens. A British Society for Antimicrobial Chemotherapy working party suggested instilling gentamicin and vancomycin into the ventricles during the operation (BSAC 1995). This approach would presumably not reduce contamination of that part of the wound outside the brain, and perhaps should be supplemented by a single immediately preoperative dose of gentamicin and/or vancomycin.

Several studies have emphasized the importance of surgical technique in reducing shunt infection rates. A French study presented a protocol that considered preoperative preparation, intraoperative precautions and postoperative care. When this protocol was implemented, the infection rate dropped from 7.75 to 0.17% (Choux et al 1992). Although this study was unable to define the relative values of the various elements of their protocol, it is clear that antibiotic prophylaxis is only part of the approach to reducing the incidence of shunt infections.

Orthopaedic surgery

Fractures

Open fractures, those where a break in the bone is accompanied by a skin wound, are associated with an infection rate that is proportional to the extent of soft tissue damage. Fractures with little soft tissue injury and a small wound less than 1 cm long have infection rates of less than 10%. When skin is missing or badly torn, or when there is extensive vascular damage and muscle injury that makes it difficult to cover the fracture, infection rates can be as high as 55%. Fixation of the fractures has been associated with increased infection rates when compared to those fractures not requiring fixation, although this may reflect the severity of the injury, and may not be an independent risk factor. Despite high infection rates in severe injuries the lack of well-conducted prospective trials of prophylaxis means that their efficacy remains uncertain. However, there is increasing evidence that antibiotics active against *Staph. aureus* reduce the rate of wound infection. The additional presence of coliforms and anaerobes in extensively damaged wounds would suggest that patients with such injuries should receive broader-spectrum antibiotics, but there is little trial evidence to support

this. When soft tissue coverage of the fracture is difficult there is a likelihood that the wound will become infected with hospital environment flora, which may be multiply-resistant to antibiotics. Broad-spectrum antibiotics may hasten this. When prophylaxis is given there is a tendency for it to be continued for up to 10 days. Where duration of prophylaxis has been studied, 24 hours' duration has been as effective as 5 days (Dellinger 1991).

Fractures that remain closed at the time of injury may be opened in the operating theatre to allow fixation, placement of prosthetic devices or osteosynthesis. Because the wound is made in a controlled, aseptic fashion the infection rate is low, usually below 10%. However, good evidence has accumulated that supports the role of prophylaxis in such surgery. Most recently, the Dutch Trauma Trial group published a randomized, double-blind, placebo-controlled trial of antibiotic prophylaxis in the operative treatment of closed limb fractures, demonstrating that a single preoperative dose of ceftriaxone significantly reduced the rate of both wound infections and other types of nosocomial infections, including respiratory and urinary tract infections, and that in the settings of the study such prophylaxis was very cost-effective (Boxma et al 1996).

Joint replacement surgery

Elective hip and knee prosthesis surgery is now a major part of orthopaedic surgery. One of the most serious and common complications is infection of the bone and soft tissue surrounding the implant. This can result from intraoperative contamination, which accounts for early infections, and haematogenous seeding, which can occur years later. Early infections can be significantly reduced by the ultra-filtration of operating theatre air, laminar air-flow ventilation, whole-body exhaust suits and strict theatre discipline to reduce movement in the theatre to the absolute minimum. Antibiotics also appear to reduce infection rates. It is not clear whether theatre effects and antibiotics are independent, and so cumulative when combined, or whether the use of one makes the other redundant. The cause of early infection is usually *Staph. aureus,* and any prophylaxis should be active against this organism. Short courses of antibiotics lasting for 12–24 hours seem to be as effective as courses lasting 7 or 14 days. An optimal approach would be to combine ultra-clean air theatres and short courses of antibiotics, for example flucloxacillin. An alternative, or additional, approach to chemoprophylaxis is to incorporate antibiotics, for example gentamicin or cefuroxime, in the bone cement, bone graft or materials to fill dead space. The limited available data do not suggest a clear role in routine prophylaxis in elective joint replacement (Anon 2001).

Late infections are predominantly caused by coagulase-negative staphylococci, which are usually assumed to infect the joint following haematogenous spread. Other bacterial species can also cause late infections, so that it is important that patients with prosthetic joints receive prompt appropriate treatment for infections at any site. Currently there is little else that can be done to avoid late infections. In particular, risk–benefit analyses show that patients with joint prostheses undergoing dental treatment should not be given prophylactic antibiotics.

Oral and maxillofacial surgery

The oral cavity is heavily colonized with aerobic α-haemolytic streptococci, anaerobic streptococci and anaerobic Gram-negative rods. Nevertheless, minor oral surgery, including most dentoalveolar surgery, has an infection rate of less than 1% and wound infection prophylaxis in healthy individuals is not indicated. However, endocarditis prophylaxis may be indicated. More invasive and extensive surgery has a higher infection rate, about 10–15%, and penicillin has been advocated as a suitable agent for prophylaxis when the transoral approach is used. When the incision involves the skin, either alone or in combination with an oral mucosa incision, staphylococcal infections are more likely, and flucloxacillin could be added. In prolonged surgery additional antibiotic doses should be administered, but there is no evidence to support prolonged postoperative courses of prophylaxis. In general, prophylaxis is recommended for contaminated/clean-contaminated head and neck surgery but not clean procedures, nose or sinus surgery or tonsillectomy.

Hand surgery

A recent investigation of infection rates following a wide range of hand surgical procedures at one unit revealed overall rates of 10.7% in elective operations and 9.7% in emergency operations (Platt & Page 1995). Further analysis showed that elective surgery patients who had received prophylactic antibiotics did not have a significantly lower wound infection rate compared with the no prophylaxis elective surgery patients. However, patients undergoing emergency surgery were at greater risk of wound infection if they were not given antibiotics prophylactically compared with emergency patients receiving antibiotics. Emergency procedures were 13.4 times more likely to become infected if the original trauma had left significant contamination, crush injuries or devascularization of tissues. *Staph. aureus* was the organism most frequently isolated from infected wounds.

Wound infections following hand surgery can have grave effects on subsequent recovery of dexterity, and it is legitimate to use prophylaxis in situations where prophylaxis provides even only a small benefit. Appropriate circumstances have included elective or emergency surgery involving percutaneous K-wires, joint prostheses and operations of 2 hours or more duration, and all emergency hand surgery on dirty wounds, open fractures or where a delay of 6 hours or more has occurred between trauma and surgery. It is possible that patients with systemic disease such as diabetes, and patients with local disease, including rheumatoid arthritis or eczema, would benefit from prophylactic antibiotics for all types of hand surgery.

Appropriate antibiotics are flucloxacillin, or clindamycin if penicillin-allergic, given before tourniquet inflation (tourniquets are used to reduce bleeding that would otherwise obscure the surgical site). One dose should be adequate for elective surgery. It may be justifiable to give treatment for 48 hours or longer if the wound is grossly contaminated, and in these circumstances the possibility of infection due to anaerobic organisms (especially if a bite or similar wound). In this event infection could be prevented by adding metronidazole or by using co-amoxiclav as a single agent.

Improving antibiotic prophylaxis

Errors in antimicrobial prophylaxis for surgery are one of the most frequent medication errors in hospitals (Burke 2001). Optimal use including case selection, agent used, dose, route of administration, timing and duration should be audited. Results of these audits need to be fed back to the whole surgical unit as appropriate use of antimicobial prophylaxis may involve several disciplines (nurses, anaesthetists, operating department assistants) and not just the prescribing physician. As well as assessing the process of administration of antibiotic(s), other objective measures such as SSI rate or other adverse outcomes such as *C. difficile* infection should be measured. Computer-based expert systems may improve prescribing. In one study the use of such a system was associated with an improvement in the timeliness of prophylaxis (in those patients in whom prophylaxis was indicated only 40% received antibiotics within 2 hours before incision in 1985; this increased to 99.1% in 1994), and a shortening in prophylaxis duration (average number of doses per patient in 1985 was 19, and 5.3 in 1994) (Pestotnik et al 1996).

Common therapeutic problems in surgical antibiotic prophylaxis are summarized in Table 37.6.

Alternative approaches

Despite optimal antibiotic prophylaxis, surgical wound infections still occur and alternative strategies have been developed. Warming patients using either a forced-air warming blanket or a non-contact radiant heat dressing have reduced infection rates in clean surgery (Melling et al 2001).

Table 37.6   Common therapeutic problems in surgical antibiotic prophylaxis

Problem	Background	Management
Antibiotics given too soon	An adequate concentration of antibiotic is required at the site of operation for them to be effective	Most surgical prophylaxis is given at induction of anaesthesia Administration of antibiotics should be audited
Antibiotics continued for prolonged periods after the operation	This increases hospital costs, promotes the emergence of resistant bacteria and may cause complications such as *C. difficile*	Antibiotic prophylaxis should be prescribed for a fixed duration
Operation involves insertion of prosthetic material	All implants have a detrimental effect on host defences and a lower bacterial inoculum is required to initiate infection	Rigorous adherence to antibiotic prophylaxis
Repeated surgical exploration	Patients exposed to antibiotics may have resistant bacterial flora so the standard antibiotic prophylaxis regimens may be inappropriate	Generally a more broad-spectrum agent is used but the choice depends on the nature of the operation and knowledge of local resistance patterns
Patient allergic to β-lactams	Unable to use certain standard regimens due to risk of anaphylaxis to penicillins and cephalosporins	Choice of agent will depend on type of surgery; aminoglycosides, fluroquinolones or clindamycin may be used

CASE STUDIES

Case 37.1

A patient with a clinical diagnosis of appendicitis is found, at operation, to have caecal carcinoma.

Question

Should any modifications be made to the prophylaxis protocol employed?

Answer

Patients undergoing appendicectomy should receive prophylaxis if the appendix is suspected or found to be perforated, and there is an argument that antibiotics should be given routinely for appendicectomy. In the patient with unsuspected caecal carcinoma there is bound to be contamination of the wound by faecal organisms during a lengthier and more difficult than expected operation. Under these circumstances, high levels of antibiotics with activity against coliforms, anaerobes and *Staph. aureus* should be maintained throughout the operation and for several hours thereafter by giving additional doses of antibiotics.

Case 37.2

The urine culture result of a patient admitted for a transurethral resection of prostate has been lost by the microbiology laboratory and the patient is due to go to theatre in 5 minutes.

Question

What antibiotics, if any, should be given as prophylaxis?

Answer

If the urine is infected, likely organisms are coliforms and *Pseudomonas aeruginosa*. Appropriate antibiotic cover could be selected from aminoglycosides (e.g. gentamicin), antipseudomonal third-generation cephalosporins (e.g. ceftazidime), fluoroquinolones (e.g. ciprofloxacin), ureidopenicillins (azlocillin or piperacillin), the monobactam aztreonam or a carbapenem (meropenem). In practice the antibiotic chosen should be the one routinely used in the hospital for urological operations in the presence of *Pseudomonas* bacteriuria. Note that although intramuscular gentamicin can be used for such operations, in this particular case there is little time for high serum levels to be achieved, and an intravenous route of administration is advisable.

Case 37.3

A patient due to have a cholecystectomy for recurrent cholangitis has already received her preoperative prophylactic antibiotics on the ward when her operation is postponed for 5 hours.

Question

Are any further doses of antibiotic prophylaxis required, and if so, where and when should they be given?

Answer

It is likely that the half-lives of the antibiotics used will not be sufficiently long to accommodate the delay in surgery, and further doses will be required at a time guided by the pharmacokinetics of the drugs involved. It is probable that this will be during surgery, and the surgeons should be aware of the need to top up the antibiotic levels. It is a good idea to routinely give preoperative antibiotics at induction, and not on the ward, in order to avoid this sort of problem.

Case 37.4

A patient has a venflon site infection due to methicillin-resistant *Staphylococcus aureus* (MRSA). He is on the waiting list for heart valve replacement surgery.

Question

Are any alterations to the standard antibiotic prophylaxis required, and if so, what should they be?

Answer

Valve replacement surgery caries a high risk of morbidity and mortality if infection of the valve or surgical wound occurs (the latter may result in mediastinitis). In this particular case it is necessary to delay the operation until the venflon site infection is treated. It is also necessary to determine the extent of colonization and try to eradicate it from these sites using topical agents such as nasal mupirocin and chlorhexidine body washes. As eradication of MRSA can be difficult, the standard prophylaxis used (flucloxacillin, cefuroxime) will have to be changed to an agent that would be reliably active against MRSA, such as a teicoplanin or vancomycin.

Case 37.5

A neurosurgical patient has been given cefuroxime for 6 days post-operatively as he has an external ventricular drain in place.

Question

Is such treatment part of standard antibiotic prophylaxis? Are there any adverse consequences of this regimen?

Answer

Most surgical antibiotic prophylaxis is given perioperatively in this patient; because of the presence of an external ventricular drain it has been continued (Prabhu et al 1999). Although cefuroxime is used in this context to prevent infection of external ventricular drains, recent studies suggest no reduction in infection rates (Alleyne et al 2000). Prolonged administration of antibiotics results in an alteration of host microbial flora; bacteria that are resistant to cefuroxime, such as MRSA or *Pseudomonas aeruginosa*, are selected out. Therefore, if the patient's external ventricular drain becomes infected, or the patient develops a hospital-acquired pneumonia, it is likely to be due to a more resistant organism. Widespread use of antibiotics in this manner contributes to the emergence of resistant organisms within the hospital. The patient may also develop a complication of antibiotic use such as pseudomembranous colitis.

Case 37.6

Following a total hip replacement, loosening of the prosthetic joint occurs and it is decided that the prosthetic joint has to be replaced.

Question

What is the standard antibiotic prophylaxis for hip joint replacement? Why may you want to alter the regimen for this patient?

Answer

Cefuroxime is frequently used as antibiotic prophylaxis for hip replacement surgery. In this particular case it is important to determine whether the loosening of the old prosthesis is due to infection. Inflammatory indices should be measured (C-reactive protein and erythrocyte sedimentation rate) and if there is evidence of infection then a two-stage procedure should be performed. Perioperative tissue/bone samples are taken and, based on microbial culture and sensitivity testing, a course of antibiotic therapy is given. After 6 weeks of treatment, if there is adequate response to therapy (reduction in CRP), a new joint may be implanted.

In some cases the prosthetic joint is found to be infected in theatre and it may be prudent to use teicoplanin or vancomycin as standard antibiotic prophylaxis if a prosthetic joint is to be replaced.

REFERENCES

Alleyne C H, Hassan M, Zabramski J M 2000 The efficacy and cost of prophylactic and periprocedural antibiotics in patients with external ventricular drains. Neurosurgery 5: 1124–1129

Anon 2001 Antimicrobial prophylaxis for orthopaedic surgery. Drugs and Therapeutics Bulletin 39(6): 43–46

Boxma H, Broekhuizen T, Patka P et al 1996 Randomised controlled trial of a single-dose antibiotic prophylaxis in surgical treatment of closed fractures: the Dutch Trauma Trial. Lancet 347: 1133–1137

British Society for Antimicrobial Chemotherapy (BSAC) 1995

Working Party on the Use of Antibiotics in Neurosurgery of the British Society for Antimicrobial Chemotherapy. Treatment of infections associated with shunting for hydrocephalus. British Journal of Hospital Medicine 53(8): 368–373

Burke J P 2001 Maximizing appropriate antibiotic prophylaxis for surgical patients: an update from LDS hospital, Salt Lake City. Clinical Infectious Diseases 33(Suppl. 2): S78–83

Choux M, Genitori L, Lang D et al 1992 Shunt implantation: reducing the incidence of shunt infection. Journal of Neurosurgery 77(6): 875–880

Classen D C, Evans R S, Pestotnik S L et al 1992 The timing of prophylactic administration of antibiotics and the risk of surgical-wound infection. New England Journal of Medicine 326: 281–286

Dellinger E P 1991 Antibiotic prophylaxis in trauma: penetrating abdominal injuries and open fractures. Reviews in Infectious Diseases 13(Suppl. 10): S847–857

Dellinger E P, Gross P A, Barrett T L et al 1994 Quality standard for antimicrobial prophylaxis in surgical procedures. Clinical Infectious Diseases 18: 422–427

Fry D E 1988 Antibiotics in surgery: an overview. American Journal of Surgery 155(5A): 11–15

Gaynes R P, Culver D H, Horan T C et al and the National Nosocomial Infections Surveillance System 2001 Surgical site infection (SSI) rates in the United States, 1992–1998: the National Nosocomial Infections Surveillance System basic SSI risk index. Clinical Infectious Diseases 33(Suppl. 2): S69–77

Horan T C, Gaynes R P, Martone W J et al. 1992 CDC definitions for nosocomial surgical site infections, 1992: a modification of CDC definitions of surgical wound infections. Infection Control and Hospital Epidemiology 13: 606–608

Infection in Neurosurgery Working Party of the British Society for Antimicrobial Chemotherapy 1994 Antimicrobial prophylaxis in neurosurgery and after head injury. Lancet 344: 1547–1551

Kogler J, Hancke E, Marklein G et al 1989 Ciprofloxacin for single shot prophylaxis during cholecystectomy. Infection 17(3): 174–175

Kreter B, Woods M 1992 Antibiotic prophylaxis for cardiothoracic operations: meta-analysis of thirty years of clinical trials. Journal of Thoracic and Cardiovascular Surgery 104(3): 590–599

Melling A C, Ali B, Scott E M et al 2001 Effect of preoperative warming on the incidence of wound infection after clean surgery: a randomized controlled trial. Lancet 358: 876–880

Pestotnik S L, Classen D C, Evans R S et al 1996 Implementing antibiotic practice guidelines through computer-assisted decision support: clinical and financial outcomes. Annals of Internal Medicine 124: 884–890

Platt A J, Page R E 1995 Post-operative infection following hand surgery: guidelines for antibiotic use. Journal of Hand Surgery 20(5): 685–690

Prabhu V C, Kaufman H H, Voelker J L et al 1999 Prophylactic antibiotics with intracranial pressure monitors and external ventricular drains: a review of the evidence. Surgical Neurology 52: 226–237

Soderquist-Elinder C, Hirsch K, Bergdahl S et al 1995 Prophylactic antibiotics in uncomplicated appendicitis during childhood – a prospective randomised study. European Journal of Pediatric Surgery 5(5): 282–285

Waddell T K, Rotstein O D 1995 Antimicrobial prophylaxis in surgery. Canadian Medical Association Journal 151(7): 925–931

FURTHER READING

Martin C. French Study Group on Antimicrobial Prophylaxis in Surgery, French Society of Anaesthesia and Intensive Care 1994 Antimicrobial prophylaxis in surgery: general concepts and clinical guidelines. Infection Control and Hospital Epidemiology 15: 463–471

Martone W J, Nichols R L, 2001 Recognition, prevention, surveillance, and management of surgical site infections. Proceedings of a Symposium Held at the Fourth Decennial International Conference on Nosocomial and Healthcare-associated Infections. Clinical Infectious Diseases 33(Suppl. 2): S67–106

Scottish Intercollegiate Guidelines Network (SIGN) 2000 Antibiotic prophylaxis in surgery. SIGN Secretariat, Royal College of Physicians, 9 Queen Street, Edinburgh EH2 IJQ

Sheretz R J, Marosok R D, Garibaldi R A et al 1992 Consensus paper on the surveillance of surgical wound infections. Infection Control Hospital Epidemiology 13: 599–605

Swedish-Norwegian Consensus Group 1998 Antibiotic prophylaxis in surgery: summary of a Swedish-Norwegian consensus conference, vol. 30; pp. 47–57

Tuberculosis 38

L. K. Nehaul

KEY POINTS

- Each year there are an estimated 8 million new cases of tuberculosis (TB) and 2 million deaths from the disease worldwide.
- One-third of the world's population is infected with the tubercle bacillus.
- Multidrug-resistant tuberculosis is a problem in many parts of the world.
- Adequate and effective treatment is essential to treat the individual, control the spread of TB, and minimize the occurrence of multidrug-resistant disease.
- Tuberculosis is caused by infection with *Mycobacterium tuberculosis*, *M. bovis* and *M. africanum*. *M. tuberculosis* accounts for over 98% of isolates in the UK.
- TB infection usually occurs by the respiratory route. Over 90% of people infected enter a latent phase from which there is a lifelong risk of reactivation.
- People with HIV infection have an increased risk of tuberculosis if coinfected.
- Certain medical risk factors increase the risk of tuberculosis.
- Two types of testing are used to confirm infection with TB: the Heaf (multiple puncture) and Mantoux tests. The Heaf test is quick and simple and preferred in BCG vaccination programmes.
- Most treatment regimens in the developed world are of 6–9 months duration and contain isoniazid, rifampicin and pyrazinamide, possibly with ethambutol or streptomycin.
- Rifampicin, isoniazid and pyrazinamide are all potentially hepatotoxic. Isoniazid may cause a dose-dependent peripheral neuropathy while ocular toxicity is the most important side-effect of ethambutol.

Tuberculosis (TB) is an important public health problem worldwide. In industrialized countries, the numbers of reported cases levelled out in the mid to late 1980s and then started increasing. This increase also occurred in countries across all continents, leading the World Health Organization (WHO) to declare tuberculosis a global emergency in 1993.

Of additional concern has been the increae in multidrug-resistant tuberculosis, with outbreaks in different parts of the world. This has been attributed to both human immunodeficiency virus (HIV) infection and inappropriate or inadequate treatment.

Adequate and effective treatment is essential, both clinically for patients and to control the spread of tuberculosis. The success of this depends on close collaboration between clinical and public health teams, and a shared understanding with primary care teams as to the role of all health professionals involved in the care of people with tuberculosis and their contacts.

Epidemiology

Tuberculosis causes about 2 million deaths worldwide each year, and one-third of the world's population is infected with the tubercle bacillus. It is becoming the leading cause of death among HIV-positive people.

Globally over 3 million cases of tuberculosis disease are notified annually although the estimated number of new cases is put at 8 million. The majority of cases occur in poor countries in the southern hemisphere, but TB is re-emerging in Eastern Europe, which experiences over a quarter of a million cases each year.

The numbers of cases reported in 1999 to the WHO, globally and by WHO region, are presented in Table 38.1. The figures do not give the full picture because of under-reporting and under-recording in all countries.

In the UK and other industrialized countries, changes have taken place in the age/sex incidence of tuberculosis in recent decades. Mortality shifted from the young to the old with the advent of chemotherapy. In the late 1950s, only 20% of notifications in Britain were from patients over 45 years of age, but by the late 1970s the proportion was 60%, with a majority of males (Christie 1987). The results of the 1988 national survey of tuberculosis indicated that 55% of cases occurred in white males more than 55 years of age.

There is a higher notification rate of tuberculosis in the UK in people from high-prevalence countries, mainly South-East Asia. The risk of tuberculosis is highest in the 5 years after arrival in the UK. The number of cases by region in England and Wales from the 1998 national tuberculosis survey are shown in Table 38.2.

Table 38.1 Number of cases of tuberculosis reported to the World Health Organization in 1999 and notification rate per 100 000 of the population in 1999 and 1994 (WHO 2001)

	Number of cases notified	Notification rate per 100 000 population	
		1999	1994
Africa	644 972	105	96.8
Americas	233 823	29	34.9
Eastern Mediterranean	156 637	32	55.2
Europe	362 532	42	33.3
South-East Asia	1 469 672	97	94.4
Western Pacific	822 177	49	45.5
Global	3 689 813	62	60.1

Table 38.2 Tuberculosis in England and Wales in 1998: number of cases and rate per 100 000 population for all regions

Region	Number of cases	Rate per 100 000 population
London	2243	31.12
West Midlands	622	11.66
North-West	656	9.93
Northern and Yorkshire	605	9.54
Trent	452	8.80
Wales	163	5.56
South-East	461	5.53
Eastern	244	4.54
South-West	212	4.33

Source: Communicable Disease Surveillance Centre (London) 1998 National Tuberculosis Survey (1999 boundaries)

Aetiology

Tuberculosis infection is caused by tubercle bacilli, which belong to the genus *Mycobacterium*. These form a large group, but only three relatives are obligate parasites that can cause tuberculosis disease. They are part of the *Mycobacterium tuberculosis* complex and include *M. tuberculosis, M. bovis* and *M. africanum*. However, generally only the first two are found in isolates from people with tuberculosis diagnosed in the UK, with *M. tuberculosis* accounting for over 98% of isolates.

The vast majority of the other members of the genus *Mycobacterium* are saprophytes and are widely distributed in the environment, often in soil, mud and water. They are often referred to as atypical to distinguish them from *M. tuberculosis*. Only about 15 are recognized as pathogenic to humans, some causing pulmonary disease resembling tuberculosis. Public health action is not required for infections caused by atypical mycobacteria, as there is no evidence of person-to-person transmission.

Infection with tubercle bacilli occurs in the vast majority of cases by the respiratory route. The lung lesions caused by infection commonly heal, leaving no residual changes except occasional pulmonary or tracheobronchial lymph node calcification (Chin 2000). Over 90% of people initially infected enter this latent phase, from which there is a lifelong risk of reactivation. In approximately 5–10% of apparently normal hosts, and as many as 50% of people with advanced HIV infection,

the initial infection may progress to pulmonary tuberculosis or, by lymphohaematogenous spread of bacilli, to pulmonary, meningeal, or other extrapulmonary involvement, or lead to disseminated disease (miliary TB). Infants, adolescents and immunosuppressed people are more susceptible to the more serious forms of tuberculosis such as miliary tuberculosis or tuberculous meningitis.

Pulmonary (respiratory) tuberculosis is more common than extrapulmonary (non-respiratory) tuberculosis, accounting for about 70% of cases in the UK. Sites of extrapulmonary tuberculosis can include the pleura, lymph nodes, pericardium, kidneys, meninges, bones and joints, larynx, skin, intestines, peritoneum and eyes. In practice in the UK the lymph nodes are the commonest site for extrapulmonary disease.

Progressive pulmonary tuberculosis arises from exogenous reinfection or endogenous reactivation of a latent focus remaining from the initial infection. If untreated, about half the patients will die within 5 years, a majority of these within 18 months. Completion of chemotherapy using drugs to which the tubercle bacilli are sensitive almost always results in a cure, even in those with HIV infection.

Symptoms include fatigue, fever, night sweats and weight loss, which may occur early, while localizing symptoms of cough, chest pain, haemoptysis and hoarseness become prominent in the advanced stages.

Abnormal radiographs with pulmonary infiltration, cavitation and fibrosis can occur before clinical manifestations.

Transmission

Transmission occurs through exposure to tubercle bacilli in airborne droplet nuclei produced by people with pulmonary or laryngeal tuberculosis during expiratory efforts such as coughing or sneezing. Laryngeal tuberculosis is rarely seen in the UK.

Incubation period

The incubation period from infection to demonstrable primary lesion or significant tuberculin reaction ranges from 2 to 10 weeks. Latent infection may persist for a lifetime. HIV infection appears to shorten the interval for the development of clinical tuberculosis.

Infectious forms of tuberculosis

Patients should be considered infectious if they have sputum smear-positive pulmonary disease, that is, where they produce sputum containing sufficient tubercle bacilli to be seen on direct sputum examination, or laryngeal tuberculosis. Patients with smear-negative pulmonary disease (three sputum samples) are far less infectious than those who are smear-positive. The relative transmission rate from smear negative compared with smear positive patients has been estimated to be 0.22 (British Thoracic Society 2000).

Risk groups

Risk groups for tuberculosis include:

- people infected with HIV
- close contacts of patients with tuberculosis, especially those with sputum smear-positive pulmonary disease
- people from countries with a high prevalence of tuberculosis (greater than 40/100 000 population)
- alcoholics and injecting drug users
- medical risk factors (Table 38.3).

Impact of HIV infection

People with HIV infection have an increased risk of tuberculosis. The estimated annual risk of tuberculosis in those with HIV infection and tuberculosis coinfection is 7–10% as opposed to a 10% lifetime chance in someone infected with tuberculosis, but not HIV.

Most cases of tuberculosis in patients with HIV infection are likely to result from the reactivation of previously acquired infection, but reinfection may be

Table 38.3   Medical risk factors for tuberculosis

Diabetes mellitus
Conditions requiring prolonged high-dose corticosteroid therapy and other immunosuppressive therapy
Chronic renal failure
Some haematological disorders, e.g. leukaemia and lymphomas
Other malignancies
Gastrectomy
Jejunoileal bypass

Source: Morbidity and Mortality Weekly Report (MMWR), 1995, vol. 44, NO RR - 11

important in populations with a high prevalence of tuberculosis.

Diagnosis

The preliminary diagnosis of tuberculosis disease is based on the symptoms and signs in the patient, in conjunction with the tuberculin reaction and radiographic appearance. Microbiological investigations can confirm the diagnosis, although this can take up to 6 weeks using routinely available techniques.

Investigations

Tuberculin reaction

Tuberculin testing is used to confirm infection. The two types of test used in the UK are the Heaf (multiple puncture) and Mantoux tests. Both use solutions of tuberculin purified protein derivative (PPD). Several strengths of PPD are available, and it is important that the correct solution is used.

The Heaf test is quick and simple. It is particularly useful where large numbers of tests are performed, such as in BCG vaccination programmes in schools. A solution of 100 000 units/ml of PPD is applied in sufficient amount to spread over the gun head and the Heaf gun, with six needles arranged in a circle, is used to puncture the skin. The result is ideally read in 7 days but can be read from 3–10 days. There are five grades of response:

Grade 0 No induration at puncture sites. Erythema only present.

Grade 1 Discrete induration at four or more needle sites.

Grade 2 Confluent areas of induration forming a ring with a clear centre.

Grade 3 A disc of induration 5–10 mm wide.

Grade 4 Solid induration greater than 10 mm. Vesiculation or ulceration may also occur.

In the UK, grade 3 and 4 reactions are considered to indicate infection along with grade 2 response in a tuberculosis contact who has not previously had the BCG (bacillus of Calmette and Guérin) vaccine. The BCG vaccine is used in many countries with a high incidence of tuberculosis to prevent the disease in people who are tuberculin-negative. Prior vaccination with BCG usually results in a positive tuberculin skin test. This is impossible to differentiate from that due to *M. tuberculosis.*

Grade 3 and 4 reactions are said to be strongly positive. Anyone Heaf tested as a TB contact, or in a vaccination programme, and found to have these reactions needs to be referred to a chest clinic for further investigation, including chest radiography.

The Mantoux test is more time-consuming and requires greater skill to administer. The PPD for routine use in this test contains 100 units/ml. (For individuals in whom tuberculosis is suspected, or who are known to be hypersensitive to tuberculin, the preparation containing 10 units/ml should be used.) In this test 0.1 ml of the appropriate solution is injected intradermally so that a bleb is produced. The results should be read 48–72 hours later, but a valid reading can be obtained up to 96 hours. A positive result consists of induration with a transverse diameter of at least 5 mm following injection of 0.1 ml of PPD 100 units/ml.

The reaction to tuberculin protein may be suppressed by infections or conditions causing immunosuppression, including:

- infectious mononucleosis
- viral infections in general
- live viral vaccines (delay tuberculin testing for 3 weeks)
- Hodgkin's disease
- sarcoidosis
- corticosteroid therapy
- immunosuppressing treatment or diseases, including HIV.

Chest radiography

The earliest change is the appearance of an ill-defined opacity or opacities, usually seen in one of the upper lobes. In the more advanced stages of the disease, the opacities are larger and more widespread and may be bilateral.

Occasionally there is extensive patchy shadowing involving the whole lobe.

An area or areas of translucency within the opacities indicates cavitation. The presence of cavitation in an untreated case usually indicates that disease is active.

Radiological changes of a pleural effusion or pneumothorax may also be seen.

Microbiological investigations

Microbiological confirmation proves the diagnosis of tuberculosis, although this may take as long as 6 weeks for the final results. It is still largely based on microscopy and culture techniques. Direct microscopy of sputum using the Ziehl–Neelsen or fluorescent rhodamine–auramine stains is the simplest and quickest method of detecting the infectious patient, although this test is said to be positive in only 60% of culture-confirmed cases (Davies 1999). However, these are much less useful in non-pulmonary and childhood disease, the diagnosis of which depends more on culture. With conventional culture methods, such as the Lowenstein–Jensen medium, growth may take up to 6 weeks.

More modern methods are now available. These include the use of liquid cultures which can produce results in 1–2 weeks. Other techniques utilize more sensitive measures to detect the bacilli. These include amplification of a defined region of DNA from a few starting copies, the polymerase chain reaction (PCR). The PCR test is used where a more rapid answer is needed to guide public health action, for example a case of suspected sputum smear-positive pulmonary tuberculosis in a school. Alternatively, identification may be performed by geneprobe on an isolate from the patient.

DNA fingerprinting is useful in detecting whether cases might be linked, i.e. due to new infection acquired from others rather than reactivation from existing endogenous infection.

Diagnosis of tuberculosis in people with HIV

Tuberculosis can occur early in the course of HIV infection and may therefore be diagnosed before the patient is known to be HIV-positive. The possibility of HIV infection in people with tuberculosis should therefore be considered, and testing for the virus should be undertaken after appropriate counselling in those with risk factors for HIV.

Early in the course of HIV disease, before serious immunodeficiency occurs, tuberculosis usually presents with upper zone changes on chest radiography, with or without cavitation, and the tuberculin test is usually positive, and acid-fast bacilli may also be seen on microscopy.

As the immunodeficiency state worsens, the presentation of tuberculosis can become increasingly non-specific and atypical. Acid-fast bacilli are often not seen on sputum microscopy, and mycobacterial culture is often negative. Chest radiographs may be unusual, with lower zone changes and diffuse or miliary shadowing; cavitation is seen less often.

Extrapulmonary manifestations, particularly lymph node disease but also disease affecting the gastrointestinal system and central nervous system, are much more common, and the tuberculin test reaction is often negative (Heaf grade 0 or 1).

Patients may appear relatively well for the degree of abnormality shown on radiography, but if the shadowing is not felt to be associated with non-mycobacterial infections or Kaposi's sarcoma, then antituberculous treatment may have to be started empirically pending results of the cultures, and the clinical process monitored.

Treatment

Traditionally, tuberculosis was treated with bed rest, isolation and open spaces in sanatoria. Although this treatment may have had some effect in non-cavitating cases, it was less effective in more advanced disease.

Tuberculosis had started to decline in the UK before the advent of chemotherapy, probably due to improved nutrition and social conditions in the population. With the advent of effective antituberculous chemotherapy, it became apparent that patients no longer needed sanatorium treatment. Results with regimens containing isoniazid together with p-aminosalicylate (PAS) or ethambutol, and sometimes streptomycin, gave excellent results. Treatment was required for 18–24 months if relapse was to be prevented. The availability of pyrazinamide and, more importantly, rifampicin made shorter courses of treatment a possibility.

Most regimens in the developed world now contain isoniazid, rifampicin and pyrazinamide, possibly with another agent such as ethambutol.

In order to eradicate the bacteria in an individual, combination antituberculous chemotherapy is always used. The choice of drug regimen is based on a number of factors, including a need to reduce the risk of resistance emerging and improve patient adherence.

In most developed countries there are firm guidelines for the treatment of tuberculosis and contacts of cases.

Bacterial characteristics

There are four environments in which tubercle bacilli live. The activities of antituberculous agents in these environments will influence the choice of regimen. Open pulmonary cavities have a plentiful supply of oxygen and will have large numbers of rapidly growing organisms. However, bacilli in closed lesions will be oxygen starved and therefore slow-growing or dormant. Intracellular tubercle bacilli will be slow-growing due to the low intracellular pH and lack of oxygen. Some bacilli may also grow intermittently as their environment changes around them.

The antituberculous agents differ in their ability to kill these different populations of bacilli. Isoniazid is effective against intracellular organisms, and rifampicin most effective against intermittently dividing bacilli. Dormant bacilli are usually found in closed lesions hidden from the effects of both the immune system and the action of drugs. These bacilli are usually eradicated from the body by encapsulation (closing off of pathological lesions within the body and fibrosis over time).

Treatment of tuberculosis

Treatment guidelines in the UK were updated by the Joint Tuberculosis Committee of the British Thoracic Society in 1998. The guidelines are summarized in Table 38.4, and the evidence-based gradings are set out in Table 38.5.

Treatment of pulmonary tuberculosis

In the UK, the Joint Tuberculosis Committee recommends a 6 month regimen consisting of rifampicin, isoniazid, pyrazinamide and ethambutol for the initial 2 months followed by a further 4 months of rifampicin and isoniazid. The fourth drug (ethambutol) may be omitted in patients with a low risk of resistance to isoniazid. Low risk patients include previously untreated white patients known to be HIV-negative, or thought likely to be HIV-negative on risk assessment, and who are not contacts of a patient with known drug resistant organisms.

Individuals who are known or suspected to be HIV positive, or from other ethnic groups, or who have had previous treatment, or are recent arrivals, such as immigrants or refugees whatever their ethnic group, have a significantly higher risk of resistance to isoniazid and other drugs and should be commenced on the four drug combination unless there are strong contraindications to the use of any one of these drugs.

If pyrazinamide is not prescribed or cannot be tolerated, then the duration of treatment in adults and children should be extended to 9 months and ethambutol given for the initial 2 months.

The doses of all drugs which should be given in a single daily dose are shown in Table 38.4. Although streptomycin dosages are shown in the table, trials have shown no loss of efficacy if it is omitted in patients with fully sensitive organisms. It is also rarely used due to its toxicity and the inconvenience of having to administer it by injection.

Table 38.4 Dosages of first-line antitubercular agents[a] (British Thoracic Society 1998)

Drug	Forms available	Dosage					Reduce dose in	
		Adults daily	Adults intermittent (doses per week)	Children daily	Children intermittent (doses per week)		Renal failure	Liver failure
Rifampicin failure	Capsules 150 mg, 300 mg[b] Liquid 100 mg in 5 ml Injection for infusion 300 mg	450 mg (< 50 kg) 600 mg (> 50 kg)	600–900 mg (3)	10 mg/kg	15 mg/kg (3)		No	Only in severe liver
Isoniazid	Tablets 100 mg[b] Injection 100 mg Mixture[c]	300 mg	15 mg/kg (3)	5 mg/kg	15 mg/kg (3)		Only in severe renal failure	In patients with acute or chronic liver disease
Ethambutol[f]	Tablets 100 mg 400 mg[b] Mixture[c]	15 mg/kg[d]		As adult dose	30 mg/kg (3) 45 mg/kg (2)		Yes	No
Pyrazinamide	Tablets 500 mg	1.5 g (< 50 kg) 2.0 g (≥ 50 kg)	2.0 g[d] < 50 kg (3) 2.5 g[a] ≥ 50 kg (3) 3.0 g (< 50 kg) (2) 3.5 g (≥ 50 kg) (2)	35 mg/kg	50 mg/kg (3) 75 mg/kg (2)		Yes	No
Streptomycin	Injection 1 g	750 mg (< 50 kg) 1 g (> 50 kg)	750 mg–1 g[e]	15–20 mg/kg			Yes	No

[a] Some of the doses quoted are not licensed but have been recommended by the British Thoracic Society (see References).
[b] Also available as combined oral-preparations (see *British National Formulary*).
[c] Mixture may be prepared extemporaneously.
[d] Doses refer to patients over 50 kg. Reduce by 500 mg for patients weighing less than 50 kg.
[e] Drug levels should be monitored to prevent toxicity.
[f] Accurate calculation is required to reduce the risk of toxicity.

Table 38.5 Grading of recommendations (British Thoracic Society 1998)

Grade	Recommendations
A	Requires at least one randomized controlled trial as part of the body of literature of overall good quality and consistency addressing the specific recommendation
B	Requires availability of well-conducted clinical studies but no randomized clinical trials on the topic of recommendation
C	Requires evidence from expert committee reports or opinions and/or clinical experience of respected authorities, but indicates absence of directly applicable studies of good quality

These regimens are too expensive for many poorer countries where tuberculosis is of high prevalence and money for public health services is short. Many regimens are used but the duration of treatment is usually increased to 12–18 months if rifampicin is not used. In spite of its unpleasant toxic effects, PAS is still used in a number of countries as it is cheap. Using unpleasant, less-effective regimens leads to non-adherence, which leads to recurrence of disease, possibly with resistant organisms, making treatment that much more difficult. The World Health Organization recommended treatment strategy is to use 'directly observed treatment, short course' (DOTS). In this approach, health workers must watch their patients swallow each dose of drugs. This supervision must continue every day for the first 2 months and, ideally, for all 6 months of treatment.

Intermittent regimens

For short-course regimens to be effective, patient adherence to the treatment regimen is essential. If this is found to be a problem, or is thought likely to be so, treatment may be given intermittently, two or three times weekly. In this way treatment can be fully supervised, ensuring that adherence is complete. This may be useful for certain groups in whom adherence is likely to be a problem, for example homeless people and those with chronic alcohol problems. In the developing world, intermittent regimens may also be of use in an attempt to overcome non-adherence. Strong consideration should be given to the use of an intermittent directly supervised regimen if there are serious doubts about adherence.

A number of trials of intermittent regimens have shown that a short course of therapy is as effective when given intermittently as when given daily. Regimens may be fully or partially intermittent. In the latter, four drugs (isoniazid, rifampicin, pyrazinamide and either

ethambutol or streptomycin) are given daily for 2 months followed by rifampicin and isoniazid two or three times weekly for the subsequent 4 months. For most drugs the doses are increased when given intermittently; these are shown in Table 38.4.

Treatment of non-pulmonary tuberculosis

There have been relatively few comparative trials of treatments for non-respiratory disease, but evidence suggests that regimens used for respiratory tuberculosis (6 months) are effective in non-respiratory disease. However, the duration of treatment may need to be extended for certain sites.

Tuberculous meningitis

Tuberculous meningitis has been treated effectively with rifampicin and isoniazid for 12 months together with pyrazinamide and a fourth drug for the first 2 months. This could be streptomycin or ethambutol but both only reach cerebrospinal fluid through inflamed meninges. Care must be exercised when ethambutol is used in unconscious patients as visual acuity cannot be assessed. Tuberculous meningitis is a serious disease and treatment must be started promptly. The factor that most affects prognosis is the stage at which the disease is diagnosed and treatment started. In view of this it is often justified to start a therapeutic trial of antituberculous drugs in the absence of a definite diagnosis. Corticosteroids are recommended in more severe disease (stage II or III).

Tuberculosis of peripheral lymph nodes

More recent trials have shown that 6 months of treatment are just as effective as 9 months, and the 6 month regimen is therefore recommended.

Bone and joint tuberculosis

Bone and joint tuberculosis is treated effectively with standard agents such as isoniazid and rifampicin for 6 months. The spine is the most common site for bone tuberculosis and occasionally surgery may also be needed to either relieve spinal cord compression or correct spinal deformities that may have occurred.

Disseminated tuberculosis

Generalized (disseminated or miliary) tuberculosis must be treated promptly as there is still appreciable mortality from delayed diagnosis and treatment. Standard regimens containing both isoniazid and rifampicin are used. If the patient is severely ill or hypoxaemic, then corticosteroids may also be used (see below).

Treatment of tuberculosis in special circumstances

Tuberculosis in children

The dose of drugs used in children are shown in Table 38.4. Doses are generally estimated to facilitate prescription of easily given volumes of syrup, or tablets of appropriate strength. Ethambutol should not routinely be used in young children who would be unable to report visual toxicity if it occurred. However, it may have to be used if toxicity or resistance to other agents occurs.

Pregnancy

Pregnant women should be given standard therapy, although streptomycin should not be used as it may be ototoxic to the fetus. Although the other first-line drugs have not been shown to be teratogenic, they are either contraindicated or must only be used with caution. It is considered safe for mothers to breastfeed while taking antituberculous agents.

Patients should be warned of the reduced effectiveness of oral or injectable contraceptives in regimens containing rifampicin.

Renal disease

Patients with renal disease may be given isoniazid, rifampicin and pyrazinamide in standard doses as these drugs are eliminated by predominantly non-renal routes. Ethambutol undergoes extensive renal elimination and therefore dose reduction is needed. Some authors have suggested monitoring serum concentrations; however, in many centres this service is not readily available. Streptomycin must be used with considerable caution if toxicity is to be prevented, and is best avoided in renal failure. Rifampicin may be given in standard doses to patients on dialysis. The doses of the other agents need to be modified. A number of different regimens have been suggested.

Liver disease

In patients who present with liver failure or in alcoholics, monitoring of liver enzymes is recommended as rifampicin, isoniazid and pyrazinamide are all known to be potentially hepatotoxic. However, increases in transaminases at the start of antitubercular treatment occur frequently. These are usually transient and not a reason for stopping treatment unless frank jaundice or hepatitis develop, in which case all drugs should be stopped. It is usually possible to restart treatment when values have returned to pretreatment levels.

Immunocompromised patients

Patients who are immunocompromised, including those with HIV infection, should be treated with normal first-line agents unless multidrug-resistant tuberculosis is suspected. Theoretically these patients have a greater risk of relapse and may need to be treated for longer than the normal 6 months. On current evidence, at the completion of treatment life-long chemoprophylaxis with isoniazid should be instituted.

Steroids

Corticosteroids have long been used in the treatment of tuberculosis, chiefly for their anti-inflammatory properties. They may be of benefit, and a dose of around 60–80 mg of prednisolone has been used. Because of enzyme induction, the dose of corticosteroids taken for other conditions should be adjusted if rifampicin is used. Steroids probably find their greatest use for pericarditis or pleural disease and endobronchial disease in children. They are also used in genitourinary tuberculosis where they help reduce the symptoms of cystitis and obstruction. In tuberculous meningitis, corticosteroids are said to improve survival and reduce sequelae.

Drug resistance

Drug-resistant tuberculosis is a considerable problem worldwide, but is not often seen in the UK. Isoniazid is the most usual agent to which resistance is seen. At least three agents to which the organisms are sensitive should be given. The UK guidelines recommend a four-drug regimen. If multiple resistance is encountered, specialist advice on treatment is usually required and treatment is based on the sensitivities of the infecting organisms. If rifampicin is not included in the regimen, then the duration of treatment will have to be increased to 12–18 months.

It is rarely necessary to resort to reserve drugs, some of which are becoming difficult to obtain in the UK. The doses and side-effects of these are shown in Table 38.6.

The fluoroquinolones, especially ciprofloxacin and ofloxacin, have been used in patients with drug resistance, as has rifabutin (ansamycin).

Monitoring treatment

In pulmonary tuberculosis, sputum examination and culture are the most sensitive markers of the success of treatment. Patients taking regimens containing rifampicin and isoniazid should be non-infective within 2 weeks. If a patient does not become culture-negative, it may be due to either drug resistance or non-adherence, the latter being most likely. Chest radiographs provide only limited information as to the progress of treatment.

Table 38.6   Reserve drugs: dosages and side-effects (British Thoracic Society 1998)

Drug (once daily)	Children	Adults	Main side-effects
Streptomycin	15 mg/kg	15 mg/kg (max dose 1 g daily)	Tinnitus, ataxia, vertigo, renal impairment
Amikacin	15 mg/kg	15 mg/kg	As for streptomycin
Capreomycin		15 mg/kg	As for streptomycin
Kanamycin		15 mg/kg	As for streptomycin
Ethionamide or protianomide	15–20 mg/kg	<50 kg, 375 mg twice a day ≥50 kg, 500 mg twice a day	Gastrointestinal, hepatitis; avoid in pregnancy
Cycloserine		250–500 mg twice a day	Depression, fits
Ofloxacin		400 mg twice a day	Abdominal distress, headache, tremulousness
Ciprofloxacin		750 mg twice a day	As ofloxacin plus drug interactions
Azithromycin		500 mg	Gastrointestinal upset
Clarithromycin		500 mg twice a day	As for azithromycin
Rifabutin		300–450 mg	As for rifampicin; uveitis can occur with drug interactions e.g. macrolides. Often cross-resistance with rifampicin
Thiacetazone	4 mg/kg	150 mg	Gastrointestinal, vertigo, conjunctivitis, rash. Avoid if HIV positive (Stevens–Johnson syndrome)
Clofazimine		300 mg	Headache, diarrhoea, red skin discolouration
PAS sodium	300 mg/kg	10 g every morning or 5 g twice a day	Gastrointestinal, hepatitis, rash, fever

PAS, p-aminosalicylate.

Good adherence is essential if treatment is to be successful, and checking adherence is not easy, especially when a patient is uncooperative. Rifampicin will colour the urine red within about 4 hours of a dose and this has been used to monitor adherence.

Drugs used and toxicities

In the UK, the first-line drugs for the treatment of tuberculosis are rifampicin, isoniazid, pyrazinamide, ethambutol and streptomycin. Other agents such as capreomycin, PAS and cycloserine are reserved for use when first-line agents fail, usually due to resistance. Ethionamide and protionamide are no longer available in the UK, but it is possible to import the latter.

The major adverse reactions of the first-line drugs are shown in Table 38.7.

With the exception of streptomycin, the first-line agents are usually administered orally. For patients who cannot take tablets or capsules, there is a liquid preparation of rifampicin. There are no commercial sources of liquid isoniazid, ethambutol or pyrazinamide in the UK although there is a BPC formulation for isoniazid elixir. Extemporaneous formulations for all three drugs have been used. The manufacturers or local medicine information centres are probably the best sources of information about these individual formulations. Rifampicin may also be given intravenously, and isoniazid by the intravenous and intramuscular routes in patients who are severely ill and cannot take oral medication. Although not commercially available, ethambutol injection has been used and may be available on request from the manufacturer.

Rifampicin, isoniazid and pyrazinamide are all potentially hepatotoxic. Transient increases in transaminases and bilirubin commonly occur at the start of treatment. However, there is no need to monitor liver function routinely in patients with normal liver function

Table 38.7 Major adverse reactions of first-line antituberculous drugs

Drug	Common reaction	Uncommon reaction
Isoniazid		Hepatitis, cutaneous hypersensitivity, peripheral neuropathy
Rifampicin		Hepatitis, cutaneous reactions, gastrointestinal reactions, thrombocytopaenic purpura*, febrile reactions, 'Flu-syndrome'
Pyrazinamide	Anorexia, nausea, flushing	Hepatitis, vomiting, arthralgia, hyperuricaemia, cutaneous hypersensitivity
Ethambutol		Retrobulbar neuritis, arthralgia

at the start of treatment. If frank jaundice or hepatitis occur, all drugs should be stopped and liver function allowed to return to normal, at which time treatment should be recommenced one drug at a time. Clinical hepatitis is rare although patients may complain of vague symptoms such as abdominal pain and malaise which may indicate impending hepatitis.

Isoniazid may also cause a dose-dependent peripheral neuropathy, probably due to depletion of vitamin B_6. This reaction is rare in recommended doses but certain patient groups, e.g. the poorly nourished, alcoholics, diabetics, uraemic patients and pregnant women, are at greater risk and should receive pyridoxine supplementation at a dose of 10–20 mg per day.

Hypersensitivity reactions or rashes may occur with any of the drugs although the most important is that due to rifampicin, which, although rare, can be quite severe. It is more prevalent during intermittent treatment and presents as a flu-like syndrome, sometimes with abdominal pain and respiratory symptoms. This usually resolves on reverting to a daily dosage. However, if more serious effects such as renal impairment or haematological abnormalities occur, the drug should be stopped and never restarted. Rashes can occur with isoniazid, pyrazinamide and streptomycin.

Ocular toxicity is by far the most important side-effect of ethambutol. It occurs in fewer than 2% of patients at the usual dosage of 15 mg/kg but is more common in the elderly and people with renal impairment. Patients may complain of changes in colour vision or visual field which may appear suddenly. The effect is usually reversible on discontinuation but permanent damage may occur if the drug is continued. It is important that visual acuity is checked before treatment. It has been recommended that regular visual checks should be performed. However, as the majority of patients only receive the drug for 8 weeks, many clinicians do not feel that this is necessary for adults, preferring to counsel patients to report any changes in visual acuity. This precludes its use in those who are unable to report such changes such as young children and the severely ill.

Disease control and prevention

Four priorities for tuberculosis control and prevention have been identified for the UK:

1. Cases of tuberculosis must be identified and treated promptly. This includes awareness of tuberculosis as a possible diagnosis in those with medical or other risk factors, who have a chronic cough, or lower respiratory tract infection not responding to antibiotic treatment. Prompt treatment ensures that patients with infectious tuberculosis become non-infectious, as soon as possible, usually within 2 weeks of starting treatment.
2. Those at increased risk of infection with *M. tuberculosis* should be investigated without delay. This includes:
   - close contacts of known cases
   - recent immigrants from high prevalence countries.
3. The possibility of HIV infection should be considered in all cases of tuberculosis.
4. All cases of tuberculosis should be notified. This ensures that examination of contacts is carried out, and local and national surveillance of tuberculosis is maintained.

Chemoprophylaxis

Chemoprophylaxis is recommended routinely for the following, who may have recently acquired infection or may be at risk of infection:

- contacts under 16 years of age with Heaf grade 2–4 or equivalent and no history of BCG, and those with grade 3 or 4 with prior BCG vaccination
- contacts in whom recent conversion to tuberculin positivity has been noted
- children under 2 years of age who are close contacts of smear-positive cases and who have not had BCG vaccination; they should receive chemoprophylaxis irrespective of their tuberculin status, followed by

BCG vaccination, where appropriate, at the completion of chemoprophylaxis
- HIV infected close contacts of a patient with smear-positive pulmonary disease.

Prophylaxis is usually with isoniazid alone for 6 months or rifampicin and isoniazid for 3 months. Both regimens are equally effective.

BCG vaccine

BCG vaccine contains a live, attenuated strain derived from *M. bovis*.

BCG vaccine does not protect against infection. Instead it prevents the more serious forms of disease such as miliary tuberculosis and tuberculous meningitis.

Patient care

It is possible to cure virtually all patients with tuberculous infection or disease provided that an adequate regimen is prescribed and the patient complies with treatment. By far the largest cause of treatment failure is non-adherence by the patient. Non-adherence has serious consequences: treatment may fail and disease may relapse, in some cases with resistant organisms. If a non-adherent patient remains infectious they will also be a public health hazard.

Factors affecting adherence

A number of studies have shown that adherence falls as the number of tablets to be taken per day increases, and falls still further if doses have to be taken frequently through the day. Ideally, the least number of tablets should be given.

Patients may fail to adhere because they feel better and do not appreciate the need to continue with their medication. Lack of clarity of instructions, written, verbal or other, may compromise adherence, particularly if the patient is confused by conflicting advice by different health care professionals. Finally, adverse effects, or symptoms perceived to be adverse effects, may reduce adherence.

Improving patient adherence

Antituberculous therapy should be prescribed once a day using as few tablets as possible. Single daily dosing enables patients to fit their medication into their daily routine. Rifampicin and isoniazid are both well absorbed when taken on an empty stomach. However, absorption is reduced and delayed when taken with or after food. It is therefore recommended that both are taken 1 hour before food to achieve rapid high blood levels. It is usually recommended that patients take their antituberculous medication before breakfast. Cueing tablet taking to a regular activity such as brushing the teeth may improve adherence in some patients.

The number of tablets to be taken each day may be reduced by using combination preparations. These also have the advantage of reducing the possibility of monotherapy and consequent resistance. There are a number of combination preparations available. Some of the preparations, for example Rifater, contain ratios of drugs that differ slightly from the dosages recommended by the British Thoracic Society. This difference in dosage is probably not clinically significant and is far preferable to potential undertreatment due to non-adherence. Mynah is a preparation available in a number of different ratios to facilitate administration of the correct dose.

Combination preparations may not be suitable for use in children as the required dose regimens differ from those of adults.

Patient education

Written instruction and/or patient information leaflets may be offered to support verbal counselling if there is any doubt as to the patient's understanding. It should be emphasized that the disease will be cured but this will take some months and the tablets will need to be taken as prescribed even if the patient feels better. Some patients will adhere initially while they are unwell, but will fail to adhere later as they begin to feel better.

The occurrence of some adverse effects may require discontinuation of a drug, but others are harmless. The patient should be told which side-effects to expect and which require referral to a member of the health care team. Again written instructions may be helpful.

A number of patients from abroad with tuberculosis have a poor command of English. It may still be possible to give written instructions on dosage as some pharmaceutical companies are able to provide pictorial material and dosage sheets in a number of languages.

Counselling points

Patients taking rifampicin should be told that the drug will cause a harmless discoloration of their urine and other body fluids, for example sweat and tears. The staining of tears is important if the patient uses soft contact lenses as these may be permanently stained. Gas-permeable and hard lenses are unaffected. Women using the oral contraceptive pill should be advised to use other non-hormonal methods of contraception for the duration of treatment with rifampicin and for 8 weeks afterwards.

Although ocular side-effects are rare when ethambutol is taken in normal dosages, patients should be warned of this potentially serious side-effect. They should be advised to stop the drug and report to their doctor if they notice any changes in vision, such as a reduction in visual acuity or changes in colour vision. This is especially important because visual changes are usually reversible on discontinuation of the drug but may be permanent if the drug is not stopped.

CASE STUDIES

Case 38.1

A man in his mid-30s is admitted to hospital with a cough productive of sputum and a fever. A chest X-ray ray indicates bilateral pneumonia with apical involvement. A sputum smear reveals the presence of acid, alcohol fast bacilli. The patient is transferred to a side room and commenced on antituberculous therapy.

Soon after admission, a history of drug misuse comes to light. The man 'absconds' from hospital on two occasions. He sometimes leaves his room, and enters the general medical ward, coming into contact with other patients.

Questions

1. What form of tuberculosis does this patient have?
2. Should he be kept in hospital for treatment, and should he be compelled to stay in hospital?
3. Does he need any other health care?

Answers

1. This man has sputum smear-positive pulmonary tuberculosis, the infectious form of the disease.
2. As he wanders onto the general ward, and in view of his habit of absconding from hospital, he poses a risk to others, particularly susceptible individuals. Therefore, he should preferably be kept in hospital for at least 2–3 weeks to help ensure adherence with treatment and so that he becomes non-infectious.

   If encouragement to comply with treatment and to avoid the main ward or leaving hospital fails, legal measures could be considered. These are set out in the Public Health (Control of Diseases) Act 1984 for England and Wales. Transfer to a specialist infectious diseases hospital or unit may be necessary.
3. Referral to a psychiatrist specializing in substance misuse could help. Where a patient presenting with tuberculosis has other health problems, it is important that all their health needs are addressed, as this may help encourage adherence with treatment.

Case 38.2

A man in his 40s is diagnosed as having tuberculosis of a lymph node in the neck, and is referred to a chest physician in the local hospital for treatment. The man fails to attend follow-up appointments at the hospital, but continues to obtain prescriptions for 4 months of quadruple therapy.

Questions

1. Should investigations other than histological examination be done to help confirm the diagnosis?
2. Should the patient have had 4 months of quadruple therapy?
3. What action should be taken if there is a suspicion the patient is not receiving the correct treatment regimen?

Answers

1. A sample of the lymph node should be sent for microbiological investigations. This will confirm the diagnosis, and drug sensitivities will be assessed.
2. The patient should only have had 2 months of quadruple therapy. If he has had ethambutol, which can affect visual acuity for longer, he should be referred for an eye test. He should therefore be advised to see his GP as soon as possible.
3. If there is a suspicion that a patient is taking drugs for longer than the recommended period it is wise to contact the prescribing doctor to inform him or her of the facts, and to ask whether that is part of the intended treatment regimen.

Case 38.3

A woman in her mid 20s is diagnosed as having sputum smear-negative pulmonary tuberculosis. Although she initially takes her antituberculous drugs, she does not attend follow-up clinics, and her condition deteriorates. Her GP collects a sputum sample from her and persuades her to attend the chest clinic. The sputum smear is now positive, and it is found she has been continuing in her job.

Questions

1. What type of treatment regimen should be offered to this patient?
2. Who should be involved in planning this treatment regimen, and what arrangements should be put in place to ensure this works?
3. Should the patient's work contacts be screened?

Answers

1. Patients like this should receive supervised treatment three times a week in a convenient setting such as at home.
2. There needs to be close collaboration between the physician responsible for treatment, the patient's general practitioner, the public health team, and the health care professionals (often district nurses or health visitors in the UK) who will supervise treatment. The patient needs to be involved in discussions about these arrangements, as treatment will not be successful without the patient's cooperation.

   The physician will need to adjust the treatment dosage in line with the three times a week regimen, inform the GP and ensure the correct prescriptions are issued. Those supervising treatment need a clear explanation of what is expected of them, including details of the drugs and dose, and duration of treatment. They also need to know what to do if the patient does not adhere.

3. The question of whether work contacts should be screened must be dealt with on an individual case basis. This usually involves the public health team informing the patient of the need to inquire into work contacts, and getting the patient's agreement to approach a supervisor or manager in the workplace. A telephone conversation will provide initial information on the working environment and should be followed up by a visit if initial inquiries indicate a possible need to screen workplace contacts.

Case 38.4

A 65-year-old man with a chest infection resulting in cough with sputum production does not improve after two courses of antibiotics prescribed empirically.

Questions

1. What investigations should be done?
2. In this patient, all three sputum specimens came back as smear (AFB) positive. Does this mean the patient has tuberculosis?
3. Should the patient be notified to the local public health team (communicable disease control)?

Answers

1. Three early morning sputum specimens should be collected and sent to the microbiology laboratory for microscopic examination for acid fast bacilli (AFB), culture for *M. tuberculosis* and *M. bovis*. In this case, as the patient has failed to respond to antibiotic treatment, a diagnosis of tuberculosis should be considered.
2. Not necessarily. He may have an atypical mycobacterial infection. He should be sent to the chest clinic for further clinical assessment of symptoms and a chest X-ray. Some atypical mycobacterial infections cause pulmonary disease resembling tuberculosis. The chest physician will make a judgement on the most likely clinical diagnosis.
3. Only if the clinician thinks the most likely diagnosis is tuberculosis. If unsure, but the patient is commenced on antituberculous therapy, he should be notified as having tuberculosis. If the culture subsequently indicates infection with atypical mycobacteria, the case can be denotified.

Acknowledgement

Permission to use material prepared for the first edition by P. J. Barker is gratefully acknowledged, as is the help from consultant physician colleagues in Gwent for the case studies.

REFERENCES

British Thoracic Society 2000 Control and prevention of tuberculosis in the United Kingdom: Code of Practice 2000. Thorax 55: 887–901

Chin J 2000 Control of communicable diseases manual. American Public Health Association, Washington DC

Christie A B 1987 Tuberculosis: non-tuberculosis mycobacteriosis. In: Infectious disease. Churchill Livingstone, Edingburgh, ch. 17.

Davies P D O 1999 Clinical tuberculosis. Chapman and Hall, London

Haslett C et al (eds) 1999 Davidson's Principles and Practice of Medicine. Churchill Livingstone, Edinburgh

Joint Tuberculosis Committee of the British Thoracic Society 1998 Chemotherapy and management of tuberculosis in the United Kingdom: recommendations 1998. Thorax 53: 536–548

Rose A M C et al 2001 Tuberculosis at the end of the 20th century in England and Wales: results of a national survey in 1998. Thorax 56: 173–179

WHO 2001 Global tuberculosis control. World Health Organization, Geneva http://www.who.int

FURTHER READING

Interdepartmental Working Group on Tuberculosis 1998 The prevention and control of tuberculosis in the United Kingdom. Department of Health Scottish Office, Welsh Office, London (www.doh.gov.uk/Ebguide.htm)

Medical Research Council Cardiothoracic Epidemiology Group 1992 National survey of tuberculosis notifications in England and Wales in 1988. Thorax 47: 770–775

Public Health Laboratory Service Communicable Disease Surveillance centre http://www.phls.co.uk/facts/index

Valway S, Watson J, Bisgard C et al 1998 Tuberculosis and air travel: guidelines for prevention and control. World Health Organization, Geneva.

Veen J, Raviglione M, Rieder H L et al 1998 Standardised tuberculosis treatment outcome monitoring in Europe. Recommendations of a Working Group of the World Health Organization (WHO) and the European Region of the International Union Against Tuberculosis and Lung Disease (IUATLD) for uniform reporting of cohort analysis of treatment outcome in tuberculosis patients. European Respiratory Journal 12: 505–510.

HIV infection 39

H. Leake Date   M. Fisher

KEY POINTS

- Untreated infection with the human immunodeficiency virus (HIV) leads to a progressive deterioration in the cellular immune response. After initial seroconversion, the infected individual may appear asymptomatic for a number of years, before developing symptomatic disease and/or acquired immune deficiency syndrome (AIDS).
- Complications arising from HIV infection can manifest in a variety of ways, usually as opportunistic infections or malignancies that are uncommon in the immunocompetent population.
- The aim of the treatment of HIV infection is to reconstitute, or prevent further deterioration of, the immune system, with the intention of improving the quality and quantity of life of the infected individual. Management of HIV-related complications primarily involves the treatment and prophylaxis of opportunistic diseases.
- Antiretroviral agents are classified by their mechanism of actions as: nucleoside analogue reverse transcriptase inhibitors (NARTIs), nucleotide analogue reverse transcriptase inhibitors, non-nucleoside reverse transcriptase inhibitors (NNRTIs), protease inhibitors (PIs) and fusion inhibitors. Drugs are given in combination (usually at least three agents) to improve efficacy and reduce the development of viral resistance.
- Treatment regimens are frequently complex and many of the drugs have significant toxicities and interactions with other drugs and with food. A high level of adherence to therapy is vital to ensure efficacy and to prevent the emergence of resistant virus. The pharmacist has a key role to play as part of the multidisciplinary team in supporting the patient in adhering to treatment.

The acquired immune deficiency syndrome (AIDS) is the state of profound immunosuppression produced by chronic infection with the human immunodeficiency virus (HIV).

Epidemiology

In June 1981, five cases of *Pneumocystis carinii* pneumonia (PCP) were described in homosexual men in the USA. Reports of other unusual conditions, such as Kaposi's sarcoma (KS), followed shortly. In each of these patients there was found to be a marked impairment of cellular immune response, and so the term 'acquired immune deficiency syndrome' or 'AIDS' was coined. In 1984 a new human retrovirus, subsequently named human immunodeficiency virus (HIV), was isolated and identified as the cause of AIDS.

Although initially described in homosexual men, it soon became apparent that other population groups were affected, including intravenous drug users and haemophiliacs. During the first decade the epidemic grew, and the importance of transmission via heterosexual intercourse and from mother to child (vertical transmission) was increasingly recognized. By 1996 the incidence of new infections in developed nations appeared to have stabilized, although more recent trends suggest that safer sexual practices may have been relaxed as a result of the perceived benefits of newer anti-HIV therapies. In the UK it is noteworthy that 1999 and 2000 were the first years in which, nationally, new diagnoses of HIV attributed to heterosexual transmission outnumbered those attributed to sex between men. The impact of recent treatment advances on the mortality from AIDS-related illnesses has been staggering, although current data indicate that rates may now have plateaued, possibly due to the failure to diagnose HIV infection among the asymptomatic population.

In the developing world (particularly Sub-Saharan Africa, South-East Asia and South America) numbers continue to increase alarmingly and prevalence rates of up to 40–50% have been reported in certain communities in Botswana and South Africa. In such resource-poor nations where the advances in medical management which will be outlined below are currently not generally accessible, the effects of HIV on the population and its economy are enormous.

The virus has been isolated from a number of body fluids, including blood, semen, vaginal secretions, saliva, breast milk, tears, urine, peritoneal fluid and cerebrospinal fluid (CSF). However, not all of these appear to be important in the spread of infection, and the predominant routes of transmission remain: sexual intercourse (anal or vaginal); sharing of unsterilized needles or syringes; blood or blood products in areas where supplies are not screened or treated; and vertical transmission in utero, during labour or through breastfeeding.

In the absence of a definitive evidence-base and given the rapidly developing nature of this field of medicine, such guidelines should be integrated wherever possible into routine patient care. As newer diagnostic techniques (such as HIV resistance assays and therapeutic drug monitoring) become routinely used, it is likely that the monitoring of therapy and the decision-making processes of when and what to switch will become increasingly complex.

Most studies evaluating triple combinations of antiretrovirals have been designed with so-called 'surrogate marker' end points, measuring the effect on laboratory parameters such as CD4 count and HIV viral load. These trials are generally smaller and shorter in duration than clinical end point studies that are powered to measure the impact on survival and disease progression. The first large clinical end point trial that demonstrated the superiority of a triple combination over dual therapy was ACTG 320 (Hammer et al 1997). Following the results of this trial, the standard of care has been, where treatment is indicated, to use a combination of at least three agents. Subsequently, the reduction in morbidity and mortality associated with HAART use has been demonstrated in routine clinical practice, as well as in trials (Palella et al 1998).

Broadly speaking, the majority of individuals are currently commenced on a combination of two nucleoside analogues (NARTIs) and a non-nucleoside reverse transcriptase inhibitor (NNRTI) or two NARTIs and one or two protease inhibitors (PIs). More recently, the use of triple nucleoside analogue therapy has been adopted by some, and newer combinations (such as triple class or nucleoside-sparing regimens) are being studied. It is likely that with newer classes in development, these approaches may well change over the next few years.

The aim of initial therapy is to achieve viral load suppression in the plasma to levels below the detection limits of available assays. Such virological suppression is almost invariably accompanied by an elevation in CD4 count and clinical evidence of immune reconstitution. While sustained suppression may be possible for some, viral rebound occurs in many and is usually accompanied by the development of resistance to one or more agents in the combination. Upon confirmed virological failure, a resistance test is usually performed which will help identify which agents the virus may have adapted to and the extent to which any such resistance mutations may confer cross-resistance to other available drugs. A second-line regimen is then constructed, wherever possible utilizing a new class of drug to which the individual has not previously been exposed. Upon virological failure of subsequent regimens, the therapeutic options available become increasingly limited and the aims of such 'salvage regimens' may not always be to achieve complete virological suppression

but rather to gain immunological and clinical benefit within acceptable tolerability and toxicity limits.

Many of the antiretrovirals, particularly the PIs and NNRTIs, exhibit a wide range of interactions, especially with other drugs that are metabolized via the cytochrome P450 enzyme system. The pharmacist has a vital role to play in the selection of appropriate drugs, avoiding significant interactions (including with herbal medicines) and ensuring that the timing and frequency of doses are compatible with the patient's lifestyle. For details of common side-effects and interactions of the currently available antiretroviral agents see Table 39.1, A and B.

Table 39.1A General prescribing and monitoring information for antiretroviral agents

- The information summarized in Table 39.1B is intended to be used as a quick reference and does not replace the full prescribing details provided by the manufacturers. The reader is encouraged to contact the local HIV team for further advice or information when managing an HIV-positive patient (particularly if the patient is taking antiretrovirals).

- Interaction and side-effect data on drugs that are on trial, compassionate release or newly licensed are often limited and are frequently updated. The absence of such information in Table 39.1B and 39.2 should be interpreted with caution. Health care workers should therefore be especially vigilant to the possibility of their occurrence.

- Adverse events should be reported to the Medicines Control Agency (MCA) via the blue card scheme. With greater exposure and longer-term use it is likely that more adverse events will be recognized. Some of these may be 'class-effects' associated with particular groups of antiretrovirals and should therefore be suspected/monitored for, even in new agents within a class. Examples include: lipodystrophy syndrome and metabolic abnormalities (e.g. dyslipidaemias and diabetes mellitus), particularly with PIs; mitochondrial myopathy/nucleoside wasting with nucleoside RTIs; rash with NNRTIs.

- Many of the newer antiretroviral agents have not been studied extensively in individuals with renal or hepatic insufficiency. Data are also limited in patients with other significant co-morbidity (e.g. diabetes, cardiac disease). Caution should therefore be exercised when prescribing for such patients and all their medical conditions should be closely monitored.

- There are limited data on the safety of many of these drugs when taken during pregnancy, or on long-term effects on babies/children. Efavirenz has been shown to be teratogenic in animal studies, but comparable data are not available for the other antiretrovirals. Caution should therefore be exercised with all agents due to the absence of data on most of them. Treatment of women who are planning conception (or who are pregnant) must be discussed with the relevant experts.

Table 39.1B Antiretroviral agents

Drug names and manufacturer	Dose and formulation	Administration	Major/common side-effects	Significant drug interactions and important pharmacokinetic information
Non-nucleoside reverse transcriptase inhibitors (NNRTIs)				

Delavirdine (DLV) (Rescriptor™)	400 mg three times a day or 600 mg twice a day
	
	100 mg + 200 mg tablets
		Can be taken with or without food
		
		Tablets can be dissolved in water or acidic drink (e.g. cola or orange juice)
		
		Avoid antacids (including DDI buffered tablets) within 1 h
			Rash (in about 18% of patients: more common if low CD4, usually in first 3 weeks; most can be successfully 'treated through' with antihistamines etc., severe rash or Stevens–Johnson syndrome (SJS) are rare and resolve on stopping drug)
			
			Reversible liver abnormalities (especially raised ALT and AST)
				Non-linear kinetics: do NOT dose adjust without discussing with HIV pharmacist/drug company
				Metabolized by CYP450 (mostly 3A). Inibits CYP450 3A4 and 2C9 (will have similar interactions to ketoconazole); inhibitory effects will wear off a few days after cessation
				Increases levels of terfenadine, erythromycin, astemizole, cisapride, etc. (all contraindicated)
				Increases levels of sildenafil (Viagra™) – avoid or start with lowest dose of sildenafil (25 mg)
				Increases levels of midazolam – avoid or start with low dose and titrate and monitor carefully; do not use in out-patients or day case attenders
				Increases levels of protease inhibitors (PIs):
				  Consider reducing indinavir dose to 400 mg three times daily or 600 mg three times daily
				  Caution with saquinavir (monitor LFTs more frequently)
				  Discuss with HIV consultant before initiating delavirdine/PI combination
				CYP450 3A4 enzyme inducers (e.g. rifampicin, rifabutin, phenytoin, carbamazepine) contraindicated (they decrease delavirdine levels)
				Adefovir significantly reduces delavirdine levels – avoid until further information available
				CYP450 3A4 inhibitors (e.g. clarithromycin, fluoxetine, ketoconazole, indinavir, ritonavir, saquinavir) can all increase delavirdine levels but no dosage adjustment required
				Nelfinavir decreases delavirdine levels (suggested dose adjustment to 600 mg three times daily). Delavirdine increases nelfinavir levels (?dose adjustment or TDM)
				?May increase warfarin levels – monitor INR
				Chronic use of anti-ulcer agents (H_2 antagonists or proton pump inhibitors) may reduce delavirdine levels and is not recommended. Antacids should not be taken within 1 h of delavirdine

Efavirenz (EFV) (Sustiva™)	600 mg once daily (usually at night) Increased to 800 mg once daily after 2 weeks with nevirapine ?Increase to 800 mg once daily with rifampicin 200 mg capsules 600 mg tablet oral solution (30 mg/ml)	Can be taken with or without food. Absorption is increased by fatty food (avoid co-administration if side effects) Taken at night to minimize sedative effect, but can be taken in morning if preferred	CNS disturbances (from sedation/feeling 'stoned'/dizzy and impaired concentration to vivid dreams, mood swings and hallucinations). Mild–moderate severity more common; most wear off after 1 month. Warn patients re not driving if affected Rash (in about 18% of adults mostly in first 2 weeks; usually successfully 'treated through' with antihistamines etc.; severe rash or SJS are rare and resolve on stopping drug) Incidence may be higher in children ↑LFTs (esp. AST and ALT). ↑GGT ?Commoner if hep B or C co-infected Monitor cholesterol/triglycerides	Metabolized by CYP450 3A4 (induces own metabolism) Plasma half-life (steady state) c 48 h Mixed inhibitor and inducer of CYP3A4 – complex interactions (not yet fully evaluated). Induces CYP2B6. Inhibits 2C9 and 2C19 (and 2D6 at high concentrations) in vitro Caution with other drugs metabolized by these enzymes, or which induce/inhibit them; use alternatives wherever possible. Avoid clarithromycin Caution with sildenafil (Viagra™) Do TDM on potentially affected drugs where indicated (e.g. phenytoin) Do NOT co-administer with terfenadine, astemizole, cisapride, midazolam or triazolam Increase indinavir dose to 1000 mg three times daily; increase lopinavir/r dose to 4 capsules (533.3 mg) twice daily Increase efavirenz to 800 mg once a day if given with nevirapine Increase efavirenz to 800 mg once a day with rifampicin; increase rifabutin to 450 mg once a day with efavirenz (recommendations based on limited data) Methadone dose may require alteration – monitor closely Do not give with saquinavir (either formulation) as sole PI Increase amprenavir dose (or add in ritonavir 100 mg twice daily) if co-administering with efavirenz (TDM advised)

Table 39.1B (continued)

Drug names and manufacturer	Dose and formulation	Administration	Major/common side-effects	Significant drug interactions and important pharmacokinetic information
Nevirapine (NVP) (Viramune™)	200 mg once daily for 1st 2 wks then 200 mg twice a day (experimental – 400 mg once daily) 200 mg tablets + oral suspension (50 mg/5 ml)	Can be taken with or without food Can be taken at night if causes sedation	Rash (in c. 15%; mostly early on, usually treat through); TEN/SJS in c. 0.5%. Do NOT ↑dose if rash; use BI s rash management guidelines Raised LFTs/hepatitis (check every 2 wks for 1st 2 months) Nausea, headache, sedation, fatigue	Metabolized by CYP450 (3A4 > 2B6). Plasma half-life (steady state) c. 24 h CYP450 inducer (2B6 > 3A4) – decreases levels of PIs (do not give with saquinavir as sole PI); increase efavirenz dose to 800 mg once a day if given concomitantly Rifampicin decreases nevirapine levels – ?increase dose by 50%. Rifabutin-induced ↓ in nvp levels may not be significant (discuss with HIV/TB team before prescribing rifamycin with nevirapine) Caution with drugs metabolized by or inducers of CYP3A4 and 2B6 (e.g. carbamazepine). ?TDM where possible
Nucleoside reverse transcriptase inhibitors (NARTIs)				
Abacavir (ABC) (Ziagen™)	300 mg twice daily 300 mg tablets and oral solution (20 mg/ml)	Can be taken with or without food	Usually well tolerated (headache, nausea etc. reported but rare) Abacavir hypersensitivity (4% incidence): see BNF/SPC for full details. Patient must NEVER be rechallenged if abacavir withdrawn due to suspected hypersensitivity. Discuss with HIV team if reaction suspected. Counsel patient Hepatic steatosis (see BNF for more details)	No clinically significant interactions noted so far Mycophenolate mofetil may increase abacavir levels – ?utility in clinical practice
Combivir™ (CBV) (zidovudine + lamivudine)	One tablet twice daily (Tablet contains 300 mg zidovudine + 150 mg lamivudine)		See entries for individual drugs	See entries for individual drugs
Didanosine (ddI) (Videx™)	If >60 kg: 400 mg once a day If <60 kg: 250 mg once daily 25 mg and 200 mg tabs; 400 mg, 250 mg, 200 mg and 125 mg e-c capsules Suspension (unlicensed)	Tablets: Must be taken on an empty stomach (>30 min before and > 2 h after food) May be taken with clear apple juice to improve tolerability Must be chewed, crushed or dispersed before taking Enteric-coated capsule must be taken >2 h before and >2 h after food	Nausea, bloating, diarrhoea (all may be reduced with e-c formulation) Pancreatitis (caution in patients with 'high' alcohol intake or history of pancreatitis) Peripheral neuropathy Hyperuricaemia Hepatic steatosis (see BNF for more details) Dry mouth	Oral ganciclovir or valganciclovir (increased ddI levels → potential ↑ risk of pancreatitis; ↓ ganciclovir levels → risk of Tx failure) – take at least 2 h apart Take dapsone (and other drugs adsorbed by antacids) at least 2 h before or after buffered formations of ddI (see 'antacids' interaction section of BNF for more details) Take indinavir > 1 h after ddI tablets (can take with e-c caps) Caution with drugs associated with pancreatitis such as i.v. pentamidine Levels increased by tenofovir – caution with concomitant use and check current recommendations with manufacturers
Lamivudine (3TC) (Epivir™)	150 mg twice daily or 300 mg once daily 150 mg and 300 mg tablets and oral solution (10 mg/ml)	Can be taken with or without food	Generally well tolerated (GI disturbances, headache, anaemia and neutropenia have been reported but not common) Hepatic steatosis (see BNF for more details) Recurrent hepatitis can occur in chronic hepatitis B carriers on discontinuation of 3TC (has anti-HBV activity)	Increased risk of neutropenia with high-dose co-trimoxazole and ganciclovir/ valganciclovir Increases trimethoprim levels Do not use with DDC
Stavudine (d4T) (Zerit™)	If > 60 kg 40 mg twice daily or 100 mg PRC once daily If < 60 kg 30 mg twice daily or 75 mg PRC once daily 15 mg, 20 mg, 30 mg and 40 mg capsules and oral solution (1 mg/ml)	Can be taken with or without food	Peripheral neuropathy (symptoms may worsen before improvement noted following discontinuation) Pancreatitis (rare) Hepatic steatosis (see BNF for more details)	Caution with drugs associated with peripheral neuropathy such as vincristine, thalidomide or isoniazid Do not use with AZT Doxorubicin may inhibit effect of stavudine (?significance) Ribavirin may reduce efficacy of stavudine: consult specialist HIV/hepatology team before co-prescribing

Table 39.1B (continued)

Drug names and manufacturer	Dose and formulation	Administration	Major/common side-effects	Significant drug interactions and important pharmacokinetic information
Trizivir™	One tablet twice daily	(Tablet contains abacavir 300 mg, lamivudine 150 mg and zidovudine 300 mg)	See entries under individual drugs N.B. Patients who have had a hypersensitivity reaction to abacavir must NEVER be rechallenged with ABACAVIR or TRIZIVIR	See entries under individual drugs
Zalcitabine (ddC) (Hivid™)	750 micrograms (0.75 mg) three times daily (Experimental: 1125 micrograms twice daily)	Can be taken with or without food	Peripheral neuropathy Pancreatitis (rare) Mouth ulcers Hepatic steatosis (see BNF for more details)	Caution with drugs associated with peripheral neuropathy such as vincristine, thalidomide or isoniazid Do not use with 3TC
Zidovudine (AZT) (Retrovir™)	Usual dose 250 mg twice daily (300 mg twice daily in Combivir and Trizivir)	Can be taken with or without food	Nausea, vomiting, headache, fatigue and muscle pain. More common in first few weeks and usually wear off. Haematological toxicities, (e.g. neutropenia, anaemia) may develop after several months (rare at doses now used) Myopathy may be associated with long-term therapy (>12 months) Hepatic steatosis (see BNF for more details)	Myelotoxic drugs e.g. ganciclovir and high dose co-trimoxazole, may worsen neutropenia. Fluconazole and probenecid may ↑ AZT levels Take > 1 h apart from clarithromycin (can ↓ AZT absorption) Monitor phenytoin levels Do not give with D4T Possible interaction with ribavirin: consult specialist HIV/hepatology team before co-precribing
Protease inhibitors (PIs)				
Amprenavir (APV) (Agenerase™)	1200 mg twice daily 150 mg capsules Oral solution (15 mg/ml) (caution: high polyethylene glycol content)	Can be taken with or without food (may reduce GI side-effects if with/after food)	Nausea, diarrhoea, abdominal discomfort Rash Taste perversion, perioral paraesthesia ?Other PI 'class side-effects' (see BNF for more details)	Metabolized by CYP450 3A (caution when given with inducers) Inhibitor of CYP450 (caution with other drugs metabolized by this route) Do NOT co-administer with terfenadine, astemizole, cisapride, triazolam, midazolam, ergotamines or rifampicin Increase dose or add in ritonavir (various experimental dose combinations) if given with efavirenz Complex interaction with Kaletra™ – seek specialist advice
Atazanavir (ATV) (unlicensed)	400 mg once daily 200 mg capsules	Take with or just after food	Hyperbilirubinaemia (may need dose ↓ or stop if ≥ grade 3 or 4) ECG changes Does not appear to ↑ lipids but otherwise may potentially cause similar side-effects to other PIs N.B. Still relatively little experience with this agent, so be particularly vigilant for possible side-effects	Mainly metabolized by CYP450 3A (caution when given with inducers) In vitro – moderate inhibitor of CYP 3A. Also competitively inhibits CYP1A2 and CYP2C9 N.B. Still relatively little experience with this agent, so be particularly vigilant for possible drug interactions (assume similar to nelfinavir)
Indinavir (IDV) (Crixivan™)	200 mg, 333 mg and 400 mg capsules 800 mg 8 hourly 1000 mg every 8 hours if on rifabutin (and halve rifabutin dose) With ritonavir (unlicensed doses): 800 mg twice daily (with 100 or 200mg twice daily RTV) or 400mg twice daily (with 400mg twice daily RTV) Reduce dose in hepatic insufficiency	Store with desiccant Drink > 1.5 l water per day (even if taking with ritonavir) Best on an empty stomach >1 h before food or >2 h after meals May take with light, low fat (<5 g fat) snacks (diet booklet available) No food restrictions if with ritonavir At least 1 h after ddl tablets (OK to take at same time as ddl e-c capsules)	Nephrolithiasis Hyperbilirubinemia Increases in AST and ALT Rash, dry skin, pruritus, hair loss Ingrown toenails Taste perversion Haemolytic anaemia Hyperglycaemia/diabetes Lipodystrophy syndrome Dyslipidaemias	Indinavir is an inhibitor of CYP450 3A and may increase levels of other drugs metabolized by this system Do NOT co-administer with: terfenadine, astemizole, cisapride, triazolam and midazolam Indinavir is metabolized by CYP450, so inducers or inhibitors of this system may respectively reduce or increase its serum level (rifampicin is contraindicated) Ketoconazole ↑ indinavir levels. Rifabutin ↓ indinavir levels and indinavir ↑ rifabutin levels (↓ dose to 150 mg once daily) Administer indinavir and didanosine tablets at least 1 h apart

Table 39.1B (continued)

Drug names and manufacturer	Dose and formulation	Administration	Major/common side-effects	Significant drug interactions and important pharmacokinetic information
Lopinavir/r (ABT 378/r) (Kaletra™)	133.3 mg lopinavir co-formulated with 33.3 mg ritonavir 3 capsules twice daily 4 capsules twice daily with efavirenz and nevirapine	Take with or after food Do NOT contain ethanol (unlike ritonavir caps)	GI side-effects (diarrhoea, nausea etc.) Hyperlipidaemia; rash; headache ↑LFT's (esp. AST and ALT) and GGT. ?Commoner if hep B or C co-infected Contains low dose ritonavir (so potentially the same range of side-effects, though likely to be less severe than with full dose) ?Other PI 'class side-effects' e.g. metabolic/lipid/body shape changes (see BNF for more details)	Metabolized by CYP450 3A4 (caution when given with inducers) Nevirapine and efavirenz reduce lopinavir levels: ↑ dose Lopinavir is a moderate inhibitor of CYP 3A4. Ritonavir is a potent inhibitor of CYP3A4 and also affects other isoenzymes (see under ritonavir for full list of interactions). Caution with other drugs metabolized by this route Do NOT co-administer with terfenadine, astemizole, cisapride, triazolam, midazolam, ergotamines or rifampicin
Nelfinavir (NFV) (Viracept™)	250 mg and 650 mg tablets 1250 mg twice daily 750 mg three times daily ?1000 mg three times daily if with nevirapine 250 mg tablets (650 mg in development)	Take with or after food to increase bioavailability (up to 2 h after full meal, or with/just after small meal/snack)	Diarrhoea and flatulence Hyperglycaemia/diabetes Dyslipidaemias Lipodystrophy syndrome	Metabolized by CYP450 and CYP450 inhibitor – potential interactions with many other drugs. Caution with other drugs metabolized by this route and CYP450 inducers Do NOT use with: astemizole, terfenadine, cisapride, rifampicin, triazolam, vincristine, ergot derivatives, amiodarone, quinidine Halve rifabutin dose and ?↑NVF dose when co-administered May reduce efficacy of oral contraceptive pill (combined and progesterone-only)
Ritonavir (RTV) (Norvir™)	100mg capsules oral solution (80 mg/ml) 600 mg twice daily Escalate dose over c.2. weeks to ↓ side-effects (e.g. 300 mg twice a day for 4 days, 400 mg twice a day for 4 days, 500 mg twice a day for 4 days then 600 mg twice a day thereafter) Various (unlicensed) dose combinations with saquinavir, indinavir and amprenavir	Do not administer liquid formulation with disulfiram or metro-nidazole (caps OK with metronidazole; ?still caution with disulfiram if on high-dose-ritonavir) Take with or after food if possible (to reduce GI intolerance). May mix oral solution with chocolate milk within 1 h of dosing Store capsules in refrigerator (Stable at <25°C for up to 28 days) Solution stored at room temperature	Asthenia Nausea, vomiting Diarrhoea Anorexia Abdominal pain Taste perversion Circumoral and peripheral parasthesias Hyperglycaemia/diabetes Dyslplipidaemias Lipodystrophy syndrome	Ritonavir is a potent partial inhibitor of several CYP450 isoenzymes and thus interacts with many other drugs Its inhibitory effect is commonly used to pharmacokinetically enhance other ARVs (e.g. saquinavir, indinavir, amprenavir, lopinavir). Care should be taken when stopping ritonavir to ensure that this does not result in subtherapeutic levels of other drugs It can cause increases or decreases in the level of other agents; the nature and extent of the interaction is not fully known for many potentially affected drugs Potent inducers of CYP450 may ↓ ritonavir levels (and enzyme inhibitors may ↑ ritonavir serum concentrations) Do NOT co-administer with: cisapride, rifabutin, pethidine, diazepam, midazolam, amiodarone, astemizole, terfenadine, dextropropoxyphene, piroxicam, quinidine, zolpidem See BNF/SPC for full list of contraindications and caution drugs before prescribing
Saquinavir (SQV) Invirase™ (hard gel capsule) Fortovase™ (soft gel capsule)	200 mg capsules Fortovase can use as sole PI 1200 mg three times daily or 1600 mg twice a day, or 400 mg twice a day with ritonavir Invirase ONLY use with CYP450 3A inhibitor (e.g. delavirdine or ritonavir)	Take with or after food (up to 2 h after a full meal) Grapefruit juice increases plasma levels (not thought to be clinically significant with Fortovase)	Diarrhoea Nausea Abdominal discomfort/wind Raised LFTs Dyslipidaemias Lipodystrophy Hyperglycaemia/diabetes	Metabolized by CYP450 3A4; inhibits CYP450 3A so can ↑ levels of drugs metabolized by this system Do NOT use with cisapride, astemizole, terfenadine, rifampicin and rifabutin May raise levels of dapsone, clindamycin, calcium channel blockers, quinidine, ergotamine and midazolam (?clinical significance) Caution: other drugs (CYP450 3A inducers) which may ↓ saquinavir levels (e.g. phenytoin, phenobarbital, dexamethasone, carbamazepine) Nevirapine should not normally be used with saquinavir unless also on ritonavir Co-administration of clarithromycin, ketoconazole, ranitidine or cimetidine may increase levels of saquinavir

Table 39.1B (continued)

Drug names and manufacturer	Dose and formulation	Administration	Major/common side-effects	Significant drug interactions and important pharmacokinetic information
Nucleotide reverse transcriptase inhibitors (NtRTIs)				
Tenofovir disoproxil (TDF) (Viread™)	245 mg tablet once daily (equivalent to 300 mg tenofovir dosoproxil fumarate)	Take with or after food	Seems generally well tolerated Diarrhoea Nausea Vomiting Headache N.B. Still relatively little experience with this agent, so be particularly vigilant for possible side-effects	Mostly eliminated unchanged in the urine Minor inducer of CYP450 IA (not usually significantly implicated in drug interactions) Possible interactions with nephrotoxic drugs that are excreted renally (e.g. cidofovir, probenecid) – avoid Increases levels of didanosine N.B. Still relatively little experience with this agent, so be particularly vigilant for possible drug interactions

BNF, British National Formulary; CNS, Central nervous system; hep B, hepatitis B; hep C, hepatitis C; SJS, Stevens–Johnson syndrome; PI, protease inhibitor; e-c, enteric coated; HIV, human immunodeficiency virus; TB, tuberculosis; GI, gastrointestinal; PRC, prolonged release capsules; SPC, summary of product characteristics; LFT, liver junction test; ALT, alanine transaminase; AST, aspartate transaminase; GGT, gamma glutamyl transferase; TEN, toxic epidermal necrolysis; BI, Boehringer Ingelheim; INR, international normalized ratio; TDM, therapeutic drug monitoring; HBV, hepatitis B virus.

HIV mutates readily, and resistance to antiretrovirals develops rapidly in the face of suboptimal treatment, for example monotherapy or subtherapeutic blood levels. Adherence to the prescribed regimen is therefore of paramount importance, (see 'adherence' in Patient care section).

Nucleoside analogue reverse transcriptase inhibitors

NARTIs are phosphorylated intracellularly and then inhibit the viral reverse transcriptase enzyme by acting as a false substrate. The NARTIs licensed in the UK include:

- abacavir (Ziagen)
- didanosine (ddI, Videx)
- lamivudine (3TC, Epivir)
- stavudine (d4T, Zerit)
- zalcitabine (ddC, Hivid)
- zidovudine (AZT, Retrovir).

In addition, there are combination formulations of nucleoside analogues, zidovudine plus lamivudine (Combivir), and zidovudine plus lamivudine plus abacavir (Trizivir), that may be used to reduce pill burden. Most antiretroviral regimens will include two NARTIs, together with a PI and/or a non-nucleoside reverse transcriptase inhibitor (NNRTI). The cytidine analogues lamivudine and zalcitabine theoretically may antagonize one another, as may the thymidine analogues stavudine and zidovudine, due to competition for the same metabolic pathway. These pairs of agents are therefore usually avoided within a combination.

Non-nucleoside reverse transcriptase inhibitors

NNRTIs inhibit the reverse transcriptase enzyme by binding to its active site. They do not require prior phosphorylation and can act on cell-free virions as well as infected cells. The NNRTIs available in the UK include:

- efavirenz (Sustiva)
- nevirapine (Viramune).

Delavirdine (Rescriptor) is not licensed in the UK, but is available on a named-patient basis.

Resistance to NNRTIs occurs rapidly in incompletely suppressive regimens and it is therefore essential that they should be prescribed with at least two NARTIs or a combination of NARTIs and PIs. Cross-resistance between these agents is high and therefore a number of second-generation NNRTIs are currently under development which may possess a different resistance profile. Efavirenz and nevirapine both have much longer plasma half-lives than PIs and NARTIs, so when stopping an NNRTI-containing combination, consideration should be given to continuing the other agents for up to 5 days after cessation of the NNRTI (this should be discussed with an HIV specialist).

Protease (or proteinase) inhibitors

PIs bind to the active site of the HIV-1 protease enzyme, preventing the maturation of the newly produced virions so that they remain non-infectious. The following PIs are currently available:

- amprenavir (Agenerase)
- indinavir (Crixivan)
- lopinavir/r (Kaletra) (lopinavir co-formulated with ritonavir)
- nelfinavir (Viracept)
- ritonavir (Norvir)
- saquinavir hard gelatin capsule (Invirase) and soft gelatin capsule (Fortovase)

PIs are usually used in combination with two NARTIs, although combinations with more than one other class are increasingly used, particularly in patients who have been exposed to prior therapy. The use of a single protease inhibitor as part of a HAART regimen has been hampered by the high pill burden and relatively poor pharmacokinetic profiles associated with most of the drugs in this class, so that, increasingly, dual protease inhibitor combinations are being prescribed. In most cases, such combinations utilize the cytochrome P450 inhibition properties of ritonavir to enable the administration of a second PI at a lower dosage and/or longer dosing interval and/or with the abolition of dietary restrictions.

Newer classes of antiretroviral agents and approaches to therapy

Various new classes of drugs are currently in both clinical and pre-clinical stages of development and are likely to increase the anti-HIV armamentarium over the next few years. These include:

- nucleotide analogue reverse transcriptase inhibitors, which, unlike nucleoside analogues, do not require the first intracellular phosphorylation step (e.g. tenofovir)
- entry inhibitors (fusion inhibitors (e.g. T20), co-receptor blockers, and attachment inhibitors)
- integrase inhibitors
- zinc finger inhibitors.

In addition, newer strategies for treating HIV are likely to be more widely studied including:

- structured treatment interruptions
- immunomodulatory therapies (including interleukin-2, pegylated interferon alpha and adjunctive vaccines).

New PIs in development include fos-amprenavir (amprenavir prodrug), tipranavir and atazanavir.

Toxicities of antiretroviral therapies

As more antiretroviral agents have become available and the duration for which patients have been exposed to them has increased, our understanding (or at least awareness) of their toxicities has grown significantly.

While there are many individual drug toxicities (outlined in the Table 39.1B), there are also a number of class-specific or therapy-related toxicities which warrant further discussion.

Mitochondrial toxicity is increasingly recognized in patients with prolonged exposure to nucleoside analogue antiretrovirals and is thought to explain such side-effects as peripheral neuropathy, myopathy, pancreatitis and lactic acidosis.

Rash and hepatitis are both recognized side-effects of the NNRTI class, although the incidence and severity of these complications appears greatest with nevirapine.

A fat redistribution syndrome or lipodystrophy has been increasingly seen in individuals on HAART. At the present time it remains unclear whether this is one syndrome or, in fact, different clinical complications. Lipoatrophy (fat loss, particularly from the face, upper limbs and buttocks), lipohypertrophy (abnormal fat deposition, particularly affecting the abdomen and neck) and hyperlipidaemia (raised cholesterol and/or triglycerides) are all well described. The aetiology of these features currently remains poorly understood and may represent a combination of drug factors, genetic predisposition and immune reconstitution (Carr et al 1999).

Opportunistic infections and malignancies
(Table 39.2)

Fungal infections

Pneumocystis carinii **pneumonia.** PCP remains one of the commonest causes of morbidity and mortality in HIV-positive individuals. Classically, patients present with an insidious onset of a non-productive cough, shortness of breath on exertion and an inability to take a deep breath. Fever, anorexia and weight loss are common accompanying symptoms. Patients are usually markedly immunosuppressed, with CD4 counts less than 200 cells/mm^3. Diagnosis is supported by desaturation on exercise and the typical chest radiographic appearance of bilateral interstitial shadowing, though in mild cases the chest X-ray may be normal. The diagnosis is confirmed by demonstration of the organism by immunofluorescence or silver staining of samples obtained by sputum induction (by nebulization of hypertonic sodium chloride) or bronchoalveolar lavage.

Table 39.2   Drugs used to treat opportunistic infections in HIV disease

Drug	Indication	Dosage, route, frequency, duration	Common or significant side-effects	Significant interactions	Monitoring	Comments
Aciclovir	Herpes simplex	5 mg/kg i.v. three times daily for 5–10 days, 200–400 mg p.o. five times daily for 5–10 days	Skin rash, increased LFTs extravasation (i.v.) renal impairment (i.v.)	Probenecid	Renal fuction	Intravenous infusion diluted to 0.5% w/v and infused over at least 1 h
	Herpes zoster	10 mg/kg i.v. three times daily for 5–10 days, 800 mg p.o. five times daily for 7 days				
	Prophylaxis/suppression of herpes infections	200–400 mg p.o. twice daily				
Amphotericin	Cryptococcal meningitis and other severe fungal infections	0.25–1.0 mg/kg i.v. once daily for up to 6 weeks	Non-infusion related: nephrotoxicity; hypokalaemia, anaemia Infusion related: fever, chills, nausea and vomiting, myalgia, thrombophlebitis	Nephrotoxic drugs antineoplastics, corticosteroids	Renal function, FBC, U + Es	Start with lower dose and gradually increase Dilute in buffered 5% glucose. Liposomal and lipid complex formulations available which may be better tolerated (higher doses needed) Pre- and posthydration with 0.9% NaCl may decrease nephrotoxicity
	Oral candida	One lozenge sucked four times daily				
Atovaquone Suspension	Treatment of mild–moderate PCP	750 mg p.o. twice daily for 21 days	Rash, fever, gastrointestinal upset, headache, insomnia, increased LFTs, increased amylase, decreased Na, anaemia	Rifampicin, metoclopramide warfarin, tetracycline	LFTs, U + Es, FBC	Variable absorption improved by taking with fatty food, reduced by reduced gastrointestinal transit time
	Treatment of toxoplasmosis[a]	750 mg p.o. three times daily for at least 6 weeks				
Azithromycin	Atypical *Mycobacterium* infections[a] toxoplasmosis[a] and PCP[a] (Adjunctive therapy or part of combination regimen.) *Cryptosporidium* diarrhoea[a]	500–600 mg p.o. daily for MAI treatment or PCP prophylaxis and *Cryptosporidium* treatment; 1200–1250 mg p.o. once weekly for MAI prophylaxis; 1200–1250 mg daily for toxoplasmosis treatment	Gastrointestinal upset, rash, ototoxicity, raised LFTs	Antacids, ergot derivatives,	LFTs, hearing (if on long-term or high-dose therapy)	Less significant drug interactions than with the other macrolides
Cidofovir	Cytomegalovirus retinitis	5 mg/kg weekly for two doses then every 2 weeks thereafter	Nephrotoxicity	Other nephrotoxic drugs, agents that are contraindicated with probenecid	Renal function FBC	Co-administer with probenecid and intravenous fluids Avoid if on tenofovir
Clarithromycin	Atypical *Mycobacterium* infections (MAI)	500 mg p.o. twice daily	Nausea, vomiting, abdominal pain, rash, increased LFTs, taste perversion	Astemizole, terfenadine, warfarin, digoxin, theophylline, Kaletra, ritonavir, efavirenz, nevirapine carbamazepine, ergot derivatives	LFTs	Taking with food may decrease gastrointestinal upset. Take 1–2 h apart from zidovudine
Clindamycin	Treatment of PCP[a]	600 mg–1.2 g i.v./p.o. four times daily for 14–21 days	Diarrhoea, gastrointestinal disturbance, rash, increased LFTs. Rarely pseudomembranous colitis, blood dyscrasias	Care with neuromuscular blocking agents	LFTs, FBC, diarrhoea	Taken with primaquine
	Toxoplasmosis treatment[a]	1.2 g i.v./p.o. four times daily for at least 4–6 weeks		Erythromycin		Taken with pyrimethamine
	Toxoplasmosis maintenance[a]	1.2 g p.o. daily in divided doses				

Table 39.2 (continued)

Drug	Indication	Dosage, route, frequency, duration	Common or significant side-effects	Significant interactions	Monitoring	Comments
Co-trimoxazole	Treatment of PCP	120 mg/kg i.v/p.o. in two to four divided doses for 14–21 days	Rash, nausea, and, vomiting, neutropenia, increased LFTs, anaemia, Stevens–Johnson syndrome, drug fever	Bone marrow suppressive therapy sulphonylureas, phenytoin, lamivudine	FBC, renal function, LFTs, rash	For infusion dilute each 480 mg with 125 ml of glucose 5% or sodium chloride 0.9% and infuse over 1.5–3 h. If fluid restricted 480 mg in 75 ml of glucose 5%
	Prophylaxis against PCP	480 or 960 mg p.o. daily or 960 mg three times per week				
Dapsone	Prophylaxis against PCP[a]	100 mg p.o. daily	Gastrointestinal disturbance, rash, anaemia, leucopenia, methaemoglobinaemia	Rifampicin, probenecid, nitrofurantoin Antacids	FBC, U + Es, LFTs	Tests for G6PD in patients of African or Mediterranean origin
Famciclovir	Treatment of herpes zoster Treatment of genital herpes	Doses for immunocompromised patients: zoster–500 mg three times daily for 10 days; genital herpes – all episodes 500 mg twice daily for 7 days, suppression 500 mg twice daily	Mild headache and nausea	?Probenecid	Renal function	
Fluconazole	Oesophageal candidiasis Oropharyngeal candidiasis Cryptococcal meningitis treatment Cryptococcal meningitis prophylaxis	100–200 mg p.o. daily for 2 weeks 50–100 mg p.o. daily for 7–14 days 400–800 mg i.v./p.o. daily for ≥8 weeks 200–400 mg p.o. daily	Gastrointestinal disturbance, rash, hepatotoxicity	Oral anticoagulants, hypoglycaemics, rifabutin, phenytoin, rifampicin	Renal function LFTs	
Flucytosine	Cryptococcal meningitis treatment	100 mg/kg daily p.o. i.v. in four divided doses for 2 weeks (with i.v. amphotericin)	Nausea vomiting, diarrhoea, rash, renal impairment, bone marrow suppression	Cytarabine	Renal function FBC, LFTs	Oral formulation is no longer licensed in the UK but can be imported on named-patient basis
Fomivirsen	Local treatment of CMV retinitis when other therapies ineffective or unsuitable	Intravitreal injection: new disease – 165 micrograms weekly for 3 weeks then every 2 weeks; previously treated disease – 330 micrograms on alternate weeks for 2 doses then every 4 weeks	Local inflammation and other ocular side-effects (including raised intraocular pressure)	Current or recent cidofovir treatment	Intraocular pressure	
Foscarnet	Cytomegalovirus retinitis treatment Cytomegalovirus retinitis maintenance Mucocutaneous Herpes simplex infection	90 mg/kg twice a day or 60 mg/kg three times per day i.v. (adjusted according to serum creatinine) over 2 h for 2–3 weeks 90–120 mg/kg i.v. once daily over 2 h for 5–7 days of each week 40 mg/kg i.v. three times daily for 2–3 weeks	Nephrotoxicity, alterations in serum calcium, potassium and other minerals, headache, thrombophlebitis, genital ulceration, anaemia, nausea	Nephrotoxic drugs, pentamidine	Renal function, serum calcium, magnesium, potassium and phosphate, FBC	Patients must be well hydrated. Electrolyte abnormalities must be corrected promptly and dose adjusted according to renal function. Advise patients to wash genital area after micturition to decrease risk of ulceration
Ganciclovir	Cytomegalovirus induction treatment Cytomegalovirus retinitis maintenance	5 mg/kg i.v. twice daily for 14–21 days 5 mg/kg i.v. once every day or 6 mg/kg i.v. once daily for 5 days of each week	Neutropenia, thrombocytopenia, abnormal LFTs, central nervous system effects	Zidovudine, imipenem, bone marrow suppressive agents	FBC renal function, LFTs	Give over 1 h preferably via central venous access

Table 39.2 (continued)

Drug	Indication	Dosage, route, frequency, duration	Common or significant side-effects	Significant interactions	Monitoring	Comments
Itraconazole	Oropharyngeal and oesophageal candidiasis (including fluconazole-resistant disease)	200 mg p.o. daily for 15 days (liquid or capsules); can increase to 200 mg BD	Nausea, abdominal pain, headache, hepatotoxicity	Rifampicin, phenytoin, astemizole, H_2 antagonists, nevirapine, antacids, indinavir, ritonavir, terfenadine, oral anticoagulants	LFTs	With or after food or with orange juice or cola (capsules). On empty stomach, 'swish and swallow' (liquid)
Ketoconazole	Oropharyngeal and oesophageal candidiasis	200 mg p.o. once or twice daily for 7–14 days	Abnormal LFTs, gastrointestinal disturbance, rash	Rifampicin, phenytoin, astemizole, H_2 antagonists, nevirapine, antacids, terfenadine, oral anticoagulants, indinavir, ritonavir	LFTs, adrenal function	With or after food (or with orange juice or cola)
Nystatin	Oral candidiasis	1–2 ml suspension, p.o. or 1 pastille (sucked) four times daily	Rarely, nausea, vomiting, diarrhoea		Not required	Combine with strict oral hygiene
Pentamidine Isetionate	PCP treatment Mild PCP treatment PCP prophylaxis	4 mg/kg i.v. once daily for 14–21 days (+ 600 mg nebulized for first 3 days) 600 mg nebulized daily for 21 days 300 mg nebulized every 4 weeks	Intravenous: nephrotoxicity postural hypotension, leucopenia, hypo/hyperglycaemia Nebulized: cough, bronchospasm	Nephrotoxic drugs, foscarnet	Renal function, blood glucose, blood pressure, U + Es	Infuse over 1 h, with patient supine Pretreat with bronchodilator if nebulized
Primaquine	PCP treatment	15–30 mg p.o. daily for 14–21 days	Methaemoglobinaemia, haemolytic anaemia, nausea	Bone marrow suppressive drugs	FBC	Test for G6PD in patients of African or Mediterranean origin
Pyrimethamine	Toxoplasmosis treatment[a] Toxoplasmosis maintenance[a]	100 mg on day 1 then 75 mg p.o. once daily for 4–6 weeks 25 mg p.o. once daily	Anaemia, rash, bone marrow suppression	Bone marrow suppressive drugs	FBC	Combined with sulfadiazine or clindamycin Consider use of folinic acid
Rifabutin	MAI prophylaxis MAI treatment	300–450 mg p.o. once daily with other drugs (consult SPC for specific details)	Abnormal LFTs, bone marrow suppression, uveitis	Clarithromycin, indinavir, saquinavir, ritonavir, fluconazole, oral contraceptives, oral anticoagulants	LFTs	Combine with at least one other drug for MAI treatment
Sulfadiazine	Toxoplasmosis treatment[a] Toxoplasmosis maintenance[a]	1–2 g i.v./p.o. four times daily for 4–6 weeks 2 g p.o. daily in divided doses	Nausea, vomiting, bone marrow suppression, crystalluria	Bone marrow suppressive drugs, ?warfarin, ?oral hypoglycaemics	Renal function, LFTs, FBC	Use with pyrimethamine Use folinic acid 15 mg p.o. during treatment phase
Valaciclovir	Herpes zoster treatment Herpes simplex treatment	1 g p.o. three times daily for 7 days 500 mg p.o. twice daily for 5–10 days (initial) or 5 days (recurrent) episodes	Mild headache and nausea (?more serious events reported in AIDS patients on 8 g/day long term)		Renal function	

Table 39.2 (continued)

Drug	Indication	Dosage, route, frequency, duration	Common or significant side-effects	Significant interactions	Monitoring	Comments
Valganciclovir	CMV retinitis	Induction treatment: 900 mg twice a day with food for 21 days. Maintenance: 900 mg once daily	Diarrhoea, nausea, neutropenia	(As for ganciclovir) Caution with myelo-suppressive or nephrotoxic drugs Avoid imipenem with cilastatin. Caution with didanosine, zidovudine and probenecid	FBC, U + Es, LFTs	

a Unlicensed treatment indication in UK.
FBC, full blood count; U + Es, urea and electrolyte determinations; LFTs, liver function tests; MAI, *Mycobacterium avium intracellulare*; G6PD, glucose-6-phosphate dehydrogenase; PCP, *Pneumocystis carinii* Pneumonia; CMV, cytomegalovirus.

Treatment is instigated in patients with a proven diagnosis, or empirically where there is a suspicion prior to confirmation. Oxygen is essential for patients with compromised respiratory function. First-line therapy is high-dose co-trimoxazole (120 mg/kg/day in divided doses), orally in mild cases and intravenously in moderate to severe disease. Nausea and vomiting commonly occur, and may be best managed pre-emptively by administration of a prophylactic antiemetic. Co-trimoxazole is usually administered in 500 ml or 1 litre of sodium chloride 0.9% or glucose 5% over 1.5–2 hours.

In cases of co-trimoxazole intolerance, several alternative therapies are available. For mild PCP a combination of oral trimethoprim (10–15 mg/kg/day in two divided doses) with dapsone (100 mg daily) may be effective. For moderate to severe disease a combination of clindamycin (600 mg four times a day, intravenous or oral, depending on severity) and primaquine (30 mg oral) is often used. Intravenous pentamidine (4 mg/kg/day) is another alternative, though its use may be associated with more significant adverse reactions. It should be infused with the patient lying down (to decrease hypotension), and patients should be warned of the possibility of the development of hypo- or hyperglycaemia, which may occur after cessation of the drug. Pentamidine should also be given in nebulized form (600 mg) via a suitable nebulizer (e.g. Respirgard II or modified Acorn System 22®) for the first 3 days, to ensure prompt attainment of adequate lung tissue levels. Oral atovaquone suspension (750 mg twice daily) can be used for mild to moderate PCP, but must be taken with food (particularly fatty food) to be effective. Intravenous trimetrexate is recommended for treating moderate to severe disease in patients who are intolerant of, or refractory to, standard therapy, but is no longer licensed in the UK.

For cases of moderate to severe PCP (Po_2 less than 8 kPa) adjunctive corticosteroid therapy is recommended (e.g. prednisolone 75 mg daily for 5 days, 50 mg for 5 days then 25 mg for 5 days). A controlled trial of 333 patients demonstrated a reduction in mortality from 43% to 19% and a decrease in the number of patients who required intubation, when corticosteroids were commenced within 72 hours of presentation with moderate to severe PCP (Bozzette et al 1990). For patients with first-episode PCP without severe coexisting medical complications, ventilatory support should be considered.

It has been clearly demonstrated that prophylactic therapy reduces both the incidence and severity of PCP in patients with either prior PCP or at risk of a first episode, and that this intervention significantly improves survival. Co-trimoxazole (Fischl et al 1988) and nebulized pentamidine (Hirschel et al 1991) have both been shown to be effective agents for the primary prophylaxis of PCP, although a survival benefit was only seen in one of the studies (Fischl et al 1988). In 1994, a retrospective analysis (1985 to 1993) was undertaken of 2646 HIV-positive homosexual men (CD4 less than 100 cells/mm^3) from the Multicenter AIDS Cohort Study (MACS) in the USA (Bacellar et al 1994). The PCP incidence rate was 12.8% in patients who were receiving both antiretroviral therapy (zidovudine or didanosine) and PCP prophylaxis, 21.5% in those who were just receiving PCP prophylaxis and 47.4% in those who were on neither.

Primary prophylaxis is recommended for those individuals with a previous AIDS-defining illness, markedly symptomatic disease or a CD4 count of less than 200–300 cells/mm^3. Co-trimoxazole is the gold standard and also confers protection against toxoplasmosis and some other bacterial infections. The optimum dose remains to be determined, but commonly used regimens with proven efficacy are 960 mg daily or three times a week or 480 mg daily. The incidence of adverse reactions to co-trimoxazole in HIV-positive individuals is higher than in the general population, although many patients who are intolerant of high-dose treatment do not experience problems at prophylactic doses. In cases of intolerance, several alternative approaches may be adopted. Desensitization may be attempted, or other agents may be used. Dapsone 100 mg daily (with or without pyrimethamine, according to toxoplasma status), is effective, as is nebulized pentamidine (300 mg every month or 150 mg every 2 weeks via appropriate nebulizer (as above), with prior nebulized or inhaled beta-2 agonist to prevent bronchospasm).

Candidiasis. Oropharyngeal candidiasis is a frequent manifestation of HIV infection and may occur early in the disease. Clinically, it is usually characterized by white plaques on the oral mucosa, but may present as erythematous patches or as angular cheilitis. If swallowing is difficult (dysphagia) or painful (odynophagia), oesophageal involvement may be suspected.

First-line therapy for mild oral candidiasis is topical and includes nystatin suspension/pastilles or amphotericin lozenges/suspension, with miconazole gel recommended for patients with dentures. Good oral hygiene should be stressed, and adjunctive therapies may be helpful, e.g. chlorhexidine or hydrogen peroxide mouthwashes. For severe cases, or for those in whom topical therapy has failed, systemic agents, such as fluconazole (50 mg daily) or itraconazole (200 mg once or twice daily) are recommended. Ketoconazole is now rarely used because of its potential for interactions with antiretroviral agents.

In cases of oesophageal candida (which is an AIDS-defining illness) systemic therapy is necessary (using higher doses of the above agents). Continuous azole therapy or frequent courses of these drugs predisposes to the development of azole-resistance. In such instances an alternative azole may be used, or occasionally higher than usual doses of the original agent, e.g. fluconazole 400 mg daily. In intractable cases, intravenous amphotericin is often required. In the era of HAART, such complications are rarely seen.

Cryptococcosis. Cryptococcus neoformans, in the context of HIV infection, causes a disseminated infection, usually with meningeal involvement. Patients present with fever and headaches, often without the characteristic symptoms of meningism (photophobia and neck stiffness). Diagnosis is normally made on the basis of CSF analysis, though serum cryptococcal antigen and blood cultures may also be indicative.

For patients who are moderately or severely unwell, intravenous amphotericin B with flucytosine (100 mg/kg/day, oral or intravenous) is the first-line therapy. Amphotericin is generally administered in 500 ml or 1 litre of buffered glucose 5% over 4–8 hours. The dose is increased from 0.25 mg/kg to 0.7–1 mg/kg as soon as tolerated. Renal function and serum electrolytes, particularly potassium and magnesium, should be monitored closely, and any abnormalities addressed promptly. 'Sodium loading' (pre- and post-amphotericin infusions of sodium chloride 0.9%) may help to reduce nephrotoxicity. Administration of corticosteroids and/or antihistamines may reduce the severity of infusion-related reactions. The usual duration of amphotericin and flucytosine treatment is 2 weeks, after which high-dose fluconazole (400 mg daily by mouth) should be continued for a further 10 weeks. Subsequent maintenance therapy with fluconazole 200 mg daily has been shown to be efficacious in reducing the incidence of relapse and should be continued for life (or until immune function is sufficiently restored).

In milder cases, fluconazole may be given for the entire duration of treatment. There are a number of liposomal or lipid-complexed formulations available, which are more expensive but less nephrotoxic, that may be considered in cases of amphotericin intolerance. Itraconazole has been used for both treatment and maintenance, but may be less effective than fluconazole.

Protozoal infections

Toxoplasmosis. T. gondii is a frequent cause of central nervous system disease in patients with AIDS. Individuals may present with headaches, fever, confusion, seizures or focal neurological symptoms/signs. Diagnosis is usually based on the appearance of ring-enhancing lesion(s) on computed tomography. Definitive diagnosis is based on brain biopsy, which is rarely performed, but is generally made presumptively after response to therapy.

First-line treatment is with sulfadiazine and pyrimethamine with folinic acid to prevent myelosuppression. Alternatives include clindamycin and pyrimethamine, atovaquone and, possibly, clarithromycin or doxycycline, although for these last three this is an unlicensed indication in the UK. Adjunctive therapy with corticosteroids or anticonvulsants may be used in cases of severe oedema or seizures, respectively.

Cryptosporidiosis. *Cryptosporidium parvum* is a ubiquitous organism and a common cause of diarrhoea in immunocompetent individuals. In patients who are immunocompromised, persistent infection may occur characterized by abdominal pain, weight loss and severe diarrhoea. Diagnosis is generally based on stool analysis.

Although many agents have been investigated for the treatment of cryptosporidiosis, none has proved effective. The mainstay of management remains symptomatic control with nutritional supplementation, adequate hydration and antidiarrhoeal agents. It may be necessary to administer up to 16 mg of loperamide per day and/or maximum doses of codeine (and even morphine or diamorphine) to control the diarrhoea. Many antibiotic agents have been investigated, but the majority of results have been disappointing. The use of octreotide or total parenteral nutrition (TPN) in this patient group remains controversial. The optimal treatment for cryptosporidiosis (and indeed the majority of chronic opportunistic infections) is to increase immunological function utilizing antiretroviral therapies.

Bacterial infections

Bacterial infections are common in the context of HIV infection. Recurrent bacterial pneumonia (particularly *Streptococcus pneumoniae*) and diarrhoeal illnesses (*Salmonella, Shigella, Campylobacter*) are particularly common. In general these are treated the same as in immunocompetent individuals, although recurrent infections and/or septicaemia occur more frequently.

Mycobacteria. In HIV-positive individuals, *M. tuberculosis* (TB) is characterized by:

- increased likelihood of reactivation of latent disease
- increased likelihood of de novo acquisition of TB
- more rapid progression to clinical disease following acquisition
- more rapid progression of HIV disease
- no increase in infectivity of TB compared with HIV-negative patients.

Definitive diagnosis is reliant on culture of the organism from biological specimens, but may be complicated by atypical clinical features and reduced response to tuberculin testing.

Treatment for pulmonary and extrapulmonary TB should follow conventional guidelines for immunocompetent individuals. Meningitis is an unusual but significant complication of TB, and its management requires expert guidance. The use of primary and secondary prophylaxis remains controversial but may be appropriate in high-incidence groups. The increased incidence of multidrug resistant tuberculosis (MDRTB) is a cause for concern, raises many infection control issues and highlights the need for antibiotic therapy driven by bacteriological sensitivities.

Mycobacterium avium-intracellulare (MAI) infection is a frequent manifestation of late-stage HIV disease, and is associated with decreased survival. Patients with disseminated infection classically present with fevers, weight loss, diarrhoea and hepatosplenomegaly. Diagnosis is sometimes made presumptively but is usually based on culture of the organism(s). In vitro sensitivities may not be good predictors of response to therapy. Therapy may need to be tailored to account for drug interactions with concomitant antiretrovirals, but usually includes azithromycin and ethambutol (with or without rifabutin). Alternative agents include the quinolones and amikacin. Corticosteroids may be useful for symptomatic control. Although rifabutin, clarithromycin and azithromycin have all been demonstrated to be effective agents for prophylaxis against MAI, their cost–benefit remains controversial, and use is not widespread in the UK.

Viral infections

Cytomegalovirus. CMV is a herpes virus that is acquired by approximately 50% of the general population and over 90% of homosexual men. Like other herpes viruses, once infection has occurred the virus remains dormant thereafter, but in individuals with advanced immunosuppression reactivation may occur and cause disease. In the context of HIV infection, the most common sites of disease are the retina and gastrointestinal tract, though neurological involvement and pneumonitis are well reported.

Diagnosis of CMV retinitis is based on clinical appearance; it may be detected in asymptomatic individuals, but usually presents with symptoms of blurred vision, visual field defects or 'floaters'. Untreated CMV retinitis progresses rapidly to blindness, and treatment substantially reduces the morbidity associated with this condition. Although previously lifelong treatment had been recommended, where immunological restoration occurs discontinuation may be possible (see below). Conventional therapeutic approaches are based upon an initial induction period of high-dose therapy for 2–3 weeks, until the retinitis is quiescent, followed by lower-dose maintenance treatment, with reinduction if disease progression occurs. The most common agent currently used for induction therapy in the UK is intravenous ganciclovir, which is usually administered via a central line over 1 hour. Significant side-effects encountered with this treatment include neutropenia, which may require colony-stimulating factor support, and thrombocytopenia. Maintenance treatment may be given either intravenously or orally. Although intravenous maintenance requires the insertion of a permanent indwelling catheter and causes greater myelosuppression, there are concerns regarding the poor efficacy of the oral formulation because of its low bioavailability. Intravitreal administration of ganciclovir is possible either by injection or by insertion of an implant device. However, such a treatment strategy is unlikely to confer any systemic protection of other organs (including the other eye) which should be considered when deciding upon which therapeutic approach to adopt.

An alternative agent to ganciclovir is foscarnet. Although it has a less favourable toxicity profile, it is usually reserved for cases of therapeutic failure with ganciclovir. Its main adverse effects are electrolyte abnormalities, which should be corrected promptly, nephrotoxicity that requires dose adjustment or cessation of therapy, and ulceration, particularly of the genitals, which may be prevented by assiduous attention to personal hygiene after micturition. No effective oral formulation is currently available.

Cidofovir is a newer anti-CMV agent that requires less frequent administration (weekly for 2 weeks for induction and fortnightly for maintenance), though intravenous administration is again required and nephrotoxicity and other metabolic disturbances are well recognized.

More recent treatment approaches include antisense-oligonucleotides (e.g. fomivirsen intravitreal injection) and a prodrug of ganciclovir (valganciclovir, recently licensed in the UK). The optimal positioning of these various treatments remains unclear and an individualized approach to patient management is recommended. However, valganciclovir, which is as effective as intravenous ganciclovir, is likely to be more widely used.

CMV disease of the gastrointestinal tract usually affects the oesophagus or colon, causing dysphagia and abdominal pain with diarrhoea, respectively. Diagnosis is based upon histological analysis of biopsy specimens. Treatment is as for CMV retinitis induction therapy; maintenance therapy is not usually given unless relapses occur. Neurological disease may present in a variety of ways, is difficult to diagnose and frequently carries a poor prognosis, even with treatment. The optimal agent, dosage and duration of therapy remain undetermined.

Wasting syndrome

Many patients with advanced HIV disease report significant weight loss, and an underlying pathogen can be identified. True wasting syndrome is characterized by loss of greater than 10% of body weight with diarrhoea and/or fever for which no other cause is found. Putative pathogenic mechanisms include hypermetabolism, hormonal imbalance and HIV infection of enterocytes, though in many cases reduced oral intake is sufficient to explain the degree of weight loss. Therapeutic interventions include appetite stimulants (including megestrol, medroxyprogesterone acetate, nabilone), anabolic agents and recombinant human growth hormone. Most of these agents are unlicensed for this indication; although there are data to support the use of growth hormone, its cost is usually prohibitive. The mainstay of management remains intensive nutritional support and effective antiretroviral therapy.

The impact of HAART on opportunistic infections

The widespread use of combination antiretroviral therapy has had a dramatic effect on the incidence, prognosis, and clinical aspects of opportunistic infections.

The management of such complications has changed in the following ways:

- *Decreased incidence of opportunistic infections.* HAART has resulted in a major reduction in the vast majority of opportunistic infections and a consequent reduction in mortality rates and requirement for hospital admissions.
- *Withdrawal of prophylaxis.* The rise in CD4 counts associated with HAART has been associated with an improvement in functional immunity: controlled trials have suggested that the withdrawal of both primary and secondary prophylaxis against PCP is safe, and case series and cohort studies suggest that similar results may be seen for toxoplasmosis, MAI, and CMV.
- *Successful treatment of opportunistic infections.* Some infections which were previously difficult to treat, notably cryptosporidiosis and microsporidiosis, appear to resolve with significant CD4 count improvements associated with HAART.

Currently, it has yet to be determined to what extent functional immunity to other opportunistic infections will improve and whether such withdrawal of prophylaxis/maintenance can be recommended routinely.

Cancers

Although there are many malignancies that are likely to be associated with HIV infection, the commonest malignant manifestations are Kaposi's sarcoma and lymphoma.

Kaposi's sarcoma. This is the commonest malignancy in people with HIV infection and may be triggered by infection with human herpes virus 8 (HHV-8). The majority of lesions affect the skin, and appear as raised purple papules. These may be single or multiple, and in severe cases may result in oedema, ulceration and infection. Visceral involvement is not uncommon, but rarely causes clinically significant disease.

In some cases, no therapeutic intervention is necessary, and cosmetic camouflage may be sufficient. Indeed, treatment of HIV per se with antiretroviral therapy results in improvement of (and in some cases complete resolution of) Kaposi's sarcoma in many patients. When individual lesions are troublesome, local radiotherapy or intralesional chemotherapy (e.g. vincristine) can be beneficial. Newer approaches using topical agents remain largely investigational. In cases of widespread cutaneous disease or significant visceral involvement, systemic chemotherapy is traditionally used. A combination of vincristine and bleomycin has traditionally been the first-line regimen. The liposomal formulations of doxorubicin and daunorubicin are arguably more effective and less toxic and many clinicians would favour their use as initial therapy despite the high cost. Etoposide has also been used either orally or intravenously in recalcitrant cases, with reported benefit, and encouraging data are emerging regarding the use of paclitaxel in recurrent or recalcitrant disease.

Since it now appears that Kaposi's sarcoma may be triggered by the presence of a herpes virus, future therapeutic strategies may include antiviral agents. It appears that HHV-8 is inhibited by ganciclovir and foscarnet but not by aciclovir. However, if malignant transformation has already occurred, the value of these antiviral drugs is questionable.

Lymphomas. The commonest lymphomas in patients with HIV infection are high-grade B cell types. Although these may affect any organ, it is notable that a high proportion are primarily central nervous system in origin, which are extremely rare in the general population. Diagnosis is based upon histological confirmation from biopsy specimens.

The optimal therapy for HIV-associated lymphomas has yet to be determined. For non-central nervous system disease, a regimen involving cyclophosphamide, doxorubicin, vincristine and prednisolone (CHOP) is often used. The outcome for patients with relatively preserved immune function is comparable to that in the general population. However, in those patients with advanced HIV disease the response to chemotherapy may be disappointing, possibly because many individuals are unable to tolerate treatment without dose modification. Lymphoma of the central nervous system is associated with an extremely poor outcome, and in many cases even palliative radiotherapy or corticosteroids confer little benefit.

The introduction of combination therapy has had a marked impact on the course of Kaposi's sarcoma, with clinical improvement of cutaneous lesions observed, and possibly of visceral disease also. The impact on lymphoma is less clear: some authors report improved survival and reduced incidence, but this remains less well-established than for the opportunistic infections.

Neurological manifestations

Neurological symptoms may be due to opportunistic infections, tumours or the primary neurological effects of HIV.

HIV encephalopathy or AIDS dementia complex (ADC) is believed to result from direct infection of the central nervous system with HIV itself. Individuals who may otherwise be physically well can be debilitated by profound cognitive dysfunction and amnesia. Although psychometric test results are usually suggestive of the underlying aetiology, it is wise to rule out any other cause with brain scanning and CSF analysis.

It appears that antiretroviral agents that penetrate the central nervous system can improve cognitive function, reduce subsequent deterioration, and lessen the likelihood of ADC occuring. This is certainly true of zidovudine, although it appears that the neuroprotective effect may not extend beyond 18 months of therapy. Many of the other currently available agents do not penetrate the central nervous system with the possible exception of stavudine. However, newer therapies (such as the NNRTIs and abacavir) may achieve high central nervous system levels, and their role in the prevention or treatment of ADC has yet to be elucidated. The role of CNS penetration in the prevention/amelioration of HIV associated neurological disease remains unclear; in general, therapies which boost immune function have all been associated with clinical advantage irrespective of proven CNS penetration capabilities.

Hepatitis/HIV co-infection

It is noteworthy that a significant minority of patients are co-infected with hepatitis virus infection (both hepatitis B and C) in addition to their underlying HIV infection. Given the improved prognosis from an HIV perspective, it is increasingly recognized that treatment of the concurrent hepatitis may be warranted. The following factors are relevant:

1. HIV impacts upon hepatitis eradication: it appears less likely that individuals will be able to eradicate hepatitis B or C infection if they are immunosuppressed.
2. HIV impacts upon progression of hepatitis: more rapid progression is described for hepatitis C and arguably slower progression for hepatitis B.
3. The response rates for therapeutic interventions for hepatitis B and C are less impressive in the context of HIV infection.

4. Response to treatment for HIV may impact either favourably or unfavourably on the concomitant hepatitis and its treatment. Some agents (notably lamivudine and tenofovir) are effective against both HIV and hepatitis B and therefore when treatment is being given for either condition, consideration must be given to the possibility of resistance development to these agents by one or both viruses.

5. Ribavirin, which is usually used as part of hepatitis C therapy, antagonizes in vitro the phosphorylation of stavudine and zidovudine, although the clinical relevance of this remains unclear.

It is likely that in the next few years clearly defined protocols/guidelines for the management of co-infection will be developed.

Issues for women with HIV

The issues for women with HIV are particularly complex. A full discussion is beyond the remit of this chapter, but the following general points should be borne in mind:

* viral load and CD4 results may need to be interpreted differently in women
* disease progression may be different from that observed in men (and gynaecological manifestations of HIV and the need for regular cervical screening must not be forgotten).

Pregnancy and contraception. In addition, the following considerations need to be made when discussing or prescribing therapy for women of childbearing potential:

* interactions with oral and injectable/depot contraceptive agents (although barrier methods should also be recommended in addition to hormonal contraception, to prevent transmission of HIV and other sexually transmitted infections)
* potential teratogenicity (recognizing the paucity of data)
* possible increased toxicity to both mother and child (notably mitochondrial toxicity)
* the use of antiretroviral agents to reduce vertical transmission of HIV.

Regarding vertical transmission, it is now well known that the use of combination antiretroviral therapy (with or without caesarean section) in combination with a non-breastfeeding strategy has reduced vertical transmission rates to almost zero in women where their HIV status is known and where antiretroviral therapies are widely available. None the less, questions remain regarding optimal therapies, risk of transmission of resistant virus to the neonate, and risk of toxicity from antiretroviral agents administered during pregnancy, particularly in the first trimester. Ideally all HIV positive women should be counselled regarding these issues before they become pregnant so that they can make informed decisions both on therapy and on timing of pregnancy.

Terminal care

Patients with advanced AIDS may be managed at home, in a hospice (either generic or HIV-specific) or in hospital, depending on the services available in the locality. The same principles of palliative/terminal care apply in this patient population as in any other. However, the notable difference in HIV infection is that patients may continue with a number of active or prophylactic therapies until they are very close to death. Common examples are ganciclovir or foscarnet to prevent blindness due to CMV retinitis and co-trimoxazole to prevent PCP. The decision to stop treatment, particularly with antiretrovirals, should be made in consultation with the patient. The impact of HAART on the requirement for such 'terminal' strategies has been remarkable. None the less, it is inevitable, given the likely limitations of current treatment strategies, that immunological failure and associated clinical progression will continue and therefore skills in complex palliation will continue to be required.

Patient care

AIDS is a multisystem disorder that presents numerous challenges to the infected individual, their loved ones and their health care workers. In addition, patients have other specific needs or characteristics to take into consideration, for example gay men, haemophiliacs, injecting drug users, asylum seekers, people who do not have English as a first language, women and children. (The management of HIV-infected children differs significantly from adults and is not addressed in this chapter.) Regardless of the manner in which they acquired HIV, all infected people should:

* be treated as individuals, recognizing the various lifestyle factors that may affect their choice of treatment and ability to adhere to it (e.g. lack of childcare facilities may prevent some women from accessing services or entering clinical trials)
* be given appropriate information to empower them to participate in their own health care decision-making processes and adhere to the chosen treatment regimen
* be monitored regularly for signs of treatment failure, low adherence and drug toxicity
* be given appropriate advice regarding prevention of transmission and reinfection (e.g. safer sex, safer drug use).

The pharmaceutical care needs of HIV-positive individuals overlap significantly with those of elderly, oncology and transplant patients, among others, and can be summarized by the acronym PANDA:

- Polypharmacy
- Adverse drug reactions
- New drugs
- Drug interactions
- Adherence.

People with HIV infection are commonly prescribed large numbers of drugs (some of which involve taking 16 capsules per day), with the attendant increased risk of interactions and side-effects. This patient group has also been reported to suffer a higher incidence of adverse reactions than the general population. In addition, the widespread use of new or experimental agents, or the prescribing of unusual doses or using drugs for unlicensed indications, raises the likelihood of a previously unreported adverse event occurring.

Adherence to therapy is crucial to the success of antiretroviral regimens and in the treatment and prophylaxis of opportunistic infections. The level of adherence that is required for a sustained successful outcome of antiretroviral treatment is arguably higher than in any other therapy area and has been the subject of much multidisciplinary research. For example, in one study of people taking their first regimen (containing nelfinavir), it was found that at least 95% adherence was required to achieve a sustained response (viral load below the limit of quantification) in the majority (78%) of patients. The chances of treatment success declined sharply as the level of adherence dropped, such that 80% of patients whose adherence was below 80% (as measured by electronic MEMScaps) experienced virologic failure. Virologic success was also found to correlate with a better clinical outcome (fewer hospitalizations, opportunistic infections and deaths) (Paterson et al 2000). Such clinical trial data have also been supported by clinical experience in the UK and elsewhere.

In other medical conditions, non-adherence has been shown to increase with the number of prescribed medications and to be more common in patients suffering from confusion or dementia. Compliance devices (such as pill boxes, timers and medication record cards) may be helpful in enabling patients (not just those with cognitive impairment) or their carers to manage their medicines safely and appropriately, but many of the commonly used products are too small to contain the number of dose units required. In addition, some of the drugs have particular storage requirements and may require refrigeration or storage with a desiccant. Significant progress has been made in the last few years in reducing some of the physical burden of therapy, for example with the development of combination tablets and the use of strategies to reduce dietary restrictions and dosing frequency. However,

practical issues are not the only barriers to adherence and consideration should be given to addressing the individual's health beliefs (particularly around HIV and antiretroviral therapy) before treatment is commenced, as these are likely to have a significant impact on outcome. Although there is little evidence to demonstrate what the optimal interventions to improve adherence are, it is likely that multidisciplinary and multiagency approaches will be necessary, in which pharmacists will have a major role to play. National recommendations for adherence support (evidence-based where such evidence exists) were launched in October 2002 as part of the ongoing standard setting for HIV services in the UK.

CASE STUDIES

Case 39.1

Ms A. is a 35-year-old heterosexual woman, who was recently diagnosed HIV-positive following a hospital admission with PCP. She has a history of previous injecting drug use and is currently maintained on a methadone programme via the local drug dependency unit (DDU). Her most recent CD4 count was 50 cells/mm³, with a plasma HIV RNA (viral load) of 500 000 copies/ml. Her current therapy is:

Co-trimoxazole 480 mg every day, Cilest™ 1 daily, multivitamin BPC 1 daily and methadone mixture 1 mg/ml 50 mg daily. On questioning, the patient also reports occasionally buying St John's wort from a health food store, although she is not currently taking it. The patient presents to pharmacy with her first prescription for antiretrovirals: Combivir™ once daily and efavirenz 600 mg at night, with metoclopramide 10 mg twice daily for the first 2–4 weeks.

Two weeks later the patient rings the clinic saying she feels her methadone is wearing off after about 18 hours (feeling shivery, aching, etc), but the DDU have refused to increase her methadone dose. She is also feeling dizzy, having difficulty concentrating while she is awake and is having nightmares and disturbed sleep. She is not sure she can continue with therapy if this carries on.

Questions

1. What are the actual and potential pharmaceutical care issues that should be addressed at the time Ms A. presents with her first prescription for antiretrovirals? Outline the main counselling points for Ms A.'s new drugs
2. What are the problems in this case and what are the possible management options? (Specify the preferred course of action.)
3. If Ms A. later confided in you that she was hoping to become pregnant at some stage, what issues would you want to consider and what advice would you give her?

Answers

1. Ms A. has been newly diagnosed with HIV so may be feeling rather overwhelmed with the implications of her

diagnosis and the amount of information she has been given (particularly around antiretroviral therapy). The main issues presenting here are to counsel her on her new medication and to resolve a number of potential drug interactions. Medication counselling should include:

- what the medication is, and how to take it
- potential side-effects and how to prevent them/what to do/who to contact about them (particularly nausea with Combivir – hence the metoclopramide, which she should take before each dose of Combivir for the first few weeks – and CNS side-effects, such as dizziness and vivid dreams with efavirenz – advise not to drive if affected)
- relevant drug interactions, including effects of recreational drugs and alcohol (also counsel to avoid St John's wort which may decrease efficacy of efavirenz and the oral contraceptive pill), the need for additional barrier contraception and the need to liaise closely with HIV team/DDU about her methadone dose, in case it requires adjustment
- what to do if she misses or is late with a dose, or if she vomits soon after taking a dose
- the importance of a high level of adherence for successful treatment and ways in which your team might be able to support her (e.g. provision of Dosette box, liaison with clinical nurse specialist, etc.).

Given the possibility of an interaction between the efavirenz and methadone, liaise with the DDU to explain that her methadone dose may need to be increased (or split). The most common time for this interaction to become noticeable to the patient is about 2 weeks into therapy.

2. The likely causes of Ms A.'s distress are:

- methadone withdrawal before the next dose is due, because of accelerated metabolism (caused by efavirenz induction of the hepatic enzymes)
- CNS side-effects of efavirenz.

Possible courses of action include:

- Liaise with the DDU to explain the methadone interaction. If patients are not on a programme of supervised administration, they may be able to manage the interaction by keeping the same total dose of methadone, but splitting the administration times (e.g. taking 30 mg twice daily instead of 60 mg once daily). If they are on a supervised programme they will only be able to receive their dose once a day and will not be allowed to keep part of the dose until later. A dose increase is the most appropriate course of action in this case. Explain to the patient that her methadone requirements will not continue to increase and that she can very soon be re-stabilized on a suitable stable dose.
- The CNS side-effects of efavirenz tend to be most pronounced in the first month of therapy and generally improve markedly after that time. Therefore, if Ms A. is able to persevere for another couple of weeks, she should notice an improvement in her symptoms; this simple reassurance may be sufficient. It may be that by resolving the problem of methadone withdrawal, Ms A. will be able to persevere with the other symptoms she is experiencing. However, other palliative options might include the short-term use of a short-acting hypnotic (which may, paradoxically, help counteract the sleep disturbances, though these might also improve with the methadone dose increase). Taking the efavirenz earlier in the evening may help to reduce the 'hangover' effect the next day (particularly if the effects do not begin until several hours after taking the dose).

3. There are many complex issues to consider if Ms A is considering pregnancy and it would be very important for her to discuss them with her HIV physician and/or a specialist in the care of pregnant women with HIV. Issues to consider include:

- the efficacy of the oral contraceptive pill may be reduced by her efavirenz, so until she is planning to conceive, she should use a barrier method as well. This will also protect her and her partner from acquiring new strains of HIV infection from each other (including drug-resistant HIV) as well as other sexually transmitted infections.
- the status of her partner – if he is HIV negative, she may be advised to conceive by artificial insemination, to prevent him becoming infected.
- her drug therapy – while antiretrovirals in the later stages of pregnancy and labour can reduce the transmission of HIV from mother to baby, the potential long-term effects on the fetus/baby of many of the drugs are unknown. Efavirenz has been shown to be teratogenic in cynomolgus monkeys, so many physicians would advise women not to conceive while taking this drug. However, similar teratogenicity studies have not been done on all the other antiretrovirals and there is now increasing 'real-life' experience of women becoming pregnant on efavirenz and other agents. In view of the complexity of the issues and the seriousness of the ramifications, Ms A. would be strongly advised to discuss this with her physician.

Case 39.2

Mr B. was diagnosed HIV positive in 1989 and commenced antiretroviral therapy in 1997, when he had a CD4 count of 126 cells/mm^3 and a viral load (plasma HIV RNA) of 98 743 copies/ml and had just recovered from an episode of cerebral toxoplasmosis. He is still taking his first antiretroviral combination: stavudine 40 mg twice daily, didanosine tablets 400 mg every day, and indinavir 800 mg every 8 hours. He is also taking sulfadiazine 500 mg four times a day, pyrimethamine 25 mg every day, and folinic acid 15 mg three times a week. His most recent blood results showed a CD4 count of 320 cells/mm^3 and a viral load of below 50 copies/ml.

When giving him his medication, you ask him how he is managing with his antiretrovirals and how many doses he has missed or been late with in the last week. He tells you that since going back to work 6 months ago, he is finding it increasingly difficult to adhere to his regimen as well as he had been previously. He admits that he has missed one dose in the last week and has been more than an hour late on one or two other occasions.

Questions

1. How might Mr B.'s treatment be simplified? Give pros and cons for each option.

2. What other strategies might you be able to offer or discuss with him to support him in adhering to his combination therapy?
3. Would your recommendation be different if he had also just been prescribed fenofibrate?

....

Answers

1. Mr B.'s current CD4 count is now well above 200, so one option would be to consider stopping his toxoplasmosis prophylaxis. No clear criteria have been established for doing this, but with a CD4 of 320 and a viral load consistently below detection, all the available evidence indicates that he is at very low risk of relapse if his prophylaxis is discontinued. In addition, his antiretroviral regimen could be simplified. His current combination involves him having to remain fasted (or restricted in what he can eat) for approximately 11 out of every 24 hours. The indinavir must be taken every 8 hours and has to be taken separately from the didanosine, so he must be taking medication on at least 4 occasions during the day. There are a number of options:

   - Change the didanosine from tablets to the enteric coated capsule formulation. Although this still has to be taken on an empty stomach, it can be taken at the same time as the indinavir, potentially reducing the period of dietary restriction and possibly the number of dose times (depending on when he takes his stavudine). Depending on his current routine and whether any of the other options are taken up, this may or may not offer a significant advantage.
   - Use low-dose ritonavir (100 mg twice daily) to pharmacokinetically enhance the indinavir, so that it can be given 12 hourly (800 mg) without any dietary restrictions. This has the advantage of making the regimen significantly simpler but does not involve a major change of drugs. However, even an apparently small change like this can have unforeseen effects (e.g. he may suffer side-effects from the ritonavir or he may get new side-effects from the indinavir, due to the increased drug exposure).
   - Change the indinavir to an alternative agent, either another PI (such as nelfinavir or Kaletra™, which can be given twice daily) or a drug from a different class (e.g. an NNRTI, such as efavirenz). There is always a potential risk when changing to a new drug (particularly of new side-effects). However, this is Mr B.'s first combination and if he is intolerant of the new agent he will not have lost anything, and can always switch back to the indinavir, or try another alternative. The NNRTIs have the advantage of lower pill burden and no dietary restrictions (and possibly a lower risk of metabolic abnormalities).

2. There may be practical support that can be offered or suggested, for example, Dosette box, alarm watch, the Wheel (personal pill planner, accessed via *www.aidsmap.com*). Discussing his changed lifestyle (since returning to work) may highlight relevant issues (e.g. confidentiality, shift work/long hours, irregular routine, difficulty scheduling drugs with dietary restrictions, etc.) which could be discussed with Mr B.
3. If Mr B. has just been started on fenofibrate, one assumes he has raised lipids. Of his current drugs, the one most likely to be the culprit is the indinavir. It may therefore be

prudent to choose a non-PI containing regimen if changes are going to be made. Efavirenz has a higher incidence of lipid abnormalities associated with it than nevirapine, but a change to either of these would probably be preferred to adding in ritonavir or switching to another PI.

Case 39.3

In 1996 a 44-year-old man, who had been diagnosed HIV-positive 6 years earlier, presented with pneumonia which was later confirmed to be PCP. He made a good response to treatment with high-dose co-trimoxazole and was subsequently commenced on dual combination therapy with zidovudine (AZT) and lamivudine (3TC). He remained on this regimen until 1998 when, after experiencing a fall in his CD4 count with a corresponding rise in viral load, he was switched to triple therapy with stavudine (d4T), didanosine (ddI), and efavirenz, on which he has remained ever since. His latest surrogate markers show a CD4 count of 648 cells/mm^3 and a viral load below the limits of detection (< 50 copies/ml). He presents to the HIV department with a 6-week history of feeling generally unwell, with nausea and vomiting for the past 5 days. His examination and initial investigations are unremarkable, except for some mild epigastric tenderness and a slightly elevated urea. His serum amylase is normal. A provisional diagnosis of gastroenteritis is given and he is asked to return 3–5 days later if there is no improvement. He reattends 36 hours later following further clinical deterioration with ongoing vomiting and anorexia. On this occasion, his amylase remains normal and his urea slightly elevated. Arterial blood gases are performed which reveal a metabolic acidosis (pH 7.2 and serum bicarbonate 12 mmol/l).

....

Questions

1. What is the most likely diagnosis for this patient?
2. With what test would you confirm it?
3. List three stages in your immediate management.
4. Are there any additional therapeutic interventions you might consider?

....

Answers

1. The most likely diagnosis is lactic acidosis secondary to nucleoside analogue therapy. This is believed to be a relatively rare though increasingly recognized complication of long-term nucleoside analogue therapy resulting from mitochondrial toxicity.
2. Serum lactate would be elevated (ideally a lactate:pyruvate ratio, but this is difficult to perform in most laboratories).
3. First, admit, since this is a potentially fatal condition and can be complicated by multi-organ failure, including hepatic steatosis.
   Second, stop nucleoside analogue therapy (in consultation with HIV physicians); in cases of simple hyperlactataemia it may be advisable to monitor carefully and continue therapy, but where acidosis is present, discontinuation is currently recommended.
   Third, commence supportive therapy with rehydration and possibly intravenous bicarbonate. Some physicians have

used haemodialysis/haemofiltration, though the place of this in routine practice is unclear.

4. The following agents have been used anecdotally and in case series as adjuvant therapies in this setting, although evidence for a definite therapeutic benefit is limited:

Riboflavin 50 mg daily. N.B. Tablets (50 mg) are unlicensed in the UK.

Nicotinamide. Use vitamin B compound strong tablets and/or Pabrinex™ injection.

Pabrinex™ (intravenous high potency vitamins B and C)

Sodium dichloroacetate (DCA). N.B. This is a laboratory grade chemical, and is not intended for human pharmaceutical use, though a favourable outcome has been reported in at least one case series.

Acetylcarnitine 1 g two or three times daily. N.B. This is unlicensed in the UK.

Case 39.4

A 38-year-old man was diagnosed HIV positive 10 years previously but has experienced no HIV-related symptoms or AIDS defining illnesses. He received 16 months of zidovudine (AZT) monotherapy during 1993/4 as part of the Delta study but subsequently remained off therapy until 1996 when, following a fall in his CD4 count to 240, he was commenced on stavudine (d4T), lamivudine (3TC), and indinavir. His response to this was excellent with a rise in his CD4 count to 520 and a viral load below detection (< 500 copies/ml) when, in 1998, following an admission to hospital with loin pain, his therapy was switched to d4T, 3TC and ritonavir plus saquinavir. Eighteen months later he remains well from an HIV perspective and indeed his most recent results show a CD4 count of 740 and viral load below detection (< 50 copies/ml). At the pharmacy when he is collecting his new prescription he reports to you that he is concerned that he has lost the muscles in his buttocks and arms, and that his face is thinner and he is developing varicose veins. You discuss this with his physician who reports that his latest results show an elevated cholesterol (9.6) and triglycerides (12.4).

Questions

1. Why was this patient's indinavir switched in 1998?
2. What is he now describing to you at the pharmacy?
3. What possible treatment options could you and his clinician discuss with him regarding this?
4. What options would you recommend to his clinician regarding interventions for his hyperlipidaemia?

Answers

1. It is most likely that his loin pain in 1998 was due to indinavir nephrolithiasis. In many cases this is treated with simple rehydration with oral or intravenous fluids, but in some cases (particularly if recurrent or with associated renal dysfunction) switching agents is recommended by some clinicians.

2. He is describing to you the classical features of lipoatrophy, which is part of the lipodystrophy 'syndrome'. It is unlikely that what he is describing is loss of muscle bulk or varicose veins, but rather that he has lost significant subcutaneous adipose tissue.

3. At present our understanding of the lipodystrophy syndrome and its aetiology is limited. The following strategies may be considered:

   a. Simple reassurance. It is believed that the body shape changes in the lipodystrophy syndrome do not impact on morbidity/mortality. However, the significance of the associated lipid abnormalities (see below) is uncertain and the impact on quality of life should not be underestimated.

   b. Switching antiretroviral agents. Numerous switch studies have been performed examining the potential benefits of protease to non-nucleoside or triple nucleoside switching. The results of these studies thus far suggest little, if any, benefit in terms of changes to the features of lipodystrophy.

   c. Stopping antiretroviral therapy. Some patients elect to take breaks from their therapy for reasons of toxicity. There are no data yet to suggest that this results in an improvement of the features of lipodystrophy, and there is a substantial risk of CD4 cell loss with associated disease progression.

   d. Other interventions. The following are currently being investigated for their potential role in the management of lipodystrophy (although none are licensed for this indication): cosmetic agents (e.g. polylactic acid injections); human growth hormone; glitazones.

4. a. Risk reduction. The usual recommendations regarding reduction of other risk factors are equally relevant in this patient group, i.e. smoking cessation, dietary advice, and exercise.

   b. Lipid-lowering agents. The major therapeutic concern is the adjunctive use of statins and antiretroviral agents that affect the cytochrome P450 system (such as, in this case, ritonavir and saquinavir). Therefore many clinicians would advocate the use of fibrates (such as fenofibrate) and possibly pravastatin (which is not P450 metabolized) as agents of choice. Other statins should only be used with caution. The use of glitazones is currently under investigation.

   c. Switching antiretroviral agents (as in answer 3, above). The data here are limited but do suggest that switching proteases to nevirapine (an NNRTI) or abacavir (a nucleoside analogue) may have a beneficial effect on serum lipid levels. However, the possible benefits of this must be weighed against the risks of losing virological control, particularly when this is not the patient's first antiretroviral treatment regimen.

   d. Stopping antiretroviral therapy (as in answer 3, above).

REFERENCES

Bacellar H, Munoz A, Hoover D R et al 1994 Incidence of clinical AIDS conditions in a cohort of homosexual men with CD4 cell counts < 100/mm³. Journal of Infectious Diseases 170: 1284–1287

Bozzette S A, Sattler F R, Chiv J et al 1990 A controlled trial of early adjunctive treatment with corticosteroids for *Pneumocystis carinii* pneumonia in the acquired immunodeficiency syndrome. New England Journal of Medicine 323: 1451–1457

Carr A, Samaras K, Thorlsdottir A et al 1999 Diagnosis, prediction, and natural course of HIV-1 protease inhibitor-associated lipodystrophy, hyperlipidaemia, and diabetes mellitus: a cohort study. Lancet 353: 2093–2099

CASCADE Collaboration 2000 Survival after introduction of HAART in people with known duration of HIV-1 infection. Lancet 355: 1158–1159

Fischl M A, Dickinson G M, LaVoie L 1988 Safety and efficacy of sulfamethoxazole and trimethoprim chemoprophylaxis for *Pneumocystis carinii* pneumonia. Journal of the American Medical Association 259: 1185–1189

Garred P 1998 Chemokine-receptor polymorphisms: clarity or confusion for HIV-1 prognosis. Lancet 351: 14–18

Hammer S M, Squires K E, Hughes M D et al 1997 A controlled trial of two nucleoside analogues plus indinavir in persons with human immunodeficiency virus infection and CD4 cell counts of 200 per cubic millimeter or less. New England Journal of Medicine 337: 725–733

Hirschel B, Lazzarin A, Choppard P et al 1991 A controlled trial of inhaled pentamidine for primary prevention of *Pneumocystis carinii* pneumonia. New England Journal of Medicine 324: 1079–1083

Jacobson M A, O'Donnell J J, Brodie H R et al 1988 Randomized, prospective trial of ganciclovir maintenance therapy for cytomegalovirus retinitis. Journal of Medical Virology 25: 339–349

Leake H, Weston R, Richardson C 1999 Optimising adherence to combination antiretroviral therapy. Hospital Pharmacist 6: 181–183

Mellors J W, Munoz A, Giorgi J V et al 1997 Plasma viral load and CD4 lymphocytes as prognostic markers of HIV-1 infection. Annals of Internal Medicine 126: 946–954

Palella F J Jr, Delaney K M, Moorman A C et al 1998 Declining morbidity and mortality among patients with advanced human immunodeficiency virus infection. New England Journal of Medicine 338: 853–860

Paterson D L, Swindells S, Mohr J et al 2000 Adherence to protease inhibitor therapy and outcomes in patients with HIV infection. Annals of Internal Medicine 133: 21–30

Sherr L 2000 Adherence – sticking to the evidence [editorial comment]. AIDS Care 12: 373–375

FURTHER READING

Bartlett J G The 2002 abbreviated guide to the medical management of HIV infection. Johns Hopkins University, Baltimore (also available online at www.hopkins-aids.edu)

USEFUL WEBSITES

www.aidsmap.com
www.medscape.com
www.hivinsite.ucsf.edu

www.hiv-druginteractions.org
www.hivpharmacology.com
www.hopkins-aids.edu

Fungal infections

40

S. J. Pedler

KEY POINTS

- The triazole antifungals fluconazole and itraconazole provide effective, orally-available treatment for oral and vaginal candidiasis, which were previously treatable only by topical therapy.
- Itraconazole and terbinafine are efficacious, non-toxic alternatives to griseofulvin when systemic treatment of dermatophytosis is required.
- Most therapy for deep-seated fungal infection in the immunocompromised host is empirical in nature due to the difficulties in reaching rapid, accurate diagnosis of systemic fungal infection.
- Lipid-complexed formulations of amphotericin offer a less toxic alternative to conventional amphotericin in the treatment of systemic fungal infection; of these, liposomal amphotericin appears to give the best combination of efficacy and lack of toxicity.
- The imidazoles miconazole and ketoconazole have almost been superseded by the triazoles.
- Fluconazole is used in the treatment of systemic candidiasis, and is an alternative treatment for cryptococcal infection in some patients; however, concerns exist about the increasing prevalence of fluconazole resistance in *Candida* species.
- Itraconazole has applications in the treatment of infections due to the 'pathogenic' fungi, and is a second-line agent in the treatment of aspergillosis.
- New agents such as voriconazole and the echinocandins are alternative antifungal agents currently under development, and the echinocandins may prove useful in the management of aspergillosis.

Fungi are extremely common organisms which are widely distributed in nature. Fortunately, only a tiny minority cause human disease. Such infections fall conveniently into two groups: superficial infections of skin or mucosal surfaces and deep (or systemic) infections.

There are a number of differences between fungi and bacteria. Fungi are eukaryotes (i.e. fungal cells have true nuclei, which bacteria do not), differ in their cell wall constituents, and may produce hyphae (long, branching tubular structures). In addition, yeasts reproduce by budding, a process in which the daughter cell grows as a small bud on the side of the parent, whereas bacteria reproduce by binary fission giving rise to two daughter cells of equal size. These differences are important because as a result fungi are resistant to the action of most antibacterial agents. Fungal cells are closer to mammalian cells than are bacteria, which also reduces the ease of development of drugs with selective toxicity towards fungal rather than host cells.

Fungi causing human disease

Fungi of medical importance can be classified as either yeasts or moulds. Yeasts are unicellular organisms with round or oval cells, while the moulds or filamentous fungi (such as those which grow on decaying organic material) produce hyphae. The hyphae grow and intertwine together producing the familiar fluffy material which is often seen on rotten food; this mass of hyphae is known as a mycelium. The true yeasts include such common yeasts as baker's yeast, while the yeast-like fungi are similar to yeasts but occasionally produce hyphae-like structures (pseudohyphae) as well. This group includes the commonest human fungal pathogen, *Candida albicans*. Finally, there is a group of 'dimorphic' fungi which can exist either as yeasts (at 37°C in the body) or as moulds.

Superficial infections

Superficial *Candida* infections

Epidemiology

C. albicans is a very common yeast-like fungus which forms part of the normal flora of the gastrointestinal tract of virtually all healthy individuals. When infection occurs it is usually endogenous (i.e. the source of the organism is the patient's own flora) although cross-infection leading to outbreaks of candidiasis have been described in hospitals. In addition, there are a number of other species in the genus *Candida*, such as *C. glabrata, C. krusei, C. tropicalis,* etc., which have become increasingly important as some of them have inherent resistance to antifungal agents such as fluconazole.

Superficial candidiasis usually presents as an oral mucositis or as a vaginitis (oral and vaginal thrush) although skin infection and occasionally nail infection may also occur. Predisposing factors for oral candidiasis include the presence of dentures and the use of inhaled steroids for the treatment of asthma. Patients with the acquired immunodeficiency syndrome (AIDS) also have a high incidence of oral candidiasis. Antibiotics (which remove the normal vaginal flora, allowing colonization by *Candida*), diabetes mellitus, pregnancy and oral contraceptives are predisposing factors for vaginal thrush. Candidiasis of the skin usually occurs in moist areas, for example in 'nappy rash', in the perianal region and in intertriginous areas such as skin folds and under the breasts.

Clinical presentation

The usual presentation of oral thrush is a sore mouth, particularly on eating. Examination shows white patches of the fungus on the oral mucosa and tongue (the presence of milk curds in babies' mouths may be similar in appearance); these can be removed leaving a raw, tender, often bleeding surface behind. Vaginal candidiasis usually presents as a vaginal discharge which classically is thick and creamy in nature, often accompanied by itching, which may be severe. Infection of the sexual partner may occur which may be asymptomatic or lead to a balanitis (inflammation of the glans penis).

Infection of the skin causes an inflamed, itching area of skin with pustules, maceration, and fissuring of the skin. Nail involvement may present as infection of the subcutaneous tissue around and under the nail (*Candida* paronychia), which is often seen in people whose hands are frequently immersed in water, or as infection of the nail itself (onychomycosis).

More severe mucosal infection may occur in immunocompromised patients, particularly in patients with AIDS in whom oesophageal candidiasis is common. This condition presents with difficulty and pain on swallowing, and endoscopy is usually required to confirm the diagnosis.

Diagnosis

The diagnosis of oral or vaginal candidiasis is usually made clinically but can be confirmed easily by taking a swab of the affected area. Microscopy of the specimen shows large numbers of yeast cells and pseudohyphae, and culture will readily yield the organism. Skin and nail infections may be confused with other infections and conditions such as eczema, and culture should always be performed. For superficial infections in immunocompetent hosts, further species differentiation and antifungal sensitivity testing is not usually required, but in immunodeficient patients or those who have been exposed to antifungals previously, this may be required in case the infecting strain possesses intrinsic or acquired resistance.

Treatment

Oral and vaginal candidiasis may be treated by either topical or systemic antifungal agents. The drugs currently available for topical use fall into two groups, the polyenes (of which only amphotericin and nystatin are used clinically) and the imidazoles, of which several are available including econazole, clotrimazole and miconazole. The two triazoles (fluconazole and itraconazole) can be given systemically by mouth. Skin infections may also be treated topically but nail infections are unlikely to respond to a topical antifungal agent and may need systemic treatment. Oesophagitis will invariably require systemic treatment.

Topical treatment. The polyenes are broad-spectrum antifungal agents which are virtually insoluble in water and which are not absorbed from the gastrointestinal tract or from skin or mucous membranes. Both nystatin and amphotericin (but particularly nystatin) are available in a wide range of formulations including pessaries, creams, gels, tablets, pastilles, etc. The choice of formulation clearly depends on the site of infection. Nystatin is also available in combination with steroids (which may be useful in relieving associated inflammation and itching in skin infections) and antibiotics such as tetracycline and bacitracin.

Very little in the way of unwanted effects occurs with these agents, but in mixed formulations the effects of the other components must also be taken into account. They are safe for use in pregnancy.

The imidazoles also have a broad antifungal spectrum and are also active against some Gram-positive bacteria. Once again, they are available in a wide variety of formulations and may be combined with steroids. Absorption when taken by mouth or from mucosal surfaces is minimal, but detectable serum levels are present after oral administration (particularly with miconazole). Unwanted effects are few; the imidazoles are fetotoxic in high doses in laboratory animals but this has never been shown to occur in pregnant women.

Is there any clinical difference between the polyenes and the imidazoles? For the therapy of oral thrush, the two groups seem equally efficacious. In vaginal candidiasis, although there are no direct comparisons in clinical trials, the imidazoles seem to be more effective (cure rates of 90% versus 80% for the polyenes have been quoted).

Systemic treatment. Two triazole agents are available for the treatment of oral and vaginal candidiasis. These compounds, fluconazole and itraconazole, are discussed in detail below.

Fluconazole is highly effective in vaginal candidiasis giving similar cure rates to topical therapy. However, many patients find oral fluconazole preferable to topical therapy for reasons of convenience, as it is given as a single dose of 150 mg. Itraconazole is also effective in vaginal candidiasis, given as two oral doses of 200 mg 12 hours apart. In oral candidiasis, fluconazole therapy would usually be considered only after failure of topical therapy or in difficult clinical conditions such as patients with human immunodeficiency virus (HIV) infection. Typical doses would be 50–100 mg daily for 7–14 days.

Candida balanitis can also be treated with topical polyenes or imidazoles, or with systemic fluconazole in the same dose as for vaginal infection. It is sometimes stated that when treating a woman with vaginal candidiasis the male partner should be treated simultaneously in order to prevent reinfection. Although there is no evidence to support this approach, it may be considered in women who suffer from repeated vaginal candidiasis.

Dermatophytosis

Epidemiology and causative organisms

Dermatophytosis, or tinea, is a condition caused by three genera of dermatophyte fungi, *Trichophyton, Epidermophyton* and *Microsporum*. Unlike *Candida* these are filamentous fungi (moulds) which have a predilection for keratinized tissue (i.e. skin, nail and hair). These fungi are very widely distributed throughout the world and may be acquired from the soil, from animals, or from humans infected with the fungus.

Clinical features

The classical clinical presentation of dermatophyte infection of the skin is ringworm, a circular, inflamed lesion with a raised edge and associated skin scaling. However, presentation is influenced by the site of infection and by the actual species of fungus causing the infection. In general, less severe lesions are produced by human fungal strains, while those acquired from animals can produce quite intense inflammatory reactions.

Dermatophytosis of the nail results in thickened, discoloured nails while in the scalp infection presents with itching, skin scaling and inflammation, and patchy hair loss (alopecia).

Diagnosis

The diagnosis of dermatophyte infection is confirmed by collecting appropriate specimens such as material from infected nails and skin. The fungi can be seen microscopically after the material is cleared in 10% potassium hydroxide. Specimens may also be cultured but sensitivity testing is not required.

Treatment

As with superficial *Candida* infections, dermatophytosis can be treated either topically or systemically.

Topical therapy. This is most appropriate for small or medium areas of skin infection. Larger areas, or nail or hair infection should be treated with a systemic agent. The most commonly used agents are the imidazoles, of which a wide variety is available, including clotrimazole, econazole, miconazole, sulconazole, and tioconazole. There is nothing to choose between these agents all of which are usually applied twice daily, continuing for up to 2 weeks after the lesions have healed. Side-effects are uncommon and usually consist of mild skin irritation. Other topical agents include amorolfine, terbinafine, and tolnaftate.

Griseofulvin. The first orally administered treatment for dermatophytosis was griseofulvin, which has now been available for over 30 years. Griseofulvin is active only against dermatophyte fungi and is inactive against all other fungi and bacteria. In order to exert its antifungal effect it must be incorporated into keratinous tissue (where levels are much greater than serum levels) and therefore it has no effect if used topically.

The usual adult dose is 500–1000 mg daily, given in one dose or divided doses if required. Griseofulvin is well absorbed and absorption is enhanced if taken with a high-fat meal. In children it may be given with milk. A 1000 mg dose produces a peak serum level of about 1–2 mg/l after 4 hours, with a half-life of at least 9 hours. There is also an ultra-fine preparation of griseofulvin which is almost totally absorbed and permits the use of lower doses (typically 330–660 mg daily). This preparation is not available in the UK. Elimination is mainly through the liver, and inactive metabolites are excreted in the urine. Less than 1% of a dose is excreted in urine in the active form but some active drug is excreted in the faeces.

The duration of treatment with griseofulvin is dependent entirely on clinical response. Skin or hair infection usually requires 4–12 weeks therapy but nail infections respond much more slowly; 6 months treatment is often required for fingernails, a year or more for toenail infections. Unfortunately the rate of treatment failure or relapse in nail infection is high, and may reach up to 60%.

Because of this high failure rate, other agents have been sought. Ketoconazole is an alternative to griseofulvin, but concern about side-effects such as hepatotoxicity and interference with testosterone synthesis has led to its replacement by itraconazole, which has been shown to be an effective, well tolerated treatment for dermatophyte infections including those in which griseofulvin therapy has failed. Compared to griseofulvin, shorter treatment courses (3–6 months) in nail infections are also possible with itraconazole.

Unfortunately it is not licensed for hair infection (tinea capitis) at present. This drug is described in more detail later in this chapter.

Terbinafine. Terbinafine is the first member of a new class of antifungal agents, the allylamines, to become available for systemic use. These agents act by inhibition of the fungal enzyme squalene epoxidase, an enzyme involved in the synthesis of ergosterol, an essential component of the fungal cytoplasmic membrane. Although terbinafine has a very broad antifungal spectrum in the laboratory, its in vivo efficacy does not correspond to its in vitro activity, and it is used only for the treatment of dermatophyte infection. About 70% of an oral dose is absorbed, and the drug appears in high concentrations in the skin. The half-life is about 16–17 hours, and therefore the drug can be given once per day. Terbinafine is metabolized in the liver and the metabolites are excreted in the urine, so that hepatic or renal dysfunction will prolong the elimination half-life. The usual dose is 250 mg once daily; the duration of treatment will vary depending on the site of infection, but as with itraconazole, in the treatment of nail infections much shorter courses of treatment can be given, compared to griseofulvin. It is not licensed for the treatment of dermatophytosis of the scalp and hair (tinea capitis) although clinical trial evidence (e.g. Caceres-Rios et al 2000) would indicate that it is at least as effective as griseofulvin. However, some authors disagree and continue to recommend griseofulvin as the treatment of choice in tinea captitis (Bennett et al 2000).

The main drug interactions with these agents are shown in Table 40.1. Side-effects are shown in Table 40.2. Griseofulvin is teratogenic in animals and is contraindicated in pregnancy and in severe liver disease.

Pityriasis versicolor

Causative organism

This is a common skin infection caused by a yeast-like fungus, *Malassezia furfur*. The organism is a member of the normal skin flora, and lives only on the skin because it has a growth requirement for medium-chain fatty acids present in sebum.

Clinical features

The condition usually appears as patches scattered over the trunk, neck, and shoulders. These patches produce scales and may be pigmented in light-skinned individuals, appearing light brown in colour. In dark-skinned patients, the lesions may lose pigment and appear lighter than normal skin.

In some patients, this yeast is also associated with dandruff and seborrhoeic dermatitis, although the exact role of the yeast in causing this condition remains uncertain. In AIDS patients, seborrhoeic dermatitis may be quite extensive and sudden in onset.

Diagnosis

The diagnosis is made by microscopy of scrapings from the lesion. The specimen is examined for the presence of yeast cells and short hyphae. Culture is not usually required for diagnosis, and since it requires special culture media is not routinely attempted.

Treatment

Pityriasis versicolor is treated with a topical agent such as 2% selenium sulphide, topical terbinafine, or a topical imidazole such as clotrimazole, econazole or miconazole. Relapses are common and treatment may need to be repeated. In severe cases, oral itraconazole (200 mg once daily for 7 days) may be given.

Fungal ear infection

Fungi sometimes infect the external auditory canal causing otitis externa, the most common causative organisms being various species of *Aspergillus* (such as *A. niger* and *A. fumigatus*) and *Candida albicans* and other *Candida* species. A variety of other fungi found in the environment can also cause this condition. The use of topical antibacterial agents in the ear may predispose to local fungal infection.

Clinical features

Fungal infection of the ear usually presents as pain and itching in the auditory canal, sometimes with a reduction in hearing due to blockage of the canal. There may be an associated discharge from the ear. Clinical examination shows a swollen red canal, and the fungal mycelium is sometimes visible as an amorphous white or grey mass.

Diagnosis

The diagnosis of a fungal infection of the external canal can be made by microscopy and culture of material obtained from the ear.

Treatment

Aural toilet with removal of obstructing debris is very important in the management of this condition. A topical antifungal agent such as nystatin, amphotericin, or an imidazole can also be applied.

Table 40.1   Interactions of antifungal agents with other drugs[a]

Drug	Interaction with	Result
Terfenadine and other antihistamines	Imidazoles and triazoles	Increased plasma concentration of astermizole and terfenadine, leading to cardiac arrhythmias
Any nephrotoxic agent	Amphotericin B	Enhanced nephrotoxicity
Cimetidine	Terbinafine	Increased plasma concentration of terbinafine
Ciclosporin	Ketoconazole, itraconazole (possibly fluconazole also, especially in doses of 200 mg per day or higher)	Increased ciclosporin concentration (due to reduced ciclosporin metabolism)
Didanosine	Itraconazole	Reduced absorption of itraconazole (avoid simultaneous administration)
Digoxin	Itraconazole	Increased plasma digoxin concentration
H_2 antagonists	Itraconazole	Reduced absorption of itraconazole
Midazolam	Ketoconazole, itraconazole, fluconazole	Increased plasma midazolam concentration leading to prolonged sedation
Oral contraceptives	Griseofulvin (possibly imidazoles and triazoles also)	Reduced contraceptive efficacy (induces liver enzymes which metabolize the oral contraceptive)
Phenytoin	Ketoconazole	Enhanced effect of phenytoin; plus possibly reduced ketoconazole concentration
	Fluconazole	Enhanced effect of phenytoin
	Itraconazole	Reduced plasma itraconazole concentration
Rifabutin	Fluconazole	Increased plasma concentration of rifabutin leading to an increased risk of uveitis
Rifampicin	Imidazoles and triazoles	Reduced plasma imidazole/triazole concentration (rifampicin induces more rapid metabolism)
Simvastatin and other statins	Imidazoles and triazoles (especially itraconazole)	Increased risk of myopathy
Sulphonylureas	Imidazoles and triazoles	Enhanced effects of sulphonylureas
Tacrolimus	Fluconazole	Inhibition of metabolism of tacrolimus leading to increased plasma concentration
Warfarin	Griseofulvin	Reduced anticoagulant effect (induces liver enzymes which metabolize warfarin)
	Imidazoles and triazoles	Enhanced anticoagulant effect (may displace warfarin from serum albumin binding sites and inhibit metabolism of warfarin)
Zidovudine	Fluconazole	Inhibition of metabolism of zidovudine leading to increased plasma concentration

[a] The table shows major interactions of the antifungal agents; however, this is not a complete list (see other sources, e.g. *British National Formulary*).

Table 40.2   Side-effects of antifungal agents

Drug	Side-effects
Griseofulvin	Mild: headache, gastrointestinal side-effects. Hypersensitivity reactions such as skin rashes, including photosensitivity Moderate: exacerbation of acute intermittent porphyria; rarely, precipitation of systemic lupus erythematosus. Contraindicated in both these conditions
Terbinafine	Usually mild: nausea, abdominal pain; allergic skin reactions; loss and disturbance of sense of taste
Amphotericin	Immediate reactions (during infusion) include headache, pyrexia, rigors, nausea, vomiting, hypotension; occasionally these can be severe. Thrombophlebitis after the infusion is very common Nephrotoxicity Anaemia due to reduced erythropoiesis Peripheral neuropathy (rare) Cardiac failure (this is exacerbated by hypokalemia due to nephrotoxicity) Immunomodulation (the drug can both enhance and inhibit some immunological functions)
Flucytosine	Mild: gastrointestinal side-effects (nausea, vomiting). Occasional skin rashes Moderate: myelosuppression. Hepatotoxicity
Ketoconazole	Mild: nausea, vomiting; occasional skin rashes Moderate: reduced testosterone levels; reduced plasma cortisol levels (but this may not be clinically significant) Severe: hepatotoxicity, although usually confined to elevated liver enzymes, can lead to frank jaundice and possibly fatal hepatotoxicity
Fluconazole	Mild: nausea, vomiting and occasional skin rashes; occasionally elevated liver enzymes (reversible)
Itraconazole	Mild: nausea and abdominal pain; occasional skin rashes

Deep-seated fungal infections

Most deep-seated or systemic fungal infections seen in the UK are the result of some breakdown in the normal body defences, which may be due to disease or medical treatment. There are however a group of fungi (often referred to rather misleadingly as the 'pathogenic' fungi) which are able to cause systemic infection in a previously healthy person. These infections, which include diseases such as histoplasmosis, blastomycosis, and coccidioidomycosis, are rare in the UK but rather more common in the USA and some other parts of the world. They will not be discussed further in this chapter.

Fungal infections in the compromised host

Epidemiology and predisposing factors

There are a large number of conditions which may predispose the individual to systemic or deep-seated fungal infection. These are summarized in Table 40.3. Fungal urinary tract infection is particularly common in catheterized patients who have received broad-spectrum antibiotics, while total parenteral nutrition (TPN) is strongly associated with fungemia, sometimes with unusual fungi such as *Malassezia furfur*, which is associated with the use of intravenous lipid infusions due to the growth requirement of this organism for fatty acids. Most cases of systemic fungal infection, however, are associated with some defect in the patient's immune system, and the nature of the organisms encountered is often related to the nature of the immunosupression. Neutropenia, for example, is usually associated with *Candida* species, *Aspergillus* and mucormycosis, while defects of cell-mediated immunity (for example HIV infection) is strongly associated with *Cryptococcus* infection.

Causative fungi

Many different fungi have been described as causing systemic fungal infection but the commonest organisms encountered and the conditions they cause are listed in Table 40.4 and of these *Candida* and *Aspergillus* are by far the most common.

Clinical presentation

Deep-seated fungal infection can present in a large number of different ways. The most common

Table 40.3 Conditions predisposing to systemic or deep-seated fungal infection

Infection	Predisposing conditions
Systemic candidiasis	Neutropenia from any cause (disease or treatment) Use of broad-spectrum antibiotics which eliminate the normal body flora Indwelling intravenous cannulae, especially when used for total parenteral nutrition Haematological malignancy Organ transplantation AIDS (particularly associated with severe mucocutaneous infection) Intravenous drug abuse Cardiac surgery and heart valve replacement, leading to *Candida* endocarditis Gastrointestinal tract surgery
Aspergillosis	Neutropenia from any cause, especially if severe and prolonged Acute leukemia Organ transplantation Chronic granulomatous disease of childhood (defect in neutrophil function) Pre-existing lung disease (usually leads to aspergillomas – fungus balls in the lung – rather than invasive or disseminated infection)
Cryptococcosis	AIDS Systemic therapy with corticosteriods Renal transplantation Hodgkin's disease and other lymphomas Sarcoidosis Collagen vascular diseases
Mucormycosis	Diabetic hyperglycaemic ketoacidosis (leading to rhinocerebral infection) Severe, prolonged neutropenia Burns (leading to cutaneous infection)

Table 40.4 The common causes of systemic and deep-seated fungal infection

Condition/organism	Common clinical presentations
Candidiasis (*Candida albicans, C. glabrata, C. krusei, C. tropicalis*, other *Candida* species),	Fungemia Colonization of intravenous cannulae Pneumonia Meningitis Bone and joint infections Endocarditis Endophthalmitis Peritonitis in chronic ambulatory peritoneal dialysis
Aspergillosis (*Aspergillus fumigatus, A. flavus*, other *Aspergillus* species)	Invasive pulmonary aspergillosis Disseminated aspergillosis Aspergilloma Endocarditis
Cryptococcosis (*Cryptococcus neoformans*)	Meningitis Pneumonia Cutaneous infection
Mucormycosis (various species of the genera *Rhizopus, Absidia*, and *Mucor*)	Rhinocerebral infection Pulmonary mucormycosis Cutaneous infection (especially in burns patients)
Malassezia furfur	Fungemia associated with total parenteral nutrition

presentation is as a fungemia, with fever, low blood pressure and sometimes the other features of septic shock. Relatively low-grade fungemias (for example, those associated with TPN) often present only with fever. Both *Candida* and *Aspergillus* infection may present as fungal pneumonia, but disseminated infection is quite common and multiple organ systems may be involved, particularly in *Candida* infection. Central nervous system infection, endocarditis, endophthalmitis, skin infections, renal disease and bone and joint infection are all well-recognized manifestations of disseminated candidiasis.

Cryptococcosis most frequently presents as a chronic, insidious meningitis and occasionally as pneumonia or skin infection (especially in AIDS patients). This condition is one of the most common and important fungal infections associated with AIDS, and relapses following treatment are common in HIV-infected patients, leading to a requirement for long-term maintenance treatment. The most common presentation of mucormycosis is as rhinocerebral infection. Initially an infection of the sinuses, it then spreads locally to the palate, orbit, and eventually into the brain, leading to encephalitis. Pulmonary infection, and in burns patients cutaneous infection, may also occur.

Diagnostic measures

Unfortunately the diagnosis of deep-seated fungal infection is difficult and is often only made post mortem. Systemic candidiasis may be diagnosed by isolation of the organism from blood culture and culture of other appropriate specimens. *Cryptococcus neoformans* grows readily on laboratory media and can be isolated from blood and cerebrospinal fluid; a simple test for the detection of cryptococcal antigen in CSF and serum is also available. Aspergillosis is rarely, if ever, diagnosed from blood culture but the organism can occasionally be isolated from sputum; however, bronchoalveolar lavage or open lung biopsy are the best techniques for the diagnosis of pulmonary aspergillosis. Although much work has been carried out in recent years on the diagnosis of both candidiasis and aspergillosis by detection of circulating antigens or metabolites, or the use of molecular biology techniques such as the polymerase chain reaction (PCR), these techniques are not yet available for use in routine microbiology laboratories. Mucormycosis is most readily diagnosed by histological examination of tissue biopsies since the organism is rarely cultured from clinical specimens.

Drug treatment

The difficulties in making the diagnosis of deep fungal infection are accompanied by a scarcity of effective antifungal agents for systemic use. At the present time only four agents are routinely available, although others are being developed. Ketoconazole should now be regarded as essentially obsolete for the treatment of systemic fungal infection, although it retains some specialized uses. The four available agents are discussed below.

Amphotericin B

General properties. Amphotericin is a member of the polyene group of antibiotics, which are obtained from various species of *Streptomyces*. There are a number of different polyenes but for various reasons (lack of stability or solubility, or excessive toxicity) only amphotericin is used systemically. Nystatin is only used topically.

The chemical structure of amphotericin is that of a macrolide carbon ring containing 37 carbon atoms and closed by a lactone bond. The molecule contains seven carbon-to-carbon double bonds (hence the name 'polyene' for this group of compounds) which are all situated on one side of the molecule while the other side contains seven hydroxyl groups. The molecule is therefore amphipathic (or amphoteric) in nature and this may be of some importance in the mode of action of all the polyenes. The polyenes all have very limited solubility in water and organic non-polar solvents such as acetone, but will readily dissolve in organic polar solvents such as dimethylsulphoxide. In water, amphotericin forms a colloidal suspension of micelles, which is rendered more stable if a surfactant such as sodium desoxycholate is added.

The mode of action of the polyenes is to increase the permeability of the cytoplasmic membrane leading to leakage of the cell contents and eventually death. This action is dependent on binding of the antibiotic to sterols present in the cell membrane and organisms (such as bacteria) which do not contain sterols are inherently resistant to the polyenes. The different polyenes have differing affinities for sterols, and amphotericin has a higher affinity for ergosterol (present in fungal cytoplasmic membranes) than cholesterol, which is found in mammalian cell membranes. This fact presumably explains the selective toxicity of amphotericin for fungal cells. Acquired resistance to amphotericin during or following treatment is rarely a clinical problem, although it has been described, and very few fungi are inherently resistant to this agent.

Amphotericin is active against almost all the fungi which commonly cause systemic mycoses. It is synergistic in vitro with other agents such as flucytosine and rifampicin and in some cases (e.g. amphotericin plus flucytosine in candidiasis or cryptococcosis) this synergistic interaction appears to be of clinical significance. The results of combination with the imidazoles is less certain, and both synergy and antagonism have been described.

Conventional amphotericin. The pharmacokinetics of amphotericin are unusual. A 50 mg dose produces a peak serum level of 0.5–3.5 mg/l, but the level cannot be related to clinical response. Amphotericin penetrates poorly into cerebrospinal fluid (CSF) and is heavily (99%) protein bound. Initial elimination of the drug occurs with a half-life of 24–48 hours, but this is followed by very slow elimination (half-life about 2 weeks) and the drug may take several weeks to disappear completely. This may result from strong binding to cell membrances with a gradual elution over a period of weeks. Repeated doses of the drug do not cause accumulation in serum. A small fraction (perhaps 3%) of a dose is excreted in the urine, so that renal dysfunction does not affect serum levels, and the rest appears to be inactivated in the body. The measurement of serum levels of amphotericin is not clinically helpful.

Amphotericin is administered by slow intravenous infusion. If the drug is added to electrolyte solutions or solutions with a low pH it will precipitate out, so it must always be given in 5% dextrose. Since some commercial dextrose solutions have a surprisingly low pH, presumably due to slight caramelization of the dextrose during manufacture, it may be advisable to add a small amount of a buffer to dextrose solutions before adding amphotericin. Several different dosage schedules have been suggested; the two schedules given in Table 40.5 have been used successfully. The doses shown are for adults and would need to be modified for children. Although the need for a test dose has been disputed, the manufacturers currently recommend that before commencing treatment, a 1 mg test dose be given in 50 ml of 5% dextrose over a 2–4 hour period and the patient monitored for serious side-effects (such as fever, rigors and hypotension) during that time. If the patient tolerates the test dose, there are two options. The first is designed to minimize serious side-effects by a gradual build-up to

Table 40.5   Suggested dosage schedules for conventional (not lipid-complexed formulations) amphotericin B

Regimen 1 For use in a patient with a non-life-threatening, deep-seated infection			
Dose	Volume of infusion	Day	Duration of infusion
1 mg (test dose)	50 ml	1	2 hours
If no intolerable side-effects or anaphylactic reaction follow 2 hours later with:			
10 mg	500 ml	1	6 hours
Then on each successive day, increase dose by 10 mg to standard 50 mg daily dose:			
20 mg	500 ml	2	6 hours
30 mg	1000 ml	3	6 hours
40 mg	1000 ml	4	6 hours
50 mg	1000 ml	5 et seq.	6 hours
Regimen 2 For use in a compromised patient with a life-threatening infection			
Dose	Volume of infusion	Day	Duration of infusion
1 mg (test dose)	50 ml	1	2 hours
If no intolerable side-effects or anaphylactic reaction follow 2 hours later with:			
25 mg	1000 ml	1	6 hours
Leave a 6 hour interval then administer the remainder of the 50 mg daily dose:			
25 mg	1000 ml	1	6 hours
50 mg	1000 ml	2 et seq.	6 hours

Notes

1. 50 mg represents a dose of about 0.7 mg/kg for a 70 kg adult. It may not be possible to achieve this dose, depending on the side-effects. In this case the highest dose which does not produce unacceptable side-effects should be given.
2. Alternate day treatment with a higher unit dose (up to a maximum unit dose of 1.5 mg/kg) may be given. This has the advantage of allowing the patient to attend for out-patient therapy. If the patient is still in hospital it will reduce the amount of time needed for amphotericin administration, which otherwise makes heavy use of intravenous access time that may be needed for other purposes.

the usual maximum daily dose of 1 mg/kg body weight, not exceeding 50 mg in total. This is satisfactory if the infection is not immediately life-threatening but would be inappropriate for fulminating infections. In such cases the dose is increased rapidly with careful monitoring of the patient by medical staff.

It is also possible to give amphotericin intrathecally in very small doses (0.1–0.5 mg) although this is rarely done since the advent of the triazoles for the treatment of fungal infections of the CNS. In catheterized patients with fungal urinary tract infection treatment is usually not indicated unless the patient is symptomatic, but, if required, amphotericin can be given as a bladder washout in a concentration of 50 mg/l.

Amphotericin is associated with a long list of toxic effects (see Table 40.2). It is possible to try to minimize the immediate side-effects during the infusion by administering 25–50 mg of hydrocortisone, and antiemetics and an antihistamine may also be given. Nephrotoxicity is the most serious side-effect of amphotericin, and is almost invariable in patients given a full course of treatment. Renal function should be monitored regularly (at least every other day) and if the plasma creatinine exceeds 250 mol/l the drug should be discontinued until the creatinine level falls below this limit. Hypokalemia is also a problem and may be severe, necessitating replacement therapy. Fortunately, renal function returns to normal in most patients unless very large total doses have been given. There is little experience of the use of amphotericin in pregnancy, but what there is indicates that the risk of fetal toxicity is small (Pedler & Orr 2000).

The duration of therapy is guided by clinical response. There is some evidence that the total dose administered is of some importance in determining response, and for an established deep-seated infection a total dose of 1.5–2 g would be appropriate. This represents at least 6 weeks of therapy at 50 mg/day. The patient may be well enough to attend for treatment on an out-patient basis, in which case the drug can be given in a higher unit dose on alternate days. However, a maximum alternate daily dose of 1.5 mg/kg should not be exceeded. For fungemia due to infected intravenous cannulae the main therapeutic action is removal of the cannula, since the use of antifungal agents cannot be relied upon to eliminate the fungus from the cannula. However, they should still be given to prevent disseminated infection elsewhere in the body. There is no consensus about the length of therapy in such patients but 1 week's treatment (full dose) has been suggested.

Amphotericin B lipid formulations. As a result of the toxicity of amphotericin B, considerable work has been carried out in the development of delivery systems in which amphotericin is encapsulated in liposomes or as a complex with lipid molecules. The advantages of these methods of delivery are that a higher unit dose may be given and there is a reduction in toxic effects. Three such preparations are currently available: liposomal amphotericin B (AmBisome), amphotericin B lipid complex (Abelcet) and amphotericin B colloidal dispersion (Amphocil).

In liposomal amphotericin B, the drug is contained in small vesicles each consisting of a phospholipid bilayer enclosing an aqueous environment. This permits the delivery of higher doses (3 mg/kg is recommended, but higher doses have been used in some centres) compared to conventional amphotericin, with very little of the immediate toxicity which is such a problem with the conventional formulation. Higher peak serum concentrations are obtained with the liposomal formulation compared to equivalent doses of the conventional drug, although it is not certain if this is clinically relevant. Liposomal amphotericin is concentrated mainly in the liver and spleen, where it is taken up by cells of the reticuloendothelial system. Concentrations in the lung and kidneys are much lower, which may or may not be clinically important.

There is reduced nephrotoxicity with this formulation, and some of the renal dysfunction which has been described in clinical trials of liposomal amphotericin may have been due to concomitant drugs. Unfortunately there is a lack of data from randomized, comparative clinical trials of liposomal amphotericin versus conventional amphotericin B, and much of the supportive evidence for liposomal amphotericin, indicating that it is effective and well tolerated in patients who have not responded to, or who have not been able to tolerate, the conventional drug, is anecdotal. The majority of the clinical trial work with this agent has been performed in febrile neutropenic patients rather than in proven fungal infection. However, currently available evidence is that the drug is at least as effective as conventional amphotericin B in confirmed or suspected systemic fungal infection, and possesses a much-reduced rate of immediate side-effects and nephrotoxicity. It is this comparative lack of toxicity which accounts for much of the popularity of this agent, despite its expense.

Amphotericin B lipid complex is not a liposomal formulation, but consists of large sheets of amphotericin combined with phospholipids. This formulation gives lower peak serum levels compared to the conventional drug because it is rapidly taken up by tissue macrophages, and patients seem to experience more immediate side-effects than with liposomal amphotericin. Again, clinical trial evidence is not abundant. Amphotericin B colloidal dispersion is a formulation consisting of tiny discs of amphotericin and cholesterylsuphate. It too produces low peak serum levels compared to the conventional drug. There is less clinical experience with this formulation than with the other two lipid preparations.

Which of these agents should be chosen for routine use? Unfortunately, there are no clinical data for comparative trials between the different lipid formulations. At the present time, the greatest clinical experience is with liposomal amphotericin B. In most centres in the UK, this is the preferred agent of the three, but a disadvantage is its cost; for that reason, its use should probably be reserved for those patients who fail to respond to conventional amphotericin (in whom the higher doses possible with the liposomal formulation might be effective) or those who suffer severe side-effects from conventional therapy. (For a detailed comparison of these agents, see Wong-Beringer et al 1998).

Flucytosine

Mode of action and spectrum of activity. Another useful agent for systemic fungal infection is flucytosine (5-fluorocytosine), a synthetic fluorinated pyrimidine analogue. The mode of action is twofold. Following uptake by the cell, which is dependent on the presence of cytosine permease, flucytosine is deaminated to 5-fluorouracil by cytosine deaminase. This in turn is incorporated into fungal RNA in place of uracil, leading to impairment of protein synthesis. Further metabolism of 5-fluorouracil leads to a metabolite which inhibits the enzyme thymidylate synthetase, in turn leading to inhibition of DNA synthesis. Mammalian cells have absent or weak cytosine deaminase activity which accounts for the selective toxicity of flucytosine.

For all practical purposes flucytosine is only active against yeasts and yeast-like fungi. Inherent resistance occurs in perhaps 10% of clinical isolates of *Candida* species and acquired resistance develops rapidly if the drug is used alone. There are several resistance mechanisms, some of which result from a single-step mutation giving a high frequency of secondary resistance in organisms exposed to the drug. For this reason flucytosine should always be given in combination with another agent such as amphotericin, with which it is synergistic.

Pharmacokinetics. Flucytosine is highly soluble in water and over 90% of an oral dose is absorbed from the gastrointestinal tract. Virtually all of the absorbed dose is excreted unchanged in the urine by glomerular filtration. The elimination half-life is about 4 hours, but this is greatly prolonged in renal failure and dosage modification is required in patients with renal dysfunction. The degree of protein binding is very low and flucytosine penetrates well into all tissues including the aqueous humour of the eye (where about 10% of the serum level is achieved) and the CSF (about 80% of the serum level).

Flucytosine is given orally or by a short intravenous infusion and the dose by either route in patients with normal renal function is 150–200 mg/kg/day in four divided doses. This must be reduced in renal failure, but the degree of reduction depends on the degree of renal impairment and it is obligatory to monitor the serum levels of flucytosine. Unfortunately flucytosine assay is now rarely carried out in routine laboratories in the UK and is usually performed in a reference laboratory. It must be remembered that flucytosine is often given in conjunction with amphotericin which will probably cause some degree of renal dysfunction. To avoid dose-related marrow toxicity (see below) the peak serum level (obtained at 1 hour after an intravenous dose or 2 hours after an oral dose) should be maintained in the range 25–50 mg/l and should not be allowed to exceed 80 mg/l. Haemodialysis readily removes flucytosine and patients on dialysis can be treated by giving a single dose of 25 mg/kg after each episode of dialysis.

Side-effects. The side-effects of flucytosine are given in Table 40.2. The most important toxic effect is a dose-related myelosuppression with neutropenia and thrombocytopenia. This is usually reversible and can be avoided by monitoring serum levels of flucytosine and adjusting the dose accordingly. Hepatotoxicity is also probably a result of high serum levels, and liver function tests should be performed regularly. The drug is teratogenic in some animals and is not recommended in pregnant women for relatively trivial infections such as fungal urinary tract infection. In cases of life-threatening fungal infection (which is very rare in pregnancy) the potential benefits of flucytosine must be weighed against the possible risks.

The imidazoles

Mode of action and spectrum of activity. Currently the only imidazole compound available in the UK for the treatment of systemic fungal infection is ketoconazole, although the related triazoles have all but replaced ketoconazole for the treatment of systemic fungal infection. The basic chemical structure of the imidazoles is the azole ring, a five-membered ring containing two nitrogen atoms. The triazoles also contain the azole ring but with three nitrogen atoms.

The main mode of action of the imidazoles and triazoles is by inhibition of the synthesis of ergosterol, which is an important component of the cytoplasmic membrane in fungal but not in mammalian cells. One of the nitrogen atoms of the azole ring binds to the iron atom of cytochrome P450 and inhibits its activation. Ergosterol synthesis is dependent on cytochrome P450 activation and as a result its production is impaired. These agents also damage the cytoplasmic membrane directly but this is only achieved at higher concentrations.

Ketoconazole has a broad spectrum of activity, including most yeasts and yeast-like fungi, the dimorphic fungi, and the dermatophytes. Filamentous fungi causing systemic infection are variable in sensitivity and in vitro activity is not always accompanied by an in vivo response. Naturally occurring resistance is rare but it can occasionally develop in patients given the drug.

Pharmacokinetics. Ketoconazole is only available in an oral preparation, but it is not soluble in water unless the pH is less than 3 and the presence of gastric acid is therefore required for optimal absorption. The concomitant use of antacids or H_2 antagonists will reduce the absorption of ketoconazole. The drug is lipophilic and absorption is improved if taken with food. Protein binding is high (99%) and since only a small amount is excreted in the urine, dose adjustment in renal failure is not required. The elimination half-life is about 8–10 hours, and the majority of a dose of ketoconazole is excreted in the faeces as active drug and inactive metabolites. The standard adult dose is 200 mg once daily, but this can be increased to 400 mg daily if required.

Side-effects. The side-effects of ketoconazole are listed in Table 40.2; the most important of these is hepatotoxicity. Abnormalities of liver function tests (LFTs) are quite common in patients receiving ketoconazole but frank hepatitis (which may be fatal) is less common (perhaps 1 in 12 000 cases). Therapy of more than 14 days duration is more frequently associated with hepatotoxicity and for this reason all patients receiving long courses of ketoconazole should have their LFTs monitored prior to treatment and at regular intervals thereafter. Treatment should be stopped if the LFTs show a progressive rise or if clinical hepatitis develops. Ketoconazole can inhibit the synthesis of testosterone and this may lead to the development of gynaecomastia in males on long-term high dose therapy.

The clinical uses of ketoconazole in the treatment of deep-seated fungal infection are now rather limited, since it has been almost superseded by the triazoles. It is occasionally used in the treatment of infections due to the pathogenic fungi, and in chronic mucocutaneous candidiasis.

The triazoles

The triazoles, fluconazole and itraconazole, have a similar mode of action to the imidazoles, but differ substantially from one another in their physical properties and in vivo activity; these are listed in Table 40.6; while the main side-effects of these agents are listed in Table 40.2.

Fluconazole. Fluconazole, which is available both orally and parenterally, is used only in the treatment and prophylaxis of infections due to yeasts. It cannot be used for the treatment of infections due to filamentous fungi. It is highly effective in the treatment of *Cryptococcus* infection, although recent authoritative guidelines (Saag et al 2000) recommend 6–10 weeks of amphotericin B plus flucytosine for CNS infection due to this organism. The authors suggest, however, that a shortened course of

Table 40.6 Properties of the triazoles

Property	Fluconazole	Itraconazole
Water solubility	High	Very low
Oral absorption	Good	Capsule preparation incompletely absorbed, but is improved by presence of food; new liquid formulation is better absorbed and not affected by food
Bioavailability	90%	55% (capsules), 75% (liquid); may be reduced in patients with renal dysfunction, those with reduced gastric acid production, and in AIDS patients
Peak plasma concentration	1.0 mg/l	0.2 mg/l (capsules), 0.5 mg/l (liquid); steady-state levels are only achieved after about 2 weeks of treatment
Protein binding	10%	99%
CSF penetration	60% of serum levels achieved	Very low
Excretion in urine	90% excreted as unchanged drug	< 1% as unchanged drug
Liver metabolism	Negligible	Extensive; metabolites appear in bile and urine

amphotericin (2 weeks) followed by 10 weeks of fluconazole is an acceptable alternative. In HIV-infected patients, maintenance treatment with fluconazole is required for life following cryptococcal infection. In immunocompetent hosts, fluconazole may be used as the primary treatment for disease not involving the CNS, such as pulmonary infection (Nunez et al 2000).

The role of fluconazole in systemic candidiasis is not quite so clear-cut. In patients with candidemia due to colonized intravenous cannulae, the most important treatment is removal of the infected cannula, but it is common practice to give a short course of antifungal therapy to prevent disseminated infection elsewhere. Fluconazole is suitable for this purpose (Kramer et al 1997). In non-neutropenic patients, some studies have shown fluconazole to have been as efficacious as, and significantly less toxic than, conventional amphotericin B. However, the comparative efficacy and toxicity of fluconazole and liposomal amphotericin has been less well studied. In neutropenic patients, amphotericin, often in a lipid formulation, continues to be the treatment of choice. Fluconazole has also been successfully used as prophylaxis against *Candida* infections in neutropenic patients and patients with AIDS, but this in turn has been associated with an increasing incidence of systemic infections with fluconazole-resistant strains.

Some units which use fluconazole extensively have noted the increasing isolation of yeasts resistant to the drug, and the prevalence of resistance is related to the extent of the use of fluconazole. Resistance in *Candida* species is mainly seen in patients who are given long-term prophylactic fluconazole, which selects out those *Candida* species (such as *C. krusei* and *C. glabrata*) which are inherently less susceptible to fluconazole. Resistance in *C. albicans*, the most common species infecting humans, is seen mainly in AIDS patients, partly due to the extensive use of fluconazole in treating severe oral and pharyngeal candidiasis in such patients, and partly due to the very large numbers of yeasts in the oropharynx of AIDS patients with candidiasis, which increases the chance of resistance due to spontaneous mutation. Fluconazole is an exceptionally useful antifungal agent, and it is clear that if it is to remain so, it must be used responsibly.

Itraconazole. Itraconazole is available both orally and intravenously. Itraconazole was originally available in capsules, but a new liquid formulation gives better absorption than the original capsule preparation leading to significantly greater bioavailability and higher serum levels. This is a broad-spectrum antifungal which is effective against yeasts, dermatophytes, the pathogenic fungi and some filamentous fungi, such as *Aspergillus*.

In deep-seated infection, itraconazole is used to treat infections due to the pathogenic fungi, but there is less published evidence of its use in the treatment of systemic candidiasis. However, it may be useful in patients who are infected with strains resistant to fluconazole, some of which may remain sensitive to itraconazole, and in patients who are for some reason unable to tolerate fluconazole. It has also been used to treat cryptococcosis, despite its poor CSF penetration, and in that condition it is an alternative to fluconazole for patients who cannot take the latter drug. However, one study comparing fluconazole and itraconazole as maintenance treatment for cryptococcosis (Saag et al 1999) was discontinued due to the high rate of relapse in the itraconazole arm. Itraconazole has also been studied extensively as a prophylactic agent for superficial and systemic fungal infections in immunocompromised patients (Smith et al 1999; Nucci et al 2000; Harousseau et al 2000).

A particular area of interest has been the treatment of aspergillosis, since itraconazole would be a less toxic and orally available alternative to amphotericin. Unfortunately the difficulty of performing clinical trials in aspergillosis, which is not a common condition and which invariably occurs in seriously ill patients, means that there is relatively little published work. One open prospective multicentre study evaluated cases of invasive aspergillosis in cancer patients, and concluded that there was no difference between initial treatment with amphotericin B (conventional or lipid formulations) and itraconazole (Denning et al 1998). However, a small study in heart transplant recipients indicated that treatment with amphotericin was superior (Nanas et al 1998). More studies of the use of itraconazole in invasive aspergillosis are still awaited, and amphotericin remains the treatment of choice for this condition (Harari 1999).

New agents

Not surprisingly, given the high morbidity and mortality of systemic fungal infection, and the restricted choice of suitable therapeutic agents, considerable research has gone into the development of new drugs. At the present time, there are several new triazoles under investigation, of which the most promising is voriconazole. This agent has a better pharmacokinetic profile than itraconazole, but a broader spectrum of activity than fluconazole.

The other main investigational agents at this time are the echinocandins, of which the drug known as MK-0991 is the furthest advanced. An earlier echinocandin, cilofungin, has been withdrawn from study. These agents act by inhibiting the synthesis of beta-glucans, an important cell wall constituent. They are principally active against *Candida* species and *Aspergillus*, but not against *Cryptococcus*.

Both voriconazole and the echinocandins are only at an investigational stage at present, although voriconazole in particular has been used on a compassionate basis in humans. More information about these agents can be found in the further reading list at the end of this chapter.

Choice of treatment

The overall picture of the treatment of deep-seated fungal infection is constantly changing, and is summarized in Table 40.7. At the present time, amphotericin B (perhaps in its liposomal form) is still the gold standard for the treatment of deep-seated infections due to filamentous fungi such as *Aspergillus,* and for systemic candidiasis in neutropenic patients. In immunocompetent patients, fluconazole is the primary treatment for cryptococcosis outside the CNS, and also perhaps for candidiasis. However, in immunocompromised patients, amphotericin is recommended for first-line treatment of all these conditions. Itraconazole is a useful agent in infections due to the so-called pathogenic fungi and possibly as a second-line agent in aspergillosis. Both fluconazole and itraconazole have a further role to play in the prophylaxis of systemic fungal infection.

CASE STUDIES

Case 40.1

Question

A 10-year-old boy with profound and prolonged neutropenia due to aplastic anaemia is waiting for a bone marrow transplant. However, the clinician responsible for the case is very worried about the possibility of systemic fungal infection developing before the transplant can be carried out. He has asked about the possibilities for antifungal prophylaxis. What options are available?

Answer

In this child, the main cause for concern is *Aspergillus* infection, which is particularly associated with prolonged episodes of neutropenia, and which has a high mortality rate. Although a variety of topical agents, such as oral nystatin, have been used to try to prevent systemic fungal infection, these will be of no use in the prevention of aspergillosis, where the fungal spores are inhaled into the lungs (or occasionally sinuses). Regular inhalation of aerosolized amphotericin has been tried, but many patients experience side-effects and it is of doubtful efficacy.

Fluconazole will not be useful in this patient as it is inactive against *Aspergillus.* The only remaining alternative at present is itraconazole. For effective prophylaxis, the steady-state serum level of itraconazole should be maintained at 0.5 mg/l or higher. This may not be achievable with the capsule form, and the liquid preparation should then be used instead.

Table 40.7   The choice of antifungal agents for common systemic infections

Condition	1st line therapy	2nd line therapy
Candidiasis[a]	Immunocompetent patients: fluconazole	Itraconazole
	Immunocompromised patients: amphotericin B (plus flucytosine in severe cases)	Fluconazole
Aspergillosis	Amphotericin B (conventional or lipid formulation)	Itraconazole
Cryptococcosis	Immunocompetent patients where the infection does not involve the central nervous system (CNS): fluconazole	
	Immunocompromised patients and CNS infection in all patients: amphotericin B plus flucytosine for 6–10 weeks[b]	
Mucormycosis[c]	Amphotericin B (the liposomal form is strongly recommended, although clinical trial evidence is anecdotal)	None

Notes
[a] In candidiasis due to colonized intravenous cannulae, the removal of the cannula is at least as important as the administration of an antifungal agent.
[b] A 2 week course of amphotericin plus flucytosine followed by 10 weeks of fluconazole is an alternative regimen.
[c] Surgery to remove necrotic tissue is an important component of the treatment of mucormycosis.

Case 40.2

Question

A 36-year-old man with AIDS has developed cryptococcal meningitis and is 3 weeks into a course of treatment with amphotericin B (conventional preparation) and flucytosine. He has responded well, but a blood sample has just shown that he is now neutropenic and that the platelet count is also low (thrombocytopenia). He is not, however, anaemic. In addition to the antifungals, he is also receiving other anti-infective agents, including co-trimoxazole for prophylaxis against *Pneumocystis carinii* infection, and a combination of anti-HIV drugs. It is suspected that a drug could be the cause of his bone marrow suppression, but could the antifungals be responsible?

Answer

Several anti-HIV drugs can cause neutropenia and thrombocytopenia, but the patient has been taking them for some time without such side-effects. Co-trimoxazole can also cause this problem, particularly in AIDS patients, but again the patient has taken it for some years without problems. Amphotericin is associated with quite a high incidence of anaemia and much less commonly with thrombocytopenia, but neutropenia is a rare complication. However, flucytosine is well known to cause myelosuppression, particularly when the serum level exceeds 100 mg/l, and this must be the most likely culprit in this patient.

Further investigation shows that the flucytosine level has not been monitored while the patient is on treatment. Although the dose prescribed was not excessive, the patient's renal function has deteriorated due to the use of amphotericin. Since flucytosine accumulates in the presence of renal dysfunction, it is particularly important to monitor the blood level when these drugs are used together.

In this case the post-dose level was found to be 118 mg/l. After discontinuing the flucytosine, the level dropped in 4 days to 27 mg/l, and the white cell and platelet count began to recover. The drug was reintroduced cautiously and given twice daily rather than four times daily, with a target post-dose level of 50 mg/l. It should also be remembered that flucytosine is efficiently removed by haemodialysis, and in cases of severe myelosuppression with high serum levels, the drug level can be brought down rapidly by dialysing the patient.

Case 40.3

Question

A 64-year-old woman recovering slowly from major abdominal surgery is being fed by total parenteral nutrition (TPN). Ten days into her course of TPN she develops a high fever and rigors. Empirical antibiotics are commenced, but after 48 hours there is no response and blood cultures have remained negative. Fungal infection is suspected, and fluconazole is commenced. This drug was chosen because by far the most likely fungal cause would be *Candida albicans* or a related species, and because amphotericin was not felt to be suitable for a frail patient with compromised renal function. Although there is some response, with the temperature coming down a little, she continues to feel unwell. The cannula is then removed, and the patient's fever returns to normal within 24 hours; she feels much better. What might have happened?

Answer

The response to the cannula removal is quite dramatic and is good evidence that a colonized cannula was responsible. Blood cultures are often positive in such cases, and culture of the cannula tip usually yields the infecting organism, but in this patient the tip grew nothing. TPN is strongly associated with fungemia, particularly with *Candida* species, and there is the possibility that this was an infection with a fluconazole-resistant strain of *Candida*. However, the other possibility is that the causative organism did not grow on conventional laboratory culture media. *Malassezia furfur* is one such organism because it has a growth requirement for fatty acids which are not present in routine laboratory media. Systemic infection with *M. furfur* is almost always, if not exclusively, associated with TPN due to the lipid infusions which are a component of parenteral nutrition. It is seen most commonly in neonates and very young children, and is rarely seen in adults (although this might be because culture for it is so infrequently attempted). In this case, culture of blood and the cannula tip on media incorporating olive oil grew an organism subsequently identified as *M. furfur*.

REFERENCES

Bennett M L, Fleischer A B, Loveless J W et al 2000 Oral griseofulvin remains the treatment of choice for tinea capitis in children. Pediatric Dermatology 17: 304–309

Caceres-Rios H, Rueda M, Ballona R et al 2000 Comparison of terbinafine and griseofulvin in the treatment of tinea capitis. Journal of the American Academy of Dermatology 42: 80–84

Denning D W, Marinus A, Cohen J et al 1998 An EORTC multicentre prospective survey of invasive aspergillosis in haematological patients: diagnosis and therapeutic outcome. EORTC Invasive Fungal Infections Cooperative Group. Journal of Infection 37: 173–180

Harari S 1999 Current strategies in the treatment of invasive *Aspergillus* infections in immunocompromised patients. Drugs 58: 621–631

Harousseau J L, Dekker A W, Stamatoullas-Bastard A et al 2000 Itraconazole oral solution for primary prophylaxis of fungal infections in patients with hematological malignancy and profound neutropenia: a randomized, double-blind, double-placebo, multicenter trial comparing itraconazole and amphotericin B. Antimicrobial Agents and Chemotherapy 44: 1887–1893

Kramer K M, Skaar D J, Ackerman B H 1997 The fluconazole era: management of hematogenously disseminated candidiasis in the nonneutropenic patient. Pharmacotherapy 17: 538–548

Nanas J N, Saroglou G, Anastasiou-Nana M I et al 1998 Itraconazole for the treatment of pulmonary aspergillosis in heart transplant recipients. Clinical Transplants 12: 30–34

Nucci M, Biasoli I, Akiti T et al 2000 A double-blind, randomized, placebo-controlled trial of itraconazole capsules as antifungal prophylaxis for neutropenic patients. Clinical Infectious Diseases 30: 300–305

Nunez M, Peacock J E, Chin R 2000 Pulmonary cryptococcosis in the immunocompetent host: therapy with oral fluconazole: a report of four cases and a review of the literature. Chest 118: 527–534

Pedler S J, Orr K E 2000 Bacterial, fungal, and parasitic infections. In: Barron W M, Lindheimer M D (eds) Medical disorders during pregnancy, 3rd edn. Mosby, St Louis, pp. 411–465

Saag M S, Cloud G A, Graybill J R et al 1999 A comparison of itraconazole versus fluconazole as maintenance therapy for AIDS-associated cryptococcal meningitis. National Institute of Allergy and Infectious Diseases Mycoses Study Group. Clinical Infectious Diseases 28: 291–296

Saag M S, Graybill R J, Larsen R A et al 2000 Practice guidelines for the management of cryptococcal disease. Clinical Infectious Diseases 30: 710–718

Smith D, Midgley J, Gazzard B 1999 A randomised, double-blind study of itraconazole versus placebo in the treatment and prevention of oral or oesophageal candidosis in patients with HIV infection. International Journal of Clinical Practices 53: 349–352

Wong-Beringer A, Jacobs R A, Guglielmo B J 1998 Lipid formulations of amphotericin B: clinical efficacy and toxicities. Clinical Infectious Diseases 27: 603–618

FURTHER READING

Barchiesi F, Schimizzi A M, Fothergill A W et al 1999 In vitro activity of the new echinocandin antifungal, MK-0991, against common and uncommon clinical isolates of *Candida* species. European Journal of Clinical Microbiology and Infectious Diseases 18: 302–304

Espinel-Ingroff A 1998 Comparison of in vitro activities of the new triazole SCH56592 and the echinocandins MK-0991 (L-743,872) and LY303366 against opportunistic filamentous and dimorphic fungi and yeasts. Journal of Clinical Microbiology 36: 2950–2956

Martin M V 1999 The use of fluconazole and itraconazole in the treatment of *Candida albicans* infections: a review. Journal of Antimicrobial Chemotherapy 44: 429–437

Nguyen M H, Yu C Y 1998 Voriconazole against fluconazole-susceptible and resistant candida isolates: in-vitro efficacy compared with that of itraconazole and ketoconazole. Journal of Antimicrobial Chemotherapy 42: 253–256

Pfaller M A, Jones R N, Doem G V et al 1999 International surveillance of blood stream infections due to *Candida* species in the European SENTRY program: species distribution and antifungal susceptibility including the investigational triazole and echinocandin agents. SENTRY Participant Group (Europe). Diagnostic Microbiology and Infectious Disease 35: 19–25

Rex J H, Walsh T J, Sobel J D et al 2000 Practice guidelines for the treatment of candidiasis. Clinical Infectious Diseases 30: 662–678

Richardson M D, Warnock D W 1997 Fungal infection: diagnosis and management, 2nd edn. Blackwell, Oxford

Stevens D A, Kan V L, Judson M A et al 2000 Practice guidelines for diseases caused by *Aspergillus*. Clinical Infectious Diseases 30: 696–709

Thyroid and parathyroid disorders

41

J. A. Cantrill J. Wood

KEY POINTS

- When diagnosing thyroid conditions, the possibility of drug-induced disease should always be considered.
- The treatment of hypothyroidism requires lifelong levothyroxine therapy.
- Levothyroxine replacement therapy should be introduced cautiously in the elderly particularly those with cardiac disease.
- Hyperthyroidism can be treated with thionamide therapy, radioiodine or surgery; the choice will largely be determined by the age of patient, the severity of the condition, local service availability and patient preference.
- Patients treated with thionamide therapy require careful counselling about the symptoms and management of agranulocytosis.
- Hypoparathyroidism can occur after thyroid surgery, and is managed with a vitamin D preparation.
- Surgery is the mainstay of treatment for hyperparathyroidism.

HYPOTHYROIDISM

Hypothyroidism is the clinical state that results from decreased production of thyroid hormones, or, very rarely, from their decreased action at the tissue level.

Epidemiology

Comparison of studies of the prevalence and incidence of hypothyroidism is difficult due to the variation in definitions and population samples. Using a uniform set of diagnostic criteria, the prevalence of previously undiagnosed, spontaneous, overt hypothyroidism has been estimated to be between 2 and 4 per 1000 of the total population worldwide. However, if all cases of previously diagnosed hypothyroidism, previous thyroid surgery and radioiodine treatment are included, this prevalence rises to approximately 10 per 1000. Primary hypothyroidism in the UK is common, occurring in more than 2% of the population and it occurs 10 to 20 times more frequently in men than in women. The question of widespread population screening for hypothyroidism is unresolved, but is probably not cost-effective unless incorporated into a screening programme for other conditions. Although the disease may occur at any age, most patients present between 30 and 60 years of age.

Aetiology

Hypothyroidism can be induced by a variety of structural or functional abnormalities. The condition can be classified in several ways. The principal classification is primary, secondary, tertiary and peripheral. Primary hypothyroidism accounts for more than 95% of adult cases, and is due to a failure of the thyroid gland itself. Secondary disease is due to hypopituitarism, and tertiary disease due to failure of the hypothalamus. Peripheral hypothyroidism is due to tissue insensitivity to the action of thyroid hormones. A more extensive classification is shown in Table 41.1.

In approximately 20% of patients, hypothyroidism results from destruction of the gland as a result of treatment for hyperthyroidism. Several other disorders are associated with primary hypothyroidism but are not directly causal. These include Addison's disease,

Table 41.1   Classification of hypothyroidism

Primary hypothyroidism
 Congenital hypothyroidism
 Antithyroid drugs
 Hashimoto's thyroiditis
 Postpartum hypothyroidism
 Spontaneous hypothyroidism in Graves' disease
 Postoperative hypothyroidism
 Hypothyroidism after radioactive iodine
 External radiation

Secondary hypothyroidism
 Hypopituitarism
 Selective thyroid-stimulating hormone deficiency

Tertiary hypothyroidism
 Hypothalamic disorders

Peripheral hypothyroidism

pernicious anaemia and diabetes mellitus Occasionally, hypothyroidism may be drug induced (Table 41.2).

Hypothyroidism can also be classified as non-goitrous or goitrous. Goitre is the term used for enlargement of the thyroid gland. This occurs as a direct result of excessive stimulation by thyroid-stimulating hormone (TSH) in response to low levels of circulating thyroid hormones. The commonest cause of goitre is Hashimoto's thyroiditis. This is characterized by diffuse enlargement and lymphocytic infiltration of the gland. This is an immunological disorder with measurable titres of circulating antibodies against the thyroid gland. Goitres may also occur from the use of certain drugs with antithyroid activity. Drugs used therapeutically in the treatment of hyperthyroidism may produce goitre if used in excessive doses.

Iodides may produce hypothyroidism in certain patients who are extremely sensitive to their ability to block the active transport pump of the thyroid gland. Iodine absorption from topical iodine-containing antiseptics has been shown to cause hypothyroidism in neonates. This is potentially very dangerous at a critical time of neurological development in the newborn infant. Transient hypothyroidism may be seen in 25% of iodine-exposed infants.

Pathophysiology

The thyroid gland consists of two lobes and is situated in the lower neck. The gland synthesizes, stores and releases two major metabolically active hormones: levothyroxine (T_4) and triiodothyronine (T_3). Regulation of hormone synthesis is by the secretion of TSH from the anterior pituitary. In turn, TSH is regulated by hypothalamic secretion of thyrotrophin-releasing hormone (TRH) (Fig. 41.1). Low circulating levels of thyroid hormones initiate the release of TSH, and possibly also of TRH. Rising levels of TSH promote increased iodide trapping by the gland with a subsequent increase in synthesis. The increase in circulating hormone levels feeds back on the pituitary and hypothalamus, shutting off TSH, TRH and further hormone synthesis.

Both T_4 and T_3 are produced within the gland. Dietary inorganic iodide is trapped by the gland and oxidized by the enzyme peroxidase to iodine. The next step is the incorporation of iodine with tyrosine molecules to form monoiodotyrosine (MIT) and diiodotyrosine (DIT).

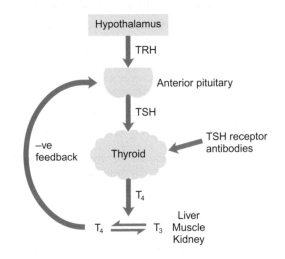

Figure 41.1 Control of thyroid hormone secretion

Table 41.2	Drug-induced thyroid disease	
Drug	Effect	Comments[a]
Amiodarone	Hypothyroidism: blocks conversion of T_4 to T_3, compensatory increase in thyroid-stimulating hormone	Affects 6–13% of patients Treatment with conventional levothyroxine replacement Monitor underlying cardiac disease
	Hyperthyroidism: due to iodine content of the drug	Affects 1–2% of patients in areas with high iodine intake Affects 12% of patients in areas with low iodine intake Drug may mask clinical features of hyperthyroidism May remit spontaneously within 6 months Reports of successful treatment with combinations of thionamide, potassium perchlorate, and/or corticosteroid therapy or surgery
Lithium	Hypothyroidism: inhibits iodine uptake and thyroid hormone release	Affects 5–15% of patients on long-term treatment Treat with conventional levothyroxine replacement
	Hyperthyroidism: paradoxical effect, mechanism unknown	Rare

[a] Suggested management assumes the drug cannot be discontinued.

Subsequently the formation of T_4 occurs as a result of the coupling of two DIT residues and of T_3 by coupling a DIT and a MIT residue. The hormones are then stored within the gland until their release into the circulation by enzymatic cleavage.

The ratio of T_4:T_3 secreted by the thyroid gland is approximately 10:1. Consequently the gland secretes approximately 80–100 micrograms of T_4 and 10 micrograms of T_3 per day. However, only 20% of circulating T_3 is derived from direct thyroidal secretion, the remaining 80% being produced by peripheral conversion from T_4. T_4 can therefore be considered a prohormone that is converted in the peripheral tissues (liver, kidney and brain) either to the active hormone T_3 or to the biologically inactive reverse T_3 (rT_3). In the circulation, the hormones exist in both the active free and inactive protein-bound forms. T_4 is 99.98% bound, with only 0.02% circulating free. T_3 is slightly less protein bound (99.8%), resulting in a considerably higher circulating free fraction (0.2%). Details of protein binding are shown in Table 41.3.

The hormones are metabolized in the periphery (kidney, liver and heart) by deiodination. T_4 and T_3 are also eliminated by biliary secretion of their glucuronide and sulphate conjugates (15–20%). The half-life of T_4 in plasma is about 6–7 days and that of T_3 24–36 hours in euthyroid adults. The apparent volume of distribution for T_4 is about 10 litres and for T_3 about 40 litres.

Clinical manifestations

The symptoms of hypothyroidism can affect multiple body systems and are usually non-specific and gradual in onset (Table 41.4). Symptoms, especially in the early stages, are frequently vague. It is not uncommon, particularly in the elderly, for symptoms to be attributed, incorrectly, by patients and their relatives to increasing age. The most common symptoms reported by patients are weakness, lethargy, cold intolerance, slowness, memory loss and weight gain (without eating more). The skin becomes dry, hair 'lifeless' and the patient may have noticed a change in voice with deepening or gruffness. The commonest conditions with which hypothyroidism are confused are obesity and depression.

Table 41.3   Protein binding of thyroid hormones (%)

	T_4	T_3
Thyroid-binding globulin (TBG)	70	77
Thyroid-binding prealbumin (TBPA)	10	8
Albumin	20	15

Effusions may occur into pericardial, pleural, peritoneal or joint spaces. Mild anaemia of a macrocytic type is quite common and responds to levothyroxine replacement. Pernicious anaemia is a frequent concomitant finding in hypothyroidism. Other, organ-specific autoimmune diseases such as Addison's disease may be associated.

Myxoedema coma

Myxoedema coma is a rare but potentially fatal complication of severe, untreated hypothyroidism. Loss of consciousness is often associated with hypothermia. Coma can be precipitated by cold weather, stress, infection, trauma and certain drugs. Respiratory depressants of any kind that are metabolized slowly in the hypothyroid patient can precipitate coma. These include anaesthetic agents, narcotics, phenothiazines and hypnotics. The condition should be treated rapidly and aggressively.

The term 'myxoedema' used to be synonymous with hypothyroidism. It is now reserved for advanced disease in which there is undue swelling of the skin and subcutaneous tissues.

Investigations

In most cases, laboratory investigation of thyroid disorders is extremely simple, due to specific radioimmunoassays

Table 41.4   Signs and symptoms of hypothyroidism

Skin and appendages	Dry, cool, flaking skin Faint yellow colour Puffy facies and eyes Coarse, brittle hair
Nervous system	Slow speech Poor memory Somnolence Carpal tunnel syndrome Psychiatric disturbance Hearing loss Depression
Muscle	Muscle pain and weakness Delayed deep tendon reflexes
Gastrointestinal	Weight gain with decreased appetite Abdominal distension Constipation
Cardiovascular	Reduced cardiac output Bradycardia Cardiac enlargement

for free T_3, free T_4 and TSH. Usually clinical assessment, combined with a single estimation of thyroid hormones and TSH, is sufficient to make the diagnosis of hypothyroidism. In primary disease, the levels of free T_4 and T_3 are low and the TSH level rises markedly. However, in the early stages or in patients who have had a subtotal thyroidectomy, the free T_4 and T_3 levels may be normal with only a modest elevation of the TSH concentration. A diagnosis of secondary or tertiary hypothyroidism is suspected on the basis of a low free T_4 and low TSH levels.

Elevation of the TSH level occurs early in the course of thyroid failure and may be present before overt clinical manifestations appear. It is important to appreciate that hypothyroidism is not one disease but a whole spectrum. Hypothyroidism can be graded according to the degree of clinical and laboratory abnormalities.

In the case of overt hypothyroidism there are clear clinical features as well as characteristic abnormalities of free T_4 and TSH. This rarely presents a diagnostic problem.

Mild hypothyroidism

The symptoms are less obvious and may be as non-specific as lack of energy. The results of thyroid function tests may be equivocal, but a normal TSH excludes the diagnosis. T_4 is probably more reliable than T_3 for early cases, because T_3 can often be decreased as a non-specific consequence of illness.

Although there is a large range of other thyroid function tests available they are only rarely required to make the diagnosis of hypothyroidism. When interpreting the results of thyroid function tests, caution may be required if the patient has other disease states and/or is taking other drugs (Tables 41.2 and 41.5).

A chest radiograph may detect the presence of effusions, and an electrocardiogram (ECG) is useful, especially in patients with angina or coronary heart disease.

Treatment

The aims of treatment with T_4 are to ensure that patients receive a dose that will restore well-being and which usually returns the TSH level to within the normal range. It is important to avoid both under- and overtreatment. All patients with symptomatic hypothyroidism require replacement therapy. T_4 is usually the treatment of choice except in myxoedema coma where T_3 may be used. Before commencing T_4 replacement the diagnosis of hypopituitarism must be excluded in order to prevent precipitation of an Addisonian crisis. If in doubt, hydrocortisone replacement should be given concomitantly until cortisol deficiency is excluded.

Drug treatment

Once the diagnosis has been established, treatment should be commenced. The condition is very rarely life-threatening, and adverse effects may result from overzealous treatment. The initial dose of T_4 will depend on the patient's age, severity and duration of disease and the coexistence of cardiac disease.

In young, healthy patients with disease of short duration, T_4 may be commenced in a dose of 50–100 micrograms daily. As the drug has a long half-life it should only be given once daily. The most convenient time is usually in the morning. After 4–6 weeks on the same dose, thyroid function tests should be checked. The TSH concentration is the best predictor of the euthyroid state, and this should be used for further dosage adjustment. Clearly a raised TSH concentration indicates either inadequate treatment or poor compliance. The majority of patients will be controlled with doses of 100–200 micrograms daily, with few patients requiring more than 200 micrograms. In adults the median dose required to suppress TSH to normal is 125 micrograms daily. However, some patients will have undetectable serum TSH levels while taking levothyroxine. In these patients, the dose should not be reduced if levels of free T_4 and T_3 are normal. In the majority of patients, once the appropriate dose has been established it remains constant. During pregnancy, an increase in the dose of levothyroxine, often by 50 micrograms daily, is needed to maintain normal TSH levels.

In elderly patients, particularly those with cardiac disease, treatment should be introduced more cautiously.

Table 41.5 Drugs and disease states affecting thyroid function
Drugs that decrease TSH secretion
Dopamine
Glucocorticoids
Octreotide
Drugs that alter thyroid hormone secretion
Decreased thyroid hormone secretion
Iodide
Aminoglutethimide
Drugs that decrease T_4 absorption
Colestyramine
Aluminium hydroxide
Ferrous sulphate
Sucralfate
Drugs that alter T_4 and T_3 metabolism
Increased hepatic metabolism
Phenobarbital
Phenytoin
Rifampicin
Carbamazepine

Some 5% of patients with long-standing hypothyroidism either complain of angina at presentation or develop it during treatment with levothyroxine. Exacerbation of myocardial ischaemia, infarction and sudden death are all well-recognized complications of T_4 replacement therapy. Patients with coronary heart disease may be unable to tolerate full replacement doses because of palpitations, angina or heart failure. Treatment should be started with 25 micrograms daily and increased slowly by 25 micrograms every 4–6 weeks. Some authorities recommend starting with 5 micrograms of T_3. The proposed advantage is that if adverse effects occur, these will be alleviated more rapidly due to the shorter half-life of T_3. During this time the patient's clinical progress should be carefully monitored. In some patients T_4 may be better tolerated if a β-blocker such as propranolol is given concomitantly.

There has been considerable recent interest in the risks of overtreatment with T_4. Although T_4 exerts an effect on many organs and tissues, it is probably the effect on bone that gives the greatest cause for concern. There is some evidence that bone density may be reduced in patients taking T_4 replacement therapy (Faber & Galloe 1994, Uzzan et al 1996). In order to minimize the risk of development of osteoporosis the dose should be carefully tailored to the needs of each individual patient.

Treatment of myxoedema coma

The treatment of myxoedema coma has been poorly studied, and the optimal regimen remains to be defined. Thyroid hormone replacement should be commenced by giving 5–10 micrograms of T_3 parenterally twice daily. Possible adrenal underactivity should be treated with parenteral hydrocortisone 100 mg three times daily. Heart failure and arrhythmias should be treated if they arise.

Sources of infection should be actively sought, particularly chest or urinary infections, and treated aggressively. The body temperature should be monitored rectally and allowed to rise slowly by keeping the patient in a warm room and wrapped in a 'space blanket' that retains heat. Urea, electrolyte and haematological assessments must be made and corrected as necessary. Even with this kind of management approach, the mortality rate exceeds 50%.

Patient care

The treatment of hypothyroidism requires lifelong treatment with T_4. Patients on long-term drug therapy are well recognized to have a low adherence with their medication regimen and these patients are no exception. Treatment with T_4 is often terminated because patients feel well and think that treatment is no longer required.

Prevention

At present nothing can be done to prevent thyroid failure from developing; however, much can be done to ensure early detection and treatment.

Careful follow-up of patients who have undergone iodine-131 treatment, subtotal thyroidectomy or completed a course of treatment for hyperthyroidism is essential. The earliest biochemical change is an increase in TSH with normal concentrations of T_3 and T_4. These should be used to diagnose hypothyroidism before the patient becomes symptomatic. Table 41.6 shows the prevalence of hypothyroidism after treatment for hyperthyroidism.

HYPERTHYROIDISM

Hyperthyroidism is defined as the production and secretion of excessive amounts of thyroid hormones.

Epidemiology

The most common cause of hyperthyroidism in the Western world is Graves' disease, which accounts for 90% of cases. This form of hyperthyroidism may affect any age group, but it is uncommon in childhood and most frequent in the third to fifth decades. Women are affected about 10 times more than men. In the UK the prevalence of overt hyperthyroidism is 20 per 1000 females and 2 per 1000 males.

Aetiology

Hyperthyroidism is a disorder of various aetiologies. The hyperthyroidism and goitre of Graves' disease are thought to result from the action of thyroid-stimulating antibodies, which mimic the effect of TSH. An uncertain

---

Table 41.6 Prevalence of hypothyroidism after treatment for hyperthyroidism

Thyroidectomy
- 6–75% hypothyroidism over their lifetime, dependent on the amount of remnant tissue. Risk highest during first year after surgery

Antithyroid drugs
- 43% relapse in the first year
- 13–21% relapse in the next 4 years

^{131}I therapy
- 24–90% develop hypothyroidism over their lifetime

proportion (perhaps 20%) of these patients will spontaneously become hypothyroid if followed for a long period of time. These immunoglobulins are now known to be antibodies to the TSH receptor on the thyroid gland. Many patients with Graves' disease have distinctive eye signs. It seems likely that these are a manifestation of a parallel but distinct immunological mechanism involving ophthalmogenic immunoglobulins. Graves' disease is a familial condition, and many studies suggest there is a genetic predisposition to the disease.

Toxic nodular goitre is another form of hyperthyroidism. For reasons that are not clear, diffuse or focal autonomous nodule formation develops in the enlarged thyroid, with associated thyrotoxicosis, which is generally of a relatively mild degree. Thyroid growth is probably stimulated by a growth receptor-stimulating antibody. Growth of new follicles outstrips local blood supply, resulting in necrosis in the centre of the growth, followed by repair and fibrosis with the formation of multiple nodules. Hyperthyroidism may also be caused by autonomous thyroid adenomas. These are benign well-differentiated tumours that secrete excessive amounts of thyroid hormones.

Hyperthyroidism of any aetiology usually suggests excessive levels of T_4. However, approximately 5% of patients will have the syndrome of T_3 toxicosis, which is probably due to preferential secretion of T_3 by the thyroid gland. Occasionally, hyperthyroidism may be drug induced (see Table 41.2).

Clinical manifestations

Hyperthyroidism is characterized by increased metabolism of all body systems due to excessive quantities of thyroid hormones. There is a wide spectrum of clinical thyroid hormone excess.

The clinical signs and symptoms reflect increased adrenergic activity, especially in the cardiovascular and neurological systems (Table 41.7). Not all manifestations will be seen in every patient. The classical presentation is a patient, usually female, complaining of palpitations, excessive sweating, fine tremor and weight loss in spite of a good or increased appetite. She may be intolerant of heat, and almost invariably admits to a preference for cooler weather.

The diagnosis of hyperthyroidism in the elderly may not be so easily made. Signs and symptoms of cardiovascular strain tend to predominate. Atrial fibrillation is frequent, and the patient may be in congestive cardiac failure. Unexplained heart failure after middle age should always arouse suspicion of hyperthyroidism. Also suggestive is failure of standard doses of digoxin to control the rapid heart rate. Other less common presentations include muscle weakness,

diarrhoea, amenorrhoea and osteoporosis. A goitre may be noted and complained of, especially if the gland is large and vascular.

Graves' disease is characterized by the typical signs and symptoms of hyperthyroidism, eye signs and, rarely, localized myxoedema. The eye signs comprise swelling of the eyelids, irritation of the conjunctivae, exophthalmos (proptosis), lid retraction and ophthalmoplegia. They may occur alone or in combination. Exophthalmos refers to the characteristic protrusion of the eyeball. Ophthalmoplegia is paresis of one or more of the extraocular muscles, and usually causes diplopia. Another extrathyroid abnormality of Graves' disease, occurring in about 5% of patients, is localized (pretibial) myxoedema. There is swelling, and sometimes tissue overgrowth, affecting the front of the shins, which may extend to the dorsum of the feet and toes.

Investigations

In any patient with suspected hyperthyroidism it is good practice to document the diagnosis with at least two sets of thyroid function tests. If the diagnosis is in doubt, treatment should be withheld. Hyperthyroidism can usually be safely observed while investigations are carried out. Plasma free T_4 levels are clearly elevated in more than 90% of patients with hyperthyroidism. A low

Table 41.7	Signs and symptoms of hyperthyroidism
Skin and appendages	Warm, moist skin Thinning or loss of hair Prominence of eyes, lid retraction Increased sweating Heat intolerance Pretibial myxoedema
Nervous system	Insomnia Irritability, nervousness Symptoms of an anxiety state Psychosis (rarely)
Musculoskeletal	Osteoporosis Muscle weakness Rapid deep tendon reflexes Tremor
Gastrointestinal	Weight loss with increased appetite Diarrhoea
Cardiovascular	Palpitations, tachycardia Shortness of breath on exertion Angina Atrial fibrillation

TSH level can also be helpful in making the diagnosis of hyperthyroidism.

In the majority of patients the combination of the clinical findings and these simple investigations is sufficient to make a firm diagnosis. If the diagnosis is still equivocal the clinical findings should be reassessed, and particular attention paid to the patient's drug history. There are a number of drugs that may modify the clinical features or interfere with the tests. If there is still doubt it is usual to assess the response of TSH to the intravenous administration of 200 micrograms of TRH. A normal response excludes hyperthyroidism. An absent or impaired response would support the diagnosis. Other diagnostic techniques may be required including isotope scan with technetium[99]m, ultrasound and needle aspiration.

Treatment

Numerous factors need to be considered when choosing the most appropriate form of therapy for an individual patient (Table 41.8). After giving these due consideration there may be more than one therapeutic option available, and the patient should be involved in the decision making. The decision may also be influenced by physician preference, which, in turn, will depend on the facilities available. Three standard forms of therapy are available: antithyroid drugs, surgery (subtotal thyroidectomy) and radioactive iodine. There is no general agreement as to the specific indications for

Table 41.8 Factors influencing choice of treatment of hyperthyroidism

Large goitre causing obstruction
Severe heart failure
Pregnancy, puerperium
Neonate
Iodide exposure
Concurrent amiodarone therapy
Previous drug side-effect
Poor compliance
Severity of symptoms
Age
Existence of complications

each form of therapy, and none of them is ideal, all being associated with both short- and long-term sequelae. One commonly agreed principle is that surgery should not be undertaken, nor iodine[131] given, while the patient is grossly thyrotoxic. The patient should first be rendered euthyroid with antithyroid drugs because there is a risk of precipitating a thyrotoxic 'storm' (the abrupt onset of symptoms of thyrotoxicosis) with iodine[131] or surgery when the patient is still thyrotoxic.

Surgery may be difficult in children and the complication rate is higher. Radioiodine is contraindicated because of the potential for development of thyroid malignancy. Surgery should also be avoided in pregnancy if the disease can be controlled with drugs. However, doses should be kept as low as possible, especially in the last 2 months of pregnancy, as excessive treatment may produce goitre in the fetus. Aplasia cutis may also occur after carbimazole therapy. Radioiodine therapy is absolutely contraindicated in pregnancy since the thyroid gland of the fetus can concentrate iodide from the third month onwards.

In patients with small goitres, relapse after a course of antithyroid therapy is less common than in those with significant gland enlargement. If surgery is contraindicated the patient should be treated medically. In patients who relapse after previous partial thyroidectomy, surgery results in distortion of local anatomy, making further operations hazardous.

Antithyroid drugs

The thionamides, propylthiouracil (PTU), thiamazole (methimazole) and its precursor carbimazole, are equally effective pharmacological therapies for hyperthyroidism. In the UK, carbimazole is usually used. These drugs prevent thyroid hormone synthesis by inhibiting the oxidative binding of iodide and its coupling to tyrosine residues. PTU, but not carbimazole, inhibits the peripheral deiodination of T_4 to T_3. In addition, the thionamides are also thought to have an immunosuppressive action.

Adverse effects

The most common serious adverse effects of antithyroid treatment are agranulocytosis and, less commonly, hepatitis, aplastic anaemia and lupus-like syndromes (Table 41.9). Overall, serious effects such as these occur in approximately 0.3% of patients treated. Skin rashes (macular or papular and itchy) occur more commonly, in approximately 5% of patients. All of these side-effects usually occur during the first 6 weeks of treatment. Cross-sensitivity between carbimazole and propylthiouracil is rare and the patient can usually be safely changed to the alternative agent if an adverse event occurs.

Table 41.9   Adverse effects of thionamides

	Adverse effect	Comments
Skin	Pruritic, maculopapular rash	Most common in first 6 weeks May disappear spontaneously with continued treatment Can be treated with an antihistamine Change to alternative agent Occurs in 5% of patients
	Rash with systemic symptoms, i.e. fever, arthralgia	Discontinue drug Alternative treatment required
Haematological	Agranulocytosis	Most common in first 6 weeks Incidence increases with age Discontinue drug Reversible Consider alternative treatment Occurs in 0.5% of patients
	Leucopenia	Transient Continue treatment Does not predispose to agranulocytosis
Other	Hepatitis Vasculitis Hypoprothrombinaemia Aplastic anaemia Thrombocytopenia	Rare Discontinue drug

Although regular monitoring of white cell counts has been advocated (Anon 1997), this is not routine practice. First, agranulocytosis is rare and second, if the condition does occur, it happens rapidly and even routine monitoring of white cell counts may miss it (International Agranulocytosis and Aplastic Anaemia Study 1988). However, patients should be warned about the onset of sore throat, mouth ulcers and pyrexia, or other symptoms, which may suggest the onset of bone marrow suppression. If they occur, treatment should be stopped and a full blood count performed.

The regimen

Carbimazole is usually given initially in doses of 20–60 mg daily, depending on the severity of the condition. It can be given as a single daily dose to aid adherence. Although the plasma half-life is short (4–6 hours) the biological effect lasts longer (up to 40 hours). Treatment should be titrated against free T_4 concentrations and checked at 4–6 week intervals until a maintenance dose of 5–15 mg daily is achieved. Some feel that this tapering regimen may not be necessary. Measuring the TSH is unhelpful in the early stages of treatment. When the patient is established on a maintenance dose, free T_4 and TSH should be measured at 3-month intervals. Failure to respond to antithyroid drugs can only mean that the initial diagnosis was incorrect or that the patient is not taking the medication.

It is important to appreciate there is a lag of 1–2 weeks between the achievement of biochemical euthyroidism and that of clinical euthyroidism. If this is overlooked, the patient may be overtreated, resulting in biochemical hypothyroidism with clinical thyrotoxicosis. For this reason, some centres routinely give initial high doses of carbimazole in combination with replacement doses of T_4. This is known as the 'block–replace' regimen. It consists of carbimazole 40 mg daily which is given to block thyroid hormone production until hypersecretion is stopped, then levothyroxine is added in at a dose of 50–150 micrograms daily to replace levothyroxine and thus prevent the development of hypothyroidism. This two-drug regimen is continued for about 1 year and patient response is monitored by measuring free T_4. The proposed advantages of the block–replace regimen are that hypersecretion is better controlled, remission rates are improved and follow-up is less onerous for patients. However, some studies have failed to confirm these benefits (Lucas et al 1997, Rittmaster et al 1998). The block–replace regimen should not be used in pregnancy as levothyroxine does not cross the placenta and fetal hypothyroidism can occur.

The optimal duration of antithyroid treatment is usually 12–24 months, but this remains a controversial issue and may depend on the presentation of the initial thyrotoxic episode (MacFarlane et al 1983, Maugendre et al 1999). Adverse effects are usually seen in the first few weeks of treatment, and there does not appear to be any additional risk from more prolonged courses of treatment. Even with prolonged courses less than 50% of patients remain in permanent remission.

All β-blockers give symptomatic relief and are useful adjuncts to carbimazole in the first few weeks of therapy. Propranolol has the theoretical advantage that it also inhibits peripheral conversion of T_4 to T_3. β-blockers are also useful in the management of patients with severe thyrotoxicosis who are awaiting surgery or radioactive iodine therapy. Small doses of a non-selective agent are usually adequate, for example propranolol 20–40 mg two to four times daily, but adherence might be improved by using a once-daily agent or a long-acting preparation of propranolol. This usually results in relief of palpitations, anxiety, sweating, tremor and diarrhoea. More severely toxic patients may require higher doses. β-blockers are not recommended for long-term use as they do not affect the underlying cause of the condition.

Patient counselling

Patients should be advised of the importance of regular clinic attendance. This is necessary to monitor both therapeutic outcome and the development of adverse effects. The development of skin rashes, mouth ulcers or a sore throat should be immediately investigated and a full blood count performed. It may be dangerous to treat these symptoms with over-the-counter medication before carrying out further investigations. If a patient presents with the symptoms described it is essential to enquire into his or her medication history.

It is important for the patient to understand the difference between specific antithyroid therapy and symptomatic treatment. The patient should also be advised about the timing of doses to aid adherence. Following completion of a course of treatment the patient should understand relapse may occur, and medical help should be sought if the initial symptoms recur (Table 41.10).

Surgery

The hyperthyroid patient to be treated surgically should first be rendered biochemically euthyroid. This may require a combination of antithyroid drugs and β-blockers, and possibly iodide.

Iodide exerts a transient inhibitory effect on the ability of the gland to trap iodide and it may also reduce the vascularity of the gland. Lithium has been used in patients hypersensitive to iodides. In doses of 800–1200 mg/day lithium has actions similar to iodides. Lithium

levels should be monitored to minimize toxicity. The dose of β-blockers should be titrated to reduce the pulse rate to below 80 beats per minute. This is usually continued for 1 week postoperatively. It is imperative that treatment is given right up to the time of operation and the operation deferred if the pulse rate is not adequately controlled. Inadequate pretreatment can result in the occurrence of thyroid 'storm' within the first day or two of operation. The pulse rate is rapid, dehydration occurs and atrial fibrillation and heart failure may develop.

Hypoparathyroidism may arise postoperatively due to interference of the blood supply to the parathyroids or their inadvertent removal during surgery. Tetany will begin shortly after the operation, and treatment should be initiated with intravenous calcium gluconate. All patients who have undergone partial thyroidectomy should have a serum calcium estimation 3 months after operation since the development of hypoparathyroidism can be delayed. Later complications of thyroidectomy include hypothyroidism and recurrent hyperthyroidism.

Radioactive iodine

Radioiodine therapy is easy to administer and effective but is contraindicated in children, in pregnancy and in women who are breastfeeding. In addition, patients with significant thyroid eye disease should not receive ^{131}I because it may result in worsening ophthalmopathy. Although there has been concern over the complications of radioiodine therapy, accumulated experience has not demonstrated any discernible genetic risk. There is a slight increase in the apparent risk of thyroid cancer in patients treated with ^{131}I, but this may be due to the underlying disease rather than the radioiodine.

The commonest complication is the development of hypothyroidism, the incidence depending on the dose given. The amount (activity) of radioiodine given should be sufficient to achieve euthyroidism in most patients

Table 41.10 Counselling points for patients on antithyroid drugs
1. Carbimazole can be given as a single daily dose
2. Anticipated duration of treatment
3. Tapering to maintenance dose
4. Use of adjuvant therapy, e.g. β-blockers
5. Report skin rashes, sore throat or mouth ulcers
6. Need for regular review
7. Management of relapse

within 2–3 months with a moderate rate of hypothyroidism thereafter.

If antithyroid drugs have been used they should be withdrawn at least 4 days before radioiodine is given and should not be restarted for at least 3 days afterwards. Drug therapy can then be withdrawn periodically to assess the effects of the radioiodine.

Treatment of complications

Treatment of eye signs

In most patients with Graves' disease, no specific treatment is required for the eyes. The commonest complaint is of 'grittiness', which can be treated with hypromellose eye drops. If lid retraction is severe the inadequate lid closure can result in early morning soreness. This can be alleviated by the short-term use of 5% guanethidine eye drops instilled each night and morning. The eyes should be monitored for any signs of infection, and treated appropriately.

Fortunately, severe eye involvement occurs in less than 2% of patients with Graves' disease. Progressive ophthalmopathy producing severe complications from proptosis, diplopia or visual failure should be treated with high-dose steroid therapy (prednisolone 60 mg daily) until symptoms resolve. Failure to respond is an indication for orbital irradiation or surgical decompression. Ciclosporin has also proved beneficial in some patients with ophthalmopathy.

Treatment of localized myxoedema

Myxoedema is usually localized to small areas and is asymptomatic. More extensive disease causes difficulty in walking and considerable discomfort. Probably the most effective therapy is the nightly topical application of steroid creams, such as betamethasone, under occlusive polythene dressings.

HYPOPARATHYROIDISM

Hypoparathyroidism is the clinical state which may arise either from failure of the parathyroid glands to secrete parathyroid hormone (PTH), or from failure of its action at the tissue level.

Epidemiology

The most common cause of hypoparathyroidism is related to surgical excision or exploration of the neck. In experienced hands, the incidence of permanent hypoparathyroidism is less than 1% for all thyroid and parathyroid surgery.

Aetiology

Hypoparathyroidism due to PTH deficiency can arise in a number of different ways, either as an idiopathic isolated autoimmune disorder or as part of a multiple endocrine deficiency. The latter is an autosomal recessive disorder characterized by hyposecretion of endocrine glands. Postoperative hypoparathyroidism is common, and follows thyroid surgery, parathyroid surgery and other neck operations. Transient hypoparathyroidism with symptomatic hypocalcaemia can occur in neonates.

Pathophysiology

Most individuals possess four parathyroid glands situated along the posterior surface of the thyroid. Ionized plasma calcium levels regulate the secretion of PTH, increased levels suppressing secretion and low levels stimulating it. PTH is an 84 amino acid residue straight-chain polypeptide that acts on hormone-specific receptors on target tissue cells. PTH acts on the renal tubular transport of calcium and phosphate and also stimulates the renal synthesis of 1,25-dihydroxycholecalciferol. PTH increases distal tubular reabsorption of calcium and decreases proximal and distal tubular reabsorption of phosphate. The effects of PTH on bone are complex. The two major cell types in bone are osteoblasts and osteoclasts. Osteoblasts are responsible for the synthesis of extracellular bone matrix and priming of its subsequent mineralization. Osteoclasts decalcify and digest the protein matrix of bone, liberating calcium. PTH stimulates osteoclast-mediated bone resorption in addition to anabolic effects on bone, with an increase in osteoblast number and function. PTH, calcitonin, vitamin D and related preparations all act to maintain plasma calcium levels within the normal range. The long-term use of phenytoin and phenobarbital stimulates the hepatic conversion of cholecalciferol and 25-hydroxycholecalciferol to biologically inactive metabolites. This increases the risk of malabsorption of calcium and development of hypocalcaemia. The risk is highest in patients on long-term therapy, those with low dietary calcium intake and patients with little sunlight exposure.

Clinical manifestations

Many of the clinical features of hypoparathyroidism are due to hypocalcaemia. The decrease in plasma calcium levels leads to increased neuromuscular excitability. The major signs and symptoms are shown in Table 41.11.

Table 41.11	Signs and symptoms of hypocalcaemia
Numbness and tingling in the extremities
Numbness and tingling around the mouth
Muscle spasm
Irritability
Cataracts (prolonged hypocalcaemia)
Positive Chvostek's sign
Positive Trousseau's sign

Investigations

Hypocalcaemia associated with undetectable or low plasma PTH levels is consistent with hypoparathyroidism. Total plasma calcium levels should always be corrected for any abnormality in the plasma albumin concentration. Hyperphosphataemia is often present. It should be noted that there are many other causes of hypocalcaemia (Table 41.12). Pseudohypoparathyroidism is easily distinguished as it is associated with excessive PTH secretion and reduced target organ responsiveness. Drugs that may produce hypocalcaemia include calcitonin, plicamycin (formerly mithramycin), phosphate, bisphosphonates, phenytoin, phenobarbital and colestyramine.

Treatment

Severe, acute hypocalcaemia with tetany should be treated with intravenous calcium gluconate. Initially, 10 ml of

Table 41.12	Causes of hypocalcaemia
Pseudohypoparathyroidism
Vitamin D deficiency
Acute and chronic renal failure
Intestinal malabsorption
Hypomagnesaemia
Drug induced
Acute pancreatitis
Medullary carcinoma of the thyroid
Hypoproteinaemia

10% calcium gluconate is given by slow intravenous injection, preferably with ECG monitoring. If the patient can swallow, oral therapy should be commenced. If further parenteral therapy is required, 20 ml of 10% injection should be added to each 500 ml of intravenous fluid and given over 6 hours. The plasma magnesium level should always be measured in patients with hypocalcaemia, and, if low, magnesium therapy instituted.

For chronic treatment, PTH therapy is not currently a practical option. The hormone has to be administered parenterally, and the current high cost is prohibitive. Maintenance treatment for hypoparathyroidism is with a vitamin D preparation to increase intestinal calcium absorption, often in conjunction with calcium supplementation. Details of the preparations available are given in Table 41.13. Ergocalciferol (vitamin D_3) can be difficult to use. It has a long pharmacological and biological half-life, takes 4–8 weeks to restore normocalcaemia, and its effect persists for 6–18 weeks following withdrawal. In contrast, calcitriol and its synthetic analogue alfacalcidol are much easier to use. Alfacalcidol restores normocalcaemia within 1 week, and its effect only persists for 1 week following withdrawal, permitting greater flexibility in dosage manipulation. The usual daily dose is 0.5–2 micrograms. Initially patients will need to be closely monitored until stable normocalcaemia is achieved. Occasionally dihydrotachysterol is used. This is a synthetic compound that is an analogue of calcitriol.

HYPERPARATHYROIDISM

Hyperparathyroidism is the clinical state that results from increased production of PTH by the parathyroid gland.

Epidemiology

Recent studies in the USA and Europe indicate an incidence rate for primary hyperparathyroidism of 25 cases per 100 000 of the population per year. The incidence is two to three times higher in women than in men, and the disease most commonly presents between the third and fifth decades.

Aetiology

The aetiology of primary hyperparathyroidism is unknown. It may occur as part of a group of familial conditions, the multiple endocrine neoplasia (MEN) syndromes.

There are several conditions associated with secondary hyperparathyroidism, including chronic renal

Table 41.13   Vitamin D preparations

Drug	Preparations	Activity
Ergocalciferol (calciferol, vitamin D$_2$)	Calciferol injection 7.5 mg (300 000 units/ml) Calciferol tablets 250 micrograms (10 000 units) and 1.25 mg (50 000 units) Calcium and ergocalciferol tablets (2.4 mmol of calcium + 400 units of ergocalciferol)	Requires renal and hepatic activation
Cholecalciferol (vitamin D$_3$)	A range of preparations containing calcium (500–600 mg) and colecalciferol (200–440 units)	Requires renal and hepatic activation
Alfacalcidol (1 α-hydroxycholecalciferol)	Alfacalcidol capsules 250 nanograms, 500 nanograms and 1 microgram Alfacalcidol injection 2 micrograms/ml	Requires hepatic activation
Calcitriol (1,25-dihydroxycholecalciferol)	Calcitriol capsules 250 nanograms and 500 nanograms Calcitriol injection 1 microgram/ml	Active
Dihydrotachysterol	Dihydrotachysterol oral solution 250 mg/ml	Requires hepatic activation

failure and vitamin D deficiency. In these conditions the excess PTH is required for a compensatory purpose. Chronic renal failure is the commonest cause, and in the early stages of the disease a rise in the plasma phosphate concentration causes a decrease in plasma calcium with compensatory stimulation of PTH. In the later stages reduced renal 1 α-hydroxylase activity and reduced intestinal calcium absorption lead to further stimulation of the parathyroid glands. Tertiary hyperparathyroidism is the term used to describe a further stage in the development of the secondary type where autonomy of the parathyroids occurs.

Pathophysiology

Primary hyperparathyroidism can result from a parathyroid adenoma, hyperplasia or carcinoma. Solitary adenoma is the commonest, occurring in over 80% of cases. Carcinoma is rare, occurring in approximately 2–3%. Metastases are relatively rare and tend to occur in the lymph nodes, liver or bone marrow.

Clinical manifestation

With increasingly early recognition of the biochemical abnormalities of primary hyperparathyroidism, largely due to automated measurement of plasma calcium, the clinical spectrum of the disease has moved towards mild or asymptomatic cases. Overt bone disease and renal stones are now relatively uncommon manifestations of the disease. Recent studies indicate that over 50% of

cases are asymptomatic at the time of diagnosis. The clinical features of primary hyperparathyroidism are shown in Table 41.14.

Although radiological evidence of bone disease is now rare in these patients, measurement of bone mineral content usually indicates that bone loss is accelerated. Thus, the risk of osteoporotic fractures later in life may be increased.

Table 41.14   Signs and symptoms of hyperparathyroidism

Anorexia, weight loss
Nausea, vomiting
Constipation
Fatigue
Proximal myopathy
Polydipsia, polyuria
Mental changes
Pruritus
Renal stones
Conjunctival and corneal deposits
Bone pain and deformity
Pathological fractures

Investigations

Fasting hypercalcaemia is the primary biochemical abnormality in primary hyperparathyroidism. It should be noted that there are many other causes of hypercalcaemia, including malignancy, drugs (thiazides, excess vitamin D), thyrotoxicosis, immobilization and sarcoidosis.

The most common cause of symptomatic hypercalcaemia is that associated with malignancy, and this diagnosis must always be excluded.

In primary hyperparathyroidism the plasma phosphate levels are often normal in mild cases but are decreased in patients with more advanced disease. PTH levels are usually elevated.

Various techniques may be required for localization of parathyroid tumours, including isotope scanning and computed tomography.

Treatment

Following the diagnosis of primary hyperparathyroidism, early surgery is normally indicated. However, the natural history of hyperparathyroidism is not fully documented. Some studies have indicated that over 50% of untreated patients with primary hyperparathyroidism show no deterioration over 5 years; but the longer-term effects on renal function and bone mass remain unknown.

The main indications for surgical treatment are persistent hypercalcaemia (> 2.75 mmol/l), symptomatic hypercalcaemia, renal impairment, recurrent renal stones and evidence of hyperparathyroid bone disease. In the postoperative period, temporary hypocalcaemia occurs in 20% of patients, particularly if there is bone involvement. In patients with bone disease, treatment with alfacalcidol should be started on the day before the operation. Approximately 10% develop permanent hyperparathyroidism.

Hypercalcaemia can be corrected by inhibiting bone resorption, increasing calcium excretion, or decreasing calcium absorption. General therapeutic measures will depend on the degree and severity of the hypercalcaemia but may include adequate hydration, mobilization, restriction of dietary calcium and avoidance of thiazide diuretics, which can decrease urinary calcium excretion. A treatment algorithm for the management of hypercalcaemia is presented in Figure 41.2.

The use of hormone therapy in hyperparathyroidism has been suggested in patients who either cannot or will

---

'Severely' raised serum calcium levels are difficult to define, but generally levels above 3.5 mmol/l need urgent reduction as they can be associated with renal dysfunction and/or cardiac arrhythmias.

Recommended treatments are as follows:

Rehydration with 0.9% sodium chloride and furosemide (frusemide), for example, 1 litre 0.9% sodium chloride 6-hourly with **furosemide (frusemide)** 40−80 mg daily

Disodium pamidronate, 30 mg, 60 mg or 90 mg, depending on severity of hypercalcaemia, according to the literature, in 0.9% sodium chloride diluted to a concentration of not more than 60 mg in 250 ml, given at a rate not exceeding 1 mg/minute. This treatment is very effective and may last for several weeks, but it takes 24−48 hours to work

In the interim rehydration should be used and **salcatonin (salmon calcitonin)** 100 units subcutaneously three times daily, used if clinically indicated for short-term use (24−48 hours) while pamidronate takes effect

Steroids are usually only effective when hypercalcaemia is related to a steroid-responsive tumour

Other treatments e.g. plicamycin (formerly known as **mithramycin**) and **dialysis** may be considered in severe and refractory cases

NB: treatment of the underlying condition e.g. malignancy, parathyroid tumour or vitamin D toxicity is vital

Figure 41.2 Treatment strategy for hypercalcaemia.

not undergo definitive surgical treatment. The limited data currently available suggest that normalization of plasma calcium is more likely to occur with oestrogen than with progestogen treatment.

Hormone therapy will have the added benefit of providing skeletal protection. Several agents have been specifically investigated for the medical management of hyperparathyroidism. β-blockers have been investigated because catecholamines have been shown to stimulate PTH secretion. However, propranolol has been ineffective, suggesting that the abnormal glands may lose their responsiveness to catecholamines. Histamine has also been shown to stimulate PTH release, leading to the use of cimetidine. Although one study found cimetidine effective, most have found it to be ineffective.

Table 41.15 outlines some of the common therapeutic problems in the management of thyroid and parathyroid disease.

CASE STUDIES

Case 41.1

Miss S. M. is a patient with known hyperthyroidism who presents with a history of heat intolerance, sweats, tremor, weight loss, severe muscle weakness and palpitations. Over the last week she has had increasing difficulty swallowing and admits that she has missed doses of her carbimazole. On examination she has a blood pressure of 180/90 mmHg, a pulse of 110 beats per minute and a diffusely enlarged thyroid gland which is about four times as large as normal. Laboratory results show an elevated free T_4 and an undetectable TSH. It is decided that thyroid surgery is indicated.

Table 41.15 Common therapeutic problems in thyroid and parathyroid disease

Thyroid disease

- Uncertainty over duration of treatment with carbimazole
- Assessing the likelihood of relapse after one episode of hyperthyroidism
- Deciding whether to use carbimazole alone or the 'block and replace' regimen
- Poor compliance with carbimazole when symptoms have resolved
- Difficulty diagnosing hypothyroidism in the elderly patient, due to lack of specific symptoms
- Initiating levothyroxine and achieving a therapeutic dose in patients with coronary heart disease, the elderly or patients with long-standing hypothyroidism

Parathyroid disease

- Compliance with and tolerability of calcium supplements
- Choosing a preparation with correct amounts of both vitamin D and calcium

Questions

1. What are the indications for surgery in patients with hyperthyroidism?
2. What adjunctive therapy would you recommend to help alleviate some of Miss S. M.'s symptoms prior to surgery?
3. What preoperative thyroid preparation is needed for Miss S. M. prior to surgery?
4. What postoperative complications are associated with thyroidectomy?

Answers

1. Surgery is considered the treatment of choice when malignancy is suspected, the patient has oesophageal obstruction and is experiencing difficulty swallowing, respiratory difficulties are present, use of thionamides, propylthiouracil or radioiodine are contraindicated or a large goitre is present which responds poorly following thionamide or radioiodine therapy.
2. β-blockers are effective in relieving many of the symptoms of thyrotoxicosis (particularly tremor, palpitations and anxiety), probably because many of these symptoms mimic sympathetic overactivity. All β-blockers are effective in alleviating symptoms but long-acting agents such as atenolol or long-acting formulations of shorter-acting agents such as propranolol are particularly useful as a once daily regimen may improve compliance. In addition, propranolol inhibits peripheral conversion of T_4 to T_3.
3. Sub-total thyroidectomy is effective and successful in over 90% of patients provided that the patient is adequately prepared for surgery. Miss S. M. should be in a euthyroid state at the time of surgery to avoid a rapid postoperative rise in T_4 levels and precipitation of thyroid storm, which carries high morbidity and mortality. Generally thionamides and propranolol are used. However, with Miss S. M. a combination of iodides and propranolol (the capsules could be opened) would be more useful, especially in view of the difficulties she has experienced with swallowing over the last week. Iodides decrease the friability of the gland and reduce its vascularity to facilitate the surgical procedure. Lugol's iodine 0.3 ml three times a day, well diluted in water or milk, should be given with propranolol for the 10–14 days before surgery.
4. In addition to the risks of anaesthesia and the surgery itself, postoperative complications include hypoparathyroidism, adhesions, laryngeal nerve damage, infection and poor wound healing. The risks of hypothyroidism are higher during the first year after surgery, although there is an insidious rise in incidence over the following 10 years. The incidence of hypothyroidism ranges from 6% to 75% and is inversely related to the amount of remnant tissue left behind.

Case 41.2

Mrs E. A. is a 66-year-old woman. She has recently been complaining of tiredness, lethargy and weight gain. Her general practitioner performed routine thyroid function tests and found she has primary hypothyroidism. She has had congestive cardiac failure for 5 years.

Her general practitioner now wishes to commence her on T_4 replacement therapy. Her current drug therapy includes:

- **captopril 12.5 mg three times daily**
- **furosemide (frusemide) 80 mg in the morning.**

Questions

1. What are the therapeutic objectives in this patient?
2. How should T_4 therapy be instituted?
3. How should the replacement therapy be monitored?

Answers

1. The therapeutic objectives should be to relieve the symptoms (tiredness, lethargy and weight gain) of hypothyroidism without producing an exacerbation of her congestive cardiac failure.
2. T_4 replacement therapy should be introduced very cautiously in this patient. Most newly diagnosed patients with hypothyroidism have a long-standing deficiency, and the rapid introduction of replacement therapy can only do more harm than good. The low circulating levels of thyroid hormones actually protect the heart from any increased metabolic demands which might worsen her cardiac failure. Mrs E. A. should be commenced on T_4 25 micrograms daily. If this is well tolerated, the dose can be gradually increased every 4–6 weeks. Older patients usually require lower maintenance doses than their younger counterparts, possibly due to a decrease in clearance of T_4 in the elderly. In older patients the daily maintenance dosage of T_4 is usually 100 micrograms or less.

   It has been suggested that T_3 should be used as replacement therapy in patients with cardiac disease. T_3 has shorter half-life than T_4, and therefore if adverse effects do develop, the effect will last for a shorter period of time. However, T_3 is more biologically active than T_4 and therefore potentially more cardiotoxic.
3. Replacement therapy should be monitored both clinically and biochemically. Symptomatic improvement of hypothyroidism should occur within 2–3 weeks of starting therapy, but maximal benefit may take considerably longer. The clinical assessment should include both symptoms of hypothyroidism and congestive cardiac failure, of which the most critical is the latter.

   The patient should be questioned about the development of any symptoms suggestive of cardiac failure; for example, ankle swelling or shortness of breath. If there is a clear exacerbation of the heart failure, the T_4 should be discontinued or the dose reduced. A temporary increase in the dose of diuretic and/or angiotensin-converting enzyme inhibitor may be required. Even when all these precautions are adhered to, it is not always possible to render the patient euthyroid. Sometimes a compromise has to be reached in which the patient is treated with sub-optimal T_4 replacement therapy but has stable cardiac status.

Case 41.3

Mr B. C. is 66 years old. He has recently been commenced on levothyroxine at a dose of 50 micrograms daily. He is now collecting his first repeat prescription for T_4. In addition he has a long-standing prescription for carbamazepine 200 mg three times daily, and ferrous sulphate 200 mg in the morning.

Question

What issues would you need to cover when counselling Mr B. C. about his medicines?

Answer

First, there are two potential drug–drug interactions within Mr B. C.'s medication regimen. Ferrous sulphate has been shown to cause a reduction in the effect of levothyroxine in patients with hypothyroidism. The mechanism is not fully understood but may be the result of the production of a poorly absorbable iron–levothyroxine complex within the gastrointestinal tract. Mr B. C. should be advised to separate his doses of levothyroxine and ferrous sulphate by 2 hours.

In addition, there have been isolated reports that the anticonvulsants carbamazepine and phenytoin increase the metabolism of thyroid hormones and decrease their serum concentrations. However, as it is normal clinical practice to monitor T_4 replacement by measurement of T_3 and T_4 concentrations, this is unlikely to be of any clinical significance. The importance of attending for regular monitoring should be stressed. It should be explained to the patient that it may be several weeks or even months before the symptoms are fully controlled. He is not yet receiving a full maintenance dose; the dose should not be increased any more frequently than every 4 weeks owing to the long half-life of T_4. Consequently, it may be several months before a full maintenance dose is achieved. Mr B. C. will also need to understand the need for lifelong therapy. It is particularly important to reinforce this when the patient has become asymptomatic from his thyroid disease.

Case 41.4

Mrs E. H., aged 55 years, has been attending the anticoagulant clinic for several years. She is on long-term anticoagulant therapy following a prosthetic heart valve replacement 3 years ago. Recently, her anticoagulant control has been difficult and she has required decreasing doses of warfarin to maintain a therapeutic international normalized level (INR). Other recent symptoms include diarrhoea and weight loss, which have been investigated by her general practitioner, as a result of which she has been found to have hyperthyroidism. Her current drug therapy is warfarin 2 mg daily.

Questions

1. How may thyroid disease influence warfarin dosage?
2. What will happen to Mrs E. H.'s warfarin requirements when her hyperthyroidism is treated?

Answers

1. Thyroid dysfunction can alter the metabolism of both oral anticoagulants and vitamin K-dependent clotting factors. The net circulating levels of vitamin K-dependent clotting factors are not usually altered in hyperthyroid patients because both the biosynthesis and catabolism of these factors are decreased. However, an enhanced anticoagulant response is seen when the warfarin-induced decrease in

clotting factor synthesis is combined with hyperthyroidism-induced increase in clotting factor catabolism.

It can be predicted that patients with hyperthyroidism will require less warfarin to produce a therapeutic INR than euthyroid patients.

2. When Mrs E. H.'s hyperthyroidism is treated, her warfarin requirements will increase. The time to stabilization will depend on which form of treatment is used. Warfarin requirements would be expected to change quickly after surgery. If drug therapy is used it usually takes several months to achieve euthyroidism but if radioactive iodine therapy is used this time period could be much longer.

Regardless of which form of treatment is used, frequent tests of anticoagulant control will need to be performed and the dose of warfarin adjusted accordingly.

Case 41.5

Mr C. J., 64 years old, visits his GP complaining of increasing lethargy and tiredness. On further questioning he has also put on 5 kg in weight over the last few months, without any change in appetite or exercise patterns. Six months ago he had a myocardial infarction and subsequently developed a ventricular tachyarrhythmia. This is now controlled on amiodarone 200 mg daily. The GP does some thyroid function tests which subsequently show a low free T_4 and a high TSH, indicating a diagnosis of hypothyroidism.

Questions

1. How common is amiodarone-induced hypothyroidism and what is the mechanism for its development?
2. The preferred management of drug-induced thyroid disease is to stop the responsible agent. If it were possible to stop the amiodarone, what would be the anticipated pattern of recovery?
3. In Mr C. J. it is not possible to stop the amiodarone. How should the hypothyroidism be managed?

Answers

1. The reported incidence of amiodarone-induced hypothyroidism varies widely, but may be as high as 13% in countries such as the UK with a high dietary iodine intake. The risk of developing hypothyroidism is independent of the daily or cumulative dose of amiodarone, but is increased in elderly and female patients. This is to be expected as autoimmune thyroid disease is the main risk factor for the development of hypothyroidism and is particularly common in these patient groups.

   Amiodarone contains pharmacological amounts of iodine and the most likely explanation for the development of hypothyroidism is an inability of the thyroid gland to escape from the acute inhibitory effects of this iodine load on thyroid hormone release and synthesis. This may reflect an unmasking of underlying thyroid disease, as hypothyroidism is a well-recognized outcome in patients with subclinical disease who are given excess iodine. In these patients, the hypothyroidism occurs relatively soon (3–12 months) after starting treatment with amiodarone.

2. The ideal approach to the treatment of this patient's hypothyroidism is to stop the amiodarone. If that is possible, many patients without pre-existing thyroid disease will become euthyroid within 2–4 months of stopping the drug although it may take longer in some patients. However, permanent hypothyroidism requiring levothyroxine replacement is common in patients with thyroid antibodies.

3. In practice, amiodarone is often used in high-risk patients or when other agents have failed to control the symptoms. In Mr C. J. amiodarone is being used to treat a life-threatening arrhythmia and stopping the drug is unlikely to be a therapeutic option. The safest, quickest and most reliable treatment is to continue the amiodarone and add in T_4. This should be done in the same way as for any other patient, increasing the dose at 4–6 week intervals until the TSH concentration is in the normal range and the patient's symptoms have resolved.

REFERENCES

Anon 1997 Drug-induced agranulocytosis. Drug and Therapeutics Bulletin 35: 49–52

Faber J, Galloe M 1994 Changes in bone mass during prolonged treatment subclinical hyperthyroidism due to L-thyroxine treatment: a meta analysis. European Journal of Endocrinology 130: 350–356

International Agranulocytosis and Aplastic Anaemia Study 1988 Risk of agranulocytosis and aplastic anaemia in relation to the use of antithyroid drugs. British Medical Journal 297: 262–265

Lucas A, Salinas I, Rius F et al 1997 Medical therapy of Graves' disease: does thyroxine prevent recurrence of hyperthyroidism? Journal of Clinical Endocrinology and Metabolism 82: 2410–2413

MacFarlane I A, Davies D, Longson D et al 1983 Single daily dose short-term carbimazole therapy for hyperthyroid Graves' disease. Clinical Endocrinology 18: 557–561

Maugendre D, Gatel A, Campion L et al 1999 Antithyroid drugs and Graves' disease: prospective randomised assessment of long-term treatment. Clinical Endocrinology 50: 127–132

Rittmaster R S, Abbott E C, Douglas R et al 1998 Effect of methimazole, with or without L-thyroxine, on remission rates in Graves' disease. Journal of Clinical Endocrinology and Metabolism 83: 814–818

Uzzan B, Campos J, Cicherat M et al 1996 Effects on bone mass of long-term treatment with thyroid hormones: a meta-analysis. Journal of Clinical Endocrinology and Metabolism 81: 4278–4289

FURTHER READING

Anon 1998 Managing subclinical hypothyroidism. Drug and Therapeutics Bulletin 36: 1–3

Beckerman P, Silver J 1999 Vitamin D and the parathyroid. American Journal of the Medical Sciences 317: 363–369

Brown A J 1998 Vitamin D analogues. American Journal of Kidney Diseases 32(2 Suppl. 2): S25–39

Hanna F W F, Lazarus J H, Scanlon M F 1999 Controversial aspects of thyroid disease. British Medical Journal 319: 894–899

Lourwood D L 1998 The pharmacology and therapeutic utility of bisphosphonates. Pharmacotherapy 18: 779–789

MacFarlane I 2000 Thyroid disease. Pharmaceutical Journal 265: 240–244

Newman C M, Price A, Davies D W et al 1998 Amiodarone and thyroid: a practical guide to the management of thyroid dysfunction induced by amiodarone therapy. Heart 79: 121–127

Woeber K 2000 Update on the management of hyperthyroidism and hypothyroidism. Archives of Internal Medicine 160: 1067–1071

Diabetes mellitus 42

J. A. Cantrill   J. Wood

KEY POINTS

- Diabetes is a chronic, incurable condition that affects 1.4 million people in the UK, over three-quarters of whom have type 2 diabetes. A further 1 million cases are thought to be undiagnosed.
- If not adequately managed; diabetes can result in a wide range of complications that have clinical, social and economic implications.
- Patients with diabetes require a wide range of educational advice, including foot care, management of intercurrent illness and hypoglycaemia.
- All patients should receive dietary advice and other appropriate lifestyle advice, for example smoking cessation.
- In addition to achieving optimal glycaemic control, it is essential that coexisting hypertension and dyslipidaemia are identified and treated. In these patients, achieving optimal glycaemic control alone will not prevent complications.
- There are a wide variety of insulins and delivery devices available, allowing regimens to be tailored to individual need.
- There are six main types of oral hypoglycaemic agents available; the initial choice of therapy in type 2 diabetes will largely be determined by the patient's renal function, age and weight.

Diabetes mellitus is a heterogeneous group of disorders characterized by varying degrees of insulin hyposecretion and/or insulin insensitivity. Regardless of cause, it is associated with hyperglycaemia.

Epidemiology

There are major ethnic and geographical differences in the prevalence and incidence of type 1 diabetes. Figures are highest in Caucasians while the disorder is rare in Japan and the Pacific area. In Northern Europe the prevalence is approximately 0.3% in those under 30 years of age. There is evidence that the prevalence is increasing. Type 1 diabetes may present at any age but there is a sharp increase around the time of puberty and a decline thereafter. Approximately 50–60% of patients with type 1 will present before 20 years of age.

Type 2 diabetes mellitus is much commoner than type 1, accounting for over 75% of all patients with diabetes in most populations. It usually occurs in patients over the age of 40 years. In the UK, diabetes affects approximately 1.4 million people, and a further million are thought to be undiagnosed. The incidence of type 2 increases with age and with increasing obesity. As with type 1, there are major ethnic and geographical variations. In general, in non-obese populations the prevalence is 1–3%. In the more obese societies, there is a sharp increase in prevalence with figures of 6–8% in the USA increasing to values as high as 30% in Hindu Tamils in South Africa. Diabetes is five times more common among Asian immigrants in the UK than in the indigenous population. World studies of immigrants have suggested that the chances of developing type 2 are between two and 20 times higher in well-fed populations than in lean populations of the same race.

Aetiology

Before considering the aetiology of diabetes it is necessary to understand the classification (Table 42.1). The two main types of diabetes are type 1 and type 2. These were formerly referred to as insulin-dependent diabetes mellitus (type 1) and non-insulin-dependent diabetes mellitus (type 2), respectively, but this terminology is no longer used.

The aetiology of type 1 has been the subject of considerable research. Genetic factors are important but do not explain fully the development of type 1. There is a strong immunological component to type 1 and a clear association with many organ-specific autoimmune diseases. Circulating islet cell antibodies (ICAs) are present in more than 70% of type 1 at the time of diagnosis. Family studies have shown that the appearance of ICAs often precedes the onset of clinical diabetes by as much as 3 years. Type 1 has been widely believed to be a disease of sudden onset, but the development now appears to be a slow process of progressive immunological damage. However, it is not currently possible to use screening methods to identify patients who will develop diabetes in the future. The

---

Table 42.1 Aetiological classification of diabetes mellitus (WHO 1999)

Type 1 (β cell destruction, usually leading to absolute insulin deficiency)
  Autoimmune
  Idiopathic

Type 2 (may range from predominantly insulin with relative insulin deficiency to a predominantly secretory defect with or without insulin resistance)

Other specific types
  Genetic defects of β cell function
  Genetic defects in insulin action
  Diseases of the exocrine pancreas
  Endocrinopathies
  Drug- or chemical-induced, e.g. nicotinic acid, glucocorticoids, high-dose thiazides, pentamidine, interferon-alpha
  Infections
  Uncommon forms of immune-mediated diabetes
  Other genetic syndromes sometimes associated with diabetes
  Gestational diabetes

---

final event which precipitates clinical diabetes may be caused by sudden stress such as an infection when the mass of the β cells of the pancreas falls below 5–10%. Studies have been carried out in which patients with newly diagnosed type 1 have been treated with immunosuppressive therapy, notably ciclosporin. Although some patients do benefit and no longer require insulin therapy, such treatment is not a safe option for long-term control.

Type 2 has a much stronger genetic relationship than type 1. Identical twins have a concordance rate approaching 100%. This suggests the relative importance of inheritance over environment. If a parent has type 2, the risk of a child eventually developing type 2 is 5–10% compared with 1–2% for type 1. The clearest association of type 2 is with obesity. Obesity is associated with hyperinsulinaemia and marked insulin insensitivity and a decrease in the number of insulin receptors. It has also been suggested that there is a selective defect in the β cell secretory mechanism that prevents it from responding normally to glucose. On average, patients with type 2 retain approximately 50% of their β cell mass. Circulating insulin levels are normal or raised when compared with normal subjects, but are inappropriately low for the degree of hyperglycaemia present.

Pathophysiology

The islets of Langerhans are the endocrine component of the pancreas, and they constitute 1% of the total pancreatic mass. Insulin is synthesized in the pancreatic β cells. It is synthesized initially as a polypeptide precursor – preproinsulin. The latter is rapidly converted in the pancreas to proinsulin, which, through the removal of four amino acid residues, forms equal amounts of insulin and C-peptide. Insulin consists of 51 amino acids in two chains connected by two disulphide bridges. In the islets, insulin, C-peptide (and some proinsulin) are packaged into granules. Insulin associates spontaneously into a hexamer that contains two zinc ions and one calcium ion.

Glucose is the major stimulant to insulin release. The response is triggered both by the intake of nutrients and the release of gastrointestinal peptide hormones. Following an intravenous injection of glucose there is a biphasic insulin response. There is an initial rapid response in the first 2 minutes, followed after 5–10 minutes by a second response that is smaller in magnitude but sustained over 1 hour. The initial response represents the release of stored insulin and the second phase reflects discharge of newly synthesized insulin. Glucose is unique; other agents, including sulphonylureas, do not result in insulin biosynthesis, only release. Once released from the pancreas, insulin enters the portal circulation. It is rapidly degraded by the liver and only 50% reaches the peripheral circulation. In the basal state, insulin secretion is at the rate of approximately 1 unit per hour. The intake of food results in a prompt five- to 10-fold increase. Total daily secretion is approximately 40 units.

Insulin circulates free as a monomer, has a half-life of 4–5 minutes and is primarily metabolized by the liver and kidneys. In the kidneys, insulin is filtered by the glomeruli and reabsorbed by the tubules, which also degrade it. In both renal and hepatic disease there is a decrease in the rate of insulin clearance, which may necessitate dosage adjustment in those who inject insulin. Peripheral tissues such as muscle and fat also degrade insulin, but this is of minor quantitative significance.

Many tissues contain receptors that are highly specific for insulin and to which it binds reversibly. The biological response to insulin can be altered by either a change in the receptor affinity for insulin, or a change in the total number of receptors. Changes in the number of receptors occur in two important clinical situations: obesity and chronic exposure to high insulin levels. Both lead to a decrease in the number of receptors, i.e. down-regulation. In obese patients, calorie restriction is associated with an increase in receptor numbers even before weight loss occurs.

The interaction of insulin with the receptor on the cell surface sets off a chain of messengers within the cell. This opens up transport processes for glucose, amino acids and electrolytes.

Acute deficiency of insulin leads to unrestrained hepatic glycogenolysis and gluconeogenesis with a consequent increase in hepatic glucose output. Glucose uptake is decreased in insulin-sensitive tissues, and hyperglycaemia ensues. Either as a result of the metabolic disturbance itself or secondary to infection or other acute illness, there is increased secretion of the counter-regulatory hormones glucagon, cortisol, catecholamine and growth hormone. All of these will further increase hepatic glucose production. At the same time the normal restraining effect of insulin on lipolysis is removed. Non-esterified fatty acids are released into the circulation and taken up by the liver, which produces acetyl coenzyme A (acetyl CoA). The capacity of the tricarboxylic acid cycle to metabolize the acetyl CoA is rapidly exceeded. Ketone bodies, acetoacetate and hydroxy-butyrate are formed in increased amounts and released into the circulation. This results in the clinical picture known as diabetic ketoacidosis (DKA).

Clinical manifestation

The symptoms are similar in type 1 and type 2, but may vary in their intensity. Common symptoms include polyuria and polydipsia, which are a consequence of osmotic diuresis secondary to sustained hyperglycaemia. Another consequence of the hyperosmolar state is blurred vision, usually due to a change in refraction. Weight loss despite normal or increased appetite is also a common feature.

Type 1 diabetes

If the diagnosis is not made when the common features of hyperglycaemia present, diabetic ketoacidosis may develop. Lowered plasma volume produces dizziness and weakness due to postural hypotension. Total body potassium loss and the general catabolism of muscle protein further contribute to the weakness. When insulin deficiency is severe and of acute onset, all of these symptoms progress in an accelerated manner. Ketoacidosis exacerbates the dehydration and hyperosmolality by producing anorexia, nausea and vomiting. As the plasma osmolality rises, impaired consciousness ensues. With progression of the acidosis, deep breathing with a rapid ventilatory rate (Kussmaul respiration) occurs as the body attempts to correct the acidosis. The patient's breath may have the fruity odour of acetone.

Type 2 diabetes

The clinical presentation of type 2 diabetes may occur in a number of different ways. Many patients with type 2 have an insidious onset of hyperglycaemia and they may have few or none of the classical symptoms. This is particularly true in obese individuals, whose diabetes may only be detected after glycosuria or hyperglycaemia is detected during routine investigation. Chronic skin infections are common, as sustained hyperglycaemia can result in severe impairment of phagocyte function. Generalized pruritus and symptoms of vaginitis are frequently the initial complaints of women with type 2. Occasionally patients will present when the complications of sustained hyperglycaemia have already developed. Retinopathy may be detected on routine ophthalmological examination or the combination of neuropathy, peripheral vascular disease and infection may manifest as foot ulceration or gangrene.

Investigations

In June 2000, the UK formally adopted a new set of World Health Organization criteria for diagnosing diabetes mellitus (WHO 1999). These new criteria, listed below, reflect research evidence on the prevention of diabetes-related complications:

1. Diabetes symptoms (i.e. polyuria, polydipsia and unexplained weight loss) plus

   - a random venous plasma glucose concentration ≥ 11.1 mmol/l
   - *or* a fasting plasma glucose concentration ≥ 7.0 mmol/l (whole blood ≥ 6.1 mmol/l)
   - *or* plasma glucose concentration ≥ 11.1 mmol/l 2 hours after 75 g anhydrous glucose in an oral glucose tolerance test.

2. With no symptoms, diagnosis should *not* be based on a single glucose determination but requires confirmatory plasma venous determination. At least one additional glucose test result, on another day with the value in the diabetic range, is essential, either fasting, from a random sample or from the 2-hour post glucose load. If the fasting or random values are not diagnostic, the 2 hour value should be used.

Current recommendations are that the diagnosis is confirmed by a glucose measurement performed in an accredited laboratory on a venous plasma sample. A diagnosis should never be made on the basis of glycosuria or a stick reading of a finger-prick blood glucose alone, although such tests are being examined for screening purposes. Glycated haemoglobin (HbA_{1c}) is also not currently recommended for diagnostic purposes.

The biochemical diagnosis of ketoacidosis is usually made at the bedside and confirmed in the laboratory. Urinalysis will show marked glycosuria and ketones. A blood glucose test strip will usually show a blood glucose level of more than 22 mmol/l. Formal laboratory measurement of glucose, urea, creatinine, electrolytes and arterial pH, Po_2 and Pco_2 (to determine the extent of the acidosis) should be carried out. Two potentially misleading laboratory results are the white blood cell count and serum sodium. The former will always be raised but correlates with the ketone body level and is not therefore a guide to infection. The serum sodium level will often be low due to the osmotic effect of glucose draining from the cells and diluting the sodium. The sodium concentration will also be spuriously low if there is marked dyslipidaemia.

Complications

Treatment aims initially to relieve the immediate signs and symptoms of diabetes (polydipsia and polyuria, weight loss, ketoacidosis). In the longer term, the main aim of treatment is to prevent the development, or slow the progression, of the long-term complications of the disease. Treatment should also aim to minimize the occurrence of hypoglycaemia.

Persistent hyperglycaemia (DCCT 1993, UKPDS 1998a, UKPDS 1998b) and hypertension (UKPDS 1998c) are the two major controllable factors that influence the development of diabetic complications. These can be divided into those caused by microvascular disease and those secondary to macrovascular disease. The main sites and forms of tissue damage are discussed below. Although they may all occur in all types of diabetes, the spectrum of incidence is different. Renal failure due to severe microvascular nephropathy is the major cause of death in type 1, whereas macrovascular disease is the leading cause in type 2. Although blindness may occur in both types, the aetiology is often different. Similarly, although neuropathy is common in both types, severe autonomic neuropathy is much more common in type 1. In countries for which there are adequate data, diabetes is the commonest cause of blindness before the age of 65 years. Where renal transplantation is offered to patients below the age of 70 years with progressive renal failure, diabetes accounts for 20–25% of referrals. Peripheral vascular disease causing ulceration or gangrene in the lower limbs is the major cause of hospital bed occupancy by patients with diabetes. It is worthwhile considering in more detail the impact of some of these chronic complications.

Eye disease

Blurring of vision is usually a benign occurrence associated with rapid changes in blood glucose control. It is most commonly reported in newly treated patients. They should be warned that this may occur and reassured that it is temporary.

Open-angle glaucoma is more common in patients with diabetes than in the general population, for reasons that are unclear. Management is the same as for patients who do not have diabetes. Cataracts are also common in patients with diabetes, past middle age.

In any population of adults with diabetes, retinopathy will be present in between 10% and 50%. It is closely related to the duration of the disease. In the early stages retinopathy may not interfere with the patient's vision, and therefore should be actively screened for. Once detected, careful attention should be paid to blood glucose and blood-pressure control. Some forms of retinopathy can be treated using laser photocoagulation. In advanced disease, surgery may be required.

Diseases of the urinary tract

Urinary tract infections are common in diabetes. Management is no different to that in the population who do not have diabetes, except that recurrence is common. The role of prophylactic antibiotics in preventing chronic renal damage is unclear.

Nephropathy is one of the potentially life-threatening complications of diabetes. Poor control of diabetes is associated with enlargement of the kidneys and a high glomerular filtration rate. These features are often present at diagnosis and resolve with effective treatment. Patients who go on to develop microalbuminuria are at risk of developing frank albuminuria and renal failure in later years. Once the serum creatinine level rises above normal, it usually increases linearly if a reciprocal plot against time is produced. When end-stage renal failure develops, standard therapy is used to treat symptoms. Continuous ambulatory peritoneal dialysis (CAPD) carries a risk of peritonitis, and blood glucose must be carefully monitored and controlled. Insulin may be given in the peritoneal infusate to cover the high carbohydrate load administered.

Nerve damage

Neuropathy can affect patients with diabetes in many different ways. The most common peripheral neuropathy is of the distal sensory type, which is particularly manifested in the feet. It is most prevalent in elderly patients with type 2, but may be found with any type of diabetes, at any age beyond childhood. Painful diabetic neuropathy can be one of the most disabling of all diabetic complications, and is a cause of considerable morbidity. In diabetic proximal motor neuropathy there is rapid onset of weakness and wasting, principally of the thigh muscles. Muscle pain is common and may require opiate analgesia. Autonomic neuropathy may affect any part of the sympathetic or parasympathetic nervous systems. The commonest manifestation is diabetic impotence. Bladder dysfunction usually takes the form of loss of bladder tone with a large increase in volume. Diabetic diarrhoea is uncommon, but can be troublesome through its tendency to occur at night. Gastroparesis may cause delayed gastrointestinal transit and variable food absorption causing difficulty in the insulin-treated patient, or it may cause vomiting. Postural hypotension due to autonomic neuropathy is uncommon, but can be severe and disabling. Disorders of the efferent and afferent nerves controlling cardiac and respiratory function are more common, but rarely symptomatic.

Cardiovascular disease

Myocardial infarction is the major cause of death in diabetes. Peripheral vascular disease is also common, and accounts for much of the morbidity associated with foot problems. Cerebrovascular events occur at an increased frequency when compared with the population who do not have diabetes. Hypertension is common, in association with both macrovascular and microvascular disease. In some populations with type 2 diabetes, the prevalence of hypertension may be as high as 50%. A further risk factor for cardiovascular disease is dyslipidaemia. Both hypertension and lipid disorders should be actively sought and treated in patients with diabetes.

Diabetic foot

Foot problems in diabetes cause more inpatient hospital bed occupancy than all the other medical problems of the diabetic patient put together. They may be, at least in part, preventable by education. Foot ulcers can be divided into three categories. Classical neuropathic ulceration occurs on the sole of the foot. The ulcers can be deep but are usually painless. Ischaemic ulcers are classically painful, usually occur on the distal ends of the toes, and are associated with signs of peripheral vascular disease and ischaemia. The most common lesions are infected foot ulcers. There are usually a number of factors involved, namely: vascular disease, neuropathy, poor foot care and poorly controlled diabetes.

Infections

Many infections are seen more frequently in diabetes, and are an indication of poor diabetic control. There is some evidence that leucocyte function is impaired by blood glucose levels above 10–13 mmol/l.

Other

There is a whole spectrum of rare complications that can also occur in diabetes. These include musculoskeletal problems (e.g. Dupuytren's contracture and Charcot arthropathy) and dermatological conditions (e.g. acanthosis nigricans and necrobiosis lipoidica). In addition to all of these chronic complications, the patient with diabetes may also be at risk of experiencing the acute complications hypoglycaemia, diabetic ketoacidosis and non-ketotic hyperglycaemic coma.

Therapy

All patients with diabetes should receive healthy living advice. This includes advice on appropriate physical activity and lifestyle modification, particularly smoking cessation and healthy eating.

Dietary therapy

Dietary control is the mainstay of treatment for type 2, and plays an integral part in the management of type 1. Dietary recommendations have undergone considerable changes in recent years. Healthy eating advice is now the same for both groups and the 'special diabetic diet' is a thing of the past. Some of the general dietary advice that patients should be given is shown in Table 42.2.

Carbohydrate

The blood glucose level is closely affected by carbohydrate intake. Daily intake should be kept fairly constant, and the amount given should be appropriate to the level of physical activity. Most active young people will require 180 g of carbohydrate per day, whereas 100 g may suffice for an elderly person. If fibre-rich foods such as wholemeal bread, jacket potatoes, etc., are eaten, the carbohydrate content of the diet may make up 50–55% of the calories. People with diabetes should limit their sugar intake, but total exclusion of sugar from the diet is unnecessary and impractical. Diets should no longer be referred to as 'sugar-free'. In addition, 'diabetic foods' are not recommended as they are often expensive and their nutritional content is not always compatible with healthy eating advice. They have been replaced in diabetes management by the reduced sugar food products, which are a feature of a general healthy diet for the whole population.

Table 42.2   Dietary advice for people with diabetes

- Eat regular meals based on starchy foods such as bread, pasta, potatoes, rice and cereals. Whenever possible, choose high-fibre varieties of these foods, e.g. wholemeal bread and wholemeal cereals.

- Try to cut down on fat, particularly saturated (animal) fats. Monounsaturated fats such as olive oil are preferred. Eating less fat and fewer fatty foods also helps to lose weight. Use less butter, margarine, cheese and eat fewer fatty meals. Choose low-fat dairy foods, e.g. skimmed milk and low fat yoghurt. Grill, steam or oven bake instead of frying or cooking with oil or other fats.

- Try to eat at least five portions of fruit and vegetables every day. This provides vitamins and fibre as well as helping to balance the overall diet.

- Cut down on sugar and sugary foods. This does not mean that the diet has to be totally free of sugar. Sugar can still be used as an ingredient in foods and baking as part of a healthy diet. However, use sugar-free, low sugar or diet squashes and fizzy drinks, as sugary drinks cause blood glucose levels to rise quickly.

- Use less salt, because a high intake of salt can raise blood pressure. Food can be flavoured with herbs and spices instead of salt.

- Drink alcohol in moderation. That is 2 units per day for a woman and 3 for a man. For example, a small glass of wine or half a pint of normal strength beer is 1 unit. Never drink on an empty stomach, as alcohol can make hypoglycaemia more likely to occur.

Fat

One major reason for increasing the proportion of calories as carbohydrate is to reduce fat intake. Since there is an increased risk of death from coronary artery disease in diabetes, it is wise to restrict saturated fats and to substitute unsaturated fats. Furthermore, obesity is a major problem in diabetes, and fats contain more than twice the energy content per unit weight than either carbohydrate or protein. About 30% of the total daily calories should be provided by fat. More severe restriction may be indicated for individuals with hypercholesterolaemia.

Fibre

Dietary fibre has two useful properties. First, it is physically bulky and increases satiety. Second, fibre delays the digestion and absorption of complex carbohydrates, thereby minimizing hyperglycaemia. For the average person with type 2, 15 g of soluble fibre (from fruit, vegetables and pulses) is likely to produce a 10% improvement in fasting blood glucose, glycated haemoglobin and low-density lipoprotein (LDL) cholesterol.

Insulin therapy in the type 1 patient

All patients with type 1 require treatment with insulin. There is a wide variety of different insulin preparations available. These may differ in species, onset of action, time to peak effect and duration of action (Table 42.3).

Species

There are three types of insulin available from different species: beef, pork and human. Beef insulin differs from human insulin in three amino acids. The slightly different chemical structure does give rise to some pharmacokinetic differences. Beef insulin is more slowly absorbed after subcutaneous injection and has a longer duration of action when compared to an equivalent pork or human formulation. Porcine insulin differs from human insulin in only one amino acid at the end of the B chain. This substitution has only minimal effect on the molecular structure of the protein, with the result that the body is much less likely to mount an antibody response to pork insulin than to beef insulin. Human insulin has been available for over 20 years but has not yet been proven to be clinically superior to pork insulin. Human insulin can be produced semi-synthetically by enzymatic modification of porcine insulin (emp). However, most human insulin is manufactured using genetic engineering. This process involves recombinant DNA technology using *Escherichia coli* (crb, prb, pyr). All insulin preparations are to some extent immunogenic in man, but immunological resistance to insulin is very rare. Human insulins should theoretically be less immunogenic, but no real advantage has been demonstrated in either trials or practice.

It is standard practice to commence all patients requiring insulin on human insulin. There is some concern patients receiving porcine insulin may develop hypoglycaemic unawareness after transfer to human insulin. Although there is little or no scientific evidence to support this, some patients request they be changed back to pork insulin. Although it may be argued that there is no proven clinical need for any insulin other than human, equally there is no proven benefit of human over pork insulin, and patients' wishes should be respected.

Insulin preparations

The onset of action, peak effect and duration of action are determined both by the insulin type and by the physical and chemical form of the insulin.

Neutral insulin is the quickest and shortest-acting of all the available insulins. It is also commonly referred to as soluble insulin. After subcutaneous injection, neutral insulin appears in the circulation within 10 minutes. The concentration rises to a peak after about 2 hours and then declines over a further 4–8 hours. This absorption curve

Table 42.3   Insulin preparations

Preparation	Origin	Onset (h)	Peak (h)	Duration (h)
Neutral insulin				
Human Actrapid (pyr)	H	0.5	2–5	8
Human Velosulin (emp)	H	0.5	1–3	8
Humulin S (prb)	H	0.5	1–3	5–7
Hypurin Bovine Neutral	B	0.5/1	2–5	6–8
Pork Actrapid	P	0.5	1–3	8
Humalog (Insulin lispro)	H	0.25	1–1.5	2–5
Neverapid (Insulin aspart)	H	0.25	1–3	3–5
Hypurin Porcine Neutral	P	0.5/1	2–5	6–8
Insumar Rapid (prb)	H	0.5	1–3	7–9
Biphasic Insulin				
Human Mixtard 10 (pyr)	H	0.5	2–12	24
Human Mixtard 20 (pyr)	H	0.5	2–12	24
Human Mixtard 30 (pyr)	H	0.5	2–12	24
Human Mixtard 40 (pyr)	H	0.5	2–12	24
Human Mixtard 50 (pyr)	H	0.5	2–12	24
Humulin M2 (prb)	H	0.5	1–9.5	14–16
Humulin M3 (prb)	H	0.5	1–8.5	14–15
Humulin M5 (prb)	H	0.5	1–8	14–15
Pork Mixtard 30	P	0.5	4–8	24
Humalog Mix 25	H	0.25	1–2	22
Hypurin Porcine 30/70	P	0.5	4–12	24
Insumar Combi 15 (prb)	H	0.5	2–4	12–20
Insumar Combi 25 (prb)	H	0.5	2–4	12–19
Insumar Combi 50 (prb)	H	0.5	1–4	12–16
Isophane Insulin				
Hypurin Porcine Isophone	P	2	6–12	24
Insumar Basal (prb)	H	1	3–4	12–20
Human Insulatard (pyr)	H	2	4–12	24
Humulin I (prb)	H	0.5	2–8	18–20
Hypurin Bovine Isophane	B	2	6–12	24
Pork Insulatard	P	2	4–12	24
Insulin zinc suspension (mixed)				
Human Monotard (pyr)	H	3	7–15	24
Humulin Lente (prb)	H	1	4–16	24
Hypurin Bovine Lente	B	2	8–12	30
Lentard MC	B/P	3	7–15	24
Insulin zinc suspension (crystalline)				
Human Ultratard (pyr)	H	4	8–24	28
Humulin Zn (prb)	H	2	6–14	20–24
Protamine zinc				
Hypurin Bovine PZI	B	4	10–20	36

Insulin preparations classified as being of human (H), beef (B) or pork (P) origin; emp, enzymatically modified pork; prb, proinsulin recombinant bacteria; pyr, precursor yeast recombinant.

can be contrasted with the physiological insulin concentration curve, where peak concentrations are reached 30–40 minutes after a meal, and decline rapidly to 10–20% of peak levels after about 2 hours. Recent years have seen the introduction of the recombinant insulin analogues insulin lispro and insulin aspart. They appear to have similar biological activity to insulin once absorbed. The differences between human insulin and these analogues lie in their pharmacokinetics. Human insulin self-associates into hexamers in neutral solutions, which then dissociate before absorption from subcutaneous tissue. Insulin analogues produce less self-association, resulting in a more rapid onset of action and shorter duration of action when compared to neutral insulin. The clinical results are higher fasting and pre-prandial blood glucose concentrations, slightly lower post-prandial concentrations and possibly slightly less hypoglycaemia. The analogues may prove to be more convenient for some patients as they can be given immediately before a meal rather than the 30 minutes recommended for human neutral insulin.

Isophane insulin is a suspension of protamine with insulin. The onset of action is usually 1–2 hours with the peak effect being seen at 4–8 hours. There is considerable inter-patient variation in the duration of action, but it usually requires twice daily administration. Isophane and neutral insulin do not interact when mixed together. As a result there is now a wide range of ready mixed (biphasic) preparations available that contain varying proportions of isophane and neutral insulin.

Lente insulin is an insulin zinc suspension that is a 30:70 mixture of an amorphous insulin and a crystalline zinc–insulin complex in suspension. Lente insulin has a slower onset of action than isophane insulin, and a longer duration of effect at the same dose. In order to maintain the integrity of the insulin crystals, all insulin zinc suspensions contain significant amounts of free zinc in solution. If mixed with neutral insulin some of the latter may be precipitated into a loose complex if they remain in contact for any length of time. Consequently it is recommended that if these two insulins are mixed, they should be injected immediately.

The longest time to peak action is seen with the crystalline form of an insulin zinc suspension and protamine zinc insulin. They are very slowly absorbed from subcutaneous tissue and have a very variable bioavailability.

The most recent development in insulin therapy is the introduction of the long-acting insulin analogue insulin glargine, which is also produced using recombinant DNA technology. When injected subcutaneously, it forms a microprecipitate at the physiological neutral pH of the subcutaneous space. Because of its stability, absorption of insulin glargine from the site of injection is delayed and prolonged, thus providing a fairly constant basal insulin supply, much like that of basal insulin secretion in non-diabetic people. The pharmacokinetic and pharmacodynamic data for insulin glargine, together with the results from clinical studies, suggest that this form of basal insulin may improve the management of type 1 diabetes.

Insulin delivery

The subcutaneous route is used for maintenance therapy. Insulin can be injected into the thigh, abdominal wall, buttocks or upper arm. Its main advantages are accessibility and that it allows most patients to administer their own insulin. However, this route cannot be regarded as physiological as it delivers insulin to the systemic rather than portal circulation. Many patients use disposable plastic syringes and insulin from a vial as their means of insulin administration. However, there are now an increasing number and variety of pen injection devices available for insulin administration. The devices are compact and do away with the need to draw up insulin from a vial. Many insulins are also available in the form of a pre-filled, disposable (but biodegradable) pen. The pen devices are not in themselves a means to improved diabetic control, but are becoming increasingly popular as they are far more convenient for patients, since there is no need to draw up doses of insulin.

Intravenous delivery should be used in the management of ketoacidosis. The short half-life of insulin means that changes in the rate of the infusion have a rapid effect on insulin action. This is not generally a satisfactory route for long-term administration.

One anticipated development in insulin delivery is the administration of insulin by the nasal route. This is likely to improve patient acceptance of insulin therapy, rather than improve clinical management.

Insulin regimens

Twice-daily injections are one of the most commonly used regimens in the UK. However, there are limited data to support an improvement in glycaemic control using three rather than two injections per day (SIGN 2001). The typical twice daily regimen may involve the use of intermediate-acting insulin alone or in combination with neutral insulin. The injections are usually given half an hour before breakfast and half an hour before the evening meal. The short-acting insulin analogues can be given immediately before a meal. The ratio of short- to intermediate-acting preparations, and the split between morning and afternoon doses varies from patient to patient. In the newly diagnosed patient who is not acutely ill, it may be simpler to start therapy at home with an intermediate-acting insulin alone, adding the short-acting preparation if and when indicated by self-monitoring.

'Multiple-injection' regimens refers to the use of neutral insulin to cover the three main meals and an intermediate- or long-acting preparation for the overnight period. Injection of neutral insulin before each meal allows greater flexibility of insulin dosage and eating habits. Many patients are taught to calculate their own dose on the basis of the pre-prandial blood glucose concentration. The injections before meals are usually given using a pen device, and the basal insulin using a conventional syringe. With this regimen the neutral insulin injections given before each meal usually comprise 60% of the total daily dosage and the longer-acting insulin 40% of the total daily dose.

Starting doses of insulin and the ratio of short- to intermediate-acting insulin are very variable. In patients who are very active (for example manual workers and those who exercise regularly) the starting dose should be kept low to reduce the risk of significant hypoglycaemia.

Adjusting the insulin dose

The information on which insulin dosage adjustment is based is derived from blood glucose self-monitoring and the incidence and timing of hypoglycaemia. On twice-daily rapid- and intermediate-acting insulin regimens, the neutral insulin may be considered as acting up to the next meal or to bedtime, while the extended-acting insulins act up to the next injection. The glucose concentration at the end of the period can be taken as a measure of the appropriateness of the relevant dose. For most patients, adjustments of insulin dose will be up or down 2–6 units at a time.

Storage of insulin

Insulin formulations are stable if kept out of light, and they are not subject to freezing or extremes of heat. Loss of potency of 5–10% occurs in vials kept at high ambient room temperatures for 2–3 months. Insulin should therefore be stored in a domestic refrigerator except for the vial(s) in current use. When pen injector devices are in use, they should never be stored in a refrigerator.

Adverse effects of insulin

Hypoglycaemia is a common major physiological complication of insulin therapy and is often a source of great anxiety to patients and carers. The signs and symptoms produced by hypoglycaemia fall into two groups, those due to adrenaline (epinephrine) release and those due to neuroglycopenia. The manifestations may occur at different blood glucose levels in different individuals. In some patients with diabetes they may occur with concentrations above 2.2 mmol/l, especially if the blood glucose level falls rapidly. The release of adrenaline (epinephrine) may result in palpitations, tremor, tachycardia, hunger and sweating. Some patients treated with β blocking agents may lose these adrenergic warning signs, with the exception of sweating, which may increase. As the neuroglycopenia ensues, restlessness and mental instability may be present as well as irritability, obstinacy and agitation. Patients also commonly complain of perioral numbness and tingling.

Thickening of subcutaneous tissues can occur at injection sites as a result of recurrent injection in a small area (lipohypertrophy). This may result in impaired and erratic insulin absorption. The solution is to rotate injection sites. Bruising is usually a sign of superficial injections. Localized skin reactions occasionally occur but usually resolve even with continued use of the same insulin preparation.

Systemic allergic reactions rarely occur with the current universal use of highly purified insulins. Though not usually species-specific, it is worthwhile trying insulin of a different species if allergy occurs.

Management of the patient with type 2

Many patients with type 2 diabetes are overweight and need advice on calorie restriction, in addition to the general healthy eating advice, in order to lose weight and achieve a body mass index (BMI) below 25 kg/m^2. Even if dietary advice and weight loss do result in good glycaemic control, the diabetes must not be regarded as cured; it may reappear in times of stress or if dietary control is lost.

However, for over 75% of these patients, dietary measures and exercise do not produce adequate glycaemic control and oral hypoglycaemic therapy is required. In practice, most patients will require oral drug therapy within 3 years of diagnosis. In the UK, the six types of agents currently available are sulphonylureas, a biguanide (metformin), repaglinide and nateglinide thiazolidinediones, an α-glucosidase inhibitor (acarbose) and guar gum. Of these, guar gum is very rarely used in clinical practice and the use of acarbose is declining. As a result of ongoing loss of β cell function, most patients will eventually need a combination of two differently acting classes of oral agent. There may also be justification for early use of two or even three different drugs early in the disease to attain good glycaemic control before β cell function deteriorates into absolute hypoinsulinaemia.

Choice of treatment

The factors used to select a particular treatment include the patient's clinical characteristics, such as their degree of hyperglycaemia, weight, age and renal function (Fig. 42.1). As a guide, patients with a fasting blood glucose of between 7 and 11 mmol/l will need dietary advice initially and exercise recommendations tailored to their capabilities. Patients with a blood glucose between 12 and 17 mmol/l may be successfully treated with diet and an oral hypoglycaemic agent initially but often require insulin in the medium term. Finally, patients whose blood glucose is consistently > 17 mmol/l in the absence of overt stress will probably need insulin, if not initially, then relatively soon after diagnosis. If it is decided that drug therapy is indicated the selection is made according to the mode of action, safety profile and potential for adverse effects of the chosen drug in the individual patient.

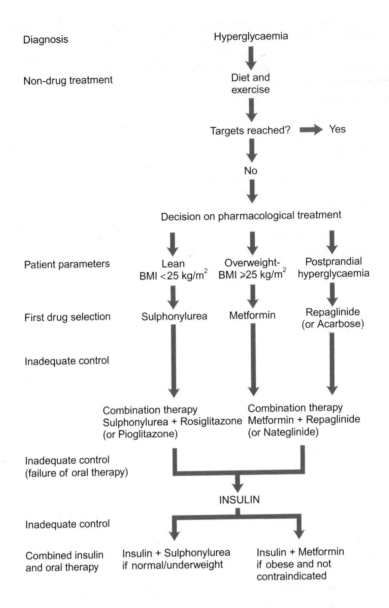

Figure 42.1   Algorithm for the treatment of type 2 diabetes.

Sulphonylureas

Mode of action.   The major actions of this class of drug rely on the ability of the pancreas to secret insulin. All sulphonylureas lower blood sugar levels by increasing pancreatic β cell sensitivity to glucose, so that more insulin is released for any given glucose load. Sulphonylurea therapy is also associated with an increased tissue sensitivity to insulin, resulting in improved insulin action. Recent studies have also suggested that sulphonylureas may promote an increased systemic bioavailability of insulin due to reduced hepatic extraction of the insulin secreted from the pancreas. Several reports have suggested that sulphonylureas may reduce platelet aggregation. However, it is likely that the antiplatelet effects are secondary to the improvement in blood glucose concentrations produced by these drugs.

Pharmacokinetics.   The pharmacokinetic parameters of the oral hypoglycaemic agents are shown in Table 42.4. Chlorpropamide is the slowest and longest-acting agent. Although glibenclamide has been shown to have a short elimination half-life, it has a prolonged biological effect, which may be explained by slower distribution and the existence of a deep compartment, possibly the islet cells.

Table 42.4 Pharmacokinetic properties of oral hypoglycaemic agents

Drug	Main route of elimination	Elimination half-life (h)	Duration of action (h)	Daily dose range	Doses per day
Sulphonyluraes					
First generation					
Tolbutamide	Hepatic	4–24	6–10	0.5–2 g	1–3
Chlorpropamide	Hepatic (80%) Renal (20%)	24–48	24–72	100–500 mg	1
Second generation					
Glibenclamide	Hepatic (40%) Biliary (60%)	2–4	16–24	2.5–15 mg	1–2
Glipizide	Hepatic	2–4	6–24	2.5–40 mg	1–3
Gliquidone	Hepatic	1–2	6–24	15–180 mg	2–3
Gliclazide	Hepatic	10–12	10–24	40–320 mg	1–2
Glimepiride	Renal (60%) Biliary (40%)	5–8	12–24	1–6 mg	1
Biguanides					
Metformin	Renal	1–5	5–8	1–3 g	2–3
Non sulphonylurea insulinotropic					
Repaglinide	Hepatic	1	4–6	1–16 mg	With each main meal
Netaglinide	Hepatic	1	3–4	180–540 mg	3 (before each main meal)
Thiazolidinediones					
Rosiglitazone	Hepatic	3–4	6–24	4–8 mg	1–2
Pioglitazone	Hepatic	5–6	16–24	15–30 mg	1

All sulphonylureas are metabolized by the liver to some degree and some may have active metabolites.

Choice of drug. There are many factors that may influence the choice of sulphonylurea. These may relate to the drug itself, the patient or the prescriber. There are few well-controlled long-term clinical comparisons between sulphonylureas. It would appear that when dosage is individualized and governed by the effect on fasting blood glucose, there is little or no difference in clinical efficacy between the different agents. In general, if a patient is not well controlled on the maximum dosage of one sulphonylurea, it is not worthwhile changing to another one, except possibly for tolbutamide.

Adverse effects. The frequency of adverse effects from sulphonylureas is low. They are usually mild and reversible on withdrawal of the drug (Table 42.5). The most common adverse effect is hypoglycaemia; this may be profound and long-lasting. Hypoglycaemia due to sulphonylureas is often misdiagnosed, particularly in the elderly. The major risk factors for the development of hypoglycaemia include: use of a long-acting agent, increasing age, inadequate carbohydrate intake and renal or hepatic dysfunction.

Other adverse effects are rare; blood dyscrasias occur in 0.1% of patients and rashes in up to 3%. Chlorpropamide can produce troublesome flushing after ingestion of alcohol, and about 5% of patients develop hyponatraemia due to its effect on increasing renal sensitivity to antidiuretic hormone (ADH). Most patients are asymptomatic with this problem but occasionally severe hyponatraemia is observed. It is not widely appreciated that patients treated with sulphonylureas often gain weight. This is unfortunate as it will exacerbate their resistance to insulin and to the sulphonylureas themselves.

Sulphonylurea dosage. The dosage should be individualized for each patient, and the lowest possible dose used to attain the desired levels of blood glucose, without producing hypoglycaemia. Treatment should start with a low dose and be increased approximately every 2 weeks. For many agents the maximum effect is seen if the dose is taken half an hour before a meal, rather than with or after food. The number of daily doses required will depend on the agent used and the total daily dose. For several drugs it becomes necessary to administer the drug two or three times daily when the dose is increased.

Table 42.5 Adverse effects of sulphonylureas

Adverse effect	Comments
Gastrointestinal	Affects approximately 2% Most commonly nausea and vomiting Dose related Advise patient to take with or after food
Dermatological	Affects 1–3% Usually occur within the first 2–6 weeks Most commonly: generalized photosensitivity, pruritus, maculopapular May require discontinuation of drug Cross-sensitivity between sulphonylureas is common Rare cases of severe allergic reactions, e.g. erythema multiforme. Stevens—Johnson syndrome
Haematological	Rare cases of fatal agranulocytosis or pancytopenia Other haematological effects usually reversible on discontinuing drug Some reports of reversible haemolytic anaemia
Hepatic	Mild, reversible elevation of liver function tests Cholestatic jaundice Usually a hypersensitivity reaction associated with fever, rash and eosinophilia
Cardiovascular	Possible excess of cardiovascular mortality in patients treated with tolbutamide (not proven)
Hypothyroidism	Association not proven May be rare cases
Alcohol flush	Rarely seen with sulphonylureas other than chlorpropamide Change to another agent
Syndrome of inappropriate antidiuretic hormone (SIADH)	Chlorpropamide, and to a lesser extent tolbutamide, enhance the effect of ADH on the kidney Results in hyponatraemia Risk factors are: increasing age, congestive cardiac failure and diuretic therapy
Hypoglycaemia	The most common adverse effect and may be severe and prolonged Highest incidence with chlorpropamide and glibenclamide All sulphonylureas and meglitinides have been implicated Risk factors include; increasing age, impaired renal or hepatic function, reduced food intake, weight loss Either decrease dose, change to a shorter-acting agent or discontinue sulphonylurea therapy

Drug interactions. Several drugs can interfere with the efficacy of sulphonylureas, by influencing either their pharmacokinetics or pharmacodynamics, or both. There is much written in the literature about displacement interactions with sulphonylureas. However, their clinical significance is doubtful. Many reported cases involve first-generation agents, which have a different protein-binding site to the second-generation agents. The first-generation agents are readily displaced from albumin by other acidic drugs, whereas the second-generation agents bind in a non-ionic fashion and are not readily displaced. Ingestion of alcohol can cause hypoglycaemia in itself and can also prolong the hypoglycaemic effect of sulphonylureas.

Biguanides

Metformin is the only biguanide available in the UK. The mechanism of action of biguanides is still poorly understood, but many theories have been proposed. These include: reduced gastrointestinal absorption of carbohydrate; inhibition of hepatic gluconeogenesis; stimulation of tissue uptake of glucose; and increased insulin receptor binding. Of these, probably the most important is the effect on hepatic gluconeogenesis. The action of metformin does not involve stimulation of pancreatic insulin secretion. The major advantage of metformin over sulphonylureas is that it does not cause either hypoglycaemia or weight gain.

Metformin has a short duration of action and is not bound to plasma proteins. It is not metabolized and is totally renally eliminated.

Adverse effects. The most common adverse effects of metformin result from gastrointestinal disturbance. These include anorexia, nausea, abdominal discomfort and diarrhoea. These effects are usually transient and can be minimized by starting with a low dose, increasing the dose slowly and administering the drug with or after food. One suggested regimen is to start with 500 mg daily for 1 week, then 500 mg twice daily for 1 week, and increasing the dosage at weekly intervals until the desired glycaemic response is achieved. Despite these precautions, a few patients are genuinely intolerant of the drug.

A rare but potentially life-threatening adverse effect is lactic acidosis. The patients at most risk are those with renal insufficiency in whom the drug accumulates, those with coexisting conditions in whom lactate accumulates, and those who are unable to metabolize lactate. In practice, metformin should not be prescribed for patients who have renal impairment, liver disease, alcoholism, uncontrolled cardiac failure or severe pulmonary insufficiency. It should also be withdrawn in a patient who develops a severe intercurrent illness, for example acute myocardial infarction or septicaemia, or who is undergoing major surgery.

Role of metformin. Metformin is useful in the obese patient with diabetes as it does not cause weight gain. If there are no contraindications it can be used in conjunction with diet as second-line therapy in patients not adequately controlled on diet alone. As it has a different mode of action to the sulphonylureas, repaglinide or the thiazolidinediones, it can be valuable when prescribed in combination.

Repaglinide

Mode of action. Repaglinide is the first in a new class of drugs, the meglitinides, to be marketed in the UK. It is a novel insulin-releasing agent which was developed from the non-sulphonylurea portion of glibenclamide. Unlike the sulphonylureas it does not inhibit pro-insulin biosynthesis and does not stimulate direct insulin exocytosis from the β cell. Repaglinide acts by mediating the closure of ATP-sensitive potassium channels in the pancreatic β cell, which causes subsequent depolarization, thereby stimulating the release of insulin from the β cells. Insulin release only occurs in the presence of glucose.

Pharmacokinetics. Although repaglinide stimulates insulin release in a similar manner to the sulphonylureas, its pharmacokinetic properties confer a rapid onset and a short duration of action. It is rapidly absorbed and reaches peak concentrations within 1 hour of administration. It is metabolized by oxidative biotransformation and direct conjugation with glucuronic acid in the liver and has a plasma half-life of less than 1 hour. It is excreted primarily by the liver and only minimally (about 8%) by the kidneys. None of the known metabolites has any hypoglycaemic effect. Repaglinide is taken immediately before main meals although the time can vary up to 30 minutes before a meal. Its pharmacokinetic profile means that repaglinide may offer some advantages in patients with poor renal function and those with irregular eating habits. The pharmacokinetic parameters of repaglinide are shown in Table 42.4.

Adverse effects. Repaglinide causes a range of side-effects; the most common include abdominal pain, diarrhoea, constipation, nausea and vomiting. More rarely hypersensitivity reactions can occur as well as elevation of liver enzymes. Repaglinide also causes hypoglycaemia.

Dosage. The recommended starting dose is 500 micrograms pre-prandially (with each meal) for patients with an $HbA_{1c} < 8\%$ (except for patients being transferred from other therapies or who have a higher HbA_{1c} where the starting dose is 1 mg pre-prandially). When transferring from another agent to repaglinide, the latter should be started on the morning of the day after the other drug has been stopped. Subsequently the pre-prandial dose is doubled at weekly intervals until a response is achieved or a pre-prandial dose of 4 mg is reached. The maximum dose is 16 mg per day.

Drug interactions. Drugs which induce or inhibit the cytochrome P450 enzyme CYP3A4 interact with repaglinide. For example, ketoconazole, itraconazole, erythromycin and fluconazole increase plasma concentrations of repaglinide, and rifampicin and phenytoin decrease plasma levels of repaglinide.

Role of repaglinide. Repaglinide is an effective first-line therapy in type 2 diabetes and may be used in combination with metformin to produce a synergistic effect. It is indicated in type 2 patients who are not controlled on diet alone or on metformin alone. It may be most beneficial in patients who experience problems with post-prandial glucose elevation and as single therapy in patients who eat at unpredictable times or have a tendency to miss meals. There appears to be no significant difference in the efficacy of repaglinide compared with glibenclamide and gliclazide but it may be more effective than glipizide. Repaglinide lowers fasting and post-prandial blood glucose by approximately 4 mmol/l and 7 mmol/l, respectively. Inter-patient variation of blood glucose with dose is high but intra-patient variation is low – the higher the glucose load, the more effectively repaglinide stimulates insulin secretion (without an increase in dose), thereby eliminating the need to vary the dose once treatment is established. Although repaglinide has been shown to be safe and effective in patients over 65 years of age it can cause hypoglycaemia and may be inappropriate for elderly patients who live alone and in those who do not experience warning signs of hypoglycaemia. Like sulphonylureas, repaglinide also causes weight gain and therefore may not be suitable for obese patients. Repaglinide requires wider clinical use and further comparative studies before its place in therapy can be clearly defined.

Nateglinide is a newer insulin secretagogue which appears to have a similar made of action and role.

Thiazolidinediones

Mode of action. The thiazolidinediones are a new class of compounds which act as agonists of the nuclear peroxisome proliferator-activated receptor-gamma (PPARG). PPARG is strongly expressed in adipose tissue and weakly in skeletal muscles, liver and some other tissues. Essentially thiazolidinediones work by enhancing insulin action and promoting glucose utilization in peripheral tissues, possibly by stimulating non-oxidative glucose metabolism in muscle and suppressing gluconeogenesis in the liver. They also have an effect on reducing insulin resistance. They have no effects on insulin secretion. The available agents in this class include pioglitazone and rosiglitazone. They act most effectively in combination with other oral antidiabetic agents including sulphonylureas and metformin.

Pharmacokinetics. Rosiglitazone is metabolized in the liver by N-demethylation and hydroxylation followed by conjugation with sulphate and glucuronic acid to form inactive compounds which are excreted mainly by the kidney but also by the liver. Pioglitazone is also metabolized extensively in the liver to both active and inactive metabolites. The pharmacokinetic parameters of both agents are shown in Table 42.4.

Adverse effects. The primary side-effect of both rosiglitazone and pioglitazone is oedema, particularly in patients with hypertension and congestive cardiac failure. As combination therapy with insulin and thiazolidinediones results in a higher incidence of oedema, use with insulin is contraindicated in the UK. Anaemia also occurs in about 1% of patients and is reflected by a small decrease in the haemoglobin concentration during the first 4–12 weeks of therapy. However, it has been postulated that this decrease is due to dilutional effects caused by an increase in plasma volume. Both agents caused weight gain of up to 3.5 kg during trials. During trials some patients also experienced headache, abdominal pain, myalgia and upper respiratory infection. Elevated liver transaminases also occur with both agents in up 0.2% of patients. Due to the association of another thiazolidinedione (troglitazone, was withdrawn from the UK market in 1997) with liver failure, it is currently recommended

with both agents that liver function is checked before initiating therapy, every 2 months for the first year, and periodically thereafter. However, liver failure caused by thiazolidinediones is not a class effect but was due to a metabolic idiosyncrasy resulting in the production of a toxic metabolite from a specific side chain in the structure of troglitazone.

Dosage. Rosiglitazone is started at a dose of 4 mg daily in combination with metformin or a sulphonylurea. This dose may be increased in patients taking rosiglitazone in combination with metformin to a dose of 8 mg daily, in single or divided doses, after a period of 6 weeks. The maximum recommended dose of rosiglitazone in combination with a sulphonylurea is 4 mg daily. Pioglitazone is started at a dose of 15 mg daily in combination with metformin or a sulphonylurea. This dose may be increased in patients taking pioglitazone in combination with either metformin or a sulphonylurea to 30 mg once daily. Administration of both agents may be either with or without food. Dosage adjustment is not necessary for either agent in patients with mild or moderate renal impairment or in the elderly. However, these agents should not be used in patients with severe renal impairment or in those with hepatic impairment.

Drug interactions. Pioglitazone is metabolized by cytochrome P450 CYP3A4. Therefore drugs which induce or inhibit this enzyme interact with pioglitazone. For example, ketoconazole, itraconazole, erythromycin and fluconazole increase serum concentrations, and rifampicin and phenytoin decrease serum levels of pioglitazone. Rosiglitazone is metabolized by CYP2C8 and 2C9, which are not major P450 pathways and therefore no clinically relevant interactions have been reported with other agents. Concurrent administration of NSAIDs may increase the risk of oedema.

Role of thiazolidinediones. Thiazolidinediones have been shown to improve glycaemic control in a range of patients, especially in those with insulin resistance, by reducing HbA_{1c} levels by up to 1.5% compared to continuing with a sulphonylurea or metformin alone. Either rosiglitazone or pioglitazone should be offered to patients in combination with metformin or a sulphonylurea if they are unable to take or have an inadequate response to metformin and a sulphonylurea in combination. This step is viewed as an alternative to transferring the patient to insulin. The combination of a thiazolidinedione with metformin is preferred to combination with a sulphonylurea, especially in obese patients. However, thiazolidinediones in combination with sulphonylureas may be useful in patients in whom metformin is contraindicated. The future of this class of agents looks promising as, unlike existing oral antidiabetic agents, both rosiglitazone and pioglitazone directly target insulin resistance and improve β cell function. They therefore tackle the two fundamental defects in type 2 diabetes and so have the potential to alter disease progression and reduce complications.

Alpha-glucosidase inhibitors

Acarbose retards carbohydrate digestion by interfering with gastrointestinal glucosidase activity. Although overall carbohydrate absorption is not significantly altered, the post-prandial hyperglycaemic peaks are markedly reduced. Acarbose is minimally absorbed in unchanged form from the gastrointestinal tract.

Adverse effects. The most common adverse effect of acarbose is abdominal discomfort associated with flatulence and diarrhoea. These symptoms usually improve with continued treatment, but can be minimized by starting with a low dose and titrating slowly.

Systemic adverse effects are rare, but high doses have been associated with idiosyncratic elevations of the levels of serum hepatic transaminases. Patients titrated to the maximum dose of 200 mg three times daily should be closely monitored, preferably at monthly intervals for the first 6 months. If elevated transaminase levels are observed, reduction in dose or withdrawal of therapy should be considered.

Role of acarbose. Acarbose is a therapeutic option in type 2 patients inadequately controlled on diet alone, or on diet and other oral hypoglycaemic agents. However, the gastrointestinal side-effects do limit the use of acarbose in clinical practice.

Insulin therapy in type 2

Patients who respond initially to oral hypoglycaemic agents for 1 month or longer, and who subsequently relapse, are referred to as 'secondary failures'. The rate of secondary failure varies from 20% to 30% in different series. These patients require treatment with insulin. Although such patients are often reluctant to change to insulin therapy, doing so can often result in considerable improvement in well-being. On the basis of glycaemic control and weight gain, no single insulin treatment regimen can be considered superior to others, although twice daily administration of fixed mixtures that contain one-third short-acting and two-thirds intermediate-acting insulin (e.g. Human Mixtard 30 or Humulin M3) are simple, cost-effective and tend to suit a significant proportion of patients. In a lean patient (BMI < 25 kg/m^2), who will be relatively sensitive to insulin, a reasonable starting dose for these fixed insulin mixtures is 12 units before breakfast and 8 units before tea. This will usually adequately control symptoms and can be adjusted to achieve appropriate glycaemic targets. Overweight patients (BMI > 25 kg/m^2) are likely to be insulin resistant and therefore their initial dose may need to be as high as 20 units before breakfast and 10 units before tea.

If overnight hypoglycaemia and unacceptable morning hyperglycaemia is a problem with this twice daily regimen, improvement may be obtained by dividing the evening insulin dose so that the soluble insulin is given before tea, and the intermediate-acting insulin is given at bedtime. This three-dose regimen is very satisfactory in a number of patients, although three injections per day may pose practical problems in some elderly patients.

Alternatively, some lean type 2 patients who are transferred from oral therapy to insulin may be successfully treated with once or twice daily isophane insulin. For example, a single daily dose of Humulin I or Human Monotard, given before breakfast, or twice daily administration of the latter, may achieve a balance between acceptable symptomatic control and convenience while reducing the risk of hypoglycaemia. Such an approach may also be appropriate in the very elderly where symptomatic control is all that is required and where a district nurse is needed to administer the insulin. However, late afternoon and evening blood glucose levels may be unacceptably high on a single daily dosing regimen but this depends on the pattern of food intake in the individual.

In type 2 patients who require temporary insulin during intercurrent illness a soluble preparation such as Humulin S or Human Actrapid can be given two or three times daily with a small dose of isophane insulin at bedtime to control blood glucose quickly and eliminate symptoms. The most commonly quoted regimen is 6 units of soluble insulin before each meal and 6 units of isophane insulin (e.g. Humulin I) at bedtime. The dose is selected initially according to the patient's previous insulin requirements, if any, and adjusted according to four times daily blood glucose measurements.

Treating hypertension

The coexistence of hypertension and diabetes dramatically increases the risk of microvascular and macrovascular complications. Most important is the increased risk of cardiovascular disease. Data from the United Kingdom Prospective Diabetes Study Group (UKPDS 1998c) suggests that tight control of blood pressure may be a more effective method of preventing complications in patients with type 2 diabetes than tight glycaemic control. The current recommendation is that both people with type 1 diabetes and those with type 2 diabetes should have a target systolic blood pressure of < 140 mmHg and a target diastolic pressure of < 80 mmHg. In type 1 diabetes, hypertension usually indicates the presence of diabetic nephropathy. If nephropathy is present the targets are a systolic blood pressure of < 130 mmHg and a diastolic pressure of < 80 mmHg, or even lower if proteinuria exceeds 1 g in 24 hours.

Many studies have examined the treatment of hypertension in patients with diabetes, using a wide range of different drug regimens. Taken together, the results suggest that it is the reduction of blood pressure, rather than the drug(s) used, which is of primary importance (Curb et al 1996, Hansson et al 1998, UKPDS 1998d). Another key message from the UKPDS is that multiple drug therapies are often required to reach the target blood pressure. The exception, in terms of drug choice, is in patients with diabetic nephropathy. In this situation, there is physiologic and clinical rationale for the preferential blockade of the renin angiotensin system with angiotensin-converting enzyme (ACE) inhibitors. There is also growing evidence that ACE inhibitors may have beneficial effects on renal function in normotensive patients (Mathiesen et al 1999) and in preventing or ameliorating other complication of diabetes (Chaturvedi et al 1998, HOPE Study Investigators 2000, SIGN 2001).

Patient care

Patient education

Diabetes is a chronic, incurable condition that has considerable impact on the life of each individual patient, whatever his or her age or type of diabetes. Patient involvement is paramount for the successful care of diabetes. The principal task of the health care team is to give each patient knowledge, self-confidence and support (Anon 2000).

The way in which education is delivered will depend upon the individual patient and the availability of local resources. Individual tuition is desirable in the early stages after diagnosis. This type of education is usually delivered by a diabetes specialist nurse. The educational aspect of care is a gradual and ongoing process. At a later stage, group education can be effectively used, especially in type 2 patients. Many such programmes are multidisciplinary and may involve doctors, nurses, dietitians, pharmacists and chiropodists. It is also essential to involve the patient's family and carers in the educational process. Patients can also obtain support and information from specialist organizations and their literature, for example Diabetes UK (formerly the British Diabetic Association). Diabetes UK provides valuable information on a wide range of diabetes-related issues, and organizes a network of local support groups providing a forum for patients to exchange ideas and discuss problems.

Patients require education and information about a wide range of subjects (Table 42.6). In particular, appropriate advice about the use of over-the-counter medications, foot care products and 'diabetic' food products is frequently requested.

Management targets

The theoretical ideal for all patients with diabetes is to achieve normoglycaemia. As this is not always possible the aim is to achieve the best possible control compatible with an acceptable lifestyle for the patient. In some patients this may mean only symptomatic control, in others this may be tight control. In making this decision the following factors should be considered: the patient's age, motivation, intelligence, understanding, likely compliance, coexisting diseases, ability to recognize hypoglycaemia, duration of their diabetes and the presence/absence/severity of complications.

Targets for pre-meal blood glucose of between 4 and 7 mmol/l and post-meal values of < 9 mmol/l may be achieved provided there is no significant hypoglycaemia. In many patients an HbA_{1C} of $\leq 6.5\%$ should be targeted. However, this may be difficult to achieve in some older patients. In the latter group a value of 7% may be more easily achieved and lead to fewer hypoglycaemic episodes. The management goals for diabetes in patients of 75 years and over may be different and more conservative than for the more motivated and otherwise

Table 42.6 Patient education in diabetes

1. The disease
   - Signs and symptoms
2. Hyperglycaemia
   - Signs, symptoms and treatments
3. Hypoglycaemia
   - Signs, symptoms and treatments
4. Exercise
   - Benefits and effect on blood glucose control
5. Diet
6. Insulin therapy
   - Injection technique
   - Types of insulin
   - Onset and peak actions
   - Storage
   - Stability
7. Urine testing
   - Glucose
   - Ketones
8. Home blood glucose testing
   - Technique
   - Interpretation
9. Oral hypoglycaemic agents
   - Mode of action
   - Dosing
   - Need for multiple therapies
10. Foot care
11. Management during illness
12. Cardiovascular risk factors
    - Smoking
    - Hypertension
    - Obesity
    - Hyperlipidaemia
13. Regular medical and ophthalmologic examinations

fit, younger elderly (those between 65 and 75 years of age) and younger adults. For example, some elderly patients will have poor vision and limited manual dexterity which may or may not be linked to a degree of cognitive impairment. Others have multiple pathology and take a number of other medications. Therefore the goals of therapy need to be both individual and realistic. In some patients they will involve only the optimization of body weight, control of symptoms and avoidance of hypoglycaemia (which has an increased risk of severe brain damage and may occur without the usual warning signs in the elderly). In others, reasonably tight control may be appropriate. Therefore, there is a difficult balance between the use of aggressive treatment with its associated risk of hypoglycaemia and the benefits of reducing complications to maintain an acceptable quality of life. Table 42.7 sets out some of the common therapeutic problems in diabetes. As the proportion of elderly people in the population rises over the next few years, management of diabetes in this age group will pose an increasing challenge.

Monitoring glycaemic control

Patients with type 1

All patients treated with insulin should, wherever possible, undertake home blood glucose monitoring (HBGM). After the capillary blood has been applied to the reagent strip a colour reaction occurs. The result can either be visually compared to a colour chart or measured using a reflectance meter. Whether the extra precision of a meter is worthwhile is largely a matter of personal preference. Strips read visually are perfectly

---

Table 42.7 Common therapeutic problems in diabetes

- Achieving normoglycaemia or HbA$_{1c}$ targets

- Achieving an acceptable balance between improving glycaemic control and minimizing episodes of hypoglycaemia

- Achieving adequate control in type 2 diabetes with diet alone, especially in patients who are overweight

- Drug-related weight gain, notably with insulin and sulphonylureas

- Achieving blood pressure targets in patients with coexisting hypertension

- Ensuring adherence as drug regimens become complex, requiring multiple drug therapies

- Making insulin therapy acceptable to patients with type 2 diabetes, inadequately controlled with oral therapies

---

adequate for most situations although the extra accuracy may be desirable in pregnancy. HBGM enables patients and carers to make a direct assessment of the effect of changes in drugs or dietary habits, exercise and patterns of illness. HBGM has the additional benefit that it can detect hypoglycaemia and, unlike urine tests, in which glycosuria may only be detected some time after changes in blood glucose have occurred, it enables more accurate calculations of insulin doses.

Patients with type 1, who are by definition ketosis-prone, should also know how and when to test their urine for ketones. This test need not be carried out as part of routine monitoring, but is essential at times of intercurrent illness, especially when the blood glucose is ≥ 17 mmol/l.

Patients with type 2

For most patients with type 2 who are treated with diet alone or with oral hypoglycaemic agents, urine glucose monitoring is adequate. This is a simple non-invasive test that can detect hyper- but not hypoglycaemia. HBGM is used by some patients with type 2, particularly if control is poor, if they are being treated with insulin or if the patient wishes to use this method.

Clinic monitoring

There are several ways in which control of diabetes can be monitored in the clinic or general practitioner's surgery. Careful monitoring of weight change is also important. In the overweight patient with type 2, weight loss may be the only form of treatment required. However, unexpected weight loss may indicate poor control. In the young patient with diabetes it is essential to ensure that normal growth and development are maintained.

The use of random blood glucose measurements in the clinic has been superseded by the monitoring of glycated proteins. Glycation of minor haemoglobin components occurs in the blood; the extent depends on both the amount of glucose present and the duration of exposure of the haemoglobin to glucose. Estimates of glycated haemoglobin (HbA$_{1c}$) provide an index of average control of diabetes over the preceding 2–3 months. HbA$_{1c}$ can be measured at any time, and levels are not normally affected by acute changes in therapy, diet or exercise. Serum fructosamine represents the glycation of all serum proteins and gives information about control over the preceding 3 weeks. As albumin is the major serum protein, the albumin concentration must be known for interpretation of fructosamine levels. However, HbA$_{1c}$ is the preferred marker for glycaemic control.

Patients should also have a comprehensive annual review and examination to look for the development of complications such as nephropathy, neuropathy and retinopathy. In patients who already have complications, review should take place more frequently.

National Service Framework

The publication of a National Service Framework (NSF) for diabetes in 2002 sets standards for diagnosis and treatment. It also describes service models, explains how the standards can be delivered and how progress can be monitored. The vision of Diabetes UK is that the NSF should ensure all patients with diabetes are treated as individuals and receive the best standards of care.

CASE STUDIES

Case 42.1

Mr G. M., 64 years old, is admitted to hospital the day before a planned operation to replace his left hip. He has had type 2 diabetes for over 20 years and has been on insulin for the last 5 years. His normal insulin regimen is Human Insulatard 30 units in the morning and 12 units in the evening.

Questions

1. What are the problems that may arise when people with diabetes undergo major surgery?
2. How should Mr G. M.'s diabetes be managed in the perioperative period?
3. When should his normal insulin regimen be resumed?

Answers

1. There is no doubt that good glycaemic control should be aimed for before, during and after surgery. Poor control may lead to severe hyperglycaemia and excess protein loss due to the postoperative catabolic state. With persistent hyperglyacemia, wound healing may be impaired and the risk of local infection increased. On the other hand, hypoglycaemia, resulting from a combination of preoperative fasting and an inappropriate insulin regimen, also poses problems. The sedated or anaesthetized patient will be unaware of hypoglycaemic symptoms and regular perioperative blood glucose measurements are essential.
2. In patients treated with a twice daily regimen of an intermediate insulin, this should be continued until the morning of surgery. Operations involving patients treated with insulin are often scheduled at the beginning of the day's operating list. This minimizes the period of preoperative fast and leaves more postoperative time to obtain laboratory tests and expert advice, if required. During surgery, insulin should be given by intravenous infusion together with potassium and glucose. Opinion is divided as to whether these should be given as a single infusion or two separate ones of insulin and a combination of potassium and glucose. The separate infusions offer greater flexibility; however, hypo- or hyperglycaemia will develop if one of the infusion lines becomes blocked. The British National Formulary gives guidance on the precise details of the insulin infusion regimen. A target whole blood glucose value of 5–10 mmol/l is recommended and measurements should be taken every hour in the perioperative period.
3. As soon as the patient feels well enough to take a light meal, they should do so. The meal should be eaten while the intravenous infusion(s) of insulin and glucose continue, to check that food is tolerated. For patients on a twice daily subcutaneous regimen, the next dose should be administered at the normal time. However, the intravenous infusion should be continued for 1 hour after the subcutaneous injection has been given, to allow time for the insulin to be absorbed. If the patient does not tolerate the meal, the insulin infusion regimen should be restarted.

Case 42.2

Mrs S. F., 62 years old, is admitted to hospital with an acute myocardial infarction. She has had type 2 diabetes for 10 years and has occasional angina on exertion.

Her treatment prior to this admission was: metformin 500 mg three times a day and a glyceryl trinitrate (GTN) spray, as necessary.

In the accident and emergency department, she is given thrombolysis, analgesia and antiemetics. She is then transferred to the coronary care unit.

Questions

1. How should Mrs S. F.'s diabetes be managed now?
2. What other treatment would you have expected Mrs S. F. to be receiving prior to her admission to hospital?
3. As part of Mrs S. F.'s routine care, her lipid levels are measured. What lipid abnormalities are commonly seen in patients with diabetes and how should they be managed?
4. The doctor considers treating Mrs S. F. with β-blockers, but decides against it as he thinks they are 'contraindicated'. What would be your response to this decision?

Answers

1. The DIGAMI (diabetes mellitus, insulin, glucose infusion acute myocardial infarction) study has shown a major advantage of improved glycaemic control during and after myocardial infarction (Malmberg et al 1999). Post-discharge mortality was significantly decreased in the intensive regimen group, compared to those who stayed on their oral hypoglycaemic regimen. The intensified regimen comprised the use of insulin and glucose infusion in hospital, followed by multiple injection insulin treatment for at least 3 months.
2. The risk of coronary heart disease in patients with type 2 diabetes is so high that many specialists feel that they should be treated as if they already have heart disease, regardless of whether or not they have symptoms. It is felt that relying on secondary prevention is not an acceptable strategy, because patients are less likely to survive a first myocardial infarct. Hence, although there are no trial data to support the recommendation, it is widely felt that all people with type 2 diabetes over the age of 50 years should be prescribed low dose aspirin, unless there are contraindications. As Mrs S. F. has diabetes and also has angina on exertion, aspirin should have been prescribed prior to this event.

3. Patients with type 2 diabetes commonly have raised plasma concentrations of low-density lipoprotein cholesterol (LDL) or triglycerides, or low plasma concentrations of high-density lipoprotein (HDL) cholesterol. Currently, there are no published results from large scale studies of lipid lowering therapy for prevention of cardiovascular disease in patients with type 2 diabetes. If this patient is found to have dyslipidaemia, the treatment should be tailored according to the abnormalities identified. In the pre-statin era, fibrates were the agents of choice for lowering triglycerides because they also helped to change fractions of LDL to the less atherogenic type. However, to date fibrates have not matched the impressive health outcomes seen with statins. It is generally acknowledged that statins should be the first-line treatment for dyslipidaemia in diabetes and that they can achieve large reductions in triglycerides. If triglycerides remain elevated on maximum doses of statins, the addition of fibrates should be considered.

4. There is compelling evidence that β-blockers reduce re-infarction and sudden death in patients with diabetes, at least as effectively and probably to a greater extent than in patients who do not have diabetes. However, studies of β-blocker usage suggest that there is a reluctance to prescribe β-blockers post myocardial infarction, even in patients who do not have diabetes. Barriers to their use may include the mistaken belief that these agents are harmful or less beneficial in patients with diabetes. Deterioration in glycaemic control or blunted counter-regulatory responses to hypoglycaemia are often cited but seldom pose clinically important problems, especially with cardioselective β-blockers. Critical limb ischaemia is an absolute contraindication, but peripheral vascular disease with intermittent claudication is not. Asthma is also an absolute contraindication, but a proportion of patients with chronic obstructive airways disease will tolerate treatment with a β-blocker. Heart failure is also often cited as a contraindication to beta blockade, but this view is now challenged by the evidence of improved morbidity and mortality with carvedilol and bisoprolol in heart failure. Mrs S. F. should be prescribed a β-blocker as the benefits clearly outweigh the risks.

Case 42.3

Mr K. S. is admitted with a small ulcer on the underside of the first joint of his second toe, which is exuding pus and smells offensive. The ulcer developed 2 days ago. His blood glucose measurements are usually between 4 and 11 mmol/l but have been over 17 mmol/l for the last 2 days. He is pyrexial and has a raised white cell count. His diabetes is usually treated with Human Mixtard 30. He takes 26 units before breakfast and 16 units before tea.

Questions

1. What are the possible causes of this patient's foot ulcer?
2. What antibiotic(s), drug(s) and dose(s) would you recommend to treat the ulcer?
3. How should Mr K. S.'s insulin be adjusted and his diabetes monitored while he has the infection?

4. What recommendations would you give to Mr K. S. with respect to foot care?

Answers

1. Mr K. S.'s foot ulcer may be ischaemic, related to trauma, neuropathic or secondary to fungal infection. Ischaemic ulcers occur as a result of circulatory problems. Ulcers may also be created following trauma to the feet, for example a pair of new shoes causing a blister on the foot. This can be a particular problem in patients who have neuropathy and have lost the feeling in their feet and are unaware of injuries until they develop a fever or until they have difficulty controlling their diabetes. The development of neuropathic ulcers is related to the loss of feeling which results from neuropathy. This leads to excessive pressure being placed on the ball of the foot, which results in callus (hard skin) formation. The latter may crack and lead directly to ulcer formation. Finally, ulcers may arise as a result of cracks forming in cases of althletes foot which subsequently become infected.

2. In patients with diabetes who develop ulcers there is a high risk of amputation if any infection is not controlled promptly. Management may also be made more difficult in patients who have poor circulation as drug penetration to the site of infection may be compromised. Therefore any ulcer which requires hospitalization should be treated aggressively with broad-spectrum antibiotics. It is important to select agents that cover *Staphylococcus* and *Streptococcus* species as these account for approximately 85% of cultures. Occasionally coliforms are also found. The presence of anaerobes is associated with a fetid odour. Although swabs should be taken and sent to microbiology for culture and sensitivities, treatment should be started without delay and modified if necessary when sensitivities become available. Therefore, initially, intravenous therapy to cover *Staphylococcus* and *Streptococcus* species should be recommended, e.g. flucloxacillin 500 mg to 1 g four times a day, amoxicillin 500 mg to 1 g three times a day and metronidazole 500 mg three times a day. The doses are selected according to the severity of the infection and likely penetration of the drug. The patient may be changed to oral therapy when the ulcer is clinically improved. This may take several days or even weeks depending on the response.

3. It is essential that the blood glucose is kept below 10 mmol/l to encourage wound healing. If the blood glucose is even mildly elevated then infection will persist as a result of impaired leucocyte function. Therefore the minimum that needs to be done is to adjust the dose of Mr K. S.'s twice-daily insulin. His insulin could be increased from 26 to 30 units in the morning and from 16 to 20 units in the evening. The blood glucose should be monitored pre-prandially four times daily over the next 24 hours. If it is still consistently greater than 11 mmol/l then the morning and evening doses should be increased by another 2 units each to 32 and 22 units respectively. However, as the patient has been adjusting his own insulin for the last 2 days without a significant improvement in his blood glucose measurements, it may be preferable to change him to four times a day subcutaneous insulin. This is usually given as three times a day rapid-acting insulin, such as Humulin S or Actrapid, before meals and isophane insulin in the evening, e.g. Humulin I. The blood glucose should be

measured pre-prandially four times daily. As Mr K. S. is currently taking 42 units of Human Mixtard 30 daily and his blood glucose levels are still high then he should be transferred to 6 units of rapid-acting insulin three times daily, 16 units of isophane insulin in the morning and 16 units of isophane insulin in the evening. The dose may then be adjusted according to his blood glucose results.

4. All patients with diabetes should be instructed not to use corn plasters, to wash and dry the feet carefully, especially between the toes (use unperfumed talc), and to make sure that the feet do not become too dry. Dryness is a particular problem in patients with neuropathy and the use of aqueous cream often helps. However, the use of cream between the toes should be avoided. Patients should also be told not to walk barefoot, to wear well-fitting shoes and to break in new shoes carefully. All patients should be instructed to see a chiropodist regularly.

Case 42.4

Mr J. O. is an 86-year-old patient with type 2 diabetes who is brought to the accident and emergency department by his grand-daughter. He normally takes glibenclamide 2.5 mg each morning for his diabetes. However, today he took his glibenclamide but did not eat his supper. His grand-daughter gave him some glucose powder at home, which appeared to revive him; however, he become drowsy again after about 30 minutes. On examination at the hospital he was still drowsy but responsive, confused and looked sweaty. His blood sugar measured 3 mmol/l.

....

Questions

1. What factors most commonly predispose a patient to drug-induced hypoglycaemia?
2. How should Mr J. O.'s hypoglycaemia have been treated initially by his grand-daughter?
3. How should his hypoglycaemia be treated if he becomes unconscious?
4. What changes would you recommend with regard to the management of Mr J. O.'s diabetes in the future?

....

Answers

1. Decreased carbohydrate intake is the most frequently reported predisposing factor in cases of drug-induced hypoglycaemia. Decreased carbohydrate intake ultimately results in depletion of liver glycogen. Because hepatic glycogenolysis is essential to the maintenance of plasma glucose concentrations in the fasting state, its depletion can cause excessive hypoglycaemia in a patient taking an oral hypoglycaemic agent. Acute decreases in carbohydrate intake, secondary to nausea and vomiting for example, are most important in individuals who have marginal glycogen stores due to irregular eating habits, for example alcoholics or elderly patients. The elderly are predisposed to hypoglycaemia because their renal function is physiologically diminished and they have a greater tendency towards irregular eating patterns. This was the case with Mr J. O.

Poor renal function also predisposes individuals to drug-induced hypoglycaemia by several mechanisms. First, endogenous and exogenous insulin clearance is impaired because the kidney is responsible for metabolic degradation of between 30% and 80% of insulin. Second, many of the drugs that induce hypoglycaemia are cleared renally as active metabolites or unchanged drug. Patients with renal failure may accumulate these active substances. Third, patients who are uraemic often become nauseated and anorectic and may voluntarily decrease their carbohydrate intake. The liver is the primary source of serum glucose during the fasting state through glycogenolysis and gluconeogenesis. Hepatic dysfunction can lead to hypoglycaemia as a result of alterations on the counter-regulatory effects. The liver is also responsible for the inactivation of drugs that induce hypoglycaemia. Alcohol is another common cause of profound and lethal hypoglycaemia coma. This is caused primarily by decreased gluconeogenesis, an important source of glucose in the fasting state. Hypoglycaemia may occur in individuals who drink large amounts of alcohol chronically, in those who binge drink, and even in those who are fasting and have only a moderate alcohol intake.

2. Most hypoglycaemic reactions are managed readily with 10–20 g of glucose. If the blood sugar still remains low after about 15 minutes then the patient should take another 10–20 g of glucose. This 'quick' source of sugar should be followed by a small complex carbohydrate snack to provide a continual source of glucose if a meal is not scheduled within the next 1–2 hours. However, in cases of hypoglycaemia induced by a long-acting oral agent the patient should be taken to a hospital accident and emergency department as severe hypoglycaemia may recur, especially if normal food intake does not resume.

3. If Mr J. O. becomes unconscious his hypoglycaemia should be treated with glucagon. One milligram of glucagon should be injected by a carer by the subcutaneous or intramuscular route. For patients in hospital the intravenous route may also be used as it can produce significantly higher blood levels within the first 5–10 minutes after injection. The patient should then be positioned face turned downward towards the floor to prevent aspiration in the event of vomiting. As soon as the patient recovers consciousness he should be fed. If glucagon is unavailable at home the patient should be taken to the accident and emergency department where a bolus dose of glucose 50% (50 ml) can be given initially and intravenous glucose continued for as long as necessary to maintain normal blood glucose until the patient is eating properly again.

4. Mr J. O. has developed hypoglycaemia secondary to his glibenclamide therapy. Hypoglycaemia is the most common and potentially severe adverse effect of the sulphonylureas, which carries a mortality of between 4% and 7%. The incidence and severity of hypoglycaemia increase with the duration of action and potency of the agent. As Mr J. O. is elderly he should ideally not be taking glibenclamide which causes prolonged hypoglycaemia in about twice as many cases as the short-acting sulphonylureas. With glibenclamide, prolonged hypoglycaemia may occur even at low doses. It is important to identify why Mr J. O. did not take his evening meal as planned. It may be related to a lack of appetite, which is common in the elderly, or to a short, self-limiting illness. However, whatever the reason, it is important to stop his glibenclamide and start him on a short-acting

sulphonylurea or, if he does miss meals occasionally, it would be safer to transfer him onto an agent such as repaglinide. Repaglinide is short-acting and is only taken when food is taken. As he has been taking a sulphonylurea he should be started on a dose of 1 mg of repaglinide pre-prandially. As soon as he is over his hypoglycaemia attack,

his repaglinide should be started on the morning of the day after the other drug has been stopped. Subsequently the pre-prandial dose may then be doubled at weekly intervals until a response is achieved or a pre-prandial dose of 4 mg is reached. The maximum dose of repaglinide is 16 mg per day.

REFERENCES

Anon 2000 Complications of diabetes: renal disease and promotion of self-management. Effective Health Care 6(1)

Chaturvedi N, Sjolie A-K, Stephenson J M et al 1998 Effect of lisinopril on progression of retinopathy in people with type 1 diabetes. Lancet 351: 28–31

Curb J D, Pressel S L, Cutler J A et al for the Systolic Hypertension in the Elderly Program Co-operative Research Group 1996 Effect of diuretic based antihypertensive treatment on cardiovascular disease risk in older diabetic patients with isolated systolic hypertension. Journal of the American Medical Association 276: 1886–1892

Diabetes Control and Complications Trial (DCCT) 1993 The effect of intensive treatment on the development and progression of long-term complications in insulin dependent diabetes. New England Journal of Medicine 329: 977–986

Hansson L, Zanchetti S Carruthers S G et al for the HOT Study Group 1998 Effect of intensive blood-pressure lowering and low-dose aspirin in patients with hypertension: principal results of the hypertension optimal treatment (HOT) randomised trial. Lancet 351: 1755–1763

Heart Outcomes Prevention Evaluation (HOPE) Study Investigators 2000 Effects of ramipril on cardiovascular and microvascular outcomes in people with diabetes mellitus: results of the HOPE study and MICRO-HOPE substudy. Lancet 355: 253–259

Malmberg K, Norhammar A, Wedel H et al 1999 Glycometabolic state at admission: important risk marker of mortality in conventionally treated patients with diabetes mellitus and acute myocardial infarction: long-term results from the Diabetes and

Insulin-Glucose Infusion in Acute Myocardial Infarction (DIGAMI) study. Circulation 99(20): 2662–2632

Mathiesen E R, Hommel E, Hansen H P et al 1999 Randomised controlled trial of long term efficacy of captopril on preservation of kidney function in normotensive patients with insulin dependent diabetes and microalbuminuria. British Medical Journal 319: 24–25

Scottish Intercollegiate Guidelines Network (SIGN) 2001 Management of diabetes. SIGN, Edinburgh www.sign.ac.uk

United Kingdom Prospective Diabetes Study (UKPDS) Group 1998a Intensive blood glucose control with sulphonylureas or insulin compared with conventional treatment and risk of complications in patients with type 2 diabetes (UKPDS 33). Lancet 352: 837–853

UKPDS Group 1998b Effect of intensive blood glucose control with metformin on complications in overweight patients with type 2 diabetes. Lancet 352: 854–865

UKPDS Group 1998c Tight blood pressure control and risk of macrovascular and microvascular complications in type 2 diabetes. British Medical Journal 317: 703–713

UKPDS Group 1998d Efficacy of atenolol and captopril in reducing risk of macrovascular and microvascular complications in type 2 diabetes (UKPDS 39). British Medical Journal 317: 713–720

World Health Organization 1999 Definition, diagnosis and classification of diabetes mellitus and its complications, part 1: Diagnosis and classification of diabetes mellitus. WHO, Geneva

FURTHER READING

Day C 1999 Thiazolidinediones: a new class of antidiabetic drugs. Diabetic Medicine 16: 179–192

Deedwania P 2000 Hypertension and diabetes: new therapeutic options. Archives of Internal Medicine 160: 1585–1594

DeFronzo R A 1999 Pharmacologic therapy for type 2 diabetes mellitus. Annals of Internal Medicine 131: 281–303

Gaster B, Hirsch L 1998 The effects of improved glycaemic control on complications in type 2 diabetes. Archives of

Internal Medicine 158: 134–140

Guidelines for community pharmacists on the care of patients with diabetes 2001 Royal Pharmaceutical Society of Great Britain, London

MacDonald T M, Butler R, Newton R W et al 1998 Which drugs benefit diabetic patients for secondary prevention of myocardial infarction? Diabetic Medicine 15: 282–289

Menstrual cycle disorders 43

K. Marshall   J. Senior   J. K. Clayton

KEY POINTS

- Girls can begin experiencing menstrual disorders once ovulatory cycles are established.
- Up to 90% of women experience some changes premenstrually, but severe premenstrual syndrome is more common in the 30–40 year age group.
- The aetiology of premenstrual syndrome is multifactorial, the symptomology complex and treatment options diverse.
- It has been estimated that 50–80% of women of child-bearing age will suffer from dysmenorrhoea at some time.
- Treatment options vary according to the type of dysmenorrhoea (primary or secondary) but include: non-steroidal anti-inflammatory drugs; combined oral contraceptive pills; and progestogen only preparations.
- Menorrhagia (excessive menstrual blood loss) affects up to 30% of menstruating women. The management of the condition depends upon the cause and can be either surgical or medical.
- Endometriosis (the presence of extrauterine endometrial tissue) can give rise to an array of symptoms including infertility. Treatment may be designed to improve fertility and manage symptoms. Medical and surgical treatments are available.

Once a girl reaches puberty, various physiological events occur, leading to the onset of menstruation, or the menarche. The average age of the menarche has decreased to around 12.5 years. This decline has been attributed to an improvement in nutrition and overall health. Even though menstruation is an event that occurs relatively late in puberty, 95% of girls reach the menarche between the ages of 11 and 15 years. Even before the first ovulatory cycle has taken place (the early cycles tend to be anovulatory), childhood ovarian activity will have gradually increased the production of oestrogen leading to the development of the secondary sexual characteristics. These events are probably initiated by the central nervous system which ultimately triggers the necessary gonadal changes that will eventually lead to the establishment of the menstrual cycle. Menstruation itself occurs as a result of cyclic hormonal variations (Fig. 43.1).

During the first half or follicular phase of the menstrual cycle the endometrium thickens under the influence of increasing levels of oestrogen (most notably estradiol, which at the peak of its preovulatory surge reaches around 2000 pmol/l) secreted from the developing ovarian follicles. Once the serum oestrogen level has surpassed a critical point it triggers, by positive feedback, the anterior pituitary to release, about 24 hours later, a surge of luteinizing hormone (up to 50 IU/l), and ovulation follows 30–36 hours after that. After ovulation, which occurs around day 14 of a 28 day menstrual cycle, and as the luteal phase progresses, the endometrium begins to respond to increasing levels of progesterone. Both progesterone and oestrogen are secreted from the corpus luteum which was formed from the remains of the ovarian follicle after ovulation. The lifespan of the corpus luteum is remarkably constant and lasts between 12 and 14 days, hence the length of the second half or the luteal phase of the menstrual cycle is between 12 and 14 days. Between days 18 and 22 of a 28 day cycle, both sex steroids peak, with levels of progesterone reaching around 30 nmol/l. As progesterone has a thermogenic effect upon the hypothalamus, basal body temperature increases by about 1°C in the second half of an ovulatory cycle (Fig. 43.2).

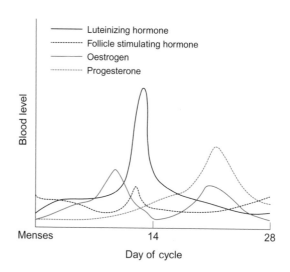

Figure 43.1 Diagram depicting the hormonal events that occur during the menstrual cycle in women.

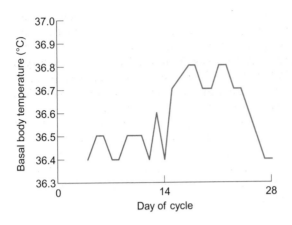

Figure 43.2 Typical temperature chart from a 28 day ovulatory menstrual cycle.

These synchronized changes mean that about a week after ovulation the endometrium is prepared for implantation, providing fertilization has taken place. If conception does not occur then luteolysis begins and steroid levels fall. This means that the endometrium cannot be maintained, and there is a loss in stromal fluid, leucocyte infiltration begins, and there is intraglandular extravasation of blood. Finally, endometrial blood flow is reduced, and this leads to necrosis and sloughing, i.e.

menstruation. Initially the blood vessels that remain intact after sloughing are sealed by fibrin and platelet plugs; subsequent haemostasis is probably achieved as a result of vasoconstriction of the remaining basal arteries. Nitric oxide may be involved in the initiation and maintenance of menstrual bleeding by promoting vasodilation and inhibiting platelet aggregation. The myometrium (the muscular layers of the uterus that contract spontaneously throughout the menstrual cycle, the frequency of these contractions being influenced by the hormonal milieu) is also more active during menstruation.

There is evidence which suggests a physiological and pathological role for the local hormones, known as prostaglandins, in the process of menstruation. Prostaglandins are 20-carbon oxygenated, polyunsaturated fatty acids, which are cyclo-oxygenase derived products of arachidonic acid. Indeed, both the myometrium and the endometrium are capable of synthesizing and responding to prostaglandins. A potential role for another family of autocoids, the leukotrienes, in the regulation of uterine function remains uncertain although it is known that leukotrienes can also be synthesized from arachidonic acid by lipoxygenase enzymes (Fig. 43.3).

Premenstrual syndrome

Premenstrual syndrome (PMS) encompasses both mood changes and physical symptoms. In primary PMS, symptoms may start up to 14 days before menstruation, although more usually they begin just a few days before and disappear at the onset of, or shortly after, menstruation. However, in secondary PMS the beginning of menstruation may not signal the complete resolution of symptoms. Severity varies from cycle to cycle, and may be influenced by other life factors such as stress and tiredness. The most severe form of PMS may be referred to as premenstrual dysphoric disorder (PMDD).

Epidemiology

Up to 90% of menstruating women experience some changes premenstrually. About 20–40% of these women actually seek medical help and about 5% are severely distressed. PMS affects young and older women alike and does not appear to be influenced by parity. Severe PMS is more common in the 30–40 year age range, and married women with young children commonly seek help. Certain events may be linked with the onset of PMS, including childbirth, cessation of oral contraceptive use (incidence of reported PMS is lower in pill users), sterilization, hysterectomy or even increasing age. PMS may be exacerbated by other stresses,

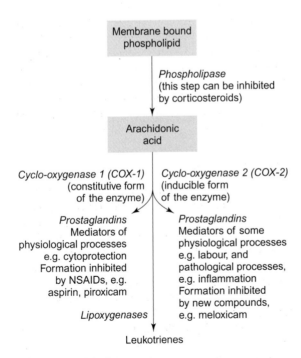

Figure 43.3 Eicosanoid biosynthesis and inhibition.

typically those associated with family life. There is also some evidence that crimes, accidents, examination failure, absenteeism and marital disturbances may be more common premenstrually.

Aetiology

PMS probably occurs as a result of several physiological changes involving ovarian hormones, mineralocorticoids, prolactin, androgens, prostaglandins, endorphins, nutritional factors (for example pyridoxine, calcium and essential fatty acids), hypoglycaemia and changes in central nervous system function (cerebral blood flow in the temporal lobes is decreased premenstrually in PMS sufferers). As symptoms vary so much from cycle to cycle, and from individual to individual, it is likely that different aetiological factors apply to different women, all of which may be affected by extenuating emotional circumstances.

Hormones

The cyclicity of PMS suggests an ovarian involvement. This is substantiated by the fact that it is still experienced after hysterectomy if the ovaries are left intact and that it disappears during pregnancy and after the menopause. One theory attributes PMS to luteal phase progesterone deficiency leading to a progesterone – estradiol imbalance, but there is no direct clinical evidence to support this in terms of serum progesterone levels. However, the problem could lie at the cellular level, i.e. a paucity of functional steroid receptors leading to differential sensitivity to hormones. Alternatively it could be a central control defect, as ovarian suppression by gonadotrophin-releasing hormone (GnRH) analogues can alleviate symptoms in some women; however, the use of these drugs is generally not recommended because of their unwanted effects associated with production of a hypo-oestrogenic state. The mineralocorticoid aldosterone may be associated with the increase in fluid retention as serum levels of this hormone are elevated in the luteal phase. However, no significant difference in blood levels of this mineralocorticoid have been found between PMS sufferers and non-sufferers. In contrast one study has found that baseline levels of cortisol were elevated during the luteal phase in PMS sufferers.

Prolactin is secreted from the decidual cells at the end of the luteal phase of the menstrual cycle as well as from the anterior pituitary. This hormone has a direct effect upon breast tissue and hence may be associated with breast tenderness. Prolactin is also associated with stress, and has an indirect relationship with dopamine metabolism and release in the central nervous system. It promotes sodium, potassium and water retention. However, there are no consistent differences in hormone blood levels of prolactin between PMS sufferers and non-sufferers. Again the differences could lie at the receptor level. Local hormones such as the prostaglandins may also be implicated in the aetiology of PMS as synthesis of these autocoids can be affected by the sex hormones as well as substrate availability. Prostaglandin imbalance in terms of increased synthesis of certain prostaglandins (e.g. PGE_2, which has antidiuretic and central sedative effects as well as promoting capillary permeability and vasodilatation) and deficiencies of others (e.g. PGE_1 which can attenuate some of the actions of prolactin) may contribute to the syndrome.

Vitamins and minerals

Pyridoxine phosphate is a co-factor in a number of enzyme reactions, particularly those leading to production of dopamine and serotonin (5-hydroxytryptamine). It has been suggested that disturbances of the oestrogen–progesterone balance could cause a relative deficiency of pyridoxine, and supplementation with this vitamin appears to ease the depression sometimes associated with the oral contraceptive pill. Decreased dopamine levels would tend to increase serum prolactin, and decreased serotonin levels could be a factor in emotional disturbances, particularly depression. There is now some evidence that premenstrual mood changes are linked to cycle-related alterations in serotonergic activity within the central nervous system and, therefore, serotonin may be important in the pathogenesis of PMS.

There are also data to suggest that a variety of nutrients may play a role in the aetiology of PMS, specifically calcium and vitamin D. Oestrogen influences calcium metabolism by affecting intestinal absorption, and parathyroid gene expression and secretion, so triggering fluctuations throughout the menstrual cycle. Disruption of calcium homeostasis has been associated with affective disorders.

Essential fatty acids

Essential fatty acids, such as GLA (γ-linolenic or gamolenic acid), provide a substrate for prostaglandin synthesis. GLA is converted into dihomo-γ-linolenic acid, which forms the starting point for the synthesis of prostaglandins of the 1 series (e.g. PGE_1). It has been suggested that women with PMS are abnormally sensitive to normal levels of prolactin and that PGE_1 is able to attenuate the biological effects of this hormone. Hence, if there is a GLA deficiency then there is less substrate for PGE_1 synthesis. Therefore, the effect of prolactin with respect to breast tenderness, fluid retention and mood disturbances may be exaggerated. Numerous other dietary factors may also be involved, including excess saturated fats and cholesterol, moderate to high alcohol consumption, zinc and magnesium deficiencies, diabetes, ageing and viral infections, all of which hinder the conversion of cis-linolenic acid to GLA. Pyridoxine, ascorbic acid and niacin also increase conversion of GLA to PGE_1, while there is some evidence to suggest that linolenic acid metabolite levels are reduced in women with PMS.

Psychological factors

PMS may not be wholly explicable in pathophysiological terms but it should not be regarded as a psychosomatic disorder as there is no simple relationship between its existence and severity with personality. It is not strictly confined to particular types of women, although there is no doubt that PMS interacts with many aspects of life, especially difficult or stressful times. The latter has been termed the 'vulnerability factor', which although not a function of the menstrual cycle can affect the way a woman reacts.

Symptoms

Symptoms occur 1–14 days before menstruation begins and disappear at the onset or shortly after menstruation begins. For the rest of the cycle the woman feels well. Symptoms are cyclical, although they may not be experienced every cycle, and can be either physical and/or psychological (Table 43.1). The lives of the 5% or so of women who are severely affected may be completely disrupted in the second half of the menstrual cycle.

Management of PMS

Self-help

The first step in the management of PMS is recognition of the problem and realization that many other women also suffer. Keeping a menstrual diary is useful and will establish any link between symptoms and menstruation, and this will provide a cornerstone for diagnosis. After a few months it will allow the patient to make predictions and help her deal with changes when they arrive. Maintenance of good general health is also important, especially with respect to diet and possible deficiencies. Smoking can exacerbate symptoms. Exercise may help, as may learning simple relaxation techniques. If fluid retention is a problem, then reducing fluid and salt intake may be of value. Increasing the intake of natural diuretics such as prunes, figs, celery, cucumber, parsley and foods high in potassium such as bananas, oranges, dried fruits, nuts, soya beans and tomatoes may all be of value. Hypoglycaemia may also be involved in premenstrual tiredness, therefore eating small protein-

rich meals more frequently may help. The effectiveness of medical intervention depends upon which symptoms are being experienced (underlining the importance of keeping a menstrual diary) and experimentation may be required.

Vitamins and minerals

Results from clinical trials have yielded conflicting results. However, some women do respond to pyridoxine and show improvement, particularly with respect to mood change, breast discomfort and headache. A typical dosage regimen would be 50 mg twice daily after meals or 100 mg after breakfast. Gastric upset and headaches have been reported at doses greater than 200 mg. High doses over long periods have also been associated with peripheral neuropathies. Pyridoxine should be commenced 3 days before symptom onset and continued for 2 days after menstruation has started.

A recent double blind placebo-controlled study of over 450 women with PMS reported that calcium

Table 43.1 Psychological and physical symptoms associated with PMS

Psychological and behavioural	Physical
Depression or feeling 'low'	Breast tenderness
Tiredness, fatigue or lethargy	Swollen/bloated feelings
Tension or unease	Puffy face, abdomen or fingers
Irritability	Weight gain
Clumsiness/poor coordination	Headaches
Difficulty in concentrating	Appetite changes
Altered Interest in sex	Acne or other skin rashes
Sleep disorders	Constipation or diarrhoea
Food cravings	Muscle or joint stiffness
Aggression	General aches and pains, especially backache
Loss of self-control	Abdominal pain/cramps Exacerbation of epilepsy, migraine, asthma, rhinitis, urticaria

supplementation was effective in reducing emotional, behavioural and physical symptoms.

γ-Linolenic acid (GLA, evening primrose oil)

Some women find that supplementation with GLA gives relief from physical symptoms, especially breast tenderness. Most of the evening primrose oil products contain 40 mg of GLA. The dosage regimen is 3–4 capsules (120–160 mg of GLA) twice a day for 8–12 weeks, after which time the dose can be reduced. Pyridoxine, niacin, ascorbic acid and zinc may also be important with respect to prostaglandin metabolism, and a number of products that contain this range of supplements are available.

Diuretics

Diuretics may be useful if the principal symptom is bloatedness, but potassium depletion could be a problem, and long-term use is not recommended.

Progestogens

This treatment is based on the hypothesis that a deficiency in the natural hormone progesterone needs to be rectified. A typical regimen would be 400 mg of progesterone daily by suppository or pessary (Cyclogest), with treatment commenced 5 days before symptom onset. However, in some women this treatment may only serve to exaggerate symptoms. Cyclogest should be used rectally by women who rely upon barrier methods of contraception. Dydrogesterone (Duphaston) 10 mg twice daily from day 12 to day 26 may also be helpful for irritability, depression and fluid retention. Possible side-effects include weight gain, nausea, breast discomfort, breakthrough bleeding and changes in cycle length. However, because of the lack of convincing trial evidence and the risk of side-effects the use of progestogens is not recommended. Problems usually arise because some synthetic progestogens, especially 19-nor compounds such as norethisterone and levonorgestrel, also display some affinity for glucocorticoid, mineralocorticoid and androgen receptors. The specificity of these synthetic agents is influenced by the substituents present on the steroid nucleus particularly at C13 – for example the third-generation progestogens that have an ethyl group at C13 (gestodene, desogestrel and norgestimate) have the least androgenic activity of all the 19-nor compounds but are still orally active. Members of the other class of synthetic progestogens are more structurally similar to natural progesterone, or its metabolite 17α-hydroxy-progesterone, but unless these agents are modified by a methyl group at C6 on the B ring to give medroxyprogesterone acetate, they are not orally active.

Combined oral contraceptive

Some women are helped by the combined oral contraceptive pill (COC) because it prevents ovulation from taking place. However, the use of exogenous oestrogen may be contraindicated because it can increase the risk of thromboembolism. The mechanism for this effect relates to the fact that oestrogen decreases blood levels of the potent natural anticoagulant antithrombin III and at the same time increases serum levels of some clotting factors. Women with other risk factors for thromboembolic disease should also avoid this form of therapy.

In October 1995 the Committee on Safety of Medicines (CSM) recommended that women should stop taking COCs containing desogestrel or gestodene after completing their current pack, because data, unpublished at the time, suggested that these progestogens might increase the risk of non-fatal venous thromboembolism (VTE). In response to this a number of trials were started to determine the facts and the underlying pharmacology about the third-generation progestogens and VTE. The results of numerous worldwide trials has revealed that there are about 15 cases of VTE per 100 000 women per year who use COCs containing second-generation progestogens and about 25 cases per 100 000 women per year who use COCs containing third-generation progestogens. It is thought that use of third-generation progestogens is associated with increased resistance to the anticoagulant action of activated protein C. Oral contraceptive treatment diminishes the efficacy with which activated protein C down-regulates in vitro thrombin formation. This is known as activated protein C resistance and is more pronounced in women using desogestrel-containing COCs than in women using levonorgestrel-containing COCs. However, it has also been recognized that women who do react to third-generation progestogens with VTE may be revealing a latent thrombophilia. There are several conditions that may be congenital or acquired that can cause thrombophilic alterations. A genetic factor known as factor V Leiden mutation is the most common inherited cause of thrombophilia and this mutation results in resistance to the effects of activated protein C. Carriers of this mutation have more than a 30-fold increase in risk of thrombotic complications during oral contraceptive use, although this has been disputed by Farmer et al (2000), who found no increase in risk of VTE with the third-generation progestogens.

In conclusion, if there is a history of thromboembolic disease at a young age in the immediate family then disturbances of the coagulation system must be ruled out before the pill is started.

Bromocriptine

Bromocriptine stimulates central dopamine receptors and thus inhibits the release of prolactin. It may be useful for breast tenderness and occasionally has beneficial effects upon fluid retention and mood changes. It should be used in small doses, for example 1–1.25 mg at bedtime with food, to avoid the side-effect of nausea and faintness due to hypotension, slowly increasing the dose to 2.5 mg twice a day if required.

Danazol

Danazol is a synthetic steroid derived from ethisterone. It is weakly androgenic and has been described as an attenuated androgen. Danazol is able to interact with androgen receptors but it also has some affinity for the progesterone receptor. It inhibits the pulsatile release of gonadotrophins from the anterior pituitary, and so abolishes cyclical ovarian activity, leading to amenorrhoea in the majority of women and subsequently a fall in serum oestrogen levels. However, it tends to be used as a last resort for relief of severe mastalgia and mood changes because of the high incidence of side-effects. These relate to the androgenicity of the compound and include nausea, giddiness, muscular pain, weight gain, acne and virilization, although these can be minimized by using low doses of 200 mg a day.

Prostaglandin synthesis inhibitors

Improvements in tension, irritability, depression, headache and general aches and pains can be seen in some women who take prostaglandin synthesis inhibitors. Most of the information available centres upon the use of mefenamic acid at doses of 250 mg three times a day 12 days before a period is due, increasing to 500 mg three times a day 9 days before the period and continuing until the third day of menstruation. Other inhibitors of prostaglandin synthesis are likely to be just as effective. For optimum effectiveness this form of therapy should be started 24 hours before the onset of symptoms. However, this starting point may be difficult to predict for women with irregular cycles.

Antidepressants

The serotonin reuptake inhibitors (SSRIs) are becoming more popular in the treatment of PMS-related depression because they are effective and well tolerated (Dimmock et al 2000). Several studies have now concluded that SSRIs are an effective first-line therapy for severe PMS and the side-effects at low doses are generally acceptable.

A small study using St John's wort has indicated that this agent may reduce the severity of PMS and that there is scope for larger randomized trials.

Patient care

In terms of treatment, self-help and perseverance will be required in the management of PMS. Because of the wide variety of symptoms a number of treatment options (Table 43.2) may have to be explored before optimal relief can be achieved.

Dysmenorrhoea

Dysmenorrhoea is usually subdivided into primary and secondary dysmenorrhoea. The former may also be referred to as spasmodic dysmenorrhoea, which is a uterine problem and is predominantly a complaint of young women. Secondary dysmenorrhoea is so called because it occurs secondary to some underlying pelvic pathology such as endometriosis or pelvic inflammatory disease.

Epidemiology

The estimates vary but epidemiological studies suggest that between 50% and 80% of women will suffer from dysmenorrhoea at some time during their reproductive life, and up to 15% of these women will be seriously debilitated by the condition, with social and economic consequences.

Primary dysmenorrhoea

Aetiology and symptoms

The incidence of primary dysmenorrhoea peaks in women in their late teens and early 20s, the pain coinciding with establishment of ovulatory cycles. A typical sufferer will usually complain of lower abdominal pain (cramping), which may radiate down into the thighs, and backache. Some women also suffer gastrointestinal symptoms (nausea, vomiting, diarrhoea), headaches and faintness. Symptoms are intense on the first day of menses but rarely continue beyond day 1 of the cycle. The severity of this form of dysmenorrhoea has been shown to be linked to a variety of factors. Factors that appear to increase the severity include young age at menarche, extended duration of menstrual flow, smoking and parity (the prevalence and severity of dysmenorrhoea is decreased in parous women). Other factors such as weight, length of menstrual cycle or frequency of physical exercise do not influence the condition.

Table 43.2   Drugs for treating premenstrual syndrome

Drug	Main symptom	Dosage	Comment
Pyridoxine	Mood changes	< 200 mg daily	Increasing dosage can lead to toxicity, e.g. neuropathy
GLA	Relieve physical symptoms especially breast tenderness	120–160 mg twice daily	May take 8–12 weeks of therapy before improvement
Diuretics	Fluid retention	E.g. bendroflumethiazide (bendrofluazide) 2.5 mg daily	Thiazides and loop diuretics can cause hypokalaemia
Progestogens	Depression?	E.g. dydrogesterone 10 mg twice daily	May cause weight gain, nausea, breast discomfort and cycle disturbances, e.g. breakthrough bleeding. No longer recommended
Combined oral contraceptives	General improvement	Taken every day for 21 days with 7 day pill-free period for withdrawal bleed	Oestrogen is contraindicated in some women because it increases coagulability of blood, increases blood pressure and is not recommended for use in women with hepatic problems or breast or genital tract carcinoma
Bromocriptine	Breast tenderness, mastalgia	Up to 2.5 mg twice daily	Patients may initially suffer from hypotension. Gastrointestinal disturbances can be minimized by taking with food
Danazol	Mastalgia	200–300 mg daily	Androgenic side-effects may outweigh advantages
NSAIDS	Headache, general aches and pains which may improve other symptoms	E.g. mefenamic acid 500 mg three times daily	Taking with food may minimize gastrointestinal problems. Use with caution in asthmatics
Antidepressants	Depression	SSRIs	Becoming a more popular choice because well tolerated. Should be withdrawn gradually

NSAID, non-steroidal anti-inflammatory drug; SSRI, selective serotonin reuptake inhibitor

In terms of the aetiology of this condition, work carried out in the 1950s and 1960s first drew attention to the possible role of the prostaglandins. Following on from this, many in vivo studies have shown that women suffering from primary dysmenorrhoea do have greater concentrations of prostaglandins, predominantly $PGF_{2\alpha}$, and to some extent PGE_2, in their menstrual fluid compared with matched control subjects. Such a prostaglandin imbalance would favour increased myometrial contractility. The effects of the prostaglandins on human myometrium are now well documented, and increased biosynthesis of prostaglandins may also account for the gastrointestinal problems encountered by some sufferers. A role for the prostaglandins is substantiated further by the fact that women whose diet contains more omega-3 fatty acids tend to suffer less. When eicosapentaenoic acid (EPA) is the substrate for prostaglandin biosynthesis, prostaglandins of the 3 series are produced (e.g. PGE_3 and TXA_3). Such local hormones are less potent stimulators of the myometrium and less effective vasoconstrictors. Other potential mediators are the endothelins, vasoactive peptides produced in the endometrium that may play a role in the local regulation of prostaglandin synthesis, and vasopressin, a posterior pituitary hormone that stimulates uterine activity and decreases uterine blood flow. The smaller branches of the uterine arteries are very sensitive to the vasoconstrictor actions of these mediators, and it is these resistance vessels that are important in the control of

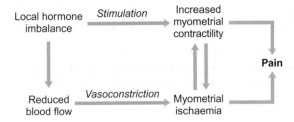

Figure 43.4 A schematic diagram indicating the interactive role of myometrial stimulants and vasoconstrictory agents in the pathway leading to pain in dysmenorrhoea.

uterine blood flow. The interrelationship between blood flow and myometrial activity is summarized in Figure 43.4.

Measurements of intrauterine pressure and myometrial activity have been made for research purposes, but there are no simple objective measurements for dysmenorrhoea.

Secondary dysmenorrhoea

Aetiology and symptoms

Secondary dysmenorrhoea tends to afflict women in their 30s and 40s, and usually occurs as a consequence of some other pelvic pathology such as endometriosis or pelvic inflammation. In terms of symptoms it differs from primary dysmenorrhoea in that the pain may actually start before menstruation begins, continue for the duration of menses and be associated with abdominal bloating and backache and a general feeling of 'heaviness' in the pelvic area. The intrauterine contraceptive device may also exacerbate menstrual pain, since it causes localized inflammation that triggers the release of prostaglandins. The prostaglandins may also be implicated in the chain of events that lead to the pain associated with secondary dysmenorrhoea. For example, if the cause is endometriosis, in which endometrial tissue is found outside the uterine cavity, then this extrauterine tissue can also synthesize prostaglandins, which may in turn disrupt normal uterine function.

Treatment

In terms of analgesia the most rational choice would be a non-steroidal anti-inflammatory drug (NSAID), as these compounds decrease prostaglandin biosynthesis by inhibiting cyclo-oxygenase. However, these preparations are not suitable for all women, and indeed some will not respond to them (it is estimated that about 30% of women will fall into this group). The lack of effect of an NSAID may be explained by pathway diversion, since the arachidonic acid that was to be converted to a prostaglandin via the action of cyclo-oxygenase can be utilized by an alternative biosynthetic route, leading to increased formation of leukotriene. However, the most likely explanation hinges on the more recent discovery of a second cyclo-oxygenase enzyme (COX-2), the formation of which is induced under pathological conditions. Many of the currently available NSAIDs are relatively poor inhibitors of COX-2, and if some of the prostaglandins in these uterine disorders are produced via the action of this form of cyclo-oxygenase then perhaps it is not surprising that the NSAIDs are not 100% effective. The development of new, selective, COX-2 inhibitors may be useful in the treatment of dysmenorrhoeic pain and at the same time spare the patient from the potential problem of gastric irritation that appears to occur as a result of COX-1 inhibition. Indeed celecoxib and rofecoxib are effective against dysmenorrhoeic pain and show a significantly lower incidence of gastrotoxicity.

It has been estimated that approximately 50% of primary dysmenorrhoea sufferers will gain relief from taking the oral contraceptive pill although, as this is a condition afflicting young girls, there may be attitudinal problems to the use of these products either in the patient or her parents. The oral contraceptive pill inhibits ovulation and thereby prevents increased luteal phase prostaglandin synthesis and so decreases uterine contractility. However, not all women are suitable candidates for combined oral contraceptive use because of the potential problems associated with exogenous oestrogen. Progestogenic preparations (for example dydrogesterone 10 mg twice daily from day 5 to 25 of cycle, norethisterone 5 mg three times daily from day 5 to 24 of the cycle) or progestogen-only pills may be useful if they actually inhibit ovulation. Antispasmodics such as butylbromide have a very limited role in the treatment of dysmenorrhoea, not least because of their poor oral bioavailability. It is also known that related compounds such as atropine and hyoscine have negligible effects upon the human uterus. A summary of the treatment options for dysmenorrhoea is presented in Table 43.3. In terms of future therapy, vasopressin antagonists may prove to be useful in preventing dysmenorrhoea. Clinical trials have shown these compounds to be well tolerated and to have no effect on bleeding patterns.

For secondary dysmenorrhoea the best treatment lies in finding the underlying cause and then taking an appropriate therapeutic route. For example, if some form of pelvic inflammatory disease is diagnosed that can be attributed to a causative organism, then antimicrobial therapy is appropriate. There is also the possibility of

Table 43.3 Summary of the treatment options for dysmenorrhoea

Drug	Side-effects
NSAIDs – preferably one with more COX-2 activity	Gastric irritation, which can be minimized by taking with or after food or using a more selective COX-2 inhibitor. Hypersensitivity reactions, particularly bronchospasm. Headache, dizziness, vertigo, hearing problems (e.g. tinnitus) and haematuria. NSAIDs may adversely effect renal function and provoke acute renal failure
Combined oral contraceptives	Many side-effects are dose related and so the development of the ultra-low-dose preparations (i.e. those containing 20 micrograms ethinylestradiol) is beneficial. The most serious potential adverse effect is the increased risk of thromboembolism due to a decrease in circulating levels of antithrombin III while increasing serum levels of some clotting factors. This risk increases with age and smoking. Analysis of current data suggests that the risk of breast cancer is not increased for most women who use the combined oral contraceptive for the major portion of their reproductive years. Use of the combined oral contraceptive also conveys several health benefits besides being an effective contraceptive. The progestogenic side-effects are discussed below
Progestogen-only preparations	Use of these agents may cause menstrual disturbances, e.g. breakthrough bleeding. Other adverse effects relate to the selectivity of the synthetic hormone, e.g. norethisterone is a first-generation progestogen and has some affinity for steroid receptors other than progesterone and so possesses androgenic, oestrogenic and antioestrogenic activity. The third-generation progestogens (gestodene, norgestimate and desogestrel) have the least androgenic activity. This should be advantageous as it is the androgenicity of the compounds that correlates with the decrease in high-density lipoproteins

surgical treatment such as hysterectomy for secondary dysmenorrhoea if the woman does not want to become pregnant.

Menorrhagia

Menstrual blood loss is usually between 35 ml and 80 ml. Blood loss is considered to be excessive if it exceeds 80 ml per period, although both women themselves and clinicians find it difficult to objectively quantify the blood loss. In practice it is defined by the woman's subjective assessment of blood loss (NICE 2000). Any change in menstruation, whether real or perceived, may be disturbing with respect to social, occupational or sexual activities, and can lead to other problems including depression and concern about an undiagnosed problem such as cancer. Physically excessive blood loss will precipitate iron deficiency anaemia (haemoglobin < 12 g/dl), which if left undiagnosed and untreated will only compound the problems outlined above.

If a patient has any intermenstrual or postcoital bleeding, then referral to a gynaecologist for endometrial biopsy is essential to exclude intrauterine pathology. Up-to-date cervical cytology is also required.

Epidemiology

In the UK about 30% of women complain of heavy menstrual bleeding, and about 1 in 20 women aged 25–44 years consult their general medical practitioner about this problem. Once referred to a gynaecologist, 60% of women will have a hysterectomy within 5 years.

Investigation and aetiology

Excessive menstrual blood loss is the commonest cause of iron deficiency anaemia in women of reproductive age. As objective measurement of menstrual blood loss is difficult, measurement of full blood count, and in particular haemoglobin concentration, gives some indication of blood loss. Thyroid function should also be assessed. If fibroids are suspected, then pelvic ultrasound may be required. Endometrial biopsy is needed if there is an associated irregularity of menstruation or if intermenstrual or postcoital bleeding is present. In the case of irregular menses, however, investigation of the uterine cavity would usually only be required in women over the age of 35 years or if medical treatment had failed to alleviate symptoms.

Table 43.4   Causes of menorrhagia (percentage frequency)

Dysfunctional uterine bleeding (60%), i.e. cause is unknown

Other gynaecological causes (30%):
    Uterine or ovarian tumours
    Endometriosis
    Pelvic inflammatory disease
    Intrauterine contraceptive devices
    Early pregnancy complications

Endocrine and haematological causes (< 5%)
    Thyroid disorders, e.g. hypothyroidism
    Platelet problems and clotting abnormalities

With respect to aetiology, menorrhagia can be divided into three categories: underlying pelvic pathology; systemic disease; and dysfunctional uterine bleeding (Table 43.4).

The typical symptoms suggestive of underlying pelvic pathology are presented in Table 43.5. Pelvic pathologies associated with menorrhagia include: myomas (fibroids, which are common benign tumours of the myometrium); endometriosis; adenomyosis (penetration of endometrial tissue into the myometrium); endometrial polyps; polycystic ovarian disease; and endometrial carcinoma (approximately 50% of sufferers will have associated menorrhagia). Very few women fall into this group, but systemic diseases from which menorrhagia may stem include: hypothyroidism; disorders involving the coagulation system such as elevated endometrial levels of plasminogen activator; and systemic lupus erythematosus. About 60% of menorrhagia sufferers have no underlying systemic or pelvic pathology and have ovulatory cycles. In these cases local uterine mechanisms appear to be important in the control of menstrual blood loss. Occasionally cycles

---

Table 43.5   Symptoms suggestive of underlying pelvic pathology

Irregular bleeding

Sudden change in blood loss

Intermenstrual bleeding

Postcoital bleeding

Dyspareunia

Pelvic pain

Premenstrual pain

---

may be anovulatory, with heavy blood losses because the endometrium has become hyperplastic under the influence of oestrogen. It should also be mentioned that use of an intrauterine contraceptive device may also increase menstrual blood loss.

The prostaglandins appear to play a role in the aforementioned local mechanisms, and have been implicated in menorrhagia. Studies have suggested an association between the type and quantity of endometrial prostaglandin synthesis and the degree of menstrual blood loss. In the mid-1970s it was discovered that women with heavy periods had raised endometrial levels of $PGF_{2\alpha}$ and PGE_2 and that blood loss could be reduced by the use of drugs inhibiting prostaglandin formation. More recent studies suggest that in menorrhagic women there is a shift towards increased biosynthesis of PGE_2 (which is known to dilate uterine vasculature) and/or increased numbers of membrane receptors for this prostanoid. The availability of arachidonic acid (a substrate for prostaglandin synthesis) is also greater in women with menorrhagia.

Treatment

The management of menorrhagia depends upon the cause of the condition. Treatment can be either surgical or medical (Table 43.6). The effectiveness of drug therapy is obviously influenced by the accuracy of the diagnosis. Drug treatment is also influenced by a woman's contraceptive needs, for example combined oral contraceptives can reduce menstrual blood loss by up to 50%, but in women over 35 years of age who smoke, this form of therapy would need careful consideration. Low dose luteal phase progestogens are no longer recommended, although long term, long-acting preparations may render a woman amenorrhoeic. Other hormonally based therapies include the gonadotrophin-releasing hormone (GnRH) analogues, although their propensity to induce a hypo-oestrogenic state with long-term use may be problematic (a 6 month course would reduce trabecular bone density by 5–6%). Because prostaglandins have been implicated in the aetiology of several forms of menorrhagia, the NSAIDs may be of use in some patients, especially if there is pain associated with menstruation. The NSAIDs appear to be most effective in women with the heaviest blood loss, for example mefenamic acid 500 mg three times daily from day 1 until heavy flow ceases. It has been found that women with menorrhagia have greater endometrial fibrinolytic activity, hence the use of antifibrinolytic drugs such as tranexamic acid, which may be useful and can reduce dysfunctional uterine bleeding by up to 50% Tranexamic acid is considered the treatment of choice (RCOG 1998), starting at 1 g three times daily on the first day of menses. Menstrual blood loss is reduced by 40–50% (Lethaby et al 2001).

Table 43.6   Summary of the drug treatment options for menorrhagia

Drug	Comments
Combined oral contraceptive	See Table 43.3. These preparations are taken for 21 days with a 7 day pill-free (or placebo) period to allow for a withdrawal bleed
Progestogen-only preparations	See Table 43.3. Compounds such as norethisterone can be used, e.g. 5 mg three times daily or 10 mg daily twice for the latter half of the cycle. Ten days of therapy should be sufficient from day 15 of the cycle in ovulatory cycles. However, if the cycles are anovulatory then a minimum of 12 days' therapy is more appropriate. Progestogens for 12 days are also required to prevent endometrial hyperplasia in peri- and postmenopausal women taking oestrogen. When progestogens such as norethisterone are used, the dosage required is higher than that used in the combined oral contraceptive pill, and the adverse effects associated with the synthetic progestogens, particularly the 19-nortestosterone derivatives, may be more pronounced
Intrauterine progestogen-only contraceptive	The levonorgestrel-releasing intrauterine device & typically releases 20 micrograms of levonorgestrel/24 hours. Unlike non-medicated IUCDs, which may increase menstrual blood loss, this device appears to reduce it, as a result of the local endometrial actions of the progestogen. The device also offers contraceptive cover without many of the side-effects associated with the non-medicated IUCDs. Progestogen-related side-effects should be minimized because of the low dose of levonorgestrel employed. Initially bleeding patterns may be disrupted, but menstrual blood loss should become lighter within three menstrual cycles
Danazol and gestrinone	These agents suppress the pituitary–ovarian axis. Side-effects include amenorrhoea, hot flushes, sweating, changes in libido, vaginitis and emotional lability. Danazol also causes androgenic side-effects such as acne, oily skin and hair, hirsutism, oedema, weight gain, voice deepening and decreasing breast size. Gestrinone appears to be better tolerated, and only needs to be taken twice a week, while danazol has to be taken daily
GnRH analogues (Gonadorelin)	After an initial period of stimulation these agents suppress the pituitary–ovarian axis. As result of inducing a hypo-oestrogenic state these compounds should only be used for 6 months because they may decrease trabecular bone density
NSAIDs	These agents only need to be taken for the first 3–4 days of menses
Tranexamic acid	This drug appears well tolerated, but can produce dose-related gastrointestinal disturbances. Patients who may be predisposed to thrombosis are at risk if given antifibrinolytic therapy. This compound is usually only taken for the first 3 days of menses

IUCDs, intrauterine contraceptive devices;
GnRH, gonadotrophin-releasing hormone

The levonorgestrel intrauterine contraceptive devices (also known as intrauterine systems) can be left in place for up to 5 years following insertion. They reduce menstrual blood loss by up to 90% after 12 months of use. The levonorgestrel-releasing intrauterine system provides relief from dysmenorrhoea, effective contraception and long-term control of menorrhagia. In addition, other slow-release progestogenic devices such as nesterone implants and vaginal rings have also been shown to reduce menstrual blood loss and promote amenorrhoea.

Hysterectomy has been the traditional surgical treatment for menorrhagia, and either an abdominal or vaginal approach can be used. Newer alternatives to hysterectomy include endometrial ablation, which can be done by transcervical resection, coagulation with a rollerball electrode, laser ablation or radiofrequency-induced thermal ablation. Endometrial ablation is less invasive than hysterectomy, but recurrence of menorrhagia frequently occurs and amenorrhoea cannot be guaranteed. However, evidence is emerging that if a single dose of goserelin (a luteinizing hormone-releasing hormone (LHRH) analogue) is administered before transcervical resection this gives a better result. This is probably because goserelin, after causing an initial stimulation of gonadotrophin release, eventually suppresses the hypothalamic pituitary axis, producing a hypo–oestrogenic state. If circulating levels of oestrogen are low, then endometrial growth will not be stimulated, thus it will be thinner, making the surgical endometrial destruction more effective.

Endometriosis

Endometriosis is a condition in which endometrial tissue is found outside the uterus. These so-called ectopic endometrial foci have been found outside the reproductive tract in the gastrointestinal tract, the urinary tract and even the lung.

Aetiology

Aetiology remains unclear, although retrograde menstruation, when shed endometrial cells migrate up through the Fallopian tubes, would appear to be involved. Endometriosis is found in women in whom the normal route for the menstrual flow is disrupted, such as when there is some genital tract abnormality. Women who have frequent and heavier periods also seem to be more likely to suffer from endometriosis. Familial predisposition may also be a factor.

Recent studies suggest that endometrium from endometriosis sufferers tends to be more invasive. This may reflect either biologic or genetic differences in the peritoneal milieu and may be explained by the up-regulation of certain types of metalloproteinase responsible for the degradation of basement membrane.

Epidemiology

Endometriosis was previously considered to be a disease affecting women in their 30s onwards, but increasing use of laparoscopy has revealed that it can occur at any time throughout a woman's reproductive life. The condition is dependent upon oestrogen stimulation and, as such, it does not occur before the menarche or after the menopause. The exact incidence of the disease is unknown but it is believed to be about 10% in the general female population of reproductive age.

Symptoms

Although not all women with endometriosis are symptomatic, the pelvis is the most commonly affected site. Consequently, most of the symptoms of endometriosis relate to this region. Symptoms take the form of dysmenorrhoea and pelvic pain although the severity of the pain does not necessarily reflect the extent of the disease since women with severe pain may have few lesions, and vice versa. Dyspareunia (often with postcoital discomfort) is also common. There may also be menstrual irregularities.

The link between endometriosis and infertility is recognized, but the mechanisms involved have not been established. If the ovaries or Fallopian tubes themselves are directly affected by the endometriotic lesions then fertility may be compromised by purely mechanical means. However, the situation is less clear when the endometriosis does not cause any anatomical distortions. In this case some of the postulated causes of infertility associated with endometriosis include: ovulation disorders such as luteinized unruptured follicle syndrome, anovulation, premature ovulation; hyperprolactinaemia; and changes in the peritoneal environment such as extrauterine endometrial material which, like normal endometrium, is subject to control by the ovarian steroids and like its uterine counterpart is also capable of producing prostaglandins. Prostaglandin levels, along with macrophage concentrations, are raised in the peritoneal fluid of women with endometriotic implants, and these may alter tubular and uterine motility within the abdomen.

Outside the reproductive tract, endometrial deposits can be found along the urinary and gastrointestinal tracts. If the former is involved then the patient may suffer from cyclical haematuria, dysuria or even ureteric obstruction. If there is gastrointestinal tract involvement, then symptoms could include dyschezia, cyclical tenesmus and rectal bleeding or even obstruction. Very occasionally the lesions are found at more distant sites such as the lungs, and could cause cyclical haemoptysis. A reduction in bone mass in women with endometriosis has also been reported.

Treatment

The aims of treatment in endometriosis are to relieve symptoms and improve fertility if pregnancy is desired. Treatment can be either surgical or medical. Surgery is increasingly performed laparoscopically, and can be employed to restore normal pelvic anatomy, and divide adhesions or ablate endometriotic tissue using either laser treatment or electrodiathermy. Medical treatment utilizes the fact that endometriotic tissue is oestrogen-dependent, and any drug therapy that will oppose the effects of oestrogen should, among other things, inhibit the growth of the endometriotic tissue. Hence the choices of drug treatment are as follows:

- GnRH analogues such as buserelin, goserelin, leuprorelin and nafarelin. These initially stimulate the hypothalamic–pituitary–ovarian axis but thereafter induce a hypo-oestrogenic state by paradoxically inhibiting follicle-stimulating hormone (FSH) and luteinizing hormone (LH) release.

- Low-dose combined oral contraceptives (20–30 micrograms of ethinylestradiol) monophasic preparations have been found to be as effective as GnRH analogues and they may slow down disease progression in young women and preserve future fertility.
- Compounds with androgenic activity such as danazol and gestrinone also inhibit pituitary gonadotrophin release by interfering with the negative feedback, and cause atrophy of endometrial tissue.
- Progestogens such as dydrogesterone, medroxyprogesterone acetate and norethisterone initially cause decidualization of the endometrial tissue followed by glandular atrophy.

None of the above drug therapies is free from side-effects. Use of the GnRH analogues may evoke menopausal symptoms such as hot flushes, decreased libido, vaginal dryness (topical vaginal lubricants may be helpful), mood changes, headache, etc. The problems associated with the hypo-oestrogenic state limit the long-term use of GnRH analogues. Although lipoprotein levels are not affected adversely, bone mass is, and this loss of bone density may not be entirely reversible after cessation of therapy. Various 'add back' hormone replacement therapies have been successfully used to minimize bone demineralization, for example low dose oestrogen/progestogen combinations used continuously. Such regimens protect against osteoporosis and other hypo-oestrogenic side-effects without apparently affecting clinical efficacy.

The androgenic compounds, because of their very nature, are associated with hirsutism, weight gain and acne. With synthetic progestogens the side-effects relate again to androgenicity, although dydrogesterone is free from virilization.

Researchers have also found that certain dietary changes may be beneficial and reduce symptoms. A decreased intake of glycaemic carbohydrates such as sugar, rice and potatoes in addition to reducing/eliminating caffeine and increasing the intake of omega-9 oils such as olive oil may also be helpful.

Total pelvic clearance, including the removal of the ovaries, is practical in women who have completed their family. This tends to be a last resort treatment but it is usually effective. However, surgery may be difficult if multiple lesions are present.

Neither surgical nor medical management is effective in all cases. Recent studies suggest that pain associated with endometriosis responds well to both surgical and medical treatment but symptoms of recurrence occur in about 50% of patients within 5 years of stopping treatment. Fertility may be increased by the use of surgery to remove endometriotic foci causing anatomical distortion. The same benefit is not associated with medical treatment.

CASE STUDIES

Case 43.1

T. M. is a 46 year old woman who is concerned about her constant tiredness. Her GP has attributed this to her heavy periods. While discussing possible management strategies her GP mentions the possibility of her having an IUD (intrauterine device) fitted. T. M. is alarmed by this. She has used an IUD in the past and it did not suit her because it made her bleed more frequently.

Questions

1. What sort of IUD will the GP be considering in this case?
2. How should this patient be counselled?

Answers

1. In this case the GP will be referring to the possible use of the intrauterine system. This is an IUD which slowly releases hormone. In the UK there is currently only one such device, namely Mirena. Mirena releases 20 micrograms of the second generation progestogen levonorgestrel every 24 hours into the uterine cavity. In terms of potential progestogenic side-effects it should be noted that this is a relatively low dose of hormone compared with that used in oral contraceptive pills.
2. T. M. should be reassured that although the medicated intrauterine system is indeed an intrauterine device, and it will offer her excellent contraceptive cover, it will eventually decrease her menstrual blood loss. The locally delivered progestogen will effectively prevent proliferation of the endometrium, reduce menstrual blood loss, and may even precipitate amenorrhoea. However, T. M. should be warned that initially she may suffer some irregular or breakthrough bleeding, but this is a tolerance effect and usually disappears within the first 3 months after device insertion. One study has estimated that levonorgestrel-releasing IUD treatment could replace approximately 75% of endometrial ablations. This also helps to contextualize the cost of devices such as Mirena (net price of about £90 for 5 years) compared with the cost of an ablation (about £1200 to £1300). Use of the intrauterine system will also provide contraceptive cover at a time when the oestrogen in the combined contraceptive may be contraindicated.

Case 43.2

Y. S. is a 16-year-old girl who presents with her mother at a pharmacy with a prescription for: Loestrin-20, 3 × 21. Mother and daughter are concerned that the doctor has prescribed a contraceptive pill when Y. S. went about her period pains. Y. S. suffers from severe cramping pains which begin just before she starts to bleed and continue for the first 3–4 hours of her period. She also seems to be more irritable and prone to tears just before her periods, which are rather irregular.

Questions

1. What is Y. S. likely to be suffering from?
2. Why has she been prescribed a combined oral contraceptive pill?

Answers

1. In this case it seems as if Y. S. is suffering from primary dysmenorrhoea, a diagnosis suggested by her age, timing of symptoms (pain) just before menses which abate once the menstrual flow is established and her description of symptoms. She is also exhibiting some symptoms of premenstrual syndrome.

2. Hormonal contraceptives that work by inhibiting ovulation such as the combined oral contraceptives may be useful in alleviating dysmenorrhoea and premenstrual syndrome in many women. Both of these conditions can begin with the commencement of ovulatory cycles, hence the ovarian steroids have been implicated, either directly or indirectly, in their aetiology. However, these drugs may be contraindicated for some women, and there may be an attitudinal problem from either the patient or her parents because they are contraceptives and parents may fear contraceptive use could lead to promiscuity. In this case it might be helpful if the pharmacist emphasized some of the non-contraceptive benefits of oral contraceptive usage such as decreased blood loss, reduced risk of developing iron deficiency anaemia, cycles regularized, and a reduced risk of developing certain cancers of the endometrium and ovary reduced.

Case 43.3

A. W. is a 36-year-old woman who, 6 years ago, was treated for endometriosis with a 6 month course of danazol. She subsequently became pregnant and her child is now 3 years old. Her symptoms have returned and are increasing in severity; the most prominent of these is dysmenorrhoea. Her pain begins around day 24 of her 30 day cycle, progressively worsening until 3 days into her menstrual bleed. A. W. would prefer to avoid danazol

treatment as she found it difficult to tolerate. She asks if there are any new treatments available. She has a BMI of 30 kg/m^3 and is a smoker.

Questions

1. What alternative therapies would be suitable for A. W?
2. Would over-the-counter analgesia be helpful for her?

Answers

1. Drug therapy (or pregnancy) rarely cures endometriosis and the condition recurs in about 50% of women within 5 years of stopping treatment. In terms of alternatives to attenuated androgens such as danazol, the combined oral contraceptives compare well with other hormonal treatments as they reduce dysmenorrhoic pain (and they are cheap). However, a combined oral contraceptive would not be suitable for A. W. because of her weight, age and smoking status. If she still requires contraception a progestogen-only contraceptive method may be an option.

   An alternative hormonal therapy would be a GnRH analogue. The hypo-oestrogenic side-effects of these compounds are generally better tolerated than the androgenic side-effects of agents such as danazol. To attenuate the use limiting side-effects of GnRH analogues on bone another steroid (e.g. tibolone) can be 'added back'. These add-back regimens do not appear to adversely affect clinical outcome but offer some protection against osteoporosis. The effects of GnRH analogues on bone density are reversed within 1 year after treatment is stopped. Women should also be alerted to the fact that they may suffer from vasomotor symptoms similar to those suffered by perimenopausal women. Other potential side-effects such as dyspareunia may be eased by use of a vaginal lubricant.

   There is also evidence to suggest that changes in diet can positively influence symptom score in endometriosis. Reducing the intake of glycaemic carbohydrates such as those found in potatoes and rice while increasing omega-9 oils (e.g. olive oil) and eliminating caffeine can help some sufferers.

2. Some women can be managed by NSAIDs alone, one study has shown that substantial analgesia was achieved in 80% of women with endometriosis after taking naproxen. The newer NSAIDs which are COX-2 selective, such as rofecoxib and celecoxib, appear helpful in the management of dysmenorrhoic pain. Over-the-counter, the most useful NSAID would be ibuprofen.

REFERENCES

Dimmock P W, Wyatt K M, Jones P W et al 2000 Efficacy of selective serotonin-reuptake inhibitors in premenstrual syndrome: a systematic review. Lancet 356: 1131–1136

Farmer R D T, Williams T J, Simpson E L et al 2000 Effect of 1995 pill scare on rates of venous thromboembolism among women taking combined oral contraceptives: analysis of General Practice Research Database. British Medical Journal 321: 477–479

Lethaby A, Farquhar C, Cooke I 2001 Antifibrinolytics for heavy

menstrual bleeding. Cochrane Review. Cochrane Library (1). Oxford: Update Software

National Institute for Clinical Excellence (NICE) 2000 Menorrhagia. National Institute for Clinical Excellence, London Royal College of Obstetricians and Gynaecologists 1998 The initial management of menorrhagia. Evidence-based clinical guidelines No. 1. Royal College of Obstetricians and Gynaecologists, London (Updates can be found at http://www.rcog.org.uk/guidelines)

FURTHER READING

Adashi E Y 1995 Long term gonadotrophin-releasing hormone 'add-back' paradigms. Keio Journal of Medicine 44: 124–132

Akerlund M 1994 Vascularization of human endometrium: uterine blood flow in healthy conditions and in primary dysmenorrhoea. Annals of the New York Academy of Science 734: 47–56

Barnhart K T, Freeman E W, Sondheimer S J 1995 A clinician's guide to the premenstrual syndrome. Medical Clinics of North America 79: 1457–1472

Brooks P M, Day R O 2000 COX-2 inhibitors. Medical Journal of Australia 173: 433–436

O'Flynn N, Britten N 2000 Menorrhagia in general practice – disease or illness? Social Science and Medicine 50: 651–661

Romer T 2000 Prospective comparison study of levonorgestrel IUD versus roller-ball endometrial ablation in the management of refractory recurrent hypermenorrhoea. European Journal of Obstetrics and Gynaecology and Reproductive Biology 90: 27–29

Thys-Jacobs S 2000 Micronutrients and the premenstrual syndrome: the case for calcium. Journal of American College of nutrition 19: 220–227 http://www.rcog.org.uk/guidelines

Menopause and hormone replacement therapy

44

K. Marshall   J. Senior   J. K. Clayton

KEY POINTS

- The menopause is signalled by the last menstrual period; this cessation of menstruation results from a loss of ovarian follicular activity.
- The problems associated with the menopause result from the ensuing loss of the female sex steroid oestrogen.
- On average, 30% of a woman's life is spent in a perimenopausal or postmenopausal state.
- Declining oestrogen levels can give rise to the following: vasomotor symptoms, localized atrophy of the genitalia, psychological problems, osteoporosis and coronary heart disease.
- In the UK only about 50% of women seek help for their symptoms.
- Hormone replacement therapy (HRT) is relatively free from side-effects.
- Contraindictions to hormone replacement therapy include undiagnosed vaginal bleeding in postmenopausal women or the presence of an oestrogen-dependent tumour.
- For women with an intact uterus, hormone replacement regimens must include a progestogenic component to prevent overstimulation of the endometrium.

The menopause

The menopause is signalled by a woman's last menstrual period and is defined as the permanent cessation of menstruation resulting from loss of ovarian follicular activity. The occurrence of the last menstruation can only be diagnosed retrospectively, and is usually taken as being final if it is followed by a 12-month bleed-free interval; such women are defined as being postmenopausal. Many women will experience erratic periods before the final cessation due to inadequate ovarian oestrogen secretion; these women are perimenopausal subjects. The problems associated with the menopause result from oestrogen deprivation. Hormone replacement therapy (HRT) reduces the effects of this deprivation and overcomes the associated symptoms. Statistics show that in developed countries the average woman lives approximately 30% of her life postmenopausally and that postmenopausal women make up about 20% of the population, thus providing a large pool of patients who could receive treatment. In the UK

only about 50% of postmenopausal women seek help for their symptoms, but the figures are rising steadily. In North America the number of women receiving treatment is probably higher due to the greater awareness among this population of the benefits to be gained from seeking help and advice about menopausal symptoms.

The menopause is one event in the anatomical, physiological and psychological changes which form the female climacteric. The major symptoms associated with oestrogen lack in postmenopausal women are listed below; they may occur in both the perimenopausal and postmenopausal states:

- vasomotor symptoms
- localized atrophy of genitalia
- osteoporosis
- coronary heart disease
- psychological problems.

Initially the symptoms are more likely to include vasomotor symptoms such as hot flushes, night sweats and palpitations, and psychological problems such as mood changes, irritability, sleep disturbance, depression and decreased libido. Many women suffer from vaginal dryness and dyspareunia, which serve to enhance the loss of libido. The urethral mucosa may become atrophied, leading to an increased incidence of urinary tract infections or urinary incontinence. In some women the urethra may eventually become fibrosed, leading to dysuria, frequency and urgency (urethral syndrome). The long-term consequences of oestrogen deprivation are often symptomless; there is a significant loss of calcium from the bones, which may give rise to frequent fractures, and there is a change in the blood lipid profile, which is associated with a rise in coronary heart disease.

Physiological changes

Ovarian

The approaching menopause is associated with loss of ovarian follicular activity. Human ovaries contain approximately 700 000 follicles at birth but these cells have a high mortality rate and fewer than 500 of them will be ovulated. This number falls progressively with increasing age so that by the time the woman reaches 50 years of age the number of follicles has fallen to zero or very few. The rate of loss of follicles is highest during the decade between 40 and 50 years of age, possibly due to an increase in the rate of degeneration (atresia) of the earliest follicles. Women over the age of 45 years who are menstruating regularly have been shown to have 10 times as many follicles as those with irregular cycles; those who have not had a period for 12 months have few follicles remaining. Thus, the size of the follicular pool is an important determinant in ovarian function.

Ovarian function includes two major roles, the production of eggs (gametogenesis) and the synthesis and secretion of hormones (hormonogenesis). Both of these functions undergo subtle changes with ageing so that fewer ova are produced and they are less readily fertilized, and the hormone levels become irregular. It is the granulosa cells in the developing follicle that normally secrete estradiol, and lack of this follicular activity results in diminishing oestrogen secretion. The diminution in the number of active follicles is followed by an increase in follicle-stimulating hormone (FSH) secretion from the anterior pituitary gland as the normal feedback mechanisms between ovarian estradiol secretion and the hypothalamus–pituitary axis become disrupted. It may be that there is an age-related decrease in sensitivity to feedback inhibition that exacerbates this increase in FSH levels. A high FSH level (above 20 U/l) and a low estradiol level (below 100 pmol/l) in the serum characterize the menopause; the low oestrogen level fails to stimulate growth of the uterine endometrium. As endometrial growth has not occurred there can be no menstruation (shedding of the endometrium) and the menopause has arrived. Since ova are not being released, the production of progesterone from the ovary also ceases, and the levels of luteinizing hormone (LH) eventually rise. Thus, perimenopausal and menopausal women are subjected to an increasing ovarian hormone deficiency, as shown in Table 44.1.

When the ovaries are conserved after hysterectomy they will usually continue to produce some estradiol, but the levels of this hormone will decline up to the age of the natural menopause. Postmenopausally, in all women androstenedione (secreted from the adrenal cortex) is converted in adipose tissue and muscle (peripheral conversion) to estrone, which becomes the major circulating oestrogen. The levels of FSH and LH remain elevated for many years if no HRT is given, but these elevated levels have no effect on the ovary since the follicles are atretic. The cessation of reproductive function in the woman and declining oestrogen production from the ovary are not the only physiological events associated with the menopause. For many years oestrogen was considered to be associated only with the genitourinary system, but its effects are more wide ranging and the major tissues affected include blood vessels, bones and the brain.

Urogenital

With the failure in ovarian oestrogen production the number of uterine endometrial oestrogen receptors occupied falls and endometrial growth is not sustained. Thus in the postmenopausal woman the endometrium becomes thin and atrophic. The oestrogen receptors in the basal layers of the vaginal epithelium are no longer stimulated to maintain the vaginal epithelium and natural lubricants from the vaginal glands. The result is vaginal atrophy and the thin, dry vagina may result in dyspareunia. Because the lower urinary tract and the lower genital tract share common embryological origin, deprivation of oestrogen can result in urethral and bladder problems. Often perimenopausal and postmenopausal women report an increase in urinary frequency, nocturia and urge incontinence.

Treatment

Hormone replacement therapy

The reasons for prescribing therapy, either perimenopausally or postmenopausally, usually depend upon relieving symptoms of oestrogen deficiency such as vasomotor symptoms, atrophy of the genitalia and psychological problems. Long-term therapy may also be given to prevent osteoporosis, cardiovascular disease

Table 44.1 Ovarian hormone secretion after the onset of the normal menstrual cycle

	Premenopausal (normal cyclic)	Perimenopausal (irregular cycles)	Postmenopausal (cessation of cycle)
Oestrogens	+++	++	+→−
Progesterone	+++	+	−
Androgens	+	+	+→−

and degenerative diseases of the central nervous system. HRT is more widely used for short-term relief of symptoms, although long-term therapy, in excess of 10 years, is now prescribed more frequently as the long-term benefits and risks are being thoroughly evaluated.

There are few contraindications to HRT, but the important ones to eliminate are undiagnosed vaginal bleeding in postmenopausal women and the presence of an oestrogen dependent tumour. The presence of liver disease, deep vein thrombosis and pulmonary embolism need careful evaluation by the physician before the use of oestrogen therapy.

Estrogen therapy

Since the symptoms and long-term effects of the menopause are due to oestrogen deprivation, the mainstay of HRT is oestrogen. This may be administered orally or parenterally but, in either case, the oestrogens used are a formulation of the naturally occurring oestrogens, estradiol or estrone:

- estradiol
- estriol
- estrone
- estropipate
- conjugated equine oestrogen (estrone sulphate 40%, equilin sulphate 60%)
- estradiol valerate.

The use of 'natural' estrogens reduces the risk of the potentially dangerous oestrogenic effects such as raised blood pressure, alteration in coagulation factors and an undesirable lipid profile, which sometimes occur with the more potent synthetic oestrogens used in the oral contraceptive agents. A 'natural' oestrogen is defined as one that is normally found in the human female and has a physiological effect. Natural oestrogens are less potent (up to 200 times) than synthetic oestrogens. Because they are naturally occurring compounds, the serum half-life of these oestrogens is similar to that of the ovarian secreted oestrogens and the duration of action is shorter than the synthetic oestrogens, such as ethinylestradiol, used in many formulations of the contraceptive pill. The serum ratio of estradiol to estrone is normally about 1:1 to 2:1, and the aim of HRT should be to preserve this ratio.

There are five routes of administration for oestrogens in HRT:

- oral
- transdermal (patches)
- gel
- subcutaneous (implants)
- vaginal

The use of oral oestrogen therapy, while convenient for the patient, does mean that the oestrogen will be subjected to conversion to estrone by the liver and gut,

thereby altering the estradiol:estrone ratio in favour of the less active oestrogen, estrone. The oral preparations have different metabolic effects due to first-pass hepatic metabolism. The levels of low-density lipoproteins (LDLs) and very low-density lipoproteins (VLDLs) are decreased, and the levels of high-density lipoproteins (HDLs) are increased, thereby giving protection against atherosclerosis, although it should be noted that triglyceride levels tend to rise in women taking oral oestrogens. A disadvantage of once-daily oral therapy is the considerable diurnal variation in the plasma oestrogen level achieved (Fig. 44.1).

More constant levels of oestrogen result from the use of transdermal patches containing estradiol, and these have the added advantage of a more physiological estradiol:estrone ratio. However, the adhesive used in these transdermal patches and the alcohol base can cause skin irritation. The patch is applied to the non-hairy skin of the lower body, and care should be taken to ensure that it is placed away from breast tissue. The patch is changed either once or twice a week, thus providing a constant reservoir of estradiol to provide a controlled release into the circulation. Estradiol is also available in a gel formulation that is applied daily to the skin over the area of a template (to ensure correct dosage), but this formulation may give erratic absorption.

The oestrogen implant gives a constant level of oestrogen from a few days after insertion for up to 6 months. This formulation maintains the best estradiol:estrone ratio and is a convenient method of administration. Because the levels of oestrogen are constantly raised there will be some increase in oestrogen receptor numbers, and this can lead to a recurrence of symptoms of oestrogen deficiency due to the presence of unoccupied oestrogen receptors. In such cases it is unwise to treat with additional oestrogen: the patient should receive counselling and perhaps a change of preparation. The disadvantage to the implant is that,

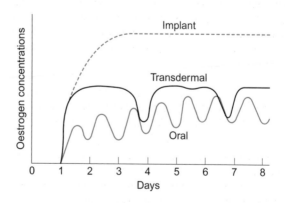

Figure 44.1 Levels of oestrogen achieved by different routes of administration.

once inserted, it cannot be removed readily, and even if it is removed the oestrogen level will take at least a month to fall. There is also evidence that the uterine endometrium (if present) remains stimulated for some time after removal of the implant. Both the transdermal and implant preparations avoid the first-pass hepatic effects of oral oestrogens and so are less likely to affect liver enzyme systems and clotting factors.

Oestrogen-containing vaginal creams are available but generally fail to produce reliable serum levels that would protect against the long-term effects of oestrogen deprivation. They do provide short-term relief from menopausal symptoms, in particular atrophic vaginitis. A vaginal ring is available that releases estradiol at a controlled rate in physiological levels for up to 3 months, and is an alternative for women who cannot tolerate the transdermal patches.

The dose of oestrogen used in HRT should be sufficient to preserve bone density: this is usually higher than that which is necessary to alleviate vasomotor symptoms. Doses that are suggested to be protective to bone density are estradiol 2 mg per day orally, 50 micrograms per day transdermally, and 50 mg every 6 months by implant. If the conjugated equine oestrogens are used the oral dose should be 0.625 mg per day. The lower doses found in vaginal creams may alleviate the vasomotor symptoms but will not protect against osteoporosis.

Oestrogens should be used alone only in women who have undergone a hysterectomy; if the uterus is present the endometrium will be stimulated, and this increase in endometrial growth may be a precursor to a malignant condition developing. Current practice is to administer progestogens with oestrogen. In the early 1970s, when oestrogen was used alone, HRT received a bad press because in women who had not undergone hysterectomy there was an increased incidence of endometrial carcinoma. In women who have undergone hysterectomy, oestrogens are usually administered continuously.

Complications of estrogen therapy. Oestrogen therapy in menopausal women causes few complications. Initial treatment may result in a reaction to the presence of oestrogen in tissues containing oestrogen receptors, such as the breast and vagina. The greater the time distance between starting HRT and the menopause the greater these effects. Other effects during initial treatment may include headache, appetite increase and calf muscle cramps. The initial effects usually resolve without intervention.

Recent studies have shown an increased risk of deep vein thrombosis (DVT) and pulmonary embolism. Oral oestrogens, because of the first-pass hepatic effects, may result in some reduction in antithrombin III but the implants and patches show smaller changes in coagulation, platelet function or fibrinolysis. Patients who have a history of deep vein thrombosis or pulmonary embolism will need careful guidance by the physician and each woman has to be considered individually and the relative risks evaluated. Other risk factors include severe varicose veins, obesity or a family history of DVT. In patients undergoing surgery or prolonged bed rest it may be necessary to withdraw HRT.

Breast cancer is one of the major worries in women who are taking HRT or in those who are considering using the therapy. It is true to say that the breast tissue is sensitive to the effect of oestrogens and that these hormones may be involved in some breast cancers; a number of studies have linked raised serum estradiol with subsequent development of breast cancer. Serum oestrogen concentrations in postmenopausal women increase with body mass index (BMI) as extra-glandular conversion of androgens (adrenal cortex origin) to oestrogens occurs in fat tissue. Thus, the relative risk of breast cancer in postmenopausal women increases with body weight. In postmenopausal women with a history of osteoporotic fracture there is a reduced risk of breast cancer, such evidence suggesting that low serum oestrogen is a factor in reducing breast cancer development. There is a positive correlation between the risk of breast cancer and the increase in bone mineral density. This evidence of natural oestrogen levels and a link with the development of breast cancer has to be considered when discussing HRT and breast cancer. There have been over 30 case–control studies involving HRT and breast cancer; the original results were mainly reassuring. Re-analysis of the epidemiological data by workers in the Collaborative Group on Hormonal Factors in Breast Cancer (1997) has made important advances. The re-analysis showed that there was a significant increase in the relative risk of breast cancer in current or recent users (last 1–4 years) of HRT. The overall risk of breast cancer diagnosis increased by 2.3% per year with an average duration of HRT use of 11 years. Thus after 10 years of HRT an extra 6 women over 50 years of age per 1000 will be diagnosed with breast cancer. This excess risk disappears in past users within 5 years of stopping the treatment. Reports on women with oestrogen-associated breast cancer suggest that these patients have a better prognosis than those women not taking oestrogen who develop the disease.

These results have encompassed a very large data set incorporating 90% of published epidemiological evidence. The difficulty in interpreting the data rests with the different treatments used in the studies, the time since menopause, the BMI and the likelihood of spontaneous cancer developing, and this is compounded by the fact that women using HRT are subjected to close scrutiny and so the pick-up rate of breast cancer may be higher than in untreated women. The results of the studies so far do not provide a reason to stop HRT but emphasize the necessity for close monitoring of women on treatment.

Progestogen therapy

The only proven reason for adding a progestogen to oestrogen therapy for HRT is to protect the endometrium in women with an intact uterus from hyperplasia and possible neoplasia. There is no evidence to date which suggests that the presence of progestogen in HRT protects against breast cancer. There are many preparations that contain progestogens added to oestrogen for a number of days per month, but to effectively prevent endometrial hyperplasia the progestogen must be taken for a minimum of 12 days. The minimum dose of progestogen required to protect against hyperplasia depends on the potency of the compound used; the progestogens commonly available in HRT preparations are either derivatives of progesterone such as medroxyprogesterone and dydrogesterone, or 19-nortestosterone substitutes such as norethisterone or levonorgestrel. All of these synthetic progestogens are active following oral administration and provide adequate protection of the endometrium against oestrogen stimulation. Some transdermal preparations also incorporate a progestogenic compound in the regimen. As with all semi-synthetic or synthetic hormones, these compounds may act on receptors other than the progesterone receptor, and the long-term consequence is not predictable.

Progesterone is the only progestogen that acts solely on the progesterone receptor, but it has poor oral bioavailability and so it is difficult to achieve satisfactory serum concentrations, although the micronized preparations are better absorbed.

Progesterone may also be administered at night in the form of a pessary or suppository or by injection in the form of a long-lasting subdermal implant. The progestogen in HRT is most commonly administered orally or transdermally and usually one of the synthetic progestogens is used.

Complications of progesterone therapy. Nortestosterone derivatives tend to have androgenic side-effects and may cause greasy skin and hair, while progesterone derivatives may cause abdominal bloating and mood changes such as irritability and depression. These effects are dose- and type-dependent, but all progestogens have a tendency to produce breast tenderness. The progestogens in general tend to attenuate some of the beneficial lipid changes seen with oestrogen treatment and are most pronounced with the androgen-derived progestogens. It is the side-effects of progestogens that usually result in poor compliance with HRT, a situation further compounded by the withdrawal bleed that accompanies most cyclical treatment with oestrogen and progestogen.

Treatment regimens combining oestrogens and progestogens

The withdrawal bleed is perceived by some postmenopausal patients to be an unacceptable side-effect of HRT and this has resulted in the development of a number of regimens (Table 44.2). In an effort to minimize this effect, formulations have been produced with which bleeding only occurs every 3 months instead of every 4 weeks, or it does not occur at all.

The use of the 70 day oestrogen preparation, while being more popular with women because bleeding only occurs every 3 months, needs further evaluation as regards endometrial protection. Bleeding can be avoided altogether if a combination of oestrogen and progestogen are given continuously throughout the treatment. Such a preparation should only be given to women who are at least 12 months postmenopausal and have an atrophied endometrium, otherwise breakthrough bleeding may occur. The incidence of endometrial hyperplasia is low with this continuous regimen, but some clinicians recommend regular endometrial biopsy in patients taking continuous oestrogen–progesterone therapy. A small proportion of women experience breakthrough bleeding (particularly in the first 6 months of therapy) even with continuous oestrogen–progesterone therapy, and the incidence of progestogenic side-effects is higher with this formulation. In patients who are changing from the cyclical therapy to the continuous combined therapy, some physicians recommend a 28 day interval between courses of treatment to allow the endometrium to become atrophic. The long-term effects of continuous oestrogen–progestogen therapy on cardioprotection remain to be evaluated, therefore these preparations should not be used in women with major risk factors from coronary heart disease; the 4 week oestrogen plus 12 day progestogen–oestrogen preparations would be the drug of choice in such patients.

Tibolone

Tibolone is a synthetic steroid that has oestrogenic, progestogenic and androgenic effects that alleviate menopausal symptoms without a monthly bleed. The

---

Table 44.2 Regimens of combined oestrogen and progestogen therapy for use in HRT

- Oestrogen 28 days + progestogen 12 or 14 days then repeat without interval (bleed every 4 weeks)

- Oestrogen 70 days + progestogen 14 days followed by 7 days placebo tablets (bleed every 3 months)

- Oestrogen + progesterone continuously (no bleed)

oestrogenic effects are weak and should not promote endometrial hyperplasia, but 10–15% of women on this treatment experience break-through bleeding. The drug is given continuously but is not suitable for women within 1 year of the menopause or immediately after oestrogen therapy; in such cases breakthrough bleeding is most likely to occur. The evidence suggests that this drug is protective against osteoporosis but the long-term cardioprotective effects remain unclear as there is some evidence of a lowering of HDL. It should also be withdrawn if signs of thromboembolic disease occur. The androgenic action of tibolone tends to increase libido. It has been reported that tibolone does have fewer breast-related adverse effects than oestrogenic or oestrogenic–progestogenic HRT regimens.

Raloxifene

This compound is a non-steroidal benzothiophene that binds to some oestrogen receptors and belongs to a class of drugs referred to as selective oestrogen receptor modulators (SERMs). These compounds act selectively on some oestrogen receptors to increase bone mineral density and antagonize oestrogen-dependent effects on breast and endometrial tissues in postmenopausal women; however, there is reported to be an increase risk of throboembolism. Raloxifene cannot be used to treat vasomotor symptoms in perimenopausal women. In fact it is reported to induce hot flushes. It has little or no stimulatory effect on the uterine endometrium and is not associated with uterine bleeding.

In summary, raloxifene is a compound that selectively stimulates one group of oestrogen receptors and may be considered a curative treatment for osteoporosis and a preventative agent in the development of oestrogen dependent breast tumors.

Treatment with hormone replacement therapy

This may be divided into two areas:

- short-term alleviation of symptoms: 6 to 12 months
- long-term prophylaxis against oestrogen deprivation: 12 years or more.

Since many women are now living into the eighth decade, the long-term consequences of oestrogen deprivation are equally as important as the shorter-term problems usually associated with the menopause.

Alleviation of symptoms

Vasomotor symptoms

Vasomotor symptoms include:

- hot flushes
- headaches
- insomnia
- giddiness and faintness.

Vasomotor symptoms occur in about 70% of women and result in physical distress in about 50%, lasting for up to 5 years in around one-quarter of the women. Flushes and sweats, particularly night sweats, indicate vasomotor instability and probably result from unoccupied oestrogen receptors on blood vessels. Oestrogens cause a rapid rise in blood flow through the blood vessels, and lack of oestrogen will render the oestrogen receptors in these vessels supersensitive to any subsequent rise in oestrogen level. During the perimenopause and menopause, oestrogen levels tend to fluctuate, and it is suggested that it is these fluctuations that result in vasomotor symptoms. The extreme sensitivity of blood vessel oestrogen receptors tends to mean that a clinical response to vasomotor symptoms is achieved with low doses of oestrogen. General advice regarding diet, for example avoiding certain foods and drinks that cause vasodilatation such as hot spicy foods and alcohol, may be helpful to some women.

Atrophy of the genitalia

These symptoms include:

- vaginal dryness and dyspareunia (painful sexual intercourse)
- vaginal discharge and bleeding
- urinary incontinence, urgency of micturition, recurrent symptoms of cystitis.

These symptoms result from oestrogen deficiency in menopausal woman and may be treated either with systemic HRT preparations or with topical applications of oestrogen incorporated into vaginal creams, pessaries and silicone vaginal rings. Such topical routes of administration do result in some systemic absorption of oestrogen through the vaginal mucosa, and, since this may be erratic, vasomotor symptoms may ensue. Absorption of oestrogen from these topical applications may also stimulate uterine endometrial development if present. Consequently, it is recommended that these treatments should not be used for more than 6 months. The dose of oestrogen required to stimulate the oestrogen receptors in the vagina and the lower urethra is about 10 micrograms per day, and the efficiency of such low doses has been demonstrated in a number of clinical trials. The effect of oestrogen on vaginal symptoms is more marked than its effect on urinary symptoms, but the incidence of urinary sensory dysfunction may be improved.

Psychological symptoms

These symptoms include:

- depression
- irritability
- exhaustion
- poor concentration and memory
- panic attacks
- lowered libido.

The role of HRT in this area has not been clearly defined although in several studies surgical menopause has been associated with depression, indicating a correlation with oestrogen lack. Many women experience psychological symptoms around the menopause, and although these may be associated with oestrogen lack they may also result from the changes in family life that often occur around this time. Disturbance of sleep pattern and sleep deprivation which are associated with the menopause are likely to contribute to the psychological symptoms. Many women find that treatment with estradiol will restore normal sleep and psychological problems are then reduced. Some of the mood changes will respond to skilled counselling and psychotropic drugs. Treatment with oestrogens at high doses (patches 100 micrograms or implants 50 mg) has been shown to improve depression scores. If a progestogen is added into the regimen then the results are less predictable since progestogen use is related to mood changes, particularly in women who have previously suffered from the premenstrual syndrome. The lowered libido experienced during the menopause is associated with lowered level of circulating androgen resulting from ovarian failure. It has been clearly demonstrated that subcutaneous implants of testosterone, 100 mg every 6 months, will increase the libido in a high proportion of patients.

Long-term health

Coronary heart disease

Women at 45 years are significantly less likely than men to die of coronary heart disease, but by the age of 60 years the death rate from the disease in both sexes is similar if women do not receive HRT. The reason for the protective action of oestrogen against heart disease is complex but relates to the changes in HDL and LDL. HDL levels are increased by oestrogen treatment and LDL levels are reduced. HDL is known to promote cholesterol efflux from macrophages in the arterial wall, thereby reducing atheromatous plaque and confering a protective effect against heart disease. Oestrogens have also been shown to be potent vasodilators by mechanisms that involve the release of nitric oxide from the endothelium and also by a direct action on the smooth muscle of the blood vessel. In addition, oestrogen modulates glucose and lipid metabolism, both of which may influence coronary heart disease. In oestrogen deficiency there is a rise in insulin resistance

resulting in weight gain. There are many published studies on postmenopausal oestrogen use and the incidence of coronary heart disease, and conflicting evidence as to the beneficial effect or otherwise has been presented. In two recent studies on HRT and the incidence of cardiovascular disease in postmenopausal women the data have shown an increase in heart attack and stroke in women taking HRT during the first 2 years of treatment, when compared to women taking a placebo. Others (Herrington et al 2000) found no cardiovascular benefit from using HRT in women with cardiovascular disease. The International Menopausal Society has developed consensus clinical recommendations regarding HRT and heart disease. The guidelines state there is no clear reason to commence treatment solely or primarily to confer cardiovascular benefit. Other recent studies claim that long term HRT may be associated with coronary benefit but there may be little or no (Simon et al 2001) increased risk of stroke. It is obvious that further long-term studies are required to clarify the relationship between HRT and coronary heart disease. The protective dose for oestrogens against coronary heart disease is similar to that required to prevent osteoporosis and is higher than that needed to treat vasomotor symptoms.

Although progestogens may negate some of the beneficial effects of oestrogens on coronary heart disease, there is strong evidence that the progestogenic dose that protects the endometrium avoids any significant impact on the lipoprotein profile.

Osteoporosis

Osteoporosis is defined as a reduced bone mass per unit volume of bone, that is, a reduction in bone density. In a woman not treated with HRT, approximately 15% of bone mass is lost within 10 years of the menopause resulting in an increased incidence of fracture, typically of the hip. Such fractures take up at least 10% of orthopaedic beds and the total cost in terms of morbidity and mortality is high. The effect of oestrogen lack is to increase osteoclastic bone resorption. There is an overall increase in bone turnover, more bone is resorbed than replaced and there is an associated increase in the rate of bone loss which may continue for 5–10 years. Oestrogens may exert effects on bone through the calcium-regulating hormones such as calcitonin and parathyroid-regulating hormones. Evidence also exists for the effect of oestrogens on the local production of bone growth factors, cytokines and prostaglandin E_2.

The greatest effect of oestrogen on bone is seen with implants, where an approximately 8% increase in vertebral bone density is seen within 1 year of treatment. Estradiol patches are the next most effective route of administration, while oral therapy only achieves an increase in bone density of about 2% per annum.

However, 5 years of oral oestrogen therapy will still achieve a lifetime reduction in femoral neck fracture by as much as 50%.

Estrogen improves the quality and quantity of bone in the postmenopausal woman. It may be started at any time after the menopause, and the benefit will continue for the duration of treatment. Bone loss will continue after treatment ceases, which leads into the controversial area of how long treatment should continue. It is recommended that to obtain maximum benefit from treatment with oestrogen the duration of the course should be at least 10 years. In women who have not undergone hysterectomy and require progestogen together with the oestrogenic treatment there is still a beneficial effect on bone density, but further studies are required to assess the effect of progestogen on the oestrogenic benefit.

Where oestrogen cannot be used or is unacceptable, usually in patients with a history of thrombosis or hormone-dependent tumour, then treatment with tibolone 2.5 mg has been shown to decrease loss of bone density when administered over a 3 year period. Further studies are needed to assess the effect of tibolone on fracture rates in women with osteoporosis. More recently raloxifene has been licensed for the prevention and treatment of osteoporosis as an alternative to HRT. Raloxifene reduces bone loss and increases bone density at the spine and hip in postmenopausal women. With its oestrogen antagonist effect on breast and endometrium raloxifene may prove to be an advance over oestrogen treatment in osteoporosis prevention and treatment in postmenopausal women.

Central nervous system

The relation between oestrogen and neurodegenerative conditions, in particular Alzheimer's disease, has received attention in the light of an observation that there is an increased incidence of the disease in older women. The development of plaques of amyloid-β, a protein that disrupts nerve cell connections in the brain, occurs more rapidly in the absence of oestrogen. This effect of amyloid-β production results in symptoms of the short-term memory loss and disorientation found in Alzheimer's disease. Hope that oestrogen treatment would halt the progression of Alzheimer's disease was not supported by a recent study (Mulnard et al 2000) that found no significant difference between the HRT group and the placebo group after 1 year. Further studies are essential to clarify the relationship between HRT and Alzheimer's disease. A trial of raloxifene (Yaffe et al 2001) demonstrated that 3 years of raloxifene treatment had no significant effect upon cognitive scores, although there was a trend toward a smaller decline in verbal memory and attention scores among women on raloxifene. However, it would as yet be premature to conclude that oestrogen replacement therapy or use of a SERM such as raloxifene have no role in preserving cognitive function.

Clinical monitoring

Before initiating HRT a detailed patient history and physical examination are essential to eliminate medical disorders and genital malignancy. Bone mineral densitometry is also necessary to set a baseline for subsequent measurements. Blood tests should include serum electrolytes and creatinine, liver function tests, haemoglobin and lipids and a full blood count. Urine analysis should also be performed. The history and findings from the physical examination may indicate other tests. The patient should have undergone routine cervical smear examination and, preferably, mammography. In women with an intact uterus any irregular vaginal bleeding should be investigated in order to exclude endometrial pathology.

After starting therapy the woman should be seen within 3 months in the first instance and then at intervals between 6 and 12 months so that symptoms may be assessed and any side-effects of therapy may be reported. Blood pressure measurements are undertaken on these routine visits: HRT is usually associated with a fall in blood pressure due to a vasodilator action of oestrogen. Hypertension is not a contraindication to treatment with HRT but does need treatment before starting on oestrogen therapy. Some women may have an elevated blood pressure on oral oestrogen but show no such effect with the non-oral route. Weight gain may occur some months after treatment has been initiated, and the patient should be advised to reduce calorie intake accordingly.

CASE STUDIES

Case 44.1

Elizabeth is a 50-year-old woman who has been on hormone replacement therapy (HRT) in the form of oestrogen/progestogen patches for the past 5 years. Before treatment with HRT she had been suffering from irregular and frequent heavy menstrual bleeding, irritability and lack of concentration. Full gynaecological and general investigation (including endometrial biopsy) at the time indicated no detectable pathology but her FSH levels were raised above normal to 35 IU/l. She is now complaining about still having monthly bleeds, although apart from this she is symptom free. She is also asking about the need to continue using a non-hormonal method of contraception.

Questions

1. What was the likely cause of Elizabeth's symptoms 5 years ago?
2. What is available to her as an alternative to the monthly bleeds?
3. Does she still need to use some form of contraception?

Answers

1. As the menopause approaches, ovarian function becomes irregular, and at 45 years of age Elizabeth was showing classical signs of ovarian changes. Since this patient had no regular cycles it was unlikely that she was still ovulating thus she was not producing ovarian progesterone. Peripheral levels of ovarian steroids fluctuate and are difficult to measure; FSH levels are a more reliable indication of ovarian activity. This patient showed moderately high levels of FSH indicating some failure of the normal FSH/oestrogen feedback mechanisms 5 years ago. The ovary was still producing oestrogen, sufficient to stimulate endometrial development, but when the oestrogen level was not sustained, the endometrium was shed, accounting for the heavy and irregular periods that Elizabeth experienced at the time. Now, after 5 years of HRT using a combined oestrogen/progesterone regimen which regularized the uterine endometrium and alleviated the symptoms, it is time to review her treatment. Because of the possibility of some ovarian activity being present at the initial diagnosis a high dose of oestrogen was required to override any remaining activity of the pituitary-ovarian pathway. The progestogen component of the treatment was included to protect the uterine endometrium from overstimulation by the oestrogen. In patients such as Elizabeth, in whom the uterus is still present, the progestogen should be used for at least 12 days in each month.
2. Now that Elizabeth is questioning the need for the monthly bleeds which she has experienced with the HRT over the past 5 years treatment must be reviewed. It is probable that the need for HRT to alleviate the menopausal symptoms will no longer be needed. A blood test to measure FSH levels once Elizabeth has stopped using the patches will determine whether there is any ovarian function. If the levels of FSH are high then it can be assumed that ovarian function has ceased and the decision about future treatment can be discussed. In the absence of any further symptoms and lack of family history of osteoporosis the decision may be stop

HRT. If the patient wishes to continue HRT and expresses concern about osteoporosis developing in later life then the possibility of using tibolone (oestrogenic, progestogenic and weak androgenic activity) could be discussed. This compound will provide protection from osteoporosis, is taken continuously and monthly bleeding will not occur.
3. Since Elizabeth has high levels of FSH (above 50 IU/l), as shown in the blood test, she will no longer be ovulating and will not need to continue with any form of contraception.

Case 44.2

Sally is a 49-year-old obese woman (BMI 31 kg/m^2) with a family history of coronary heart disease. She underwent a total hysterectomy 10 years ago as she was suffering from endometriosis and has since been treated with HRT in the form of oestrogen implants. Her general practitioner is concerned about her raised blood pressure that is reasonably controlled with lisinopril 20 mg daily. She has raised serum cholesterol and her LDL cholesterol is greater than 3 mmol/l. Her GP suggests stopping the oestrogen implants but Sally has read that HRT is useful in older women with heart disease.

Questions

1. Sally has hypercholesterolaemia. Should she continue with the HRT?
2. What advice should be given to Sally about her lifestyle?

Answers

1. Oestrogens tend to reduce blood pressure and show beneficial effects on serum cholesterol. Since this patient is in need of drug treatment for her high blood pressure and her cholesterol level is raised, the oestrogen implants are ineffective in controlling her cardiovascular symptoms and should be discontinued. Sally should be counselled that the current thinking is that HRT is not the best means of controlling or protecting against heart disease. She should continue to take lisinopril but in addition she will need a statin to control her raised LDL and serum cholesterol level.
2. Since Sally will no longer have any exogenous oestrogen she may lose a little weight spontaneously as patients on oestrogen treatment tend to have a feeling of well-being and an increase in appetite. She will need to have counselling about her diet to reduce her weight and her risk of cardiac disease. She should also be encouraged to take weight-bearing exercise to reduce her long-term risk of osteoporosis. Sally should also be told that the 10 years of treatment with oestrogen that she has already received would be protective against the future development of osteoporosis.

Case 44.3

Diana is suffering from vasomotor symptoms, lack of concentration, irritability and panic attacks. She is 45 years old, weighs 60 kg, has no history of menstrual problems but seeks advice because the hot flushes and night sweats are making life unbearable. Her colleagues at work encouraged her to go the menopause clinic as she was unable to perform effectively in her career and was making life difficult for them. She is normotensive and has no known medical problems. She has read about natural oestrogens and wonders if this could be the answer to her problems as she is unwilling to undertake a prolonged course of HRT.

Questions

1. What do you understand by the term 'natural oestrogens' and would they be effective in this case?
2. What alternatives are there to natural oestrogens for Diana?

Answers

1. Natural oestrogens or phyto-oestrogens are diphenolic compounds derived from plants and they are converted into oestrogens in the gastrointestinal tract. The term refers to a wide variety of compounds including isoflavones, lignans and coumestans. The low incidence of hot flushes in Asian women has been attributed to their diet being rich in natural oestrogens. From the data available about natural oestrogens it appears that they may act as SERMs but they may act by mechanisms other than through the oestrogen receptor. One study has shown that women on a soy-rich diet had large increases in urinary isoflavone concentrations and oestrogenic changes in vaginal cytology. There is some evidence that soy products may provide cardiovascular protection and population studies suggest they may provide some protection against breast cancer. Until controlled studies provide firm data it would be unwise to draw conclusions about the benefits of natural oestrogens (Ginsburg and Prelevic 2000). However, if Diana wishes to include natural oestrogens in her diet there is no reason to discourage her and her symptoms may be reduced. They are marketed as dietary supplements and not as drugs, and many recipes are published for phyto-oestrogen cakes and biscuits.
2. Since Diana is seeking advice about short-term treatment for menopausal symptoms and is reluctant to embark upon any prolonged HRT it may be possible for her to get symptomatic relief by using an oestrogen vaginal preparation for a period of 6 months. The amount of oestrogen absorbed from the vaginal preparations is insufficient to provide prophylaxis against osteoporosis but sufficient to be effective against vasomotor symptoms and mood changes.

Case 44.4

Geraldine is a 54-year-old solicitor with three children and a busy lifestyle. She is 1.6 m tall and weighs 53 kg, has never smoked or drunk alcohol, but she tends to have a small appetite and to take meals when she can. She spends much of her working day sitting at her desk and does not take regular exercise. Her periods ceased 2 years ago and she has not suffered from any menopausal symptoms. At a recent routine cervical smear examination she raised the question of using HRT to prevent osteoporosis as her mother had suffered from recurrent fractures in later life. She was referred for investigation and all her investigations and tests were normal except for her bone densitometry, which was 2 standard deviation units below normal and her FSH level, which was above 50 IU/l.

Questions

1. What risk factors does Geraldine have for osteoporosis and how could these be minimized?
2. What would be a suitable preparation for starting HRT in the patient and how long should her duration of treatment be?

Answers

1. Geraldine has the following risk factors for osteoporosis:
   - female gender
   - perimenopausal oestrogen deficiency
   - low bone density
   - family history of osteoporosis
   - takes little exercise
   - haphazard dietary intake.

   She probably has an inadequate calcium intake in her diet, and three pregnancies will have reduced her calcium stores. On the plus side she does not smoke or take alcohol. She should be advised to ensure she receives at least 1000 mg of calcium daily either from her diet or by the addition of calcium supplements. (If she does not take HRT she will need 1500 mg of calcium daily.) The richest sources of dietary calcium can be found in dairy products such as:
   - 0.5 l of skimmed milk 750 mg
   - 60 g of cheddar cheese 420 mg
   - A small pot of yogurt 250 mg.

   Calcium supplements are available as either over-the-counter medicines or on prescription, and Geraldine should be recommended to take one of these. She should also be recommended to take regular meals and some form of weight-bearing exercise.
2. Geraldine is clearly postmenopausal since her FSH level is high and this suggests that no viable follicles are remaining in the ovary. Since she has a tendency towards osteoporosis she would benefit from oestrogen therapy, which should be continued for at least 10 years. An alternative drug that has more recently become available is raloxifene. Raloxifene shows oestrogenic activity in bone but antagonistic activity in the breast and endometrium as well as favourable lipid profiles. The risks of thromboembolism are similar to those seen with oestrogen. If Geraldine is concerned about the risk of breast cancer with oestrogen therapy this may well prove to be an effective alternative in her case. Non-hormonal treatment for osteoporosis is available with the biphosphonate drugs.

REFERENCES

Collaborative Group on Hormonal Factors in Breast Cancer 1997 Breast cancer and hormone replacement therapy: collaborative reanalysis of data from 51 epidemiological studies of 52705 women with breast cancer and 108411 women without breast cancer. Lancet 350: 1047–1059

Ginsburg J, Prelevic G M 2000 Lack of significant hormonal effects and controlled trials of phyto-oestrogens. Lancet 355: 163–164

Herrington D M, Reboussin D M, Brosnihan K B et al 2000 Effects of estrogen replacement on the progression of coronary-artery atherosclerosis. New England Journal of Medicine 343: 522–529

Mulnard R A, Cotman C W, Kawas C et al 2000 Estrogen replacement therapy for treatment of mild to moderate Alzheimer disease. Journal of the American Medical Association 283: 1007–1015

Simon J A, Hsia J, Cauley J A et al 2001 Postmenopausal hormone and risk of stroke. Heart and Estrogen-progestin Replacement Study (HERS). Circulation 103: 638–642

Yaffe K, Krueger K, Sarkar S et al 2001 Cognitive function in postmenopausal women treated with raloxifene. New England Journal of Medicine 344: 1207–1213

FURTHER READING

Hlatky M A, Boothroyd D, Vittinghoff E et al 2002 Quality-of-life and depressive symptoms in postmenopausal women after receiving hormone therapy: results from the heart and estrogen/progestin replacement study (HERS) trial. Journal of the American Medical Association 287(5): 591–597

Kleerekoper M, Lindsay R, Lees B et al 2001 Effect of hormone replacement therapy on fractures and height loss. American Journal of Medicine 111(9): 735–736

Ewies A A 2001 A comprehensive approach to the menopause: so far, one size should fit all. Obstetric & Gynaecological Survey 56(10): 642–649

Grant E C G 2002 Hormone replacement therapy and risk of breast cancer. Journal of the American Medical Association 287(18): 2360–2361

Mosca L 2000 The role of hormone replacement therapy in the prevention of postmenopausal heart disease. Archives of Internal Medicine 160: 2263

Pines A, Bornstein N M, Shapira I 2002 Menopause and ischaemic stroke: basic, clinical and epidemiological considerations. Human Reproduction Update 8(2): 161–168

Nanda K, Bastian L A, Schulz K 2002 Hormone replacement therapy and the risk of death from breast cancer: a systematic review. American Journal of Obstetrics and Gynecology 186(2): 325–334

Panidis D, Rousso D, Kourtis A et al 2001 Hormone replacement therapy at the threshold of the 21st century. European Jounal of Obstetrics Gynecology and Reproductive Biology 99(2): 154–164

Fylstra D L 2002 Postmenopausal hormone replacement therapy: does the progestin make a difference? Journal of the American Medical Association 287(5): 591–597

Drugs in pregnancy and lactation

45

D. J. Woods   S. B. Duffull

In 1961, following numerous reports of severe anatomical birth defects in children born to mothers who had taken the hypnotic drug thalidomide early in pregnancy, the drug was withdrawn from the UK market. Consequently, it was realized that drugs have the potential to cross the placenta and harm the developing fetus.

There is now a greater appreciation of the risks of drug therapy during pregnancy and a realization that drug therapy during pregnancy should be avoided or minimized. Nevertheless, it has been estimated that over 90% of expectant mothers take three or four drugs at some stage of pregnancy. Indications for drug use range from chronic illnesses such as epilepsy, depression and rheumatoid arthritis to those commonly associated with pregnancy, in particular hypertension, urinary tract infections and gastrointestinal complaints. A significant number of women are taking medication at the time their pregnancy is detected.

Besides drug effects in utero, neonates can experience drug withdrawal effects that may also require management.

Drug use in pregnancy

Prenatal development

The human gestation period is 38 weeks and is conventionally divided into the first, second and third trimesters, each lasting 3 calendar months. The stages of development are: pre-embryonic, embryonic and fetal. The pre-embryonic stage is when the fertilized ovum consolidates; this lasts for 17 days postconception. The major organ systems are formed during the embryonic stage (18–56 days), with maturation, development and growth continuing during the fetal stage (8–38 weeks). It is common practice to describe drug exposure at any stage during pregnancy as fetal exposure, and for simplicity this convention is followed in this chapter.

Dysmorphogenesis and teratogenicity

A teratogen is an agent that interferes with the normal growth and development of the fetus, and the term is used to describe drugs or chemicals that cause major or gross birth defects. Dysmorphogenesis literally means the development of ill-shaped or otherwise malformed body structures, but the term is applied generally to include all structural and functional defects. A congenital anomaly is a non-reversible birth defect caused by genetic predisposition or other factors, such as drug exposure, that may adversely effect the development of the fetus. Congenital anomalies such as spina bifida and hydrocephalus are obvious at birth, but some defects may take many years to develop or be identified. Examples of delayed anomalies are behavioural and intellectual disorders associated with in utero alcohol exposure and the development of vaginal cancer in young women following maternal intake of diethylstilbestrol for the prevention of miscarriage. Approximately 2% of all live births are associated with a congenital anomaly, and it has been estimated that about 5% of these (0.1% of all live births) are caused by drugs. Examples of drugs that are known to be human teratogens are shown in Table 45.1.

Drug effects on the fetus

Placental drug transfer

Most drugs diffuse easily across the placenta and thus enter the fetal circulation to some extent, but for drugs with a large molecular weight such as heparin, transfer is negligible. Lipophilic, unionized drugs cross the placenta more easily than polar drugs, and weakly basic drugs may become 'trapped' in the fetal circulation due to the slightly lower pH compared with maternal plasma. Some drugs are metabolized by the placenta or fetus, but these effects are usually negligible. Occasionally, drugs are administered to pregnant women to treat fetal disorders. Flecainide, for example, has been used to resolve fetal tachycardia.

The extent of placental drug transfer as predicted by physicochemical properties is seldom employed to evaluate the safety of a drug when given during pregnancy. Knowledge of the pharmacology, toxicity and experience of use of the drug in pregnancy are much more important.

Pharmacological effects

Drugs crossing the placenta may exert a direct pharmacological effect on the fetus, for example high doses of corticosteroids (>10 mg of prednisolone daily) taken during pregnancy can cause fetal adrenal suppression. The fetus may also be indirectly affected by pharmacological effects on the maternal circulation. This is seen with some antihypertensive drugs that can cause fetal hypoxia secondary to maternal hypotension.

Table 45.1 Drugs known or suspected to be human teratogens	
Androgens	Lithium
Cytotoxic drugs (some)	Penicillamine
Carbimazole (thiamazole methimazole)	Phenytoin
Diethylstilbestrol	Tetracyclines
Ethanol	Thalidomide
Etretinate	Vitamin A
Isotretinoin	Warfarin
Leflunomide	

Pharmacological effects are usually dose related and to some extent predictable.

Idiosyncratic effects

The effects of some drugs on the fetus are less predictable and seemingly unrelated to the dose. These idiosyncratic effects are caused by complex mechanisms usually involving fetal genetic predisposition. For some drugs there may be an unknown threshold dose above which drug-induced dysmorphogenicity is more likely to occur. This theory further justifies the use of the lowest effective dose during pregnancy.

Pharmacological effects on the fetus are by far the most common drug effects during pregnancy, and the consequences are often minor and reversible. Conversely, idiosyncratic effects usually lead to major irreversible congenital anomalies.

Timing of drug exposure

The stage of pregnancy at which a drug is administered can determine the likelihood, severity or nature of any adverse effect on the fetus. Drug effects on the fetus are usually described in terms of the trimester of risk, and some drugs can present a different risk according to the trimester of exposure. An example is phenobarbital, which can cause congenital anomalies if given in the first trimester and neonatal bleeding if given in the third trimester.

Drug exposure during the pre-embryonic stage is understood to elicit an all-or-nothing response leading to either death of the embryo or complete recovery and normal development. Dysmorphogenesis is thus unlikely unless the half-life of the drug is sufficient to extend exposure into the embryonic stage.

Organogenesis occurs predominantly during the embryonic stage, and, with the exception of the central nervous system, eyes, teeth, external genitalia and ears, formation is complete by the end of the 10th week of pregnancy. Exposure to drugs during this period represents the greatest risk of major birth defects by interfering with organ formation. The general principle, whenever possible, is to avoid or minimize all drug use in the first trimester.

In the second and third trimesters, organ systems continue to develop and mature, and there is continued susceptibility to some drug effects. This is especially the case with the central nervous system, which can be damaged by exposure to some drugs (e.g. ethanol) if given at any stage of pregnancy. The external genitalia continue to form from the seventh week until term, and consequently danazol, which has weak androgenic properties, can cause virilization of a female fetus if given in any trimester. Conversely, because of their antiandrogenic properties, spironolactone and cyproterone acetate have the potential to cause feminization of the male fetus. The pharmacological effects of angiotensin-converting enzyme (ACE) inhibitors given in the second and third trimesters can result in fetal renal dysfunction and oligohydramnios (small amount or absence of amniotic fluid), and sulphonamides and thiazides can cause neonatal haemolysis and thrombocytopenia, respectively, when given in the third trimester. Another important group of drugs that can cause problems specifically in the third trimester are the non-steroidal anti-inflammatory drugs (NSAIDs). These drugs inhibit prostaglandin synthesis in a dose-related fashion, and when given late in pregnancy can cause closure of the fetal ductus arteriosus, fetal renal impairment, bleeding disorders and delay labour and birth. Regular use of NSAIDs should therefore be avoided during the third trimester.

Drug dosing in pregnancy

As a general principle, the dose of a drug given at any stage during pregnancy should be kept as low as possible to minimize toxic effects to the fetus. Drug therapy that is considered essential during pregnancy can be tapered to the lowest effective dose either before conception or during the first trimester. The doses of drugs that have the potential to cause neonatal withdrawal effects such as antidepressants and antipsychotics can be reduced as term approaches. However, pharmacokinetic changes are common in pregnancy, and these may dictate a dosage increase. Pregnancy itself can cause a temporary worsening or amelioration of some diseases and thus influence drug dosages.

Pharmacokinetic changes

Clearance. Within the first few weeks of pregnancy the glomerular filtration rate increases by approximately 50% and remains raised until after delivery. Consequently the clearance of drugs that are excreted unchanged mainly by the kidneys (e.g. lithium, some β-lactam antibiotics) are increased, and higher maintenance doses may be required. The hepatic metabolism of many drugs is increased during pregnancy, possibly due to enzyme induction by endogenous progesterone, but the effects on individual drugs are inconsistent and difficult to predict. The metabolism of methadone and phenytoin are often significantly increased in the third trimester, requiring higher maintenance doses. Conversely, in some women, metabolism of theophylline is reduced, and a reduction in the maintenance dose is required.

Volume of distribution. The weight gain of pregnancy is significant and consists of the fetus and increases in total body water and fat. These factors increase the volume of distribution of many drugs such that increased loading doses may be required. This may be important when a rapid drug effect is required or if the magnitude of the effect is proportional to the peak plasma concentration.

Protein binding. Albumin is the main plasma protein responsible for binding acidic drugs such as phenytoin and salicylates and α_1-acid glycoprotein (AAG) predominantly binds basic drugs including β-blockers and opioid analgesics. Plasma albumin concentrations fall significantly in pregnancy, and this leads to an increase in the fraction of unbound drug. Clinical effect is related to the concentration of unbound drug, which usually remains unchanged even though the total plasma concentration is decreased. Thus, a fall in the total plasma concentration does not always require an increase in dose. Phenytoin is bound to albumin and exhibits these effects, but the situation is further complicated by increased hepatic metabolism or worsening seizure control that may necessitate a dose increase. Consequently, therapy can only be reliably guided by clinical assessment or measurement of unbound rather than total plasma concentration.

Effects of drugs on the neonate

The neonate can be adversely affected by maternal drug therapy. It is only at birth that signs of fetal distress due to in utero drug exposure or the effects of abrupt discontinuation of the maternal drug supply are observed. The capacity of the fetus or neonate to eliminate drugs is minimal, and this can result in significant accumulation of some drugs, leading to toxicity. The doses of antidepressants and neuroleptics should be slowly reduced close to parturition to minimize neurological disturbances due to direct toxicity in the neonate and to minimize drug withdrawal effects. Tapering off the dose is not always practical with some drugs such as methadone and lithium, which may actually need to be increased in dose to maintain symptom control in the mother. Neonatal withdrawal effects can be very distressing, and symptoms often require treatment with sedatives or drug replacement. Morphine oral solution is used to wean babies off methadone, and its use can often be anticipated before birth. Idiosyncratic drug effects (unpredictable and not related to dose) in the fetus and neonate are possible but occur rarely compared with pharmacological effects.

Drug safety and selection

There are few, if any, drugs for which safe use in pregnancy can be absolutely assured, but only a handful of drugs in current clinical use have been conclusively shown to be teratogenic. Animal studies are not necessarily predictive of drug safety in human pregnancy, and there are species differences in the sensitivity to dysmorphogenic effects. In general, drugs which have been used extensively in pregnant women without apparent problems should be selected in preference to new drugs for which there is less experience of use. Methyldopa, for example, has a long history of safe use for the treatment of hypertension in pregnancy but is gradually being superseded by atenolol or labetalol as more experience is gained with the newer agents. A frequent recommendation is that the benefits of drug treatment should outweigh any possible risk to the fetus, but this analysis is sometimes difficult to perform with certainty. Some countries use pregnancy risk categories, which can be helpful in summarizing the available information on a particular drug. These categories are referred to in major specialized texts and drug information databases. The *British National Formulary* provides limited information on drug safety, but specialist advice should be sought if more details are required.

Much of the data on the risks associated with drug use in pregnancy are based on retrospective studies or voluntary reporting databases where the rate of anomalies may be erroneously elevated as normal outcomes may be under-reported. Individual case reports are also difficult to interpret as the denominator of drug exposure is unknown. More recently, prospective controlled trials have been utilized where the pregnancy outcomes of a defined cohort of women exposed to the drug are compared with outcomes in a matched control group. Complete follow-up of each pregnancy and postnatal monitoring is an essential feature of this type of investigation. For some new drugs, pregnancy registries have been initiated that record all reported drug exposures and follow up the outcome of the pregnancy. These registries are cumulative and work on the basis that specific anomalies would be identified relatively quickly and that there will eventually be sufficient statistical power to detect the magnitude of any increased risk relative to the general population. The safety data for aciclovir have largely been derived from a pregnancy registry. All studies have inherent methodological problems and require critical review, but in general the most recent investigations provide the most reliable data.

Preconception advice

All women planning pregnancy should be offered advice to minimize the risk of congenital anomalies. General advice includes the avoidance of all drugs, alcohol, smoking and vitamin A products (teratogenic) and beginning daily supplementation with 400 micrograms of folic acid to reduce the risk of neural tube defects. Folic acid is taken from before conception until the end of the first trimester, and the daily dose should be increased to 4 or 5 mg daily in women who are taking anticonvulsants or who have had a previous child with a neural tube defect. Women with chronic illness requiring drug treatment should be offered specialist counselling before conception, and the options explored to reduce or change drug therapy to a safer agent. Epilepsy is an example when, if continued drug treatment is necessary, attempts are made to stabilize treatment with a single drug at the lowest effective dose.

Drugs and lactation

All drugs distribute into human milk. What we need to know is how much drug passes into the milk, and what will be the likely effects of this amount when ingested by the suckling infant.

It should always be remembered that the infant is an innocent bystander. The possible risks to the child must therefore be considered carefully when a mother takes a drug while breastfeeding. In some instances, when the drug is given as a one off, for example sumatriptan for migraine, it is usually not too inconvenient for the mother to avoid breastfeeding for a short time after the dose, assuming no safety data are available. If, however, the drug is being used to treat a chronic condition such as epilepsy, then the risks of ongoing infant exposure must be considered. In addition, if the drug has been used chronically throughout pregnancy then the relative exposure of the infant to the drug via the milk must be considered with respect to the probable exposure in utero. In general, the fetal exposure to the drug during pregnancy will be considerably greater than the infant exposure from breastfeeding. The risks associated with infant exposure during breastfeeding would therefore be considered less.

There is a significant body of information available regarding the safety of drugs during breastfeeding. Unfortunately some of this information is prone to misinterpretation. This can adversely restrict the range of therapeutic agents available to the practitioner. A notable example involved indometacin, which, in a single report in 1978, was associated, although not causally, with seizures. Since this report, two well-controlled clinical trials have given indometacin a clean bill of health. However, many references still quote indometacin as contraindicated during breastfeeding. Unfortunately the literature is littered with such conflicting reports and inappropriate conclusions.

Transfer of drugs into milk

The transfer of drugs into milk is almost always by passive diffusion. Several factors will affect the rate and extent of passive diffusion. These include: maternal pharmacokinetics, the physiological nature of milk, and the physicochemical properties of the drug. Maternal pharmacokinetics alters the passage of drug into the milk phase simply by determining the amount of drug that is available for passage.

The physiological composition of milk determines which physicochemical characteristics of the drug will influence its passive diffusion. Milk differs from plasma in that it has a lower pH, lower protein-binding capacity, and higher concentrations of lipids. It can be surmised, therefore, that the following characteristics will affect the extent of drug transfer:

1. pK_a. This can be used as a measure of the fraction of drug that is ionized at a given pH (e.g. physiological pH). For basic drugs a greater fraction of the total amount will be ionized at acidic pH values, and therefore the milk phase will tend to 'trap' weak bases. In contrast, acidic drugs are more ionized at higher pH values, and will tend to be trapped in the maternal plasma.
2. *Protein binding*. Drugs that are highly protein bound in plasma will be trapped in the maternal plasma because there are fewer proteins in the milk. Milk concentrations of these drugs are usually low.
3. *Lipophilicity*. Drugs that are highly lipophilic will dissolve into the lipid content of the milk. This may increase both the extent and rate of drug transfer.

The profile of a drug that passes minimally into milk would therefore be an acidic drug that is highly protein bound and has low to moderate lipophilicity (e.g. a non-steroidal anti-inflammatory drug). In contrast, a weakly basic drug that has low plasma protein binding and is relatively lipophilic will achieve higher concentrations in the milk phase (e.g. sotalol).

It should be noted that the composition of milk varies between mothers and within the same mother. Milk production during the first few weeks postpartum is termed colostrum; this contains more proteins and fewer lipids compared to mature milk. Even during a single period of lactation the milk content changes; early milk is termed fore milk, and late milk hind milk. These changes in milk composition are, however, quantitatively less important than the physicochemical characteristics of the drug.

Estimating infant exposure

The infant exposure may be calculated either from a knowledge of the likely transfer of a drug into the milk phase, or from observational data. Observed data, while preferable, are not without pitfalls. The only data that can be used for accurate estimation of the likely infant exposure are from studies in which the milk is collected over a complete dose interval and the total infant dose calculated (Fig. 45.1).

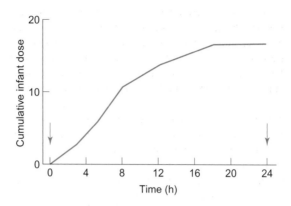

Figure 45.1 The cumulative dose received by the infant is plotted against time. The arrows represent the maternal dose times. This type of study is undertaken by the mother expressing all the milk, from both breasts, at usual times. An aliquot of milk is taken and assayed for the drug. The volume of milk is measured and the total amount of drug at each time is calculated as the product of concentration and volume. This type of study must be undertaken at steady state.

Unfortunately this type of study is seldom performed. Information must therefore be obtained from less than ideal conditions. The use of paired milk and plasma samples is an example of commonly reported data that may be misleading. Estimating the milk:plasma (M:P) ratio from simultaneous collections of mothers' milk and plasma requires that both concentration–time profiles are synchronous. This is seldom the case, and calculations based on these assumptions are likely to be erroneous (Fig. 45.2). However, a calculation of the M:P ratio

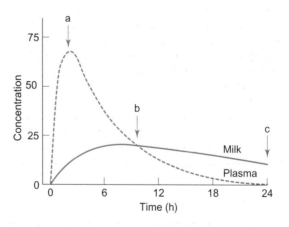

Figure 45.2 A diagrammatic representation of a drug concentration–time profile in the maternal plasma and milk phases after a single oral dose. The points a, b and c illustrate simultaneous sampling times from both phases. Sampling at 'a' would yield an estimated M:P value of 0.2, at 'b' a value of 1.0, and at 'c' a value of 9.3. All are erroneous. The true M:P ratio calculated by the AUC method is 1.2 when extrapolated to infinity.

using the area under the curve (AUC) of the drug in maternal plasma and milk over the same dose interval is a useful and accurate method. Using the example in Figure 45.2, it is seen that the M:P AUC ratio gives a value of 1.2, which is significantly different from the simultaneous sampling methods, and obviously more accurate.

If the M:P ratio is known, or can be estimated from the physicochemical characteristics of the drug, the likely infant dose (D_{inf}) can be calculated:

$$D_{inf} = Cp_{mat} \times M{:}P \times \text{volume of milk}$$

where Cp_{mat} is the average maternal plasma drug concentration. Although the volume of milk is not known, it is usual to estimate that an infant will ingest 150 ml/kg per day of milk. Reported values for M:P ratios are normally between 0.1 and 1.5, and only rarely do they exceed this range, although values of up to 5.0 have been reported. The above equation simplifies if actual milk concentration data are available, i.e. concentration multiplied by volume.

The likely infant plasma drug concentration (Cp_{inf}) can be calculated by:

$$Cp_{inf} = \frac{F \times D_{inf}}{Cl_{inf}}$$

where F is oral availability and Cl_{inf} is the infant clearance. Unfortunately, neither parameter is known accurately for drugs in infants, and estimation of the likely steady state average plasma drug concentration will be very approximate. Infant clearance values (on a weight-adjusted basis, i.e. l/h/kg) are often significantly less than adult values in the early stages of life. Estimates for clearance values in newborns are given in Table 45.2. It is worth remembering that drugs which are not absorbed orally in adults are also not likely to be absorbed by the infant. Therefore, drugs such as aminoglycosides, vancomycin, heparin, and insulin are, in most circumstances, considered safe to use in the breastfeeding mother.

Given the difficulty in estimating infant plasma drug concentrations, the relative infant dose is often used as a surrogate of exposure. To give some basis for comparison, the likely infant dose from milk can be compared with an infant therapeutic dose. In the absence of a clearly defined range of infant doses it is common to compare the dose to the maternal dose (D_{mat}). This can be done using the following equation:

$$\% \text{ dose} = \frac{D_{inf}(\text{mg/kg/day})}{D_{mat}(\text{mg/kg/day})} \times 100$$

For the great majority of drugs this calculation yields infant doses in the order of 0.1–5% of the weight-adjusted maternal dose.

What is a safe level of exposure?

While there is no simple way of determining a safe level of infant exposure, it is possible to devise guidelines that account for differing possibilities. What needs to be considered are the possible effects that the dose of the drug in question might have on the infant. If we consider that drugs are part of a continuous spectrum based on their toxicity profiles, then in theory all drugs could be presented on a line. If we then attempt to estimate the level of exposure that would be tolerable for a given intrinsic toxicity we might achieve a graph such as that shown in Figure 45.3.

At one end we would have drugs of low intrinsic toxicity (e.g. ascorbic acid), and at the other end we would have highly toxic drugs (e.g. cytotoxic agents). Considering this picture we would tolerate a significant '% dose' exposure to ascorbic acid while, in contrast, we would tolerate absolutely no exposure to cyclophosphamide. Most drugs fall between these two extremes, and each must be considered in light of its own merits. As a guideline for drugs of a low to moderate order of toxicity, which is by far the majority of drugs, an exposure of less than 10% of the weight-adjusted maternal dose is considered acceptable. This figure is arbitrary and may require modification if the infant is expected to clear the drug slowly. Hence for a premature neonate, whose clearance is likely to be a tenth that of an adult (on a l/h/kg basis), a maximum exposure (% dose) of only 1% might be considered appropriate. To reduce further the likely infant exposure the dose may be administered immediately after the infant has fed, thereby avoiding feeding during the period of maximum milk drug concentration (this assumes the maximum concentration in milk occurs at a similar time to the maximum concentration in plasma).

Assuming the arbitrary cut-off of 10% (ignoring intrinsic toxicity) there are only a small number of drugs that must be avoided during lactation. Examples are given in Table 45.3.

Table 45.2 Clearance by age	
Age group	Fraction of adult clearance[a]
2–3 months preterm	0.1
Term	0.33
1–2 months	0.5
3–6months	0.66
> 6 months	1.0

[a] Expressed as an approximate fraction of the typical adult clearance values on a weight-adjusted basis.

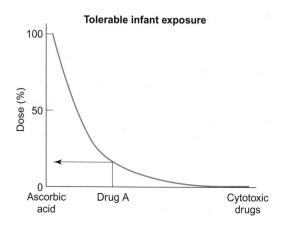

Figure 45.3 Intrinsic drug toxicity is given on the *x* axis. Infant exposure, as weight-adjusted maternal dose (% dose), is given on the *y* axis. The curve represents the maximum tolerable infant exposure over the range of drugs. Drug A is an example of a drug of relatively low toxicity where the infant might tolerate a dose of up to 15% of the weight-adjusted maternal dose.

Variability

To complicate matters further, there will be significant variability between and within individuals in the values used to estimate infant exposure (i.e. D_{inf}, F, CI_{inf}, where D_{inf} is itself a function of the estimated parameters Cp_{mat}, M:P, volume of milk). Some of this variability will systematically change over time due to developing organ function in the maturing baby and part will be unexplained variability. In addition to this pharmacokinetic variability there will be variability in the response of the infant to any given concentration of

Table 45.3 Examples of drugs that give high infant exposure
Amiodarone
Carbimazole
Ethosuximide
Isoniazid
Lithium
Metronidazole
Phenobarbital
Theophylline
Propylthiouracil

the drug. It is fortunate that most drugs seem to fall readily into 'safe' (i.e. << 10%) and 'not safe' (i.e. >> 10%) categories based on expected exposure. However, care should be taken for drugs that fall between these two extremes when variability in the estimates of the parameters used may have great impact on the prediction of their safety. This is especially true for those circumstances when initial estimates of these parameters are less precise (for example, for neonates).

Special situations

Idiosyncratic drug effects

There remains the possibility of an allergic reaction occurring in an infant to a drug ingested from the mother's milk, such as a rash from antibiotics. Allergic reactions are by nature unpredictable and a clear dose–response relationship is often not observed. Even minimal exposure of the infant to a drug through the milk may therefore confer a significant underlying risk. To date only isolated cases have been reported that document an allergic reaction occurring in an infant subsequent to the ingestion of a drug in the milk. Given the lack of reporting, the incidence of this type of reaction must be very low, and need not be considered in normal practice. As with all rules, exceptions exist. A case in point is the situation in which an infant has already experienced an allergic reaction to a given drug when previously exposed in a therapeutic setting. In this case, subsequent maternal use should be discouraged, or breastfeeding avoided.

The other main circumstance when adverse reactions may occur to small amounts of drug present in the milk is in infants with glucose-6-phosphate dehydrogenase (G6PD) deficiency. G6PD is an enzyme present in erythrocytes and is responsible for maintaining the antioxidant compound glutathione in its active form. Deficiency of this enzyme makes the erythrocyte more susceptible to oxidative stress, resulting in haemolysis. Typically only small amounts of drug are needed to precipitate such a reaction. Breastfeeding should be avoided if the infant has a known or suspected G6PD deficiency and the mother is taking drugs that have been reported to cause oxidative stress (Table 45.4).

Radiopharmaceuticals

Radiopharmaceuticals confer a special precaution for the breastfeeding mother. Although it was formerly generally believed distribution of these compounds into the milk presented a significant risk to the nursing baby, more recent reports suggest this may be true for only about half of the radiopharmaceuticals commonly used. However, for some compounds (e.g.[131]I) the milk exposure may reach values as high as 200 rad thereby

Table 45.4	Drugs associated with haemolysis in G6PD deficiency
Aspirin
Chlorpromazine
Nitrofurantoin
Quinine
Quinolones
Sulphonamides

posing a significant risk to the nursing baby. To complicate matters further there is also considerable between-patient variability in the distribution and elimination of these compounds. It is therefore not possible to arrive at a single specific recommendation regarding this diverse range of compounds. On a positive note though, it is possible to measure the presence of the compounds in the milk, which could provide the basis for clinical judgement.

Recreational drug use

Recreational drug use is widespread, variable, and probably under-reported. Many drugs may be being taken at any one time, and doses used vary widely between individuals and within the same individual. It is not appropriate to use the 10% 'cut off' rule in these circumstances since doses used are not standardized. Information from studies of recreational drug use is difficult to interpret due to the questionable accuracy of dosing history or the measurement of the M:P ratio, and the confounding of residual effects due to in utero exposure. Available data suggest that the infant exposure, as a percent of dose, for caffeine, ethanol and nicotine is approximately 10–20%. Opioid agonists, however, are poorly distributed into milk, and the percent dose found in milk is usually less than 5%. The data on the active component of marijuana, Δ^9-tetrahydrocannabinol (Δ^9-THC), and cocaine are incomplete, and assessment of infant exposure is not possible. Both nicotine and Δ^9-THC may reduce milk supply by up to 50%.

Drug effects on lactation

Only a few drugs have been demonstrated to have detrimental effects on milk production. Milk production is controlled by prolactin and any decrease in circulating prolactin or reduction in receptor binding will decrease milk production. In the main, only two groups of drugs significantly affect prolactin: hormonal agents and those that have dopamine activity. The most commonly used hormonal drugs that affect milk production are oestrogens. These agents, while distributing only minimally into milk, suppress milk production during the early stages, probably due to inhibitory effects at the prolactin receptor. Progestogen-only contraceptives are therefore used in preference to combined oral contraceptives during the early period of milk production. Drugs that act as agonists at dopamine receptors, such as bromocriptine, decrease milk production, while dopamine antagonists, for example metoclopramide, increase milk production. Both bromocriptine and metoclopramide have been used therapeutically for their effects on milk production, although recently the safety of bromocriptine has been questioned. Thiazide diuretics and serotonin antagonists, such as cyproheptadine, may also inhibit milk production.

CASE STUDIES

Case 45.1

A 28-year-old woman with a bipolar illness is currently taking lithium 800 mg daily for prophylaxis. She has decided to have a child but is concerned about the possibility of birth defects due to lithium exposure during pregnancy.

Questions

1. What risks are associated with lithium treatment during pregnancy?
2. How can these risks be minimized?
3. What other monitoring is indicated?

Answers

1. Lithium exposure during the first trimester may double the risk of birth defects compared with that of the general population. In particular, lithium is associated with Ebstein's anomaly, a rare congenital heart defect. Lithium exposure throughout pregnancy can cause neonatal goitre, and lithium toxicity can occur in the neonate as a result of placental drug transfer. The initial information used to estimate the teratogenic risk of lithium was derived from potentially biased retrospective reports where the number of normal outcomes following lithium exposure were not reliably known. More recent prospective studies, where each pregnancy was followed throughout gestation and postnatally, have consistently demonstrated a much lower teratogenic risk. It is estimated that about 95% of pregnancies where lithium exposure has occurred will have a normal outcome. The decision to continue lithium treatment during pregnancy depends on the severity of the illness. Poorly controlled illness presents significant risks to both mother and fetus.

2. There are a number of possibilities. If the clinical situation allows, the lithium can be gradually tapered and stopped before conception. Alternatively, the lithium can be continued at the lowest effective dose and stopped immediately the pregnancy is diagnosed to minimize the period the patient is not taking lithium. Lithium should be avoided in the first trimester if possible, and the drug reintroduced in the second or third trimester if necessary. It may be possible to cover lithium-free periods in the first trimester with short-term use of neuroleptic drugs. Lithium freely crosses the placenta, and the lowest effective dose should be used to avoid fetal and neonatal toxicity.

3. Plasma lithium concentrations should be monitored throughout pregnancy, and doses often need to be increased due to more rapid renal clearance. The necessity of a dose increase has to be carefully weighed against the associated increase in fetal plasma levels, which is exacerbated by the immature renal clearance.

   If lithium is taken in the first trimester, heart defects can be diagnosed by fetal echocardiography and high-resolution ultrasound performed at 16–18 weeks' gestation.

Case 45.2

A woman who is approximately 6 weeks pregnant has been diagnosed with clinical depression. She has been having at least three alcoholic drinks daily for the last few months.

Questions

1. Is fluoxetine safe to treat her depression?
2. What alternative drug treatment is available?
3. What is the significance of this woman's alcohol intake?

Answers

1. Experience of the use of the selective serotonin reuptake inhibitor (SSRI) fluoxetine in pregnancy is increasing. Tricyclic antidepressants such as amitriptyline or imipramine have been used extensively in pregnancy and are considered relatively safe. Animal studies with fluoxetine have revealed no evidence of teratogenicity in doses over 10 times the maximum human dose but these results are not predictive of human response. However, several prospective studies of pregnant women exposed to fluoxetine, including first trimester exposure, have identified no evidence of teratogenic effects. From current evidence the safety of fluoxetine in pregnancy is similar to that of the tricyclic antidepressants. Treatment should be guided by clinical response and if a tricyclic antidepressant is ineffective or contraindicated, the use of fluoxetine can be considered. It is preferable to avoid or minimize drug exposure during the first trimester. The lowest effective dose should be used throughout pregnancy and an attempt made to slowly reduce the dose approaching term to avoid neonatal withdrawal effects. Fluoxetine is the most extensively studied SSRI in pregnancy. More limited data suggest the other SSRIs (e.g. paroxetine) are also relatively safe. However, the SSRIs are a chemically diverse group of drugs and safety data cannot be extrapolated from

fluoxetine to other drugs in this class. Fluoxetine would usually be the first choice SSRI in pregnancy.

2. Experience of using drugs such as venlafaxine and nefazodone and monoamine-oxidase inhibitors (MAOIs) including moclobemide in pregnancy is limited. The use of these drugs is best avoided until more data are available.

3. Alcohol is teratogenic and it is now considered that total abstinence during pregnancy is the safest approach. The fetal alcohol syndrome (FAS) includes low birth weight, facial dysmorphogenesis and retarded mental development. Two standard drinks daily can induce mild FAS, and the severe form is usually seen with consumption of four or five drinks daily. The severity of FAS is related to the daily amount and duration of alcohol intake, thus there would be very real benefits in this case if the woman were to stop drinking immediately.

Case 45.3

A mother comments that her full-term 3-day-old baby is experiencing excessive shrill crying, jitteriness, shaking and poor suckling. She is worried the paroxetine she is taking may be crossing into her milk and causing these effects. Her medical team can find no other cause for these effects. The mother has been taking paroxetine 20 mg per day throughout pregnancy.

You note from a specialist textbook the likely infant exposure, expressed as percent weight-adjusted maternal dose is 1%. Paroxetine is a basic drug, 95% protein bound and has a half-life in adults of approximately 24 hours.

Questions

1. What is the most likely drug-related explanation?
2. Is it safe for the mother to continue to breastfeed while taking paroxetine?

Answers

1. It is most likely that these effects are caused by paroxetine due to its prolonged elimination from the infant after exposure during pregnancy. The half-life in adults is 24 hours and this will be longer in a neonate. In almost all cases drug exposure during pregnancy is greater than via breastfeeding. Studies on paroxetine have shown that the likely infant exposure via milk is low and typically 1% of the weight-adjusted maternal dose. In these studies no adverse effects were seen in the infant and the concentration of paroxetine in the infant's plasma was below the limit of detection in almost all cases. These findings are supported by the physicochemical properties of the drug which, due to its basic nature and high protein binding, support minimal passage into milk.

2. The mother should be reassured the effects are not likely to be due to the passage of excessive amounts of paroxetine into her milk. They are most likely to be due to a 'carry-over' effect from taking the drug during pregnancy. These effects should resolve naturally within the week as her baby eliminates the remaining drug. If they persist then she should seek further medical advice.

Case 45.4

A woman who has been breastfeeding for 1 month develops diarrhoea following a visit to a farm. After a few days the mother visits her community doctor, who suggests she has giardiasis, and decides to initiate treatment while waiting for the results of a stool sample. The mother is prescribed metronidazole 200 mg three times daily for 5 days.

Data

The mother weighs 60 kg.
The average steady state plasma metronidazole concentration following a 200 mg dose given three times daily is 10mg/l.
Metronidazole passes freely into milk, achieving concentrations similar to those in the maternal circulation.

Questions

1. What is the calculated percent dose exposure in this infant?
2. Would it be safe for the mother to breastfeed her child during the course?
3. Would a single, initial dose of 2000 mg be preferable? Would this change your assessment of the risk:benefit ratio?

Answers

1. The dose is 15%. Since the mother's dose is 200 mg three times per day and she weighs 60 kg, then this calculates to a total dose of 10 mg/kg/day. If the infant ingests 150 ml of milk/kg/day and the average milk concentration is 10 micrograms per ml, then the infant dose would be 10 × 150 micrograms/kg/day = 1500 micrograms/kg/day. As a percent of the weight-adjusted maternal dose it is (1.5 mg/kg/day ÷ 10 mg/kg/day) × 100 = 15%.

2. The infant exposure is greater than the generally recommended cut-off of 10%. It is necessary to consider the possible toxicity of metronidazole which is known to cause gastrointestinal side-effects in approximately 12% of those exposed to it. There have also been rare reports of neuropathies, and metronidazole is described as mutagenic with unknown long-term effects. Despite these potential effects, it is not contraindicated in breastfeeding mothers; however, it would be prudent for the mother to watch her baby for excessive vomiting or diarrhoea during the treatment course. If the dose was 400 mg three times daily then it would be recommended to alternate breastfeeding with bottle feeding, or to abstain from breastfeeding for the duration of the treatment course.

3. While the infant exposure would still be 15% of the weight-adjusted maternal dose, the absolute exposure would be 10 times greater. It is recommended that breastfeeding should be avoided for the 24 hours following the dose.
Metronidazole has a half-life of 8 hours. Consequently, after three half-lives only 12.5% of the drug would be left, which is similar to the amount achieved after a 200 mg dose.

FURTHER READING

Bennett P N (ed) 1988 Drugs and human lactation. Elsevier, Amsterdam

Briggs G G, Freeman R K, Yaffe S J 1994 Drugs in pregnancy and lactation, 4th edn. Williams and Wilkins, London

Ilett K F, Kristensen J H, Wojnar-Horton R E, Begg E J 1997 Drug distribution into human milk. Australian Prescriber 20: 84–85

Wright A, Walker J 2001 Drugs of abuse in pregnancy. Best Practice and Research. Clinical obstetrics and Gynaecology 15: 987–998

Wisner K L, Gelenberg A J, Leonard H et al 1999 Pharmacological treatment of depression during pregnancy. Journal of the American Medical Association 282: 1264–1269

American Academy of Pediatrics 2001 The transfer of drugs and other chemicals into human milk. Pediatrics 108: 776–789

Benign prostatic hyperplasia

46

R. L. Gower

KEY POINTS

- Benign prostatic hyperplasia (BPH) is a common condition which becomes increasingly common with age.
- The enlarging prostate compresses the urethra and produces lower urinary tract symptoms (LUTS) and bladder outflow obstruction (BOO).
- Surgical treatments such as transurethral incision of the prostate (TURP) are effective, but less invasive procedures such as thermotherapy and laser therapy are commonly used.
- α adrenoceptor blocking drugs are effective in reducing symptoms within 6 weeks.
- Drugs which block α_{1A} adrenoceptors are believed to have more specific activity on the prostate and produce fewer systemic adverse effects.
- 5-α reductase inhibitors such as finasteride reduce prostate size, improve symptoms and urinary flow rates over a period of about 6 months and are most effective in men with larger size prostates.

Benign prostatic hyperplasia (BPH) is the most common benign tumour in men and is responsible for urinary symptoms in the majority of men over the age of 50 years. At present, of those men who live to 80 years, 20–30% will have their prostate surgically removed to alleviate the symptoms of prostatism.

Epidemiology

BPH has a prevalence of 615 per 1000 in men aged 40–49 years, increasing to 889 per 1000 in men aged 70–79 years. By the age of 80 years virtually all men have symptoms.

From puberty to the third decade of life there is considerable expansion in the size of the prostate gland. It has been estimated that the time for it to double in size between the ages of 31 and 50 years is 4.5 years, and between 51 and 70 years it is 10 years. Theoretically there is very little increase in size of the male prostate after 70 years.

BPH is undoubtedly related to ageing, and is a phenomenon seen in all races; however, the overall size of the prostate does vary from race to race.

Pathophysiology

The prostate is a part glandular, part fibre–muscular structure about 3.5 × 2.5 cm in size surrounding the first part of the male urethra at the base of the bladder (Fig. 46.1). It develops at the 12th week of embryonic life, under the influence of androgenic fetal hormone from outpouchings of the urethra.

Simplistically the prostate can be divided into an inner and an outer zone. The inner zone is generally the site of benign hypertrophic changes, and the outer zone the site of malignant change.

The aetiology of BPH is undoubtedly multifactorial, but it is well recognized that prostatic hypertrophy is directly related to the ageing process and to hormone activity. Within the prostate, testosterone is converted by 5 α-reductase to dihydrotestosterone (DHT). Ongoing exposure to DHT leads to enlargement and hyperplasia.

Histologically the hypertrophied prostate can vary, depending on the predominance of the type of prostatic tissue present, from stromal, fibromuscular, muscular, fibroadenomatous and fibromyoadenomatous enlargement.

The enlarging prostate does not produce any constitutional change in its own right, other than that mediated by its effect on the urethra of the lower urinary tract (Fig. 46.2). As the prostate enlarges, it tends to elongate and compress the urethra, and this together with increased adrenergic tone leads to outlet obstruction. Clinical BPH therefore comprises benign clinical enlargement (BPE), bladder outflow obstruction (BOO) and lower urinary tract symptoms (LUTS).

Symptoms

LUTS can be divided into symptoms of failure of urine storage (irritative) and those caused by failure to empty the bladder (obstructive).

Obstructive

- poor flow
- hesitancy in initiation of micturition

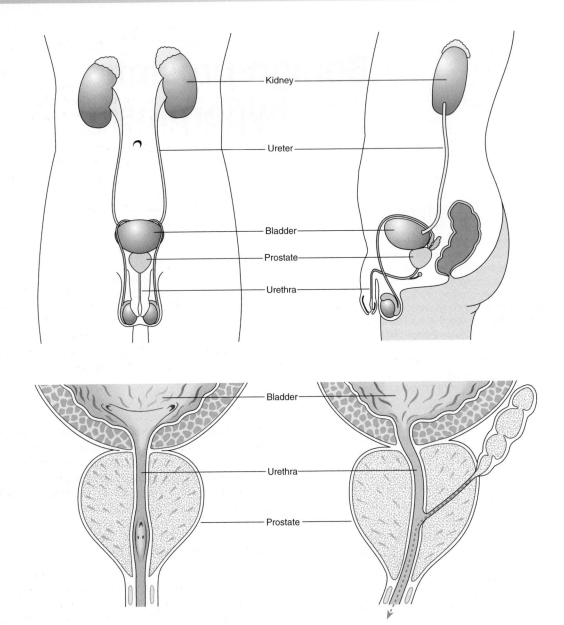

Figure 46.1 Male urinary system and prostate.

- postmicturition dribble
- sensation of incomplete emptying
- occasionally acute retention of urine – requiring emergency treatment.

Irritative

- frequency
- nocturia
- urgency and urge incontinence.

LUTS can be quantified by various scoring systems such as the international prostate symptom score (I-PSS), though each system has its limitations. Other scores measure flow rate, residual volume, prostate size and quality of life.

A digital rectal examination is essential to reveal the presence of a tumour. The measurement of protein specific antigen (PSA) is controversial but may be offered if the diagnosis of cancer would change the treatment plan (see Chapter 4, Laboratory data).

BPH can produce haematuria, but the presence of a large bladder that does not empty and leads to chronic renal failure is potentially serious. This often happens in relatively young patients without any other prostatic symptoms. Fortunately the vast majority of cases can be easily reversed by decompressing the bladder.

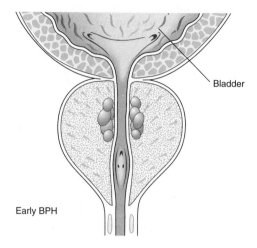

Early BPH

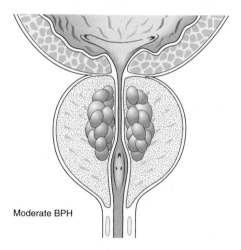

Moderate BPH

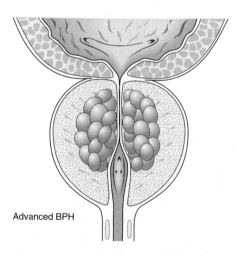

Advanced BPH

Figure 46.2 Diagrammatic representation of the impact of prostate hyperplasia on the urethra.

Examination and investigations

All patients who present with suspected BPH should undergo a rectal examination. An enlarged bladder can be palpated, and the size of the prostate determined although it has no direct relationship to the severity of symptoms. The most important reason for doing a rectal examination is to detect prostate cancer.

Further investigations include simple urinalysis, urine for culture if infection is considered, serum assessment of renal function to ascertain upper tract damage and the measurement of serum levels of prostate-specific antigen to detect the presence of a carcinoma of the prostate.

Urodynamic assessment

Urodynamic measurements include simple uroflow through to cystometry and pressure flow studies. In most cases a simple uroflow is enough, where the peak flow and average flows are recorded. Most young men should void at a peak flow of 25 ml/s, while a flow of less than 12 ml/s strongly suggests outflow obstruction.

Imaging

Simple digital ultrasound scanning of the bladder is sufficient to detect and measure a residual volume. Upper tract imaging by means of an ultrasound scan and intravenous urography is no longer routinely done unless indicated by the presence of haematuria, impaired renal function or infection.

Flexible cystoscopy

An evaluation of the bladder using a fibre-optic telescope inserted into the urethra and advanced into the bladder under topical anaesthetic is invaluable in the assessment of the type of prostatic obstruction. If the prostate has grown in such a way that there is intravesical extension where the prostatic tissue can be imagined to hinge at the bladder neck, then each time the patient tries to void, the internal urethral meatus is obstructed by this ball valve effect. This type of tissue requires surgical removal, whereas simple lateral lobe enlargement may well respond to non-surgical measures.

Prostatic ultrasound scan

This is invaluable in accurately documenting the size of the prostate and detecting malignant change. In institutions where it is freely available it gives the confidence of diagnosis and the ability to more accurately predict the outcome of various treatment options.

Treatment

Most men over the age of 50 years have some symptoms of BPH. The big problem, therefore, is who should be treated and when. With improved anaesthetic techniques the majority of operations can be done under regional anaesthesia, considerably reducing the operative risks and complications. This, together with the development of less invasive surgical procedures and the refinement of medical treatments, offers a range of management options for the individual with BPH.

Surgery

Transurethral resection of the prostate (TURP)

TURP is a common and effective procedure which achieves a high level of improvement in symptoms and flow rate and only requires a short hospital stay. Sections of prostate are removed using electrical loops attached to a telescope. Removed material is collected for histological assessment.

There is a small incidence of perioperative mortality and complications such as bleeding, urinary tract infections and epididymitis. Long-term complications include stress incontinence, urethral and bladder neck strictures and impotence.

Open prostatectomy

This procedure is performed infrequently now. It requires a longer hospital stay than TURP and is associated with a higher incidence of bleeding and other complications.

Minimally invasive techniques

Various treatment modalities have been tried as alternatives to TURP in order to reduce the risks associated with resection. Thermotherapy and laser technology are the most commonly used.

Thermotherapy

Thermotherapy uses techniques such as electrovaporization (heating the prostate using bipolar diathermy to cause vaporization of the tissue) and transurethral microwave thermotherapy (using radiative heating).

Laser therapy

Various types of laser energy can be used to destroy prostatic tissue. It has the advantage of desiccating the tissue so that it is less likely to bleed.

Although alternative measures for surgical intervention give the surgeon a choice in management, transurethral resection still gives the best result for the patient and provides samples for histological assessment.

Non-invasive treatment

In some men, BPH does not progress significantly and one management option is that of so called 'watchful waiting'. However, where medical treatment is indicated, the two principal options are α adrenoceptor blocking drugs and inhibition of 5 α-reductase.

α-adrenoceptor blocking drugs

The prostate gland is very responsive to adrenergic stimulation and it has been found that about half of the prostatic outlet obstruction in BPH arises from an increase in adrenergic tone (Chapple et al 1989) the other half being due to the hypertrophied bulk of the gland. This increase in sympathetic tone is potentially reversible by drugs. α_1-receptors predominate in the prostate and mediate the contraction of the gland's smooth muscle. At least three subtypes of this receptor exist (α_{1A}, α_{1B} and α_{1D}) and it is believed that α_{1A} is the dominant receptor in the prostate, although its role clinically has still to be confirmed. The search for drugs which selectively inhibit this receptor subtype has led to the introduction of several new agents in recent years.

The antihypertensive drug prazosin was the first α-blocking drug used to relieve the symptoms of BPH but it lacks relative selectivity for α_{1A} receptors and caused many adverse affects such as drowsiness, weakness, headache and postural hypotension (especially after the first dose). It has been replaced in use by other drugs.

Tamsulosin. This drug is a selective inhibitor at the α_{1A} adrenoceptor. It increases urinary flow rates and reduces LUTS in men with BPH within 8 hours and one week respectively as well as improving quality of life scores (Lepor 1998, O'Leary 2001). Tamsulosin has an elimination half life of about 10 hours which allows once daily dosing and there is no requirement to titrate the dose upward when initiating treatment. It is well tolerated but can cause dizziness, headache, asthenia and syncope.

It interacts with cimetidine which reduces its clearance by 25%.

Alfuzosin. In isolated human tissue, alfuzosin displays a higher selectivity for the prostate over vascular tissue compared with tamsulosin and doxazosin (Eckert et al 1999). It has a half life of five hours but is available as a once-daily formulation. It has a rapid onset of action, good tolerability and a sustained effect on quality of life (Stephenson et al 1994, Debruyne et al 1998, The Italian Alfuzosin Co-operative Group 2000).

Indoramin. Indoramin is in common use in the UK. Ramdonized clinical trials have been small and of short duration. Adverse effects are similar to those described above.

Doxazosin. Doxazosin is licensed for use as an antihypertensive agent as well as for the management of BPH. Its long half life of about 20 hours allows for once daily dosing but the dose requires titrating to limit postural hypotension. It has relatively less selective activity on the prostate specific α adrenoceptors, but has been found to improve symptoms and peak flow rates (Roehrborn & Siegel 1996).

Terazosin. Like doxazosin, terazosin is used once daily but requires dose titration. Apart from this, it is a safe and effective treatment for BPH.

5α-reductase inhibitors

Finasteride. The primary androgen responsible for the development and progression of the prostate gland to BPH is DHT. There are two isozymes of 5α-reductase and the prostate expresses mainly type 2. Finasteride is a Type 2, 5α-reductase inhibitor which regulates prostate growth. It has been shown to reduce prostate size by about 30%, improve symptom scores and increase urinary flow rates by 2.2 ml per second (Ekmann 1998). Meta-analysis has shown that changes in symptoms and peak urinary flow rates were greatest in men with prostate volumes greater than 40 ml (Boyle et al 1996). It may take 6 months before symptomatic benefit is felt by the patient, but once attained it may continue for several years with continued treatment. Finasteride has been shown to reduce the number of men who develop acute urinary retention and require surgical intervention (Roehrborn et al 2000).

Side-effects include decreased libido, impotence, reduced ejaculatory volume and reversal of male pattern baldness. Serum concentrations of PSA may be reduced by 50% in the first year of treatment with finasteride, a fact which must be taken into account if a patient has or is suspected of having prostate cancer.

It is possible that combining finasteride with an α-blocking drug may be beneficial, but studies have failed to show any benefit over monotherapy. However, in such studies the prostate size was less than 40 ml which is below the size at which finasteride has been shown to have a significant effect.

A new agent, dutasteride, is thought to inhibit both isozymes of the converting enzyme and could have a faster onset of action than finasteride.

Phytotherapy

A number of plant extracts are reputed to be effective in the management of symptoms of BPH. They include Saw palmetto berry *(Serenoa repens)*, African plum tree *(Pygeum africanum)* and stinging nettle *(Urtica dioica)*. Many of the trials are uncontrolled and until placebo-controlled, double blind studies are forthcoming, it is difficult to assess their efficacy meaningfully. The proposed mechanisms of action include an anti-inflammatory effect (by inhibition of prostaglandins) and inhibition of 5α-reductase.

Patient care

The patient generally seeks treatment for BPH because of the impact of symptoms on quality of life. In patients with troublesome bladder-filling symptoms such as frequency, urgency and urge incontinence, formal bladder training may be appropriate, using a frequency–volume chart that records intake and output over several days. This bladder training may involve asking the patient to go longer between voiding and increasing the volume voided. Keeping a chart may also help the patient better regulate fluid intake, particularly before retiring, and raise awareness of the need to minimize the intake of drinks containing caffeine or alcohol to reduce symptoms.

Bladder training may be undertaken as part of a watch and wait approach or concurrently with drug therapy. For those patients in whom drug therapy is appropriate the choice lies between an α_1 or α_{1A} adrenoceptor antagonist and a 5α-reductase inhibitor, and each, in turn, requires its own specific information to be given to the patient.

Table 46.1 lists some common therapeutic problems in the management of benign prostatic hyperplasia.

Table 46.1 Common therapeutic problems in benign prostatic hyperplasia

Problem	Solution
Patients taking α-blockers still are symptomatic	Patients should be advised that it may take 2–6 weeks before symptomatic relief is seen
Patient taking an α adrenoceptor blocker complains of cardiovascular adverse effects such as dizziness, syncope, palpitations, tachycardia or angina	These side-effects are more likely in elderly patients. They are most common after the first dose and reflect the hypotensive effects of the drugs. They can be reduced by titrating the dose or using more uroselective drugs such as tamsulosin
Sexual dysfunction	Decreased libido or impotence can occur in patients taking finasteride. Abnormal ejaculation can be caused by α-blockers. Patients should be forewarned when discussing treatment options
Patient taking finasteride has a sexual partner of childbearing age	Exposure to semen should be avoided since finasteride can cause abnormalities to genitalia in a male fetus

CASE STUDIES

Case 46.1

A 64-year-old man presents with complaints of poor urinary flow and having to visit the toilet at least twice during the night to pass urine. He is taking no medicines.

Question

What investigations are appropriate and how should this patient be managed?

Answer

This patient should undergo a full clinical examination including measurement of prostatic specific antigen (PSA) and residual volume of urine within the bladder after micturition.

If the PSA is within the normal range and the residual volume is less than 100 ml, a watch and wait policy may be the most appropriate management initially. If this is unacceptable, then the patient should be offered treatment with an α-blocking drug. If he is not hypertensive, then a uroselective drug such as tamsulosin should be considered. This should have few systemic side-effects and requires no titration of doses initially. If he is hypertensive, a less specific α-blocker may be more appropriate which will serve a dual purpose as an antihypertensive as well as treating his urinary symptoms. Careful dose titration may be necessary initially to counter any potential postural hypotension.

Case 46.2

A 50-year-old man requests treatment from his GP for a 'bladder infection'. On questioning he describes symptoms of urinary frequency, urgency and urge incontinence, but fever is absent.

Question

How should this patient be treated?

Answer

The lay person may well interpret the symptoms as representing a urinary tract infection, but in the absence of fever, this is unlikely. The patient should be referred for a full clinical assessment, culminating in a full urodynamic assessment including filling and voiding cystometry, ultrasound scan of the upper urinary tract, measurement of PSA and assessment of renal function. It is likely that this patient has an outflow obstruction which has given rise to secondary instability of the detrusor muscle in the bladder, causing involuntary contractions of the bladder resulting in incontinence. The obstruction may be due either to prostate enlargement or to a narrowing of the bladder neck due to an unrelated cause. In either case, treatment with an α-blocking drug is appropriate to reduce the outflow resistance. Should the flow be adequate, but symptoms of incontinence persist, then concurrent treatment with an antimuscarinic drug may be necessary to inhibit the cholinergic mediated contractions of the detrusor. Examples are oxybutynin, tolterodine and propiverine.

Case 46.3

An 80-year-old man presents with severe symptoms of outflow tract obstruction and initial haematuria. A rectal examination reveals a large prostate.

Question

What is the optimal treatment for this man?

Answer

A full clinical assessment is necessary to eliminate a diagnosis of cancer. If the diagnosis is BPH, then surgery may be considered necessary. If it is decided that surgery is not an option initially, because of the patient's age or patient preference, then treatment with finasteride would be appropriate to reduce bleeding over 3–6 months, as well as to reduce prostatic size which will improve the outflow symptoms. If successful, treatment may be continued indefinitely with finasteride. If, however, finasteride does not give satisfactory remission, consideration should be given to TURP with concurrent finasteride to reduce excessive surgical bleeding.

Case 46.4

A middle-aged man complains of lower abdominal swelling and feeling tired. On questioning, he admits to poor urinary flow and bedwetting.

Question

What is the optimal treatment for this man?

Answer

Full clinical examination and renal function tests should be arranged urgently. If the abdominal swelling is thought to be caused by a large bladder and laboratory tests show the renal function is deranged, the patient should be urethrally catheterized and the urine drained. The catheter should be left in situ to allow the renal function to recover before proceeding to surgical prostatectomy. Outflow tract obstruction with renal impairment requires urgent management.

REFERENCES

Boyle P, Gould L, Roehrborn C G 1996 Prostate volume predicts outcome of treatment of BPH with finasteride. Urology 48: 398–405

Chapple C R, Aubry M L, James S et al 1989 Characterisation of human prostatic adrenoceptors using pharmacology receptor binding and localisation. British Journal of Urology 142: 438–444

Debruyne F M, Jardin A, Colloi D et al 1998 Sustained release alfuzosin, finasteride and the combination of both in the treatment of benign prostatic hyperplasia. European Urology 34: 169–175

De Mey C 1999 α_1 – blockers for BPH: are there differences? European Urology 36(Suppl. 3): 52–63

Eckert R E, Schreier U, Alloussi S et al 1999 Prostate selectivity of alpha 1-adrenoceptor blockers. Journal of Urology 161(Suppl. 4): 233

Ekmann P 1998 Maximum efficacy of finasteride is obtained within six months and maintained over six years. European Urology 48: 398–405

Italian Alfuzosin Co-operative Group 2000 Safety, efficacy and impact on patients' quality of life of a long-term treatment with the α_1 blocker alfuzosin in symptomatic patients with BPH. European Urology 37: 680–686

Lepor H 1998 Phase III multicenter placebo-controlled study of tamsulosin in benign prostatic hyperplasia. Urology 51: 892–900

O'Leary M P 2001 Tamsulosin: current clinical experience. Urology 58(6A): 42–48

Roehrborn C G, Siegel R L 1996 Safety and efficacy of doxazosin in benign prostatic hyperplasia: a pooled analysis of three double-blind, placebo controlled studies. Urology 48: 406–415

Roehrborn C G, Bruskewitz R, Nickel G C et al 2000 Urinary retention in patients with BPH treated with finasteride or placebo over four years. European Urology 37: 528–536

Stephenson T P, Jensen R D and the PRANALF Group 1994 A placebo-controlled study of the efficacy and tolerability of alfuzosin and prazosin in the treatment of benign prostatic hypertrophy (BPH). In: Proceedings of the XI Congress of European Association of Urology. July 13–16, Berlin, Abstract 48

FURTHER READING

Anon 1999 α_1-adrenoceptors as targets for therapeutic agents in urology. XIIIth International Congress of Pharmacology, Munich, July 26–31, 1998. European urology 36(Suppl. 1): 1–20

Blute M L, Jacobsen S J, Kaplan S A et al 2001 Evaluation and management of benign prostatic hyperplasia: proceedings of a thought leader conference held March 31st, 2001: introduction. Urology 58(6A): 1–4

Buzelin J M, Hebert M, Blondin P and the PRAZALF Group 1993 Alpha-blocking treatment with alfuzosin in symptomatic benign prostatic hyperplasia: comparative study with prazosin. British Journal of Urology 72: 922–927

Kirby R S, Pool J C 1997 Alpha adrenoceptor blockade in the treatment of benign prostatic hyperplasia: past, present and future. British Journal of Urology 80: 521–532

Anaemia 47

C. Acomb

KEY POINTS

- Anaemia is a common condition which is caused by a number of different pathologies.
- Iron deficiency causes a microcytic, hypochromic anaemia. Once the primary cause has been corrected, ferrous iron is the standard treatment.
- Folate deficiency results in a macrocytic anaemia and is treated with replacement therapy.
- Lack of intrinsic factor prevents absorption of vitamin B_{12} and leads to a macrocytic anaemia. Treatment with parenteral B_{12} reverses the blood picture but does not always alleviate the accompanying neuropathy.
- Haemolytic anaemias include the genetic disorders of sickle cell anaemia, thalassaemia and glucose-6-phosphate dehydrogenase deficiency. In these diseases, abnormal forms of haemoglobin cause damage to the structure of the red cells and haemolysis.
- Sideroblastic anaemia is a rare anaemia in which haem synthesis is impaired owing to an enzyme deficiency.

Anaemia is not one disease. It is a condition that results from a number of different pathologies. Anaemia can be defined as a reduction from normal of the quantity of haemoglobin in the blood. The World Health Organization defines anaemia in adults as haemoglobin levels less than 13 g/dl for males and less than 12 g/dl for females. However, there are apparently normal individuals with levels lower than this. The low haemoglobin level results in a corresponding decrease in the oxygen carrying capacity of the blood.

Epidemiology

Anaemia is possibly one of the most common conditions in the world and results in significant morbidity and mortality, particularly in the developing world. Worldwide, over 50% of pregnant women and over 40% of infants are anaemic. In Britain 14% of women aged 55–64 and 3% of men aged 35–64 years have been found to be anaemic.

Aetiology

Anaemia results from two different mechanisms:

1. Reduced haemoglobin synthesis, which may be due to lack of nutrient or bone marrow failure. This leads to either reduced proliferation of precursors or defective maturation of precursors or both (Table 47.1).

Table 47.1 Examples of conditions that cause reduced haemoglobin synthesis	
Reduced proliferation of precursors	Defective maturation of precursors
Iron deficiency	Vitamin B_{12} deficiency
Anaemia of chronic disease	Folate deficiency
Anaemia of renal failure	Iron deficiency
Aplastic anaemia (primary)	Disorders of:
Aplastic anaemia (secondary to drugs, etc.)	Globin synthesis (thalassaemias)

Infiltration of the bone marrow:
  Leukaemia or lymphoma
  Myelofibrosis
  Metastases
	Iron metabolism (e.g. sideroblastic)
	Myelodysplastic syndrome

2. Increased haemoglobin loss due to haemorrhage (red cell loss) or haemolysis (red cell destruction).

It is not unusual to find more than one cause in a patient.

This chapter will cover some of the more common anaemias that involve drug therapy: iron deficiency anaemia, megaloblastic anaemia (folate deficiency and vitamin B_{12} deficiency), sideroblastic anaemia and haemolytic anaemia (sickle cell disease, thalassaemia and glucose-6-phosphate dehydrogenase deficiency anaemia).

Normal erythropoiesis

It is thought that white cells, red cells and platelets are all derived from a common cell known as the pluripotent stem cell found in the bone marrow. As these cells mature they become committed to a specific cell line. (Figure 47.1) The cells mature through the various stages, during which time they synthesize haemoglobin, DNA and RNA. Reticulocytes are found in the peripheral circulation for 24 hours before maturing into erythrocytes. Reticulocytes are released into the peripheral circulation prematurely during times of increased erythropoiesis.

Erythropoietin is a hormone produced by the cells of the renal cortex. The kidney responds to hypoxia and anaemia by increasing the production of erythropoietin. The red cell progenitors BFU-E and CFU-E have receptors on their surface. When erythropoietin binds to these receptors it promotes differentiation and division, and consequently increased erythropoiesis. Patients with end-stage renal disease fail to produce appropriate amounts of erthropoietin and so develop anaemia.

Erythropoietin production is also impaired in other conditions such as rheumatoid arthritis, cancer and sickle cell disease, though the impairment is not as great as in renal disease.

Each day approximately 2×10^{11} erythrocytes enter the circulation. Normal erythrocytes survive in the peripheral circulation for about 120 days. Abnormal erythrocytes have a shortened lifespan. At the end of their life the red cells are destroyed by the cells of the reticuloendothelial system found in the spleen and bone marrow. Iron is removed from the haem component of haemoglobin and transported back to the bone marrow for reuse. The pyrole ring from globin is excreted as conjugated bilirubin by the liver and the polypeptide portion enters the body's protein pool.

Clinical manifestations

In its mildest form, anaemia results in tiredness and lethargy; at its most severe it results in death unless treated. There is some suggestion that even mild anaemia may inhibit physical exercise and result in reduced mental performance. The reduced oxygen carrying capacity of the blood leads to reduced tissue oxygenation and widespread organ dysfunction.

A rapid blood loss, such as haemorrhage, produces shock, with collapse, dyspnoea and tachycardia. Anaemia that develops over a period of time allows the body to partially compensate. As the anaemia becomes worse, so more and more signs and symptoms may develop (Table 47.2).

Although the amount of haemoglobin in anaemia is reduced, all the blood that passes through the lungs is fully oxygenated. Increasing the respiratory rate or

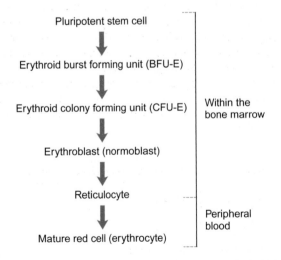

Figure 47.1 Simplified diagram of some of the stages within erythropoiesis.

Table 47.2 Non-specific signs and symptoms associated with anaemia
Tiredness
Pallor
Fainting
Exertional dyspnoea
Tachycardia
Palpitations
Worsening angina
Worsening cardiac failure
Exacerbation of intermittent claudication

increasing the FiO$_2$ (fraction of inspired oxygen) will not improve tissue oxygenation. When the haemoglobin falls below 7 or 8 g/dl there is almost always a compensatory increase in cardiac output.

Investigations

It is essential to find the cause of anaemia; there is no place for 'blind' treatment. In most patients anaemia is a consequence of a reduced concentration of haemoglobin in each red cell and/or a reduced number of red cells in the peripheral circulation. However, in certain situations, such as pregnancy and heart failure, the haemoglobin concentration may appear falsely low because of an increased blood volume. Splenomegaly and signs of heart failure are sure signs of an increased blood volume. A blood transfusion in such a patient would precipitate left ventricular failure.

The most important parameter to assess anaemia is the haemoglobin concentration of the blood. It is also usual to count the number of red cells. In addition, the size, shape and colour all contribute to the investigation (Table 47.3). The mean corpuscular volume (MCV) is also a useful parameter that helps determine the type of the anaemia. However, care must be taken since the MCV indicates the *average* size of the cells. If there are two pathologies, where one causes large cells and one causes small cells, the MCV may appear normal or be misleading. Following on from this baseline other investigations may be required. Bone marrow examination by either aspiration or trephine may be needed to make a diagnosis.

Iron deficiency anaemia

Epidemiology

Iron deficiency anaemia is the commonest form of anaemia worldwide and may be present in up to 20% of the world's population. A diet deficient in iron, parasitic infestations, for example hookworm (causing blood loss), and multiple pregnancies contribute to its high prevalence in developing countries. Even in Western societies it has been reported that as many as 20% of menstruating females show a rise in haemoglobin levels during iron therapy.

Aetiology

In Western societies the commonest cause of iron deficiency is blood loss. In women of childbearing age this is frequently due to menstrual loss. Among adult males the most likely cause is gastrointestinal bleeding. Other causes of blood loss associated with iron deficiency anaemia include haemorrhoids, nosebleeds or postpartum haemorrhage. A loss of 100 ml of blood represents the amount of iron normally absorbed from a Western diet over 40 days. The major causes of iron deficiency are listed in Table 47.4

Pathophysiology

The elimination of iron is not controlled physiologically so the homeostasis is maintained by controlling iron absorption. Iron is absorbed mainly from the duodenum and jejunum. Absorption itself is inefficient; iron bound to haem (found in red meat) is better absorbed than iron found in green vegetables. The presence of phosphates and phytates in some vegetables leads to the formation of unabsorbable iron complexes, while ascorbic acid increases the absorption of iron. In a healthy adult, approximately 10% of the dietary iron intake will be absorbed.

Anaemia may result from a mismatch between the body's iron requirements and iron absorption. The demand for iron varies with age (Table 47.5). Diets deficient in animal protein or ascorbic acid may not provide sufficient available iron to meet demand. Poor nutrition in children in inner cities in the UK frequently leads to anaemia. Milk fortified with iron given to inner city infants up to the age of 18 months has been shown to increase haemoglobin levels and improve developmental performance compared to unmodified cow's milk (Williams et al 1999). There have been calls to make iron-fortified milk free of charge for inner city children.

Table 47.3   Anaemia classified by size and colour of red cells

Hypochromic microcytic
  Iron deficiency
  Sideroblastic
  Thalassaemia

Normochromic macrocytic
  Folate deficiency
  Vitamin B$_{12}$ deficiency

Polychromatophilic macrocytic
  Haemolysis

Table 47.4   Major causes of iron deficiency anaemia

Inadequate iron absorption
  Dietary deficiency
  Malabsorption

Increased physiological demand

Loss through bleeding

Table 47.5	Typical daily requirements of iron
Infant (0–4 months)	0.5 mg
Adolescent male	1.8 mg
Adolescent female	2.4 mg
Adult male	0.9 mg
Menstruating adult female	2.0 mg
Pregnant female	3–5 mg
Postmenopausal female	0.9 mg

Malabsorption of iron has been reported in patients with coeliac disease and in 50% of patients following partial gastrectomy. Tetracyclines, penicillamine and fluoroquinolines bind iron in the gastrointestinal tract and reduce the absorption of iron from supplements. They probably do not affect the absorption of dietary iron.

During pregnancy there is an increase in red cell mass but there is also a proportionally bigger increase in plasma volume, which results in a physiological dilutional anaemia. It is thought that the gut increases its ability to absorb iron during pregnancy to meet the additional demands of fetal red cell production. Some of the increased demand is met by the stopping of menstruation. If, however, there is inadequate iron absorption, then anaemia may result.

Clinical manifestations

In addition to the general symptoms of anaemia, various other features may be present (Table 47.6). The colour of the skin is very subjective and often unreliable. Patients at risk of heart failure may present with breathlessness when anaemic. Koilonychia, dysphagia and pica are

Table 47.6	Features of iron deficiency anaemia
Pale skin and mucous membranes	
Painless glossitis	
Angular stomatitis	
Koilonychia (spoon shaped nails)	
Dysphagia (due to pharyngeal web)	
Pica (unusual cravings)	
Atrophic gastritis	

found only after chronic iron deficiency and are relatively rare.

A full blood count is an essential screening test. The cells of the peripheral blood are microcytic and hypochromic with poikilocytes (often pencil shaped) and occasional target cells (abnormal thin erythrocytes which when stained show a dark centre and peripheral ring).

Three parameters help establish the iron status of the patient: the serum iron, the total iron binding capacity (TIBC) and the serum ferritin. The serum iron exhibits diurnal variation, being higher in the morning. Iron is transported around the body bound to a serum protein called transferrin. Normally this protein is only one-third saturated with iron. The parameter TIBC is the sum of the serum iron and the unsaturated iron binding capacity (UBIC) of the iron transport proteins in the blood. The serum iron and TIBC vary with iron status (Fig. 47.2). The serum ferritin level is low in iron deficiency anaemia and markedly raised in iron overload.

Investigations

The aim of treatment is to correct the anaemia and replenish iron stores. Although the treatment of iron deficiency anaemia is relatively simple, it should not be embarked upon lightly. It is important to resolve the underlying cause as far as possible. Over-the-counter sales of iron should be discouraged except in those patients who have been fully investigated. It is not unknown for patients to be given iron unnecessarily, resulting in iron overload. Also, giving iron therapy to a

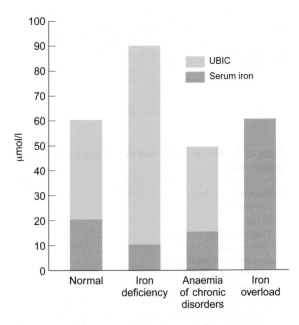

Figure 47.2 Typical examples of serum iron and UBIC.

patient who is continuing to bleed from the gastrointestinal tract is not helping to resolve the underlying problem.

Treatment

Prophylaxis of iron deficiency anaemia was formerly widely used in pregnancy, together with folic acid. However, it is now only used for women who have additional risk factors for iron deficiency, such as poor diet. Prophylaxis may also be used in menorrhagia, after partial gastrectomy and in some low birth-weight infants, for example premature twins.

Oral iron in the ferrous form is cheap, safe and effective in most patients. Depending on the state of the body's iron stores it may be necessary to continue treatment for up to 6 months to both correct the anaemia and replenish body stores. The standard treatment is ferrous sulphate 200 mg three times a day. It typically takes between 1 and 2 weeks for the haemoglobin level to rise 1 g/dl. An earlier indication of the patient's response can be seen by looking at the reticulocyte count, which should start to rise 2–3 days after starting effective treatment. Nausea or abdominal pain trouble some patients and this tends to be related to the dose of elemental iron. Giving the iron with food makes it easier to tolerate but tends to reduce the amount absorbed. Alternative salts of iron are sometimes tried; these tend to have fewer side-effects simply because they contain less elemental iron (Table 47.7). Taking fewer ferrous sulphate tablets each day would have the same effect. A change in bowel habit (either constipation or diarrhoea) is sometimes reported and this is probably not dose related. During the early stages of treatment the body absorbs oral doses of iron better. Absorption is commonly about 15% of intake for the first 2–3 weeks but falls off to an average of 5% thereafter. Recently it has been shown that for some patients eradication of *Helicobacter pylori* aids recovery from iron deficiency anaemia (Annibale et al 1999).

There are a number of modified-release oral preparations available. They have no clear therapeutic advantage over ferrous sulphate and are not recommended. Indeed, the modified-release characteristic may cause the oral iron to be carried into the lower gut, which is much poorer at absorbing iron than the duodenum. Modified-release preparations may be more likely to exacerbate diarrhoea in patients with inflammatory bowel disease or diverticulae.

There is little place for parenteral iron; it should be reserved for patients who fail on oral therapy, usually because of poor adherence and intolerable gastrointestinal side-effects. For most patients, when equivalent doses of oral and parenteral iron are used there is no difference in the rate at which the haemoglobin level rises. Patients who have lost blood acutely may require blood transfusions. The need for a rapid rise in haemoglobin is not an indication for parenteral iron. However, some patients with chronic renal failure appear to have a functional iron deficiency that responds to intravenous iron. These patients, despite receiving oral iron and epoetin (recombinant human erythropoietin), do respond with a rise in haemoglobin when given regular intravenous iron sucrose (Silverberg et al 1996).

There is a risk of anaphylactoid reactions with iron sucrose but this appears to be lower than with the older product iron dextran (now unlicensed). Patients given intravenous iron sucrose should have a test dose and there should be facilities for cardiopulmonary resuscitation available. In iron deficiency the dose of iron sucrose can be calculated depending on the haemoglobin level. In renal patients a regular weekly dose is often given and the patient's serum ferritin monitored to check for iron overload. In the UK, iron sorbitol is the only licensed product suitable for intramuscular injection. The maximum individual dose is 100 mg, so frequently a series of painful and time-consuming injections are required. The injections have to be given by deep intramuscular injection using a technique to prevent leaking of the solution down the needle track.

Patient care

It is usual practice to advise patients to take iron products with or after meals as this probably reduces the incidence of nausea. Patients should be told that their faeces may become darker and that this is nothing to worry about. This is important in patients who have had melaena since they may associate their dark stools with the bleed and worry that they are still bleeding from the gastrointestinal tract. The length of treatment and adherence should be discussed and an explanation given that iron stores need to be replenished and that this takes time.

Table 47.7 Elemental iron content of common oral preparations

Preparation	Approximate iron content
Tablets	
Ferrous sulphate 200 mg	65 mg
Ferrous gluconate 300 mg	35 mg
Ferrous fumarate 200 mg	65 mg
Oral liquids	
Ferrous fumarate 140 mg in 5 ml	45 mg
Ferrous glycine sulphate 141 mg in 5 ml	25 mg
Sodium feredetate 190 mg in 5 ml	27.5 mg

Megaloblastic anaemias

The megaloblastic anaemias are macrocytic anaemias (raised MCV). There is an abnormality in the maturation of haematopoietic cells in the bone marrow. In addition to abnormal red cells the white cells and platelets may be affected. The two major causes are folate deficiency and vitamin B_{12} deficiency. Pernicious anaemia is a specific disease caused by malabsorption of vitamin B_{12}.

Epidemiology

Folate deficiency anaemia

Much of the world's population has a marginal dietary intake of folate. Body stores are low, and as soon as there is a decrease in dietary intake or there is increased folate demand, deficiency readily occurs.

Vitamin B_{12} deficiency anaemia

Strict vegans, for example Hindus, commonly have low vitamin B_{12} levels due to their dietary deficiency though actual anaemia is rarer. All patients who have had a total gastrectomy and 6% of those with a partial gastrectomy will develop vitamin B_{12} deficiency anaemia.

Pernicious anaemia

Pernicious anaemia (reduced vitamin B_{12} absorption due to a lack of intrinsic factor) is found most commonly in people of Northern European descent. In Britain the incidence is about 120 per 100 000, being higher in Scotland than in the south of England. Pernicious anaemia is usually a disease of the elderly, the average patient presenting at 60 years of age.

Aetiology

Folate deficiency anaemia

Folate is readily available in a normal diet. Fruit, green vegetables and yeast all contain relatively large amounts of folate. Despite this relative abundance of folate in many foods, dietary deficiency is common, either as the sole cause of the folic acid deficiency anaemia or in conjunction with increased folate utilization.

Vitamin B_{12} deficiency anaemia

Deficiency occurs from inadequate intake or malabsorption. The only dietary source of vitamin B_{12} (cyanocobalamin) is from food of animal origin. It is present in meat, fish, eggs, cheese and milk. Cooking does not usually destroy vitamin B_{12}. Daily requirements are between 1 and 3 micrograms. Deficiency arises either from inadequate intake over a prolonged period or, more commonly, in Western Europe, from impaired absorption.

Malabsorption occurs if the distal ileum is removed; it may also occur with certain intestinal pathologies, particularly stagnant loop syndrome, tropical sprue and fish tapeworm infestation. Passive absorption does take place in the jejunum, but this is very inefficient and usually accounts for less than 1% of an oral dose.

Pathophysiology

The common biochemical defect in all megaloblastic anaemias is the inhibition of DNA synthesis in maturing cells.

Folate deficiency anaemia

The folate found in food is mainly conjugated to polyglutamic acid. Enzymes found in the gut convert the polyglutamate form to monoglutamate, which is readily absorbed. During absorption the folate is methylated and reduced to methyltetrahydrofolate monoglutamate. This travels through the plasma and is transported into cells via a carrier specific for the tetrahydrofolate form. Within the cell the methyl group is removed (in a reaction requiring vitamin B_{12}) and the folate is reconverted back to a polyglutamate form (Fig. 47.3). It has been suggested that the polyglutamate form prevents the folate leaking out of cells. The folate eventually acts as a co-enzyme involved in a number of reactions including DNA and RNA synthesis. Defective DNA

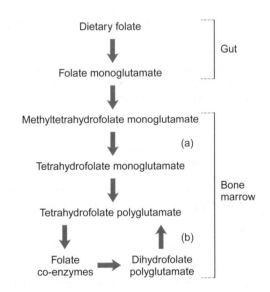

Figure 47.3 Simplified pathway of folate metabolism. (a) Vitamin B_{12} is required as a co-enzyme for this reaction; (b) the enzyme dihydrofolate reductase converts inactive dihydrofolate back to the active tetrahydrofolate.

synthesis mainly affects cells with a rapid turnover, such as gastrointestinal cells and precursors of red blood cells in bone marrow, hence the sore tongue and anaemia seen in folate deficiency. During DNA synthesis the folate co-enzyme is oxidized to the dihydrofolate form, which is inactive and has to be reactivated by the enzyme dihydrofolate reductase. This is the enzyme inhibited by methotrexate and to a lesser extent by trimethoprim and pyrimethamine. Co-trimoxazole has been shown to increase the severity of megaloblastic anaemia.

Vitamin B_{12} deficiency

Absorption of vitamin B_{12} is mainly by an active process. Enzymes in the stomach release vitamin B_{12} from protein complexes. One molecule of vitamin B_{12} then combines with one molecule of a glycoprotein called intrinsic factor. The intrinsic factor protects the vitamin B_{12} from breakdown by micro-organisms. There are specific receptors in the distal ileum for the intrinsic factor–vitamin B_{12} complex. The vitamin B_{12} enters the ileal cell and is then transported through the blood attached to transport proteins. Intrinsic factor does not appear in the blood.

Since intrinsic factor is only produced by the gastric parietal cells, a total gastrectomy always leads to vitamin B_{12} deficiency. Approximately 10–15% of patients who have had a partial gastrectomy also develop deficiency. The onset of anaemia is usually delayed because the body typically has stores of 2–3 mg, which is sufficient for 2–3 years. Vitamin B_{12} is a co-enzyme for the removal of a methyl group from methyltetrahydrofolate. Lack of vitamin B_{12} traps the folate as methyltetrahydrofolate, and prevents DNA synthesis. The exact mechanism by which vitamin B_{12} deficiency causes neuropathy is not clear but may be due to a defect in the methylation reactions needed for myelin formation.

Pernicious anaemia

Pernicious anaemia is probably autoimmune in origin. Patients typically have a gastric atrophy and no, or virtually no, intrinsic factor secretion. Two different intrinsic factor antibodies have been found in the serum of patients with pernicious anaemia. Gastric parietal cell antibodies are found in 90% of pernicious anaemia patients.

Clinical manifestations

In addition to the general features of anaemia, megaloblastic anaemia, of which folic acid deficiency and B_{12} deficiency anaemia are the two most common examples, has certain characteristics (Table 47.8).

Folate deficiency anaemia

Alcoholics and the elderly are particularly prone to nutritional deficiency. Elderly people living alone on tea and toast are typical examples of at-risk patients. Many alcoholics develop deficiency due to their poor diet; although some beers contain small amounts of folate, spirits contain none. A number of drugs have been implicated in causing folate deficiency (Table 47.9). Actual megaloblastic anaemia from drug therapy is uncommon and the exact mechanism(s) has not always been established. Serious malabsorption can occur in tropical sprue and coeliac disease. Reduced absorption is seen in Crohn's disease and following partial gastrectomy and jejunal resection.

There is a physiological increase in folate utilization during pregnancy. There may be an increased utilization in various pathological conditions, in association with

---

Table 47.8   Features of megaloblastic anaemia

Glossitis (sore, pale, smooth tongue)
Angular stomatitis
Altered bowel habit (diarrhoea or constipation)
Anorexia
Mild jaundice
Insidious onset
Sterility
Bilateral peripheral neuropathy (mainly vitamin B_{12} deficiency)
Melanin skin pigmentation (rare)
Fever (mainly vitamin B_{12} deficiency)

Table 47.9   Drugs implicated in causing folate deficiency

Malabsorption
Phenytoin
Barbiturates
Sulfasalazine
Colestyramine
Oral contraceptives
Impaired metabolism
Methotrexate
Pyrimethamine
Triamterene
Pentamidine
Trimethoprim

inflammation or in a number of chronic haemolytic anaemias, particularly thalassaemia major, sickle cell disease and autoimmune haemolytic anaemia. Chronic folate deficiency probably predisposes a patient to thrombosis, depression and neoplasia (Green & Miller 1999).

Vitamin B$_{12}$ deficiency anaemia

The megaloblastic anaemia caused by vitamin B$_{12}$ deficiency has similar features to folate deficiency (see Table 47.8). In addition to the macrocytosis, anisocytosis and poikilocytosis, there is often mild thrombocytopenia. The spleen may be slightly enlarged and there may be a slight fever. Mild jaundice may be present due to the increased breakdown of haemoglobin found in the abnormal red cells. The onset is slow and insidious so patients often present late or are diagnosed during other investigations. The feature that separates vitamin B$_{12}$ deficiency from the other megaloblastic anaemias is progressive neuropathy. It is symmetrical and affects the legs rather than the arms. Patients notice a tingling in their feet and a loss of vibration sense. Occasionally patients have difficulty in walking or experience frequent falls.

Investigations

Folic acid deficiency anaemia

Many patients are symptomless initially, and the diagnosis is made following a full blood count carried out for another reason. The peripheral blood reveals large oval red cells. Anisocytosis and poikilocytosis are common. Some of the neutrophils are hypersegmented, and thrombocytopenia may be present. The red cell folate concentration accurately reflects folate stores and is a preferable parameter to the serum folate concentration, which is subject to changes in diet and does not correlate as closely with anaemia.

Vitamin B$_{12}$ deficiency anaemia

Following the recognition of megaloblastic anaemia from the full blood count, one of the first investigations will be the determination of the serum vitamin B$_{12}$ level. The red cell folate or serum folate level is normally obtained at the same time. The serum vitamin B$_{12}$ level is low in mild anaemia and may be very low if there is marked megaloblastic anaemia or neuropathy. If there is no concurrent folate deficiency the serum folate level tends to be raised while the red cell folate level falls, possibly due to a failure of folate polyglutamate synthesis in cells.

Oral vitamin B$_{12}$ absorption can be measured by a number of techniques, the most common test being the Schilling test. The test is based on giving a radiolabelled oral dose of vitamin B$_{12}$ and an unlabelled parenteral dose that saturates the vitamin B$_{12}$-binding proteins. The amount of labelled vitamin in the urine gives a measure of absorption. The test can be repeated by giving the radiolabelled oral dose with intrinsic factor. The absorption should now be approaching normal if the patient has intrinsic factor deficiency but remains low if there is ileal disease.

Although 90% of patients with pernicious anaemia have parietal cell antibodies, their presence is not diagnostic because 50% of patients with gastric atrophy without pernicious anaemia also have the antibodies present.

Treatment

It is necessary to establish whether the patient with megaloblastic anaemia has vitamin B$_{12}$ deficiency or folic acid deficiency, or both. Treatment of vitamin B$_{12}$ deficiency with folic acid may lead to the resolution of the haematological abnormalities but does not correct the neuropathy, which continues to deteriorate. If it is not possible to delay until a definitive diagnosis is made, both folic acid and vitamin B$_{12}$ may be given.

Folate deficiency anaemia

Folate deficiency is usually managed by replacement therapy. The duration of the treatment depends on the cause of the deficiency. Changes in dietary habits or removal of any precipitating factor should also be considered.

The normal daily requirement of folic acid is approximately 100 micrograms a day; despite this, the usual treatment doses given are 5–15 mg a day. Even in malabsorption states, because of these large doses, sufficient folate is usually absorbed. Therefore parenteral folic acid treatment is not normally required. Treatment for 4 months will normally be sufficient to ensure that folate deficient red cells are replaced.

Large doses of folic acid can produce a partial haematological response in patients with vitamin B$_{12}$ deficiency. The blood picture appears nearly normal but the neurological damage due to the vitamin B$_{12}$ deficiency continues. Folic acid therapy should not be started until vitamin B$_{12}$ deficiency has been excluded. It has also been suggested that patients on long-term folic acid therapy should have their vitamin B$_{12}$ levels checked at regular intervals, for example yearly.

Pregnancy

The folate requirement increases in pregnancy and is higher in twin pregnancies. Folate deficiency regularly occurs in patients with a poor diet who do not take supplements. Prophylaxis with folate (350–500 micrograms daily) is now frequently given in pregnancy, often in combination with iron. It is important that these products with low doses of folate are not used to treat megaloblastic anaemia. In addition, although low dose folate should be started before conception to prevent first occurrence of neural tube defect, higher doses (5 mg daily) are required in women with a history of neural tube defects (DoH 1992).

Vitamin B$_{12}$ deficiency anaemia

The majority of patients with vitamin B$_{12}$ deficiency require lifelong replacement therapy. Occasionally specific therapy related to the underlying disorder may be all that is necessary, for example treatment of fish tapeworm.

Since the anaemia has developed slowly, the cardiovascular system does not tolerate blood transfusions very well and is easily overloaded. Transfusions should not normally be given. In severe cases where emergency transfusion is deemed necessary, packed cells may be given slowly while blood (mainly plasma) is removed from the other arm. Diuretics may also need to be given, especially if the patient has congestive heart failure and poorly tolerates fluid overload.

For most patients a definite diagnosis is made before treatment is started. The standard treatment is hydroxocobalamin 1 mg intramuscularly repeated five times at 3 day intervals to replenish body stores. This is followed by a maintenance dose, usually 1 mg intramuscularly every 3 months. US texts recommend cyanocobalamin rather than hydroxocobalamin because of the fear that some patients appear to develop antibodies to the vitamin B$_{12}$ transport protein complex in the serum. In the UK, hydroxocobalamin is the treatment of choice. It is retained in the body longer than cyanocobalamin, and reactions to it are very rare. The haematological response to both is probably identical. A small amount of passive absorption of vitamin B$_{12}$ does take place from the gastrointestinal tract. An oral dose of 1 mg every day is worth trying in patients who are unable to have injections.

Because potassium is an intracellular ion and is used in the production of new cells, hypokalaemia may develop during the initial haematological response. Potassium supplements may be needed in the elderly and patients receiving diuretics or digoxin. The serum iron level also falls as it is incorporated into haemoglobin. The more severe the anaemia the more likely it is to see a fall in the serum potassium or iron level.

Not only is it very gratifying to follow the response to treatment, it is also important to monitor the response to ensure that the patient returns to normal without any attendant problems. There is often a subjective improvement before an objective one. Typically the patient feels better within 24–48 hours and yet there may be no discernible haematological response. The first haematological change in the peripheral blood is a rise in the reticulocyte count starting around day 3 or 4 and peaking after 7–8 days. The more severe the anaemia, the higher the peak reticulocyte count. The reticulocyte count should remain raised while the haematocrit is less than 35%. Failure to remain raised during this time indicates the need for further evaluation. The arrest or slowing down of erythropoiesis may be due to inadequate stores of other essential factors, such as iron, or may be due to coexisting disease such as hypothyroidism or infection.

The red cells return to normal and the platelet count rises to normal, or even higher, after 7–10 days. The haemoglobin takes much longer to return to normal. It should rise by approximately 2–3 g/dl each fornight. Neurological damage may be irreversible. Peripheral neuropathy of recent onset often partially improves but any spinal cord damage is irreversible even with optimum therapy.

Patient care

Folic acid deficiency anaemia

In patients who have a dietary component to their deficiency, appropriate nutritional advice should go alongside their folic acid therapy. If the cause of the deficiency has been eliminated, patients can expect to receive folic acid for approximately 4–6 months. In patients with a continuing requirement, as in haemolytic anaemia, patients can expect lifelong treatment. Those starting out on folic acid therapy can anticipate feeling better after a few days but should be informed that their blood picture will take much longer to return to normal.

Vitamin B$_{12}$ deficiency anaemia

Patients feel subjectively better very shortly after their first hydroxocobalamin injection. They can be told that their sore tongue will start to improve within 2 days and be back to normal after 2–4 weeks. Patients need to be informed that they require regular injections, usually every 3 months. Surprisingly, some patients say that they feel they are ready for this injection as they approach their appointment time and feel better after the injection. Adherence is not usually a problem.

Sideroblastic anaemias

Epidemiology

Sideroblastic anaemias are a group of conditions that are diagnosed by finding ring sideroblasts in the bone marrow. There are both hereditary and acquired forms. The hereditary forms are rare, while some of the acquired forms are relatively common with as many as 30% of alcoholics admitted to hospital having sideroblastic anaemia.

Aetiology

In the majority of hereditary forms there is an X chromosome linked pattern of inheritance. Both autosomal dominant and autosomal recessive families have been described. The main defect is a reduced activity of the enzyme 5-aminolevulinate synthase (ALAS) which is involved in haem synthesis.

The acquired forms include idiopathic forms, forms associated with myeloproliferative disorders and forms secondary to the ingestion of drugs (Table 47.10). Regardless of the cause, there is impaired haem synthesis.

Pathophysiology

An examination of the bone marrow typically shows a number of erythroblasts that have iron granules surrounding the cell nucleus. These cells are known as ring sideroblasts. In the hereditary forms there are low levels of ALAS. This mitochondrial enzyme is involved in the first step in the synthesis of haem and requires pyridoxal phosphate as a co-factor. Pyridoxine is a precursor for pyridoxal.

Drugs and toxins

Alcohol can lead to the formation of ring sideroblasts. In this scenario, the ethanol is metabolized to acetaldehyde which subsequently lowers the levels of ALAS and pyridoxal. In slow acetylators isoniazid reacts with pyridoxal and the resulting product is then rapidly

excreted. Doses of chloramphenicol over 2 g per day invariably lead to sideroblasts. This is thought to be due to the inhibition of mitochondrial protein synthesis.

Clinical manifestations

The hereditary forms typically develop in infancy or childhood. The anaemia can be severe or mild. There may be splenomegaly, which can lead to mild thrombocytopenia. The idiopathic acquired forms tend to develop insidiously, usually in middle age or later. Many patients may be asymptomatic for long periods. In the forms associated with other disorders the clinical picture tends to be dominated by the underlying diseases.

Investigations

In the hereditary form the red cells in the peripheral blood are hypochromic and microcytic. Despite this there are frequently increased iron stores in the bone marrow. The serum iron and ferritin may also be high. In the acquired forms the peripheral blood has hypochromic cells, which may be either normocytic or macrocytic. The common finding is the presence of sideroblasts in the bone marrow.

Treatment

In patients with the hereditary forms, large doses of pyridoxine (200 mg daily) reduce the severity of the anaemia. Long-term high dose pyridoxine has been associated with peripheral neuropathy and so lower maintenance doses are sometimes tried. There have been case reports of patients responding to parenteral pyridoxal-5-phosphate after failing to respond to pyridoxine. Patients with an acquired form occasionally respond to high dose pyridoxine, and a 2–3 month trial may be helpful in symptomatic patients. The response tends to be slow and only partial. The investigational agent haem arginate has been shown to increase the red cell count and decrease the number of ring sideroblasts in some patients with acquired sideroblastic anaemia. In common with other conditions where an increased turnover of cells in the bone marrow is a feature, folate supplements are often necessary.

Inevitably some patients fail to respond to these treatments and frequent blood transfusions are required. This leads to the complications of iron overload and sensitization and the risk of blood borne virus transmission. The chelating agent desferrioxamine is given either by intravenous or subcutaneous infusion. It binds free iron and iron bound to ferritin. Therapy should be considered when the serum ferritin level reaches 1000 micrograms/l. Patients with very high ferritin levels may need daily infusions. Daily subcutaneous infusions using a disposable infusor or small infusion pump are suitable

---

Table 47.10 Acquired sideroblastic anaemia

Associated with other disorders
 Myelodysplastic syndromes
 Myeloid leukaemia
 Myeloma
 Collagen diseases

Associated with drugs and toxins
 Alcohol
 Isoniazid
 Chloramphenicol
 Penicillamine
 Pyrazinamide
 Cycloserine
 Progesterone (single case report)
 Copper deficiency

for home use. Published evidence suggests that for an equivalent dose, a longer infusion time results in increased iron excretion. Intravenous infusions can be given whenever the patient comes into hospital for a blood transfusion. Oral vitamin C increases the effectiveness of desferrioxamine but also increases its cardiotoxicity. Desferrioxamine should not be given concurrently with prochlorperazine as prolonged unconsciousness may result. More recently an oral agent, deferiprone, has been introduced. It has been shown to be beneficial (Al-Refaie et al 1995) but it is reported to cause reversible neutropenia in some patients and so currently is reserved for patients intolerant of desferrioxamine.

Although the peripheral blood cells are frequently hypochromic and microcytic, the condition is associated with increased iron stores, therefore iron supplements should be avoided. The drugs and toxins (see Table 47.10) tend to cause a reversible anaemia. Removing the offending agent usually resolves the anaemia.

Ascorbic acid also increases the tissue toxicity of iron in patients with iron overload.

Patient care

Few patients with hereditary or the idiopathic acquired forms have completely reversible anaemia. Patients need to be aware that pyridoxine may take several months before there is any sign of improvement. They should be advised not to purchase over-the-counter iron or vitamin supplements (particularly ascorbic acid or pyridoxine) without seeking medical advice first.

Haemolytic anaemias

In the haemolytic anaemias there is a reduced lifespan of the erythrocytes. If the rate of destruction of the erythrocytes exceeds the rate of production, then anaemia results. There are a wide range of haemolytic anaemias with both genetic and acquired disorders (Table 47.11). Only sickle cell anaemia, thalassaemia and glucose-6-phosphate dehydrogenase deficiency will be discussed.

Epidemiology

Sickle cell anaemia

Sickle cell disease is a hereditary condition of which several different variants of exist. It is found in a number of ethnic groups, mainly in populations originating from tropical regions. In the UK approximately 5000 people, largely from the Afro-Caribbean population, have sickle cell disease.

Thalassaemias

The β thalassaemias occur mainly in populations from around the Mediterranean, North and West Africa, the Middle East and the Indian subcontinent. More than 100 β thalassaemia mutations have been identified and they tend to produce severe anaemia. The α thalassaemias are more common but the milder variants do not cause severe anaemia while the severe homozygotes lead to death in utero or infancy.

Glucose-6-phosphate dehydrogenase deficiency anaemia

About 300 million people in the world are affected by glucose-6-phosphate dehydrogenase (G6PD) deficiency. There are more than 300 different forms of G6PD deficiency, only some of which cause anaemia. The most common form of G6PD deficiency is found in 15% of black Americans. It causes anaemia when the individual is exposed to a trigger factor. A more severe form is the Mediterranean variant of G6PD deficiency. Some of these individuals may have chronic haemolytic anaemia, even in the apparent absence of exposure to a precipitating factor.

Aetiology

Sickle cell anaemia

Patients with sickle cell disease have a different form of haemoglobin. Those with the most common variant of sickle cell disease have haemoglobin S (Hb S) (normal haemoglobin is usually designated Hb A). Haemoglobin S has valine substituted for glutamic acid as the sixth amino acid in the β-polypeptide compared with normal haemoglobin. Patients with homozygous Hb S develop many problems including anaemia.

Table 47.11 Examples of haemolytic anaemias

	Examples
Genetic disorders	
Membrane	Hereditary spherocytosis Hereditary ovalcytosis
Haemoglobin	Sickle cell anaemias Thalassaemias
Energy pathways	Glucose-6-phosphate dehydrogenase deficiency
Acquired disorders	
Immune	Rh or ABO incompatibility Autoimmune
Non-immune	Infections (parasitic, bacterial) Drugs and chemicals Hypersplenism

Sickle cell trait is where a person is a carrier of the gene (heterozygous for the sickle cell gene). These people are usually asymptomatic. The offspring from a father with trait and a mother with trait has a 1 in 4 chance of having sickle cell disease (Fig. 47.4).

Thalassaemias

In α thalassaemia there is either no α chain production (α^0 thalassaemia) or reduced production of a chain (α^+ thalassaemia). Heterozygotes are usually symptomless while homozygotes are more severely affected, as are compound heterozygotes in which there is a thalassaemia gene and a gene from another haemoglobin variant (e.g. Hb S).

G6PD deficiency

There are a large number of variants of G6PD activity found in different populations and ethnic groups. G6PD is an erythrocyte enzyme that is indirectly involved in the production of reduced glutathione. Glutathione is produced in response to, and protects red cells from, oxidizing reagents.

Pathophysiology

Sickle cell disease

The membrane of red cells containing Hb S is damaged, which leads to intracellular dehydration. In addition, when the patient's blood is deoxygenated, polymerization of Hb S occurs, forming a semisolid gel. These two processes lead to the formation of crescent-shaped cells known as sickle cells. Sickle cells are less flexible than normal cells (flexibility allows normal cells to pass through the microcirculation). The inflexibility leads to impaired blood flow through the microcirculation, resulting in local tissue hypoxia. Anaemia results from an increased destruction of red cells. Some red cells in patients with sickle cell disease contain fetal haemoglobin (Hb F). These cells do not sickle.

Thalassaemias

In β thalassaemias there is a reduced or absent production of the globin β chain. This leads to a relative excess of α chain which, when unpaired, become unstable and precipitates in the red cell precursors. There is ineffective erythropoiesis and those mature cells that reach the circulation have a shortened life span.

In α thalassaemias the pathology is slightly different. The deficiency of α chains leads to an excess of γ or β chains. This time erythropoiesis is less affected but the haemoglobin produced (haemoglobin Bart's or Haemoglobin H) is unstable when the cells are in the circulation and precipitates as the cells grow older. This leads to a shortened lifespan with the spleen trapping many of the cells. Haemoglobin Bart's and haemoglobin H are also physiologically useless.

G6PD deficiency

G6PD is essential for the production of the reduced form of phosphorylated nicotinamide-adenine dinucleotide (NADPH) in erythrocytes. If there is a deficiency in G6PD this decreases the production of NADPH. NADPH is needed to keep glutathione in a reduced form. Reduced glutathione maintains haemoglobin in a reduced form and helps erythrocytes deal with oxidative stress. Hence in G6PD deficiency, if the erythrocytes are exposed to an oxidizing agent, the haemoglobin becomes oxidized and forms what are known as Heinz bodies. The cell membrane is damaged and some of the red cells haemolyse and others have their Heinz bodies removed by the spleen to form 'bite cells'.

Clinical manifestations

Patients with acute haemolytic anaemia commonly complain of malaise, fever, abdominal pain, dark urine and jaundice. They have haemoglobulinaemia, hyperbilirubinaemia, reticulocytosis and increased urobilinogen levels in the urine. Patients with chronic haemolytic anaemia also usually have splenomegaly. Their anaemia is usually normochromic and normocytic.

Sickle cell anaemia

Patients with severe variants of the disease have chronic anaemia, arthralgia, anorexia, fatigue and splenomegaly.

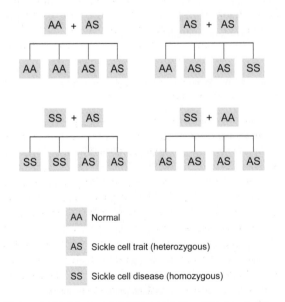

Figure 47.4 Inheritance patterns in sickle cell trait and sickle cell disease.

They have crises more frequently than other variants of the disease. A crisis can be precipitated by infection and fever, dehydration, hypoxia or acidosis. A combination of these factors is sometimes present. The clinical manifestation of a crisis can vary, the most common being an infarct crisis. Infarction of the long bones and larger joints or an infarction of a large organ (e.g. the liver, lungs or brain) may all occur. Severe pain is a common feature, depending on the site of the infarction. Destructive bone and joint problems are frequently seen.

Thalassaemias

The anaemia causes erythropoietin production to increase and results in expansion of the bone marrow. In severe disease this causes bone deformity and growth retardation. The spleen is actively involved in removing the abnormal mature cells from the circulation and becomes enlarged.

G6PD deficiency

Clinically the two most important types of G6PD deficiency occur in the black population and in people originating from the Mediterranean area. The black population has a milder form that results in an acute self-limiting haemolytic anaemia following exposure to an oxidizing agent, for example infection, acute illness, fava beans or drugs (Table 47.12). The haemolytic anaemia is self-limiting because the young cells produced by the bone marrow have higher levels of G6PD activity than old cells. Following exposure to the oxidizing agent, the old cells are haemolysed but the new cells produced in response are more capable of tolerating the insult (until they grow old). In the Mediterranean form of the disorder, the enzyme activity is very low, haemolysis is not usually self-limiting and, indeed, some

---

Table 47.12 Common drugs implicated in causing haemolysis in G6PD deficiency
Drugs to be avoided in all variants
Ciprofloxacin (and probably other quinolones)
Dapsone
Methylthioninium chloride (methylene blue)
Primaquine (reduced dose may be used in milder variants)
Nalidixic acid
Sulphonamides (including co-trimoxazole)
Drugs to be avoided in more severe variants
Aspirin (low dose used under supervision)
Chloramphenicol
Chloroquine (may be acceptable in acute malaria)
Menadione
Probenicid
Quinidine
Quinine (acceptable in acute malaria)

---

patients have a chronic haemolytic anaemia despite the absence of an obvious causative factor.

Investigations

Sickle cell disease

The common form usually presents in the first year of life. From then on the patient has a chronic haemolytic anaemia interspersed with crises. Abnormal haemoglobin can be detected using electrophoresis. The proportion of Hb S is a useful monitoring parameter. Regular serum ferritin determinations identify the need for desferrioxamine therapy and are used to monitor progress.

Thalassaemia

For β thalassaemia the diagnosis is relatively straightforward: haemolytic anaemia from infancy and racial background. Haemoglobin electrophoresis is used to determine the amounts of abnormal haemoglobin.

G6PD deficiency

The history and the clinical findings steer the diagnosis, which is then confirmed by measuring G6PD activity. Care must be taken during the acute phase since there are increased numbers of young cells with higher levels of activity that may be misleading The increased numbers of young cells result from the selective destruction of older cells and the increased production of reticulocytes.

Treatment

Many patients with chronic haemolytic anaemia will have an overactive bone marrow to compensate for the chronic haemolysis. This increases demand for folate, and folic acid supplements are often required, particularly for patients with a poor diet.

Sickle cell anaemia

Patients with sickle cell disease have a high incidence of pneumococcal infections and a number of studies have shown the benefit of prophylactic antibiotics. Penicillin V (phenoxymethyl penicillin) 250 mg twice a day is usual for adults, erythromycin being used for patients allergic to penicillin. Administration of pneumococcal vaccine and *Haemophilus influenzae* vaccine is now common.

Attempts have been made to increase the proportion of Hb F and reduce the proportion of Hb S in the circulation. Several drugs (Table 47.13) have been shown (some only in animal models) to stimulate fetal haemoglobin production (Charache et al 1995).

Hydroxycarbamide (hydroxyurea) is effective and may reduce the frequency of crises but is limited by its

Table 47.13 Drugs that may increase fetal haemoglobin production

5-Azacytidine
Cytarabine
Vinblastine
Hydroxycarbamide (hydroxyurea)
Erythropoietin
Short-chain fatty acids (butyrates, valproate)

cytotoxicity. Erythropoietin has been shown to increase Hb F in some animal models, but this has yet to be fully demonstrated in humans. Transfusions and exchange transfusions have also been used to decrease the proportion of Hb S. This is limited by the usual complications of chronic infusions: iron overload, the risk of blood-borne virus transmission and sensitization.

Sickle cell crises require prompt and effective treatment. Removal of the trigger factor, hydration and effective pain relief are the mainstays of treatment. Appropriate antibiotic therapy should be started at the first signs of infection. Strong opioids are required for pain relief. Traditionally many patients have been given frequent intramuscular injections of pethidine. However, pethidine is not ideal since it is short-acting, not very potent and repeated injections lead to the accumulation of metabolites that have been associated with seizures. Morphine is a more logical choice of opioid, and some centres are having success with morphine in a patient-controlled analgesia system (PCAS).

Thalassaemia

There is currently no effective treatment for thalassaemia. Many patients with severe forms are transfusion-dependent from an early age, which inevitably leads to iron overload. Desferrioxamine and deferiprone are routinely needed (see the section on sideroblastic anaemia, p. 733 above, for details). Splenectomy helps some patients. Prevention is actively explored with genetic counselling programmes in Italy and Greece, and antenatal screening in a number of countries.

As in sickle cell disease, much attention is being placed on the idea of switching the bone marrow to the production of fetal haemoglobin rather than the defective adult haemoglobin of β thalassaemia but these therapies are still in the early stages of development. It is likely that a combination of drugs, hydroxycarbamide (hydroxyurea) and erythropoietin, will provide some clinical improvement.

G6PD deficiency

In cases of acute haemolytic anaemia the causative oxidizing agent should be stopped and general supportive measures adopted. In chronic haemolytic anaemia most patients become reasonably well adjusted to their anaemia. They need to avoid known precipitating factors to prevent acute episodes occurring on top of their chronic haemolytic anaemia.

There is no specific drug treatment for this disorder. During acute episodes the patient should be kept well hydrated to ensure good urine output, thus preventing haemoglobin damaging the kidney. Blood transfusions may be necessary. Vitamin E (an antioxidant) appears to have little clinical benefit in preventing haemolysis.

Patient care

In those patients requiring regular desferrioxamine, advice is required on the most appropriate regimen and delivery system.

Sickle cell disease

Patients need to be encouraged to take their prophylactic penicillin and folic acid therapy regularly between crises. During a crisis some health professionals worry about the patient developing opioid addiction. While this may happen, it is also important to recognize that crises are extremely painful and the patient requires effective analgesia.

Thalassaemia

Currently drug therapy does not play a large part in treatment. However, if hydroxycarbamide (hydroxyurea) becomes the standard treatment, there will be a need to educate the patient regarding its cytotoxic nature.

G6PD deficiency

Since drug therapy does not play a large part in the management of these patients, little drug specific advice can be given. Patients can be given a list of drugs to avoid but since most of these are prescription-only medicines it is important that patients remind health care professionals of their condition.

Table 47.14 summarizes some of the common therapeutic problems in the management of anaemia.

Table 47.14   Common therapeutic problems in anaemia

Problem	Possible cause/solution
Patient with iron deficiency anaemia is not responding to treatment	Check primary cause, e.g. is the patient bleeding? Check that there has been a response in the reticulocyte count Are drugs interfering with iron absorption? Is the patient taking an appropriate formulation (i.e. not modified release)?
Patient taking iron therapy for long time	Iron stores return to normal in 3 months and therapy need only be continued for a further 3 months. If anaemia persists, investigate primary cause
Patient with macrocytic anaemia is not responding to treatment	Check whether any concurrent drugs are interfering with folate metabolism In patients treated with folate, check B_{12} levels
Patient has bowel disturbance	Iron can cause both diarrhoea and constipation. Treat symptomatically
Patient is alcoholic	Check for folate deficiency and/or variceal or gastric bleeding causing iron deficiency anaemia
Serum potassium is low in a patient with B_{12} deficiency	Give potassium supplementation in early stages of treatment

CASE STUDIES

Case 47.1

Mr H. A., a 62-year-old single, unemployed man, was admitted to hospital for investigation of anaemia. He presented with a 6-month history of lethargy, chest pain, dizziness and falls, and a past history of having a partial gastrectomy 16 years ago. The drug history taken by the junior doctor showed that Mr H. A. was taking diazepam and a GTN spray on admission.

Review of systems revealed no vomiting and no melaena. He complained of some indigestion after meals and reported his appetite as 'fine if someone else cooks'. On examination he was pale, with a blood pressure of 140/80, a pulse of 90 and a haemoglobin level of 2.5 g/dl (normal range 13.5 to 18.0 g/dl). A gastroscopy was normal, and a biopsy showed no evidence of coeliac disease. A barium enema was normal and faecal occult bloods (FOBs) negative.

Over the first 3 days he was transfused with 8 units of blood and was given furosemide (frusemide) 40 mg with alternate bags. On day 7 he was started on ferrous sulphate 200 mg three times a day, folic acid 5 mg twice daily and ascorbic acid 200 mg three times daily.

Questions

1. How might a full drug history taken by a pharmacist help this patient?
2. Comment on the use of vitamin C in Mr H. A.
3. How long should Mr H. A. remain on ferrous sulphate?

Answers

1. Although all Mr H. A.'s prescribed drugs were documented, it is possible that Mr H. A. was taking purchased medication. On admission he complained of indigestion over the last 3 months, and on questioning revealed that he was self-medicating with aluminium hydroxide mixture. From a theoretical point of view, antacids may reduce the amount of iron absorbed by increasing the pH of the stomach and by reducing the solubility of ferrous salts. It is unlikely that this contributed significantly to the development of his anaemia, but if he intends to continue using an antacid after discharge it would be better not to take a dose of antacid after within 1–2 hours of his ferrous sulphate. It would be also worth checking to see if he has been self-medicating with a purchased aspirin- or ibuprofen-based product; both drugs have been implicated in causing gastrointestinal blood loss, though in this case his gastroscopy was normal and the OBs negative.
2. Ascorbic acid slightly increases the absorption of iron in some patients. It probably keeps iron in solution either in the ferrous form or by forming a soluble chelate with the emic form. In most patients this is of little clinical benefit. It may have an advantage in Mr H. A. since he appears to have had a poor diet and may be vitamin C deficient. He may also benefit from a short course of multivitamins.
3. Mr H. A. needs to continue iron therapy until he has at least replenished his iron stores. This may take up to 6 months, after which time he should be reassessed, taking into account whether he is now having a suitable diet. In practice, since his haemoglobin was dangerously low on admission it may be quite reasonable to leave him on iron for the rest of his life.

Case 47.2

Mr W. K., a 46-year-old mechanic, was referred to hospital by his general practitioner. He gave a history of diarrhoea and vomiting a week ago and now was complaining of headaches and feeling 'lousy'. His general practitioner had given him metoclopramide and ferrous sulphate. Mr W. K. did not appear jaundiced although he said he had noticed his urine was unusually dark a few days ago. On examination he was obese, with a blood pressure of 120/80 mmHg and a pulse of 80. Rectal examination revealed black stools. He had a normal gastroscopy and three negative FOBs. His serum biochemistry showed a normal level of alanine transaminase and a slightly raised total bilirubin level. Mr W. K.'s reticulocyte count was 13.5% (normal range 0.5–1.5%). Mr W. K. was diagnosed as having G6PD deficiency, probably triggered by an infection.

Questions

1. How do you explain Mr W. K.'s dark urine and dark stools?
2. Would Mr W. K. benefit from any medication following his admission?
3. Why would it be necessary to repeat his red cell G6PD after 2 months?

Answers

1. Mr W. K.'s dark urine was a consequence of his haemolytic anaemia. Bilirubin is a breakdown product of haemoglobin that is transported to the liver and conjugated before being excreted in the bile. Bacteria in the intestine convert this to urobilinogen, most of which is excreted in the stool. Small amounts of urobilinogen are reabsorbed, and some of this appears in the urine. Urobilinogen is oxidized to urobilin, which is coloured. During episodes of haemolysis, erythrocytes are destroyed faster than normal, and hence there is an increase in the formation of bilirubin and increased excretion of urobilinogen in the urine. Also during haemolysis, free haemoglobin may be released into the blood. If the haemolysis is severe enough the normal mechanism for removing haemoglobin from the circulation is overcome and haemoglobin may appear in the urine.
   Dark stools may indicate melaena and upper gastrointestinal bleeding. In Mr W. K.'s case his gastroscopy was normal and he had three negative FOBs. His dark stools were due to the ferrous sulphate prescribed by his general practitioner prior to admission.
2. His raised reticulocyte count indicates he is rapidly replacing his lost red cells. Erythropoiesis consumes folate and iron and since his folate is towards the lower end of the reference range it may be worth giving him a short course of folate supplements.
3. Young red cells tend to have higher levels of enzyme activity than more mature cells. Determining G6PD levels during the acute phase may be misleading since there is a relatively high proportion of young cells. Mr W. K.'s result 2 months later would more accurately represent his normal state.

Case 47.3

Miss P. R., a grey-haired, 58-year-old lady, was admitted from casualty. She had fallen over and bruised herself but had not broken any bones. The casualty officer thought Miss P. R. appeared pale with possibly a lemon-yellow tinge to her skin, she was slightly confused and had paraesthesiae of the feet and fingers. She had a past history of heart failure and was taking furosemide (frusemide) and amiloride. She was admitted for investigation and discovered to have a macrocytic anaemia. Pernicious anaemia was suspected. Folate levels, vitamin B_{12} levels and a Schilling test were carried out before commencing treatment.

Questions

1. What are the features that may lead you to consider pernicious anaemia as a diagnosis?
2. Can Miss P. R. have a blood transfusion after samples have been taken for folate and vitamin B_{12} levels?
3. The red cell folate is reported as 150 mg/l (reference range 160–640 mg/l). Would Miss P. R. benefit from folate therapy?

Answers

1. Macrocytic anaemia and paraesthesiae are typical features (though not diagnostic) of pernicious anaemia. Patients may be mildly jaundiced, which is often described as lemon-yellow in colour. Interestingly, pernicious anaemia is more common in women than men and is associated with blue eyes and early greying of the hair. Miss P. R. may have other features of pernicious anaemia, which include glossitis, angular stomatitis and altered bowel habit.
2. Patients with pernicious anaemia develop their anaemia over a long period of time and tend not to tolerate increases in blood volume very well. A transfusion may result in fluid overload and precipitate heart failure. Miss P. R. already has heart failure so, unless she becomes severely compromised by the anaemia, a transfusion should not be given. In patients who have such a pronounced anaemia that an urgent transfusion is required, an exchange transfusion of a small volume of packed cells may be appropriate.
3. In vitamin B_{12} deficiency, folate tends to leak from cells and the red cell folate is often low (serum folate is sometimes raised). Many patients initially require both folate and vitamin B_{12} although the folate can usually be stopped after a short course. Folate therapy must never be given to patients who have not been fully investigated for vitamin B_{12} deficiency. If vitamin B_{12} deficient patients are given large doses of folate without hydroxocobalamin, the full blood count can appear to improve but the peripheral neuropathy from the vitamin B_{12} deficiency progresses.

Case 47.4

Mrs G. N., a 76-year-old retired textile factory worker was seen by her general practitioner, complaining of tiredness. She had been seen 2 months earlier and started on ferrous sulphate for a microcytic anaemia. Initially she had felt better but the tiredness soon returned. A bone marrow aspiration revealed increased erythropoiesis, iron stores and red cell precursors.

A diagnosis of sideroblastic anaemia was made and it was decided to give her monthly transfusions. She was also started on pyridoxine 50 mg three times a day in addition to the ferrous sulphate.

Questions

1. What are the potential problems of Mrs G. N.'s treatment?
2. After 3 months there appeared to be little benefit to show from the pyridoxine. How might the management be improved?

Answers

1. Mrs G. N.'s bone marrow aspiration and serum ferritin level showed that she had high levels of stored iron. Repeated monthly transfusions will also contribute to further iron accumulation. In sideroblastic anaemia the bone marrow appears to be inefficient at incorporating iron into haem. The administration of iron leads to iron overload which may result in damage to the heart, liver and endocrine organs. The ferrous sulphate must be stopped iron accumulation remains a problem, desferrioxamine therapy may be tried.
2. Pyridoxine does not always improve the blood picture in patients with sideroblastic anaemia. Doses up to 400 mg a day have been used. In the case of Mrs G. N. an increase in dose should be tried. Patients with sideroblastic anaemia often do not realize that pyridoxine is not just a simple vitamin but a specific treatment for anaemia. Counselling the patient may improve compliance. Some patients also benefit from folate and this should be tried especially if Mrs G. N.'s serum folate level was found to be low.

Case 47.5

Mrs R. O., a 70-year-old retired teacher, presented with a history of increasing tiredness over the last 6 weeks. She had a past history of a partial gastrectomy 4 years ago. On questioning, her relevant symptoms include 'pins and needles' in her toes and loose bowels. She said that she had never been a good eater but ate red meat twice a week.

Questions

1. Why was it 4 years after her gastrectomy before Mrs R. O. developed vitamin B_{12} deficiency?
2. How long will it take for Mrs R. O. to respond to treatment?
3. What long-term therapy will Mrs R. O. require?

Answers

1. Vitamin B_{12} requires intrinsic factor produced by the stomach for absorption. Patients who have had a total gastrectomy, and some with a partial gastrectomy, malabsorb vitamin B_{12} Most patients have good body stores and even with no new vitamin B_{12} entering the body (e.g. following a total gastrectomy) it takes at least 2 years to deplete the stores.
2. Many patients feel better within days of starting hydroxocobalamin and before a change in their haemoglobin concentration can be detected. Mrs R. O.'s blood picture may take a number of weeks to return to normal, but the 'pins and needles' may be a sign of peripheral neuropathy, which is frequently irreversible and may not respond to the hydroxocobalamin treatment.
3. Mrs R. O. will need lifelong replacement therapy with hydroxocobalamin. This is usually given at a dose of 1 mg i.m. every 3 months.

REFERENCES

Al-Refaie F N, Hershko C, Hoffbrand A V et al 1995 Results of long term deferiprone (L1) therapy: a report of the International Study Group on Oral Chelators. British Journal of Haematology 91: 224–229

Annibale B, Marignani M, Monarca B et al 1999 Reversal of iron deficiency anaemia after *Helicobacter pylori* eradication in patients with asymptomatic gastritis. Annals of Internal Medicine 131: 668–672

Charache S, Terrin M L, Moore R D et al 1995 Effect of hydroxyurea on the frequency of painful crises in sickle cell anaemia. New England Journal of Medicine 332: 1317–1322

Department of Health (DOH) 1992 Folic acid and the prevention of neural tube defects: report from an expert advisory group. Department of Health, London.

Green R, Miller J W 1999 Folate deficiency beyond megaloblastic anaemia: hyperhomocysteinemia and other manifestations of dysfunctional folate status. Seminars in Haematology 36(1): 47–64

Silverberg D S, Blum M, Peer G et al 1996 Intravenous ferric saccharate as an iron supplement in dialysis patients. Nephron 72: 413–417

Williams J, Wolff A, Daly A et al 1999 Iron supplemented formula milk related to reduction in psychomotor decline in infants from inner city areas: randomised study. British Medical Journal 318: 693–698

Leukaemia

48

G. Jackson   G. Stark

KEY POINTS

- Leukaemias are uncommon malignancies.
- Acute lymphoblastic laeukaemia (ALL) is the commonest malignancy in childhood.
- With the exception of ALL, leukaemias are more common in the elderly.
- Age is one of the most important prognostic factors in the treatment of leukaemia. With the exception of neonates, older patients are less likely to be cured than younger patients.
- The treatment of leukaemia is continually improving with the introduction of more focused therapy and with improvements in supportive care.
- The use of bone marrow transplantation in the treatment of all forms of leukaemia is increasing. Some of the results are very exciting but the short-and long-term problems of this type of intensive treatment need to be borne in mind.

Leukaemias, together with lymphoma, are the main haematological malignancies. Although rare, they are of particular interest in that dramatic improvements in the prognosis for patients with these cancers have been achieved through the use of chemotherapy, and cure is now a possibility in a significant number of cases.

Many forms of leukaemia exist, but they are all characterized by the production of excessive numbers of abnormal white blood cells. The leukaemias can be broadly divided into four groups:

- acute myeloblastic leukaemias (AMLs)
- acute lymphoblastic leukaemias (ALLs)
- chronic myelocytic leukaemias (CMLs)
- chronic lymphocytic leukaemias (CLLs).

The leukaemias were formerly defined as either acute or chronic on the basis of the patient's life expectancy and on how quickly they initially become unwell. They are now classified on the basis of cell morphology, maturity, surface antigens and cytogenetics. The adjectives 'myeloid' and 'lymphoid' refer to the predominant cell involved, and the suffix -cytic or -blastic to mature or immature cells, respectively.

Epidemiology

Together the haematological malignancies account for only 5% of all cancers; of these, CLL is the most common form of leukaemia in Europe and the USA (Figures for the UK are given in Table 48.1). CLL mainly affects an older age group: 90% of patients are over the age of 50 and nearly two-thirds are over 60 years old at diagnosis. It rarely occurs in young people and is twice as common in men as in women. CML is primarily a disease of middle age with the median onset in the 40–50-year age group, but it can occur in younger people.

Acute leukaemia is rare, with a total annual incidence of approximately 4 per 100 000 of the population. The more common form of the disease is AML, which accounts for 75% of cases of acute leukaemia. The incidence of AML rises steadily with age, occurring only rarely in young children. In contrast, ALL is predominantly a childhood disease, with the peak incidence in the 3–5-year age group, and is the most common childhood cancer.

Aetiology

In common with other cancers, the aetiology of leukaemia is not fully understood. Leukaemia is thought to result from a combination of factors that induce

Table 48.1 Incidence of leukaemia in the UK (Leukaemia Research Fund 2000)

	New cases/year	Incidence per 100 000 of the population
CLL	2700	4.58
CML	500	0.85
ALL	600	1.00
AML	1600	2.71

genetic mutations in cells or allow mutated cells to proliferate. However, epidemiological studies have identified a number of specific risk factors for the development of leukaemia, which are described below.

Radiation

The association between ionizing radiation and the development of leukaemia is evident from nuclear disasters such as Hiroshima and more recently Chernobyl. Long-term follow-up of survivors of Nagasaki and Hiroshima has shown an increase in all forms of leukaemia other than CLL. The link is also apparent for patients who received radiotherapy for the treatment of malignant and non-malignant conditions such as Hodgkin's disease or ankylosing spondylitis. However, the effect of chronic low-level exposure to radiation is less certain.

Exposure to chemicals and cytotoxic drugs

There is a small but definite risk of acute leukaemia occurring in patients successfully treated for other malignancies with cytotoxic and immunosuppressive agents. The combination of chemotherapy, especially alkylating agents such as cyclophosphamide, and radiotherapy presents the highest risk. This has practical implications as an increasing number of patients achieve a 'cure' as a result of combination therapy, while occupational exposure of health professionals to these agents is also an area of concern. Occupational exposure to paint, insecticides and solvents, in particular the aromatic solvent benzene, have all been associated with the development of leukaemia.

Viruses

Human T cell lymphotrophic virus, an RNA retrovirus endemic in Japan and the West Indies, has been linked to a rare T cell leukaemia/lymphoma.

Genetic factors

Down's syndrome, constitutional trisomy of chromosome 21, is associated with an increased risk of developing leukaemia. Disorders that predispose to chromosomal breaks such as Fanconi's anaemia and ataxia telangiectasia are also associated with an increased risk of developing acute leukaemia. These alterations may permit the expression of oncogenes, which promote malignant transformation.

Haematological disorders

Many patients with other haematological disorders have a greatly increased risk of developing leukaemia,

particularly AML. These disorders include the myelodysplastic syndromes, the non-leukaemic myeloproliferative disorders, aplastic anaemia and paroxysmal nocturnal haemoglobinuria.

Pathophysiology

In leukaemia the normal process of haemopoiesis is altered (Fig. 48.1). Transformation to malignancy appears to occur in a single cell, usually at the pluripotential stem cell level, but it may occur in a committed stem cell with capacity for more limited differentiation. Accumulation of malignant cells leads to progressive impairment of the normal bone marrow function and bone marrow failure.

Acute leukaemias

In acute leukaemia the normal bone marrow is replaced by a malignant clone of immature blast cells derived from the myeloid (AML) or lymphoid (ALL) series. More than 30% of the cellular elements of the bone marrow are replaced with blasts. This is usually associated with the appearance of blasts in the peripheral circulation accompanied by worsening pancytopenia. In ALL the blasts may infiltrate lymph nodes and other tissues such as liver, spleen, testis and the meninges, in particular. In AML blasts tend to infiltrate skin, gums, liver and spleen.

Classification of AML

AML may be subdivided according to the French–American–British (FAB) classification (Bennett et al 1976), depending on the predominant differentiation pathway and the degree of maturation (Table 48.2). M0 is an AML which shows no evidence of differentiation. For the M1, M2 and M3 classifications, granulocytic differentiation is predominant; for M4, differentiation is mixed granulocytic and monocytic; for M5 monocytic; for M6 erythroid; and for M7 differentiation is predominantly along the megakaryocytic lineage.

Classification of ALL

A FAB classification based on cell morphology also exists for ALL, but the disease is usually classified immunologically, based on the presence or absence of B cell or T cell markers (Table 48.3). Each subtype displays different clinical presentations, response to treatment and ultimately, prognosis, with pre-B having the best prognosis and B-ALL the worst. It is worth noting that B-ALL (Burkitt's type) seems to be a

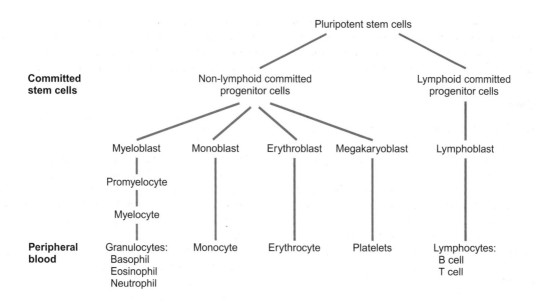

Figure 48.1 Haemopoiesis.

Table 48.2 French–American-British (FAB) classification of AML

Classification	Leukaemia type	Adult distribution (%)
M0	Undifferentiated	1–2
M1	Myeloblastic with differentiation	20
M2	Myeloblastic	30
M3	Promyelocytic	10
M4	Myelomonocytic	25
M5	Monoblastic	10
M6	Erythroleukaemic	5
M7	Megakaryoblastic	< 1

Table 48.3 Classification of ALL

Pre-B ALL	Possessing the common ALL antigen CD 10
B cell type	B-ALL of Burkitt's type
T cell type	T-ALL
Null	Non-B, non-T and lacking the common ALL antigen CD 10

morphologically and biologically distinct form of leukaemia.

Chronic leukaemias

In chronic leukaemia the normal bone marrow is replaced by a malignant clone of maturing haemopoietic cells.

CLL

CLL is characterized by a clonal expansion of morphologically mature lymphocytes, which are usually of B cell origin. These cells accumulate in the peripheral blood and give rise to a lymphocytosis which may be very marked. Lymphocytes accumulate in lymph nodes and spread to the liver and spleen, which become enlarged. The bone marrow is progressively infiltrated. Although the cells appear morphologically normal they are functionally deficient.

CML

The characteristic feature of CML is the predominance of maturing myeloid cells in blood, bone marrow, liver, spleen and other organs. CML was the first cancer to be associated with a specific chromosomal abnormality: the Philadelphia chromosome translocation (Ph), seen in over 90% of cases. This is a translocation of genetic material between the long arms of chromosome 22 and chromosome 9. This results in the apposition of the BCR gene (chromosome 22) and the ABL gene (chromosome 9). This novel BCR-ABL gene encodes a fusion protein which has tyrosine kinase activity. This genetic event is believed to be crucial in the pathogenesis of, or perhaps even to initiate the development of, CML since overactivity of the tyrosine kinase results in the uncontrolled growth characteristic of leukaemic cells (Faderl et al 1999).

Clinical manifestations

Acute leukaemia

Most of the clinical manifestations of acute leukaemia are related to bone marrow failure. Symptoms of infection, anaemia and bleeding are common and life-threatening presenting problems. Bleeding may be particularly severe in one subtype of AML (M3) where disseminated intravascular coagulation (DIC) is common. Some patients develop symptoms and signs due to infiltration of major organs by leukaemic cells. The disease commonly presents with a short history, and left untreated it is rapidly fatal.

The involvement of other tissues such as spleen, liver, lymph nodes and meninges is more common in ALL than AML. Involvement of the central nervous system (CNS) gives rise to headaches, vomiting and irritable behaviour. CNS disease is rare at presentation, but develops in up to 75% of children with ALL unless specific prophylactic treatment is given. Less commonly patients present with features of hypermetabolism, hyperuricaemia or generalized aches and pains.

Chronic leukaemia

CML

Patients with CML commonly present with non-specific symptoms, such as malaise, weight loss and night sweats. The main physical sign is an enlarged spleen that may give rise to abdominal discomfort. Hepatomegaly is also detected in approximately 40% of newly diagnosed patients. Neutropenia and thrombocytopenia are uncommon at presentation. Thus, unlike the acute leukaemias, patients with CML rarely present with symptoms of infection or haemorrhage. In up to 30% of cases, patients are asymptomatic and the disease is detected as a result of a routine blood test performed for other reasons.

CML is a triphasic disease. The initial chronic phase may last from several months to 20 years; the median is around 5 years. During this time treatment can alleviate symptoms and reduce the white blood count (WBC) and spleen size, allowing patients to lead near normal lives. An accelerated phase eventually occurs where the disease becomes more aggressive with progressively worsening symptoms: unexplained fevers, bone pain, anaemia, thrombocytopenia or thrombocytosis. Finally, after a period of weeks or months a blast crisis occurs, resembling fulminating acute leukaemia. In a small percentage of patients this occurs abruptly.

CLL

An increasing number of patients are diagnosed as having CLL by chance, when a full blood count is performed for an unrelated reason. Symptomatic patients often suffer with B symptoms; these are night sweats, unexplained fever and weight loss. At diagnosis, findings may include generalized lymphadenopathy and some enlargement of the liver and spleen. The course of CLL is variable; in some patients the disease may remain indolent for many years while others experience a steady deterioration in their health. Survival varies from 2 to 20 years depending on the extent of disease. Patients are immunocompromised with a reduction in serum γ-globulin and are at increased risk of bacterial and viral infections. There is an increased susceptibility to autoimmune disease, particularly immune haemolytic anaemias and thrombocytopenia. With progressive disease bone marrow failure becomes apparent, resulting in fatigue, infection and bleeding and the disease becomes less responsive to treatment. Patients with CLL also have an increased risk of developing a more aggressive malignancy such as high-grade non-Hodgkin's lymphoma or prolymphocytic leukaemia.

Investigations

Examination of peripheral blood and bone marrow are the key laboratory investigations carried out in cases of suspected leukaemia. However, some additional investigations can help in the diagnosis and classification of this group of diseases. Some of the main findings at diagnosis are presented in Table 48.4.

In acute leukaemia, leukaemic blast cells are usually seen on the peripheral blood film. The blasts of ALL and AML are distinguished using morphology, cytochemical stains, cytogenetics and cell surface antigen analysis. In CML the principal feature is a leucocytosis with WBC ranging from 30×10^9 to 250×10^9/l comprising the complete spectrum of myeloid cells. In CLL it is lymphocytes in particular which are increased, with levels exceeding 10×10^9/l. Non-random chromosome abnormalities are increasingly being identified in patients with leukaemia. The information obtained from cytogenetic analysis of bone marrow or peripheral blood cells can be used to confirm the diagnosis and classification of leukaemia and may provide a guide to the likely response to treatment and prognosis.

Table 48.4   Findings at diagnosis in leukaemia

	AML	ALL	CML	CLL
WBC	↑ in 60% may be N or ↓	↑ in 50% may be N or ↓	↑↑ commonly 100×10^9–250×10^9/l	Commonly ↑
Differential WBC	Mainly myeloblasts	Mainly lymphoblasts	Granulocytes ↑ ↑, especially neutrophils, myelocytes, basophils and eosinophils < 10% blasts present	Lymphocytes > 10×10^9/L
RBC	Severe anaemia	Severe anaemia	Anaemia common	Anaemia in 50% of patients, generally mild
Platelets	↓↓	↓↓	Usually ↑, may be N or ↓	↓ in 20–30%
Bone marrow aspiration and trephine	Predominantly blasts	Predominantly blasts	Hypercellular Blasts < 15%	Lymphocytic infiltration
Cytogenetic analysis	Important abnormalities detected	Important abnormalities detected	Presence of Ph chromosome	
Lymphadenopathy	Rare	Common	Rare	Common
Splenomegaly	50%	60%	Usual and severe	Usual and moderate
Other features	DIC, high urate	High urate, CNS involvement	↑ serum uric acid	Immuneparesis

N, normal; ↓, reduced; ↑, increased

Treatment

Although significant progress has been made in the treatment of leukaemia, work continues to further improve prognosis. As leukaemias are rare malignancies the most important studies are undertaken on a national or international basis and in the UK many of these are coordinated by the Medical Research Council (MRC).

In addition to the specific anti-leukaemia treatment, general supportive therapy is vital, to manage both the disease and the complications of therapy.

Acute leukaemia

At the outset, intensive combination chemotherapy is given in the hope of achieving a complete remission (CR). This initial phase of treatment is termed induction or remission induction chemotherapy. A CR can only be achieved by virtual ablation of the bone marrow, followed by recovery of normal haemopoiesis. If two cycles of therapy fail to induce CR an alternative drug regimen can be used. If this is unsuccessful it is unlikely that CR will be achieved. The subsequent duration of the first remission is closely linked to survival.

Remission is defined as the absence of all clinical and microscopic signs of leukaemia, less than 5% blast forms in the bone marrow and return of normal cellularity and haemopoietic elements. Despite achieving CR, occult residual disease will persist and further intensive therapy is given in an attempt to sustain the remission. This postremission consolidation therapy may be chemotherapy, or the combination of chemotherapy, radiotherapy and bone marrow transplantation.

Acute lymphoblastic leukaemia

Treatment of ALL in childhood has been one of the success stories of the last three decades. Over 80% of children will achieve a remission lasting > 5 years (Niemeyer & Sallan 1993). Unfortunately the results in adults are not so impressive. The combination of vincristine, prednisolone, anthracyclines and asparaginase induces complete remission in about 90% of children with ALL and 80% of adults, though sadly relapse is far commoner in adults (Table 48.5). Other active drugs in the treatment of ALL include methotrexate, 6-mercaptopurine, cyclophosphamide, and mitoxantrone (mitozantrone).

Patients with ALL are at a high risk of developing central nervous system infiltration. Cytotoxic drugs penetrate poorly into the central nervous system which thus acts as a sanctuary site for leukaemic cells. For this reason all patients with ALL receive central nervous system prophylaxis. Cranial irradiation plus intrathecal methotrexate or high-dose systemic methotrexate can be used.

Maintenance treatment is important to sustain a complete remission. It is usually milder than induction or consolidation chemotherapy, but is carried on for at least 18 months. Treatment usually consists of weekly methotrexate and daily 6-mercaptopurine with intermittent vincristine and prednisolone.

The treatment of relapsed disease varies with the site of relapse. Isolated central nervous system or testicular relapse may be successfully treated with radiation and reinduction therapy. Cure can still be achieved for some patients. Bone marrow relapse is much more difficult to cure, especially if it occurs early.

Acute myeloblastic leukaemia

As for ALL, the treatment of AML involves induction and consolidation chemotherapy. In AML therapy,

however, the chemotherapy regimens used to achieve remission are much more myelotoxic, and patients require intensive supportive care to survive periods of bone marrow aplasia (Fig. 48.2). The pyrimidine analogue cytarabine has formed the basis of treatment for AML for 20 years. The addition of daunorubicin and oral thioguanine has achieved a CR rate of 75% in patients under the age of 60 years. and about 50% in those over 60 years (Löwenberg et al 1999). The precise dose and scheduling of these agents is continually being refined in order to improve the response rates. Despite the numbers of patients who achieve CR following induction therapy, the majority relapse, with only about 25% becoming long-term disease-free survivors (Webb 1999). Thus, in common with ALL, additional postremission therapy is required. Intensive consolidation chemotherapy with high-dose cytarabine and daunorubicin or amsacrine appears to improve survival rates to approximately 50% after 3 years, with even more encouraging results being obtained in patients under 25 years of age (Löwenberg et al 1999). There is generally no role for maintenance therapy in AML. Similarly, central nervous system prophylaxis is not routinely indicated though patients thought to be at particularly high risk of CNS disease (e.g. M5 subtype) do receive prophylactic therapy.

It has been shown that the AML subtype M3 is sensitive to all-trans retinoic acid (ATRA), which induces blast maturation and remission when used as a

---

Table 48.5 Treatment of ALL (adapted from MRC protocol)

	Dose	Route	Regimen
Induction (4 weeks)			
Vincristine	1.5 mg/m^2	i.v.	Weekly for 4 weeks
Prednisolone	40 mg/m^2	oral	Daily for 4 weeks
L-Asparaginase	6000 u/m^2	i.m.	3 × weekly for 3 weeks
Daunorubicin	45 mg/m^2	i.v.	Daily for 2 days
Intensification (1 week)			
Vincristine	1.5 mg/m^2	i.v.	1 dose
Daunorubicin	45 mg/m^2	i.v.	Daily for 2 days
Prednisolone	40 mg/m^2	oral	Daily for 5 days
Etoposide	100 mg/m^2	i.v.	Daily for 5 days
Cytarabine	100 mg/m^2	i.v.	2 × daily for 5 days
Thioguanine	80 mg/m^2	oral	Daily for 5 days
CNS prophylaxis (3 weeks)			
Cranial irradiation	24 Gy		
Methotrexate	i.t. weekly for 3 weeks also given during induction and intensification		
Maintenance therapy (2 years)			
Methotrexate	20 mg/m^2	oral	Weekly
6-Mercaptopurine	75 mg/m^2	oral	Daily
Prednisolone	40 mg/m^2	oral	5 days/month
Vincristine	1.5 mg/m^2	i.v.	Monthly

i.m., intramuscular; i.v., intravenous; i.t., intrathecal; MRC, Medical Research Council; ALL, acute lymphoblastic leukaemia

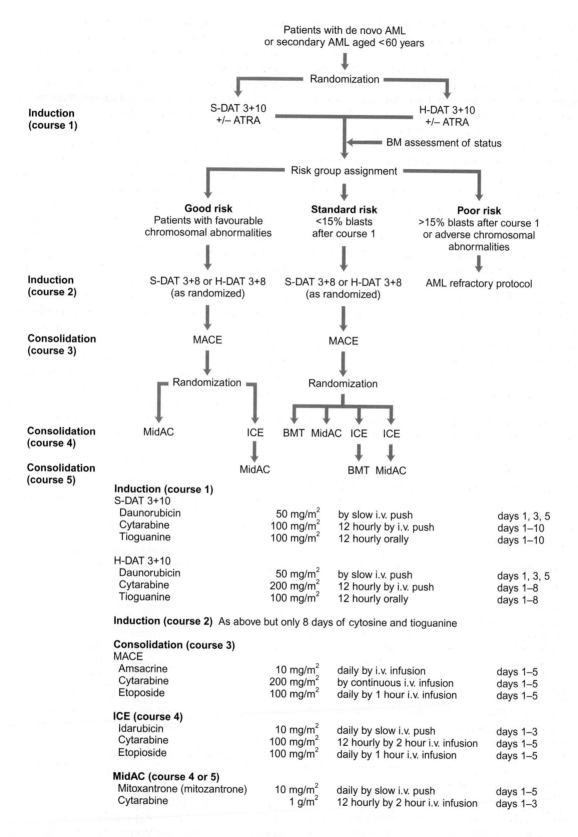

**Induction
(course 1)**

Patients with de novo AML
or secondary AML aged <60 years

Randomization

S-DAT 3+10
+/– ATRA

H-DAT 3+10
+/– ATRA

BM assessment of status

Risk group assignment

Good risk
Patients with favourable
chromosomal abnormalities

Standard risk
<15% blasts
after course 1

Poor risk
>15% blasts after course 1
or adverse chromosomal
abnormalities

**Induction
(course 2)**

S-DAT 3+8 or H-DAT 3+8
(as randomized)

S-DAT 3+8 or H-DAT 3+8
(as randomized)

AML refractory protocol

**Consolidation
(course 3)**

MACE

MACE

Randomization

Randomization

**Consolidation
(course 4)**

MidAC

ICE

BMT MidAC ICE ICE

**Consolidation
(course 5)**

MidAC

BMT MidAC

Induction (course 1)
S-DAT 3+10
  Daunorubicin   50 mg/m^2 by slow i.v. push   days 1, 3, 5
  Cytarabine   100 mg/m^2 12 hourly by i.v. push   days 1–10
  Tioguanine   100 mg/m^2 12 hourly orally   days 1–10

H-DAT 3+10
  Daunorubicin   50 mg/m^2 by slow i.v. push   days 1, 3, 5
  Cytarabine   200 mg/m^2 12 hourly by i.v. push   days 1–8
  Tioguanine   100 mg/m^2 12 hourly orally   days 1–8

Induction (course 2) As above but only 8 days of cytosine and tioguanine

Consolidation (course 3)
MACE
  Amsacrine   10 mg/m^2 daily by i.v. infusion   days 1–5
  Cytarabine   200 mg/m^2 by continuous i.v. infusion   days 1–5
  Etoposide   100 mg/m^2 daily by 1 hour i.v. infusion   days 1–5

ICE (course 4)
  Idarubicin   10 mg/m^2 daily by slow i.v. push   days 1–3
  Cytarabine   100 mg/m^2 12 hourly by 2 hour i.v. infusion   days 1–5
  Etopioside   100 mg/m^2 daily by 1 hour i.v. infusion   days 1–5

MidAC (course 4 or 5)
  Mitoxantrone (mitozantrone)   10 mg/m^2 daily by slow i.v. push   days 1–5
  Cytarabine   1 g/m^2 12 hourly by 2 hour i.v. infusion   days 1–3

Figure 48.2   Example of acute myeloblastic leukaemia (AML) treatment protocol (adapted for Medical Research Council trial). This example is a summary only. Details of treatment are available from the full protocol.

single agent (Tallman et al 1997). In combination with standard chemotherapy, remission rates are significantly better than those seen when chemotherapy is used alone. In contrast to other subtypes of AML, studies have shown that inclusion of ATRA as part of a maintenance strategy significantly increases the long-term survival of patients with this subtype of AML.

An alternative approach to postremission therapy is stem cell transplantation. In patients under 40 years of age allogeneic bone marrow transplantation has resulted in disease-free survival of 45–65% at 5 years post-transplant. These patients are considered cured of their disease. Only about 10% of patients are suitable for allogeneic bone marrow transplants and there is little evidence to suggest that autologous stem cell transplantation improves the outcome for patients with AML in first complete remission. It is always worth remembering that AML is most common in the elderly, and intensive intravenous chemotherapy regimens are not always appropriate for this population of patients.

Treatment of AML in relapse is difficult and the prognosis is generally poor. Encouraging results have been seen using a combination of fludarabine, cytosine arabinoside and G-CSF (granulocyte-colony stimulating factor). Novel approaches in AML therapy are often piloted in this group of poor risk patients. A combination of anti-CD33 antibody, which targets myeloid blasts, with calicheamicin, an anthracycline antibiotic, is a promising and effective approach (Sievers et al 1999). Arsenic trioxide has potent and specific activity against AML M3 blasts and may be useful for patients who have relapsed.

Chronic leukaemia

Chronic myelocytic leukaemia

Until recently the treatment of CML has been essentially palliative, producing modest increases in survival, but with the main aim of keeping patients asymptomatic by maintaining the WBC below $50 \times 10^9/l$. Hydroxycarbamide (hydroxyurea) is the most widely used drug in the management of CML in chronic phase. Treatment with hydroxycarbamide (hydroxyurea) is initiated at a dose of 1.5–2 g/day, and usually brings the WBC under control within 1–2 weeks. The dose can then be reduced to a maintenance dose of 0.5–2 g/day. Withdrawing or reducing the dose abruptly can cause a rebound increase in WBC. The side-effects of hydroxycarbamide (hydroxyurea) are generally mild but include rashes and gut disturbances.

Interferon can control symptoms of CML but in addition it is the first agent shown to modify the disease process. It promotes the expression of suppressed normal haemopoiesis at the expense of the malignant clone. Recent studies have shown that α-interferon therapy prolongs the chronic phase and improves the median survival of patients with CML (Sawyers 1999).

Another approach is the use of allogeneic stem cell transplantation in selected patients under 50 years of age for whom a suitable donor can be found. There is a high risk of mortality with this procedure (10%) and 5–10% of patients relapse within the first 3 years, but there are now long-term survivors who can be considered cured. Patients who relapse following allogeneic bone marrow transplantation may go into remission after an infusion of lymphocytes from the donor. To date allogeneic transplantation is the only proven curative therapy in CML.

STI 571 (GLIVEC™) is a novel and exciting anti-cancer agent. It has been specifically designed to target the abnormal tyrosine kinase product of the BCR-ABL fusion gene. Although results are preliminary, exceptionally good results have been seen with this oral agent (Drucker et al 1999). Clinical trials continue but it is likely that STI 571 will significantly modify the natural history of CML.

Transformation of CML into acute leukaemia can be treated in the same manner as de novo acute leukaemia, in an effort to achieve a second chronic phase. Treatment is slightly more successful if transformation is lymphoid rather than myeloid. In general remissions are rare and the median survival is less than 6 months.

Chronic lymphocytic leukaemia

We are currently unable to cure CLL. All treatment is, therefore, considered palliative. There is no evidence that early treatment of asymptomatic patients improves outcome. Indications for treatment are:

- rapidly increasing white blood cell count (WBC)
- increasing or troublesome lymphadenopathy
- systemic symptoms
- marrow failure
- autoimmune complications.

The alkylating agents chlorambucil and cyclophosphamide are commonly used. Prednisolone can reduce the lymphocyte count without contributing to myelosuppression and is given for autoimmune phenomena such as haemolytic anaemia and immune thrombocytopenia. The use of purine analogues, particularly fludarabine, has been an exciting development in the treatment of CLL. Although complete remissions are unusual, good responses are seen even in patients whose leukaemia is resistant to alkylating agents. With regard to initial therapy of CLL, fludarabine-treated patients show a higher response rate than chlorambucil-treated patients but no survival advantage for the use of fludarabine has been demonstrated (Rai et al 2000). Splenic complications may necessitate splenectomy or splenic irradiation.

Radiotherapy can also be used to control localized painful lymphadenopathy. Combination chemotherapy, such as CHOP (Chapter 49) used in lymphoma may be beneficial in advanced disease.

Patients with CLL are particularly prone to infection. Herpes viruses, in particular herpes zoster, can cause significant problems.

Stem cell transplantation

The potential role of stem cell transplantation is increasingly being explored in the management of all types of leukaemia.

The basic principle

This technique provides a means of rescuing the patient from the potentially lethal effects on the bone marrow of ablative therapy given in an attempt to eradicate all traces of disease (Fig. 48.3). The conditioning regimen most commonly used is a combination of high-dose cyclophosphamide and total body irradiation. Other conditioning regimens include high-dose melphalan, etoposide or cytarabine.

Following administration of conditioning therapy, 2–3 days elapse to allow its elimination from the body, then previously harvested stem cells are reinfused peripherally. The stem cells will return to and repopulate the marrow, restoring normal haemopoiesis. Peripheral blood counts recover in 2–4 weeks. Throughout this time patients require intensive supportive care and the

procedure, particularly allogeneic stem cell transplantation, causes significant morbidity and has a mortality rate of 5–15%.

The source of stem cells

In allogeneic stem cell transplantation (allograft) stem cells are obtained from a human leucocyte antigen (HLA) matched donor. These stem cells can be removed directly from the bone marrow, under general anaesthetic, or harvested from the peripheral blood. Under certain circumstances, in the absence of a matched sibling donor, an autologous bone marrow or peripheral blood stem cell transplant (autograft) can be performed. Following conditioning, the patients receive their own cryopreserved marrow or peripheral blood stem cells, previously harvested from them while in complete remission. There is a potential risk, however, that stem cells obtained in this way may contain undetected, residual disease. Attempts have been made to purge the bone marrow of disease in vitro but these have generally been unsuccessful.

Peripheral blood stem cell transplantation

This relatively new technique for rescuing bone marrow following ablative conditioning therapy is increasingly used to restore haemopoiesis (Russell 1998). Patients receive the haematopoetic growth factor G-CSF, either alone or following an infusion of high-dose chemotherapy such as high-dose cyclophosphamide. Patients receive G-CSF for a period of about 7 days. This stimulates the release of stem cells into the peripheral

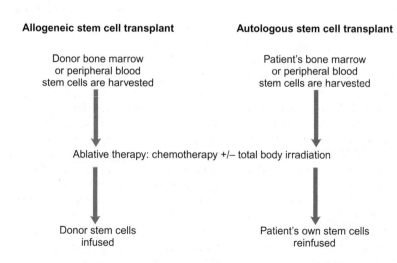

Allogeneic stem cell transplant

Donor bone marrow
or peripheral blood
stem cells are harvested

Autologous stem cell transplant

Patient's bone marrow
or peripheral blood
stem cells are harvested

Ablative therapy: chemotherapy +/– total body irradiation

Donor stem cells
infused

Patient's own stem cells
reinfused

Figure 48.3   Stem cell transplantation.

circulation. Stem cells are then harvested from the peripheral circulation by a process of cell pheresis. The harvested cells can then be reinfused, fresh, into the patient following conditioning therapy or frozen and stored for later use. Peripheral stem cell transplantation offers some advantages over conventional bone marrow transplant techniques; collection of peripheral stem cells negates the need for general anaesthesia and it has been found that the haemopoietic recovery period following transplantation is shortened by 5–10 days. This technique can also be used to harvest stem cells from allogeneic donors. In this case G-CSF is used alone to stimulate stem cell release into the peripheral circulation.

Complications

Infection is almost inevitable in patients undergoing bone marrow transplantation. Other significant complications of allografts include interstitial pneumonitis and hepatic veno-occlusive disease, but the major life-threatening complication is acute graft-versus-host disease (GVHD). The likelihood of GVHD occurring increases with age, with the result that allografts are largely restricted to patients under 45 years of age. GVHD is caused by T lymphocytes in the donated marrow reacting to host tissues. The severity of the reaction ranges from a mild maculopapular rash to multisystem organ failure with a high mortality rate. Acute GVHD occurs within 100 days of the bone marrow transplantation and typically presents with fever, rash, diarrhoea and liver dysfunction. Prophylactic therapy is routinely given with methotrexate or ciclosporin, alone or in combination, for 6–12 months post-transplant. Should acute GVHD develop, high-dose methylprednisolone, ciclosporin, antithymocyte globulin and more recently, anti-cytokine monoclonal antibodies, e.g. anti-TNF (tumour necrosis factor) antibodies, have been used to treat the condition.

Thalidomide has been used successfully in the treatment of chronic steroid refractory GVHD. Chronic GVHD can occur in the 3–18 months following bone marrow transplantation. It is a multisystem disorder associated with chronic hepatitis, severe skin inflammation and profound immuno-suppression. Treatment is successful in approximately 50% of patients and consists of immunosuppression with azathioprine and prednisolone together with prophylactic antibiotics. Ciclosporin can also be used. The main cause of death is infection.

The place of stem cell transplantation

The place of stem cell transplantation in the management of a particular form of leukaemia depends very much on the prognosis of patients treated with conventional chemotherapy (Table 48.6). For example, the results of intensive chemotherapy in children with ALL are good

and bone marrow transplantation is generally only considered for children who have relapsed and in whom a second remission can be achieved. However, conventional treatment of adults is less successful and allogeneic bone marrow transplantation may be offered to adults in first remission.

Patient care

Supportive care

The treatment of CLL and CML is largely carried out on an out-patient basis, with patients taking oral medication at home, or attending out-patient clinics on a weekly or monthly basis for injections of chemotherapy. Patients are routinely monitored to follow the progress of disease and to observe treatment-related side-effects. Supportive therapy such as blood transfusions can also be given on an out-patient basis. In contrast, the intensity of induction and consolidation regimens used in the management of patients with acute leukaemia renders them pancytopenic. Therapy is usually given on an in-patient basis with patients often remaining in hospital following treatment for 3–4 weeks until their bone marrow recovers sufficiently. This is in contrast to therapy for most solid tumours where, following administration of treatment, patients are often well enough to remain at home until their next cycle of chemotherapy is due.

Advanced leukaemia, bone marrow transplants and aggressive chemotherapy for acute leukaemia all result in pancytopenia. Red cell transfusions are given to patients to maintain their haemoglobin above 9–10 g/dl. Evidence of bleeding includes petechial haemorrhages in skin and mucous membranes, and patients receiving aggressive treatment must be examined daily for any of the above signs. Platelet concentrates are given to thrombocytopenic patients who have signs of bleeding

Table 48.6 Indications for allogeneic stem cell transplantation in leukaemia

AML	First remission[a]
CML	Chronic phase
ALL	First remission in adults
	Second remission in children
CLL	Not appropriate

[a] Autologous bone marrow transplantation may be considered in acute leukaemia in the absence of a suitable donor

and may be given prophylactically should platelets fall below $10 \times 10^9/l$. The probability of infection developing rises as the WBC, specifically the neutrophil count, falls. With an absolute neutrophil count of below $0.5 \times 10^9/l$, patients are at high risk of infection, the risks are even greater if the period of neutropenia is prolonged.

Chapters 49 and 50 examine many of the non-haematological toxicities which result from the use of cytotoxic drugs and these are clearly pertinent to haematology patients. The major contributors to morbidity and mortality in patients with leukaemia are relapsed disease and infection.

Infection in the immunocompromised patient

A number of intrinsic and extrinsic factors all contribute to the risk of infection in this vulnerable group of patients (Fig. 48.4).

While cross-infection can occur via staff, other patients or contaminated objects, the main sources of infection in this group of patients are endogenous, arising from commensal gut and skin organisms. The normal host defences to infection are broken down; damage to mucous membranes, particularly in the gastrointestinal tract, occurs with chemotherapy and radiotherapy, allowing infecting organisms to enter the bloodstream. Most infections in neutropenic patients arise from three main sites: the gastrointestinal and respiratory tracts, and the skin. Table 48.7 lists the main pathogens responsible for infection in this group of patients.

Preventive measures

Oral hygiene. Mouth care is important in all patients receiving chemotherapy but particularly neutropenic patients. Patients are generally asked to use mouthwashes regularly and prophylactic antifungal therapy may also be given. Although it is important to avoid any sort of trauma to the oral mucosa, teeth should be cleaned regularly using a soft toothbrush. Attention must also be paid to the care of dentures. Patients require careful counselling on mouth care, stressing the importance of oral hygiene.

Prophylactic anti-infectives. In general, prophylactic antibiotics are avoided because of the possible development of resistant organisms, but they may have a place in the management of periods of prolonged myelosuppression following chemotherapy and bone marrow transplantation. Prophylactic antifungal agents are often given and patients undergoing bone marrow transplantation and therapy for ALL require prophylaxis against herpes virus and *Pneumocystis carinii* (Table 48.8).

Gut decontamination. Gut decontamination using a combination of non-absorbable oral antibiotics and antifungal agents reduces the population of potentially pathogenic organisms in the intestine. One such combination includes neomycin sulphate, colistin sulphate, nystatin and amphotericin. However, opinions are divided over this practice, as gut decontamination can lead to the overgrowth of resistant organisms.

Growth factors. An exciting development in the care of patients with leukaemia has been the production of haematopoietic growth factors using recombinant DNA technology. The first of these, G-CSF, given daily by subcutaneous injection or intravenous infusion after

Table 48.7 Pathogens commonly causing infection in neutropenic patients

Gram-negative bacteria	*Pseudomonas* spp. *Escherichia coli* *Klebsiella* spp. *Enterobacter* spp. *Proteus* spp. *Serratia* spp. *Legionella pneumophilia*
Gram-positive bacteria	*Streptococcus* spp. *Staphylococcus epidermidis* *Staphylococcus aureus*
Anaerobes	*Clostridium difficile* *Clostridium perfringens* *Bacteroides* spp.
Fungi	*Candida* spp. *Aspergillus* spp.
Viruses	Herpes simplex Herpes zoster Cytomegalovirus Hepatitis
Protozoa	*Pneumocystis carinii*

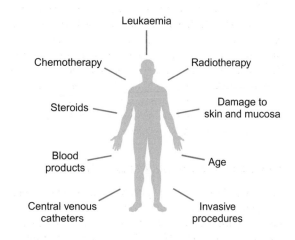

Figure 48.4 Infection risk in immunocompromised patients.

Table 48.8   Prophylactic anti-infectives

Gram-negative bacteria	Ciprofloxacin
Candidiasis	Nystatin
	Fluconazole
	Itraconazole
Herpes simplex	Aciclovir
Pneumocystis carinii	Co-trimoxazole

completion of chemotherapy, stimulates neutrophil production and may reduce the duration of neutropenia by up to 7 days. The cost of these compounds is a major issue and results of studies investigating the effects of G-CSF on morbidity and mortality, following chemotherapy, have been disappointing (Hann 1995).

Aseptic technique.   Careful attention should be paid to the care of intravenous cannulae, particularly central venous catheters. The increased incidence of staphylococcal infection in immunocompromised patients can largely be attributed to their use. Invasive procedures, such as venepuncture, must be carried out using strict aseptic technique. Similarly, urinary catheters are a major source of infection and their use should be avoided if at all possible.

Protective isolation.   Reverse barrier isolation during periods of neutropenia, nursing in strict sterile environments and HEPA (high-efficiency particulate air) filtration have been used in an attempt to reduce infection rates. This is extremely demanding for staff and patients alike and is generally only appropriate following bone marrow transplantation.

Treatment of infection

Commonly, neutropenic patients show no signs of focal infection; they are unable to form pus. The only clinical manifestations of septicaemia might be general malaise, fever or hypotension. A patient's condition can deteriorate very rapidly, with collapse occurring within hours of the first signs of infection. Treatment should be instigated as soon as infection is suspected. Following a clinically serious febrile episode (temperature 38°C for more than 1 hour or 39°C or more on a single reading) samples are taken for culture, these may include blood, urine, sputum and stool cultures along with line and throat swabs. Intravenous antibiotics must be started empirically, without delay (Viscoli & Castagnola 1998). Standard empirical therapy varies from unit to unit but may involve the combination of an aminoglycoside with an antipseudomonal penicillin such as piperacillin to provide broad-spectrum bactericidal cover. In penicillin-allergic patients ceftazidime or cefotaxime may be substituted, but local resistance patterns are of paramount importance. Antibiotics with a broad spectrum of activity, such as ciprofloxacin, have been used as single agents.

Vancomycin or teicoplanin are often prescribed if an infected central venous catheter is suspected, to provide additional cover against Gram-positive organisms. Microbiological advice should be sought in cases of methicillin-resistant *Staphylococcus aureus* (MRSA) infection. Metronidazole may be added to the antibiotic regimen to cover anaerobes if the clinical presentation suggests the source of the infection may be oral, perineal or gut. Anti-infective therapy should subsequently be modified on the basis of cultures but in the majority of neutropenic patients a causative organism is never identified.

If the pyrexia persists for more than 3 days in spite of broad-spectrum antibiotics, or if the patient's condition is deteriorating, systemic fungal infection should be suspected. Intravenous amphotericin is generally the first choice to ensure *Aspergillus* and *Candida* are covered. The main limitation of amphotericin is its toxicity, in particular nephrotoxicity. Lipid-based amphotericin may be appropriate in patients with pre-existing renal impairment or in cases where conventional amphotericin has induced nephrotoxicity. It also allows the dose of amphotericin to be escalated in those patients with life-threatening fungal infection who have failed to respond to conventional amphotericin.

Table 48.9 lists some of the common problems encountered in the treatment of the leukaemias.

Table 48.9 Common therapeutic problems in the leukaemias

Problem	Cause	Solutions
Mucositis and oral ulceration	Chemotherapeutic agents directly toxic to mucosal epithelium	Regular mouth toilet including use of antibacterial mouthwash
	Radiotherapy is directly toxic to the mucosa and also reduces saliva production by salivary glands	Prophylactic use of antiviral and antifungal agents for patients in whom myelosuppression is likely to be prolonged
	Vulnerable mucosa is likely to be attacked by infective agents, e.g. herpes simplex, candida	
Fever in neutropenic patients	Infection predominantly caused by bacteria and/or fungi	Broad-spectrum antibiotics must be commenced as soon as blood cultures have been taken. A strategy of planned progressive therapy including use of an antifungal agent in non-responsive fever is appropriate
Graft-versus-host disease (GVHD)	T lymphocytes from the donor react against host tissues	Use a sibling donor if possible
		Use the donor most closely HLA matched to the patient
		Consider T cell depletion of graft (though this may increase the risk of disease relapse)
		Prophylactic therapy with methotrexate and ciclosporin
		Treat GVHD with corticosteroids, ciclosporin, antithymocyte, globulin, FK 506, anticytokine monoclonal antibodies
		Irradiate all blood products
Late complications of treatment	Risks of haemopoietic malignancy and non-haemopoietic malignancy are increased post-chemotherapy	Aim to tailor therapy to the underlying disease, i.e. do not overtreat and do not undertreat
	Late cardiotoxicity secondary to anthracyclines	Do not exceed maximum cumulative doses of anthracyclines
		Liposomal anthracyclines may be useful in the future

CASE STUDIES

Case 48.1

Mrs R. Y. is a 40-year-old woman undergoing an allogeneic bone marrow transplant for chronic myelocytic leukaemia. Post-transplant she experienced severe mucositis and gastrointestinal toxicity. She was unable to eat and so take in adequate nutrition and in view of this was commenced on total parenteral nutrition. On day 16 she had a temperature, and antibiotic therapy was initiated with gentamicin and piperacillin. The fever had not resolved 72 hours later and blood cultures remained negative. Daily blood counts taken to monitor the fall and recovery of her peripheral blood count revealed she was still pancytopenic. In patients such as Mrs R. Y., with persistent fever not responding to adequate antimicrobial therapy, there is a high possibility of systemic fungal infection, most commonly with *Candida* species. In light of this, therapy was commenced with intravenous amphotericin B.

Questions

1. What advice would you give to nursing and medical staff on the preparation and administration of amphotericin?
2. How might the need for venous access be met?

Answers

1. Amphotericin injection should be reconstituted with water for injection and added to glucose 5% infusion. It must not be administered with sodium chloride as solutions containing electrolytes will disrupt the colloidal suspension. The glucose should have a pH greater than 4.2 and phosphate buffer

may be added to ensure this. The infusion should pass through an in-line filter with a mean pore diameter greater than 1 μm to retain any aggregates of amphotericin which may form. It should also be protected from light. A final concentration less than 0.1 mg/ml reduces the chance of aggregate formation and minimizes thrombophlebitis. Nephrotoxicity is the most serious adverse effect of amphotericin therapy and the dose of amphotericin is increased gradually to minimize this problem. A number of dosing schedules have been adopted, but in a critically ill patient such as Mrs R. Y. treatment may be started with 0.5 mg/kg/day and increased each day by 0.25 mg/kg to a maximum dose of 1 mg/kg/day. Hypersensitivity reactions can also occur and a test dose of 1 mg may be administered before starting treatment. Other acute toxicities of amphotericin include fever, chills, nausea, vomiting, headache, myalgia and arthralgia. If fever does occur patients can be given hydrocortisone and chlorphenamine (chlopheniramine) prior to subsequent doses. Toxicity is also minimized by administering the drug over at least 6 hours. Mrs R. Y.'s renal function and electrolytes (including magnesium levels) must be carefully monitored throughout the course of treatment with amphotericin. The risk of renal toxicity is increased when other nephrotoxic agents, such as aminoglycosides, are prescribed concurrently. Patients frequently develop hypokalaemia during amphotericin therapy and potassium levels must be carefully monitored; oral or parenteral potassium supplements are commonly required.

Novel formulations of amphotericin have been developed to overcome the toxicity of the existing amphotericin preparation. Liposomally encapsulated amphotericin enables much higher doses of amphotericin to be administered without the usual toxicities, especially nephrotoxicity. This allows the use of amphotericin in patients with pre-existing renal disease or patients who have experienced amphotericin-induced nephrotoxicity. The new formulations also permit the dose to be escalated over 1 mg/kg in cases of life-threatening infection which could not be eradicated with conventional doses.

2. For most patients with acute leukaemia, venous access eventually becomes a problem. Peripheral veins become thrombosed with repeated injections of chemotherapy and other agents. Patients can also become increasingly distressed by repeated venepunctures. At the outset of treatment most patients will have a central venous catheter inserted. The tip of the catheter is inserted into the superior vena cava, via the cephalic vein and exits through a subcutaneous tunnel in the chest wall. This is usually performed under a general anaesthetic. The line can have up to three lumens and this allows the administration of drugs, parenteral nutrition, blood products and access for sampling blood. Provided the line is placed correctly, vesicant drugs can also be safely given via a central line without fear of them causing soft-tissue damage. The major complication with central venous lines is the risk of infection; local soft-tissue infection of the subcutaneous tunnel or more serious bacteraemia or septicaemia. To lessen this risk, local policies should be implemented which lay down specific procedures for catheter care. Infection rates are minimized by reducing manipulation of the line. Handling of central venous catheters is frequently restricted to designated trained personnel. Where appropriate, patients may be trained to look after their lines themselves.

Case 48.2

A 35-year-old woman recently diagnosed with chronic myelocytic leukaemia attends the haematology clinic to discuss the options for treatment.

Questions

1. Which treatment options are available?
2. Which treatment is likely to be the best choice for this patient?

Answers

1. There are clearly a number of potential treatment options but it is often very difficult, in these circumstances, to determine the optimal treatment option for an individual patient. It is vitally important to fully inform patients regarding their condition and its prognosis, and about treatment options and their potential advantages and disadvantages. Only by providing this patient with all of the necessary information can she decide on the treatment option that is most appropriate/acceptable to her individual circumstances.

   The various treatment options are:

   - palliative therapy with hydroxycarbamide (hydroxyurea) to control cell counts
   - interferon alfa
   - interferon alfa and cytosine
   - allogeneic matched sibling transplant
   - matched unrelated donor (MUD) transplantation if a matched sibling is not available
   - entry into a clinical trial, possibly involving STI 571, the tyrosine kinase inhibitor.

2. A purely palliative approach is unlikely to be acceptable to a young patient but hydroxycarbamide (hydroxyurea) can still be used acutely to control high cell counts. There is no doubt that use of interferon alfa alone results in cytogenetic remission in a small percentage of patients and this effect is enhanced by the addition of cytosine. The side-effects of interferon alfa include flu-like and affective symptoms. The addition of cytosine increases myelosuppression and risk of mucositis. Although these treatments can induce cytogenetic remission, the duration of such responses is unclear and only a minority of patients respond completely. Currently the only proven curative therapy for CML is allogeneic stem cell transplantation. Results are better for sibling than for MUD transplants as the degree of immunosuppression and risk of GVHD are lower in the former group. Results for all types of transplantation are better if they are performed in chronic phase and within 1 year of diagnosis.

   It is probably true at this time that this patient's best chance of cure is with an allogeneic transplant procedure but the patient must be aware of the risks involved. With transplantation there is a trade off between potential long-term cure against significant risks of morbidity and mortality in the short term. The mortality rate of transplantation is approximately 20%.

   The situation has been made more exciting but more complicated by the advent of tyrosine kinase inhibition. STI 571 produces promising responses in CML with minimal complications as compared to transplantation, though there are limited follow-up data. The haematology team must clearly be available to guide the patient through the decision making process, but given the variety of philosophies of approach available the patient should be fully involved at all stages of the process.

mouth. In addition ATRA can cause a severe and life-threatening sterile pneumonitis. It is important to recognize this syndrome quickly as it often responds to high dose dexamethasone and if left untreated leads to respiratory failure and death.

Case 48.3

A 37-year-old dental technician presented with acute promyelocytic leukaemia (APML). He had a number of bleeding problems at presentation. He was commenced on oral all-trans retinoic acid (ATRA) followed by chemotherapy with daunorubicin, cytosine arabinoside and tioguanine. Within 4 weeks he had achieved a complete remission. He went on to receive a further two courses of intensive chemotherapy followed by maintenance therapy with 6-mercaptopurine, methotrexate and ATRA.

Question

Why is ATRA used in this circumstance and what are its side-effects?

Answer

Acute promyelocytic leukaemia is a variant of AML which presents with coagulation defects, low platelet counts and severe bleeding. Patients are at risk of severe haemorrhage at presentation but have a relatively good prognosis with chemotherapy. ATRA can rapidly correct the coagulopathy found at presentation. This agent also increases the likelihood of the patient entering remission, when combined with standard high dose chemotherapy. It is also used as a maintenance agent and when used with 6-mercaptopurine and methotrexate increases the number of patients who remain in a long-term remission. The side-effects of ATRA include dry eyes and a dry

Case 48.4

A 57-year-old man with a 6 year history of chronic lymphocytic leukaemia presented with a rising white cell count, worsening lymphadenopathy and hepatosplenomegaly. He had previously been treated with six courses of chlorambucil. Treatment was commenced with fludarabine 25 mg/m^2 daily for 5 days. The treating physician commenced co-trimoxazole 960 mg on alternate days and also ordered irradiated blood products for transfusion.

Question

Why did the physician take the precautions outlined above?

Answer

Fludarabine is an exciting new agent available for the treatment of CLL. It is usually used as a second-line agent although many haematologists are now considering its use as a first-line therapy. It can be given either orally or intravenously. This agent is very immunosuppressive and patients treated with this drug are at high risk of developing *Pneumocystis* pneumonia. It is important that patients are given prophylaxis against this severe infection.

As patients are immunosuppressed they are also at risk of developing transfusion-related graft-versus-host disease, a complication of blood product transfusion which is frequently fatal. This complication can be prevented by irradiation of blood products prior to transfusion.

REFERENCES

Bennett J M, Catovsky D, Daniel M T, et al 1976 Proposals for the classification of the acute leukaemias (FAB cooperative group). British Journal of Haematology 33: 451–458

Druker B J, Talpaz M, Resta D et al 1999 Clinical efficacy and safety of an ABL specific tyrosine kinase inhibitor as targeted therapy for chronic myelogenous leukaemia. Blood 19(Suppl. 1): 368a

Faderl S, Talpaz M, Estrov Z et al 1999 The biology of chronic myeloid leukaemia. New England Journal of Medicine 341(3): 164–172

Hann I M 1995 Haematopoietic growth factors and childhood cancer. European Journal of Cancer 31a: 1476–1478

Leukaemia Research Fund 2000 Facts and statistics. Available online http://www.Irf.org.uk. (accessed 1 May 2002)

Löwenberg B, Downing J R, Burnett A 1999 Acute myeloid leukaemia. New England Journal of Medicine 341(14): 1051–1062

Niemeyer C M, Sallan S E 1993 Acute lymphoblastic leukaemia. In: Nathan D G, Oski F A (eds.) Haematology of infancy and childhood, 4th edn. W B Saunders, Philadelphia

Rai K R, Peterson B L, Appelbaum F R et al 2000 Fludarabine compared with chlorambucil as primary therapy for chronic lymphocytic leukaemia. New England Journal of Medicine 343: 1750–1757

Russell N H 1998 Developments in allogeneic peripheral blood progenitor cell transplantation. British Journal of Haematology 103: 594–600

Sawyers C L 1999 Medical progress: chronic myeloid leukaemia. New England Journal of Medicine 340: 1330–1340

Sievers E L, Appelbaum F R, Speilberger R T et al 1999 Selective ablation of acute myeloid leukaemia using antibody-targeted chemotherapy: a phase 1 study of anti-CD33 calicheamicin immunoconjugate. Blood 93: 3678–3684

Tallman M S, Andersen J W, Schiffer C et al 1997 All-trans-retinoic acid in acute promyelocytic leukaemia. New England Journal of Medicine 337(15): 1021–1028

Viscoli C, Castagnola E 1998 Planned progressive antimicrobial therapy in neutropenic patients. British Journal of Haematology 102: 879–888

Webb D K H 1999 Management of relapsed acute myeloid leukaemia. British Journal of Haematology 106: 851–859

FURTHER READING

Gordon-Smith T, Marsh J 2000 Haematology. In: Medicine International. Medicine Publishing, London Company, 28(3)

Heslop H E, Brenner M K, Krance R A 1999 Bone marrow transplantation. In: Hoffbrand A V, Lewis S M, Tuddenham E G D (eds.) Postgraduate haematology, 4th edn. Butterworth Heinemann, pp: 530–549

Hoffbrand A V, Pettit J E 1993 Essential haematology, 3rd edn. Blackwell Science, Oxford

Howard M R, Hamilton P J 1997 Haematology: an illustrated colour text. Churchill Livingstone, Edinburgh

Provan D, Heuson A 1998 ABC of clinical haematology. BMJ Publishing, London

Lymphomas 49

M. Maclean   D. Blake

The lymphomas are malignant tumours of lymph nodes or other lymphatic tissues. The primary cancerous cell of origin is the lymphocyte; as a result there is often considerable overlap between lymphomas and lymphoid leukaemias. The lymphomas are divided into two major groups, namely Hodgkin's disease (HD) and the non-Hodgkin's lymphomas (NHLs).

Hodgkin's disease

Hodgkin's disease (HD), described by Thomas Hodgkin in 1832, has an incidence in the UK of 2.2 per 100 000 for women and 3.3 per 100 000 for men. It is predominantly a disease of young adults, having a peak incidence between the ages of 15 and 40 years.

Aetiology and risk factors

The aetiology is unclear although both a genetic susceptibility and an underlying viral infection, possibly the Epstein–Barr (glandular fever) virus, have been proposed as causative factors. There are no well-defined risk factors for the development of HD. Certain associations have been identified which suggest genetic predisposition or a role for an infectious or environmental agent. For example, same sex siblings of patients with HD have a 10 times higher risk of developing the disease.

Signs and symptoms

HD usually presents with painless enlargement of lymph nodes, often in the neck. About 40% of patients will present with fever, night sweats and/or weight loss. These have prognostic significance, and are designated B symptoms; others include malaise, itching (25%) or pain at the site of enlarged nodes after drinking alcohol. Bone pain may result from skeletal involvement. Primary involvement of the gut, central nervous system or bone marrow is rare. There is often a disturbance of immune function due to a progressive loss of immunologically competent T-lymphocytes with patients becoming particularly prone to viral and fungal infections.

Laboratory findings

Laboratory findings include normochromic, normocytic anaemia, a raised erythrocyte sedimentation rate and eosinophilia. One-third of patients have a leucocytosis due to an increase in neutrophils. Advanced disease is associated with lymphopenia. Serum LDH (lactate dehydrogenase) is raised in 30–40% of patients at diagnosis and has been associated with a poor prognosis.

Histopathology

The diagnosis is made by lymph node biopsy. The diagnostic feature of HD is the identification of the giant binucleate Reed–Sternberg cell. The disease is subclassified into four histological types:

- nodular sclerosing, which is the commonest type in the UK and commoner in women
- mixed cellularity, which is commoner in older males and carries a poor prognosis
- lymphocyte depleted
- lymphocyte predominant (which may be a form of NHL).

Investigations and staging

Once the diagnosis has been made on biopsy, further investigations are needed to assess disease activity and the extent of its spread through the lymphoid system or other body sites. This is called staging and is essential for assessing prognosis, with cure rates for localized tumours (stage I or II) being much higher than those for widespread disease (stage IV). The Cotswolds staging classification (Table 49.1) is commonly used for Hodgkin's disease (Lister et al 1989). The most effective ways of staging are by chest X-ray and computed tomography (CT) or magnetic resonance imaging (MRI).

Table 49.1 The Cotswolds staging classification for Hodgkin's disease

Stage	Defining features
I	Involvement of a single lymph node region or lymphoid structure
II	Involvement of two or more lymph node regions on the same side of the diaphragm
III	Involvement of lymph nodes regions or structures on both sides of the diaphragm: III$_1$ – with or without involvement of splenic, hilar, coeliac or portal nodes III$_2$ – with involvement of para-aortic, iliac or mesenteric nodes
IV	Involvement of extranodal site(s) beyond that designated E
Modifying characteristics	A: no symptoms B: fever, drenching sweats, weight loss X: bulky disease > one-third width of the mediastinum >10 cm maximal dimension of nodal mass E: involvement of a single extranodal site, contiguous or proximal to known nodal site CS: clinical stage PS: pathological stage

Other useful tests include erythrocyte sedimentation rate, serum lactate dehydrogenase and liver function tests. Rarely, a laparotomy with liver biopsy and splenectomy is required for accurate staging.

Non-Hodgkin's lymphoma

The non-Hodgkin's lymphomas (NHLs) are a heterogeneous group of lymphoid malignancies ranging from indolent, slow-growing tumours to aggressive, rapidly fatal disease. Paradoxically, the more aggressive NHLs are more susceptible to anticancer therapy. The overall incidence of NHL in the UK is 11 per 100 000 per year; it is slightly more common in men than in women (1.5:1). The disease is rare in subjects under 30 years of age and increases steadily in incidence with increasing age. Childhood non-Hodgkin's lymphoma is commoner in developing countries than in developed nations.

Aetiology and risk factors

The aetiology is unclear although immunosuppression, for example following organ transplantation, may predispose to the development of lymphoma, possibly in association with Epstein–Barr virus infection. Infection with the human immunodeficiency virus (HIV-1) is associated with an increased incidence of lymphoma, and there is an increased risk among survivors of atomic explosions. There is some evidence that Burkitt's lymphoma, an aggressive B-cell lymphoma common in West African children, is caused by an interaction between Epstein–Barr virus infection and malaria. The human T-lymphotrophic virus type 1 (HTLV-1) is associated with a rare type of T-cell lymphoma.

Signs and symptoms

B symptoms such as fever, weight loss and night sweats may be present, as well as fatigue and weakness. These are more commonly seen in advanced or aggressive NHL but may be present in all stages and histological subtypes.

Low grade lymphomas

Patients present with a long history of disease, sometimes reporting a waxing and waning of enlarged lymph glands. Spontaneous regression of enlarged nodes can occur causing low grade lymphoma to be confused with an infectious condition.

Intermediate and high grade lymphomas

The majority of patients present with lymphadenopathy, and more than one-third with extranodal involvement.

The gut, bone marrow or nervous system are common sites of presentation. B symptoms are more common, occurring in about 30–40% of patients. T-cell lymphomas commonly present with skin infiltration.

Laboratory findings

Laboratory examinations may reveal anaemia, a raised erythrocyte sedimentation rate and a raised serum lactate dehydrogenase level. There may be a reduction in circulating immunoglobulins, and a monoclonal paraprotein may be seen in a small number of cases. The immune disruption caused by the disease may also result in an increased susceptibility to viral infection or autoimmune haemolytic anaemia or thrombocytopenia.

Histopathology and classification

There have been many attempts to classify the NHLs into histological categories that have clinical significance. Despite this, many problems and areas of confusion remain. Approximately 85% of true NHLs are of B-cell origin while 15% are of T-cell origin or are unclassifiable.

There are three classification systems in common use: the Kiel classification, which divides them into high grade lymphomas and low grade lymphomas; the Working formulation of 1982 which adds a third group, intermediate grade; and, more recently, the revised European-American lymphoma (REAL) classification

system and its subsequent modification and acceptance by the World Health Organization (Table 49.2). The REAL/WHO classification incorporates some diagnosis not included in the Working formulation and is gaining acceptance.

Diagnosis

In addition to routine imaging, other recommended investigations include bone marrow aspirate and trephine. Cerebrospinal fluid (CSF) examination should be performed where the risk of central nervous system (CNS) involvement is thought to be significant.

Definitive diagnosis of NHL can only be made by biopsy of pathologic lymph nodes or tumour tissue. An expert histopathologist may need to utilize more sophisticated techniques such as immunophenotyping or genotyping in order to obtain a more accurate subclassification.

Chromosomal abnormalities may also be of diagnostic importance; for instance, African Burkitt's lymphoma is invariably associated with a specific translocation between chromosomes 8 and 14. In addition, the (14:18) translocation, which encodes the BCL oncogene, is found in follicular lymphoma.

Staging

Determining the extent of disease in patients with NHL provides prognostic information and is useful in

---

Table 49.2 REAL classification of non-Hodgkin's lymphoma

Grade	B-cell	T-cell
Indolent (low grade)	Small lymphocytic lymphoma	Sezary syndrome/mycosis fungoides
	Lymphoplasmacytic lymphoma/Waldenstrom's macroglobulinaemia	Smouldering/chronic adult T-cell leukaemia/lymphoma

	Marginal zone lymphomas
	    Extranodal, mucosa-associated lymphoid tissue
	    Splenic lymphoma with villous lymphocytes
	    Monocytoid B-cell lymphoma	

	Follicular lymphoma (grades I and II)	
Aggressive (intermediate grade)	Mantle cell lymphoma	Peripheral T-cell lymphoma (unspecified)
	Follicular lymphoma (grade III)	Angioimmunoblastic lymphoma
	Diffuse large B-cell lymphoma	Angiocentric lymphoma
	Primary mediastinal B-cell lymphoma	Interstinal T-cell lymphoma
		Anaplastic large cell lymphoma
Aggressive with high risk of CNS disease (high grade)	Precursor B lymphoblastic	Precursor T lymphoblastic
	Burkitt's lymphoma	Adult T-cell leukaemia/lymphoma

treatment planning. Patients with extensive disease usually require different therapy to those with limited disease. The NHLs used to be staged according to the Ann Arbor classification formerly used for HD but without the use of the A (without B symptoms) or B (with B symptoms) suffixes. Staging is, however, less relevant than with HD as prognosis is influenced more by histological subtype.

Nodal enlargement can be assessed by computed tomography. Bone marrow trephine biopsy will detect bone marrow involvement, which is more common than in Hodgkin's disease. Erythrocyte sedimentation rate, serum lactate dehydrogenase and serum β_2-microglobulin levels may indicate disease activity and can be of prognostic importance.

Treatment

HD and NHLs are aggressive diseases that are rapidly fatal if untreated. The objective of treatment is to achieve eradication of the disease and thus affect a cure. The management of HD and NHL is different and they will therefore be discussed separately (Figs. 49.2 and 49.3). Strategies for treatment are subject to much research, with new data being published all the time. The aim is to improve cure rates, increase survival and reduce toxicity. Many patients diagnosed with lymphoma in the UK will be entered into one of the ongoing national or European trials.

Hodgkin's disease

HD is, in general, sensitive to radiotherapy and chemotherapy. The treatment plan for individual patients is based on the stage of disease (See Table 49.1) at presentation.

Early stage disease

Patients with stage IA and IIA HD with small-volume disease are generally treated with radiotherapy alone. A recent meta-analysis (Specht et al 1998) of involved field radiotherapy vs. more extensive radiotherapy vs. radiotherapy plus chemotherapy found that the more intensive treatment approaches did not improve survival over involved field radiotherapy. Where disease is confined to above the diaphragm the mantle field is used (Fig. 49.1). The inverted Y is employed when the disease is confined below the diaphragm (Fig. 49.1). This group of patients have relapse-free survival rate of 80% at 5–10 years. Those that do relapse after treatment generally respond well to chemotherapy.

Intermediate disease

Patients with stage I or II presenting with bulky disease, B symptoms or with more than two sites of disease are considered to be poor risk if treated with radiotherapy alone. These patients are usually treated with combination chemotherapy (Table 49.3) and radiotherapy to sites of bulk disease.

Advanced disease

Patients with advanced disease (stages III and IV) are treated with combination chemotherapy. A number of regimens have been shown to be effective (Table 49.3). The ABVD regimen is considered the current gold standard treatment for advanced disease. Most patients who respond to therapy will receive six cycles of treatment, but a small proportion may require further cycles.

Canellos et al (1992) compared three chemotherapy regimens in 361 patients with newly diagnosed advanced HD: MOPP (chlormethine (mustine), Oncovin (vincristine), procarbazine, prednisolone), ABVD (Adriamycin (doxorubicin), bleomycin, vinblastine, dacarbazine) and MOPP alternating with ABVD. Overall survival at 5 years was not significantly

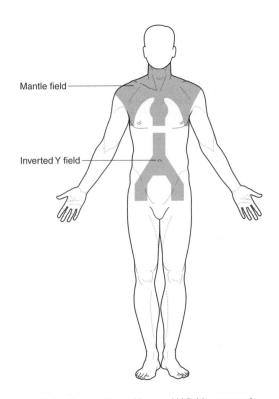

Figure 49.1 The mantle and inverted Y fields commonly employed in the treatment of HD. From Souhami & Tobias (1998, p. 437) with permission from Blackwell Science.

Table 49.3 Combination chemotherapy regimens effective in the treatment of HD

Regimen	Dose and route	Frequency
ABVD (4-week cycle)		
Doxorubicin	25 mg/m^2 i.v.	Days 1 and 15
Bleomycin	10 000 IU/m^2 i.v.	Days 1 and 15
Vinblastine	6mg/m^2 i.v.	Days 1 and 15
Dacarbazine	375 mg/m^2 i.v.	Days 1 and 15
ChIVPP/EVA (4-week cycle)		
Vincristine	1.4 mg/m^2 (max. 2 mg if > 60 years)	Day 1
Etoposide	75 mg/m^2 p.o.	Days 1 to 5
Chlorambucil	6 mg/m^2 p.o.	Days 1 to 7
Procarbazine	90 mg/m^2 p.o.	Days 1 to 7
Prednisolone	50 mg p.o. (flat dose)	Days 1 to 7
Doxorubicin	50 mg/m^2 p.o.	Day 8
Vinblastine	6 mg/m^2 i.v.	Day 8
ChIVPP/PABlOE (7-week cycle)		
Chlorambucil	6 mg/m^2 p.o.	Days 1 to 14
Vinblastine	6 mg/m^2 i.v.	Days 1 and 8
Procarbazine	100 mg/m^2 p.o. (max. 200 mg)	Days 1 to 14
Prednisolone	40 mg/m^2 p.o. (max. 60 mg)	Days 1 to 14
Doxorubicin	40 mg/m^2 i.v.	Days 29
Vincristine	1.4 mg/m^2 i.v. (max. 2 mg)	Days 29 and 36
Prednisolone	40 mg/m^2 p.o. (max. 60 mg)	Days 29 to 38
Etoposide	200 mg/m^2 p.o.	Days 29,30 and 31
Bleomycin	10 000 IU/m^2 i.v.	Days 29 and 36

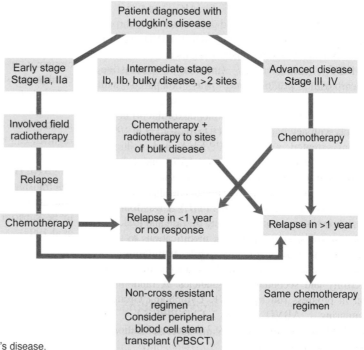

Figure 49.2 Treatment algorithm for Hodgkin's disease.

Table 49.4 Chemotherapy regimens effective in the treatment of NHL

Drug	Dose and route
CHOP (21-day cycle)	
Cyclophosphamide	750 mg/m^2 i.v., day 1
Doxorubicin (hydroxydaunorubicin)	50 mg/m^2 i.v., day 1
Vincristine (Oncovin)	1.4 mg/m^2 (max. 2 mg) i.v., day 1
Prednisolone	100 mg p.o. daily for 5 days
PAdriaCEBO (used in elderly patients)	
Prednisolone	50 mg p.o. daily for 4 weeks, then alternate days from week 5 to treatment end, then reduce and stop
Doxorubicin (Adriamycin)	35 mg/m^2 i.v., day 1
Cyclophosphamide	300 mg/m^2 i.v., day 1
Etoposide	150 mg/m^2 i.v., day 1
Vincristine	1.4 mg/m^2 (max. 2 mg) i.v., day 8
Bleomycin	10 000 IU/m^2 i.v., day 8
Cycle to be repeated at 2-weekly intervals for 8–16 weeks (4–8 cycles)	
PMitCEBO (used in elderly patients)	
Prednisolone	50 mg p.o. daily for 4 weeks, then alternate days from week 5 to treatment end, then reduce and stop
Mitoxantrone (mitozantrone)	7 mg/m^2 i.v., day 1
Cyclophosphamide	300 mg/m^2 i.v., day 1
Etoposide	150 mg/m^2 i.v., day 1
Vincristine	1.4 mg/m^2 (max. 2mg) i.v., day 8
Bleomycin	10 000 IU/m^2 i.v., day 8
Cycle to be repeated at 2-weekly intervals for 8–16 weeks (4–8 cycles)	

intensive combination chemotherapy and CNS prophylaxis. Although relatively infrequent in adults, high grade lymphomas constitute the majority of NHLs in children.

Lymphoblastic lymphomas

Lymphoblastic lymphomas comprise about 2% of adult NHLs. Patients are often treated with leukaemia-type regimens. Despite a very high rate of complete responders, long-term survival remains poor. Patients who fail after first-line chemotherapy have a long-term disease-free survival of less than 10%.

High dose chemotherapy in NHL

Patients who relapse following initial therapy generally have a poor prognosis and the results of treatment with conventional dose chemotherapy are unsatisfactory. There is now widespread acceptance of the use of high dose chemotherapy in such patients. Extended remissions are possible, but the long natural history of

low grade lymphoma makes it difficult to assess at present if conventionally 'incurable' patients are being cured. Patients with intermediate/high grade NHL who relapse following conventional chemotherapy may be salvaged using an alternative regimen, followed by high dose chemotherapy plus peripheral blood stem cell transplant (PBSCT) or autologous bone marrow transplant (ABMT). Such an approach has been shown to be superior in terms of survival to salvage with chemotherapy alone (Philip et al 1995); the multicentre phase III PARMA study compared the role of ABMT to salvage with chemotherapy alone. Two hundred and fifteen patients with relapsed NHL were treated with two courses of conventional chemotherapy. Responding patients were then randomly allocated to receive either four further courses of chemotherapy plus radiotherapy or radiotherapy plus high dose chemotherapy with ABMT. Of the original patients, 58% responded to conventional chemotherapy. The response rate following further treatment was 84% in the ABMT group and 44% in the further conventional therapy group. At 5 years the event-free survival rate was 46% in the ABMT group and 12% in the conventional chemotherapy group. The overall survival rates were 53% and 32%, respectively.

Several randomized studies are investigating the role of high dose chemotherapy and transplantation as initial treatment in poor risk patients with intermediate/high grade NHL. High dose chemotherapy is discussed in more detail in Chapter 50 (Solid tumours).

Patient care

The chemotherapy regimens used to treat HD and NHL (see Tables 49.3 and 49.4) are usually administered on an out-patient basis with the patient visiting the clinic regularly for assessment and treatment. The patient is monitored by full blood counts carried out before each cycle of chemotherapy and at the 'nadir' between cycles. The nadir is when the blood count is at its lowest point, usually 10–14 days after the first day of chemotherapy. The interval between each cycle of chemotherapy enables normal body cells to recover before further treatment. Disease response to treatment is monitored by repeating some of the diagnostic investigations, such as CT, at suitable intervals. If there is little or no response to treatment a different chemotherapy regimen will need to be used or a decision made to withdraw from active therapy and provide best supportive care.

Counselling and support

Counselling is an essential part of the care of the cancer patient: it involves more than the explanation of drug therapy and investigations, and includes the psychological support of the patient and his or her family. Prior to treatment with chemotherapy, the patient will be counselled by the doctor, chemotherapy nurse and, increasingly, by oncology pharmacists. It is necessary to explain how the chemotherapy is to be given and discuss both potential and inevitable side-effects. The probability of successful treatment must be weighed against the prospect of serious and life-threatening adverse effects.

The support available to the cancer patient, to help cope with both the illness and its treatment, has improved dramatically in recent years. Multidisciplinary teams working within specialized units have become skilled in anticipating the problems of lymphomas and their treatment. The oncology pharmacist is an important member of those teams. Also, many charities provide care, support and advice, for example BACUP (British Association of Cancer United Patients), Macmillan Cancer Relief and the Lymphoma Association.

Patient-specific treatment modifications

The selection of appropriate therapy must also take into consideration the individual patient. Considerations include the patient's age, renal and hepatic function and underlying medical conditions, such as heart disease, diabetes or chronic pulmonary disease. The patient's tolerance of side-effects and complications of therapy may then be predicted. The decision is based on an understanding of the pharmacodynamics and pharmacokinetics of the drugs being used as well as the clinical condition of the patient. The pharmacist can advise on potential problems in patients on concurrent medication for underlying medical conditions, dosage alterations in impaired hepatic and renal function and pharmaceutical aspects of administration.

Supportive care

During a course of chemotherapy the patient requires supportive care to minimize the adverse effects of treatment. The common adverse effects of the chemotherapy regimens discussed in this chapter are outlined in Table 49.5. These will occur to varying degrees depending on the combination of drugs and the doses used as well as individual patient factors.

Nausea and vomiting

Nausea and vomiting following chemotherapy is the most distressing and most feared adverse effect of chemotherapy. Its effect on the patient should not be underestimated and its treatment is an important part of supportive care. The severity will depend on the combination of drugs used. For example, oral chlorambucil is generally well tolerated by almost all patients and requires no antiemetic cover. Regimens such as PMitCEBO and ABVD, which are moderately and highly emetic respectively, will make most patients vomit if no antiemetics are given. The control of chemotherapy-induced nausea and vomiting is discussed in Chapter 32 and in Case 49.1. For further reading see the end of the chapter. The patient should be counselled on the appropriate use of the antiemetics prescribed (see Table 49.5).

Tumour lysis syndrome

The lymphomas are, in general, highly sensitive to chemotherapy, and the resulting lysis of cells may lead to hyperuricaemia, hyperkalaemia and hypercalcaemia in patients with bulky disease, and may result in urate nephropathy. The patient should be encouraged to maintain a high fluid intake, and renal function and serum urate levels should be monitored. Allopurinol must be commenced before chemotherapy and continued for 3–4 weeks until the tumour load has reduced and serum urate levels are normal. The patient should be counselled on the importance of a high fluid intake and regular allopurinol therapy until told to stop by the doctor.

Table 49.5 Adverse effects associated with chemotherapy regimens used in the lymphomas with supportive measures and counselling points

Adverse effect	Cytotoxics implicated	Supportive measures	Counselling points
Bone marrow suppression	Chlorambucil Cyclophosphamide Dacarbazine Etoposide Vinblastine Prednisolone	Blood transfusion Platelet transfusions Mouth care Antibiotic therapy for febrile episodes Growth factors	Expect tiredness Report bleeding or unusual bruises Importance of good personal hygiene Adhere to mouth care regimen Avoid people with infections Monitor temperature Report febrile episodes or signs of infection **immediately**
Nausea and vomiting	Cyclophosphamide Doxorubicin Procarbazine Dacarbazine	Antiemetic therapy	Emphasize regular use – a short course is more effective than 'as required' Take tablets before meals Report episodes of vomiting (especially if taking oral cytotoxics) For dexamethasone, emphasize short course **not** to be continued
Mucositis	Doxorubicin	Mouth care regimen	Importance of good oral hygiene, instruct how mouthwashes are used, stress importance of regular use
Tumour lysis syndrome	High tumour load sensitive to chemotherapy	Hydration Allopurinol	Stress importance of regular allopurinol until appropriate to stop Drink plenty of fluids
Alopecia	Cyclophosphamide Doxorubicin Etoposide	Provision of wig if wanted	Hair usually regrows on completion of therapy
Impaired gonadal in function	Alkylating agents Procarbazine Doxorubicin (to a lesser degree)	Sperm storage	Refer to doctor, depends on regimen, reversible some cases
Neuropathy	Vincristine	Discontinue use or substitute vinblastine	Report tingling sensations or difficulty with buttons, jaw pain or stiffness, constipation (do not self-treat – refer to doctor)
Cardiomyopathy	Doxorubicin		Report breathlessness, tiredness
Lung fibrosis	Bleomycin		Report breathlessness

Mucositis

Chemotherapy may cause mucositis, which is inflammation of or damage to the surface of the gastrointestinal tract. In the mouth this may lead to painful ulceration, local infection and difficulty in swallowing. Disruption of the mucosal barrier will allow bacteria and fungi to have easier systemic access. A mouth care regimen should, therefore, be instituted with myelosuppressive therapy. This involves good oral hygiene with regular use of an antiseptic mouthwash such as 0.2% chlorhexidine or 0.1% hexetidine and an antifungal mouthwash or lozenges, usually nystatin or amphotericin.

Bone marrow suppression

Myelosuppression is usually the dose-limiting factor with these regimens, and it is necessary to carry out full blood counts before treatment to confirm that recovery has occurred. If the platelet count is below $100 \times 10^9/l$ and/or the absolute neutrophil count is less than $1 \times 10^9/l$, the subsequent dose may be reduced or treatment delayed by a week.

Anaemia is treated with blood transfusions as necessary and thrombocytopenia with platelet transfusions. Prolonged thrombocytopenia is not usually a problem with the regimens described in this chapter.

Neutropenia is the most life-threatening acute toxicity; the neutropenic patient is at constant risk from infections. Seemingly minor infections such as cold sores can spread rapidly, and infections not seen in the normal population, such as systemic fungal infections, can occur. Supportive measures involve reducing the risks and the aggressive treatment of any infectious episodes. The patient is counselled to avoid contact with people with infection or who may be carriers. Most infections, however, are from an endogenous source such as the gut or skin. The patient is educated on the importance of good personal hygiene, mouth care (as discussed earlier), how to monitor body temperature and to report any febrile episodes immediately. Co-trimoxazole 960 mg may be prescribed as prophylaxis against *Pneumocystis* pneumonia in patients receiving chemotherapy for lymphomas, particularly in patients receiving a fludarabine-containing regimen. Antifungal prophylaxis is used by some centres.

Febrile neutropenia

A febrile episode in the neutropenic patient is an indication for immediate treatment with broad-spectrum intravenous antibiotics. The patient is assessed to determine, if possible, the site of infection. Blood cultures and any other appropriate cultures are taken and then antibiotic therapy is commenced. Gram-negative septicaemia is probable in this situation, and therefore first-line therapy is usually a third-generation cephalosporin or antipseudomonal penicillin with gentamicin. If the patient does not respond to this combination within 48 hours, second-line therapy, which includes a glycopeptide for Gram-positive cover, is substituted. If positive microbiological cultures are found, the appropriate antibiotic can be prescribed on the basis of sensitivities; however, if the patient is responding to empiric therapy the antibiotics should not be changed. Only one-third of suspected infections are ever confirmed, and the pathogen may not be isolated or the febrile episode may not be due to infection. Non-infectious causes include blood transfusion and underlying disease.

Growth factor support

Patients with persistent neutropenia or those who have repeated admissions for neutropenic sepsis may be supported with granulocyte colony-stimulating factor (G-CSF). There is evidence that patients with lymphomas receiving a reduced dose of chemotherapy as a consequence of myelosuppression have a worse prognosis when compared with patients who receive full doses. G-CSF has been investigated as a prophylactic measure to ensure that patients receive full doses of chemotherapy, on schedule, however despite increases in remission rates no difference in overall survival has been observed (Fridrik et al 1997, Gisselbrecht et al 1997).

CASE STUDIES

Case 49.1

Miss A. is 20 years old and is receiving a course of ChIVPP/PABIOE (see Table 49.3) for stage IIb Hodgkin's disease. She has no other medical problems and has normal renal and hepatic function. She received her first cycle of ChIVPP 4 weeks ago and and presented to the out-patient pharmacy with a prescription for her oral chemotherapy and metoclopramide 20 mg three times daily when required, to take home.

Four weeks later she attended the chemotherapy clinic for a cycle of PABIOE. Her full blood count had recovered sufficiently for her to receive this cycle. She tolerated the ChIVPP combination reasonably well, complaining only of mild nausea that started 2 days after starting the course and continued while she was taking the oral cytotoxics. She took the metoclopramide initially but experienced jaw spasm, which resolved when she stopped taking the tablets.

....

Questions

1. What are the key counselling points for the oral chemotherapy drug procarbazine?
2. Comment on the use of metoclopramide in this patient.
3. What antiemetic regimen would you recommend for future courses of ChIVPP?
4. What antiemetic regimen would you recommend with the PABIOE?

....

Answers

1. Procarbazine often causes nausea and occasionally vomiting. Nausea can be reduced by taking the capsules in divided doses. If she vomits she should inform the hospital, especially if she has brought up any of her chemotherapy doses. This is particularly important for Miss A., who should receive optimum doses as the aim of her treatment is cure. Procarbazine is a mild monoamine oxidase (MAO) inhibitor but dietary restriction is not considered necessary. Some centres, however, do recommend avoiding tyramine containing foods or trying small amounts and then waiting an hour to see if a reaction occurs. The symptoms of a reaction include headache, flushing, pounding heart, sweating and occasionally vomiting.
The patient should be counselled to avoid alcohol as disulfiram-like reaction may occur. She should inform her doctor if she develops a rash.
2. Metoclopramide is the most widely used antiemetic in cancer chemotherapy; however, it can cause disturbing dystonic reactions, drowsiness, restlessness and diarrhoea. Patients under 30 years of age and women are more likely

to experience dystonic reactions. Miss A. falls into both these categories.

The jaw spasm Miss A. described is one form of dystonic reaction. Because of her age and sex it is not surprising that she was unable to tolerate the metoclopramide. Severe dystonic reactions can be reversed with an intravenous anticholinergic agent such as procyclidine.

3. Miss A. should be prescribed an alternative antiemetic such as domperidone 20 mg four times daily. Domperidone, although a dopamine anatgonist similar to metoclopramide, does not cross the blood–brain barrier and is therefore rarely associated with extrapyramidal side-effects. This should be taken regularly for the duration of the regimen. She should be advised to take these tablets 30 minutes before meals and at night.

4. Doxorubicin is moderately emetogenic; etoposide and vinblastine are rarely emetogenic. Half an hour before administration of the intravenous doses Miss A. should receive domperidone 20 mg and dexamethasone 4 mg orally. The antiemetics should continue, with domperidone 20 mg four times daily. Patients receiving moderately emetic regimens would normally receive a short course of oral dexamethasone, for example 4 mg twice daily for 2–3 days, with the domperidone. Miss A. is, however, taking prednisolone as part of her regimen, so the oral dexamethasone should be omitted.

If this regimen fails, a single dose of a 5-HT$_3$ antagonist should be given with dexamethasone prior to the intravenous doses and domperidone as above for delayed nausea and vomiting. There is no evidence that a 5-HT$_3$ antagonist is any better than domperidone and dexamethasone for delayed nausea and vomiting, and should be reserved as a third-line option.

For further information read the American Society of Clinical Oncology Practice Guidelines (Gralla et al 1999).

Case 49.2

Mrs B. is a 72-year-old widow who has been newly diagnosed with low grade NHL. She has been seen in the out-patient haematology clinic and has brought a prescription to the pharmacy for chlorambucil 10 mg daily for 14 days. When she hands in her prescription she expresses concern about the side-effects of the tablets. The doctor who saw her had spent a lot of time talking to her about her treatment but she feels confused with all the information given.

Questions

1. What are the side-effects of chlorambucil?
2. How would you counsel this patient?

Answers

1. Chlorambucil, an alkylating agent, is generally well tolerated. The major side-effect is bone marrow suppression. Other side-effects are uncommon, and include nausea and vomiting, rash, mucositis and diarrhoea. Hepatotoxicity and jaundice have been reported. Mrs B. is an elderly patient and is thus more likely to experience

toxicity because of deteriorating renal and hepatic function and underlying medical conditions.

2. Mrs B. may be distressed by her diagnosis and may not have been able to absorb all the information she was given in the clinic. She may also be seeking confirmation of information.

Mrs B. should be counselled to complete the course of tablets as prescribed. She should be told that she will probably feel tired and be more prone to infection because the tablets lower the blood count and resistance to infection. She should be advised to inform the haematologist if she feels unwell. Chlorambucil is unlikely to make her feel nauseous, but if this occurs she should inform the doctor, who will be able to prescribe an antiemetic.

Case 49.3

Mr C. is 56 years old and was diagnosed with stage III high grade NHL over 10 weeks ago. Since then he has received three cycles of CHOP (see Table 49.4) and has come to the hospital for his nadir blood count. He complains of painful mouth ulcers and a sore throat. On examination he has mucositis and oropharyngeal candidiasis. He has a white blood cell count (WCC) of 3.2 (normal range 3.5–11 × 109/l) with 25% neutrophils (normal range 30–75%). When questioned about mouth care he revealed that he had been prescribed 0.2% chlorhexidine (10 ml four times daily) and nystatin (1 ml four times daily) and has been using these regularly as counselled.

Questions

1. How would you treat Mr C.'s *Candida* infection?
2. Would you alter his mouth care regimen?
3. How would you counsel this patient?

Answers

1. Mr C. has an absolute neutrophil count (ANC) of 0.8 × 10^9/l (25% of WCC) and is therefore neutropenic (ANC < 1.0 × 10^9/l). Localized candidal infections can spread rapidly in the immunosuppressed patient, so local therapy with an antifungal mouthwash will be inadequate therapy. A course of fluconazole (100 mg daily for at least 7 days) should be prescribed. Therapy should continue for a further 7 days if Mr C. is still neutropenic or if the thrush has not completely resolved.

2. Chlorhexidine mouthwash should be continued as before. Nystatin can be restarted when the fluconazole has stopped. As Mr C. is complaining of pain, an analgesic should be added. Benzydamine mouthwash, a locally acting analgesic, could be prescribed initially. If this does not give adequate pain relief, then systemic analgesics such as paracetamol or dihydrocodeine should be given.

3. Regular mouth care reduces the risk of infection but does not entirely remove it. It is not necessarily a reflection of how well the patient has adhered to his mouth care regimen. Mr C. should continue his mouth care regimen as before. Chlorhexidine mouthwash should be used first, held in the mouth as long as possible, ensuring the entire mucosa is covered before spitting out. The nystatin should then be used in the same manner but swallowed. The

mouthwashes should be used after meals and at bedtime. He should not eat or drink for at least half an hour after using the mouthwashes.

The benzydamine should be used before meals as Mr C. will probably find eating painful. He should be advised to use a soft toothbrush, to eat soft foods and to avoid hot and spicy dishes. He may be reassured that once his blood count recovers his mouth ulcers should resolve and that the fluconazole should relieve his sore throat.

Case 49.4

Mr D., 38 years old with advanced HD, is admitted to the haematology ward as an emergency. He had a temperature of 39°C that morning, feels generally unwell but has no specific symptoms. It is 12 days since he started his third cycle of ABVD (see Table 49.3). On admission he is taking the following medication:

- Co-trimoxazole 960 mg twice daily on three days a week
- 0.2% chlorhexidine mouthwash 10 ml four times daily
- Nystatin mouthwash 1 ml four times daily.

Blood cultures are taken, and ceftazidime 2 g i.v. three times daily and gentamicin 480 mg i.v. once daily are prescribed to be commenced immediately. Blood biochemistry results are normal; his full blood count was Hb 10.8 (normal range 13.5–18.0 g/dl for men), WCC 2.5 (normal range 3.5×10^9 to 11×10^9/l), neutrophil count 0.6 (normal range 1.5×10^9 to 7.5×10^9/l) and platelets 150 (normal range 150×10^9 to 400×10^9/l). Mr D. weighs 86 kg and is 186 cm tall.

Questions

1. Comment on the rationale for the antibiotic therapy prescribed.
2. How would you monitor this patient?
3. What would be an appropriate second line regimen if he remains pyrexial?
4. What modifications would need to be made to subsequent cycles of chemotherapy?

Answers

1. Mr D.'s full blood count is probably at its nadir following his last course of chemotherapy. He is neutropenic and febrile: fever is often the only sign of infection in neutropenic patients. Immunosuppression is also a feature of HD and contributes to susceptibility to infection. Treatment should commence immediately after cultures have been taken, as infection can be rapidly fatal in these patients. The antibiotics selected should provide broad-spectrum cover and follow local policy as there are institutional variations in predominant pathogens and antimicrobial sensitivities. The organisms responsible for infectious episodes are constantly changing: in the 1970s, Gram-negative infections predominated, now Gram-positive organisms account for 65% of positive cultures. As Gram-negative infections are more rapidly fatal, first-line therapy should be biased towards these infections. Ceftazidime, a third-generation cephalosporin, and gentamicin are, therefore, an appropriate combination to use in this patient.

The dose of ceftazidime is appropriate. Infection is considered to be severe in these patients as signs and symptoms are often muted. Single daily dose gentamicin is at least as effective as multiple dosing and less nephrotoxic: it is more convenient and cost-effective and overcomes deficiencies of the traditional method such as subtherapeutic dosing and inadequate monitoring. The dose is 5–7 mg/kg, and has been calculated correctly for Mr D. He has normal renal function, so no dose modifications are necessary.

2. Monitor temperature, pulse and blood pressure and any patient symptoms for signs of improvement or deterioration. Blood biochemistry should be checked daily to detect any deterioration in renal function. Microbiology reports should be checked and antibiotics reviewed if any micro-organisms have been cultured. However, no change should be made to antibiotics if the patient is showing signs of improvement. The administration of gentamicin should be monitored, checking both administration and sampling time for drug levels. The results should be checked and recommendations for dose modification made where appropriate using a method such as the Hartford nomogram.

3. If the patient remains pyrexial 48 hours after the first-line antibiotics have been commenced they should be replaced with second-line therapy, again following local policy. This should be a combination of a glycopeptide (vancomycin or teicoplanin) and a second broad-spectrum antibiotic to provide Gram-negative cover (e.g. ciprofloxacin). If blood cultures show growth – found in only 30–40% of neutropenic patients – the choice of antibiotics should be on the basis of sensitivities. It is important to note that febrile episodes lasting several days may involve more than one infecting organism.

The patient's full blood count should start to recover from day 14 but may be delayed by this infection. It is unusual for patients on conventional chemotherapy for HD to require more than one change to antibiotic therapy, and clinical improvement is often seen with recovery of neutrophil count. If he is still pyrexial at 96 hours then the likelihood of fungal infection must be considered and intravenous amphotericin commenced if appropriate. The incidence of fungal infection is increasing in patients with prolonged neutropenia. Mr D.'s neutropenia is short-lived, so he is more likely to have a bacterial infection.

4. A dose reduction for subsequent cycles of chemotherapy may be considered. However, as this patient is being treated with curative intent, it may be more appropriate to give GCSF and maintain the dose intensity.

Case 49.5

Mrs E. is 52 years old and has just been diagnosed with stage IV high grade NHL. She is a non-insulin-dependent diabetic stabilized on glibenclamide 10 mg daily. She is prescribed her first course of CHOP (see Table 49.4) as an in-patient. She is 161 cm tall and weighs 78 kg, giving a surface area of 1.85 m². Her prescription chart is as follows:

Cyclophosphamide   1390 mg i.v. day 1
Doxorubicin   92 mg i.v. day 1

Solid tumours 50

J. So

KEY POINTS

- Although cancer is a disease which predominantly affects the elderly, it is the leading cause of death in adults aged under 65.
- Superior outcomes are seen when treatment is supervised by, or given at, a specialized cancer centre.
- Before treatment, patients must be carefully staged to establish the type and extent of disease.
- Dependent on the disease, treatment goals may be cure, prolongation of survival or palliative symptom control.
- Cancer chemotherapy is the main treatment against disseminated disease.
- Optimum patient management with cytotoxic chemotherapy relies on anticipating the adverse effects of these agents and providing effective pharmaceutical care.
- There is an explicit, acknowledged role for the oncology pharmacist in the management of the cancer patient.

The term 'cancer' is used to describe more than 200 different diseases including the leukaemias, lymphomas and those cancers affecting discrete organs which collectively may be described as solid tumours. It is important to remember that some tumours are benign and mainly harmless but this chapter will focus on the management of patients with solid malignancies which require some form of treatment. Although a solid tumour can affect any organ, half of all new cases present as lung, breast, colorectal or prostate cancer. Treatment is best carried out in specialized cancer centres (or units which have close links with cancer centres) and may include surgery, radiotherapy, chemotherapy or a combination of these. Care of the cancer patient demands a broad range of services involving multidisciplinary collaboration provided by teams across the hospital, community and hospice network.

Epidemiology

Cancer is a common disease, affecting up to one in three of the UK population, and one in four will die from it. Mortality statistics for 1998 show that in the UK, 154 730 people were registered as dying from a malignancy. Although male lung cancer death rates continue to fall, it is still the commonest cause of male cancer death at 27%, followed by cancer of the prostate (12%) and large bowel (11%), together accounting for half of male cancer deaths. For women, despite the decline in breast cancer deaths, breast cancer is still the leading cause of female cancer death (18%), closely followed by lung cancer (18%) and large bowel cancer (11%). The number of female deaths from lung cancer continues to rise and in some parts of the UK there are already more deaths from lung cancer in women than from breast cancer. Figures 50.1 and 50.2 show the ten commonest causes of cancer death in men and women respectively in the UK in 1998, excluding non-melanoma skin cancers.

Although more than a quarter of a million people develop cancer each year in the UK, it is predominantly a disease of old age with over 66% of all new cancers diagnosed in people aged over 65 years. However, in adults under 65 years, 34% of deaths are caused by cancer, outnumbering those caused by heart disease; and when the sexes are looked at separately, nearly 50% of deaths in women under 65 are due to cancer.

Aetiology

The causes of cancer may be broadly classed as either environmental or genetic, although these may be interrelated and the causes of some cancers are multifactorial.

Environmental factors

Lifestyle and environmental factors play a large part in the development of many cancers with cigarette smoking having been identified as the single most important cause of preventable disease and premature death in the UK. Overall, one-third of all cancer deaths are linked to tobacco use, which causes over 90% of lung cancer deaths (Cancer Research Campaign 2000). Smoking is also a well-established risk factor for other cancers including stomach, bladder (Castelao et al 2001) and possibly breast cancer (Johnson 2001), and cervical cancer is twice as common in women who smoke regularly compared to those who are non-smokers. The

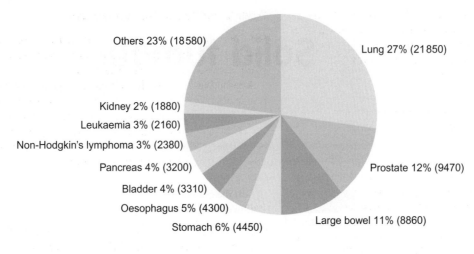

Others 23% (18580)

Lung 27% (21850)

Kidney 2% (1880)

Leukaemia 3% (2160)

Non-Hodgkin's lymphoma 3% (2380)

Pancreas 4% (3200)

Bladder 4% (3310)

Oesophagus 5% (4300)

Stomach 6% (4450)

Prostate 12% (9470)

Large bowel 11% (8860)

All malignant neoplasms – 80 440

Figure 50.1 The 10 most common causes of cancer death in men in the UK in 1998 (with kind permission from Cancer Research Campaign 2000).

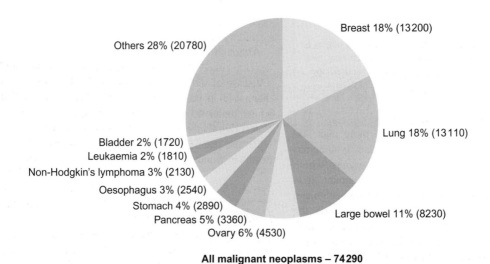

Others 28% (20780)

Breast 18% (13200)

Bladder 2% (1720)

Leukaemia 2% (1810)

Non-Hodgkin's lymphoma 3% (2130)

Oesophagus 3% (2540)

Stomach 4% (2890)

Pancreas 5% (3360)

Ovary 6% (4530)

Lung 18% (13110)

Large bowel 11% (8230)

All malignant neoplasms – 74290

Figure 50.2 The 10 most common causes of cancer death in women in the UK in 1998 (with kind permission from Cancer Research Campaign 2000).

most important lifestyle factor for bowel cancer is likely to be diet. High dietary salt, nitrites/nitrosamines and gastric colonization by *Helicobacter pylori* have all been implicated in gastric cancer. Several studies have shown a significant positive association between being overweight and oesophageal adenocarcinoma (Maric & Cheng 2001). Recreational exposure to sunlight is associated with an increased risk of melanoma, while cervical cancer is caused by infections with oncogenic strains of the sexually transmitted human papillomavirus.

Environmental causes include exposure to ionizing radiation and carcinogens such as asbestos and aniline dyes.

Genetic factors

A number of rare tumours are known to be associated with an inherited predisposition. Examples include the paediatric malignancies Wilms' tumour of the kidney and bilateral retinoblastoma, a rare cancer of the eye. Some commoner cancers such as breast, ovary and colon may also show a familial link. A woman's risk of developing breast cancer is increased if her mother, sister or daughter has had premenopausal or bilateral breast cancer in which case referral to a breast family history clinic may be advised.

Screening and prevention

Screening

Screening (secondary prevention) programmes aim to detect preclinical cancer in asymptomatic individuals in the general population in order to provide earlier, and thus more effective, treatment. Any screening test must be simple, reliable, highly specific (to exclude healthy individuals) and highly sensitive (detection 90–95%). To date, screening has been of proven value in cancers of the breast and cervix, while screening tests are being assessed for use in colorectal and prostate cancer. Genetic testing for the BRCA2 gene, for example, is used as a predictive diagnostic test for breast cancer.

Prevention

The strong associations between cancer risk and environmental factors means there is great potential for the primary prevention of cancer through healthier eating, moderate drinking, limiting exposure to sunlight and avoiding smoking; current public health programmes therefore target these lifestyle changes.

Chemoprevention

Women at high risk of breast cancer are being targeted for participation in trials of the drug tamoxifen which may help protect them from developing the disease. Similarly, individuals at high risk of colon cancer are being targeted for participation in trials using non-steroidal anti-inflammatory drugs (NSAIDs) where the evidence suggests they can reduce the incidence of precancerous lesions.

Cancer at the cellular level

The normal cell and the role of p53

In the normal cell, there are genes associated with tumour suppression, notably the p53 gene which acts as a regulator of cell growth and proliferation. Agents which damage DNA cause p53 to accumulate. This switches off replication of abnormal cells, arresting them in the cell cycle allowing them time to repair. If repair fails, p53 may trigger cell suicide by apoptosis. Thus p53 controls and halts the proliferation of abnormal cell growth.

Transformation of the normal cell

If a normal cell loses p53 function or the latter becomes impaired, then uncontrolled growth may result which is more likely to produce malignant clones.

Alternatively, cells in which oncogenes (genes responsible for malignant transformation) such as c-*myc* are activated may also give rise to malignant clones. Cancer arises from the transformation of a single normal cell. Most cancers require a series of genetic mutations in a cell before an invasive tumour results.

The cancer cell

Cancer cells differ from normal cells in that they function differently. Inherently unstable, they may display different protein or enzyme content and chromosomal abnormalities (such as translocations or deletions) which may differ in their susceptibility to chemotherapy or radiotherapy. Also their changed appearance (visible under light microscopy) from normal cells allows them to be more easily detected.

Tumour growth

A solid tumour represents a population of dividing and non-dividing cells. The time it takes for a tumour mass to double in size is known as the doubling time. The latter will vary dependent on tumour type but for most solid tumours is about 2–3 months. In most solid tumours the growth rate is very rapid initially (exponential growth) and then slows as the tumour increases in size and age, a pattern described as Gompertzion growth. The growth fraction is the percentage of actively dividing cells in the tumour and this decreases with tumour size.

This pattern of tumour growth kinetics has implications for chemotherapy treatment. Generally chemotherapy is most successful when the number of tumour cells is low and the growth fraction high, which is the situation in the very early stages of cancer.

Tumour spread

As a primary tumour grows and invades normal tissue, malignant cells often infiltrate blood vessels and the lymphatic system. Malignant cells are thereby transported to other organs of the body where they can subsequently form secondary cancers or metastases. The pattern of spread tends to be predictable for different tumour types. Breast cancer usually metastasizes to the lungs and central nervous system while prostate cancer tends to metastasize to bone, in particular to the lumbar spine. Generally, the larger the tumour mass, the more likely it has metastasized to other sites.

Patient management

Clinical assessment

Presentation

The clinical features of cancer vary with tumour type. However, patients most commonly present with non-specific complaints which include weight loss, bleeding, malaise, pain, or the presence of a painless lump. In general, solid tumours are clinically detectable when there are approximately 10^8–10^9 tumour cells present. The patient is usually in the terminal stages of the disease when there are 10^{12} cells present. This means that unless a tumour is detected by chance during a routine physical examination or by screening, the disease at presentation is usually at an advanced stage.

Before treatment, each patient must undergo a thorough assessment to establish diagnosis, stage of disease and general fitness level. These factors will influence the choice of treatment and give a guide to prognosis.

Diagnosis

An accurate diagnosis is usually made from a sample of tissue. This sample may be obtained invasively as a biopsy, for example during bronchoscopy when lung cancer is suspected, or, as in the case of a patient presenting with a breast lump, aspiration through a fine needle is possible.

Malignant tumours vary in their sensitivity to chemotherapy. For example, there are two major groups of lung cancer: small cell and non-small cell lung cancer. Each of these groups is treated with different combinations of chemotherapy drugs, so precise histopathology is important.

Tumour markers

A number of biological markers have been found which can help confirm the diagnosis of particular tumours (Table 50.1) as well as assist in monitoring response to treatment, or they may be the first sign of early relapse after complete remission.

Staging investigations

Since the cancer is often disseminated at the time of presentation, it is absolutely vital that patients undergo thorough staging investigations to establish the extent and nature of disease. This will determine the most appropriate treatment offered to the patient. Baseline investigations range from clinical examination, blood tests, liver function tests, diagnostic imaging such as chest and skeletal X-rays, ultrasound, computed tomography (CT), magnetic resonance imaging (MRI) and positron emission tomography (PET), depending on the disease type and likely pattern of spread.

Table 50.1 Tumour markers

Tumour marker	Indicative cancer type
α-fetoprotein (AFP) β human chorionic gonadotrophin (β-HCG)	Testicular tumours
Ca125	Ovarian cancer
5-hydroxyindole acetic acid (5-HIAA)	Carcinoid tumours

Staging classification

Most tumours are classified into three or four stages, denoted I, II, III and IV. In general, the higher the stage the more advanced the disease and the poorer the prognosis. For some diseases, including breast cancer, a more complex staging classification is used, the TNM (tumour–nodes–metastases) system where T (0–4) indicates the size of the primary tumour, N (0–4) the extent of lymph node involvement and M (0–1) the presence or absence of distant metastases.

Performance status

The patient's general level of fitness (performance status) at the time of diagnosis is often a good indicator of prognosis and will help determine if they are likely to withstand intensive chemotherapy and therefore influence the choice of treatment. A number of physical rating scales have been devised to assess performance status, including the Karnofsky performance index and the World Health Organization (WHO) performance scale (Table 50.2).

Prognostic factors

These are factors that can predict outcome in individual patients. Table 50.3 lists prognostic factors used in lung cancer (Hoffman et al 2000).

Treatment

Treatment goals

After the diagnosis of cancer has been confirmed and the extent of disease fully investigated, the goals of treatment have to be considered. The primary goal is to cure. Patients are said to be 'cured' of cancer when they are completely disease-free and have a normal life

Table 50.2   Performance status scales

Karnofsky performance index	WHO performance scale
100 Normal, no complaints, no evidence of disease	
90 Able to carry on normal activity, minor signs or symptoms of disease	0 Able to carry out all normal activity without restriction
80 Normal activity with effort, some signs or symptoms of disease	
70 Cares for self, unable to carry on normal activity or do active work	1 Restricted in physically strenuous activity but ambulatory and able to carry out light work
60 Requires occasional assistance but is able to care for most of own needs	
50 Requires considerable assistance and frequent medical care	2 Ambulatory and capable of all self-care but unable to carry out any work; up and about more than 50% of waking hours
40 Disabled, requires special care and assistance	
30 Severely disabled, hospitalization is indicated, although death is not imminent	3 Capable of only limited self-care; confined to bed more than 50% of waking hours
20 Very sick, hospitalization necessary, active supportive treatment is necessary	
10 Moribund, fatal processes progressing rapidly	4 Completely disabled; cannot carry on any self-care; totally confined to bed or chair
0 Dead	

Table 50.3   Prognostic factors in patients with lung cancer

Tumour stage
Performance status
Degree of weight loss
Sex (women fare better)
Serum lactate dehydrogenase
Presence of bone/liver metastases

expectancy. The smaller the tumour bulk when treatment is given, the greater the opportunity of achieving cure.

If cure is not feasible, then the goal is to prolong survival while maintaining patient quality of life.

The third goal of cancer therapy is palliative care with relief of symptoms such as pain.

The decision is influenced by factors such as the pace and extent of the disease as well as coexisting symptoms and concurrent medical conditions, performance status and, importantly, the patient's wishes (Grunfeld et al 2001).

The possibility of cure or long-term survival justifies aggressive treatment, but with palliative therapy it is particularly important that the toxicity of treatment is carefully weighed against the potential benefits.

Treatment guidelines

Consensus on the best approach to managing each particular type of cancer is continually evolving, based on the evidence of clinical research gleaned from randomized trials conducted by cancer centres either nationally or internationally. National guidelines promote equity for patients and ensure a consistent treatment approach. In the absence of clinical consensus, patients should be encouraged to participate in clinical trials.

Treatment methods

Three main options are available for the treatment of patients with solid tumours: surgery, radiotherapy and chemotherapy. Each type of treatment may play a number of roles, either alone or in combination, depending on the disease.

Role of surgery

Surgery can be curative when solid tumours are localized or confined to one primary anatomical site or region as in localized disease. It can also be used to remove isolated metastatic masses. Surgical techniques may be used to support chemotherapy administration when given by continuous infusion or by the intraperitoneal/intrahepatic routes. Surgery may also play a role in diagnosis through tissue biopsy or in staging to ascertain the extent of tumour involvement such as in ovarian cancer. In the latter it may also be used to debulk or reduce the size of the tumour to effect pain relief or to improve the effectiveness of subsequent radiation or chemotherapy. However, with more widespread disease, systemic treatment becomes necessary, with chemotherapy playing a major role.

Although chemotherapy encompasses cytotoxic drugs, endocrine (hormonal) therapy and cytokines (such as interferon), the remainder of this chapter will focus on cytotoxic drugs.

Cytotoxic chemotherapy

Childhood malignancies, choriocarcinoma and testicular tumours in adults are most responsive to chemotherapy and these patients are regularly cured, even with advanced disease. However, for most patients treated with chemotherapy, cure is unlikely and treatment will be to prolong survival or be purely palliative.

Chemotherapy regimen

Although chemotherapy may infrequently be administered as a single agent it is more usual to combine two or more drugs to achieve additive or synergistic effects. Generally, drugs used in combination should have established efficacy as single agents, different mechanisms of action and differing toxicity profiles to allow their use at optimal doses.

Chemotherapy scheduling

Because chemotherapy is not specific to malignant cells, any actively proliferating normal cell will be at potential risk of damage, in particular the cells of the bone marrow. With many cytotoxic drugs, the white blood cell count is at its lowest level or nadir by around 10 days after treatment. Recovery generally occurs by day 20 post-treatment, and therefore treatment is repeated every 3–4 weeks. (With agents such as melphalan and mitomycin, haematological recovery may be delayed for 42–50 days following treatment, in which case the interval between treatment cycles needs to be increased.) In most cases, a course of treatment will comprise a maximum of six cycles of chemotherapy.

Chemotherapy dose

The dose of most chemotherapy agents is calculated using the patient's body surface area (BSA) and is usually given in the form of mg per square metre. BSA may be calculated from the height and weight of the patient using a nomogram and may need to be recalculated for subsequent cycles of chemotherapy if the patient experiences significant weight changes. Table 50.4 gives an example of a chemotherapy regimen for use in breast cancer.

Rationale at the cellular level

An understanding of cell cycle kinetics has helped in designing chemotherapy regimens and schedules. Within a solid tumour a proportion of non-dividing cells will die while others are in a resting phase of growth. Since dividing cells are most responsive to chemotherapy, resting cells should ideally be encouraged into the cell cycle, a process called recruitment. Recruitment may follow an initial reduction in the tumour cell population and should increase the proportion of cells killed by successive cycles of treatment.

Some cytotoxic drugs are phase-specific in that they affect cells at defined stages in the cell cycle. In these cases, treatment should ideally be scheduled to target the maximal number of cells in the drug-sensitive phase of the cell cycle. For example, fluorouracil is phase-specific. It also has a very short plasma half-life of less than 15 minutes. Administration of fluorouracil by prolonged continuous infusion, rather than by bolus

Table 50.4 Example of a chemotherapy regimen: CMF (cyclophosphamide, methotrexate, fluorouracil) in adjuvant and advanced breast cancer

Drug	Dose	Route
Cyclophosphamide	600 mg/m^2	i.v.
Methotrexate	40 mg/m^2	i.v.
5-Fluorouracil	600 mg/m^2	i.v.

All on day 1
Repeat every 3 weeks for six cycles

injection or short infusion, should theoretically increase the cell kill. In practice this has been shown to translate into an improved clinical response and survival advantage in patients with gastrointestinal cancer (Advanced Colorectal Cancer Meta-Analysis Project 1998).

Adjuvant chemotherapy

Historically, chemotherapy was used solely in the treatment of recurrent or advanced widespread disease when it was not likely to yield cure. Chemotherapy is now also used in the treatment of localized disease as adjuvant therapy postoperatively or following radiotherapy, in an attempt to eradicate any undetected metastatic disease and increase the likelihood of cure. Only patients whose cancers have a high or intermediate risk of recurrence are selected for adjuvant chemotherapy since it is not desirable to expose patients whose disease may already have been cured by surgery or radiotherapy to the toxicity and unpleasantness of cytotoxic chemotherapy.

In colorectal cancer for example, the role of adjuvant chemotherapy is well established for Dukes' C carcinoma where several large trials have shown a reduction in the recurrence and death rate. In patients with Dukes' B or less advanced disease the benefit of adjuvant chemotherapy is less well defined.

Neo-adjuvant chemotherapy

In neo-adjuvant chemotherapy, chemotherapy is given before local therapy, often preoperatively, in order to reduce tumour size and facilitate surgical removal. The use of neo-adjuvant chemotherapy has been found of particular value in Ewing's sarcoma, one of the most common bone tumours, when it allows limb-sparing surgery as an alternative to amputation.

High dose chemotherapy

In vitro studies have demonstrated a clear dose–response relationship for chemotherapy-sensitive tumours; however, the profound toxicity of chemotherapy, in particular permanent or prolonged myeloablation, has been the major obstacle to delivering high dose chemotherapy and exploiting this phenomenon.

A technique has now been developed where patients are treated with chemotherapy and haemopoietic growth factors (such as lenograstim or filgrastim) which cause the release of progenitor or stem cells (from the bone marrow) into the peripheral blood. These peripheral blood stem cells (PBSC) can then be harvested or removed from the circulation and stored for subsequent re-infusion into the patient as a means of haemopoietic rescue following high dose chemotherapy. Clinical trials are still ongoing to determine their optimal role and scheduling in the treatment of subgroups of patients with solid tumours.

Synchronous chemoradiation

The use of chemotherapy alongside radical radiotherapy has been investigated in several cancers, including those of the cervix, head and neck and lung. Studies to date have indicated superior results compared to either radiation alone or radiation followed by chemotherapy. It is thought that synchronous chemotherapy may act chiefly as a radiosensitizer and allow shortening of radiation therapy time. Further studies using more intensive radiation or chemotherapy programmes will be needed to determine its future role (Tobias & Ball 2001).

Adverse effects of cytotoxic drugs

Most cytotoxic drugs have been developed because of their effect on dividing cells, and as a result rapidly proliferating normal tissue is at risk. Myelosuppression is frequently the dose-limiting toxicity with these compounds. Neutropenia and thrombocytopenia place patients at risk of life-threatening infection and bleeding, respectively.

The other acute adverse effects occurring most frequently include nausea and vomiting, mucositis, anorexia and alopecia. Individual drugs will also give rise to specific adverse effects, some of which may not be reversible on stopping treatment. Cardiotoxicity, nephrotoxicity and pulmonary toxicity, which are specific to the chemotherapeutic agent or class, may depend on cumulative drug exposure, the schedule of administration and previous therapy. Long-term side-effects include infertility due to suppression of ovarian and testicular function and occasionally the induction of a secondary malignancy.

Chemotherapy-related toxicity is an important issue. Not only can it result in prolonged hospitalization and a reduction in patients' quality of life, but also successful treatment can be compromised. A reduction in dose intensity, the dose of cytotoxic delivered for unit time, because of dose reductions or treatment delays, can result in reduced response rates and survival.

Drug analogues

Significant progress has been made in reducing the morbidity of cytotoxic drugs. One approach has been to develop analogues of existing agents which have an improved toxicity profile. Carboplatin, an analogue of cisplatin, is not associated with the severe nephrotoxicity and neurotoxicity seen with the parent compound. However, it is itself more likely to give rise to myelosuppression.

Drug formulations

Liposomal formulations of existing drugs have also been used with some success, notably a Stealth liposome of the anthracycline doxorubicin. The advantage is that nearly all the drug remains encapsulated within the liposome which means reduced plasma levels of free drug and therefore fewer adverse effects compared to conventional doxorubicin. Preferential uptake into tumour cells also results in less toxicity, with notably reduced cardiotoxicity.

Chemo-specific adjunctive treatments

Both ifosfamide and cyclophosphamide are metabolized to the inactive acrolein which is responsible for bladder toxicity. The co-administration of mesna, a sulphydryl-containing compound which binds to acrolein, has reduced the incidence of haemorrhagic cystitis associated with ifosfamide and high dose cyclophosphamide.

Calcium leucovorin or folinic acid is a reduced form of folic acid. Competing directly with methotrexate for transport into cells, folinic acid is effectively used as a form of rescue when high doses of methotrexate are used.

Drug resistance

Failure to achieve cure or long-term survival with chemotherapy commonly results from resistance within the tumour cell population.

Clones of cells can be inherently resistant at the outset (intrinsic resistance), while other tumour cells appear to acquire resistance after several treatment cycles. Furthermore, resistance may involve more than one drug, when it is termed multidrug resistance.

In the laboratory, malignant cells have demonstrated a variety of methods of resisting the effect of cytotoxic drugs. Cells may develop the ability to reduce intracellular concentration of cytotoxic drug via the membrane pump, p-glycoprotein. Some cells show the ability to deactivate the drug enzymatically. In other instances the cells develop a mechanism for repairing damaged DNA.

A number of strategies have been pursued in an attempt to overcome the problem of drug resistance including developing new (non cross-resistant) agents and using different dosages and schedules of administration.

Pharmaceutical care of patients receiving chemotherapy

The role of the oncology pharmacist was made explicit by the publication of national cancer service standards in England (Department of Health 2000). Alongside the safe preparation of cytotoxic drugs which includes dose verification for the individual patient, pharmacists have a clear and acknowledged role in assisting the production of evidence-based guidelines or protocols for drugs plus an increasing role in the prescribing of supportive drugs used in symptom control.

Prescription verification

Table 50.5 summarizes the key factors which need to be taken into consideration to ensure optimal treatment for patients. Although each cytotoxic drug varies in its particular spectrum of toxicity, some general precautions can be taken to minimize the risk of predictable adverse effects occurring.

Cumulative dosing

The use of doxorubicin is limited by a dose-dependent cardiomyopathy. A number of other factors have been implicated, including treatment schedule, patient age and pre-existing cardiac disease, but dose is the most important. The maximum recommended cumulative dose is 550 mg/m^2 or 400 mg/m^2 for patients who have received radiotherapy to the mediastinum, and the pharmacist will have to monitor treatment closely to make sure this cumulative dose is not exceeded throughout the patient's lifetime.

Dose modification or delay

Appropriate investigations must be carried out before treatment to ensure that patients are fit for chemotherapy; in particular, the patient's haematological, renal and hepatic function should be investigated. For some cytotoxic drugs it may be necessary to adjust the dose in the presence of renal or hepatic impairment to ensure that delayed excretion or reduced metabolism does not result in toxicity (Table 50.6).

If the bone marrow does not recover sufficiently between cycles of treatment then a dose reduction or a delay in treatment may be necessary. In general, patients with a white cell count below 3×10^9/l or a platelet count below 100×10^9/l should not be given myelosuppressive cytotoxics.

Drug interactions

Prescriptions for cancer chemotherapy are often complex, involving combinations of both parenteral and oral cytotoxic drugs, intravenous fluids and other supportive therapies. The potential for drug interactions to arise is considerable. However, care is required when assessing the clinical significance of potential drug interactions. A documented interaction does not

Table 50.5   Pharmaceutical care: monitoring chemotherapy

Diagnosis	• Is prescription in accordance with treatment protocol/established regimen?
Protocol	
Regimen	
Weight/height	• Calculate body surface area • Verify dose • Calculate total exposure to drugs with cumulative toxicity

Clinical factors:
    Age
    Haematological status
    Renal/hepatic function
    Concurrent disease
    Allergy
    Toxicity from previous cycle
	• Is dose adjustment required?
	
	• Are there any contraindications to planned therapy?

Administration	• Is the route appropriate? • Does the patient have suitable venous access? • Has treatment been scheduled correctly?
Interactions	• Concurrent medication? • Pharmaceutical interactions with intravenous drugs or infusion fluids?
Supportive care	• Has appropriate supportive therapy been prescribed? • Ensure appropriate monitoring is completed
Documentation	• Has treatment been accurately documented?

necessarily imply that drugs should not be used together but will necessitate close monitoring of the patient.

Patient information and counselling

All patients must be provided with basic information about their treatment, including any anticipated side effects. Some patients will wish to receive more detailed information, others will not (Leydon et al 2000). Careful counselling is required, particularly with adolescents, to encourage compliance with oral chemotherapy. Clear written information must also be provided alongside supplementary verbal counselling. Patients must understand the different medications, specific use and duration of treatment. The last point is particularly important to patients and other health care professionals in order to prevent highly potent cytotoxic medicines from being inadvertently continued beyond their intended course.

Symptom control

Nausea and vomiting

Nausea and vomiting are probably felt by most patients to be the most distressing side-effects of chemotherapy, and in extreme cases poor symptom control can result in patients refusing further treatment. In selecting an appropriate antiemetic regimen, relevant factors include the emetogenic potential of the chemotherapy drugs prescribed (Table 50.7), the putative mechanism(s) of inducing emesis, and the likely onset and duration of symptoms. Individual patient characteristics also have to be taken into consideration. For example, sickness in pregnancy and travel sickness are well recognized predisposing factors which increase a patient's susceptibility to emesis following chemotherapy treatment. Differences in the severity of emesis can also occur between patients receiving the same type of chemotherapy and even between treatment cycles in the same patient.

The 5-hydroxytryptamine type 3 ($5\text{-}HT_3$) receptor antagonists granisetron, ondansetron and tropisetron have become the gold standard in the management of acute chemotherapy-induced nausea and vomiting when treating patients with highly emetogenic chemotherapeutic regimens such as those including cisplatinum. They are most effective in dealing with acute emesis (less than 24 hours duration) when combined with dexamethasone. It is important to achieve optimal control of nausea and vomiting at the outset to

Table 50.6 Cytotoxic drugs requiring monitoring or dose adjustment depending on organ dysfunction

	Monitoring or dose adjustment required	
	Renal	Hepatic
Bleomycin	✓	
Carboplatin	✓	
Cisplatin	✓	
Cyclophosphamide	✓	
Dacarbazine		✓
Dactinomycin		✓
Docetaxel		✓
Doxorubicin		✓
Epirubicin		✓
Etoposide	✓	
Gemcitabine	✓	✓
Ifosfamide	✓	
Irinotecan	✓	✓
Methotrexate	✓	
Mitomycin		✓
Mitoxantrone (mitozantrone)		✓
Nitrosoureas	✓	
Paclitaxel		✓
Raltitrexed	✓	✓
Vinca alkaloids		✓
Vinorelbine		✓

Pain control

Drug therapy remains the cornerstone of effective pain management but appears undertreated (Mayor 2000), thus highlighting the importance of regular patient assessment and appropriate dose or drug treatment changes. For example, patients experiencing intolerable side-effects to morphine may be transferred to transdermal fentanyl skin patches. Analgesia should be prescribed both regularly and for breakthrough pain, and laxatives should be prescribed to prevent constipation.

The route of administration is also important. When patients are unable to manage oral medication, it is important to assess the use of alternative routes such as the rectal, subcutaneous, epidural and transdermal routes.

Bone marrow suppression

Myelosuppression following chemotherapy is common, and for some patients profound. The risk of systemic infection can be reduced by good oral hygiene and mouth care using antiseptic mouthwashes and antifungal prophylaxis (prophylactic antibiotics are not routinely indicated). Patients must be advised to immediately report symptoms of infection and bruising. Platelets may be required, but fever or other evidence of infection occurring in a neutropenic patient, where the neutrophil count is less than $0.8 \times 10^9/l$, must be aggressively treated with broad spectrum intravenous antibiotics to prevent overwhelming infection developing.

The duration and depth of neutropenia can be dramatically reduced by the administration of haemopoietic growth factors which stimulate neutrophil

avoid anticipatory symptoms which can prove very difficult to treat.

The route of administration for antiemetics is an important consideration. With intravenous chemotherapy it may be simpler to administer all treatments by the intravenous route. Alternative routes other than oral which may be useful when vomiting occurs include the rectal and buccal route. Because of the risk of bleeding, the rectal route should be avoided when patients are thrombocytopenic.

Table 50.7 Emetogenic potential of cytotoxic drugs

High	Moderate	Low
Cisplatin	Carboplatin	Bleomycin
Dacarbazine	Carmustine	Etoposide
Ifosfamide	Cyclophosphamide	Fluorouracil
Chlormethine (mustine)	Dactinomycin	Gemcitabine
	Docetaxel	Methotrexate
	Doxorubicin	Vinblastine
	Epirubicin	Vincristine
	Irinotecan	Vindesine
	Melphalan	Vinorelbine
	Mitomycin	
	Mitoxantrone (mitozantrone)	**Oral**
		Chlorambucil
	Paclitaxel	Cyclophosphamide
	Raltitrexed	Melphalan

production and in cases of severe neutropenia, effectively rescue the patient. Once the patient's neutrophil count has recovered sufficiently, their use may be safely discontinued. These agents may also be used prophylactically in patients with a high risk of febrile neutropenia before receiving chemotherapy.

Blood transfusions are commonly required by patients at some stage of their treatment due to anaemia. Alternatively, erythropoietin may be useful in some patients receiving platinum-containing chemotherapy to shorten the period of anaemia and improve the patient's quality of life.

Extravasation

Extreme care must be taken when administering cytotoxic drugs parenterally.

Extravasation – the accidental leakage of an intravenous drug into the surrounding tissue – can cause pain, erythema and severe local necrosis, resulting in permanent tissue damage. The patient must be asked to immediately report any pain or a stinging sensation at the injection site since the degree of damage is determined by the amount of drug extravasated and the speed at which it is detected. If extravasation is suspected, the administration of further chemotherapy must stop and remedial treatment commenced as soon as possible. Drugs most likely to cause problems on extravasation are listed in Table 50.8.

In-patient versus out-patient setting

The majority of patients receive chemotherapy in the out-patient clinic or day care setting, where cytotoxics are administered by intravenous bolus injection or short intravenous infusion at 3 or 4 week intervals. More complex treatment, such as cisplatinum-containing regimens, which require pre-hydration with intravenous fluids and aggressive use of antiemetics, will require in-patient treatment.

Domiciliary treatment

Oral cytotoxic drugs can be taken at home, but consideration must be given to the possibility of poor compliance or reduced bioavailability from impaired absorption or vomiting. Drugs such as interferon can also be given at home with many patients coping well with their self-administered subcutaneous injections.

Ambulatory or home chemotherapy

The development of indwelling central venous catheters has enabled suitable patients to receive continuous ambulatory chemotherapy via a portable pump or infusion device in the home environment. The range of devices has grown but one of the most patient friendly is the disposable elastomeric pump or infusor. Housing a balloon reservoir which is filled with drug (usually 5-fluorouracil), it infuses the chemotherapy at a predetermined rate over a period of up to 7 days. Although patients still visit the out-patient clinic at regular intervals, it allows them the freedom to receive most of their treatment at home. As patients are taught how to change and manage their infusor devices, patient counselling becomes crucial since patient confidence and skill in handling infusors at home needs to be discussed with each individual. Figure 50.3 shows a typical infusor device.

Monitoring anticancer therapy

As well as desirable outcomes, treatment with chemotherapy may result in a variety of undesirable outcomes; both require careful monitoring.

Monitoring toxicity

The toxicity resulting from treatment is routinely assessed following each cycle of chemotherapy, and may result in therapy being modified on subsequent cycles, for example a dose reduction, a delay in treatment or, in some cases, an alternative treatment. A number of international rating scales are available for rating predictable acute reactions arising from chemotherapy, including that of the World Health Organization (Table 50.9). Standardizing the assessment of treatment-related toxicity in this way allows comparison to be made between published reports of clinical trials.

Table 50.8 Classification of drugs according to their potential to damage tissue if extravasated	
Vesicant drugs	Irritant drugs
Amsacrine	Carboplatin
Actinomycin D	Etoposide
Carmustine	Methotrexate
Dacarbazine	Mitoxantrone (mitozantrone)
Doxorubicin	
Epirubicin	
Idarubicin	
Mitomycin C	
Chlormethine (mustine)	
Paclitaxel	
Vinca alkaloids	
Vinorelbine	

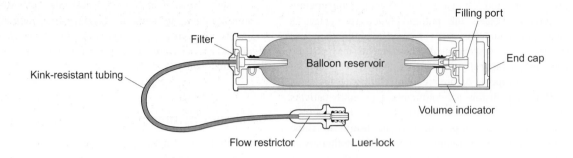

Figure 50.3 Baxter infusor pump (with kind permission from Baxter Healthcare Ltd.; Allwood et al 1997, p. 82).

Monitoring response to treatment

Throughout treatment, the response to therapy is closely monitored, noting changes in performance status, symptoms and objective measurements of the tumour. This may necessitate repeating some or all of the initial staging investigations. Should the initial treatment prove ineffective an alternative can then be considered without delay. Assessment of response should be formally documented before proceeding to further therapy.

Definitions of response. These have been standardized by the World Health Organization as follows:

- *Complete response or remission (CR):* disappearance of all recognizable tumour masses and/or biochemical changes directly related to the tumour and resolution of symptoms determined by two observations at least a month apart.
- *Partial response (PR):* decrease by 50% or more in all tumour masses, measured by the product of the longest × the widest perpendicular diameters for at least a month.
- *Stable disease (SD) or no change (NC):* changes smaller than those described above for PR or less than for PD for at least a month.
- *Progressive disease (PD):* occurrence of any new lesion or increase in the longest × widest perpendicular diameters of measurable disease by at least 25%.

Again, this allows comparison of results between different reported studies. An update of the WHO guidelines has been published (Therasse et al 2000) called RECIST, or, Response Evaluation Criteria in Solid Tumours. To avoid confusion it is clearly important to stipulate in trial protocols which system is to be used. Although clinical response indicates tumour sensitivity, it may not necessarily predict long-term survival nor does it measure other benefits such as quality of life.

Quality of life

Quality of life assessments can be used to quantify the subjective benefits of treatment. Although not routinely used in clinical practice, they form an important part of the evaluation process of new drugs or new regimens. Quality of life is particularly important when a prolongation of survival is not anticipated. Patient questionnaires should generally be completed before, during and after treatment. Commonly used questionnaires include that used by the European Organization for Research and Treatment of Cancer (EORTC QLQ-C30).

Acknowledgement

I gratefully acknowledge the work of Geoff Saunders, Principal Pharmacist, Clinical Services, Christie Hospital, Manchester, UK, in assisting me by producing the case studies and answers that follow.

Table 50.9   World Health Organization grading of acute and subacute toxicity

	Grade 0	Grade 1	Grade 2	Grade 3	Grade 4
Nausea/vomiting	None	Nausea	Transient vomiting	Vomiting requiring therapy	Intractable vomiting
Diarrhoea	None	Transient < 2 days	Tolerable, but > 2 days	Intolerable, requiring therapy	Haemorrhagic dehydration
Constipation	None	Mild	Moderate	Abdominal distension	Distension and vomiting
Oral	No change	Soreness/erythema	Erythema, ulcers; can eat solids	Ulcers; requires liquid diet only	Alimentation not possible
White blood cells ($\times 10^9$/l	> 4.0	3.0–3.9	2.0–2.9	1.0–1.9	< 1.0
Patelets ($\times 10^9$/l)	> 100	75–99	50–74	25–49	< 25
Haemoglobin (g/dl)	> 11.0	9.5–10.9	8.0–9.4	6.5–7.9	< 6.5
Hair	No change	Minimal hair loss	Moderate patchy alopecia	Complete alopecia, but reversible	Non-reversible alopecia

CASE STUDIES

Case 50.1

Mr D. K., a 71-year-old gentleman with metastatic carcinoma of the colon, was admitted for his fourth cycle of second-line chemotherapy. Between cycles he has been well, his appetite has been good, his bowels have not given him any problems, and his weight has been stable. The treatment planned for Mr D. K. is as follows:

Atropine 250 Micrograms S. C.
Sodium chloride 0.9% 250 ml   irinotecan 350 mg i. v. 90 min
Dextrose 5%   250 ml   l-folinic acid 175 mg i. v. 2hr
Sodium chloride 0.9% 100 ml   5FU   800 mg i.v. 15min
Sodium chloride 0.9% 1000 ml   5FU   1800 mg i.v.   15hr
Sodium chloride 0.9% 1000 ml   5FU   1800 mg i.v.   15hr
Sodium chloride 0.9% 1000 ml   5FU   1800 mg i.v.   15hr

Questions

1. Comment on the use of atropine as premedication before the chemotherapy.
2. What medications will Mr D. K. require on discharge and what counselling points would you include?

Answers

1. Irinotecan can cause an acute cholinergic syndrome in 9% of patients. This occurs during or within the first 24 hours after irinotecan infusion and is characterized by early diarrhoea and other symptoms such as sweating, abdominal cramping, lachrymation, myosis and salivation. These symptoms resolve after administering atropine 250 micrograms s.c. Atropine should not routinely be administered to all patients due to receive irinotecan; however, the prophylactic use of atropine is recommended with subsequent doses of irinotecan in patients who have suffered an acute and severe cholinergic reaction.

2. In addition to antiemetics, Mr D. K. should receive a quantity of loperamide and a broad spectrum antibiotic together with instructions for their use should they become necessary. All patients should be made aware of the risk of developing delayed diarrhoea which can occur at any time between 24 hours after the irinotecan infusion and the start of the next cycle. At the first sign of diarrhoea Mr D. K. should commence loperamide 2 mg every 2 hours continuing for at least 12 hours after the last episode of diarrhoea. In addition he should drink large amounts of fluids such as water, soda water, soup or rehydration fluids. If the diarrhoea persists for 48 hours or if he develops a fever then Mr D. K. should contact the hospital so that he can be instructed to commence the course of antibiotics and how to further manage his condition.

Case 50.2

Mr M. M., a 68-year-old man with non-small cell lung cancer has been admitted for his first course of MIC (mitomycin, ifosfamide, cisplatin) chemotherapy. Currently he feels well in himself although it is noted he has a glomerular filtration rate (GFR) of 50 ml/min, indicating mild renal impairment. His body surface area is 1.92 m². The treatment planned for Mr M. M. is as follows:

Mitomycin C 6 mg/m² = 11 mg
Ifosfamide 3 g/m² = 5.5 g with mesna
Cisplatin 50 mg/m² = 95 mg

Questions

1. What dose adjustments if any would you recommend?
2. How would you counsel the patient about the expected side-effects of the chemotherapy?

Answers

1. Cisplatin is potentially nephrotoxic. It is usually administered at full dose only if the patient's GFR is above 60 ml/min. If the GFR is below 60 ml/min cisplatin should be used with extreme caution and the individual protocol consulted for dosage modifications. Between 60 and 40 ml/min cisplatin can be dosed at 1 mg for every 1 ml/min clearance; if the GFR is below 40 ml/min cisplatin it is not generally used, and alternative agents are prescribed. Mr M. M.'s GFR is 50 ml/min so a more appropriate dose for him is 50 mg. No dosage adjustments are necessary for ifosfamide or mitomycin C at this level of renal function.

2. Mr M. M. needs to be counselled about the general side-effects of chemotherapy as well as the more specific ones he is likely to encounter. In general all patients receiving a course of chemotherapy are at risk from the effects on the bone marrow so he needs to know that he may be more prone to infection and if he develops a sore throat, cough, fever or a temperature above 37.5°C then he should contact the hospital without delay. Other adverse effects on the bone marrow can cause anaemia with excessive tiredness and sometimes breathlessness, or if the platelet count is lowered then he may develop nose bleeds, bruising or bleeding gums. Nausea and vomiting can usually be controlled with antiemetics. However, if, despite this, he continues to feel sick, he should contact either his GP or the hospital so that the antiemetic regimen can be reassessed.

   Side-effects specific to the MIC regimen include hair thinning, tingling or numbness in fingers and toes, cystitis, lethargy, tinnitus, mouth ulcers, and taste disturbances. It should be pointed out that all these effects are temporary and should disappear after treatment is completed.

Case 50.3

Mr M. B., a 30-year-old man, was admitted for his third course of 3-day BEP (bleomycin, etoposide, cisplatinum) chemotherapy (bleomycin 30 000 i.u. $d_{1,8,15}$, etoposide 165 mg/m^2d_{1-3}, cisplatin 50 mg/m^2 d_{1+2} for treatment of his good-prognosis testicular teratoma. After his last treatment he was slightly constipated, his backache was better but he had indigestion post chemotherapy. For the last week he has been an in-patient at his local district general hospital and on discharge had a low neutrophil count. On examination his general condition was good, his acne had increased, he had increased pigmentation on his back and complained of swelling and tenderness of his finger tips. It was decided to continue BEP chemotherapy as planned and follow this up with a course of granulocyte-colony stimulating factor (G-CSF).

Questions

1. What adjustments should be made to the chemotherapy regimen?

2. Comment on the appropriateness of the use of G-CSF.
3. What is the likely cause of the patient's indigestion post chemotherapy and how might it be avoided in the future?

Answers

1. The most serious delayed effect of bleomycin is interstitial pneumonia. Although this toxicity is dose related and limiting, lifetime exposure to bleomycin reduces the risk of developing pulmonary changes, some patients may develop changes at an early stage. Skin pigmentation and hyperkeratosis are both signs of bleomycin toxicity and, while in themselves not harmful, they are an indication that the patient is at increased risk of developing pulmonary changes. The planned bleomycin treatment should be cancelled with an alternative agent substituted if appropriate.

2. Both filgrastim and lenograstim are forms of recombinant human granulocyte-colony stimulating factor (G-CSF) that are licensed for the reduction of the incidence and severity of neutropenia post chemotherapy. Prophylactic use of G-CSF is warranted where the likelihood of developing neutropenic sepsis is greater than 40%. As Mr M. B. had an episode of neutropenia requiring hospitalization after his last course of chemotherapy, prophylactic use of G-CSF at a dose of approximately 150 micrograms/m^2 is justified.

3. Standard antiemetic regimens for cisplatin-based chemotherapy contain a 5-HT$_3$ antagonist combined with a corticosteroid. While the majority of patients will tolerate this combination, some will develop the gastric side-effects typical of corticosteroids, particularly if the course of chemotherapy has been given over a number of days. Mr M. B. would have been given corticosteroids for at least 5 days precipitating his symptoms of indigestion. Further use of corticosteroids should be covered with concomitant use of either an H$_2$ antagonist or a proton pump inhibitor.

Case 50.4

Mrs R. H., a 54-year-old lady with stage III poorly differentiated adenocarcinoma of the ovary, has been admitted for her second cycle of carboplatin and paclitaxel 175 mg/m^2 treatment. She has been generally well for the last 3 weeks with some nausea in the first few days post chemotherapy and pains in the backs of her legs, especially in the last week. Mrs R. H. is 1.68 m in height, weighs 62 kg and has a GFR of 73 ml/min.

Questions

1. What has caused Mrs R. H.'s leg pains and how might they be treated in the future?
2. Calculate the dose of paclitaxel and carboplatin to be given.
3. What antiemetic regimen would be appropriate for this patient?

Answers

1. Paclitaxel causes arthalgia or myalgia in 60% of patients and is severe in 13% of patients. Most commonly patients complain of pain in the calf muscles occuring up to 2 weeks after chemotherapy treatment. These pains often respond to

treatment with a non-steroidal anti-inflammatory agent and do not usually recur once treatment with paclitaxel is completed.

2. In common with most cytotoxic agents, the dose calculation of paclitaxel is usually based on the patient's surface area. In Mrs R. H.'s case, her surface area works out as 1.7 m^2 giving a dose of 297.5 mg (round off to 300 mg) paclitaxel. The dose of carboplatin can be individualized according to the patient's renal function using the Calvert formula where the dose in mg equals the glomerular filtration rate (GFR) in ml/min plus a non-renal constant of 25 multiplied by the target area under the curve (AUC), i.e. (GFR + 25) × AUC. For example, if the target AUC was 5, then in Mrs R. H.'s case the dose would be (73 + 25) × 5 = 490 mg.

3. The antiemetics that Mrs R. H. requires should be chosen according to the expected emetogenicity of the chemotherapy regimen she is receiving. This choice should be further refined according to her response to antiemetic therapy. Carboplatin will cause emesis in approximately 60–90% of patients in the absence of effective antiemetic prophylaxis; similarly paclitaxel will cause emesis in 10–30% of patients without effective prophylaxis. The combined emetogenicity of the two drugs will cause emesis in > 90% of patients without adequate prophylaxis. Mrs R. H. must receive a 5-HT$_3$ antagonist in combination with a corticosteroid, for example ondansetron 8 mg twice daily or granisetron 1 mg up to twice daily combined with dexamethasone up to 8 mg twice daily for 48 hours.

REFERENCES

Advanced Colorectal Cancer Meta-Analysis Project 1998 Efficacy of intravenous continuous infusion of fluorouracil compared with bolus administration in advanced colorectal cancer. Journal of Clinical Oncology 16: 301–308

Allwood M, Stanley A, Wright P 1997 The cytotoxics handbook, 3rd edn. Radcliffe Medical Press, Oxford

Cancer Research Campaign 2000 CRC CancerStats: mortality – UK July 2000. Cancer Research Campaign

Castelao J E, Yuan J-M, Skipper P L et al 2001 Gender and smoking-related bladder cancer risk. Journal of the National Cancer Institute 93: 538–545

Department of Health 2000 Manual of cancer service standards, December 2000. Department of Health, London

Grunfeld E A, Ramirez A J, Maher E J et al 2000 Chemotherapy for advanced breast cancer: what influences oncologists' decision-making? British Journal of Cancer 84(9): 1172–1178

Hoffman P C, Mauer A M, Vokes E E 2000 Lung cancer. Lancet 355: 479–485

Johnson K C 2001 Risk factors for breast cancer. British Medical Journal 322: 365

Leydon G M, Boulton M, Moynihan C et al 2000 Cancer patients' information needs and information seeking behaviour: in depth interview study. British Medical Journal 320: 909–913

Maric R N, Cheng K K 2001 Overweight and adenocarcinoma of the oesophagus. British Medical Journal 322: 366

Mayor S 2000 Cancer pain still undertreated. British Medical Journal 321: 1309

Therasse P, Arbuck S G, Eisenhauer E A et al 2000 New guidelines to evaluate the response to treatment in solid tumours. Journal of the National Cancer Institute 92: 205–216

Tobias J S, Ball D 2001 Synchronous chemoradiation for squamous carcinomas. British Medical Journal 322: 876–878

FURTHER READING

Allwood M, Stanley A, Wright P 1997 The cytotoxics handbook, 3rd edn. Radcliffe Medical Press, Oxford

Chung-Faye G A, Kerr D J 2000 ABC of colorectal cancer: innovative treatment for colon cancer. British Medical Journal 321: 1397–1399

Department of Health 2000 The NHS cancer plan September

2000. Department of Health, London

Devita V T, Hellman S, Rosenberg S A 1997 Cancer – principles and practice of oncology, 5th edn. Lippincott, Philadelphia

Finley R S, Balmer C (eds.) 1998 Concepts in oncology therapeutics, 2nd edn. American Society of Health-System Pharmacists, Bethesda, MD

Rheumatoid arthritis and osteoarthritis

51

A. Alldred   E. A. Kay

KEY POINTS

Rheumatoid arthritis

- About 2% of men and 5% of women over the age of 55 years have rheumatoid arthritis (RA).
- The cause of RA is unclear.
- The aims of treatment are to relieve pain and inflammation, prevent joint destruction and preserve functional ability.
- Non-steroidal anti-inflammatory drugs (NSAIDs), including COX-2 NSAIDs, are the major group of drugs used for the relief of pain and inflammation in RA. COX-2 NSAIDs may reduce the incidence of gastrointestinal adverse events associated with these drugs.
- Patients with RA should be treated early and aggressively with disease modifying antirheumatic drugs (DMARDs). Combination therapy may be useful in patients unresponsive to monotherapy.
- Biological tumour necrosis factor (TNF) blockade therapies are a major advance in the management of RA. They are particularly useful in patients with resistant disease.
- Patients with RA must be educated and counselled appropriately.

Osteoarthritis

- Osteoarthritis (OA) is uncommon in people aged less than 45 years, but the prevalence increases up to the age of 65 years when at least 50% of the population have radiographic evidence in at least one joint.
- A wide variety of factors predispose to and promote OA, including genetic factors, age and joint loading.
- Lifestyle changes such as maintaining optimal weight and undertaking regular exercises are an essential part of treatment.
- Regular simple analgesics are affective. Oral NSAIDs may be of value in some patients.
- Intra-articular corticosteroids and hyaluronic acid derivatives may be useful in patients with OA of the knee.

RHEUMATOID ARTHRITIS

Rheumatoid arthritis (RA) is one of the most common chronic inflammatory conditions, affecting the population worldwide. It is a progressive disease of the synovial lining of peripheral joints characterized by symmetrical inflammation leading to potentially deforming polyarthritis and a wide spectrum of extra-articular features (Table 51.1). The disease is classified according to the 1987 revised American College of Rheumatology (ACR) criteria for the classification of RA.

Epidemiology

Approximately 1% of the worldwide adult population is affected by RA, with about twice as many female sufferers as male (Markenson 1991). The increased frequency in women is more pronounced in the UK with a female to male ratio of 3:1. The prevalence of RA increases with age in both sexes with nearly 5% of women and 2% of men over 55 years of age affected. The age of onset is typically around 30–50 years, and reaches its peak in the fourth decade. Some ethnic variation has also been observed in the prevalence of RA. Among rural black Africans the prevalence is low, about 0.1%, compared to 3% in Caucasians. Comparative studies among urban and rural populations suggest that environmental factors associated with modern urban life may also be important.

Table 51.1   Extra-articular features of rheumatoid arthritis

Common	Uncommon
Anaemia	Pleural effusion
Nodules	Pulmonary fibrosis
Muscle wasting	Pericarditis
Dry eyes (Sjögren's syndrome)	Scleritis
Depression	Systemic vasculitis
Osteoporosis	Mitral valve and conduction defects
Episcleritis	
Carpal tunnel syndrome	
Leg ulcers	
Lymphadenopathy	
Nail-fold vasculitis	
Peripheral sensory neuropathy	

Socio-economic impact of RA

RA is a disease that is associated with major socio-economic implications for the population it affects. The articular and extra-articular progressive nature of RA leads to both significant patient morbidity and mortality. Patients with RA have six times the probability of severe limitation of activity, four times as many restricted days and 10 times the work disability rate of the general population. Over a period of 6 years the average earnings of a patient with RA will be reduced by approximately 60% and after 10 years of disease duration more than 50% of patients are unable to work at all (Wolfe 1990). Survival rates among patients with RA are lower than those in the general population. Median life expectancy is reduced by 7 years for men and 3 years for women. These reduced survival rates are similar to those observed for Hodgkin's disease, diabetes and stroke.

Aetiology

The cause of RA remains unclear. Although there is abundant evidence that RA is immune-mediated, it is still not clear whether it is primarily an autoimmune disease. It is possible that many different arthritogenic stimuli activate the immune response in the susceptible host. Whether the initiating agent is an infection, a self-antigen or an environmental factor remains unproven (Buckley 1997).

Epidemiological data support the case for both environmental and genetic factors causing RA. Research in twins and other genetic studies suggest the genetic component is at best 30% (Hazes & Silman 1990). However, RA does not tend to aggregate in related families, indicating genetics play only a small role in disease susceptibility (Markenson 1991). The evidence of an association between the antigen HLA-DR4 and RA is much stronger. The relative risk for an individual with HLA-DR4 to develop the disease is between 2.0 and 6.0. In American whites, 60–70% of RA patients are positive for HLA-DR4. This seems to be particularly important in severe forms of the disease. The frequency of HLA-DR4 among Dutch patients with severe extra-articular disease is greater than 90%.

The similarity of RA to other arthritides such as Lyme disease for which an infectious agent has been identified has prompted the search for similar candidates. Epstein–Barr virus has been linked to RA for over 10 years. Of patients with RA, 80% have a circulating antibody directed against antigens specific for Epstein–Barr virus, and the autoantibody response in RA enhances the response to these antigens. Parvoviruses (small DNA viruses that cause disease in many species),

particularly B19, have been linked to RA. Mycobacteria have also been linked to RA because these bacteria express heat shock proteins, which are the arthritogenic factors of adjuvant arthritis in rats.

Pathophysiology

RA is characterized by the infiltration of a variety of inflammatory cells into the joint. The synovial membrane becomes highly vascularized, synovial fibroblasts proliferate and inflammatory cells release numerous cytokines and growth factors into the joint. These agents subsequently cause synovial cells to release proteolytic enzymes resulting in destruction of bone and cartilage (Cawston 1998).

The current view is that chronic inflammation is initiated by antigen induced activation of T lymphocytes which accumulate within the joint (Cawston 1998). Mast cells, macrophages and synovial fibroblasts are also released which produce inflammatory mediators such as tumour necrosis factor (TNF) and interleukin-1 (IL-1). TNF is closely linked with the proinflammatory cytokine network in RA. These mediators can induce matrix-degrading activities that eventually lead to joint destruction. These activities include the activation of synovial fibroblasts to produce collagenases and metalloproteinases to break down collagen. Other cytokines such as IL-6 and granulocyte macrophage colony stimulating factor also participate in the inflammatory cascade. There is a paucity of CD8-positive suppressor T lymphocytes and natural killer cells, whose function it is to 'turn off' the immune response, and there is a deficiency of lymphokines (e.g. interleukin-2), which suggest that both the humoral and cellular responses are incomplete. The initiating antigen thus triggers an aberrant response, which becomes self-perpetuating, long after the offending antigen has been cleared.

Sustained inflammation leads to hypertrophy of the synovium, and the formation of 'pannus', which spreads over the surface of the joint causing erosive destruction of the cartilage and bone. The presence of persistent synovitis causes an effusion consisting of synovial fluid rich in proteins and inflammatory cells. The extra-articular features of the disease may be due to systemic circulation of these immune complexes.

Clinical manifestations

The diagnosis of RA is based on criteria first developed by the American Rheumatism Association in 1958, and subsequently modified in 1988 (Table 51.2). These criteria were designed principally for disease classification, and differences in their interpretation may partly explain variable incidence figures.

Table 51.2   Classification of rheumatoid arthritis

1. Morning stiffness	Duration > 1 h lasting > 6 weeks
2. Arthritis of at least three areas	Soft tissue swelling or exudation > 6 weeks
3. Arthritis of hand joints	Wrist, metacarpophalangeal joints or proximal interphalangeal joints lasting > 6 weeks
4. Symmetrical arthritis	At least one area, lasting > 6 weeks
5. Rheumatoid nodules	As observed by physician
6. Serum rheumatoid factor	As assessed by a method positive in less than 5% of control subjects
7. Radiographic changes	As seen on anteriposterior films of wrists and hands

Presence of four of the above criteria = diagnosis of rheumatoid arthritis

The course of RA is highly variable, and although it is primarily a disease of the synovial joints it can affect many organ systems. The disease is characterized by flares and remissions. Approximately 20% of patients achieve remission after a short illness with no further disease activity, 25% obtain remission with mild residual disease, 45% have persistent activity with variable progressive deformity, and 10% progress to complete disability.

Early symptoms of RA are non-specific and consist of fatigue, malaise, diffuse musculoskeletal pain and stiffness. Joint pain and loss of function are the most obvious symptoms of RA. The peripheral joints of the hands and feet are usually involved first and are usually symmetrical. The metacarpophalangeal and proximal interphalangeal joints of the hands and the metatarsophalangeal joints of the feet are affected, but the distal interphalangeal joint is usually spared. Ultimately any of the diarthrodial joints can be affected. Synovial hypertrophy and effusion cause swelling, and the affected joints are warm and tender. Affected joints cannot be fully extended or fully flexed due to tenosynovitis. Erosive changes give rise to joint instability and subluxation. Characteristic deformities include ulnar deviation, swan neck and boutonnière deformities (Fig. 51.1). The most serious long-term disability is associated with damage to the larger weight-bearing joints. Patients usually experience prolonged morning stiffness, which improves during the day, only to return at night.

The extra-articular features of RA (Table 51.1) occur in approximately 75% of seropositive patients, and are often associated with a poor prognosis.

A number of factors have been shown to be associated with a poor prognosis in RA (Table 51.3).

Investigations

The diagnosis of RA is made on presenting signs, symptoms and some biochemical investigations. The most useful of these are the inflammatory markers, for example erythrocyte sedimentation rate (ESR), C-reactive protein (CRP) and plasma viscosity (PV),

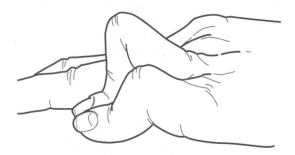

Figure 51.1   Typical Boutonnière deformity with flexion of the proximal interphalangeal joint and extension of the distal interphalangeal joint.

Table 51.3   Predictors of poor prognosis in rheumatoid arthritis

- Male with disease onset before age 50
- Disease duration > 5 years before treatment
- Number of affected joints > 20
- Lack of formal education
- Lower socioeconomic status
- Functional disability within 1 year of onset
- Extra-articular involvement
- Several co-morbidities
- Sero-positive disease
- HLA-DR4 positive

rheumatoid factor and antinuclear antibodies (ANA). A raised inflammatory marker simply confirms the presence of an inflammatory condition and is present in many disease states. A normal inflammatory marker, however, does not preclude active disease. Although these markers are not specific to RA they may be used to assess response to drug treatment as they are usually raised when the disease is active.

Rheumatoid factors are autoantibodies directed against the host immunoglobulin. Routinely performed tests only detect IgM rheumatoid factor. Rheumatoid factor is present in approximately 80% of patients with RA (sero-positive disease) and 5% of normal subjects. Extra-articular features of RA are much more common in patients with a high titre for rheumatoid factor. Antinuclear antibodies are investigated to rule out the possibility of other connective tissue disorders such as systemic lupus erthymatosus (SLE). Antinuclear antibodies are raised in 80% of patients with SLE. Neither rheumatoid factor nor antinuclear antibodies are universal diagnostic tools, but assist with the overall diagnostic picture. Other abnormal laboratory tests include an elevated alkaline phosphatase, an elevated platelet count, a decreased serum albumin level and a normochromic, normocytic anaemia.

Radiographs, mainly of the hands and feet, are used to establish the diagnosis of RA and to follow its progression. Erosions can be seen at the joint margins and loss of joint space due to erosion of cartilage and bone may be identified. In severe long-standing disease the dominant features include subluxation and deformity. The synovial fluid is not routinely analysed to establish the diagnosis of RA but typically it is yellow, watery and turbid due to a high white blood cell count, and has a low glucose content.

Treatment

The goals of management of RA are to:

- relieve pain and inflammation
- prevent joint destruction
- preserve or improve a patient's functional ability,
- maintain a patient's normal lifestyle.

Treatment of RA should begin as soon as possible as there is evidence that most patients develop joint destruction within the first 2 years of their disease (Fuchs et al 1989). Such early treatment may be realized by the use of early arthritis clinics in which patients are often seen within 2 weeks of referral from their general practitioner.

The multidisciplinary approach to treating RA patients is important. Physiotherapists, occupational therapists, clinical nurse specialists, podiatrists, social workers and pharmacists all have a crucial role. Education of patients is an important aspect of treatment. The patient should have a knowledge of the disease process, the likely prognosis and treatment strategies. Psychological aspects of the disease should also be covered. Such education is best carried out by the multidisciplinary team and should reinforce the importance of adherence to all aspects of the treatment plan.

The treatment for each patient is individualized and based on factors such as age, occupation and family responsibilities. Other considerations include the degree of disease activity and joint function, and the patient's response to previous therapy.

Non-drug treatment

Physiotherapy is a vital part of treating RA, both in acute flares of disease and in the chronic state. Heat, cold and electrotherapy help to reduce pain and swelling, and a programme of exercise strengthens joints to prevent disuse atrophy, mobilize joints to minimize deformity and increase the range of movement and functions. Occupational therapy educates patients to protect joints with the use of appliances and splints. Surgical techniques ranging from carpal tunnel decompression to major joint replacement can be effective in relieving pain and restoring function. With more aggressive and effective drug treatments becoming available, surgical intervention is likely to be less frequent.

Drug treatment

Traditionally, treatment for RA was introduced in a stepwise 'pyramidal' manner. First-line agents such as analgesics and non-steroidal anti-inflammatory drugs (NSAIDs) were used to relieve symptoms. Then second-line (e.g. sulfasalazine) and third-line (e.g. azathioprine) disease-modifying anti-rheumatic drugs (DMARDs) were added when symptoms were not adequately controlled. Used in this way, DMARDs suppress markers of disease activity and improve function but their impact on long-term disability is disappointing. The ultimate aim of treatment is to induce disease remission. This, in conjunction with the evidence of early joint destruction, has led to the much earlier use of DMARDs in RA. There is also increasing evidence that the degree and severity of joint damage is linked to corresponding levels of inflammation. Thus, treatment that suppresses underlying inflammation should produce improvements in function and bone erosions. Reduction in previously elevated CRP levels has correlated with better preservation of joint function.

Although complete disease remission is rarely achieved, assessment of CRP gives a good indication of disease activity and correlates with preservation of function, and should therefore be kept as near normal as possible.

Simple analgesics

Paracetamol, paracetamol combinations and dihydrocodeine are all useful for simple pain relief. Although they have no anti-inflammatory properties, and do not affect the disease process, they do have a place in both early and late stages of the disease. They may help with referred pain associated with muscle weakness and the general soreness associated with RA.

Non-steroidal anti-inflammatory drugs (NSAIDs)

The major pharmacological agents for the relief of pain and inflammation in rheumatic diseases are the NSAIDs. These agents have replaced the use of high-dose aspirin, as they are less toxic, longer acting and have better adherence. Their pharmacokinetic profiles are presented in Table 51.4. Although the NSAIDs differ in chemical structure, they all have similar pharmacological properties in terms of antipyretic, anti-inflammatory and analgesic action and are involved in essentially similar drug interactions (Table 51.5). The main exception to

this is the lack of antiplatelet effect with the new COX-2 NSAIDs rofecoxib and celecoxib. Short-term treatment with these agents does not inhibit platelet aggregation or prolong bleeding times.

Patient response to NSAIDs is highly variable, and therapeutic trials with several NSAIDs may be necessary to determine the best agent. Despite numerous clinical trials, differences between NSAIDs in objective measures of efficacy have not emerged. It is estimated that 60% of patients will respond to any one NSAID. If a patient does not respond it may be necessary to try several other NSAIDs before the most appropriate agent is found. It is recommended that the drug should be changed after 1 week of non-response if an analgesic effect is the desired outcome or 3 weeks if an anti-inflammatory effect is required. Aproximately 10% of patients will not find any NSAID beneficial. This variability in response may be partly explained by the differing individual effects on the inflammatory pathways, although other factors are clearly important. Patient preference and adherence are the best indicators of success. Factors that should be considered in choosing

Table 51.4 Pharmacokinetic parameters of NSAIDs

Drug	T_{max} (h)	V_d (l/kg)	$t_{1/2}$ (h)	Renal excretion (%)
Short half-life				
Aspirin	1–2	0.15	0.25	< 2
Diclofenac	1–3	0.12	1.1	> 1
Aceclofenac	1.25–3	0.25	4	66
Etodolac	2		3	
Fenoprofen	1–2	0.10	2.5	2–5
Flurbiprofen	1–2	0.10	3–4	< 15
Ibuprofen	0.5–1.5		2.1	1
Indometacin	1–2	0.12	4.6	< 15
Ketorolac	1	0.11–0.33	4–6	50–60
Ketoprofen	0.5–2	0.11	1.8	< 1
Dexketoprofen	0.25–1	0.24	2	
Long half-life				
Azapropazone	3–6	0.16	15	62
Diflunisal	1–2	0.10	5–20	< 3
Fenbufen	1–2		11	4
Meloxicam	1–2	0.16	20	3
Nabumetone	3–6	0.11	26	1
Phenylbutazone	2	0.17	50–100	1
Piroxicam	2	0.12	28	10
Sulindac	1		7 (sulindac) 16 (active sulphide)	7
Tenoxicam	1–2	0.12	60	< 1
Celecoxib	2–3	7.14	11	
Rofecoxib	2–4	1.55	17	

T_{max}, time to maximum serum concentration; V_d volume of distribution; $t_{1/2}$ elimination half-life.

Table 51.5 Drug Interactions of NSAIDs

Affected drug	Drug causing effect	Effect
Oral anticoagulants	NSAIDs	Aspirin enhances hypoprothrombinaemic effect All increase risk of gastrointestinal bleed, all have antiplatelet effects
Hypotensive agents	NSAIDs	Decreased hypotensive effect
Diuretics	NSAIDs	Decreased diuretic effect
Potassium-sparing drugs, e.g. angiotensin-converting enzyme (ACE) inhibitors, potassium-sparing diuretics	Indometacin	Hyperkalaemia
Lithium	Most NSAIDs	Increased lithium levels
Methotrexate	All NSAIDs	Increased methotrexate levels
Most NSAIDs	Probenecid	Increased NSAID concentration

a specific NSAID are relative efficacy, toxicity, concomitant drugs, concurrent disease states, patient age, renal function, dosing frequency and cost.

There is no evidence of synergism or reduced toxicity with the use of more than one NSAID. In fact there is evidence that two NSAIDs may increase the risk of gastrointestinal (GI) toxicity (Corte et al 1999). Only one agent should therefore be prescribed at a time, although a short-acting drug may be used during the day with a longer-acting preparation at night.

The NSAIDs can broadly be divided into those with a long or short plasma half-life. The site of action for NSAIDs is assumed to be within the joint space, and thus synovial fluid pharmacokinetics may be more important for efficacy than plasma kinetic profiles. However, in synovial fluid, prostaglandin concentrations remain suppressed long after an NSAID becomes undetectable. Studies on synovial fluid kinetics demonstrate that drug concentrations are more sustained and show less variability than plasma concentrations. This means that many short half-life NSAIDs need only be given twice daily to reduce pain and stiffness, while many long half-life NSAIDs take more time to reach a steady state and remain in the synovial fluid longer after treatment withdrawal. The half-lives of NSAIDs are shown in Table 51.4.

Mechanism of action of NSAIDs. The main mechanism of action of NSAIDs (Fig. 51.2) is believed to be the inhibition of the enzyme cyclo-oxygenase (COX). COX converts the fatty acid arachidonic acid into endoperoxidases, prostaglandins and thromboxanes in a cell specific manner. These prostanoids have a diverse variety of physiological functions, including protection of the GI tract, renal homeostasis, platelet aggregation, contraction of uterine smooth muscle, etc., and are widely implicated in pathological states associated with inflammation.

Initially, NSAIDs were thought to function by inhibition of a single COX. However, over the years it has been shown that there are two isoforms of COX, COX-1 and COX-2. COX-1 is thought to function mainly as a physiologic enzyme producing the prostaglandins critical for maintaining normal renal function, gastric mucosal integrity and haemostasis. COX-2 is virtually undetectable in most tissues under physiologic conditions. However, COX-2 is induced by certain inflammatory stimuli, including interleukin-1 (IL-1) and tumour necrosis factor (TNF). Marked increases in levels of COX-2 have been found at sites of inflammation in musculoskeletal disease such as rheumatoid arthritis.

NSAIDs act by direct inhibition of COX-1 and COX-2, via blockade of the COX enzyme site. The subsequent inhibition of prostaglandins reduces inflammation but also results in additional activities on platelet aggregation, renal homeostasis and gastric mucosal integrity. In addition NSAIDs interfere with a variety of other processes which may contribute to their effects. These include leukotriene synthesis, superoxide generation, lysosomal enzyme release, neutrophil function, lymphocyte function and cartilage metabolism.

NSAIDs differ in the extent and manner in which they inhibit COX-1 and COX-2 (Table 51.6). This is often expressed as the COX-2:COX-1 selectivity ratio. This ratio shows significant variation according to the source enzyme/type of cells used for the assays. Valid comparisons cannot therefore be made between different assays. It is also unclear how these ratios translate into

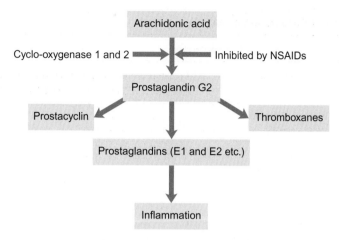

Figure 51.2 Mechanism of action of NSAIDs.

clinical practice. Having said this, the older traditional NSAIDs inhibit COX-1 and COX-2 to similar a degree. Etodolac and meloxicam inhibit COX-2 up to 50 times more than COX-1, and newer agents celecoxib and rofecoxib are even more COX-2 selective. Those NSAIDs inhibiting both COX-1 and COX-2 non-selectively would be expected to decrease joint inflammation but also cause increased bleeding tendency, gastric ulcers and renal dysfunction. NSAIDs which are more COX-2 selective might be expected to decrease inflammation but not cause increased bleeding due to gastric ulceration.

Adverse effects. NSAIDs are widely used for the treatment of inflammatory conditions. They are also the drugs most often reported to the various regulatory authorities as being responsible for adverse effects. They are associated with significant morbidity and mortality. Gastrointestinal complications are the most important adverse reactions, with other serious reactions including renal impairment, angiodema, urticaria, hepatic dysfunction, hematological abnormalities and bronchospasm.

Gastrointestinal adverse events. Gastric damage appears to require a direct mucosal effect as well as inhibition of prostaglandin biosynthesis. Impairment of mucosal defensive factors (mucus and bicarbonate secretion, mucosal blood flow) also plays a major role. Gastrointestinal (GI) adverse reactions range from superficial damage, with minor symptoms such as dyspepsia, abdominal pain, and diarrhoea, to duodenal and gastric ulceration and potentially fatal complications. Patients generally complain of nausea and indigestion, but some of those presenting with bleeding or perforation will have no history of dyspepsia or peptic ulceration. Finding the true incidence of gastrointestinal side-effects due to NSAIDs is difficult. Short- and long-term treatment with aspirin and other NSAIDs is known to induce dyspeptic symptoms in up to 60% of cases and gastroduodenal lesions in 30–50% of patients. Others report the incidence of GI side-effects to be between 8% and 34%. The prevalence of symptomatic ulcers has been reported to be between 14% and 31%, with gastric ulcers most prevalent. Serious gastrointestinal haemorrhage or perforation can be expected in 1% and may be associated with a mortality rate in excess of 10%, especially in the elderly. Less than half these patients will experience dyspeptic symptoms before the serious event.

Strategies to reduce risk of NSAID-induced ulcers

Corte et al (1999) have described major risk factors that contribute to NSAID-induced ulcers. These can be classified according to NSAID factors and patient factors (Table 51.7).

Table 51.6 COX-2 selectivity of common NSAIDs

NSAID	Ratio
Indometacin	1.78
Ibuprofen	1.69
Etodolac	0.11
Celecoxib	0.11
Rofecoxib	0.05

Expressed as a ratio of the 50% inhibitory concentration of COX-2 to the 50% inhibitory concentration of COX-1 in whole blood.

Table 51.7   Major risk factors that contribute to NSAID-induced ulcers

NSAID factor	Patient factor
Choice of NSAID	Age: older patients are at intrinsically-increased risk of ulceration
High dose NSAID	Previous history of GI damage, e.g. perforation, ulceration
Two NSAIDs e.g. low dose aspirin + NSAID	Concurrent ulcerogenic medication, e.g. steroids
Use of NSAID plus anticoagulant	Presence of chronic disease, e.g. cardiovascular disease, rheumatoid arthritis

The presence of one factor elevates the risk of GI complications but the presence of more than one risk factor is even more deleterious. In a recent meta-analysis, significant risk factors included: age > 60 years, previous history of GI complications and concomitant corticosteroid use. Patients treated with corticosteroids and NSAIDs are 15 times more likely to suffer from peptic ulcer disease than patients taking neither drug.

A number of strategies have been proposed to reduce the morbidity associated with the risk of ulcer development with NSAID treatment. These strategies are summarized below:

Choice of NSAID. A review of 12 controlled epidemiological studies examining 14 different NSAIDs, has shown there is a differential risk of GI complications between drugs (Henry et al 1996). The work demonstrated that ibuprofen (dose 1.2 g/day) has the lowest risk of GI complications and azapropazone the highest. Diclofenac also ranks low, though higher than ibuprofen, with indometacin and piroxicam intermediate risk (Table 51.8). The risk of GI gastrointestinal complications with NSAIDs is dose related and ibuprofen may be no safer than those NSAIDs defined as intermediate risk.

Table 51.8   Relative risk of major gastrointestinal complications with various NSAIDs (combined data from 12 controlled studies)

Drug	Mean rank (relative risk)
Ibuprofen	1.0
Diclofenac	2.3
Naproxen	7.0
Indometacin	8.0
Piroxicam	9.0
Azapropazone	11.7

Preventive therapy.   Preventive therapy cannot be recommended to all patients receiving NSAIDs on cost effectiveness grounds. However, in high-risk patients preventive therapy should be considered (Corte et al 1999). High-risk patients include those 65 years and over, those on concomitant medication known to increase the likelihood of upper gastrointestinal adverse events (e.g. low dose aspirin, corticosteroids and warfarin) those with serious co-morbidity (e.g. cardiovascular disease, renal or hepatic impairment, diabetes and hypertension), a previous history of gastroduodenal ulcer, gastrointestinal bleeding or gastroduodenal perforation, and those requiring prolonged use of maximum recommended doses of standard NSAIDs (NICE appraisal No 27).

Various agents have been used to reduce the incidence of NSAID-induced GI adverse effects:

- *Misoprostol* is effective in the prevention of NSAID-induced gastric and duodenal ulcers, as well as the reduction of serious upper GI complications. It has been shown to reduce serious GI complications by 40 to 50% compared to placebo.
- *Omeprazole* is also effective in the prevention of NSAID-induced GI complications. The omeprazole vs. misoprostol for NSAID-induced ulcer management (OMNIUM) study has shown that omeprazole is more effective than misoprostol in maintaining patients in remission (61% of patients treated with omeprazole vs. 48% misoprostol; Hawkey et al 1998).
- *Lansoprazole* has recently been licensed for the prophylaxis of NSAID-associated benign gastric and duodenal ulcers following a large, randomized, multicentre trial of lansoprazole vs. misoprostol and placebo in the prevention of NSAID ulcers. At 12 weeks 83% of patients on lansoprazole 30 mg remained healed compared with 79% on lansoprazole 15 mg, 88% on misoprostol and 46% on placebo.
- *Ranitidine* is the most extensively tested H_2 receptor antagonist used in the prevention of NSAID-induced GI toxicity. Ranitidine protects against NSAID-induced chronic duodenal ulceration but does not

produce a significant benefit in the prophylaxis of NSAID-induced gastric ulceration.

Use of COX-2 selective NSAIDs. COX-2 selective NSAIDs clearly have a theoretical advantage over standard NSAIDs with respect to a reduction in GI side-effects. Meloxicam, a more preferential COX-2 selective NSAID, appears to have a reduced incidence of symptomatic GI adverse events than its comparators at a dose of 7.5 mg per day. At doses of 15 mg per day, meloxicam caused GI mucosal injury intermediate between placebo and piroxicam 20 mg per day. Newer COX-2 selective NSAIDs such as rofecoxib and celecoxib are much more selective than the preferential COX inhibitors:

- *Rofecoxib.* In studies comparing rofecoxib with comparator NSAIDs, significant differences in GI toxicity were not reported from individual studies. However, by pooling the results, a lower incidence of confirmed GI ulcers, bleeds and perforations could be demonstrated compared to the other NSAIDs. Rofecoxib has been compared to naproxen in a large randomized double blind study, (Bombardier et al 2000). Over 8000 patients with rheumatoid arthritis were randomized to receive rofecoxib or naproxen. In this study rofecoxib reduced the risk of clinically important upper GI events (ulcers, perforations, obstructions and bleeds) by 54% compared with naproxen. There was a higher incidence of myocardial infarction in the rofecoxib group compared to the naproxen group. Patients taking low dose aspirin were excluded from this study. It is suggested these differences may be due to a positive protective effect of naproxen, rather than an increased incidence of myocardial infarction with rofecoxib and that these patients should have been on aspirin.
- *Celecoxib.* Celecoxib has also shown significant improvements in the incidence of gastroduodenal ulcers compared to naproxen and diclofenac. Compared to naproxen, celecoxib showed a reduction of gastroduodenal ulcers of about 20%. In a study comparing celecoxib and diclofenac there were significantly more gastroduodenal ulcers in the diclofenac group than the celecoxib group. The prevalence of gastroduodenal ulcers was 4% with celecoxib compared to 15% with diclofenac. The CLASS study randomized over 8000 patients with osteoarthritis or RA to celecoxib, ibuprofen or diclofenac (Silverstein et al 2000). Aspirin for cardiovascular protection was permitted. In all patients, celecoxib reduced the incidence of upper GI ulcer complications alone and with symptomatic ulcers compared with comparator NSAIDs. In the subgroup of patients taking aspirin, however, there was no difference between celecoxib and naproxen in the incidence of upper GI complications alone or combined with symptomatic ulcers. This suggests that

the benefit of using a COX-2 NSAID may be lost in patients taking concomitant aspirin therapy. There was no difference in the incidence of cardiovascular events between celecoxib and NSAIDs, irrespective of aspirin use.

Current data suggest that COX-2 selective NSAIDs are not always appropriate as first-line therapy in patients with arthritis. When an NSAID is required, ibuprofen remains a suitable first choice. Co-prescription with a gastroprotective agent is recommended if treatment with an NSAID is essential in older patients, those with a history of GI ulceration, bleeding or perforation, or receiving systemic corticosteroids or anticoagulant therapy. Treatment with a COX-2 selective NSAID needs to be evaluated against this approach in managing such high-risk patients. Further studies may answer such questions.

Other adverse events. Most NSAIDs can reduce creatinine clearance and produce a non-oliguric renal failure, possibly as a result of inhibition of prostaglandin synthesis in the kidney. This effect tends to be relatively minor, usually reversible and associated with long-term therapy. Those patients with impaired renal function, hepatic cirrhosis or circulatory volume depletion are most at risk. Indometacin is the most commonly reported cause of NSAID-induced renal failure and fenoprofen the NSAID most commonly associated with interstitial nephritis and nephrotic syndrome.

Asthmatic patients may develop wheezing following administration of NSAIDs. It is known that aspirin will provoke or worsen asthma in approximately 5% of patients.

Although perhaps theoretical, some NSAIDs have been shown to affect chondrocyte function in vitro in animal models. This has led to the suggestion that NSAIDs may prevent regeneration of articular cartilage and hasten the development of osteoarthritis. Other possible adverse effects of NSAIDs involve the skin, liver and bone marrow. Indometacin, in particular, can cause headache, dizziness and psychiatric disturbances. Common drug interactions are listed in Table 51.5.

Disease-modifying anti-rheumatic drugs (DMARDs)

DMARDs have a major role in managing rheumatoid arthritis, and although they have very different chemical structures and different mechanisms of action, each shows activity in managing this disabling condition.

The DMARDs currently used in clinical practice include methotrexate, sulfasalazine, injectable/oral gold, antimalarials, ciclosporin, penicillamine, azathioprine and leflunomide. The choice of DMARD by individual clinicians depends upon the balance between adverse effects and efficacy. All the DMARDs possess a slow onset of action, with response to treatment usually expected within 4–6 months.

The dose of a DMARD should generally be titrated upwards as long as side-effects allow. When the maximum recommended dose has been reached and response is inadequate an additional DMARD may be added, or the initial DMARD stopped and switched to an alternative.

The developing knowledge and understanding of the pathophysiology of RA has radically altered the therapeutic approach and use of disease modifying therapy. As stated previously, the standard approach traditionally included the use of the 'pyramid', where patients were treated first with NSAIDs, with introduction of the more toxic DMARDs at a later stage.

However, this pyramidal approach clearly failed to prevent the erosive changes and joint destruction associated with RA and has subsequently been replaced with a more aggressive approach (Machold et al 1998). The knowledge that disease progression is rapid within the first few years of onset has led to the much earlier use of DMARDs. This early use of DMARDs has also been accompanied by an increasing use of combination therapy although the evidence of benefit is unclear.

In practice initial treatment of RA is generally with a single agent. If a satisfactory response is not achieved after a 3–6 month trial with monotherapy, then combination treatment is usually given. This is most likely to be a combination of sulfasalazine and methotrexate. Patients who fail to respond will be offered other therapeutic options such as leflunomide, before finally being offered TNF blockade therapy (Fig. 51.3).

Comparison of the relative efficacy of DMARDs using a wide variety of disease symptoms and laboratory markers have been carried out over the years, although the results are inconclusive. A more useful comparison is the continuation rates of the different DMARDs. Toxicity, loss of efficacy or both, tend to limit continuation of therapy, frequently to less than 2 years. Methotrexate and sulfasalazine have the highest 5-year continuation rates of approximately 50–60%. For parenteral gold and penicillamine, 5-year continuation rates are only about 20%, and the rate for oral gold is as low as 5%.

Sulfasalazine and methotrexate are generally regarded as first-line therapies due to their improved efficacy profile (approximately 40% response rates) and high continuation rates compared to the other DMARDs.

Mechanism of action of DMARDs. The precise mechanism of action of these drugs is unclear. All the DMARDs inhibit the release of, or reduce the activity of, inflammatory cytokines. Activated T lymphocytes appear to be particularly important in this process and it is known that methotrexate, leflunomide and ciclosporin all inhibit T cells. Cytokines, which appear to be

important in the inflammatory cascade, include tumour necrosis factor (TNF) and the interleukins, IL-1, IL-2, and IL-6. There is good evidence that DMARDs inhibit these cytokines in vitro and in vivo. Leflunomide has also been shown to inhibit the proliferation of B cells with a subsequent inhibition of antibody production.

Several new biological therapies have been designed to expressly target T cells or specific cytokines. The most recent of these therapies to be used in clinical practice are the anti-TNF agents. These include the monoclonal antibody infliximab which neutralizes the activity of TNF and the soluble TNF receptor etanercept which binds to TNF and renders it biologically inactive. Interleukin-1 antagonists are also being developed for use in rheumatoid arthritis.

Use of DMARDs, including toxicity. Most DMARDs require some form of monitoring to ensure safe therapy. The majority of DMARDs can cause bone marrow and hepatic toxicity and the monitoring requirements are set out in Table 51.9.

Patient information sheets and booklets are recommended for patients taking DMARDs. Counselling should reinforce the need for adherence to monitoring requirements, the expected onset of action, potential toxicity and action to take in the event of adverse effects.

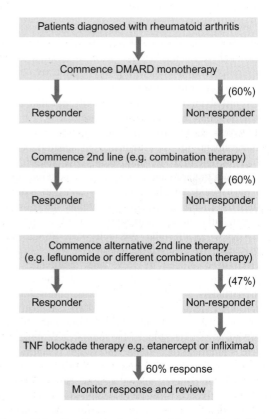

Figure 51.3 Algorithm for treatment of rheumatoid arthritis.

Table 51.9 Dosage, side-effects and monitoring guidelines for DMARDs

Drug	Dose schedule	Adverse effects	Monitoring
Sulfasalazine	Initially 500 mg once daily, Increasing in weekly steps of 500 mg to 1 g twice daily	Nausea, reversible male infertility, rashes, marrow suppressions, hepatitis	FBC fortnightly LFTs 4-weekly for 12 weeks then 3–6 monthly
Methotrexate	5–25 mg once weekly	Rashes, nausea, stomatitis, marrow suppression, hepatitis, pneumonitis	FBC fortnightly for 12 weeks then monthly LFTs monthly
Sodium aurothiomalate (gold i.m.)	10 mg test dose, then 50 mg weekly until signs of remission, then reduce frequency to monthly	Rashes, stomatitis, marrow suppression, proteinuria	FBC and urinalysis prior to each injection
Penicillamine	250–750 mg once daily (on empty stomach)	Rashes, taste disturbance, nausea, proteinuria, myasthenia, myositis, marrow suppression	FBC fortnightly until stable dose, then monthly Weekly urinalysis
Ciclosporin	2.5 mg/kg per day	Hirsutism, gingival hyperplasia, hypertension, renal impairment	Fortnightly U & E, blood pressure and urinalysis for 2 months, then 1–2 monthly. Use baseline creatinine to alter dose
Leflunomide	Loading dose 100 mg daily for 3 days then maintenance dose of 10–20 mg per day	Gastrointestinal disturbance, alopecia, liver abnormalities, hypertension, marrow suppression	FBC, U&E, LFTs and BP fortnightly during first 6 months then at least every 8 weeks thereafter
Azathioprine	1.5–2.5 mg/kg day	Nausea, hepatitis, cholestatic jaundice, marrow suppression	FBC, U & E and LFTs fortnightly for 2–3 months, then 1–2 monthly

FBC, full blood count, LFT, liver function test; U & E, urea and electrolytes.

Sulfasalazine is the most commonly prescribed DMARD in the UK due to its favourable risk–benefit ratio. Sulfasalazine has a high continuation rate, a low rate of serious adverse effects and has been shown to slow disease progression. It is often used in mild to moderate disease. The monitoring requirements are less arduous than most other DMARDs, conveying a significant benefit for patients. In order to reduce the problems of nausea, the dose is usually titrated from 500 mg daily, increasing at weekly intervals up to 1 g twice daily.

Methotrexate usage is increasing in the UK, fast becoming first-line therapy in most centres. It is generally used in patients with moderate to severe disease, especially in those with poor prognosis (Table 51.3). Methotrexate is probably the most effective DMARD. It has a high 5-year continuation rate and a low incidence of adverse effects at low weekly doses. It has a relatively rapid onset of action of 4–6 weeks and is easy to administer as a single weekly dose. It has a relatively high response rate of 40–50% and has been

shown to improve quality of life and reduce joint destruction.

Hepatic fibrosis and liver toxicity do, however, occur in a significant proportion of patients, and appear to be enhanced by a high alcohol intake. Patients should therefore be encouraged to either avoid alcohol while on methotrexate, or at the very least restrict it to special occasions. Liver function tests must be frequently monitored (Table 51.9). Severe alveolitis can be a serious and sometimes fatal adverse event with methotrexate therapy, and requires urgent medical treatment. Any patient experiencing increasing dyspnoea should be advised to stop methotrexate and seek medical help immediately.

Nausea and stomatitis can be managed by the addition of folic acid to methotrexate therapy. The optimal dose has yet to be discovered but ranges from 5 mg weekly to 5 mg daily. A number of centres omit the folic acid on the day methotrexate is administered. Until recently it was thought the addition of folic acid did not reduce the efficacy of methotrexate therapy, although a recent study has cast doubt over this assertion. Intramuscular methotrexate, although not licensed for use in RA may prove useful when side effects (particularly nausea and vomiting) impede use. Intramuscular methotrexate may also be useful in patients with poor response despite high dose oral therapy, especially in those with suspected poor oral absorption.

Perhaps one of the greatest concerns with methotrexate therapy is the potential for bone marrow suppression. This is of particular concern either in overdose or in patients on too high a maintenance dose. Bone marrow suppression includes neutropenia, thrombocytopenia and lymphopenia and can be fatal. This usually occurs in patients who inadvertently take methotrexate daily rather than weekly and is not uncommon in the elderly population. Patients must be clear that they should take methotrexate only once per week, on the same day each week. Any sign of infection such as unexplained fever or sore throat, etc., must be reported immediately. Patients should also be advised to avoid contact with people who may have chickenpox.

Sodium-aurothiomalate (gold injection), is a long-established DMARD, and is a very effective agent in the treatment of RA. The use of injectable gold is, however, limited by its side-effect profile. Patients are most likely to stop gold therapy due to toxicity, compared to any other DMARD. Important adverse events include rashes, stomatitis, proteinuria, leucopenia and thrombocytopenia. Despite this, injectable gold can provide benefit to some patients for many years and it may be a useful agent in those with progressive disease who have failed to respond to other therapies.

Patients may be instructed to test their own urine for proteinuria. If significant protein is detected, the gold therapy should be withheld, urinary tract infection excluded and the proteinuria quantified by means of a 24-hour urine collection. Patients on gold injections should also be asked to report new side-effects such as rashes or mouth ulcers.

Auranofin (oral gold) is a completely different drug entity to sodium aurothiomalate and although less toxic is generally less effective. It is now seldom used. Adverse effects are similar to injectable gold but less frequent. The troublesome diarrhoea experienced with oral gold may be improved by a high-bulk diet.

Penicillamine is now seldom used due to problems with toxicity and poor long-term efficacy. There is no evidence that penicillamine reduces joint erosions. It is initiated at a daily dose of 125 mg with monthly increases until a response is demonstrated. There is little benefit to increasing the dose above 750 mg as efficacy appears to have a ceiling effect. Penicillamine should be taken on an empty stomach as absorption is reduced by up to 50% when taken with food. The common adverse events include thrombocytopenia, proteinuria, taste disturbances and rashes. Less common is neutropenia

and, rarely, autoimmune side-effects such as myositis and drug induced lupus may occur.

Ciclosporin is an immunosuppressive agent used in RA. It has proven efficacy in early and late disease but long-term data on reducing joint destruction are lacking. Because of this and the potential for toxicity, ciclosporin is reserved for patients who have failed to respond to conventional therapies. Ciclosporin can cause nephrotoxicity and hypertension, which may have significant long-term consequences, and patients with a history of these are generally excluded from therapy. Treatment is initiated at a dose of 2.5 mg/kg/day and increased up to a maximum of 4.5 mg/kg dependent upon tolerance. There is no requirement to monitor ciclosporin blood levels in RA. Prior to commencing therapy, patients must have baseline blood pressure and creatinine measured, and both should be carefully monitored. Other side-effects include hirsutism, tremor and gum hyperplasia.

Hydroxychloroquine and other antimalarials are the least toxic of all the DMARDs. However, they are also the least effective and are generally reserved for less severe forms of the disease, or in combination regimens. Hydroxychloroquine generally requires little monitoring, and gastrointestinal toxicity is the main adverse effect. Retinopathy is thought only to occur after high cumulative doses, and the need for and frequency of eye tests are still a matter of debate. The typical dose is about 400 mg/day, although this has been increased up to 800 mg/day with the aim of achieving earlier efficacy.

Azathioprine is thought to have a steroid-sparing effect and is of particular use when treating RA refractory to other agents.

Cyclophosphamide is a potent cytotoxic agent that can be used either orally or as intravenous pulse therapy in the management of rheumatoid vasculitis.

Both azathioprine and cyclophosphamide have the potential to cause infertility and the development of malignancies. The risks must therefore be carefully balanced against intended clinical improvement.

Combination DMARD therapy. Many clinicians believe that combination therapy with different DMARDs is more likely to achieve a clinical improvement. Monotherapy has frequently been disappointing. It has not always adequately controlled inflammation and side-effects are common with the high doses that are often required to control symptoms.

Combination therapy may therefore offer better symptom control, particularly combining agents with different modes of action. To date the evidence supporting the efficacy of combination therapy is conflicting. Some studies have shown no improvement in efficacy compared to monotherapy, but with higher toxicity. Others have shown impressive benefits. A triple regimen of hydroxychloroquine, methotrexate and sulfasalazine has shown significant improvements compared to monotherapy with the individual agents. This combination regimen was also well tolerated.

A 'step-down' approach, where DMARD therapy is given in combination from the outset of treatment and then tapered down, has shown improvements in disease activity. Sulfasalazine, methotrexate and prednisolone have been used in this way with some success. A more common approach in the UK is to use the 'step-up' regimen. Here, treatment is commenced with monotherapy, and a second agent added if the first is ineffective or if there is a partial response. Methotrexate in combination with ciclosporin has been shown to be effective in this way, as has methotrexate and sulfasalazine.

Corticosteroids

Systemic corticosteroids have long been used in the management of RA and were the first drugs to result in reversibility of the disease. However, their place in therapy is still not agreed. Corticosteroids suppress cytokines and produce a rapid improvement in signs and symptoms of the disease. They have a potent anti-inflammatory effect and recent studies have suggested a slowing of radiological progression. However, side-effects associated with long-term high-dose therapy such as osteoporosis, diabetes mellitus and hypertension have severely limited the long-term role of corticosteroids in RA. As such, the dosage, duration and stage of disease that corticosteroids should be used is still open to debate.

Oral prednisolone may be used to provide temporary relief until a DMARD becomes effective, or in patients with aggressive disease who cannot be adequately controlled with a combination of DMARDs ('step-up' or 'step-down' approach). Once commenced, systemic corticosteroids can be difficult to withdraw as the disease tends to flare with dose reductions. In order to minimize side-effects, a daily maintenance dose of 7.5 mg of prednisolone or less should be used, given as a single dose in the morning. Prophylaxis against osteoporosis is recommended in patients likely to be on long-term therapy.

Intra-articular steroid administration (i.e. methylprednisolone acetate, triamcinolone acetonide or triamcinolone hexacetonide) can effectively relieve pain, increase mobility and reduce deformity in one or more joints. The duration of response to intra-articular steroids is variable and triamcinolone hexacetonide may produce the greatest response. The dose used is dependent upon the joint size, with methylprednisolone acetate 40 mg or triamcinolone hexacetonide 20 mg appropriate for large joints (e.g. knees). The frequency at which injections may be given is controversial, but repeated injections are usually given at intervals of 1–5 weeks or more, depending on the degree of relief obtained from the first injection. If repeated injections are required, then the dose of DMARD may need to be increased. Intramuscular steroids may be useful in patients with an acute flare of disease, and intravenous pulses of methylprednisolone are particularly helpful in controlling rheumatoid vasculitis.

New developments in rheumatoid arthritis

Despite new approaches in the use of conventional DMARDs, there are still many limitations to their use. The response rate to either mono or combination therapy is at best around 40–60%. This results in over half the patients treated with DMARDs experiencing an insufficient response.

This poor response and high rate of toxicity with conventional DMARD therapy has led to the search for new therapeutic strategies. Apart from better use of monotherapy and a greater use of combination therapy, several new agents are now available for the management of RA.

Leflunomide. Leflunomide is a new, oral DMARD for the treatment of RA. It is a novel isoxazole derivative, which has shown both anti-inflammatory and immuno-modulatory properties. Leflunomide primarily acts by inhibiting the synthesis of DNA and RNA in immune response cells,, particularly activated T cells. It also inhibits the production of the pro-inflammatory cytokines, TNF and, interleukin-1 (IL-1). Leflunomide appears to be equivalent to sulfasalazine and methotrexate in short-term studies. It has shown significant improvements in functional disability and quality of life and slows radiographic progression of RA. It has a rapid onset of action (within 4 weeks) which is significantly faster than sulfasalazine and it appears well tolerated. The commonest side-effects are gastrointestinal disturbances, reversible alopecia, rash, hypertension and abnormal liver function tests. Most of these are mild to moderate and resolve without any complications.

Leflunomide is likely to be used in two groups of patients with RA. The first will be patients who cannot tolerate their current DMARDs because of serious adverse effects. For this group, leflunomide will be used as an alternative to their current DMARD. The second group of patients will be those who have either partial response or no response to their current DMARD. In this group, leflunomide is likely to be used either as an alternative DMARD, or in a subgroup with severe disease as combination therapy.

Etanercept and infliximab. Tumour necrosis factor (TNF) is a pro-inflammatory mediator that contributes to the pathogenesis of synovitis and joint destruction in RA. The discovery of TNF led to the development of TNF blockade therapy in an attempt to antagonize the biological effects of TNF in rheumatoid arthritis. The first two of these therapies were etanercept and infliximab.

Etanercept is a recombinant human soluble TNF receptor. The mechanism of action of etanercept is competitive inhibition of TNF, binding to cell surface receptors and preventing TNF-mediated cellular responses. It is administered as a twice weekly subcutaneous injection. It is generally well tolerated with the commonest adverse event being the development of injection site reactions (approximately 40% incidence). These are often mild, transient, resolve with time and do not usually necessitate suspension of treatment. Upper respiratory tract infections (rhinitis, sinusitis, etc.) have also been reported. There have also been reports of demyelinating disorders (including multiple sclerosis) in patients treated with etanercept.

Infliximab is a chimeric human-murine monoclonal antibody administered by slow I.V. infusion, every 4–8 weeks at a dose of 3 mg/kg. It must be given with oral methotrexate to prevent the development of murine antibodies. Infliximab neutralizes the biological activity of TNF. It is generally well tolerated with infusion-related events such as headache, diarrhoea, rash, fever, chills, urticaria and dyspnoea being the most common side-effects.

Serious infections and sepsis have been reported in some patients treated with both etanercept and infliximab. These reports have included some fatalities and have occurred mainly in patients predisposed to infections. These agents must not be used in patients with active infection.

TNF blockade has significant advantages over existing DMARD treatments. The efficacy of both products is similar with response rates in the region of 60–70% compared to 40% with other therapies. Both agents have been shown to significantly reduce disease activity and to improve quality of life. There is also radiological evidence that infliximab halts disease progress.

Both agents are expensive, costing in the region of £7500 to £12 000 per patient per year. On the basis of available data, it appears that those patients who currently have a suboptimal response to methotrexate therapy at adequate doses (either orally or intramuscularly) are the best candidates for TNF blockade treatment.

Given the lack of available data comparing TNF blockade with other standard DMARDs at any stage of the disease, and the potential cost of treatment, their use will be restricted to specific groups of patients. These are patients in whom there are no other reasonable treatments and those with unacceptable levels of fatigue and a poor quality of life (Fig. 51.3).

It is recommended that TNF blockade therapies are used in patients with highly active disease who have failed an adequate trial (at least 6 months) of at least two standard DMARDs. Patients at high risk of infection must be excluded from treatment.

Patient care

Education of the patient with rheumatoid arthritis is vital. The patient should have a knowledge of the disease process, the likely prognosis and treatment strategies. Psychological aspects of the disease should also be covered.

Hospital inpatients may find self-medication particularly valuable. In general, NSAID preparations should be taken with or after food, and patients should be warned of potential adverse effects and what to do if these occur. Patients must be warned not to supplement their prescribed NSAIDs with purchased ibuprofen or aspirin and should be careful of consuming additional 'hidden' paracetamol.

Patient information sheets for DMARDs are very useful, but counselling must reinforce the need to comply with monitoring requirements and explain the time delay before a response is seen, potential toxicity and action to take in the event of adverse effects.

A number of common therapeutic problems that may be encountered are presented in Table 51.10.

OSTEOARTHRITIS

Osteoarthritis (OA) is a chronic disease and the most common of all the rheumatological disorders. It is the most common joint problem in individuals over the age of 65 years and is the major cause of hip and knee replacements in developed countries. OA is painful and disabling and represents a major challenge to health resources. Until recently, OA was generally considered to be an inevitable consequence of ageing. However, research in the last decade has led to the view that OA is an active disease with potential for treatment.

Epidemiology

The prevalence of OA increases with age. Generally OA is uncommon in people aged less than 45 years with a prevalence of just 2%. This increases in people aged over 65 years to 68% of women and 58% of men. OA occurs in all populations irrespective of race, climate, or geographical location. Most forms of the disease are more common and severe in women. Ethnic origin contributes to the pattern of the disease, for example hip disease is less common in Chinese and Asians than in those of Western origin. Obesity has been shown to be associated with the development of OA, especially in women and particularly with OA of the knee. The proportion of OA attributable to obesity is estimated to be 63%. A strong genetic component is thought to be

Table 51.10 Common therapeutic problems in rheumatoid arthritis

Problem	Solution
Lack of efficacy of NSAID effect	Patient response at best around 60% thus change after 2–3 weeks if lack of consider adding simple/weak opiod analgesia
Intolerance to NSAID, e.g. dyspepsia	Consider changing NSAID If mild, treat with antacid If patient at high risk of GI morbidity consider gastroprotection Consider COX-2 selective NSAID If dyspepsia with COX-2 NSAID, treat with antacid
Need to reduce GI morbidity with NSAID	Avoid NSAID if possible and use simple/weak opioid analgesia Consider lowest risk NSAID at lowest possible dose if NSAID required Use gastroprotection in high risk patients Consider use of COX-2 NSAID with caution
Patient unwilling to commence DMARDs, especially in early disease	Counsel as to early irreversible joint destruction in first 2 years of disease Reassure as to adverse events with DMARDs
Lack of effect with DMARD	Ensure adequate trial of at least 12 weeks given Consider changing DMARD Consider combination DMARD therapy
Management of resistant RA	Consider addition of corticosteroids Consider triple DMARD therapy Consider TNF blockade therapy
Intolerance of DMARD	Titrate dose slowly Consider changing DMARD Treat mild side-effects symptomatically Consider changing route of administration e.g. parenteral methotrexate
Nausea and vomiting with methotrexate	Add folic acid Consider splitting the dose Consider changing to parenteral route Treat with antiemetics pre and post administration

present, particularly in women. Heberden's nodes are three times more common in sisters with OA than in the general population. An inherited defect in type II collagen genes is linked with the development of early onset polyarticular OA.

Aetiology

OA is a complex disease involving both cartilage and bone and is generally believed to result from an imbalance in erosive and reparative processes. The disease process is not a simple wear-and-tear mechanism as inflammatory components may also be present. Osteoarthritis is multifactorial in aetiology and a wide variety of factors predispose an individual to this condition (Table 51.11). Other aetiological factors include mechanical overloading of joints, failure in the bone remodeling process, synovial and vasuclar changes, crystal deposition and catabolic enzyme secretion.

Pathogenesis

The pathogenesis of OA has been classified into four stages:

1. initial repair
2. early stage OA

Table 51.11 Predisposing factors for the development of osteoarthritis

- Increasing age
- Race
- Genetic predisposition
- Gender   < 45 years more common in males
            > 55 years more common in females
            OA knee more common in females
- Obesity
- Systemic disorders, e.g., hypertension
- Physical and occupational factors

3. intermediate stage OA
4. late stage OA.

Initial repair is characterized by proliferation of chondrocytes synthesizing the extracellular matrix of bone. Early stage OA results in degradation of the extracellular matrix as protease enzyme activity exceeds chondrocyte activity. There is net degradation and loss of articular cartilage. Intermediate OA is associated with a failure of extracellular matrix synthesis and increased protease activity, further increasing cartilage loss. Finally, late stage OA will result in extreme or complete loss of cartilage with joint space narrowing. Bony outgrowths (osteophytes) appear at joint margins and there is general bone sclerosis. Clinically this stage manifests with pain and reduced joint movement.

Clinical manifestations

OA is characterized by joint pain, reduced joint movement, stiffness and joint swelling. The signs and symptoms are dependent upon the affected joints. The most commonly affected are the distal interphalangeal, proximal interphalangeal and first metacarpophalangeal joints, the knees, hips and the cervical and lumbar spine. Muscle weakness or wasting is usual. Pain, worsened by loading and movement but eased by rest is the primary symptom. Pain is usually localized to the affected joint, although it may be referred away from its origin (e.g. hip pain may be felt at the knee). Pain is often worse at the end of the day. Stiffness and reduced joint movement generally become worse as the day progresses, and are particularly troublesome after a long period of rest. Swelling, caused either by synovitis or osteophyte formation, and joint deformity restrict the range of joint movement and may lead to loss of function. The degree of disability depends on the site involved. Hip and knee disease are the most significant causes of morbidity associated with OA. Crepitus may be heard in affected joints upon passive or active movement.

Investigations

OA is primarily diagnosed on the clinical presentation. Confirmation and evaluation of progression can be achieved using radiography. The presence of bone sclerosis, osteophyte formation and joint space narrowing are usually evident on radiography. There is, however, lack of association between symptoms and radiographic changes. On arthroscopy normal cartilage is smooth, white and glistening, while OA cartilage is yellowed, irregular and ulcerated. Synovial fluid analysis, for crystals, should be carried out to determine if pseudogout is present. In OA the ESR/plasma viscosity and C-reactive protein levels are usually normal, and there is no extra-articular disease.

Treatment

The objectives in treating OA are to:

- reduce pain
- increase mobility
- reduce disability
- minimize disease progression.

A variety of treatment options are available and include both non-drug and drug strategies (Fig. 51.4).

Non-drug treatment

Non-drug treatment, particularly patient education, plays an important role in the management of OA. Patients should be advised to protect joints through modification of daily living and reduction in weight. Physiotherapy may help patients regain muscle strength and improve the range of movement of affected joints. An exercise programme, heat, cold, ultrasound, diathermy and other aspects of physical therapy will support this strategy. Exercise regimens should encourage 'little and often' physical activity to improve muscle strength and resting tone. Occupational therapy may also help to protect joints and preserve function especially with the use of physical aids and splints. Transcutaneous electrical nerve stimulation (TENS) and nerve blocks should be considered for severe pain and may also be assisted with orthopaedic surgery such as arthroplasty.

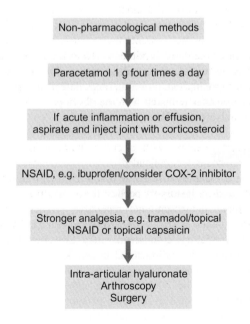

Figure 51.4 Algorithm for the management of osteoarthritis.

Drug treatment

Most patients with OA have pain as a result of the damage to bone and cartilage. In the absence of inflammation, simple analgesia and joint protection are often sufficient for the treatment of mild to moderate disease. The American College of Rheumatology (2000) has recommended simple analgesia as first-line therapy in patients with osteoarthritis of the hip and knee.

Paracetamol is safe and as effective as NSAID therapy in mild to moderate OA. It is usually given at a dose of 1 g four times daily. This is often taken 'as required', although a regular regimen is frequently more successful. Addition of codeine or dextropropoxyphene to paracetamol may result in a slight increase in benefit although this must be assessed against an increased incidence of adverse effects (Eccles et al 1998).

There may be an associated inflammatory component to OA. In these situations, NSAIDs may provide more effective pain control than simple analgesics. The evidence for the use of NSAIDs in the management of OA is conflicting. Compared to simple analgesia, NSAID treated patients have significantly reduced pain at rest and on movement. However, other studies have shown that paracetamol and ibuprofen have comparable efficacy in mild to moderate pain with ibuprofen being superior where there is severe pain. As such, patients should be given a trial of paracetamol as initial therapy before switching to NSAID therapy.

The choice of NSAID should be made after evaluation of risk factors for serious upper gastrointestinal and renal toxicity. Many OA patients will be elderly and female and particularly susceptible to gastrointestinal side-effects. A NSAID such as ibuprofen may be a suitable choice in such patients, and a 2-week trial should give an indication of its efficacy. The use of NSAIDs should be reviewed regularly and, if possible, restricted to short courses.

Gastroprotection with a proton pump inhibitor or misoprostol is recommended in patients at high risk of gastrointestinal events. These will include patients aged > 65 years, a history of peptic ulcer or gastrointestinal bleeding, concomitant steroids, concomitant anticoagulants or the presence of co-morbidity. COX-2 selective NSAIDs have been found to be more effective than placebo and comparable to standard NSAIDs in the management of OA. These agents may provide an alternative NSAID strategy in patients at high risk of gastrointestinal events, although there is no evidence comparing these drugs to a standard non-selective NSAID with a gastroprotective agent.

Topical NSAIDs, topical capsaicin or simple rubefacients may be of use when pain is localized or if systemic therapy is not recommended. Use of NSAIDs via the topical route can, however, produce systemic side-effects.

An alternative approach to the use of oral agents is the use of intra-articular injections. Intra-articular steroids may be of benefit in patients with acute inflammation or joint effusion. It has been recommended that repeat injections should not be given more often than every 3 months for a given joint. The duration of symptomatic improvement following intra-articular injection may range from a few days to 1 month or longer. Intra-articular hyaluronic acid derivatives (visco-supplementation) may prove useful in some patients. These agents have been shown to be more effective than placebo and equivalent to intra-articular steroids and oral NSAIDs in reducing pain associated with OA of the knee. Intra-articular hyaluronic acid derivatives are expensive and are indicated for patients who have failed non-drug treatment, simple analgesia, NSAIDs, strong analgesia and intra-articular corticosteroids (Fig. 51.4).

Finally, tramadol is a centrally acting opioid agonist which inhibits re-uptake of noradrenaline (norepinephrine) and serotonin. It has been shown to be comparable to ibuprofen in OA and may be used as adjunct therapy in patients who are inadequately controlled with NSAIDs.

New developments

Several chondroprotective agents or similar drugs have been proposed for the management of OA. Chondroitin and glucosamine compounds are the most common. While some studies support the use of these agents in OA, it is generally believed there are insufficient data to support widespread use. A recent meta-analysis investigating the use of glucosamine in OA concluded that while there may be some symptomatic benefit, there is no evidence that glucosamine offers a long-term cure in OA. However, McAlindon (2001), in a large 3 year study, has suggested that glucosamine is a safe and beneficial disease-modifying agent in OA.

Depression and anxiety are common and should be treated to reduce the impact of pain and disability associated with OA. Social support is essential for most patients.

CASE STUDIES

Case 51.1

Mrs J. M. is an 85-year-old lady with RA affecting multiple joints. She has a history of congestive cardiac failure. Mrs J. M. has recently complained of dyspepsia and nausea since commencing naproxen. This was recently changed from diclofenac which had been stopped due to lack of effect. She currently takes naproxen 500 mg twice a day, prednisolone EC 5 mg once daily, furosemide (frusemide) 40 mg once daily and aspirin 75 mg once daily.

Questions

1. Should Mrs J. M. be prescribed a gastroprotective agent? Explain your rationale.
2. If so, which gastroprotective agent would you recommend?
3. What is the role of COX-2 NSAIDs in a patient such as Mrs J. M.?

Answers

1. Mrs J. M. should be prescribed a gastroprotective agent as she is at high risk for NSAID-induced gastric ulceration. She has a number of risk factors, i.e. age, concomitant corticosteroids, concomitant low dose aspirin, co-morbidity (RA and CCF) and she is female. The presence of one risk factor elevates the risk of GI complications, but more than one risk factor is even more deleterious. In a recent study, significant risk factors included age > 60 years, previous history of GI complication and concomitant corticosteroid use. Patients treated with corticosteroids and NSAIDs are 15 times more likely to suffer from peptic ulcer disease than non-users of either drug. In the misoprostol ulcer complications outcomes safety assessment trial (MUCOSA), four risk factors were identified: age > 75 years, history of previous peptic ulcer, history of GI bleeding and cardiovascular disease. At 6 months patients with none of these risk factors had a risk of NSAID-induced GI complication of 0.4%. In patients with one risk factor the risk was 1% and in patients with all four risk factors, the risk was 9%. These studies conclude that these patients are at high risk of experiencing NSAID-induced GI effects and should therefore be offered preventative therapy.

2. Various agents have been used to reduce the incidence of NSAID-induced GI adverse effects. Misoprostol is effective in the prevention of NSAID-induced gastric and duodenal ulcers and has shown a reduction of 40–50% in serious GI complications compared to placebo. Misoprostol is licensed for the prophylaxis of NSAID-induced peptic ulcer disease at a dose of 200 micrograms two to four times daily. Omeprazole is also effective in the prevention of NSAID-induced GI complications. The omeprazole vs. misoprostol for NSAID-induced ulcer management (OMNIUM) study has shown that omeprazole (20 mg per day) is significantly more effective than misoprostol (200 micrograms twice a day) in maintaining patients in remission (61% of patients treated with omeprazole vs. 48% misoprostol). Lansoprazole has recently been licensed for the prophylaxis of NSAID-induced ulceration. In a large randomized multicentre trial in patients with NSAID-induced ulcers, 83% of patients on lansoprazole 30 mg remained healed compared with 79% on lansoprazole

15 mg, 88% on misoprostol and 46% on placebo. Ranitidine is the most extensively tested H_2 antagonist in the prevention of NSAID-induced GI toxicity. A meta-analysis of six placebo controlled studies has shown that ranitidine protects against NSAID-induced duodenal ulceration but not gastric ulceration. Misoprostol 200 micrograms two to four times daily, lansoprazole 15–30 mg per day or omeprazole 20 mg per day are the drugs of choice in the prevention of NSAID-induced GI complications. Proton pump inhibitors are often considered first choice in most patients due to the high incidence of diarrhoea and abdominal colic in a significant number of patients treated with misoprostol.

3. COX-2 selective NSAIDs may have an advantage over standard NSAIDs with respect to a reduction in GI side-effects. In the VIGOR study over 8000 patients with RA were randomized to receive rofecoxib or naproxen. Rofecoxib reduced the risk of clinically important upper GI events (ulcers, perforations, obstructions and bleeds) compared with naproxen by 54%. Patients taking low dose aspirin were excluded from this study. Celecoxib has also shown significant improvements in the incidence of gastroduodenal ulcers compared to standard NSAIDs. In the CLASS study over 8000 patients were randomized to celecoxib, ibuprofen or diclofenac. Low dose aspirin was permitted. In all patients, celecoxib reduced the incidence of upper GI ulcer complications alone and with symptomatic ulcers. In the subgroup of patients taking aspirin, however, there was no difference between celecoxib and naproxen in the incidence of upper GI complications alone or combined with symptomatic ulcers. This suggests that the benefit of using a COX-2 NSAID may be lost in patients taking concomitant aspirin therapy.

There is evidence therefore that COX-2 selective NSAIDs cause less serious GI adverse events than standard NSAIDs. However, there is currently no evidence comparing COX-2 NSAIDs against a standard NSAID and a gastroprotective agent. Current data therefore suggest that COX-2 selective NSAIDs should not be used as first-line therapy. Co-prescription with a gastroprotective agent is recommended if treatment with a NSAID is essential in older patients, those with a history of GI ulceration, bleeding or perforation, or receiving systemic corticosteroids or anticoagulant therapy. Treatment with a COX-2 selective NSAID needs to be evaluated against this approach. It also appears the benefit of COX-2 NSAIDs is lost in those patients taking concomitant low dose aspirin. These patients should be offered a gastroprotective agent.

Case 51.2

Mrs A. N. is a 54-year-old lady suffering from sero-positive RA for the last 10 years. She has resistant disease which has not responded to, or she has failed to tolerate, sulfasalazine, methotrexate, intramuscular gold, ciclosporin and azathioprine. She is currently being treated with diclofenac 50 mg three times daily, prednisolone 5 mg once daily, lansoprazole 30 mg once daily and paracetamol. She is admitted with an acute flare of disease.

Questions

1. What treatment options are available for the management of the acute flare in this patient?

2. What disease modifying options are available for Mrs A.N.?
3. Is TNF blockade therapy indicated in a patient such as Mrs A.N.? If so which agent would you recommend?

Answers

1. Mrs A. N.'s acute flare will require a multimodal approach to treatment. This will include bed rest, physiotherapy, hydrotherapy and drug treatment. The therapeutic options include intra-articular injections if a small number of joints are affected e.g. knees, shoulders. Alternatively a depot intramuscular corticosteroid, e.g. methylprednisolone 80–120 mg, may be used if the flare involves numerous joints, especially small joints such as the hands and feet. Oral prednisolone 20–30 mg in short courses may be an alternative, although this is usually reserved for those patients in whom injections are not appropriate. Finally, supplemental analgesia, e.g. dihydrocodeine, may be helpful for managing background/referred pain.

2. Disease modifying options for Mrs A. N. include increasing the oral prednisolone dose. Corticosteroids suppress the disease process and have an anti-inflammatory effect. However, this must be balanced against the long-term side-effects common with oral steroids. It is also extremely difficult to reduce a patient's steroid dose, due to exacerbations of disease, once the dose has been increased. Combination DMARD therapy seems a reasonable approach in Mrs A. N. She has failed numerous monotherapy strategies and the combination of agents, which she has either not tried, or those stopped due to lack of effect, may offer an alternative approach. Using combination therapy with those DMARDs stopped due to lack of effect often results in synergism. Those agents stopped due to toxicity are generally avoided in combination. Leflunomide may also offer a new disease modifying option in Mrs A. N. Leflunomide is likely to be used in two groups of patients with RA, those who cannot tolerate their current DMARD because of serious adverse effects and those who have either partial or no response to their current DMARD. It is proving to be a useful addition in these patients and is given as 100 mg per day for 3 days followed by a maintenance dose of 10–20 mg per day. Hypertension appears to be the most serious limiting problem to date.

3. TNF blockade has significant advantages over existing DMARD treatments. The efficacy of both etanercept and infliximab is similar with response rates in the region of 60–70% compared with 40% for existing therapies. Both agents have been shown to significantly reduce disease activity and improve quality of life. There is also radiological evidence that infliximab halts disease progress. It is recommended TNF blockade is used in patients with highly active disease, failing an adequate trial (at least 6 months) of at least two standard DMARDs. Mrs A. N. is therefore eligible for TNF blockade therapy. However, both agents are expensive and cost in the region of £7500 to £12 000 per patient per year. On the basis of the available data so far, particularly the lack of available data comparing TNF blockade with other standard DMARDs, initial therapy is likely to be targeted to a specific group of patients. These are patients in whom there are no other reasonable treatments and patients with unacceptable levels of fatigue and poor quality of life. Most rheumatologists will therefore reserve TNF blockade for those patients in whom combination therapy or leflunomide have failed or not been

tolerated. In these circumstances it is unlikely Mrs A. N. would as yet be a candidate for this option. Since Mrs A. N. is not taking methotrexate, etanercept would be the anti-TNF agent of choice. Infliximab must only be given to patients receiving concomitant methotrexate in order to prevent the development of murine antibodies.

Case 51.3

Mrs V. B. is a 65-year-old lady with a 4-year history of RA, who presents to her GP with month ulcers, general lethargy, a sore throat, raised temperature and general bruising. Her current medication includes methotrexate 15 mg once each week, folic acid 5 mg three times per week, diclofenac SR 75 mg twice daily and a recent course of co-trimoxazole 2 tablets twice daily for a urinary tract infection.

Questions

1. What is the side-effect profile of methotrexate?
2. What is the probable cause of the symptoms described by Mrs V. B.?
3. What treatment options are available for the management of Mrs V. B.'s symptoms?

Answers

1. Methotrexate is a dihydrofolate reductase inhibitor, which is increasingly being used as the first line DMARD for the management of RA. It is generally well tolerated, especially at the low weekly doses employed in RA. The main side-effects with methotrexate include GI toxicity, bone marrow toxicity, liver toxicity and pulmonary toxicity. GI side-effects include nausea, vomiting and diarrhoea. Haematological side-effects include bone marrow suppression, particularly thrombocytopenia and neutropenia. Regular full blood count monitoring is required and patients should be advised to report any signs of infection, especially sore throat, to their doctor. Methotrexate can cause liver toxicity, especially cirrhosis. Regular liver function test monitoring is required. Pulmonary toxicity includes dyspnoea and pulmonary fibrosis or alveolitis. Patients should be advised to report any sudden shortness of breath to their doctor. Mouth ulcers, stomatitis, alopecia, rash and bruising can also be troublesome adverse effects.

2. The probable cause of the signs and symptoms described by Mrs V. B. is methotrexate toxicity. She describes the classical symptoms of this syndrome. Methotrexate toxicity is a serious and potentially fatal event and should be managed accordingly. There are a number of risk factors for toxicity and these include age, reduced renal function, high dose therapy, concomitant anti-folate drugs, concurrent NSAIDs, etc. Mrs V. B. has recently had a course of co-trimoxazole for a urinary tract infection. Co-trimoxazole is also an anti-folate agent and concomitant therapy can increase the risk of methotrexate toxicity. The same is true with trimethoprim, and these combinations should be avoided. NSAIDs can reduce renal perfusion, thereby reducing methotrexate excretion and hence increasing toxicity. In clinical practice this is rarely significant and most

patients are maintained on their NSAID plus methotrexate. However, in a patient with reduced renal function this combination should be avoided. A common cause of methotrexate toxicity is inadvertent daily rather than weekly administration. Patients must be counselled as to the weekly regimen. Careful risk analysis should be undertaken especially in elderly patients with the potential for confusion. Mrs V. B.'s methotrexate toxicity is probably due to a multitude of factors, principally the anti-folate co-trimoxazole, concomitant diclofenac and possibly reduced renal function secondary to her age.

3. The most effective therapy for methotrexate toxicity is calcium folinate (calcium leucovorin). This is used to diminish the toxicity and counteract the folate antagonist action of methotrexate. The dosage depends on the severity of the leucopenia. In mild to moderate toxicity it is given in a dose of 15 mg every 6 hours for 48–72 hours. In more severe cases up to 120 mg is usually given in individual doses over 12–24 hours by intramuscular injection, intravenous bolus or infusion. Measures to ensure prompt excretion of methotrexate are also important, and include alkalinization of urine to a pH greater than 7.0 and maintenance of increased urine output. In cases where leucopenia is severe, treatment with granulocyte-colony stimulating factor may be required. It can induce marked increases in peripheral blood neutrophil counts within 24 hours of administration. A subcutaneous dose of 500 000 units/kg/day may be given and should be continued until the neutrophil count is greater than 1.5×10^9/l. Topical agents such as anti-inflammatory mouthwashes (benzydamine), analgesic gels (choline salicylate), protective agents (carmellose) or corticosteroids (hydrocortisone lozenges, Eriamcinolone in oral paste) may all be useful in managing mouth ulcers and stomatitis.

Case 51.4

A 68-year-old man with inflammatory osteoarthritis, particularly of the knees, presents at a hospital rheumatology clinic. He complains of worsening pain and mobility despite regular intra-articular corticosteroids, analgesia and NSAIDs. His current therapy includes tramadol MR 100 mg twice daily, rofecoxib 12.5 mg once daily, paracetamol 1 g four times daily and fluoxetine 20 mg once daily. The visco-supplementation agent Synvisc® is prescribed.

Questions

1. What is visco-supplementation?
2. What is the place of visco-supplementation in the management of OA and in which patients would you advise therapy?
3. What are the contraindications and adverse reactions associated with visco-supplementation therapies?
4. How might you monitor the effectiveness of this therapy?

Answers

1. In joints affected by OA the synovial fluid's capacity to lubricate and absorb shock is reduced. These changes are partly due to the reduction in the size and concentration of hyaluronic acid molecules in the synovium. A new approach in the management of OA of the knee is to inject hyaluronic acid or its derivatives into the joint. Hyaluronan is a polysaccharide composed of repeating disaccharide units of glucuronic acid and N-acetyl glucosamine. When these molecules are very long they make a highly visco-elastic solution that is lubricant at low shear and shock absorbing at high shear. When injected into a joint this is known as visco-supplementation.

2. The published evidence suggests that intra-articular hyaluronic acid derivatives are better than placebo and in some cases comparable to NSAIDs in the management of pain on movement associated with OA of the knee. A summary of the relevant trials concludes that although these products are expensive, and available published data supporting their effectiveness are limited, there may be situations in which they have a role. This is likely to be in a small number of patients who meet the following criteria: OA of the knee, daily pain, failure of adequate doses of stepwise analgesia, failure of tramadol and/or NSAIDs, failure of an adequate trial of physiotherapy and either failure of two separate intra-articular injections of corticosteroids or intolerance or contraindication to corticosteroids (Failure in this context is when pain relief is not achieved after 4 weeks of treatment). They may also be indicated if surgery is either not appropriate or contraindicated, including patients too young for surgery, and failed the above measures. In practice this is a large number of resistant patients with osteoarthritis.

3. Intra-articular hyaluronic acid derivatives should not be injected if there is venous or lymphatic stasis or into severely inflamed or infected joints. Transient redness, pain, warmth and swelling of the injected joint may occur in about 10–40% of patients treated. There have been a small number of reports of severe synovitis following injection of hyaluronic acid requiring intra-articular corticosteroids. There have also been anecdotal reports of pseudogout following injection. Hyaluronic acid derivatives should not be used if there is a large intra-articular effusion whilst some preparations should not be used in patients who are hypersensitive to bird proteins because they contain small amounts of avian protein. Anaphylactic like reactions has been reported following intra-articular Hyalgan® injections.

4. It is unclear which patients will respond to visco-supplementation. All patients should receive close follow-up to evaluate this. The Western Ontario and McMasters Universities (WOMAC) index is a useful measure for determining response. It is a patient completed questionnaire which evaluates pain, stiffness and functionality. WOMAC is the standard outcome measure used in OA of the hip and knee. It is well validated and accepted worldwide. Patients can be monitored using the WOMAC prior to treatment and at three months (response defined as a 10–20% reduction in the pain subscale of WOMAC), with the use of supplemental analgesia and a physician assessment of response.

Case 51.5

Mrs A. H. is a 58-year-old lady with a long history of severe RA. She presents to the hospital rheumatology clinic with severe pain in her left foot. On examination, three toes are

found to be discoloured, and appear ischaemic. A large ulcer is also found on the heel of the same foot. She is diagnosed as having rheumatoid vasculitis.

Questions

1. What is rheumatoid vasculitis and what is its aetiology?
2. What is the role of cyclophosphamide and methylprednisolone in the management of this patient?
3. What precautions should be taken with cyclophosphamide use?
4. What other treatment options are available for Mrs A. H.?

Answers

1. Rheumatoid vasculitis is a severe, often life-threatening condition that may present as a complication of RA. Severe inflammation of blood vessels occurs, commonly producing pain and ulcers in the extremities. Many organs may be affected, particularly the kidneys. The primary aetiology is immune complex deposition in blood vessels.
2. Cyclophosphamide and methylprednisolone have been used effectively in rheumatoid vasculitis for their potent immunosuppressive actions. Regimens do vary, but intravenous pulses every 3–6 weeks are often used. Methylprednisolone at a dose of 500 mg to 1 g over an hour or more (to prevent cardiac arrhythmia or ischaemia) gives a rapid and intense anti-inflammatory action as well as immunosuppressive activity. Once the condition improves, oral steroids may be considered. Such an improvement may be seen by monitoring laboratory indices such as ESR, renal function and urine protein content. Patients usually tolerate cyclophosphamide although prophylactic antiemetics should be given and the possibility of fertility suppression should be discussed with patients.
3. Prior to administration of cyclophosphamide, patients should have a full blood count, urea and electrolytes, and creatinine measured. A full medical examination should also be carried out to exclude intercurrent illness or evidence of infection. A high fluid intake (at least 2.5 l on the infusion day) should be maintained to reduce the risk of haemorrhagic cystitis, possibly with the addition of intravenous fluids. Mesna is sometimes also given, although there is little clinical evidence that it is needed with such moderate doses of cyclophosphamide. Extravasation of cyclophosphamide is unlikely to be serious if infusion is promptly discontinued, and ward staff should be familiar with the extravasation procedure.
4. Administration of iloprost has been used in rheumatoid vasculitis to improve vasculitic ulcers and reduce peripheral ischaemia although it is unlicensed for use in this condition. Iloprost is a prostacyclin analogue, which is a potent vasodilator and inhibitor of platelet aggregation. It is given either as an intravenous infusion over 6–8 hours for 3–6 days or, in severe peripheral ischaemia, as a continuous 24-hour infusion for up to 5 days. Infusion rates are titrated according to patient response and tolerance. Pulse and blood pressure should be monitored regularly as hypotension can occur and it is therefore usual practice to withhold any medication that might potentiate this, e.g. nifedipine. Doses of 2–10 micrograms/hour are usually employed.

REFERENCES

Rheumatoid arthritis

Bombardier C, Laine L, Reicin C et al 2000 Comparison of upper gastrointestinal toxicity of rofecoxib and naproxen in patients with rheumatoid arthritis. For the VIGOR study group. New England Journal of Medicine 343: 1520–1528

Buckley C D 1997 Treatment of rheumatoid arthritis. British Medical Journal 315: 236–238

Cawston T E 1998 Mechanisms of joint destruction and therapeutic approaches. Medicine International 26: 4–9

Corte L C, Caselli M, Castellino G et al 1999 Prophylaxis and treatment of NSAID-induced gastroduodenal disorders. Drug Safety 20: 527–543

Fuchs H A, Kaye J J, Callahan L F et al 1989 Evidence of significant radiographic damage in rheumatoid arthritis within the first 2 years of disease. Journal of Rheumatology 16: 585–591

Hawkey C J 1998 Progress in prophylaxis against non-steroidal anti-inflammatory drug associated ulcers and erosions. Omeprazole NSAID Steering Committee. American Journal of Medicine 104: 67S–74S; discussion 79S–80S

Hawkey C J, Karrasch J A, Szczepanski L et al 1998 Omeprazole compared with misoprostol for ulcers associated with nonsteroidal antïnflammatory drugs. Omeprazole versus Misoprostol for NSAID-induced Ulcer Management (OMNIUM) Study Group. New England Journal of Medicine 338: 727–734

Hazes J M W, Silman A J 1990 Review of UK data on the rheumatic diseases, + 2. Rheumatoid arthritis. British Journal of Rheumatology 29: 310–312

Henry D, Lim L L, Garcia Rodriguez L A et al 1996 Variability in risk of gastrointestinal complications with individual anti-inflammatory drugs: results of a collaborative meta-analysis. British Medical Journal 312: 1563–1566

Machold K. P, Eberl G, Leeb B F et al 1998 Early arthritis therapy: rationale and current approach. Journal of Rheumatology 25; suppl 53: 13–19

Markenson J A 1991 Worldwide trends in the socio-economic impact and long-term prognosis of rheumatoid arthritis. Seminars in Arthritis and Rheumatism 21: (Suppl. 1)4–12

National Institute for Clinical Excellence (NICE). 2001 Guidance on the use of cyclo-oxygenase (COX) II selective inhibitors, celecoxib, rofecoxib, meloxicam and etodolac for osteoarthritis and rheumatoid arthritis. NICE Appraisal no. 27. NICE, London

Silverstein F E, Faich G, Goldstein J L et al 2000 Gastrointestinal toxicity with celecoxib versus nonsteroidal anti-inflammatory drugs for osteoarthritis and rheumatoid arthritis. The CLASS study: a randomised controlled trial. Journal of the American Medical Association 284: 1247–1255

Wolfe F 1990 Fifty years of anti-rheumatic therapy: the prognosis of rheumatoid arthritis. Journal of Rheumatology 17:(Suppl. 22): 24–32

Osteoarthritis

American College of Rheumatology Subcommittee on Osteoarthritis Guidelines 2000 Recommendations for the medical management of osteoarthritis of the hip and knee.

Arthritis and Rheumatism 43: 1905–1915

Eccles M, Freemantle N, Mason J 1998 North of England evidence based guideline development project: summary guideline for non-steroidal anti-inflammatory drugs versus basic analgesia in treating the pain of degenerative arthritis. British Medical Journal 317: 526–530

McAlindon T 2001 Glucosamine in osteoarthritis: dawn of a new era? Lancet 357: 251

FURTHER READING

Brooks P M 1998 Rheumatoid arthritis: aetiology and clinical features. Medicine International 26(6): 28–32

Li E, Brooks P, Conaghan G 1998 Disease modifying anti-rheumatic drugs. Current Opinion in Rheumatology 10: 159–168

Wernick R, Campbell S M 2000 Update in Rheumatology. Annals of Internal Medicine 132: 125–133

Cicuttini F, Spector T D 1998 Osteoarthritis. Medicine International 26(6): 68–71

Gout and hyperuricaemia

52

E. A. Kay   A. Alldred

KEY POINTS

- Asymptomatic hyperuricaemia is common.
- Serum uric acid may not always be raised at the time of an acute attack of gout.
- As hypouricaemic therapy will be lifelong for the majority of patients, it is important to consider the risks and benefits of starting prophylactic therapy.
- Prolonged therapy to lower serum urate should be considered when:
  - there have been recurrent attacks
  - there is evidence of tophi or chronic gouty arthritis
  - there is associated renal disease
  - the patient is young with high serum uric acid and family history of renal or heart disease
  - normal levels of serum uric acid cannot be achieved by lifestyle changes.
- Allopurinol or uricosuric agents should not be started until the acute attack has settled for 2–3 weeks.
- Allopurinol is the drug of choice for prophylaxis due to its convenience and the low incidence of side-effects.
- Before allopurinol is commenced, renal function should be checked.
- Lower doses of allopurinol should be used when renal function is impaired.

'Gout' is a term that represents a heterogeneous group of diseases usually associated with hyperuricaemia. The hyperuricaemia may be due to an increased rate of synthesis of the purine precursors of uric acid or to a decreased elimination of uric acid by the kidney or both.

Hyperuricaemia is a biochemical condition, while gout is a clinical diagnosis. Prolonged hyperuricaemia is necessary but not sufficient for the development of gout.

Gout is characterized by recurrent episodes of acute arthritis due to deposits of monosodium urate in joints and cartilage. Formation of uric acid calculi in the kidneys (nephrolithiasis) may occur.

Epidemiology

The prevalence of gout in the UK is approximately 2.6 cases per 1000. In about 10% of these cases gout is a secondary manifestation, with diuretics being the most frequent causative factor. Figures for the incidence of gout vary between populations, and its prevalence is known to change with environmental and dietary factors in the same population over a short period of time.

Gout is a condition that most frequently affects middle-aged men, with only approximately 5% of cases occurring in women. Most women with gout have a family history of the disease, although studies in men have failed to detect a significant genetic component. The risk of acute gout occurring secondary to hyperuricaemia is approximately equal for both sexes but hyperuricaemia is many times more common in men.

The incidence and prevalence of gout increases with the level of serum uric acid – the risk of developing gout rises from about 0.5% per annum in men with serum urate of 0.42 mmol/l to 5.5% per annum at a serum urate of 0.54 mmol/l (Nuki 1998).

Aetiology

Uric acid is the end product of purine metabolism in humans, who lack the enzyme uricase (which degrades uric acid to allantoin in most mammals).

The development of gout is primarily related to the degree and duration of hyperuricaemia. Concentrations of urate in synovial fluid correlate closely with serum levels. A rigid definition of hyperuricaemia is not possible, but in general terms the upper limit of normal is 0.47 mmol/l for men, 0.40 mmol/l for postmenopausal women and 0.37 mmol/l for premenopausal women.

Overproduction of uric acid

Overproduction of uric acid may result from excessive turnover of nucleoproteins (as, for example, in type 1 glycogen storage disease, neoplastic diseases and myeloproliferative disorders), excessive dietary purines, or excessive synthesis of uric acid due to rare enzyme mutation defects (e.g. Lesch–Nyhan syndrome). Diet plays a minor role in this condition and thus dietary restrictions, with the exception of limiting alcohol intake, have a minor role to play.

Two-thirds of the urate formed each day is excreted by the kidneys and one-third is eliminated via the gastrointenstinal tract.

Underexcretion of uric acid

Underexcretion of uric acid results from a defect in renal excretion. Uric acid is filtered at the glomerulus, and almost completely reabsorbed in the proximal tubule. Of the reabsorbed uric acid, 50% is secreted distal to the proximal tubular reabsorption site and approximately 75% of this secreted urate is reabsorbed. In the hyperuricaemic state, large loads are filtered and urate reabsorption increases to avoid the dumping of poorly soluble urate into the urinary tract. Tubular urate secretion is not influenced by serum urate concentrations, and it is probably the impaired urate secretion that is responsible for the hyperuricaemia.

Another cause of gouty arthritic attacks can be physical stress. Factors such as tight shoes, hill walking and hiking have been reported to cause acute attacks in the great toe. A history of joint trauma may also subsequently be associated with attacks of gout.

Clinical manifestations

The natural history of gout has four stages:

- asymptomatic hyperuriceamia
- acute gouty arthritis
- intercritical gout
- chronic tophaceous gout.

Acute gout is traditionally considered monoarticular, with the great toe most frequently affected. Approximately 80% of patients with gout have the initial attack in the great toe (podagra). The majority of patients will have podagra at some time during the course of the disease. Other joints frequently affected are small joints of the feet or ankles, the hands (distal interphalangeal joints), elbows and knees. The initial presentation of the disease may be polyarticular and low-grade inflammation may be present in many joints.

The patient with acute gouty arthritis complains of severe pain with a hot, red, swollen and extremely tender joints. The weight of the bedclothes or the jar of a person walking on the floor is said to be agony to the sufferer, and weight-bearing is impossible. The affected joint has overlying erythema and signs of marked synovitis. The patient may be pyrexial with a leucocytosis (total white cell count in excess of 11×10^9/l) and elderly patients may be confused. Untreated attacks last days or weeks before subsiding spontaneously, and resolution may be accompanied by pruritis and desquamation of the overlying skin.

Chronic tophaceous gout is associated with the presence of tophi and renal disease. In time, with treatment, the tophi disappear although the renal function will probably remain static.

Premature atherosclerosis, cardiovascular disease and nephropathy are associated with gout but whether these are a consequence of hyperuricaemia remains unclear. In asymptomatic individuals gout, hypertension and coronary artery disease occur more commonly than in matched control groups. The half-lives of platelets in patients with gout are much shortened and thus platelet adhesiveness is increased. A number of studies have suggested that hyperuricaemia may be an independent risk factor for hypertension and atherosclerotic disease, while an association between hyperuricaemia and hypertriglyceridaemia has also been proposed. Obesity and alcohol excess are common factors to both these latter disorders rather than a direct causal mechanism for hyperuricaemia.

Gouty nephropathy is a form of chronic interstitial nephritis that occurs typically in patients who have had hyperuricaemia for many years. This is associated with hyperexcretion of urate and urine hyperacidity. Crystals are deposited around the renal tubules and incite an inflammatory response. The renal medulla becomes infiltrated with mononuclear cells and fibrosis occurs. Clinically this is manifested by proteinuria and/or renal impairment.

Events provoking acute gouty arthritis

Events provoking acute gouty arthritis are listed in Table 52.1. Diuretics are most frequently implicated.

Table 52.1   Events provoking acute gouty arthritis
• Trauma
• Unusual physical exercise
• Surgery
• Severe systemic illness
• Severe dieting
• Dietary excess
• Alcochol
• Drugs Diuretics Initiation of uricosuric or allopurinol therapy Initiation of B$_{12}$ in pernicious anaemia Following drug allergy Cytotoxic drug therapy

These patients are characterized by the presence of tophi which often develop in Heberden's nodes (gelatinous cysts or bony outgrowths on the dorsal aspects of the distal interphalangeal joints). Patients affected rarely have acute attacks, and the condition usually responds to withdrawal of the diuretic. If the diuretic is essential, allopurinol may be used to lower uric acid levels.

Radiotherapy and chemotherapy in patients with leukaemias and lymphomas may lead to hyperuricaemia. Uric acid nephropathy may occur in association with acute increases in uric acid production, and this is the most common cause of acute renal failure in patients with leukaemia. This can be treated prophylactically with allopurinol commencing 3 days pre-therapy and continuing for the duration of remission-inducing chemotherapy. Other measures that can be adopted to prevent urate nephropathy in this situation include alkalinization of the urine and vigorous fluid intake.

Investigations

The diagnosis of acute gout can only be made through examination of synovial fluid aspirated from the inflamed joint. Monosodium urate crystals are needle shaped and are negatively birefringent under a polarizing microscope. Aspirated synovial fluid also contains large numbers of polymorphonuclear leucocytes.

Sudden onset of acute inflammatory monoarthritis, particularly in the foot or ankle, should always raise the suspicion of gout; however, in 10% of patients acute gouty arthritis is polyarticular.

Hyperuricaemia alone is not diagnostic of gout as many hyperuricaemic patients never develop symptomatic gout and some patients with acute gout have a normal serum uric acid concentration. Attacks of gout tend to be precipitated by changes in uric acid concentration, and the absolute level may have fallen back to normal during an attack. The diagnosis of gout is thus confirmed only by microscopic examination of synovial fluid aspirated from the affected joint.

Differential diagnosis

The differential diagnosis in acute gouty arthritis must include infection. Patients with gout commonly present with acute swelling and tenderness of the joint with a fever, raised plasma viscosity and leucocytosis, with no previous history of arthritis. Patients with joint sepsis are usually more ill and have other systemic signs of infection such as a swinging fever and severe malaise. Large joints are most frequently infected, and the joint is hot, tender and swollen with effusion and marked limitation of movement.

Treatment

Patient education and an understanding of the basis for therapy is critical for successful management.

In an acute attack of gout the primary goal is to relieve pain and inflammation. Others include termination of the acute attack, prevention of further attacks and consideration of long-term hypouricaemic therapy.

Gout is a disease that is often associated with obesity, hypertriglyceridaemia, hypertension and high alcohol intake. A subgroup of patients (usually elderly women) taking diuretics has been recognized.

Acute attacks

Rest and prompt treatment with full doses of non-steroidal anti-inflammatory drugs (NSAIDs) are first-line management in acute attacks. Aspirin and its derivatives (choline salicylate, benorilate) should be avoided as these agents compete with uric acid for excretion and can worsen an acute attack. NSAIDs will relieve pain and inflammation and they can abort an attack if commenced early. An alternative, but second-choice, agent is colchicine. There are no controlled studies comparing colchicine with NSAIDs in matched patients.

Agents that decrease the serum uric acid level (allopurinol or uricosuric agents such as probenecid and sulfinpyrazone) should not be used in an acute attack. Patients generally have been hyperuricaemic for several years, and there is no need to treat the hyperuricaemia immediately. In addition, agents that decrease serum uric acid concentrations may cause mobilization of uric acid stores as the serum level falls. This movement of uric acid may prolong the acute attack or precipitate another attack of gouty arthritis. However, if the patient is already stabilized on allopurinol at the onset of the acute attack, it should be continued.

Non-steroidal anti-inflammatory drugs (NSAIDs)

NSAIDs are effective first-line therapy for otherwise healthy patients presenting with acute gout. NSAIDs should be administered in high dosage for the first 1–3 days or until the pain has settled. Lower doses should be continued until all symptoms and signs have resolved, usually after 7–10 days. Indometacin is commonly prescribed for an acute attack of gouty arthritis initially at a dose of 75–100 mg twice a day. This dose should be reduced after 5 days as the acute attack settles. NSAIDs usually take between 24 and 48 hours to work, although complete relief of gouty signs and symptoms is usually seen after 5 days of treatment. Adverse effects of indometacin will include headaches, mental changes and gastrointestinal upset, although these will resolve with

Safety of Medicines has restricted azapropazone to acute gout only when other NSAIDs have been tried and failed, and its use is contraindicated in patients with a history of peptic ulceration, in moderate to severe renal impairment, and in the elderly with mild renal impairment. A maximum dose of 1.8 g of azapropazone in divided doses may be given until symptoms subside, followed by 1.2 g/day in divided doses until symptoms resolve. Adequate fluid intake must be ensured throughout treatment. In mild renal impairment or the elderly, 1.8 g in divided doses can be given for 24 hours, followed by 1.2 g daily reducing to a maximum of 600 mg daily in divided doses as soon as possible.

Uricosuric agents

Most patients with symptomatic hyperuricaemia underexcrete uric acid, and these patients can be managed with uricosuric agents.

Uricosuric agents such as probenecid (500 mg to 1 g twice daily) and sulfinpyrazone (100) mg three or four times a day) offer an alternative to allopurinol. These agents should be avoided in patients with urate nephropathy and those who overproduce uric acid. They are ineffective in patients with poor renal function (creatinine clearance of less than 20–30 ml/min).

Probenecid is well absorbed orally with a serum half-life of 6–12 hours. Therapy should be initiated with a dose of 250 mg twice daily, increased to 500 mg twice daily after 2 weeks, with a further increase up to 2 g daily if required. An initial low dose of uricosuric agent helps to prevent precipitation of an acute attack along with prophylactic therapy against an acute attack using an NSAID or colchicine for about 3 months. This also decreases the risk of stone formation in the kidney. Patients should be advised to maintain a high fluid intake (at least 2 litres per day) to minimize the risk of stone formation.

Approximately 5–10% of patients receiving long-term probenecid suffer nausea, heartburn, flatulence or constipation. A mild pruritic rash, drug fever and renal disturbances can occur.

Its major limiting factor is a lack of efficacy due to poor compliance, concurrent low dose salicylates or renal insufficiency.

The serum level of probenecid is elevated by concomitant indometacin, and aspirin inhibits the uricosuric actions of probenecid and sulfinpyrazone. Other common drug interactions are listed in Table 52.3, and the pharmacokinetic profile of the drugs used in the management of gout are presented in Table 52.4.

Benzbromarone

This unlicensed agent may be used at 100 mg daily, on a named patient basis in patients with moderate renal

Table 52.3   Common drug interactions associated with therapy for gout and hyperuricaemia

Interacting drug	Affected drug	Effect
Allopurinol	Azathioprine	Increased levels of azathioprine
Allopurinol	Mercaptopurine	Increased levels of mercaptopurine
Allopurinol	Anticoagulants	Enhanced anticoagulant effect
Aspirin (low dose)	Uricosurics	Decreased hypouricaemic effect
Probenecid	Indometacin	Increased indometacin levels
Probenecid	Ketoprofen	Increased ketoprofen levels
Probenecid	Naproxen	Increased naproxen levels
Probenecid	Methotrexate	Increased methotrexate levels
Probenecid	Zidovudine	Increased zidovudine levels
Probenecid	Cephalosporins	Increased cephalosporin levels
Probenecid	Dapsone	Increased dapsone levels
Probenecid	Aspirin	Increased aspirin levels
Sulfinpyrazone	Anticoagulants	Enhanced anticoagulant effect

Table 52.4 Pharmacokinetic parameters for drugs used in the management of gout

Agent	$t_{1/2}$(h)	T_{max}(h)	V_d(l/kg)	Protein binding	Clearance, hepatic (l/h)
Allopurinol	1–3[a]	2–6	–	0–4.5	46
Colchicine	20	2	1–2	31	36
Probenecid	4–12[b]	4	0.12–0.18	85–95	1.4
Sulfinpyrazone	1–2	3	0.06	98–99	1.4

[a] Active metabolite 12–30 h.
[b] 3–8 h (0.5g); 6–12 h (2 g).

impairment when other uricosuric agents are ineffective or allopurinol is precluded owing to hypersensitivity.

Prophylactic treatment of asymptomatic hyperuricaemia

It is unnecessary and excessive to treat all patients with hyperuricaemia with urate-lowering drugs although individuals with high serum uric acid levels are more likely to develop gout. The risk of hyperuricaemia causing renal disease is controversial although the consensus appears to be that hyperuricaemia alone does not have a deleterious effect on renal function. The presence of hyperuricaemia does seem to be a risk factor for development of cardiovascular disease although the evidence is not sufficiently strong at the moment for prophylactic therapy to be considered necessary. Obese patients should lose weight gradually and their blood pressure and renal function should be monitored annually.

Drug-induced gout

Hyperuricaemia and gout occur with diuretics, especially thiazides. Where possible an alternative agent should be used (e.g. vasodilator for hypertension), but where this is not possible, allopurinol should be used to lower urate levels. Other drugs that reduce renal urate excretion include low-dose aspirin and alcohol. Ciclosporin-induced hyperuricaemia and gout has been reported, especially in men, after an average of 24 months. The condition did not seem to be related to serum ciclosporin concentrations. Acute gout associated with omeprazole has also been reported.

Other drugs may interfere with renal excretion of uric acid including ethambutol, pyrazinamide, niacin and didanosine (Agudelo & Wise 1998).

Radiotherapy and chemotherapy in patients with neoplastic disorders can cause hyperuricaemia. This can be treated prophylactically with allopurinol, commencing 3 days before therapy.

Patient care

Patients with gout should be advised about factors that may contribute to hyperuricaemia, such as fasting, obesity and alcohol excess. If these are avoided or corrected, drug treatment may not be needed. Asymptomatic hyperuricaemia need not be treated, but renal function can be checked to ensure that it is not deteriorating.

Patients at risk of recurrent gouty attacks should receive a supply of NSAIDs. They must be adequately informed to commence treatment at the first signs of an attack. This should abort the attack in most patients. Patients must be told the correct manner and dose in which NSAIDs should be used, the potential side-effects and the action to take if side-effects occur. They should be advised to avoid aspirin and instead use paracetamol for analgesia.

Patients receiving allopurinol should be informed of the need to continue single daily dose treatment in the absence of any symptomatic response. They must be warned of potential side-effects and told to report any adverse skin reactions.

Patients receiving uricosuric agents should be recommended to maintain a good fluid intake to reduce the risk of renal calculus formation. Urine flow of at least 2 litres per day is required.

A therapeutic algorithin for the management of gout is presented in Figure 52.1. Common therapeutic problems are listed in Table 52.5.

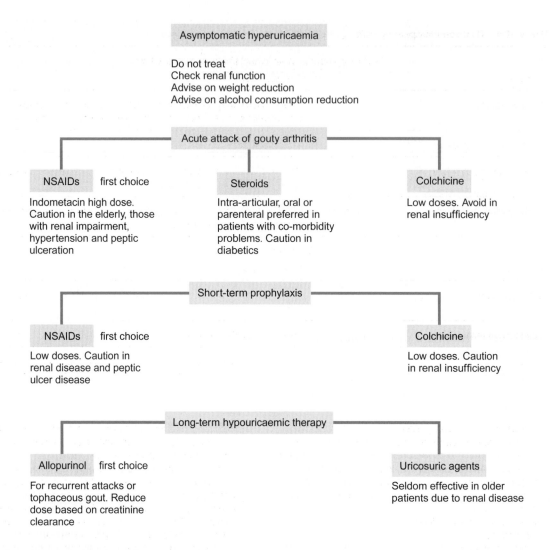

Asymptomatic hyperuricaemia

Do not treat
Check renal function
Advise on weight reduction
Advise on alcohol consumption reduction

Acute attack of gouty arthritis

NSAIDs first choice

Indometacin high dose.
Caution in the elderly, those
with renal impairment,
hypertension and peptic
ulceration

Steroids

Intra-articular, oral or
parenteral preferred in
patients with co-morbidity
problems. Caution in
diabetics

Colchicine

Low doses. Avoid in
renal insufficiency

Short-term prophylaxis

NSAIDs first choice

Low doses. Caution in
renal disease and peptic
ulcer disease

Colchicine

Low doses. Caution
in renal insufficiency

Long-term hypouricaemic therapy

Allopurinol first choice

For recurrent attacks or
tophaceous gout. Reduce
dose based on creatinine
clearance

Uricosuric agents

Seldom effective in older
patients due to renal disease

Fig. 52.1 Algorithm for the management of gout.

CASE STUDIES

Case 52.1

Mr H. C. is 70 years old and weighs 75 kg. He presents
with symmetrical polyarticular arthritis and fever. He has
very painful red and swollen metacarpophalangeal joints,
proximal interphalangeal joints, wrists, elbows and knees.
On admission he was taking digoxin 125 micrograms day,
furosemide (frusemide) 40 mg/day, warfarin 3 mg/day and
isosorbide mononitrate 20 mg twice daily. He is a non-
smoker, who enjoys a glass of wine. The house officer has
commenced azapropazone 600 mg twice daily. The results
of his investigations are as follows: temperature 38° C,
serum creatinine 140 mol/l (62–133mol/l), ESR 60 mm in
1st hr, rheumatoid factor 12 (<12 international normalized
units), serum urate 0.55 mmol/l (0.15–0.51 mmol/l),
synovial fluid analysis from knee and elbow–urate
crystals. The diagnosis is a first attack of acute gout.

Questions

1. What factors predispose this patient to gout?
2. Comment on the treatment started and possible alternatives
   (drug, dose, duration and monitoring requirements).
3. What advice would you give regarding correction of the
   hyperuricaemia?

Answers

1. Mr H. C. has gout which may be related to both
   overproduction and underexcretion of uric acid. He has
   hyperuricaemia and mild renal impairment (creatinine
   clearance 46 ml/min). The male:female incidence of gout is
   2–7:1 and obesity is strongly associated with
   hyperuricaemia, reflecting excess dietary intake. The
   hyperuricaemic actions of thiazide and loop diuretics are
   frequently encountered in clinical practice. The mechanism
   is related to extracellular fluid contraction. The typically

Table 52.5   Common therapeutic problems in the treatment of gout

Treatment of acute attacks and short-term prophylaxis	
Problem	Possible solution
Elderly patients	These patients may not tolerate NSAIDS. Colchicine in low doses or corticosteroids are an option, but care with co-morbidity (see below)
Patients with renal failure	Avoid NSAIDS
Patients with heart failure	Use colchicine in low doses and with caution. Corticosteroids may be an option, but use with care in diabetic patients
Patients with a history of gastrointestinal problems	NSAID with a gastroprotective agent such as proton pump inhibitor or misoprostol. Consider colchicine
Long-term prophylaxis	
Problem	Possible solution
Elderly patients	Uricosuric agents are rarely effective in the elderly due to reduced renal function
Patients with renal failure	Uricosuric agents are not effective. Allopurinol dosage should be reduced
Recurrent attacks	Allopurinol dosage should be reduced if creatinine clearance is reduced

affected patient is usually elderly and female, with a long history of continuous diuretic ingestion. Diuretic-induced gout may present as classic acute synovitis but sometimes takes the form of a generalized arthritis that can be misdiagnosed as osteoarthritis or rheumatoid arthritis. Other factors which may predispose to gout in this particular patient include:

- hereditary enzyme defects
- hypertension
- hyperlipidaemia
- diabetes
- myeloproliferative disorders
- haemolytic anaemia
- excess alcohol intake.

2. The goal of treatment is to relieve the pain and inflammation of acute gout. This is an atypical presentation of gout. Classically it presents as rapid onset with excruciating pain and swelling in a single joint (first metatarsophalangeal joint in 90% of cases), and systemic features are mild or absent. In this patient, presentation could be confused with rheumatoid arthritis, but urate crystals confirm gout.

   The treatment options for Mr H. C. are NSAIDs, colchicine or intra-articular steroids. Allopurinol or uricosuric agents should not be started at this stage. Lowering of urate levels is not urgent and the patient is likely to have been hyperuricaemic for some time. These agents cause mobilization of uric acid stores which may prolong or precipitate an acute attack. However, if the patient is already taking an antihyperuricaemic agent, it should be continued at the same dose. NSAIDs are effective in relieving symptoms and have a quicker onset of action than colchicine (at 2 hours as opposed to 6 hours). NSAIDs are effective if used in high dosage for 1–3 days then reduced and continued for a further 7–10 days.

The potential problems in this patient are aggravation of heart failure due to sodium and water retention and aggravation of existing renal impairment.

NSAIDs, especially azapropazone, interact with warfarin. Most NSAIDs enhance the risk of bleeding by antiplatelet effects, but do not have a significant effect on the international normalized ratio (INR). Azapropazone causes significant displacement of warfarin from protein binding sites and inhibits hepatic enzyme activity leading to increased levels of free warfarin and an increase in INR. Further, elderly patients share an increased risk of gastrointestinal side-effects. The azapropazone should be stopped and treatment with colchicine begun. Colchicine is effective for acute gout, commencing with 1 mg initially followed by 500 micrograms every 3 hours until pain is reduced or side-effects occur or until a maximum dose of 6 mg is reached. Colchicine does not interact with warfarin and will not aggravate existing heart failure. The potential problems in this patient include gastrointestinal toxicity, as approximately 80% of patients are affected by vomiting, diarrhoea and abdominal pain. If renal function deteriorates to less than 10 ml/min creatinine clearance the dose should be reduced.

Intra-articular steroids are effective and work within 12–24 hours, but the differential diagnosis of joint infection must be made carefully. Intra-articular steroids are unlikely to affect this patient's heart failure and these are safe in renal impairment.

3. The feasibility of discontinuing the diuretic or changing to bumetanide should be considered. The dietary and alcohol issues to consider include a low fat diet to help reduce weight and hyperlipidaemia and a reduction in alcohol consumption which leads to increased uric acid production and reduced excretion.

Anti-hyperuricaemic drugs should not be commenced until the acute attack has settled completely. Anti-hyperuricaemic drugs are usually only considered for recurrent gouty attacks, with radiological evidence of joint damage, tophaceous deposits or nephrolithiasis, and therefore are probably not indicated at this stage. The patient should continue on colchicine at a prophylactic dose of 500 micrograms twice daily to minimize the risk of acute attack, and continue for 1 month after correction of urate level. The treatment of choice in this patient would be allopurinol. This will inhibit xanthine oxidase enzyme required for uric acid production and therefore is a logical choice for overproducers. Allopurinol will reduce serum urate levels after 2 days and the levels should be monitored after 2–3 weeks.

In patients with renal impairment the dose should be reduced, and a suitable dose in this patient would be 150 mg daily. The allopurinol may interact with warfarin and increase the INR, which should be monitored after 1 week. Probenecid and sulfinpyrazone increase uric acid excretion, but are not suitable where overproduction is the major cause of hyperuricaemia. These agents are ineffective where the creatinine clearance is less than 50 ml/min and a high fluid intake is needed to reduce the risk of renal stone formation. The potential problems in this patient are that these agents may be ineffective due to renal impairment. The sulfinpyrazone may aggravate heart failure owing to sodium and water retention and may enhance the effect of warfarin. Probenecid may impair the excretion of NSAIDs. On balance, allopurinol, at a suitably reduced dose combined with INR monitoring, will probably be the most effective treatment for the future.

Case 52.2

Mr J. D. is 57 years old and is admitted to hospital with a deep-vein thrombosis. He is known to have recurrent attacks of gout and takes a 300 mg allopurinol tablet each day as well as occasional analgesics.

Questions

1. It is decided to prescribe warfarin for Mr J. D.'s deep vein thrombosis. What are the problems with using a standard loading dose of warfarin (day 1, 10 mg; day 2, 5 mg; day 3, 5 mg) to treat his deep-vein thrombosis?
2. Allopurinol has a half-life of 2 hours but is given once a day, why is this?

Answers

1. Warfarin is highly protein bound and has a long plasma half-life. The administration of a 10 mg loading dose will reduce the time for the drug to reach a steady state, but in this patient the dose is excessive. Patients more than 60 years of age or weighing less than 60 kg or with a serum albumin level less than 35 g/dl, all require a reduced loading dose. Although Mr J. D. does not fulfil any of these criteria, he is taking allopurinol. Allopurinol inhibits the metabolism of warfarin by inhibiting the oxidative metabolic pathway. The dose of warfarin should therefore be reduced by approximately 50% for the loading dose. The usual

maintenance dose will also require a reduction of approximately 50%. In the early stages of therapy the INR should be checked every few days until it has stabilized at twice normal.
2. Allopurinol has no activity on xanthine oxidase. Allopurinol undergoes hepatic conversion to its active metabolite, oxipurinol. The half-life of allopurinol is approximately 2 hours. Oxipurinol is excreted renally and undergoes net reabsorption in the renal tubule as does urate itself. The half-life of oxipurinol is 13–18 hours in patients with normal renal function. For this reason, allopurinol may be successfully administered with a single daily dose.

Case 52.3

Mr K. F. is a 47-year-old factory worker who weighs 75 kg. He has a history of gout controlled with one 300 mg tablet of allopurinol each day. He was admitted to hospital after collapsing with chest pain while running to catch a bus. On admission he was diagnosed as having suffered a myocardial infarction and was treated with diamorphine, streptokinase, heparin and low-dose (150 mg) aspirin.

Questions

1. What effect will the aspirin have on Mr K. F.'s gout?
2. Should Mr K. F.'s management be changed because of his history of gout?

Answers

1. Mr K. F. is already taking allopurinol as prophylaxis against further attacks of gout. In this situation the addition of aspirin to his drug regimen is probably of no consequence. His gout is already controlled with allopurinol.
   The administration of aspirin 300 mg or more can lead to elevation of serum urate levels, by inhibition of tubular secretion, and thus predispose patients to acute attacks of gout. In contrast, high-dose salicylate therapy acts in a similar manner to the uricosuric agents by inhibiting tubular reabsorption of urate, which leads to an increased excretion and a fall in serum levels.
   As a general principle therefore, low-dose aspirin should be avoided in patients with gout. In the case of Mr K. F., low-dose aspirin has been demonstrated in many studies to decrease mortality following myocardial infarction and for this reason treatment should continue, probably lifelong.
2. No changes in the management of Mr K. F. should be made because of his history of gout. It would be appropriate to counsel him over his risk factors for ischaemic heart disease and gout. He should be advised to stop smoking, reduce his alcohol intake and adopt a low fat diet.

Case 52.4

Mrs C. is an 80-year-old woman who presented to the accident and emergency department with a red, painful and swollen index finger. She had experienced two previous gouty attacks in the past 6 months. Her previous medical history included atrial fibrillation, congestive heart failure, hypertension and hyperlipidaemia. Her alcohol

intake was about 25 units/week and her medication included amiodarone 200 mg daily, furosemide (frusemide) 80 mg daily, enalapril 15 mg daily and simvastatin 20 mg at night. Her investigation revealed serum urate 0.6 mmol/l (0.15–0.55 mmol/l), serum creatinine 80 μmol/l (62–133 μmol/l), and her calculated creatinine clearance was 42 ml/min.

The diagnosis was acute gout of a recurrent nature and she was started on colchicine 500 micrograms daily.

Questions

1. What risk factors does Mrs C. have which predispose her to gout?
2. Is colchicine an appropriate choice for the acute management of gout in Mrs C?
3. What treatment option would you recommend for Mrs C. for prophylaxing her gout?

Answers

1. Her risk factors include hypertension, hyperlipidaemia, excess alcohol intake, furosemide (frusemide), high urate level, reduced renal function and being an elderly woman on a diuretic.
2. Colchicine is a good choice for Mrs C. as it will not exacerbate her other medical conditions. However, the dose is too low at 500 micrograms daily. The initial dose should be 1 mg, followed by 500 micrograms every 2–3 hours up to a maximum dose of 6 mg or until diarrhoea. In elderly frail patients, the dose may be reduced to 500 micrograms three times a day.

Another therapeutic choice, NSAIDs, would be unsuitable for Mrs C. as she has congestive heart failure and hypertension and NSAIDs can worsen both conditions. She also has a high risk for gastrointestinal adverse reactions with NSAIDs therapy, and therefore NSAIDs are best avoided.

Intra-articular steroids would not be suitable as the finger joints are small, difficult to inject and painful. There is also the risk of infection.

Oral steroids have a slow onset of action and can cause multiple side-effects in the elderly.

3. The choice of prophylactic agents include allopurinol, uricosuric agents or colchicine. Allopurinol is the treatment of choice. Sulfinpyrazone may worsen her heart failure by increasing sodium and water retention. Colchicine does not reduce hyperuricaemia and therefore reduce renal impairment, but it may prevent the symptoms of gout if allopurinol cannot be tolerated. Probenecid is unlikely to be effective owing to the renal impairment. Allopurinol is effective for recurrent gouty attacks. The initial dose should be 100 mg daily because of renal impairment. This should control the symptoms of gout and help to protect against further deterioration in Mrs C.'s renal function.

REFERENCES

Ahem M J, Reid C, Clardon T P et al 1987 Does colchicine work? Results of the first controlled study in gout. Australian and New Zealand Journal of Medicine 17: 301–304

Agudelo C A, Wise C M 1998 Crystal associated arthritis. Clinics in Geriatric Medicine 14: 495–513

Emmerson B T 1996 The management of gout. New England Journal of Medicine 334: 445–450

Graham W, Robert J B 1983 Intravenous colchicine in the management of gouty arthritis. Annals of the Rheumatic Diseases 12: 16–19

Gray R G, Tenenbaum J, Gottlieb N L 1981 Local corticosteroid injection treatment in rheumatic disorders. Seminars in Arthritis and Rheumatism 10: 231–254

McDonald J, Fam A G, Paton T et al 1988 Allopurinol hypersensitivity in a patient with coexistent systemic lupus erythematosus and tophaceous gout. Journal of Rheumatology 15: 865–868

Northridge D B, Almack P M 1986 Allopurinol desensitisation. British Journal of Pharmacy Practice 8:200

Nuki G 1998 Metabolic and endocrine arthropathies. Medicine 263: 54–59

Peterson G M, Boyle R R, Francis H W et al 1990 Dosage prescribing and plasma oxypurinol levels in patients receiving allopurinol therapy. European Journal of Clinical Pharmacology 39: 419–421

Singer J Z, Wallace S L 1986 The allopurinol hypersensitivity syndrome: unnecessary morbidity and mortality. Arthritis and Rheumatism 29: 82–87

Wallace S L, Singer J Z 1988 Systemic toxicity associated with the intravenous administration of colchicine – guidelines for use. [Review] Journal of Rheumatology 15: 495–499

Wood J 1999 Gout and its management. Pharmaceutical Journal 262: 808–811

FURTHER READING

Conaghan P G, Day R O 1994 Risks and benefits of drugs used in the management and prevention of gout. Drug Safety 11: 252–258

Scott T, Clarke F 1996 Acute and long-term management of gout. Prescriber 7(17): 41–53

Snaith M L 1995 Gout, hyperuricaemic and crystal arthritis. British Medical Journal 310: 521–524

Star V L, Hochberg M C 1993 Prevention and management of gout. Drugs 45: 212–222 [table]

Glaucoma 53

L. C. Titcomb   S. D. Andrew

KEY POINTS

- Glaucoma is a large group of disorders with widely differing clinical features.
- Primary open-angle glaucoma (POAG) is a chronic progressive disease of insidious onset.
- The aim of treatment in POAG is to reduce the intraocular pressure (IOP), preventing further damage to the nerve fibres and the development of further visual field defects.
- A wide range of drugs is used to treat POAG. Surgery may be undertaken if maximally tolerated medical therapy fails to control the IOP.
- POAG is a symptomless disease until well advanced. Concordance with therapy is an important issue.
- Acute primary angle closure glaucoma (PACG) is a medical emergency that must be treated rapidly to prevent blindness.
- The aim of medical treatment in acute PACG is to reduce the IOP in preparation for surgery.
- A wide range of drugs can provoke an attack of PACG in susceptible individuals.

The term 'glaucoma' does not represent a single pathological entity. It consists of a large group of disorders with widely differing clinical features. It is therefore difficult to attempt a single definition of the term, but it may be generally defined as those conditions in which the intraocular pressure (IOP) is too high for the normal functioning of the optic nerve head.

Epidemiology

The diseases which make up the group known as glaucoma are usually classified according to the manner in which aqueous humour outflow is impaired.

Primary open-angle glaucoma

Primary open-angle glaucoma (POAG), also referred to as chronic simple glaucoma, is associated with a relative obstruction to aqueous outflow through the trabecular meshwork, and is a chronic progressive disease of insidious onset, usually affecting both eyes. It is the most common type of glaucoma, and affects approximately 1 in 200 of the population over the age of 40 years. POAG is responsible for about 20% of all cases of blindness in the UK, and affects both sexes equally. It is frequently an inherited condition, with approximately 10% of first-degree relatives of POAG sufferers eventually developing the disease (Pitts-Crick 1994).

Primary angle closure glaucoma

Primary angle closure glaucoma (PACG), or closed-angle glaucoma, is a condition in which closure of the angle by the peripheral iris results in a reduction in aqueous outflow. It occurs in predisposed eyes and is frequently unilateral. The disease affects approximately 1 in 1000 adults over the age of 40 years, and occurs in four times as many females as males.

Two conditions similar to POAG are normal-tension glaucoma, where the IOP is not raised on initial screening although signs of damage are present, and ocular hypertension, where signs of damage do not accompany the raised IOP.

Secondary glaucomas can arise for a number of reasons, including inflammation, intraocular tumour, raised episcleral venous pressure, or congenitally due to developmental abnormalities.

Aetiology

The factors that determine the level of IOP are the rate of aqueous humour production and the resistance encountered in the outflow channels. A fine balance between these is necessary to keep the pressure within the eye in the range of 16–21 mmHg.

Production of aqueous humour occurs in the ciliary epithelium by two mechanisms: secretion due to an active metabolic process, independent of the level of IOP, and ultrafiltration influenced by the level of blood pressure in the ciliary capillaries and the level of IOP.

Outflow of aqueous humour occurs by two routes. Approximately 80% of total outflow is through the trabecular meshwork into the canal of Schlemm and into the venous circulation via the aqueous veins. The uveoscleral pathway account for the remaining 20%: through the ciliary body into the suprachoroidal space, to be drained into the ciliary body, choroid and sclera via the venous circulation.

Pathophysiology

The primary site of damage is thought to be the optic nerve head, rather than any other point along the nerve axon. This most easily explains the progressive loss of visual field. Studies of axoplasmic flow show a vulnerability of the nerves to elevated IOP as they pass through the optic disc.

In POAG increased resistance within the drainage channels causes the rise in IOP. It is thought that the main route of resistance to aqueous outflow lies in the dense juxtacanalicular trabecular meshwork, or the endothelium lining the inner wall of Schlemm's canal.

In PACG the rise in IOP is caused by a decreased outflow of aqueous humour, due to closure of the chamber angle by the peripheral iris. It occurs in predisposed eyes, and the predisposing factors can be anatomical or physiological. The anatomical characteristics are lens size, corneal diameter and axial length of the globe. The lens continues to grow throughout life. This brings the anterior surface closer to the cornea. Slackening of the suspensory ligaments increases this movement. Both factors occur very gradually and lead to a progressive shallowing of the anterior chamber. The depth of the anterior chamber and width of the chamber angle are related to corneal diameter, and those eyes predisposed to PACG are observed to have a corneal diameter less than that seen in normal eyes. A short eye, which is frequently also hypermetropic, has a small corneal diameter and a thick and relatively anteriorly located lens.

The physiological precipitating factors of PACG in predisposed eyes are not fully understood. Two theories currently exist. The dilator muscle theory suggests that contraction of the dilator muscle causes a posterior movement, which increases the apposition between the iris and anteriorly located lens and the degree of physiological pupillary block. The simultaneous dilatation of the pupil renders the peripheral iris more flaccid, and causes the pressure in the posterior chamber to increase and the iris to bow anteriorly. Eventually the peripheral iris obstructs the angle, and the IOP rises (Fig. 53.1).

The sphincter muscle theory postulates that the sphincter of the pupil precipitates angle closure. The pupillary blocking force of the sphincter is greatest when the diameter of the pupil is about 4 mm.

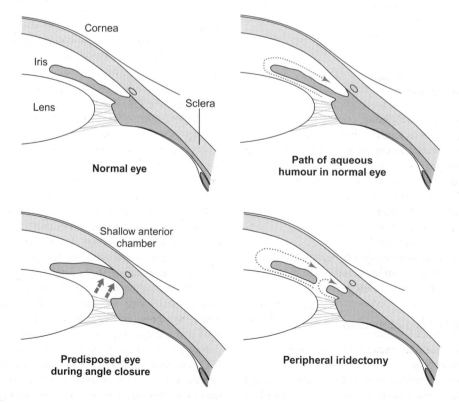

Figure 53.1 Changes to the eye seen during closed-angle glaucoma.

Clinical manifestations

POAG is characterized by the following: an IOP greater that 21 mmHg, an open angle, glaucomatous cupping and visual field loss. Because of its insidious onset, POAG is usually asymptomatic until it has caused a significant loss of visual field. In some eyes, subtle signs of glaucomatous retinal nerve damage can be detected prior to development of pathological cupping and detectable field loss. The earliest clinically significant field defect is a scotoma, which is an area of depressed vision within the visual field. Patients with POAG frequently show a wider swing in IOP than normal, therefore a single pressure reading of 21 mmHg or less does not exclude the diagnosis. It may be necessary to measure IOP at different times of the day, or at periodic intervals.

Acute PACG is due to a sudden closure of the angle and a severe elevation in IOP. The symptoms include rapidly progressive visual impairment, periocular pain and congestion of the eye. In severe cases nausea and vomiting may occur. The signs include injection of the limbal and conjunctival vessels giving a 'ciliary flush'. The IOP usually lies between 50 and 80 mmHg and causes corneal oedema with epithelial vesicles. The anterior chamber is shallow and iridocorneal contact can be observed. The pupil is vertically oval and fixed in a semidilated position. It is unreactive to light and accommodation. The fellow eye usually has a shallow anterior chamber and a narrow angle. The optic nerve head is oedematous and hyperaemic.

Investigations

Intraocular pressure may be measured by tonometry, such as indentation tonometry in which a plunger is applied to the cornea and the amount of indentation on the eye reflects the pressure within it. Tonography is a technique used to measure the outflow of aqueous humour from the eye, resulting from indentation of the eye, using a tonometer. Gonioscopy is used to estimate the width of the chamber angle, with the aid of a slit lamp. Perimetry is important for both the diagnosis and management of glaucoma by detecting early scotomata and larger changes in visual field.

In patients with POAG, cupping of the optic disc becomes progressively apparent, and is used in both diagnosis and assessment of the efficacy of treatment. The increased intraocular pressure appears to push the optic disc back into an excavation. This is known as glaucomatous cupping.

The colour of the optic disc will be observed to change from a creamy pink colour due to the rich capillary network seen in the healthy eye to increased pallor with advancing disease as the optic nerve tissue progressively atrophies (Infield & O'Shea 1998).

Treatment

The aim of treatment in POAG is to reduce the raised IOP, preventing further damage to the nerve fibres and the development of further visual field defects. The key to effective treatment is careful and regular follow-up including measurement of visual acuity, tonometry, gonioscopy, evaluation of the optic disc, and perimetry (of primary importance).

The actual safe level of IOP is unknown, the importance of disc and field assessment being underlined by evidence that IOP does not rise above the 'normal' range in up to 50% of glaucomas (normal-pressure glaucomas). However, in many cases maximal retardation of disease process is achieved if the IOP is maintained in the lower teens. The effect on the visual field and the appearance of the optic disc are the only indications that IOP is being controlled at a safe level. A raised IOP without field or disc changes may not require treatment but will need regular review.

The initial treatment of POAG is usually medical. Topical administration is the preferred type of therapy and there is a wide range of preparations available (Table 53.1). The chosen drug should be administered at its lowest concentration and as infrequently as possible to obtain the desired effect. A drug with few potential side-effects should be chosen, with oral therapy retained as the final option. In most cases the initial topical treatment is with a β-blocker or latanoprost. If this is ineffective, the strength of the β-blocker may be increased, another prostaglandin prostamide substituted or a carbonic anhydrase inhibitor, or a sympathomimetic added. Pilocarpine is usually reserved for those patients not controlled by a combination of the drugs listed above. Oral therapy with carbonic anhydrase inhibitors is usually reserved for use as the final stage of treatment in those complex glaucomas awaiting surgery (Fig. 53.2).

If maximum medical management fails to control the IOP, surgery will be performed, using filtration surgery (trabeculectomy) to create a fistula to act as a new route for aqueous outflow. Occasionally argon laser trabeculoplasty to promote increased aqueous humour outflow may be employed, but this tends to be reserved for elderly subjects with moderate glaucoma and an IOP of less than 30 mmHg. It is important to realize that the effect of laser trabeculoplasty may rapidly reverse, and therefore constant vigilance is necessary. Laser ciliary ablation to reduce aqueous humour production is used for some intractable glaucomas (Khaw 1994).

The medical management of acute PACG is essentially to prepare the eye for surgical treatment. The aim of treatment is to decrease the IOP and associated

Table 53.1 Drugs used in the treatment of primary open-angle glaucoma

Therapeutic category	Primary mechanisms of action
Topical β-blocking agents	Decrease aqueous formation
Topical miotics	Increase aqueous outflow
Topical adrenergic agonists	Increase aqueous outflow and decrease aqueous formation
Topical carbonic anhydrase inhibitors	Decrease aqueous formation
Oral carbonic anhydrase inhibitors	Decrease aqueous formation
Topical prostaglandins	Increase aqueous outflow
Topical prostamides	Increase aqueous outflow

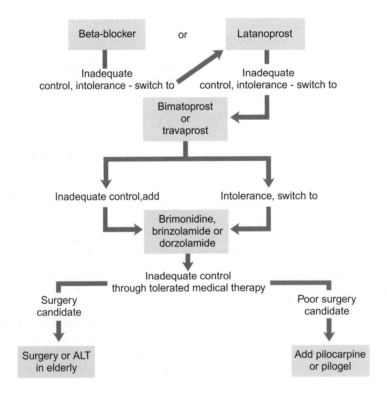

Figure 53.2 Topical therapy for primary open-angle glaucoma (POAG). ALT, argon laser tabeculoplasty.

inflammation. Analgesics and antiemetics are sometimes needed, dependent on symptom severity, to make the patient comfortable. It is usual to treat the unaffected eye prophylactically with miotics (Fig. 53.3).

Paralysis of the iris sphincter usually occurs at an IOP of more than 60 mmHg, due to ischaemia. Therefore, intensive miotic therapy, previously the treatment of choice in many cases of PACG, is usually ineffective,

and the IOP needs to be lowered by drugs that reduce aqueous humour production rather than by trying to pull the peripheral iris away from the angle with miotics. An intravenous loading dose of acetazolamide followed by oral treatment, sometimes in combination with corneal indentation, to physically force aqueous humour to the peripheral anterior chamber and artificially open the angle, should allow the IOP to drop sufficiently to

Time

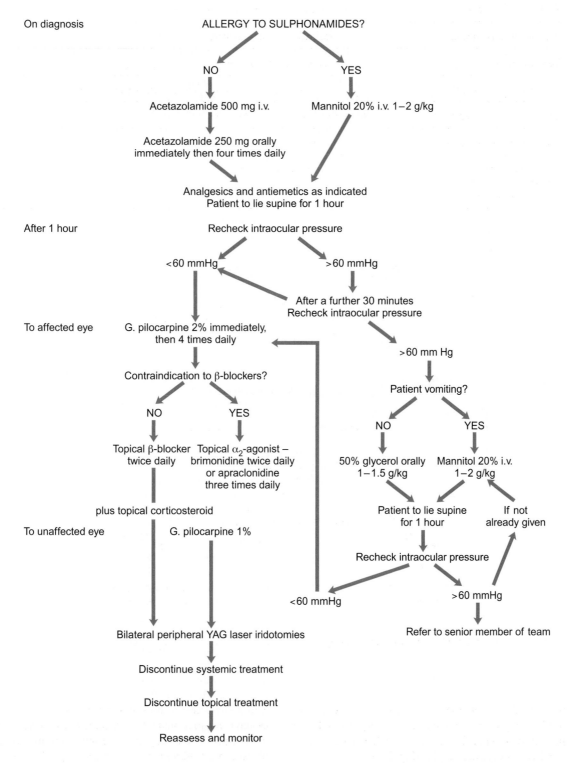

On diagnosis — ALLERGY TO SULPHONAMIDES?

NO → Acetazolamide 500 mg i.v. → Acetazolamide 250 mg orally immediately then four times daily

YES → Mannitol 20% i.v. 1–2 g/kg

Analgesics and antiemetics as indicated
Patient to lie supine for 1 hour

After 1 hour — Recheck intraocular pressure

<60 mmHg

>60 mmHg → After a further 30 minutes Recheck intraocular pressure → >60 mm Hg

To affected eye — G. pilocarpine 2% immediately, then 4 times daily

Contraindication to β-blockers?

NO → Topical β-blocker twice daily

YES → Topical α₂-agonist – brimonidine twice daily or apraclonidine three times daily

plus topical corticosteroid

To unaffected eye — G. pilocarpine 1%

Patient vomiting?

NO → 50% glycerol orally 1–1.5 g/kg

YES → Mannitol 20% i.v. 1–2 g/kg

Patient to lie supine for 1 hour

If not already given

Recheck intraocular pressure

<60 mmHg

>60 mmHg

Refer to senior member of team

Bilateral peripheral YAG laser iridotomies

Discontinue systemic treatment

Discontinue topical treatment

Reassess and monitor

Figure 53.3 Algorithm for the treatment of primary angle closure glaucoma (PACG). YAG, yttrium aluminum garnet.

relieve iris ischaemia and allow the sphincter to respond to pilocarpine therapy.

If corneal indentation and acetazolamide fail to decrease IOP, hyperosmotic agents may be required. Once the IOP has been reduced medically the condition is usually treated surgically, either by surgical peripheral iridectomy or laser iridotomy, to remove an area of the peripheral iris to allow flow of aqueous humour through an alternative pathway (see Fig. 53.1). Filtration surgery is indicated if a large proportion of the angle has been permanently closed by adhesions between the iris and the cornea.

β adrenoceptor antagonists

The exact mechanism of action of β adrenoceptor antagonists (β-blockers) in lowering IOP has not been fully established but they have been shown to reduce aqueous humour formation rather than increase outflow. Five drugs are available in the UK for topical administration: betaxolol, carteolol, levobunolol, metipranolol and timolol (Table 53.2). β-blockers have a number of important properties in addition to β adrenoceptor blockade. These include intrinsic sympathomimetic activity (ISA), cardioselectivity and membrane stabilizing activity, which are all of importance when considering the side-effects seen with these agents (Table 53.3).

The property of membrane stabilization is relevant to the incidence of ocular side-effects. The absence of anaesthetic properties reduces the number and severity of foreign body and dryness sensations, anaesthesia of the cornea and dry eye syndrome.

Ocular side-effects of topically administered β-blockers are shown in Table 53.4.

It has been suggested that those β-blockers that show ISA are less likely to produce bronchospasm and peripheral vascular side-effects. Carteolol is the only commercially available drug that shows ISA. The selectivity of cardioselective β-blockers diminishes with increasing dosage, even within the therapeutic range. Betaxolol is the only commercially available topical β-blocker that demonstrates cardioselectivity.

A degree of bradycardia and hypotension is commonly seen with all β-blockers, although it is more marked with non-selective agents. These may be of clinical significance and should be monitored, particularly if the patient is known to suffer cardiac disease or hypertension, for there may be a tendency to underestimate this particular problem.

The precipitation of bronchospasm in susceptible patients can occur with the administration of as little as one drop of timolol. Those β-blockers that show cardioselectivity or ISA are less likely to cause bronchoconstriction, although it has been demonstrated that respiratory function improved in patients whose treatment was changed from timolol to betaxolol or an adrenergic agonist, these same patients having previously been asymptomatic.

All topical β-blockers have been reported to cause bronchospasm, hence 'at risk' patients with a tendency to airway disease who require treatment for glaucoma should be treated with extreme caution.

The Committee on Safety of Medicines (CSM) has advised that β-blockers, even those with apparent cardioselectivity, should not be used in patients with asthma or a history of obstructive airways disease unless no alternative treatment is available. In such cases the risk of inducing bronchospasm should be appreciated and appropriate precautions taken.

Ocular β-blockers are generally not contraindicated in diabetes although a cardioselective agent may be preferable. However, they are best avoided in patients who suffer frequent hypoglycaemic attacks as they do produce a slight impairment of glucose tolerance.

Systemic side-effects of topically administered β-blockers are shown in Table 53.5.

The long-term benefits of β-blockers on visual function preservation have been shown to be less than would be expected. This may be due to adverse effects on the ocular microcirculation whereby the β-blockers

Table 53.2	Examples of ophthalmic β-blockers		
Drug	Brand name	Strength (%)	Daily dosage frequency
Betaxolol	Betoptic solution	0.5	2
	Betoptic suspension[b]	0.25	
Carteolol	Teoptic	1	2
		2	2
Levobunolol	Betagan[b] and generic form	0.5	1–2
Metipranolol[a]	Minims[c]	0.1	2
		0.3	2
Timolol	Timoptol[b] and generic form	0.25	2
	Cosopt (with dorzolamide 2%)	0.5	2
	Xalacom (with latanoprost 0.005%)	0.5	1
	Timoptol-LA	0.25	1
		0.5	1

[a] Metipranolol multidose marketed as Glauline was withdrawn in 1990 due to the occurrence of granulomatous anterior uveitis.
[b] Available in unit-dose and multidose forms.
[c] Available in unit-dose form only.

Table 53.3 Pharmacological profile of ophthalmic β-blockers

	β-blocking potency[a]	ISA	Cardioselectivity	Membrane stabilizing activity
Betaxolol	3–10	–	++	+
Carteolol	30	++	–	–
Levobunolol	6	–	–	–
Metipranolol	2	–	–	+
Timolol	5–10	–	–	+

[a] Propranolol = 1.

Table 53.4 Ocular side-effects of topical β-blockers

Allergic blepharoconjunctivitis

Burning and itching

Blurred vision

Conjunctival hyperaemia

Corneal anaesthesia

Dryness

Foreign body sensation

Macular oedema

Pain

Punctate keratitis

Uveitis[a]

[a] Granulomatous anterior uveitis has been reported with metipranolol.

Table 53.5 Systemic side-effects of topical β-blockers

Vascular
  Hypotension
  Arrhythmias
  Reduced stroke volume
  Bradycardia
  Peripheral vasoconstriction

Respiratory
  Bronchoconstriction
  Dyspnoea

Gastrointestinal
  Nausea
  Diarrhoea

Endocrine
  Hypoglycaemia (insulin induced)

Central nervous system
  Anxiety
  Depression
  Irritability
  Fatigue
  Hallucinations
  Sleep disturbances

interfere with endogenous vasodilation and cause optic nerve head arteriolar vasoconstriction. The various β-blockers demonstrate marked differences in their vasoconstrictive effect, with betaxolol possibly demonstrating the least vasoconstriction.

Betaxolol

In theory, because of its cardioselectivity, betaxolol should have fewer adverse effects on the pulmonary and cardiovascular systems. However, it is probably less effective than other β-blockers as an ocular hypotensive agent. On initiation of treatment the fall in IOP is slower than with other topical β-blockers.

When betaxolol is used in conjunction with adrenaline (epinephrine) it leads to a greater reduction in IOP than that achieved with timolol and adrenaline (epinephrine), while the addition of dipivefrine also increases the efficacy of betaxolol. The 0.25% suspension is as effective as the 0.5% solution and is better tolerated by the patient (Weinreb et al 1990).

Carteolol

It has been suggested that because of the ISA of carteolol, smaller changes are seen in pulmonary and cardiovascular parameters than are seen with the non-cardioselective β-blockers without ISA. Carteolol is generally well tolerated and has been shown to be as effective as timolol at lowering IOP in the majority of patients.

At present, it is the least lipophilic of the topical β-blockers and consequently is likely to show a lower incidence of central nervous system side-effects.

Levobunolol

This non-cardioselective β-blocker without ISA is reported to be as effective or slightly more effective than timolol at lowering IOP and more effective than betaxolol or metipranolol. It is one of the two β-blockers to be licensed for once daily use, and is as effective with once daily dosing as the usual twice daily regimen. It is reported to cause more stinging on administration than betaxolol and metipranolol but to be equal in patient comfort to timolol.

Metipranolol

This is a non-cardioselective β-blocker without ISA. The multidose form was discontinued following reports of anterior uveitis associated with its use. It is now restricted to patients allergic to preservatives or those wearing soft contact lenses. Patient tolerability of the product is poor, stinging and dry skin around the eye being common complaints.

Timolol

This non-cardioselective β-blocker without ISA was the first to be introduced, and as such is the agent against which all newer β-blockers are compared. It is effective in the long-term treatment of glaucoma, often in conjunction with other antiglaucoma therapy in terms of IOP lowering. The presentation of timolol in a prolonged-release formulation (a polysaccharide-based, gel-forming solution) leads to a prolonged corneal contact time and increased penetration of timolol into the eye. This permits once daily administration while maintaining the ocular hypotensive effect achieved with the usual twice daily administration of previously available timolol solutions (Shedden 1994). Timolol is available in combination products with the carbonic anhydrase inhibitor dorzolamide and the prostaglandin analogue latanoprost (see Table 53.2).

Sympathomimetic agents

Adrenaline (epinephrine)

Adrenaline (epinephrine) is an α and β-adrenoreceptor agonist. It decreases IOP by reducing aqueous inflow via an alpha-mediated vasoconstriction in the ciliary body and increased outflow due to a dilatation of the aqueous and episcleral veins. Adrenaline (epinephrine) is a mydriatic and therefore its use is contraindicated in PACG and in patients who show a shallow anterior chamber because of the risk of precipitating angle closure. Adrenaline (epinephrine) can cause ocular surface inflammation, which may affect subsequent surgery, and if used in the aphakic eye (i.e. without the lens), and perhaps the pseudophakic eye, it can result in cystoid maculopathy (usually reversible on cessation).

Ocular side-effects of topically administered adrenaline (epinephrine) are shown in Table 53.6 and these limit its usefulness. Systemic side-effects are shown in Table 53.7, illustrating that adrenaline (epinephrine) should be used with caution in patients with hypertension and heart disease.

Commercially-available forms of adrenaline (epinephrine) were discontinued in late 2002.

Dipivefrine

In an attempt to decrease the dose of adrenaline (epinephrine) administered, a prodrug, dipivalyl adrenaline (dipivefrine), was developed.

Dipivefrine is converted to adrenaline (epinephrine) after absorption by esterases present in the eye. It passes

Table 53.6 Ocular side-effects of topical adrenaline (epinephrine)
Allergic blepharoconjunctivitis
Adrenochrome deposits
Conjunctival hyperaemia
Corneal oedema
Macular oedema (aphakic eyes)
Pain

Table 53.7 Systemic side-effects of topical adrenaline (epinephrine)
Arrhythmias
Cerebrovascular accident
Hypertension
Myocardial infarction
Tachycardia

more rapidly through the cornea than adrenaline (epinephrine), and the effects of a 0.1% solution are comparable with a 1% solution of adrenaline (epinephrine). This lower concentration causes fewer local and systemic side-effects.

Apraclonidine

Apraclonidine (a derivative of clonidine) was the first of the selective adrenergic agonists to be introduced. This drug, which acts predominantly on α_2 but also α_1 receptors, reduces the rate at which aqueous humour is produced. Eye drops containing apraclonidine 1% are used to control or prevent postoperative elevation of IOP following anterior segment laser surgery, while eye drops containing a 0.5% solution are used for the short-term adjunctive treatment of patients with chronic glaucoma not adequately controlled by other drugs while awaiting surgery.

Topical and systemic side-effects of α_2 agonists are shown in Tables 53.8 and 53.9.

Brimonidine

More α_2 selectivity is seen with brimonidine. This α_2 selectivity results in no mydriasis and absence of vasoconstriction in microvessels. Brimonidine is as effective as timolol at peak but significantly less effective at trough (Schuman 1996); it is more effective at both peak and trough than betaxolol (Serle et al 1996).

Brimonidine may be used as monotherapy to lower IOP in patients with open-angle glaucoma or ocular hypertension, who are intolerant of β-blockers, or in whom β-blockers are contraindicated, as there is no effect on pulmonary function and only minimal cardiovascular effect with brimonidine (David 2001). It may also be used as an adjunctive therapy in those patients whose IOP is not adequately controlled with a topical β-blocker. However, brimonidine is contraindicated in patients receiving MAOIs or antidepressants which affect noradrenergic transmission and there is the possibility of brimonidine potentiating or causing an additive effect with CNS depressants.

Adrenergic neurone blockers

Commercially-available preparations of sympathomimetic agents are shown in Table 53.10.

Miotics

Miotics act to increase the outflow of aqueous humour by a stimulation of ciliary muscle and an opening of channels in the trabecular meshwork. Miotics are directly acting parasympathomimetic agents that act at muscarinic receptors and include pilocarpine and carbachol.

The pharmacological profiles of the miotic agents are shown in Table 53.11. Miosis is an unwanted incidental effect, and can cause considerable difficulties to patients. Reduced visual acuity, especially in the presence of central lens opacities, spasm of accommodation, accompanied by severe frontal headache (browache) and diminished night vision may cause poor adherence in many patients.

Table 53.8 Ocular side-effects of topical α_2 agonists

Ocular pruritus
Discomfort
Tearing
Hyperaemia
Conjunctival and lid oedema
Lid retraction / Conjunctival blanching / Mydriasis — Reported after perioperative use of apraclonidine

Table 53.9 Systemic side-effects of topical α_2 agonists

Dry mouth/nose
Headache
Asthenia
Bradycardia
Depression

Table 53.10 Available ocular products containing sympathomimetic agents

Drug	Trade name	Strength	Daily dosage frequency
Dipivefrine	Propine	0.1%	2
Apraclonidine	Iopidine	1%	1 h prior to surgery and on completion
	Iopidine	0.5%	3
Brimonidine	Alphagan	0.2%	2

Table 53.11 Pharmacological profile of miotic agents

	Time to onset (min)	Duration of action (h)	Daily dosage frequency
Pilocarpine	20	3–4	4
Carbachol	40	8–12	3
Ecothiopate[a]	10–45	24	1–2

[a] Now only available on a named-patient basis for use under expert supervision.

Table 53.13 Commercially available miotic products

Drug	Trade name	Strength	Daily dosage frequency
Pilocarpine	Pilocarpine	0.5–4%	4
	Minims	1, 2 and 4%	4
	Pilogel	4%	1
Carbachol	Isopto Carbachol	3%	3–4

Ocular side-effects of topically administered miotic agents are shown in Table 53.12.

In eyes with narrow angles, PACG may be precipitated by an aggravation of pupillary block.

Systemic side-effects are due to parasympathetic stimulation, and include anxiety, bradycardia, diarrhoea, nausea, vomiting and sweating.

Pilocarpine is the more commonly used miotic in the treatment of POAG, and advances have been made to reduce its inconvenient four times a day dosage regimen (Table 53.13). A slow-release gel preparation, Pilogel, has been introduced in which a single daily application administered at bedtime allows low intraocular pressure

Table 53.12 Ocular side-effects of topical miotic agents

Allergic conjunctivitis
Ciliary/conjunctival injection
Lens changes
Lid twitching
Myopia
Pain
Pigment epithelial cysts
Poor night vision
Posterior synechiae
Pupillary block
Retinal tear/detachments
Uveitis
Vitreous haemorrhage

to be maintained for 24 hours, with the patient sleeping through the more troublesome ocular side-effects, i.e. blurred vision.

Carbonic anhydrase inhibitors

Carbonic anhydrase is the enzyme involved in aqueous humour production in the ciliary body. By inhibiting its action, secretion is reduced.

Acetazolamide

There is only one systemic carbonic anhydrase inhibitor available in the UK, acetazolamide. Although this agent is amongst the most potent ocular hypotensive agents available, it has limited use in the long-term management of glaucoma due to poor patient adherence following occurrence of side-effects. The systemic side-effects are shown in Table 53.14.

Paraesthesia occurs in almost all patients on commencement of therapy but usually disappears on continued therapy. The malaise complex can include fatigue, depression, weight loss and decreased libido.

Acetazolamide is also available in injection form, and given either intramuscularly or, preferably, intravenously is useful in the preoperative/emergency treatment of closed-angle glaucoma.

Topical carbonic anhydrase inhibitors: dorzolamide and brinzolamide

The topical carbonic anhydrase inhibitors dorzolamide and brinzolamide are useful alternatives to acetazolamide in glaucoma management. They are licensed for use in patients resistant to β-blockers or those in whom use of β-blockers is contraindicated. Dorzolamide is used either alone three times a day or alongside a β-blocker twice daily, while the licence for brinzolamide states that the drug can be used two or three times a day as monotherapy. Mean changes in intraocular pressure with brinzolamide administered

Table 53.14   Side-effects of systemic carbonic anhydrase inhibitors

Acidosis
Diarrhoea
Drowsiness
Elevated uric acid
Hypokalaemia
Nausea/vomiting
Malaise complex
Paraesthesia
Sulphonamide crystalluria
Sulphonamide sensitivity
Transient myopia

twice daily and three times a day and dorzolamide administered three times a day are equivalent, but less than those seen with timolol 0.5% twice daily (Silver 1998). Side-effects similar to those of systemic sulphonamides may occur and should be watched for, but the most common side-effects and the most frequent causes of patient discontinuation are local, as shown in Table 53.15. Of the two topical carbonic anhydrase inhibitors, brinzolamide appears to cause less burning and stinging on instillation (Silver 1998, Sall 2000). A combination of timolol 0.5% and dorzolamide 2%,

Table 53.15   Side-effects of topical carbonic anhydrase inhibitors

Ocular	Systemic
Blurred vision	Fatigue
Burning/stinging	Headache
Itching	Dry mouth
Tearing	Nausea
Conjunctivitis	Dyspnoea
Ocular discharge	Taste perversion
Eyelid pain/discomfort	

Cosopt (see Table 53.2), has been shown to be well tolerated and as effective as its components when administered separately (Strohmaier et al 1998, Boyle et al 1998). The combination has a number of advantages such as abolition of the potential for dilution and washout that can occur when two drugs are used concomitantly in separate formulations and a lower exposure to preservative.

Prostaglandins and prostamides

Prostaglandin analogues such as latanoprost and travoprost, lower IOP with a once daily application at night, primarily by increasing the uveoscleral outflow with no significant effect on other parameters of aqueous humour dynamics.

The prostamide bimatoprost is thought to increase outflow through both trabecular and uveoscleral outflow pathways.

Latanoprost

Latanoprost appears to be generally well tolerated by patients and is relatively free of systemic side-effects but has some interesting local effects. Pigmentation of the iris occurs in patients with mixed colour (green-brown or blue-brown) irides after 3–6 months of use and is a result of increased deposition of melanin in the melanocytes. An increase in the length and thickness of the eyelashes and pigmentation of the palpebral skin are side-effects recognized during post-marketing surveillance.

It is licensed for the reduction of elevated IOP in patients with POAG and OHT. Latanoprost doubles the outflow of aqueous humour through the non-conventional or uveoscleral route and has been shown to be at least as effective as, or more effective than, timolol (Camras et al 1996, Mishima et al 1996).

Travoprost

Travoprost is an ester pro-drug, converted to its active acid form by corneal hydrolytic enzymes as it is absorbed through the eye. Travoprost acid is a potent full agonist for FP receptors with lower affinity for the other prostanoid receptors responsible for pain, etc. It appears to be generally well tolerated by patients and is relatively free of systemic side effects but has the local effects associated with all the topical prostaglandin analogues. It is licensed for the treatment of patients with POAG and OHT who are intolerant or insufficiently responsive to other agents. Travoprost has been found to be equal or superior to latanoprost and superior to timolol in lowering intraocular pressure in patients with POAG or OHT (Netland et al 2001, Goldberg et al 2001). Travoprost is instilled once daily at night.

Bimatoprost

Bimatoprost is a synthetic prostamide which enters the eye unchanged. The receptors responsible for the increased outflow through both trabecular and uveoscleral outflow pathways are yet to be structurally identified. The peak IOP lowering effect occurs 8 to 12 hours after administration and the effect is maintained for at least 24 hours. Bimatoprost is licensed for the reduction of elevated IOP in POAG and OHT as monotherapy in patients insufficiently responsive or intolerant of first line therapy, in those in whom first line therapy is contra-indicated and as adjunctive therapy to β-blockers. In patients with elevated IOP, the IOP-lowering effect of bimatoprost has been shown to be superior to that of timolol. (Sherwood et al 2001). In patients with glaucoma and ocular hypertension it was found to be similar to that of latanoprost, with more patients reaching target IOPs with bimatoprost than with latanoprost (Gandolfi et al 2001). Systemic side effects reported in clinical trials include hypertension (1.7%) and elevated liver function tests (3%). However, review of the cases showed that 75% of patients with hypertension already had a history of hypertension and in all the cases of elevated liver function tests, the abnormality could be explained by concurrent disease or medication known to cause such a rise. Bimatoprost causes similar ocular side effects to latanoprost and travoprost. It is administered once daily at night.

Hyperosmotic agents

Hyperosmotic agents are of great value during PACG emergencies due to their speed of action and effectiveness. The most commonly used agents are oral glycerol and intravenous mannitol, although isosorbide and urea have both been used in the past. Hyperosmotic agents act by drawing water out of the eye, and therefore lower IOP. The maximal effect of glycerol is seen within 1 hour and lasts for about 3 hours, while mannitol acts within 30 minutes with effects lasting for 4–6 hours.

Glycerol

Glycerol is given orally, usually as a 50% solution in water, the dose being 1–1.5 g/kg body weight given as a single dose. It is not a strong diuretic but may cause nausea and vomiting. Although it is metabolized to glucose in the body, it may be given to diabetics who are well controlled.

All practitioners should be aware of the difference in dose in ml required for a 50% solution of glycerol formulated as a 50% w/v solution and one formulated as a 50% v/v solution (Table 53.16).

Mannitol

Mannitol is given as a 20% solution in water for intravenous administration. The dose is 1–2 g/kg body weight up to a maximum of 500 ml given over 30–40 minutes at a rate not exceeding 60 drops per minute. It is a strong diuretic, and as large volumes are required, it may cause problems due to cardiovascular overload, pulmonary oedema and stroke.

Patient care

Primary open-angle glaucoma

When the condition is first diagnosed, patients should be told that the disorder cannot be cured but only controlled by the regular use of the prescribed treatment. As POAG is, until far advanced, as symptomless disease, the result of non-adherence with treatment should be made clear and the importance of regular attendance at clinics stressed.

The existence of the patients' self-help group, the International Glaucoma Association, should be brought to the patient's attention.

The patient's technique for instillation of eye drops should be checked and corrected if necessary with emphasis on the dose (one drop), the position of instillation, into the temporal side of the lower conjunctival sac, and the importance of punctal occlusion to minimize systemic side-effects.

The preferred times for administration of topical medication should be discussed with the patient, with a 12-hourly regimen for twice-daily drugs, 8-hourly for drugs given three times a day and as near a 6-hourly regimen as practical for pilocarpine. Prostaglandins and prostamides are best administered at bedtime.

The importance of allowing a reasonable interval between drops should be underlined. Sometimes the order of instillation of different types of eye drop is important for pharmacological or practical reasons. For example, the instillation of pilocarpine should always precede that of a sympathomimetic to prevent pain in the eye resulting from a strong miosis following a weak mydriasis. The instillation of aqueous eye drops that remain in the conjunctival sac for a maximum of 10 minutes should precede that of viscous eye drops, for example hypromellose eye drops, or suspensions, for example dexamethasone 0.1% eye drops, with which the contact time is prolonged.

Eye drops containing benzalkonium chloride should not be instilled with soft contact lenses in situ. The patient should be instructed to remove the lens immediately before instillation and replace it approximately 30 minutes later. Patients using adrenaline (epinephrine) eye drops should adopt the same procedure, as the oxidation products of this drug will stain the contact lens.

Table 53.16   Doses of hyperosmotic agents in the treatment of primary angle closure glaucoma

Oral glycerol 50% at 1 g/kg				i.v. Mannitol 20% w/v[a]		
50% w/v solution		50% v/v solution				
Weight (kg)	Dose (ml)	Weight (kg)	Dose (ml)	Weight (kg)	Dose at 1 g/kg (ml)	Dose at 2 g/kg (ml)
40	80	44.5	70	40	200	400
50	100	50.8	80	50	250	500
60	120	57.2	90	60	300	–
		63.5	100	70	350	–
70	140	69.9	110	80	400	–
		76.2	120	90	450	–
80	160	82.6	130	100	500	–
90	180	88.9	140			
		95.3	150			
100	200	101.7	160			
For each additional 5 kg	Add 10 ml	For each additional 6.4 kg	Add 10 ml			

[a] Maximum dose 500 ml

As POAG is a hereditary disorder, patients should be told to advise first-degree relatives to be screened. Such people over the age of 40 years are entitled to free eye tests by their optician.

Primary angle closure glaucoma

Patients found to have shallow anterior chambers and narrow angles are normally promptly listed for peripheral iridectomies. However, if the procedure is delayed, they should be advised of the symptoms of an attack of acute PACG and details of the factors that are likely to precipitate an attack so that they can be avoided. They should be advised that there are a number of prescription and non-prescription drugs that they should not take. When visiting the doctor and purchasing medicines from a pharmacy, the patient should always remember to mention his or her condition, and the prescriber should ensure that the drug is appropriate for a patient prone to angle closure. Drugs contraindicated in this condition are listed in Tables 53.17 to 53.20. Note that the order of the drugs listed is purely alphabetical.

Following an attack of angle closure and surgical treatment of the disorder, the patient should be told that the drugs previously contraindicated can be safely taken provided that iridectomy/iridotomy remains patent.

Patient adherence

The patient is more likely to comply with the prescribed treatment if the drug or drugs prescribed can be

Table 53.17   Topically administered ophthalmic drugs contraindicated in narrow-angle glaucoma

Anticholinergics	Sympathomimetics with α adrenergic activity
Atropine	Adrenaline (epinephrine)
Cyclopentolate	Cocaine
Homatropine	Dipivefrine
Hyoscine	Ephedrine
Lachesine	Guanethidine
Oxyphenonium	Hydroxyamphetamine
Tropicamide	Naphazoline
	Phenylephrine
	Xylometazoline

Table 53.18 Systemically administered anticholinergic drugs contraindicated in narrow-angle glaucoma and suitable alternative drugs	
Contraindicated drug	Alternative therapies
Drugs used in the treatment of parkinsonism and drug-induced parkinsonian side-effects	
Trihexyphenidyl (benzhexol)	Amantadine
Benzatropine	Bromocriptine
Biperiden	Lisuride
Methixene	Pergolide
Orphenadrine	Selegiline
Drugs used as antispasmodics	
Ambutonium	Alverine
Belladonna	Mebeverine
Dicycloverine (dicydomine)	Peppermint oil
Homatropine methylbromide	
Hyoscine	
Mepenzolate	
Poldine	
Propantheline	
Drugs used in the treatment of motion sickness	
Hyoscine	Cinnarizine
Cyclizine	
Dimenhydrinate	
Promethazine theoclate	

Table 53.19 Systemically administered drugs with anticholinergic side-effects contraindicated in narrow-angle glaucoma and suitable alternative drugs	
Contraindicated drug	Alternative therapies
Antidepressants	
Amitriptyline	Fluoxetine
Amoxapine	Flupentixol
Butriptyline	Fluvoxamine
Clomipramine	Paroxetine
Desipramine	Sertraline
Dasulepin (dothiepin)	Trazodone
Doxepin	Viloxazine
Imipramine	Monoamine-oxidase inhibitors
Iprindole	Lithium salts (but caution if used in conjunction with acetazolamide, which increases excretion)
Lofepramine	
Maprotiline[a]	
Mianserin[a]	
Nortriptyline	
Protriptyline	
Trimipramine	
Antipsychotics	
Chlorpromazine	Benperidol
Fluphenazine	Droperidol
Loxapine	Haloperidol
Pericyazine	Flupentixol
Perphenazine	Fluspirilene
Pipotliazine	Oxypertine
Prochlorperazine	Pimozide
Promazine	Sulpiride
Thioridazine	Zuclopenthixol
Trifluoperazine	
Antihistamines	
Azatadine	Acrivastine
Cyproheptadine	Astemizole
Mequitazine	Cetirizine
Loratadine	
Terfenadine	
Antiarrhythmics	
Disopyramide	Other antiarrhythmics, but caution with amiodarone and verapamil if topical β-blockers used concurrently as this combination can lead to bradycardia and atrioventricular block

[a] Tetracyclic antidepressants – monitor in narrow-angle glaucoma.

administered according to a simple, infrequent dosage regimen and cause no, or few, local or systemic side-effects.

Thus a patient treated with a once daily or twice daily β-blocker, or the once daily prostaglandin analogues, would be expected to adhere to the regimen better than someone treated with pilocarpine with its unfortunate side-effects and inconvenient four times a day dosage regimen. Common side-effects of topical and systemic medication should be fully discussed with the patient so that the headache and the effects of miosis encountered with pilocarpine and the paraesthesia with acetazolamide are not unexpected, leading to premature discontinuation of therapy.

As glaucoma is predominantly a disease of elderly people, physical disability may prevent successful treatment, however conscientious the patient. For example, rheumatoid arthritis may reduce the patient's ability to squeeze the bottle of eye drops, while the tremor of Parkinson's disease can make correct positioning of instillation difficult. Various aids have been introduced to help with correct positioning and squeezing of eye drops and these should be made available to patients so disabled. Patients with poor visual acuity can be helped by colour coding of eye drop labels and supplying bottles labelled with large print.

Certain manufacturers have endeavoured to enhance adherence by including dose-reminder caps (on brimonidine, dipivefrine and levobunolol) and facilitate instillation by supplying aids to open the bottle

Table 53.20 Systemically administered sympathomimetic drugs with α-adrenergic activity contraindicated in narrow-angle glaucoma

Ephedrine
Isometheptene
Phenylpropanolamine
Pseudoephedrine
Levodopa

(latanoprost), position the bottle (timolol) or make their eye drop containers easier to squeeze (dorzolamide, Cosopt).

Where self-medication is impossible, a simple infrequent dosage regimen is more likely to be achieved when a relative, a neighbour or the district nursing service becomes responsible for administration of the medication. In these cases, a drug administered once daily, such as Timoptol-LA or a prostaglandin analogue or bimatroprost, has an obvious advantage over one that should be administered at 12-hourly intervals. If pilocarpine is required and bedtime administration is possible, the prescribing of Pilogel will be more practical than pilocarpine eye drops, the administration of which is totally impractical for anyone other than someone living with the patient.

Common therapeutic problems in glaucoma are listed in Table 53.21.

CASE STUDIES

Case 53.1

Mr A. C. is a 70-year-old widower with primary open-angle glaucoma. He is currently prescribed Minims Metipranolol 0.1% twice daily and G. dorzolamide 2% twice daily. He is finding it increasingly difficult to adhere to his prescription due to the worsening of his rheumatoid arthritis which is making it impossible for him to administer his drops correctly. He asks you if there is anything his GP can provide which may help.

Question

What advice would you give to Mr A. C.?

Answer

There are two issues here:

Table 53.21 Common therapeutic problems in glaucoma

Problem	Comments
Lack of adherence	Treatment perceived to be worse than disease Complex multiple drug regimens Frequency of dosing Inability to differentiate between different types of medication Inability to instill medication
Contraindication to therapy	Pilocarpine in uveitis β-blockers in asthma, bradycardia, heart block, uncontrolled heart failure Dipivefrine, prostaglandin analogues and prostamides in aphakia Dipivefrine and a wide range of other topical and systemic drugs in shallow anterior chamber α_2 agonists in depression Carbonic anhydrase inhibitors in renal failure
Intolerance to drug	Miosis and ciliary spasm with pilocarpine Red eye with dipivefrine Bronchospasm with β-blockers Paraesthesia with acetazolamide
Use outside licensed indications	Paediatric patients Pregnant women Nursing mothers
Hypersensitivity	To active drug To preservative in multidose formulations

- the appropriateness of Mr A. C.'s prescription
- the ease of administration.

Metipranolol in the treatment of chronic open-angle glaucoma is now restricted to those patients allergic to preservatives or to those wearing soft contact lenses. Neither of these applies to this patient for he is using another eye drop containing preservatives and does not wear contact lenses. Therefore another β-blocker, and one that is available in a bottle, would be more appropriate as it would be easier for the increasingly arthritic Mr A. C. to hold and use than Minims.

As Mr A. C. is coprescribed a β-blocker and carbonic anhydrase inhibitor, it would seem logical to prescribe Cosopt, a combination of timolol 0.5% and dorzolamide 2%, so that he would have only one drop to administer twice daily with the added benefit of the patient-friendly bottle.

Several different types of compliance aids are available and these may also be useful to Mr. A. C. to help him to administer his eye drops. Another option would be to enlist the services of the district nurse who would be able to administer the twice daily eye drops for Mr A. C. if he still has problems with administration using the compliance aids.

Case 53.2

Ms F. S. is a 45-year-old teacher and has recently suffered from a bout of flu. Following on from this she had complained of severe nasal congestion for which the GP had suggested pseudoephedrine tablets 60 mg three times daily.

Ms F. S. had bought a bottle of Sudafed™ tablets over-the-counter at her local pharmacy and had taken them as recommended for the last 2 days. She presents on the third day complaining of nausea, vomiting, severe ocular pain and loss of vision and asks could the tablets be causing the problem and what should she do?

Questions

1. What would you recommend that Ms F. S. do?
2. What could be the possible cause of Ms F. S.'s condition?

Answers

1. Anyone presenting with ocular pain and loss of vision should be referred immediately to the local accident and emergency department (ophthalmic if available). Since these symptoms are accompanied by nausea and vomiting in a woman over the age of 40, this is probably an acute attack of PACG and will need treatment with intravenous acetazolamide, with or without oral hyperosmotic agents.
2. Pseudoephedrine is a sympathomimetic drug with α-adrenergic activity which is contraindicated in narrow-angle glaucoma and so may well have precipitated this attack. If the patient is aware of her condition, she should always remember to mention it when visiting the doctor and purchasing medicines from a pharmacy. There are a large number of prescription and non-prescription drugs that should not be taken by patients with shallow anterior chambers prone to PACG.

Case 53.3

Mr B. W. is a 65-year-old retired librarian with a history of asthma and hypertension who suffers from glaucoma. He is currently prescribed G. latanoprost 0.005% at night in both eyes, but is having problems tolerating the drops, complaining of terrible burning and itching, however his IOP is well controlled.

His concurrent medication is an inhaled short acting β₂-stimulant as required, a regular standard inhaled corticosteroid, a regular modified dose release oral theophylline and modified release oral verapamil once daily.

His wife is concerned that he will stop using his drops and asks if there are any other drops that he could use.

Question

What advice would you give Mr B. W.?

Answer

Mr B. W.'s intolerance to the latanoprost eye drops could be due to either the active ingredient or the preservative. The other common first line treatment for glaucoma is topical β-blockers; however, with Mr B. W.'s medical history β-blockers are contra-indicated, both because of his history of asthma but also because of the possible drug interaction with verapamil taken for his hypertension.

There are currently no preservative free forms of prostaglandin analogues but as his IOP is well controlled it may be appropriate to try travoprost 0.004% or bimatoprost 0.03% at night. Both these preparations contain less preservative than latanoprost.

However, if the side effects continue to be troublesome, then what alternative treatments are available?

The patient could be started on brimonidine, a sympathomimetic with no effect on pulmonary function and only minimal cardiovascular effect, used twice daily or a carbonic anhydrase inhibitor such as dorzolamide three times a day or brinzolamide, twice daily.

Case 53.4

Mrs C. L. is a 60-year-old widow, weight 60 kg, who presents at her local accident and emergency department complaining of a sudden loss of vision accompanied by severe ocular pain. On examination she is found to have a 'ciliary flush', a pupil unreactive to light and an IOP of 72 mmHg. The diagnosis is an acute attack of PACG but on taking Mrs C. L.'s drug history it is found that she suffered an allergic reaction to co-trimoxazole 2 years ago when it was prescribed for an acute exacerbation of chronic bronchitis.

Question

The accident and emergency docotr telephones for advice regarding appropriate treatment for Mrs C. L. What treatment would you recommend and what would be the appropriate dose?

Answer

If a patient presents with an acute attack of PACG and is not allergic to sulphonamides, then the first step is usually treatment with intravenous acetazolamide.

In the case of Mrs C. L., who is sensitive to sulphonamides, the first-line treatment would be intravenous mannitol 20% due to its rapid onset of action (approximately 30 min), the dose being 1–2 g/kg. As Mrs C. L. weighs 60 kg the dose would be 60–120 g mannitol, which equates to 300–600 ml of the 20% w/v solution. However, the maximum volume of the 20% solution to be administered by slow intravenous infusion is 500 ml and a dose of 1 g/kg should therefore be used (or the maximum volume of 500 ml).

Mrs C. L. should then lie supine for 1 hour after which time her IOP should be measured. If her IOP is still greater than 60 mmHg she should be left supine for a further 30 minutes and her IOP should then be rechecked. If her IOP falls below 60 mmHg then topical treatment with β-blockers and/or α_2 agonists, and topical corticosteroids can be commenced.

However, if her IOP remains above 60 mmHg, alternative steps must be taken. At this point it is necessary to determine whether Mrs C. L. is nauseous or vomiting. If this is the case then a repeat dose of intravenous mannitol 20% should be administered. If no nausea or vomiting is present then oral glycerol 50% should be given at a dose of 1–1.5 g/kg bodyweight.

For Mrs C. L. this would be a dose of 60 g of glycerol at 1 g/kg. For glycerol formulated as a 50% v/v solution the amount of glycerol required by Mrs C. L. would be 94.4 ml. However, for glycerol formulated as a 50% w/v solution the dose would be 120 ml. It is therefore imperative that the glycerol preparation available is ascertained and the correct dosage recommended.

Case 53.5

Mr H. J. is a 63-year-old widower who lives alone and suffers from POAG. He is well controlled on twice-daily timolol, twice daily dorzolamide and four times a day pilocarpine. However, he has recently been diagnosed with cataracts and is finding it increasingly difficult to differentiate between his eyes drops. He enquires whether anything can be done to help him.

Questions

1. Simplifying Mr H. J.'s regimen would help. What simpler treatment regimens could you suggest?
2. How can the differentiation issue be addressed?

Answers

1. There are two simpler alternatives to twice daily timolol eye drops: the once daily timolol gel and the only topical β-blocker licensed for once daily use, levobunolol. Dorzolamide, a carbonic anhydrase inhibitor, is only licensed for twice daily usage in conjunction with a β-blocker; however, it is available in a combination product with timolol 0.5% as Cosopt for twice daily administration.

An alternative to four times a day pilocarpine would be the once daily Pilogel applied at night.

As the co-instillation of two long-acting gels is inappropriate, the practical alternatives to Mr H. J.'s current regimen are:

- A twice daily regimen with current drugs: timolol eye drops 0.5% twice a day, at 10 a.m. and 10 p.m., dorzolamide 2% twice a day at 10.10 a.m. and 10.10 p.m and Pilogel 4% at night at 10.20 p.m.

OR

- Cosopt twice a day, at 10 a.m. and 10 p.m. and Pilogel 4% at 10.10 p.m.

2. Regarding the differentiation problem between eye drop preparations, if Mr H. J. is prescribed Cosopt and Pilogel, then this should not be a problem because the combined β-blocker/dorzolamide preparation is in a bottle while the gel is in a tube. However, if he were to continue with his two separate drops and the gel, then the two bottles might be difficult to distinguish. The dispensing pharmacy could use larger print labels and distinguish the different preparations by easily visible means such as colour coding, or use tactile differentiation methods such as applying raised shapes on the base of the bottle or simply winding an elastic band around one of the bottles.

REFERENCES

Boyle J E, Ghosh K, Gieser D K et al 1998 A randomized trial comparing the dorzolamide-timolol combination given twice daily to monotherapy with timolol and dorzolamide. Ophthalmology 105: 1945–1951

Camras C B, United States Latanoprost Study Group 1996 Comparison of latanoprost and timolol in patients with ocular hypertension and glaucoma. Ophthalmology 103: 138–147

David R 2001 Brimonidine (Alphagan): a clinical profile four years after launch. European Journal of Ophthalmology 11(Suppl. 2): S72–77

Gandolfi S, Simmons S T, Sturm R et al 2001 Three-month comparison of bimatoprost and latanoprost in patients with glaucoma and ocular hypertension. Advances in therapy 18 No. 3: 110–121

Goldberg I, CunhaVaz J, Jakobsen J E et al 2001 Comparison of topical travoprost eye drops given once daily and timolol 0.5% given twice daily in patients with open-angle glaucoma or ocular hypertension. Journal of Glaucoma 10: 414–422

Infield D A, O'Shea J G 1998 Glaucoma: diagnosis and management. Postgraduate Medical Journal 74: 709–715

Khaw P T 1994 The surgical treatment of glaucoma. Optician 208: 26–29

Mishima H K, Masuda K, Kitazawa Y et al 1996 A comparison of latanoprost and timolol in primary open angle glaucoma and ocular hypertension: a 12-week study. Archives of Ophthalmology 114: 929–932

Netland P A, Landry T, Sullivan E K et al 2001 Travoprost compared with latanoprost and timolol in patients with open-angle glaucoma or ocular hypertension. American Journal of Ophthalmology 132: 472–484

Pitts-Crick R 1994 Epidemiology and screening of open-angle glaucoma. Current Opinion in Ophthalmology 5: 3–9

Sall K, Brinzolamide Primary Therapy Study Group 2000 The efficacy and safety of brinzolamide 1% ophthalmic suspension (Azopt®) as a primary therapy in patients with open-angle glaucoma or ocular hypertension. Survey of Ophthalmology 44(Suppl. 2): S155–S162

Schuman J S 1996 Clinical experience with brimonidine 0.2% and timolol 0.5% in glaucoma and ocular hypertension. Survey of Ophthalmology 41(Suppl. 1): S27–37

Serle J B, Brimonidine Study Group 1996 A comparison of the safety and efficacy of twice daily brimonidine 0.2% versus betaxolol 0.25% in subjects with elevated intraocular pressure. Survey of Ophthalmology 41(Suppl. 1): S39–47

Shedden A H 1994 Timolol maleate in gel-forming solution: a novel formulation of timolol maleate. Chibret International Journal of Ophthalmology 10: 32–36

Sherwood M, Brandt J 2001 Six-month comparison of

bimatoprost once-daily and twice-daily with timolol twice-daily in patients with elevated intraocular pressure. Survey of Ophthalmology 45 (Suppl. 4): S361–368

Silver L H, Brinzolamide Primary Therapy Study Group 1998 Clinical efficacy and safety of brinzolamide (Azopt™), a new topical carbonic anhydrase inhibitor for primary open-angle glaucoma and ocular hypertension. American Journal of Ophthalmology 126: 400–408

Strohmaier B S, Snyder E, DuBiner H et al 1998 The efficacy and safety of the dorzolamide-timolol combination versus the concomitant administration of its components. Ophthalmology 105: 1936–1944

Weinreb R N, Caldwell D R, Goode S M et al 1990 A double-masked three-month comparison between 0.25% betaxolol suspension and 0.5% betaxolol ophthalmic solution. American Journal of Ophthalmology 110: 189–192

FURTHER READING

Choong Y F, Irfan S, Menage M J 1999 Acute angle closure glaucoma: an evaluation of a protocol for acute treatment. Eye 13: 613–616

Cordeiro F, Wells T (Section curators) Glaucoma ophthalmology. eTextbook (online).
http://www.eyetext.net/members/main/glaucoma/Glaucoma.html

Hitchings R A (ed) 2000 Fundamentals of clinical ophthalmology glaucoma. BMJ Publishing Group, London

Titcomb L C 1999 Eye disorders: treatment of glaucoma, part 1. Pharmaceutical Journal 263: 324–329

Titcomb L C 1999 Eye disorders: treatment of glaucoma, part 2. Pharmaceutical Journal 263: 526–530

Drug-induced skin disorders 54

P. Magee

Drug-induced skin eruptions are likely to be among the most frequent adverse reactions seen by pharmacists, since approximately 30% of all reported adverse drug reactions involve the skin. Only nausea, tiredness, diarrhoea and headache are reported more often. The tendency for drugs to cause rashes is very variable; some drugs seldom if ever cause rashes (e.g. digoxin, potassium chloride and ferrous sulphate), while up to 5% of patients given co-trimoxazole, ampicillin or carbamazepine develop a rash.

The evidence for these observations does not come from clinical trials designed to establish incidence of adverse reactions as this would be unethical. Adverse drug reactions are identified from the systematic review of single case reports and information from clinical trials which are in fact looking at therapeutic efficacy. However, most evidence results from post-marketing surveillance, either spontaneous reporting (Committee on Safety of Medicines, Yellow Card Scheme) or post-marketing studies. For example, an assessment of co-trimoxazole-induced skin disorders can be found in a study of the General Practice Research Data Base (Jick & Derby 1995).

Diagnosis

It is often difficult to determine the cause of a drug-induced eruption because:

- almost any drug can affect the skin
- unrelated drugs produce similar reactions
- the same drug may produce different reactions in different patients
- many reactions cannot be distinguished from naturally occurring eruptions.

Moreover, new drugs continue to be marketed and many drugs are prescribed as combined preparations. The possibility of a food additive or a pharmaceutical excipient causing a skin reaction must not be overlooked as re-exposure is likely and cross-reactivity can occur, for example aspirin-sensitized patients may also be sensitized to tartrazine.

If a patient presents with a rash and is currently taking or has recently finished medication, it is important to:

- check that the rash is not due to a specific skin disease such as endogenous eczema or scabies
- take an accurate drug history
- ascertain the time course of the eruption in relation to drug use
- note whether the appearance of the rash is typical of any classic drug-induced eruption.

It may then be possible to assess if a drug is the likely cause.

Rechallenge remains the most useful method of confirming a diagnosis. However, rechallenge is not possible for severe cutaneous reactions and even prick and patch testing are not without risk.

Treatment

Not all cutaneous reactions are serious but the implicated drug should usually be stopped, although in some cases a dosage reduction may be sufficient if an alternative treatment is not appropriate.

In most cases the rash will disappear within a few days and the patient can be treated symptomatically with oral antihistamines and calamine lotion.

Erythematous eruptions

An erythematous or exanthematous eruption is the most common type of drug-induced skin reaction (Table 54.1).

The rash is characterized by erythema (abnormal flushing of the skin) and may be morbilliform (resembling measles) or maculopapular, consisting of macules (distinct flat areas) and papules (raised lesions conventionally less than 1 cm in diameter). The rash is usually bright red in colour and the skin may feel hot, burning or itchy. The whole of the skin surface can be involved, though the face is often spared. Sometimes the rash may disappear even though the drug is continued, but if itching is marked it is less likely that the rash will clear. In some severe cases erythroderma may follow an erythematous reaction. Here the erythema persists with continual scaling, which may be associated with lymphadenopathy, pyrexia, thirst and shivering with heat and fluid loss from the skin.

Most erythematous eruptions are probably allergic reactions but other mechanisms may sometimes be involved. Allergic reactions can occur early or late in therapy. Early reactions are more usual and start within 2–3 days of drug administration and occur in previously sensitized patients. In the late type of reaction the hypersensitivity develops during administration but the rash may not manifest itself until around the ninth day and can occur as late as 3 weeks after starting treatment and may also appear up to 2 weeks after cessation of therapy.

A distinct reddish-coloured morbilliform rash may be caused by ampicillin, its derivative amoxicillin and its esters bacampicillin, pivampicillin and talampicillin. The reaction will occur in almost all patients with infective mononucleosis (glandular fever) and is not always an indicator of true penicillin allergy although patients often self-report penicillin sensitivity as a result of this reaction. A high incidence of this reaction also occurs in patients with cytomegalovirus. These are often transplant patients taking immunosuppressive drugs or patients with leukaemia.

Treatment of an erythematous eruption involves drug withdrawal and treatment for any associated itching. Measures should be taken to ensure that the patient is not re-exposed to the drug. A note of the suspected sensitivity should be made in medical records, and a personal card with the same information should be given to the patient.

A high incidence of erythematous rashes can be expected during or following treatment with penicillin or chemically related antibiotics, with gold salts and with non-steroidal anti-inflammatory drugs (NSAIDs). Sulphonamides are a frequent cause and more common in patients with AIDS (de Raevel et al 1988).

Pruritus

Pruritus (itching) can have many causes. Commonly these are systemic or psychological. However, drugs can induce pruritus either as a symptom of other cutaneous

Table 54.1 Drugs causing erythematous eruptions

Allopurinol
Antituberculous drugs, especially rifampicin and second-line agents
Antidepressants, e.g. tricyclics, maprotiline
Barbiturates
Captopril
Carbamazepine
Cimetidine
Diuretics: thiazides, furosemide (frusemide)
Gold salts
Lincomycin
Nalidixic acid
Nitrofurantoin
NSAIDs
Penicillin
Phenothiazines
Phenylbutazone, oxphenbutazone
Phenytoin
Oral retinoids
Ranitidine
Streptomycin (less common with other aminoglycosides)
Sulphonamides
Sulphonylureas
Ampicillin rashes do not necessarily indicate penicillin hypersensitivity.

reactions or with itching as the only clinical manifestation. In either condition the itch can be so intense that the scratching this induces will cause lesions so that it is not always possible to know if there was originally an underlying rash.

For most drugs the mechanism for inducing pruritus is not known but it is likely that both central and peripheral mechanisms are involved. Drug-induced pruritus is usually generalized but local anal pruritus can follow antibiotic-induced candidiasis. It can also be produced as a contact allergy following the local administration of ointments and suppositories. Drugs with autonomic activity may produce sweating and prickly heat followed by pruritus.

To treat pruritus the itch–scratch–itch cycle must be broken once the drug cause has been eliminated. Topical steroids and occlusive dressings help to prevent scratching.

Urticaria

Drug-induced urticaria is common and accounts for approximately 28% of all drug-induced skin disorders (Table 54.2).

An urticarial rash, often referred to as 'hives' or nettle rash, is an acute or chronic allergic reaction in which red weals develop. The weals itch intensely and may last for hours or days. Giant urticaria or angio-oedema is a severe form of urticaria involving swelling of the tongue, lips and eyelids, and requires urgent medical attention. Laryngeal oedema is the most serious complication.

Only acute urticaria is likely to be drug induced. It occurs immediately or shortly after the administration of

the drug in a sensitized patient, and can be regarded as the cutaneous manifestation of anaphylaxis. Chronic urticaria is rarely caused by a drug unless the patient is continually exposed, for example to trace amounts of penicillins in milk and dairy products. However, aspirin and codeine can exacerbate idiopathic chronic urticaria.

Erythema multiforme

Erythema multiforme can follow an infection, for example with herpes simplex, although drugs are also a common cause (Table 54.3). It accounts for approximately 5% of drug reactions involving the skin.

Erythema multiforme is a serious, sometimes fatal, skin disease.

As the name implies, it can present in a variety of patterns. The usual erythematous lesions occur in crops on the hands and feet more often than on the trunk. Each maculopapular lesion increases in size, leaving a cyanotic centre that produces an 'iris' or 'target' lesion. The lesions appear over a few days, reaching a diameter of 1 or 2 cm within 48 hours. They may blister and can reach a size of up to 10 cm. They usually fade within 1

Table 54.3 Drugs causing erythema multiforme and the Stevens–Johnson syndrome

| Barbiturates |
| Carbamazepine |
| Cimetidine |
| Dapsone |
| Ethosuximide |
| Gold salts |
| Isoniazid |
| Lamotrigine |
| NSAIDs |
| Penicillins |
| Phenytoin |
| Propranolol |
| Rifampicin |
| Sulphonamides (especially long-acting compounds) |
| Sulphonylureas |
| Nearly 200 other drugs have also been implicated (Litt & Pawlak 1997). |

Table 54.2 Drugs causing urticaria

| Aspirin |
| Barbiturates |
| Imipramine |
| Indometacin |
| Iodine |
| Paracetamol |
| Penicillins |
| Ranitidine |
| Serum, toxoids, pollen vaccines |
| Sulphonamides |
| Tartrazine |

or 2 weeks of stopping the drug. Healing occurs without scarring although hyperpigmentation may persist for a long time. Involvement of the mucous membranes is common, and the mouth, eyes and genitalia may be affected to varying degrees. If the blistering and mucosal lesions are severe the disease is termed the Stevens–Johnson syndrome. There is also systemic involvement, with fever, malaise, polyarthritis and diarrhoea. There have been case reports of haematuria and renal failure.

Drugs are the most common cause of the Stevens–Johnson syndrome, and all suspected drugs should be stopped as the disease has a mortality rate of approximately 15% without treatment. Rechallenge is never justifiable. Treatment with systemic steroids produces a rapid response in both erythema multiforme and the Stevens–Johnson syndrome.

Toxic epidermal necrolysis (TEN) – Lyell's syndrome

This is a rare condition but with a high mortality rate of approximately 33%. The main cause of TEN in adults is drug therapy (Table 54.4). In children it is a phage type II staphylococcal infection, referred to as the staphylococcal scalded skin syndrome. A higher incidence of TEN is reported in immunocompromised patients with systemic lupus erythematosus (SLE) and HIV.

Lyell's syndrome frequently has a prodromal phase of malaise sometimes accompanied by a sore throat and fever. The skin reaction starts with large areas of erythema involving most of the skin surface and is followed by a bullous (a large blister containing serous fluid) phase in which the epidermis peels off. This stage

Table 54.4 Drugs causing toxic epidermal necrolysis
Allopurinol
Barbiturates
Dapsone
Gold salts
Lamotrigine
Penicillins
Phenolphthalein
Phenylbutazone
Phenytoin
Sulphonamides

is complicated by fluid loss, septicaemia and bronchopneumonia. Mucous membrane involvement may precede the skin eruption by 10–14 days, giving a clinical appearance similar to the Stevens–Johnson syndrome.

Diagnosis is made clinically and from a skin biopsy. In drug-induced TEN there is separation of the basal layer of the epidermis. In staphylococcal scalded skin syndrome, separation occurs in the granular layer without necrolysis. Drug rechallenge is never used to confirm a diagnosis. The patient with TEN will require full intensive care support and antibiotic treatment. Corticosteroids are not indicated as these may increase mortality (Schopf et al 1991).

Eczematous eruptions – dermatitis

An eczematous eruption may occur during systemic drug therapy, or it may develop as a result of allergy to a topical preparation (allergic contact dermatitis) or by direct contact with a primary irritant (contact dermatitis) (Table 54.5).

The skin lesions are characterized by redness with widespread exfoliation (peeling) and intense itching. Small blisters can develop, especially in contact dermatitis, that burst and weep exudate.

Primary irritant dermatitis is essentially a major public health problem although certain topical drugs (e.g. tar and dithranol) are primary irritants. However, allergic contact dermatitis is a common complication of topical therapy, for example persistent dermatitis from medication or dressings used to treat leg ulcers. Allergic contact dermatitis is a major complication of topical treatment. It can be caused by the drug or any of the excipients of the preparation. Patch testing of all ingredients of a topical preparation is used to find the causative agent.

Cross-sensitivity reactions can occur when an eczematous eruption or anaphylaxis develops after administration of a systemic drug in a patient previously sensitized by topical application. Cross-sensitivity is one of the major reasons for not using topical antibiotics. Cases of cross-sensitivity have also been reported in patients and medical staff who handle systemic formulations of known sensitizers such as chlorpromazine.

Patch testing can be used to confirm a diagnosis of drug-induced dermatitis and treatment is the same as that used for idiopathic eczema: emollients and topical steroids.

Vesicular and bullous eruptions

Vesiculobullous eruptions are termed 'pemphigoid' unless they are associated with specific skin conditions (e.g. erythema multiforme).

Table 54.5 Drugs causing eczematous eruptions
Local anaesthetics
Antibiotics, especially neomycin, streptomycin, chloramphenicol
Antihistamines
Antiseptics
Atropine
Captopril
Carbamazepine
Ethylenediamine (in aminophylline)
Gold salts
Imidazole antifungal drugs
Lanolin
Preservatives in creams and ointments
Methyldopa
Phenothiazines
Phenylbutazone
Phenytoin
Quinine, quinidine
Sulphonamides
Sulphonylureas
Thiazide diuretics

Table 54.6 Drugs causing vesicular and bullous eruptions
Azapropazone
Barbiturates (may be associated with drug-induced coma)
Captopril
Furosemide (frusemide)
Iodides
Nalidixic acid (phototoxic)
Penicillamine
Phenylbutazone
Rifampicin
Salicylates
Sulphonamides

A vesicle is a blister filled with serum with a diameter up to 0.5 cm. If larger than this it is termed a bulla.

Pemphigoid reactions can be autoimmune or drug-induced (Table 54.6). When drug-induced they can be part of a fixed drug eruption or generalized, as for example the large bullae that are seen in patients with barbiturate poisoning. The eruptions will resolve with drug withdrawal although they can persist for up to 2 years.

Lichenoid eruptions

Drug-induced lichenoid eruptions (Table 54.7) closely resemble lichen planus, occurring as flat mauve lesions, but they may be atypical, showing marked scaling. The lesions are found mainly on the forearms, neck and on the inner surface of the thighs. The mouth may be involved, and hair loss can occur.

The pathogenic mechanism is unknown. It is not allergic and is probably dose-dependent.

The eruptions resolve with drug withdrawal, with or without topical steroids, but hyperpigmentation may remain. There is also a possibility of late malignancy (Bauer 1981).

Erythema nodosum

The lesions seen in erythema nodosum are painful subcutaneous nodules usually limited to the extremities. Transient erythema may precede the lesions.

Erythema nodosum is usually a complication of infection and is not commonly drug-induced. However, it has been observed in women taking oral contraceptives and with other drugs such as sulphonamides, salicylates, penicillins and gold salts.

Purpura

Purpura is a rash resulting from bleeding into the skin from capillaries. It can be caused by drug-induced thrombocytopenia or result from drugs that damage blood vessels (non-thrombocytopenic or vascular purpura). It can also occur with the hypocoagulation associated with reduced circulating clotting factors. In the latter case, drug interactions with the anticoagulants can be a cause.

Table 54.7 Drugs causing lichenoid eruptions
Aspirin
ACE inhibitors
β-blockers
Carbamazepine
Chloroquine
Ethambutol
Gold salts
Mepacrine
Methyldopa
NSAIDS
Penicillamine
Phenothiazines
Quinidine
Quinine
Sulphonylureas
Thiazide diuretics

Table 54.8 Drugs causing psoriasiform eruptions
Aspirin
β adrenoceptor blockers, most frequently atenolol, oxprenolol and propranolol
Chloroquine
Iodides
Lithium
NSAIDs
Withdrawal of topical steroids

Table 54.9 Drugs causing fixed drug eruptions
Barbiturates
Chlordiazepoxide
Dapsone
Dichloralphenazone
Griseofulvin
Indometacin
Meprobamate
Phenolphthalein
Phenylbutazone
Phenytoin
Quinine
Salicylates
Sulphonamides
Tetracyclines

Psoriasiform eruptions

Drugs can either exacerbate psoriasis in pre-disposed patients or induce psoriasiform rashes in previously unaffected patients (Table 54.8).

The psoriasiform eruptions mimic psoriasis and are characterized by itchy, scaly red patches on the elbows, forearms, knees, legs and scalp.

Fixed drug eruptions

Fixed drug eruptions are characterized by the fact that they tend to occur at the same site in a particular patient each time the drug is administered. Drugs causing fixed drug eruptions are listed in Table 54.9.

The lesions are flat and purplish brown in colour but may be raised in the acute stage. They take between 2 and 24 hours to develop following drug ingestion. On the first drug exposure there is usually only one lesion, but subsequent exposure can result in multiple lesions. The eruption usually involves the limbs rather than the trunk and often occurs on mucous membranes.

Once the drug has been stopped the lesions heal with scaling followed by pigmentation, which may be the only physical sign at the time the patient presents.

The fixed drug eruption is possibly the only case of a drug-induced cutaneous reaction where oral rechallenge can be safely used to confirm the diagnosis and patch testing at the site of the eruption, but not elsewhere, is often positive (Alanko 1994).

Systemic lupus erythematosus (SLE)

Syndromes indistinguishable from SLE may occur following drug administration (Table 54.10). It is not clear if drugs cause this by initiating the disease or by triggering it in predisposed patients.

The cutaneous manifestation of drug-induced SLE is the characteristic butterfly-shaped rash on the face. There may also be a rash on the neck and back of the hands. Laboratory tests for antinuclear factor and lupus cells may be positive and the erythrocyte sedimentation rate may be elevated. Cerebral and renal involvement is rare. In some cases antinuclear antibodies occur without clinical manifestations.

Clinical manifestations of the SLE syndrome are predominant in women but the occurrence of antinuclear antibodies shows no preference for gender. The syndrome is usually reversible if the drug is withdrawn, although the antinuclear factor may persist for several months.

Acneform eruptions

Acne is a common complaint but is rarely drug-induced.

Drugs can, however, produce acne-like eruptions or aggravate existing acne (Table 54.11). The lesions are usually papular, but no comedones (blackheads) are present.

Skin necrosis

Necrosis can follow the extravasation of irritant drugs, particularly cytotoxic agents. Anticoagulants, both oral and heparin, can produce a severe haemorrhagic skin necrosis. Other causes of necrosis include the severe impairment of skin circulation which is occasionally produced by β adrenoceptor blockers, the synergistic effects of certain antitumour drugs with radiotherapy, and the topical application of gentian violet and brilliant green.

Photosensitivity

Drug-induced photosensitivity can be either phototoxic or photoallergic and can result from systemic or topical therapy (Table 54.12).

Phototoxic reactions resemble severe sunburn, and can progress to blistering. They are dose-dependent for drugs and sunlight, occur within a few hours of taking the drug and subside quickly on drug withdrawal.

Photoallergic rashes are usually eczematous, lichenoid, urticarial, bullous or purpuric. They are not dose-dependent and can be delayed in onset. Recovery is slow following drug withdrawal. In some cases photoallergy can persist for years after the drug was taken.

Patients receiving photosensitizing drugs should be counselled to avoid strong sunlight and to use a total sun block that contains a reflective substance such as titanium oxide. This is because most absorbed sunscreens only provide protection against medium-wavelength radiation (UVB), while it is the long-wavelength radiation (UVA) that is responsible for photosensitive reactions.

Table 54.10 Drugs causing systemic lupus erythematosus
Antiepileptics, e.g. phenytoin, primidone, ethosuximide
β adrenoceptor blockers
Chlorpromazine
Griseofulvin
Hydralazine
Isoniazid
Lithium
Methyldopa
Oral contraceptives
Penicillamine
Procainamide
Propylthiouracil
Sulfasalazine

Table 54.11 Drugs causing acne
Androgens (in women)
Corticosteroids and ACTH (inlcuding inhaled preparations)
Ciclosporin
Ethambutol
Isoniazid
Lithium
Oral contraceptives
Phenobarbital
Phenytoin
Propylthiouracil (resembling acne rosacea)
Topical corticosteroids (perioral dermatitis)
Quinine, quinidine (papular eruptions)

Table 54.12	Drugs causing light-induced eruptions

Topical preparations
  Antihistamines
  Antiseptics: bithionol, hexachlorophene
  Coal tar derivatives
  Sunscreens

Systemic drugs
  Amiodarone
  Antihistamines
  Cinoxacin
  Diuretics: thiazides, furosemide (frusemide)
  Griseofulvin
  Nalidixic acid
  NSAIDs
  Phenothiazines
  Psoralens – used therapeutically
  Sulphonamides
  Sulphonylureas
  Tetracyclines
  Tricyclic antidepressants

Table 54.13	Drugs causing skin pigmentation
Drug	Pigmentation
Amiodarone	Blue-grey
Anticonvulsants (hydantoin derivatives)	Brown
Antimalarials	Blue-grey
β adrenoceptor blockers	Brown
Imipramine	Blue-grey
Methyldopa	Brown
Oral contraceptives	Brown spots/ patches
Phenothiazines	Brown/blue-grey
Psoralens	Brown
Tetracyclines	Blue-black

Pigmentation

Hyperpigmentation, hypopigmentation or discoloration can all be drug induced (Table 54.13). Pigmentation can be widespread or localized and can occasionally occur in internal organs.

The mechanism of drug induction is not always known. In some cases the drug itself may be responsible or it may induce a disturbance in melanin pigmentation.

Nail changes

Nail discoloration can be drug induced. Blue nails can result from therapy with mepacrine and blue-black nails from cytotoxic drugs and minocycline. Potassium permanganate solutions will dye nails brown, and white nails can result from therapy with antitumour agents.

Photo-onycholysis (separation of the nail from the nail plate associated with UVA radiation) can be exacerbated by oral contraceptives and tetracyclines. Cytotoxic agents may also induce onycholysis by direct toxicity to the matrix (Creamer et al 1995).

Drug-induced psoriasis may cause nail pitting.

Hair disorders

Drug-induced alopecia (Table 54.14) may be partial or complete and can involve sites other than the scalp. The most severe loss usually occurs with cytotoxic therapy; it begins shortly after administration of the drug and the effect is dose-dependent and fortunately reversible. The hair loss in patients receiving paclitaxel has unique characteristics. Hair loss is sudden and complete and many patients experience loss of all body hair, including axillary and pubic hair, eyelashes and eyebrows (Gore et al 1995). The loss of body hair often occurs with cumulative therapy and is more severe after longer infusion times. Interferons have also been reported to produce hair loss; however, this is probably secondary to the influenza-like symptoms (Tosti et al 1994).

Hirsutism is excessive hairiness, especially in women, in the male pattern of hair growth, while hypertrichosis is the growth of hair at sites not normally hairy. Both conditions can be drug-induced and in some cases the same drug can produce both patterns of hair growth (Table 54.14). If it is not possible to withdraw the drug and there is no suitable alternative, then these patients should have this fully explained to them and be advised to use a depilatory cream if necessary. This particular side-effect of minoxidil has been exploited in the treatment of alopecia.

Some drugs can induce both alopecia and hirsutism. For example, the hydantoin anticonvulsants can cause alopecia of the scalp and hirsutism of the body. This occurs mainly in young women.

Skin malignancy

Skin malignancy is an increasing concern. Its growing prevalence is associated with exposure to sunlight, but also with increased immunocompromised populations, for example HIV patients.

Immunosuppressive drugs will facilitate the development of malignant and pre-malignant skin lesions. Azathioprine was believed to have a specific risk in organ transplantation because ultraviolet light leads to

Table 54.14   Drugs causing hair disorders

Alopecia
Acetretin
Anticoagulants
Anticonvulsants
Antithyroid drugs
β adrenoceptor blockers
Withdrawal of oral contraceptives
Cytotoxic drugs
Etretinate
Gold salts
Lithium
Sodium valproate
Tacrolimus

Hirsutism
Acetazolamide
Anabolic steroids
Androgens
Corticosteroids (topical and systemic)
Ciclosporin
Danazol
Diazoxide
Dihydrotestosterone
Minoxidil
Nifedipine
Oral contraceptives
Penicillamine
Phenytoin
Tamoxifen
Verapamil

breakdown of the drug into mutagenic products. However, it has been shown that patients treated with ciclosporin but not azathioprine have a similar risk of skin malignancy (Shuttleworth et al 1989). This suggests the skin cancer risk is mainly a result of reduced immune surveillance and human papilloma virus infection.

Malignancy shows significant latency, and caution has been expressed over the use of the very potent new generation of immunosuppressive agents such as the anti-TNF alpha drugs. However, these drugs are proving to be very effective in otherwise highly disabling disease.

Immunosuppressive drugs are not directly photoallergic. However, all patients receiving immuno-suppressive therapies should be counselled on the risk of malignancy and advised to avoid exposure to sunlight, and those on long-term therapy should be monitored for skin lesions.

Patient care

All adverse effects to drugs should be taken seriously. Rashes, even the less serious with no systemic involvement, are distressing, often irritant and

disfiguring. Their presence can be indicative of drug allergy which can become more significant on drug rechallenge.

It is therefore important to find the drug cause so patients are made aware and can report and avoid the sensitivity.

Treatment is symptomatic with oral antihistamines, calamine and corticosteroids (unless the patient is immunocompromised). Patients should be reassured about the self-limiting nature of the disorder, and that disfigurement is unusual.

CASE STUDIES

Case 54.1

A 6-year-old patient with poorly controlled epilepsy is prescribed lamotrigine 25 mg twice daily.

Questions

1. What adverse event would you be concerned about and what would increase the risk of this happening?
2. What therapy would you recommend for this child?

Answers

1. This child would be at risk of a serious skin rash, including Stevens–Johnson syndrome and toxic epidermal necrolysis. This risk is higher:

   - in children: with a frequency of 1:300 to 1:100
   - with concomitant use of valproate, which interacts to increase plasma levels of lamotrigine
   - if initial dosing of lamotrigine is high
   - if the dose is rapidly escalated.

2. Lamotrigine is not recommended as monotherapy in children under 12 years of age. It is therefore likely that the lamotrigine is add-on therapy. The dose given is too high as initial therapy. If the child is on valproate the initial dose should be 150 micrograms/kilogram daily. Whereas if the child is taking enzyme-inducing drugs but not valproate the initial dose is 600 micrograms/kilogram daily in two divided doses. In both cases the dose should be slowly increased in line with the licensed dose recommendations.

Case 54.2

Miss A. F. is a 15-year-old, 6 weeks post renal transplant patient. She is very distressed about the growth of facial hair and the worsening of acne.

Questions

1. What are the possible causes of Miss A. F.'s skin complaints?
2. How might these conditions be treated?

Answers

1. It is likely that Miss A. F. is receiving transplant immunosuppression that includes ciclosporin and prednisolone. The ciclosporin is most likely to have caused the growth of facial hair. The prednisolone could have worsened the acne, or this may be normal adolescent acne made worse by Miss A. F.'s improved health. Ciclosporin could also be a causative agent for her acne.

2. Hirsutism was a side-effect of ciclosporin that many young transplant patients had to cope with and depilatory creams had to be used. It is now possible that a switch to tacrolimus could be considered if the patient finds this side-effect distressing. The prednisolone is low dose in transplantation. It will eventually be reduced to a maintenance dose, and could be stopped in most cases if acne were still a problem. Topical acne preparations and, if necessary, oral antibiotics can be used to treat the acne.

Case 54.3

Mr H. W. is HIV positive and was initiated on antiretroviral therapy 6 weeks previously, after his CD4 count fell and his viral load increased. He has been receiving triple therapy with two nucleoside reverse transcriptase inhibitors, zidovudine and lamivudine, as the combination Combivir, and a non-nucleoside reverse transciptase inhibitor, nevirapine. Mr H. W. has also been taking co-trimoxazole prophylaxis. He is admitted to hospital by his consultant when he develops an extensive erythematous rash with maculopapular lesions and severe blistering of the mouth.

Questions

1. What type of reaction does Mr H. W.'s history suggest?
2. What is the likely causative agent? Suggest alternative drug therapy.

Answers

1. The features of Mr H. W.'s rash are suggestive of erythema multiforme and the involvement of the mucous membrane may indicate Stevens–Johnson syndrome.

2. It is likely that the skin reaction is drug-induced, and the causative drug must be stopped immediately. Co-trimoxazole is a common cause of Stevens–Johnson syndrome in HIV patients. However, the non-nucleoside reverse transcriptase inhibitor nevirapine is associated with a high incidence of rash, inlcuding Stevens–Johnson syndrome, and must also be stopped. The antiretroviral choice for this patient would then be to add one or possibly two (quardruple therapy) protease inhibitors in place of nevirapine, and also to add pentamidine for *Pneumocystis carinii* (PCP) prohpylaxis. Although these choices have significant side-effect profiles, antiretroviral therapy should be continued and may be subject to constant change due to adverse events and resistance.

REFERENCES

Alanko K 1994 Topical provocation of fixed drug eruption: a study of 30 patients. Contact Dermatitis 31: 25

Bauer F 1981 Quinacrine hydrochloride drug eruption (topical lichenoid dermatitis): its early and late sequelae and its malignant potential. Journal of the American Academy of Dermatology 4: 239

Creamer J J, Mortimer P S, Powles T J 1995 Mitozantrone-induced onycholysis: a series of five cases. Clinical and Experimental Dermatology 20: 459

de Raevel L, Song M, van Maldergen L 1988 Adverse cutaneous drug reactions in AIDS. British Journal of Dermatology 119: 521

Gore M, Levy V, Rusitn G et al 1995 Paclitaxel (Taxol) in relapsed and refractory ovarian cancer: the UK and Eire experience. British Journal of Cancer 72: 1016–1019

Jick H, Derby L E 1995 Is co-trimoxazole safe? Lancet 345: 118–119

Litt J Z, Pawlak W A 1997 Drug eruption reference manual. Parthenon Publishing, New York, p. 490

Schopf E, Sluhmer A, Razny B et al 1991 Toxic epidermal necrolysis and Stevens–Johnson syndrome: an epidemiological study from West Germany. Archives of Dermatology 127: 839

Shuttleworth D, Marks R, Griffin P J A et al 1989 Epidermal dysplasia and ciclosporin therapy in renal transplant patients: a comparison with azathioprine. British Journal of Dermatology 120: 551

Tosti A, Misciali C, Piraccin B M et al 1994 Drug induced hair loss and hair growth: incidence, management and avoidance. Drug Safety 10: 310

FURTHER READING

Buxton P K 1988 ABC of dermatology. British Medical Association, London

Davies D M, Ferner R E, de Glanville H (eds) 1998 Davies's Textbook of adverse drug reactions, 5th edn. Oxford Medical Publications, Oxford

Dukes M N G, Aronson J K (eds) 2000 Meyler's side effects of drugs, 14th edn. Elsevier, Amsterdam

de Groot A C, Weyland J W, Nater J P (eds) 1994 Unwanted effects of cosmetics and drugs used in dermatology, 3rd edn. Elsevier, Amsterdam

Eczema and psoriasis 55

M. M. Carr

Eczema and psoriasis are common inflammatory skin disorders that have some similarities and may sometimes be difficult to distinguish from each other in practice. Both may respond to some of the same treatments, and both can be functionally and socially disabling. However, they are distinct diseases with different causes, occurring in different groups of people.

Eczema

The terms 'eczema' and 'dermatitis' may be used interchangeably and describe the same clinical and histological entity. Both words are derived from the Greek: 'eczema', meaning 'to boil', describes the characteristic tiny blisters of the condition, and 'dermatitis' means 'inflammation of the skin'. There are several patterns of the condition. A common convention is to describe as 'eczema' those that are endogenous or constitutional and as 'dermatitis' those that are exogenous or due to contact.

Pathophysiology and clinical features

The histological features of eczema/dermatitis are similar, regardless of aetiology, and differ in the acute and chronic phases. In the acute stage, fluid escapes from dilated dermal blood vessels to produce oedema in the epidermis. This collects into vesicles or tiny blisters, particularly where the skin is thick, as in the palms and soles. These vesicles may coalesce into larger blisters. Where the skin is thinner they tend to rupture onto the skin surface, causing exudation and crusting. The chronic stage shows less oedema and vesiculation and more thickening of the epidermis and horny layers, produced by prolonged rubbing and scratching by the sufferer. Both stages are accompanied by a heavy inflammatory cell infiltration of the dermis and epidermis. These histological features are mirrored by the clinical picture; the different types of eczema/dermatitis have a number of features in common, although they vary in other ways according to their cause, site and severity.

Acute eczema/dermatitis

Acute eczema/dermatitis is characterized by a progression through a number of stages:

- red, hot, swollen and itchy skin
- papules and tiny blisters, sometimes coalescing to form large ones (called pompholyx on the palms and soles)
- exudation and crusting
- scaling.

Chronic eczema/dermatitis

In addition to the features listed above, chronic eczema/dermatitis may show:

- drier skin, becoming more scaly
- lichenification (i.e. dry, thickened, leathery skin with exaggerated skin markings, due to rubbing and scratching) (Fig. 55.1)
- painful fissures.

Clinical types

Atopic eczema

Atopic eczema is a common condition affecting about 15% of children, the majority of whom recover before

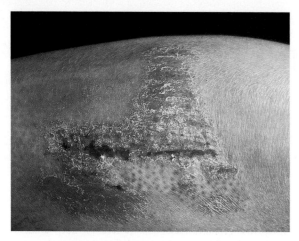

Figure 55.1 Dry, excoriated, lichenified chronic eczema.

their teens (Kay et al 1994). The tendency to this type of eczema is genetically determined, with 70% of sufferers having a family history of atopy (one or more of eczema, asthma, hayfever or urticaria), but the disease is regarded as being multifactorial. Between 30% and 50% of eczema patients will also develop asthma or hayfever. Atopic eczema is typically symmetrical in distribution and affects particularly the face and flexures (fronts of the elbows and wrists, backs of the knees; Fig. 55.2), although it may also affect the hands and feet or become generalized (erythroderma). The flexures tend to become lichenified as the child becomes older, and the skin is generally very dry and itchy. On the palms and soles, where the skin is naturally thick, an intensely itchy sago-like eruption known as pompholyx may occur, consisting of numerous tiny intact vesicles.

Atopics produce antigen-specific cirulating IgE antibodies to such allergens as the house dust mite,

pollens and other inhalants, and foods such as dairy products. Scratch or prick testing to these allergens is unreliable; there is a high false-positive rate with this method, and it is rarely carried out. A more reliable method of detection is by RAST (radioallergosorbent) testing, although here too false-positive tests are common, and not necessarily relevant to the state of an individual's eczema; they may be a better reflection of allergies related to asthma or hayfever. For these reasons, allergy testing is not carried out routinely on atopics.

Provoking factors. A number of factors may aggravate atopic eczema, but none should be regarded as the sole cause of the problem:

- Dryness and extremes of temperature may increase itch, and so cause scratching.
- Inhalant and food allergens can produce similar effects.
- Irritants such as soap and water may have their effect, either by increasing dryness or by a direct effect on skin cells, having penetrated through fissures.
- Allergic contact dermatitis may complicate atopic eczema as loss of the natural lipid barrier function makes the entry of allergens into the skin easier.
- In older children, teenagers and adults stress is a common exacerbating factor.
- Probably the single most potent cause of a sudden deterioration in atopic eczema is infection, either bacterial or viral; atopics have impaired cell-mediated immunity, making the affected area prone to this problem. Particularly troublesome organisms are *Staphylococcus aureus,* herpes simplex virus and varicella. Milder viral infections such as warts and molluscum contagiosum are also very common. (Figs 55.3, 55.4.)

Contact dermatitis

Two types of contact dermatitis exist: the first is where the rash is caused by an allergy to an external substance (cell-mediated immune or type IV reaction); in the second type the cause is wear and tear and irritation.

Allergic contact dermatitis. A large number of compounds found in daily life, both in the home and at work, may be responsible for allergic contact dermatitis. Common culprits are:

- metals (e.g. nickel)
- topical medicaments (including antibiotics, antihistamines and local anaesthetics), ointment bases and preservatives
- dyes
- plants
- rubber compounds
- in industry, resins, plastics and cement frequently cause problems (Fig. 55.5).

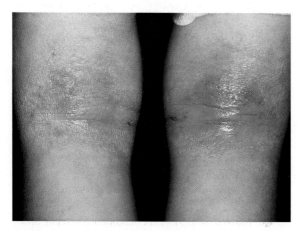

Figure 55.2 Flexural eczema in childhood.

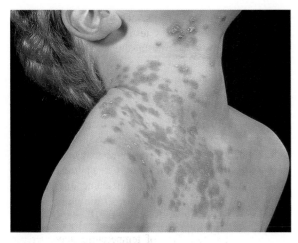

Figure 55.3 Impetigo complicating atopic eczema.

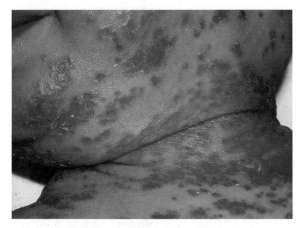

Figure 55.4 Typical 'punched-out' lesions of eczema herpeticum in an atopic baby.

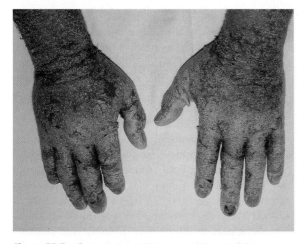

Figure 55.5 Contact dermatitis to cement in a building worker.

The dermatitis rarely starts after the patient's first exposure to the allergen, and there may be months or years of contact before the reaction occurs.

The first and most important step in the diagnosis of contact allergy is to take a detailed history and note the pattern and distribution of the rash; this will frequently establish the cause. Common patterns include dermatitis under metal fastenings in clothes such as zips and jeans studs (nickel allergy) and under rubber gloves. A rash around the eyes may indicate airborne allergens from plants, nail varnish or strike-anywhere matches (phosphorus sesquisulphide vapour), or allergens in local applications of medicaments. Make-up allergy is surprisingly uncommon. If the allergy is severe or uncontrolled, the dermatitis may extend to other areas of the skin and occasionally become generalized.

If confirmation or further investigation is required patch testing may be useful, unlike skin tests in other types of eczema. A battery of possible allergens is applied to uninvolved skin (usually the back) in small quantities at the appropriate concentration and in the correct vehicle. The skin is examined for an eczematous reaction under the test patches at 48 hours and 96 hours, which would indicate delayed hypersensitivity.

Once an allergy has been confirmed the patient must avoid the allergen, since this type of allergy is lifelong and the dermatitis is likely to persist as long as contact continues.

Primary irritant dermatitis. This is the commonest cause of hand eczema, and is seen particularly in housewives, nurses, hairdressers and those who work with oils and greases in industry. Contact with anything that dehydrates the skin, particularly water, detergents and soaps, and degreasers, removes the natural protective oils from the skin, allowing evaporation of water and penetration of irritants. The longer the skin is exposed to such treatment, the more likely is the development of dermatitis. Atopics are particularly prone to this problem, especially on the hands.

No allergy is involved in this type of dermatitis and therefore patch testing is not usually indicated unless a coexiting allergy is suspected or needs to be excluded.

Other eczemas

Seborrhoeic eczema. This involves the areas of the body with a high density of sebaceous glands, i.e. the face, scalp and upper trunk, and occurs after puberty, when these glands become active (Fig. 55.6). It is due to an overgrowth of *Pityrosporum ovale,* a yeast that is a normal commensal on the skin. The skin is red, with greasy yellow scales, and the scalp shows severe dandruff.

An infantile version of the disease may occur in the first months of life, causing 'cradle cap' on the scalp and

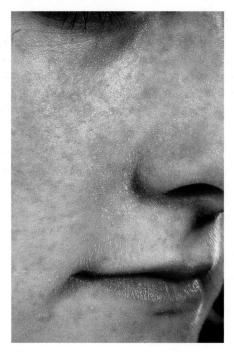

Figure 55.6 Seborrhoeic eczema in a teenager.

a shiny red rash in the folds of the skin and in the napkin area. This recovers in a few weeks or months.

Discoid eczema. As the name suggests, this occurs in circular patches. These characteristically occur on the forearms and lower legs, and are intensely itchy. As a result, they are frequently excoriated, and become secondarily infected.

Varicose/stasis eczema. This is usually the result of varicose veins, venous stasis and oedema in the lower leg, particularly around the ankle, and may progress to varicose ulceration. The patient with varicose eczema is particularly at risk of developing allergic contact dermatitis to topical medicaments such as antibiotics and vehicles, and to rubber in compression bandages.

Asteatotic eczema. This means 'lacking in oil', and is typically found in the elderly, in whom the skin becomes over-dry, perhaps aggravated by the use of soap.

Treatment

The same basic principles of treatment apply regardless of the type of eczema.

Emollients

The mainstay of eczema treatment is the use of liberal quantities of moisturizers as, in all types, the basic problem is the loss or deficiency of the skin's lipid layer. Adequate use of emollients will reduce the requirement for topical steroid, both in quantity and potency. Soap should be avoided if at all possible, and a soap substitute such as aqueous cream should be applied before, during and after bathing or showering. In addition, a bath oil or emulsifying ointment added to the water may be very helpful in hydrating the skin. Despite this long-established clinical experience, there have been very few controlled trials to confirm the effectiveness of emollients (Charman 2000).

If the patient is prone to secondary infection of the skin, reinfection via the emollient tub may be avoided by supplying a proprietary preparation in a pump dispenser.

It is very important that sufficient quantities of moisturizer be supplied; the minimum weekly requirement for an infant is 50 g, for a 10-year-old 100 g, and for an adult 200 g.

Topical corticosteroids

Eczema is an inflammatory condition, so specific treatment must be anti-inflammatory, which in practice means corticosteroids, normally used topically.

Topical steroids have been developed over the past 40 years and have revolutionized the treatment of inflammatory dermatoses, particularly the eczemas. Modification of the first compound, hydrocortisone, has produced large numbers of more potent drugs. Unfortunately, with time and increasingly extensive usage of topical fluorinated steroids, it became apparent that the greater the potency of the steroid, the greater its potential for adverse effects. Epidermal atrophy (thinning), telangiectasia (prominent surface blood vessels), striae (stretch marks), and premature ageing due to collagen loss, rosacea and exacerbation of skin infection are frequently seen. Rarely, pituitary–adrenal axis suppression may occur, and reduced growth rates in children after prolonged use have been reported. As a result of publicity in both the medical and popular press in the 1970s and 1980s, general practitioners and their patients are now only too well aware of the potential hazards of steroid usage, with the result that some patients may receive inadequate treatment. Others may have inappropriate treatment through using topical steroids as emollients. The aim of topical steroid therapy should be to control the eczema using a potent application if necessary, under close medical supervision, and then to maintain that control using a drug of the lowest effective potency.

Choice of preparation. *Potency.* Topical steroids are classified by potency into four groups: very potent (group 1), potent (group 2), moderately potent (group 3) and mildly potent (group 4). The clinical potency generally correlates with the frequency and severity of adverse effects after prolonged usage. The newer potent steroids appear to have lower potential for systemic absorption, and may produce fewer long-term side-effects, but this has yet to be fully evaluated in long-term studies. They do have the advantage of being effective in once-daily applications, which is convenient for the user. Group 4 steroids are most suitable for use on thin skin, such as the face and flexures, and on children's skin for maintenance therapy Preparations of increased potency may be needed to control acute exacerbations of the eczema and on areas where the horny layer and epidermis are naturally thicker, for example on the palms of the hands and soles of the feet.

Base. Topical steroids are available in ointment, cream and oily cream formulations and as aqueous or alcoholic lotions, gels and mousse for use on the scalp. In general, dry eczemas should be treated with ointments and weeping areas with creams. Where the scalp is inflamed or excoriated an alcoholic lotion may be uncomfortable and the use of a cream or mousse preparation preferred.

Allergies. Some constituents of the bases occasionally cause allergic reactions; propylene glycol and lanolin in ointments, and parabens, ethylene diamine and chlorocresol in creams are the commonest culprits. Allergy to the steroid molecules is also being increasingly recognized. These factors must be taken into account when choosing a preparation for a particular patient.

Antibiotic/antiseptic additives. Chronic low-grade infection is common in eczema and dermatitis, and this may be exacerbated by using a steroid alone. Significant infection is best managed with oral antibiotics; topical steroid/antibiotic combinations should be avoided as the topical antibiotics can prove to be potent sensitizers. An exception is chlortetracycline. Chronic infection can be controlled using a topical steroid/clioquinol combination of appropriate potency, which is antiseptic rather than antibiotic.

Quantities. It is important to monitor the topical steroid consumption of the patient, to ensure that there is not overusage and, equally, that treatment is adequate. In many cases only localized areas of the body need treatment, but in a widespread eczema, an adult may need up to 170 g per week for a twice-daily application, and an infant 35 g (Table 55.1).

Table 55.1 Minimum quantity (grams) of topical application required for twice-daily treatment for 1 week

Age	Whole body	Trunk	Both arms and legs
6 months	35	15	20
4 years	60	20	35
8 years	90	35	50
12 years	120	45	65
Adult (70 kg)	170	60	90

Antibiotics

Wherever possible, swabs should be taken from infected skin before starting oral antibiotics. The antibiotic of choice to cover *Staph. aureus* is normally erythromycin or flucloxacillin, which should be given for a minimum of 10 days. Chronic infection may occasionally require long-term treatment.

Herpes simplex virus infection should be treated promptly with aciclovir, orally if the problem is widespread or the patient is ill, to prevent a marked deterioration of atopic eczema.

Drying agents

In vesicular or weeping eczema the blisters and oozing areas are dried using potassium permanganate baths, soaks or wet compresses. Crystals or tablets are added to warm water to produce a purplish-pink colour, and the skin soaked for at least 15 minutes if possible. This seems to have an astringent and antiseptic effect.

Antihistamines

Pruritus is often the most distressing feature of eczema, and the patient may benefit from the short-term use of a sedative antihistamine at night. The newer, non-sedative antihistamines have little value in this situation. Topical antihistamines are potent sensitizers and have no place in the management of eczema.

Coal tar preparations

Although less cosmetically acceptable than other topical preparations, tar is an effective antipruritic. It is chiefly used in impregnated bandages to occlude the limbs in atopic children at night, both for symptomatic relief and to prevent scratching. Ichthammol is used in the same way.

Tar creams and ointments are useful in the treatment of discoid eczema, which is often resistant to topical steroids.

There has recently been concern about the safety of tar, based on animal testing and experience in industry, but this has not so far been borne out in clinical practice.

Bandaging

In children with atopic eczema, occlusion with bandages has long been useful to prevent scratching and to keep ointments and creams in contact with the skin. The recent technique of wet wrapping, involving the application of emollients and steroids under a double layer of conforming tubular bandage, and keeping the inner layer moist, can be very effective, and the cooling effect of evaporation very soothing. Parents can be trained to apply these dressings at home.

Compression bandaging or graduated support stockings may be the single most effective method of control of varicose eczema, once the acute phase has been treated.

Other treatments

Topical imidazoles. Ketoconazole as a shampoo or cream will reduce the population of *Pityrosporum ovale* on the skin, and thus control seborrhoeic eczema and dandruff. The disease runs a chronic, relapsing course, so regular or intermittent use is usually necessary. Other imidazoles can also be used.

Systemic steroids. Oral corticosteroids are used as a short-term measure in the treatment of acute eczemas, to bring the condition rapidly under control. Acute exacerbations of atopic eczema, acute allergic contact dermatitis and erythrodermic eczema, where the skin is red and hot all over the body, may require this type of management.

With the advent of other immunosuppressive agents, the need for long-term treatment with oral steroids for eczema is now very rare.

Ciclosporin. This drug is extremely effective in the treatment of chronic severe eczema (Camp et al 1993) and at present is used mainly in adult patients, although its use in children is increasing. The therapeutic range is 2–5 mg/kg. The eczema tends to relapse when the drug is stopped, but intermittent courses can be very useful in keeping the condition manageable. It is an immunosuppressant, so patients must be carefully monitored for signs of infection. The main adverse reactions are hypertension and renal impairment but these are reversible if the dose is reduced or the drug stopped. A number of drugs interact with ciclosporin and must be used with caution (Table 55.2). There are concerns about the long-term risks of developing skin cancers on light-exposed areas of the body, underlining the importance of using this drug for short-term treatment wherever possible.

Topical preparations of ciclosporin have so far proved disappointing in treating eczema due to poor skin penetration.

Table 55.2   Interactions with drugs used in the treatment of psoriasis and eczema

	Interacting drug	Outcome
Methotrexate	Aspirin NSAIDs Probenecid	Increased serum concentration and toxicity of methotrexate
	Phenytoin Sulphonamides Trimethoprim	Increased bone marrow toxicity
Azathioprine	Allopurinol	Enhanced effect and toxicity of azathioprine
	Warfarin	Inhibition of anticoagulant effect
	Cimetidine Indometacin	Enchanced myelosuppression
Ciclosporin	NSAIDs Aminoglycosides Co-trimoxazole Ciprofloxacin	Increased risk of nephrotoxicity
	Ketoconazole Itraconazole Erythromycin Oral contraceptives Calcium channel blockers	Increased serum concentration of ciclosporin
	Phenytoin Carbamazepine Rifampicin	Decreased serum concentration of ciclosporin
Acitretin	Methotrexate	Increased serum concentration of methotrexate

NSAID, non-steroidal anti-inflammatory drug.

Azathioprine. This antimitotic drug is used as a steroid-sparing agent, or alone, in cases of severe resistant eczema, at a dose of 50–150 mg per day. It acts more slowly than ciclosporin, but is widely used for long-term treatment. It suppresses the bone marrow and the immune system and patients must be monitored, with regular blood tests.

Other immune modulators. Interferon gamma has been used in cases of severe refractory eczema, but has unpleasant flu-like side-effects. Methotrexate has also been used in unresponsive, adult atopic eczema, but has never been evaluated in clinical trials.

Evening primrose oil. This has proved disappointing in clinical trials, but may occasionally have a place in the treatment of resistant eczema, especially where extreme dryness is the major problem (Munn 1999).

Phototherapy. Some atopic patients benefit from the use of PUVA (the combination of oral psoralen and ultraviolet A) or UVB, particularly in the dry, chronic stages (Krutmann 2000). Narrow-band UVB therapy is now becoming widely available, and may be as effective and safer than PUVA. Potential side-effects of all types of phototherapy include burning, premature ageing of the skin and increased risk of skin cancer. Patients attend for 2–3 treatments per week, usually for several weeks, and courses may be repeated at intervals.

Diets. These are not used routinely in the management of atopic eczema as they are of value only in a very few cases. They should only be used under the supervision of a dietitian.

Chinese herbal medicine. Traditional Chinese herbal medicines are prescribed and made up on an individual basis for the patient. A standardized form has been devised by a Chinese practitioner in collaboration with Great Ormond Street the Hospital for Sick Children in London. The active principle and constituents are unknown, and the treatment is therefore only available on a named-patient basis. It has been shown to be effective in atopic eczema (Sheehan & Atherton 1994) but possible side-effects include liver disturbance, so patients are monitored regularly with blood tests, as all patients receiving individual prescriptions should be. The treatment is still undergoing close scrutiny and conflicting results have been obtained (Fung et al 1999).

Alternative therapies. These include psychotherapy, hypnotherapy, yoga and reflexology, which may help individual, usually adult, atopic patients.

Therapies for the future. Tacrolimus is an immunosuppressive drug used in organ transplantation. It is more potent than ciclosporin and has greater skin penetration. The topical form has been shown to be effective in short-term treatment of atopic eczema (Ruzicka et al 1997). Topical SDZ ASM 981 is another immunosuppressant being developed in topical form. It has shown early encouraging results in adult atopic eczema

(Van Leent et al 1998). Antagonists of inflammatory mediators may also hold possibilities for the future.

None of these drugs is yet available on prescription in the UK.

Patient care

It is important to recognize that eczema affects many aspects of a patient's life and has considerable effects on the family. Apart from the appearance and discomfort of the rash, the irritability and loss of sleep, there may be considerable limitations on the patient's activities, and assistance in treating and overcoming the problems may be needed from general practitioners, dermatologists, nurses, pharmacists and teachers. Advice and help through contact with other sufferers and their families and information on the latest dressings, treatments, clothing, etc. can be obtained from the local branch of the National Eczema Society.

The parents of atopic children need to understand that the prescribed treatments are designed to control the condition, not to cure it, and that the majority of atopics gradually improve during childhood and need to be treated until their eczema naturally resolves. They should not be afraid to use prescribed topical steroids, as they are necessary and used under medical supervision.

Cool cotton clothing is the most suitable for eczema sufferers, and while soap powders are probably not a problem if used in a modern washing machine with an efficient rinsing programme, leave-in fabric conditioners are best avoided. House dust mite precautions are advisable in many atopics, particularly if they also suffer from asthma or allergic rhinitis. In cases of allergic contact dermatitis, avoidance of the known allergen is the treatment of choice, as continued exposure will result in persistence of the rash, despite medication.

Eczema patients should aim to lead as normal a life as possible, and schools and employers can help to achieve this. Emollients applied regularly at breaktimes, with assistance if necessary, make an enormous difference to the state of the skin. Encouraging other children to accept the eczema, and not to regard it as infectious, can boost a child's self-image greatly.

It is worth discussing careers at an early stage with atopics and their parents so as to avoid disappointment later. Even if the eczema has apparently settled, exposure to water, detergents, oils, greases and degreasers may result in a recurrence of the problem, particularly on the hands, which may ultimately result in the loss of a job. For this reason, nursing, hairdressing, catering and handling machinery are unwise occupations for an atopic, who should consider a clean, dry job in preference.

A treatment flow chart for eczema is outlined in Figure 55.7.

ECZEMA

History and examination

Atopic eczema			Contact dermatitis		Seborrhoeic dermatitis	Asteatotic eczema	Discoid eczema	Varicose eczema
Acute, exuding	Dry, chronic lichenified	Infected	Irritant	Allergic				

Emollients for all

Drying agents Mild–moderate topical steroid ointment or cream	Moderate–strong topical steroid ointment	Antibiotics (oral) Aciclovir	Avoid irritants Protection (topical steroids)	Avoid allergens Protection Topical steroids	Imidazote shampoo/ cream	± Mild–moderate topical steroid ointment	Tar Strong topical steroid ointment	Mild–moderate topical steroid cream/ ointment

Review after 2–4 weeks of treatment. If no improvement, consider 2nd line therapy

Systemic steroids	Ciclosporin	Azathioprine	Phototherapy

A treatment flow chart for eczema.

Aetiology

Psoriasis is a chronic condition which may affect the skin and joints. In the skin it is seen as a red scaly rash that affects about 2% of the population in Europe and North America. The cause is still not known, but there is a genetic predisposition to the disease; over 70% of patients have a family history. HLA typing shows a preponderance of certain antigens, including DR7 and CW6. The nature of the genetic defect is unknown, but certain non-hereditary factors appear also to contribute by precipitating an attack. These include the following:

Infection

Streptococcal infections, particularly in the upper respiratory tract, may be followed 10–14 days later by an attack of psoriasis. This is particularly common in children, and may be the first presentation of the disease, in a typical guttate pattern (see below).

Patients with psoriasis who develop the acquired immune deficiency syndrome (AIDS) may have a severe flare of the rash.

Koebner phenomenon

An injury to the skin, for example a cut, burn, scratch or operation scar, may cause psoriasis subsequently to develop at that site, which may later spread further.

Lithium, chloroquine and β-blockers

These drugs, given for depression, rheumatological disorders and cardiovascular disease, respectively, may provoke a flare of psoriasis in susceptible patients.

Stress

An association between stress, either emotional or physical, and psoriasis is frequently claimed, but is difficult to confirm or refute.

Alcohol and smoking

Excess alcohol consumption may aggravate psoriasis, and psoriasis is known to be associated with high rates of alcoholism; it may be difficult to establish cause and effect. There is also a high correlation between smoking and psoriasis of the palms and soles, of the pustular variety.

Pathogenesis

Many changes occur in the skin in psoriasis, which may be either the cause or effect of the disease.

Histologically, the epidermis is thickened (acanthosis), the granular layer is absent and epidermal cell nuclei are seen persisting in the horny layer (parakeratosis). In the dermis, the dermal capillaries are dilated and tortuous and closer to the surface of the skin than normal.

Large numbers of inflammatory cells are present in all layers of the skin; granulocytes are predominant, and form microabscesses in the epidermis. Langerhans' cells and lymphocytes are also increased.

In dynamic terms, the main abnormality is increased epidermal cell turnover – about 10 times the normal rate. The histological changes described above have led to a number of hypotheses as to the way in which this hyperproliferation is brought about. The presence of lymphocytes and Langerhans' cells has suggested an immunological cause, with mediators known as cytokines being released by these cells, recruiting more inflammatory cells to the process and thus stimulating epidermal cell turnover at an increased rate. Some studies suggest that epidermal cells themselves produce the cytokines that promote their own proliferation, and attract lymphocytes. Changes in the structure of the dermal blood vessels also occur, possibly as a result of mediator activity. None of these observations or theories is mutually exclusive, but their relationship to the underlying genetic defect is as yet unknown.

Clinical features

The typical psoriatic lesion is a red, scaly, sharply demarcated plaque, which may be of any size, and may affect any part of the body. However, the commonest sites are the extensor surfaces of the elbows (Fig. 55.8) and knees, the sacrum and the scalp. Hands and feet are frequently involved. The scale is silvery, and easily scraped off, revealing tiny bleeding points.

Psoriasis is not characteristically itchy, but may be when very inflamed, rapidly spreading or involving the palms and soles.

The natural history of psoriasis is that it tends to appear for the first time in young adults, although it may start in infancy or old age, and it runs a chronic, relapsing course. Treatment is aimed at control of the current attack, not cure, and will not influence the future progress of the disease.

A number of different patterns of psoriasis occur, and these are described below.

Guttate psoriasis (Fig. 55.9)

This means 'drop-like', describing the multiple small plaques all over the body which occur particularly in children, after streptococcal sore throats. This type is usually self-limiting after a few weeks.

Chronic plaque psoriasis

Medium or large plaques occur on the trunk and limbs, and may be very persistent.

Psoriasis of the scalp (Fig. 55.10)

Involvement of the scalp may be as demarcated plaques or may involve the whole scalp, extending into the hairline. The scale is white, thick and chalky, and hair loss may occur when the scalp is thickly scaled. This should recover if the scale is cleared and kept under control.

Psoriasis of the nails

The nails are frequently affected in psoriasis and this may be the only evidence of the disease in some cases.

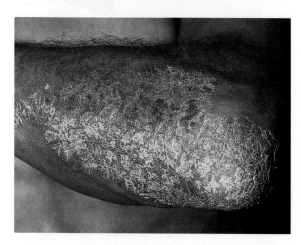

Chronic scaly plaque psoriasis on an elbow.

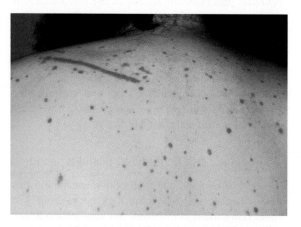

Guttate psoriasis showing Koebner phenomenon in scratch mark.

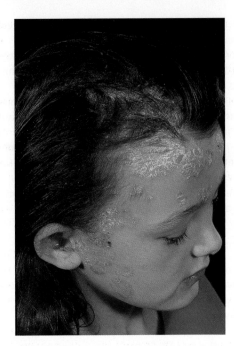

Figure 55.10 Chalky scaling of scalp psoriasis extending on to the face.

The changes include pitting, onycholysis (separation of the nail from its bed) and hyperkeratosis under the nail, and can be uncomfortable and disfiguring in some patients. The changes in psoriatic nails are very resistant to treatment.

Psoriasis of the palms and soles (Fig. 55.11)

At these sites there is sharp demarcation of the involved areas, which are inflamed and very scaly and may contain sterile pustules of large pin-head size. These dry up into brown macules and the affected skin then becomes hyperkeratotic and fissuring. As a result, secondary infection, with accompanying itch and pain, is common.

Flexural psoriasis

When psoriasis occurs in the flexures, such as the axillae, groins, submammary areas and genitalia, the demarcation is still present, but the affected areas are glazed rather than scaly, and bright red.

Erythrodermic and generalized pustular psoriasis

These are severe and potentially life-threatening forms of the disease, and are fortunately uncommon. The whole skin surface is involved, and very inflamed, and the patient is sick; the pustules are sterile and may coalesce to form sheets of pus.

Psoriatic arthropathy

The arthritis associated with psoriasis occurs in about 5% of psoriatics. It is of a similar type to rheumatoid arthritis but the rheumatoid factor is negative. Several patterns are recognized.

Distal arthritis. This involves the terminal interphalangeal joints of the fingers and toes, and is associated with nail changes.

Large joint involvement. Here a single large joint may be involved, and the arthritis is destructive.

Sacroiliitis/spondylitis. The changes here are similar to ankylosing spondylitis, with the sexes equally affected; there is a strong association with HLA-B27.

Treatment

Many patients with psoriasis need very little treatment, as their disease is minimal. Emollients may be all that is necessary to prevent drying and fissuring of the elbows and knees. Other patients may simply prefer not to treat their skin, as the process is laborious, time-consuming and frequently messy.

Many of the treatments still used today are historical, and therefore empirical, and have never been subjected to controlled trials. More modern therapies, which are all directed at reducing epidermal cell turnover, have been more critically tested. Different types of psoriasis may respond best to different treatments.

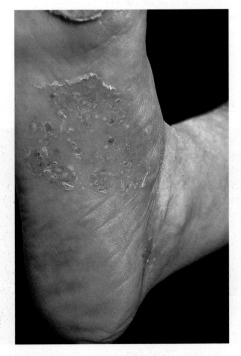

Figure 55.11 Pustular psoriasis of the sole.

Topical therapy

Emollients. These may be all that is needed in very mild cases. Rest and soothing applications are essential in the management of erythroderma, although the patient may also need systemic therapy.

Topical steroids. These are widely and probably overused in the treatment of psoriasis. They are of most value in acutely inflamed plaques, where they control the inflammation, preparing the way for other treatments. They are not as effective on chronic scaly plaques.

Mild, group 4 steroids are helpful on the face and on flexures, where dithranol, tar and calcipotriol may be irritant. More potent steroids are frequently used on the hands and feet, possibly in combination with clioquinol if the skin is fissured, or with salicylic acid if there is hyperkeratosis. Potent steroid preparations are commonly used on scalp psoriasis, often with unsatisfactory effect. This is because lotions and creams will not penetrate thick scale efficiently, and the scalp should be prepared with a keratolytic such as salicylic acid first. Aqueous and alcoholic lotions will cause stinging and burning on inflamed scalps, and a cream, ointment or mousse may be preferable. The use of potent topical steroids on large areas of psoriasis, although anti-inflammatory in the short term, may result in a rebound flare when the steroid is discontinued. This results in continuation of the steroid, and, ultimately, unwanted side-effects.

Dithranol. For many years, dithranol has been the mainstay of in-patient treatment of psoriasis. It has a number of disadvantages that until recently made it impractical to use as an out-patient therapy. It burns the skin, especially the clinically normal skin surrounding the psoriatic plaques, and it stains skin, clothing and bath fittings. It is usually unsuitable for use on the face, flexures or acutely inflamed psoriasis.

Ingram regimen. This is still the standard inpatient treatment regimen for psoriasis in most centres in the UK. Dithranol is applied in Lassar's paste, a stiff vehicle designed to prevent dithranol from spreading onto uninvolved skin, starting at a concentration of 0.1%, and increasing the strength every few days if no burning occurs, normally up to 2%. The paste is covered with stockinette tubular dressings, left on for 24 hours, then washed off in a bath with a coal tar additive. This is followed by treatment with UVB (short-wave ultraviolet light). Daily treatment will clear most psoriasis in 2–3 weeks.

Short-contact regimens. Since 1980, it has been known that sufficient dithranol penetrates the skin in 20–30 minutes to have a similar effect to 24-hour applications. When applied for a short time, higher concentrations can be used with less burning and staining, so that it is not so critical to keep the dithranol off normal skin. These factors have made it possible for some patients to use a cream formulation of dithranol at home, applied for 20–30 minutes per night, and then bathed or showered off. The starting concentration is usually 0.5%, increasing every 5 days, if tolerated, to 3%.

Coal tar. This has been used in numerous mixtures over the years, in combination with emollients, salicylic acid and topical steroids, but is less popular in most centres than once it was, as cleaner, less smelly treatments have become available. In addition, restrictions on manufacturing in hospital and community pharmacies have greatly reduced the number and variety of preparations available. Attempts to purify coal tar to make it more cosmetically acceptable have resulted in loss of potency. Coal tar compounds are now mostly used on guttate and scalp psoriasis, and localized pustular psoriasis of the palms and soles.

The efficacy of tar in psoriasis is enhanced when used with UVB; the tar may be used as a bath additive before irradiation.

There are theoretical risks of carcinogenesis from the long-term use of tar preparations, although these do not appear to be borne out in clinical practice, despite the long-established use of tar in dermatology. There is however, little published data on the subject.

Salicylic acid. This is useful to reduce scale, in preparation for other treatments, and can be mixed with dithranol (as in Lassar's paste), coal tar, emollients, steroids and shampoos.

Vitamin D analogues. Calcipotriol is a popular out-patient treatment for psoriasis, available as an ointment, cream or scalp lotion. It is colourless, odourless and does not stain. It is more effective than tar, but may be more irritant, and more effective than short-contact dithranol cream, with less staining and burning. It seems to have similar efficacy in psoriasis to 0.1% betamethasone ointment; it causes more irritation but no long-term skin atrophy. It should not be used on the face, where it may cause dermatitis. It does not cause hypercalcaemia provided that the weekly dose does not exceed 100 g. A newer vitamin D analogue, tacalcitol, is used for the once-daily treatment of chronic plaque psoriasis (Van de Kerkhof et al 1996) and is suitable for use on the face, as it is less irritant than calcipotriol.

The efficacy of topical vitamin D_3 analogues may be enhanced by combination with a topical steroid or with UVB.

Ultraviolet light (UVB). Many patients report that they are better in the summer or after a sunny holiday. Artificial UVB (wavelength 290–320 nm) is therefore used therapeutically, usually in combination with tar, and also in conjunction with short-contact dithranol in out-patient dressings units in some dermatology departments.

Recently, narrow-band UVB (wavelength 311–313 nm) has been introduced in a number of units, and appears to be more effective than conventional UVB, and possibly as effective as PUVA (see below); there may be fewer long-term side-effects. This is currently being evaluated.

Topical treatment of psoriasis at special sites.

Scalp. Mild scalp psoriasis may be controlled simply by using a tar shampoo regularly. More thickly scaled scalps may require overnight application to the hair roots of an ointment or cream containing salicylic acid; one of the most effective is based on coconut compound ointment. On the following day the scales are loosened with a toothcomb and then shampooed out with a coal tar shampoo, or suitable detergent. This regimen is messy but more effective than aqueous or alcoholic lotions, and usually more comfortable. It does, however, require considerable time and commitment from the patient or the family.

Nails. Once fungal infection of the nails has been excluded as the main differential diagnosis, there is little treatment that can be offered. Intralesional steroid injections into the nail bed and phototherapy have both been tried, with disappointing results. If the patient is on systemic therapy for psoriasis there may be some improvement in the nails. However, in most cases any improvement is most likely to be spontaneous.

Systemic therapy

Indications for the use of systemic therapy include severe and widespread psoriasis, failure or intolerance of topical treatment and rapid relapse of psoriasis after clearance.

PUVA. PUVA (Psoralen plus UVA) was developed to bridge the gap in therapy between traditional messy applications and toxic systemic drugs and it still has a valuable role in the treatment of moderate to severe chronic plaque psoriasis, despite increasing evidence of long-term side-effects. Psoralens are drugs that are activated by long-wave ultraviolet light (UVA, wavelength 320–400 nm) to interfere with DNA synthesis, and thus reduce epidermal cell turnover. Two psoralens are available for PUVA treatment in the UK, 8- and 5-methoxypsoralen; neither has a product licence, so patients are treated on a named-patient basis. The psoralen is either taken by mouth 2 hours before exposure to UVA, when the drug has reached maximum concentration in the skin, or applied topically, usually in a bath containing the drug immediately before exposure. The initial exposure time is calculated by previous light testing, and the time increased as tolerated by the patient as the course progresses; the treatment is normally given twice weekly until clearance or significant improvement is achieved, usually in about 6 weeks. This is accompanied by a tan. Unless the psoriasis is severe and relapsing maintenance therapy is avoided to minimize long-term side-effects. Further courses can be given

subsequently, if necessary, and total cumulative dosage of UVA carefully monitored (British Photodermatology Group 1994)

Adverse effects. PUVA should be avoided in pregnancy. Nausea is the commonest side-effect, and is worst on the day of treatment. Pruritus and drying of the skin are also frequent problems. Ageing of the skin and the development of melanoma and non-melanoma skin cancer are the major long-term risks; this depends on the skin type of the patient (fair, type 1 skins suffer most) and the total cumulative dose of UVA. Those on past or present immunosuppressant therapy are also at increased risk.

The eyes are always protected with suitable UVA-screening spectacles from the time of taking the tablet until 12 hours after UVA treatment, to avoid the possibility of developing cataracts.

In some units bath PUVA is preferred as this avoids the systemic side-effect of nausea and makes the wearing of sunglasses unnecessary.

Cytotoxic drugs. These drugs all have toxic effects on the bone marrow and the germ cells, and must be avoided in pregnancy. Their use should be supervised by a dermatologist.

Methotrexate. This folic acid antagonist is the most popular cytotoxic drug in use for severe psoriasis, including acute generalized pustular psoriasis, and is the most effective treatment for psoriatic arthritis. It is given in a once-weekly, low-dose regimen, usually orally but occasionally intramuscularly to avoid side-effects, following a test dose of 2.5 mg. The therapeutic dose is normally up to 30 mg weekly (Roenigk et al 1988).

Some patients complain of nausea and other gastrointestinal side-effects, together with fatigue and lassitude, for up to 48 hours after the weekly dose, but this may be eased with regular metoclopramide, and folic acid 5 mg per day on the non-methotrexate days can also be very helpful.

Acute toxic effects occur due to the effect on the folic acid metabolism of the rapidly dividing cells in the bone marrow and gastrointestinal tract, resulting in marrow suppression or gastrointestinal bleeding. They can be reversed by folinic acid rescue (120 mg of folinic acid over 12–24 hours intravenously or intramuscularly in divided doses, followed by 15 mg/kg orally every 6 hours for 48 hours) which opposes the folate antagonist effect of methotrexate. These adverse effects are more likely to occur in the elderly with poor renal function, so a creatinine clearance test should be performed before the start of treatment and the dose reduced if renal function is impaired. The full blood count should be monitored regularly.

Liver toxicity, producing a hepatitic pattern in the liver function tests, may occur and progress to fibrosis and cirrhosis in the long term unless the drug is reduced or stopped. Regular liver function tests are therefore performed, together with procollagen III levels, and a liver biopsy is recommended if there are sustained or significant abnormalities. Patients are strongly advised to abstain from drinking alcohol while they remain on the drug.

Several commonly used drugs interact with methotrexate (see Table 55.2), so a careful drug history is necessary, and the patient and the general practitioner should be warned of contraindicated medication.

Hydroxycarbamide (hydroxyurea). This drug has similar effects on the bone marrow and germ cells to methotrexate, but not the hepatic toxicity. It needs to be used continuously, as relapse occurs when the drug is stopped. Previous treatment with hydroxycarbamide (hydroxyurea) appears to increase the risks of development of skin cancer in patients receiving PUVA.

Immunosuppressant drugs.

Ciclosporin. This is an effective teatment for severe psoriasis in doses lower than those used to prevent rejection of transplanted organs; it is used in a range 2–5 mg/kg daily (Ellis et al 1991). Renal function and blood pressure are monitored regularly, and any rise in creatinine or blood pressure reversed by a reduction in dosage, or cessation of the drug. Relapse may occur when the drug is stopped, but intermittent therapy is preferred to maintenance, as this should reduce the long-term risks of skin cancers, lymphomas and solid tumours. Patients should also be warned to avoid overexposure to the sun, and should not receive concurrent PUVA or UVB therapy.

Systemic corticosteroids. These have little place in the treatment of psoriasis, except in the management of life-threatening erythroderma. In fact, systemic steroids, or their withdrawal, may provoke an acute generalized pustular psoriasis.

Acitretin.

This is a second-generation oral retinoid used in the treatment of severe resistant psoriasis, acute pustular psoriasis and palmoplantar psoriasis. It is available on hospital prescription only, due to its teratogenic effects and women of child-bearing age must use effective contraception during treatment and for 2 years after its cessation. It is probably better to find an alternative in this group of patients if at all possible. Acitretin enhances the action of PUVA and allows a reduction in UVA dosage while providing a protective effect against malignant change in the skin. This combination therapy is known as Re-PUVA. Acitretin may cause abnormalities in liver function tests and serum lipids, and these are monitored and adjustments in dosage or advice about a low-fat diet given. There may be effects on bone maturation, so acitretin is avoided if at all possible in children.

All patients develop dry skin, especially on the lips, as the most common adverse effect, and the mucous membranes of the eye and nose may also be affected. There may be considerable hair loss, but this and all the other side-effects are dose-related and reversible.

Photodynamic therapy.

This is a new treatment which involves the application of a photosensitizing drug, 5-aminolaevulininc acid (ALA), which causes a local accumulation of protoporphyrin IX. This compound is then activated by irradiation with visible light, and causes tissue destruction. Studies have shown this to be effective for localized plaque psoriasis (Boehncke et al 1994); side-effects seem to be confined to a burning sensation at the site of treatment.

Therapies for the future. Research for the future is targeted at immunotherapy for psoriasis; T cells, antigen-presenting cells, cytokines and adhesion molecules all appear to play important roles in the pathogenesis of psoriasis, and drugs for the future, either topical or systemic, will be designed either to suppress or block their actions. Tacrolimus and ascomycin appear at present to be promising.

Psoriasis is a chronic disease, which in its mild form is little more than a nuisance. In moderate and severe cases it may be distressing for the patient and socially unacceptable. The patient becomes very conscious of the appearance of the rash and the fact that it leaves a trail of silvery scales in its wake. This is probably at its worst when the patient undresses, causing a 'snowstorm' of scales, which increases the dusting and vacuuming required at home. When the joints are involved there is pain, often severe, and later deformity of the joints concerned. If the skin of the hands and feet is affected, fissuring and resultant infection and pain may make work impossible, either because of exacerbation by the friction of manual work or because of the health risks in catering, nursing or personal contact. In some cases the embarrassment is just too great for the sufferer to stay at work.

Psoriatics can be greatly helped by doctors, nurses, pharmacists and other health professionals. An explanation that the disease is inherited and not infectious is often helpful; although there is no cure the disease can be controlled so that the individual can lead a normal life. It may be reassuring to know that if things are out of control an admission to hospital or a course of daily treatment in an out-patient therapy unit may be available.

It must be emphasized that a responsibility lies with the patient to apply or take any treatment regularly to ensure maximum benefit, and to attend regularly for follow-up and monitoring in a clinic if the treatment is systemic. It may be helpful for those whose psoriasis tends to clear in the summer months to take advantage of any natural sunshine.

Information on the entitlement to benefits to replace clothing ruined by ointments or washing machines worn out by constant use is available, and the Psoriasis Association provides an excellent local service in this and many other ways, together with practical advice from fellow sufferers on day-to-day problems.

Figure 55.12 is a treatment flow chart for psoriasis.

Table 55.3 outlines some common therapeutic problems in the management of eczema and psoriasis.

CASE STUDIES

Case 55.1

A 3-year-old child was brought to the clinic with widespread, dry atopic eczema, from which she had suffered from the age of 6 months. She had always been a poor eater and restless sleeper due to the itch of her eczema, and had been treated repeatedly for bacterial infection of her skin. Her normal skin treatment was 1% hydrocortisone cream. Her parents had been advised to keep bathing to a minimum, because of the discomfort it caused. They were very keen to have tests performed, to identify the cause of the eczema, and to decide on a cure.

Question

What advice could be given to the child's parents?

Answer

Time should be spent explaining to the parents that eczema is a disease whose cause is not known, but which is likely to improve spontaneously through childhood, probably leaving the child with little more than dry skin by the teens. Skin tests will therefore not contribute to the management in childhood and

may cause discomfort which may frighten the child. It should be emphasized that the eczema will be controllable if a suitable regimen of regular treatment is developed. The emphasis is on bathing with plenty of emollient on the skin and in the water, which makes the process comfortable, with additional applications of emollient as necessary. A topical steroid ointment of moderate potency, with an antiseptic added if the eczema is infected, should control the eczema, and the potency can subsequently be reduced for maintenance. Systemic antibiotics may also help.

If this regimen does not produce a marked improvement in 2 weeks, a short admission to hospital or daily visits to a treatment unit may help both the child and the parents, who can be given advice and tuition in methods of topical treatment application and bandaging.

Case 55.2

A 17-year-old girl was referred to the clinic with a 6-month history of severe hand dermatitis. She had been a trainee hairdresser since leaving school, and the problems with her hands had started within a few months of commencing work. Her hands were now dry, fissured, painful and itchy, but improved when she had more than a week's holiday from work. As a child, she had mild atopic eczema and asthma, which had appeared to improve when she was about 8 years old.

Question

What is the cause of this girl's problems, and how can they be managed?

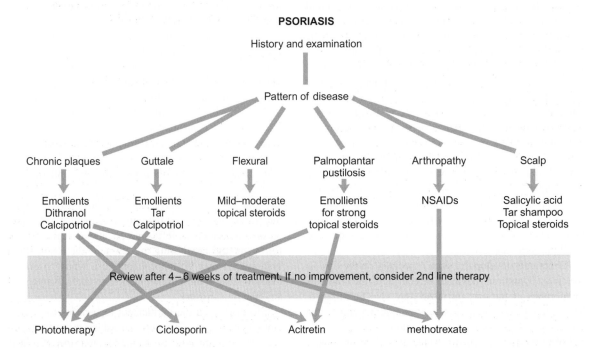

PSORIASIS

Figure 55.12 A treatment flow chart for psoriasis.

Table 55.3 Common therapeutic problems in eczema and psoriasis

Problem	Result
Topical treatments are frequently messy and sticky	Patients are reluctant to use them
Water-based creams contain preservatives and may cause stinging on inflamed skin	Children will resist their use, and become distressed at treatment time
Topical treatment is time-consuming for patients and their families/carers	Treatments may be missed
Methods of application and amount to use often not well explained	Treatment is inadequate
Patients or parents may be frightened by publicity about the side-effects of topical steriods	Treatment may be inadequate or non-existent
Dithranol stains skin, fabric and hardware a purple-brown colour	Bathrooms may be ruined if short-contact therapy is used carelessly
Emollients may not emulsify completely with water	Outflow from bath or shower may become blocked, and washing-machines damaged
Topical treatments are hard work and may take many weeks to show results	Patients become discouraged
Systemic therapies all have significant side-effects blood	Patients have to attend clinics regularly for monitoring of tests, blood pressure, etc.

Answer

This girl is an atopic, and should have been advised at an early stage that a career in hairdressing would be very risky in terms of development of dermatitis. She will be prone to both irritant and allergic contact dermatitis, which may be caused by water, shampoos and perming and colouring chemicals. She needs to be patch tested to try to determine the cause, although both types of reaction may be involved.

She should stop work, as this has been shown to improve her condition, and her hands should be treated intensively with emollients and barrier creams. Potent topical steroid ointment may be necessary until the dermatitis is under control, and thereafter emollients alone should continue.

Most important, she should be encouraged to change occupations to a clean, dry job where her hands will be at less risk from ongoing dermatitis. In future she will have to protect her hands from domestic chores with cotton-lined rubber gloves.

Case 55.3

A 32-year-old man with lifelong eczema is working under great pressure as a management executive, and his eczema has been deteriorating steadily over several months. He has used emollients and topical steroids in adequate quantities and has had several courses of oral antibiotics when the eczema appeared to be secondarily infected. None of this has had a sustained effect, and he cannot afford time off work to be admitted for in-patient treatment. His sleep is disturbed and tiredness is beginning to affect his daily activities.

Question

What are the options for treatment for this man?

Answer

This patient needs effective treatment before the eczema becomes erythrodermic. Systemic medication should bring the problem under control, and three might be considered: first, as a short course, high dose systemic steroids should have a rapid effect and can be tailed off over a week or two. If it is anticipated that a few weeks or months of treatment may be needed, since his stress is ongoing, ciclosporin would be a better choice as the side-effects can be monitored and detected at an early stage with blood pressure readings and blood tests. This treatment can be tailed off when the situation seems to be under control. If long-term systemic management is necessary, azathioprine might be considered; however, it takes much longer than the other two drugs to take effect, and it may be at least a month before any relief of symptoms is obvious, so treatment might initially be combined with prednisolone. In the long-term, however, azathioprine will not cause hypertension, renal impairment, obesity, osteoporosis or skin atrophy, and it can be monitored with simple blood tests.

A 55-year-old woman presents at the clinic with a history of chronic plaque psoriasis from the age of 16; she has never been clear of the disease in that time. She has had numerous topical treatments over the years, none of which has been particularly effective. She was markedly intolerant of dithranol. Over the previous 2 years she has gradually developed arthritis in her finger joints, with early signs of deformity. She has tried a number of pain-killers and non-steroidal anti-inflammatory drugs (NSAIDs) but these have not relieved her pain and stiffness.

Question

What would be the best treatment for this patient's problems?

Answer

Providing that there are no contraindications, methotrexate would be the most suitable single treatment to control this lady's psoriasis of both the skin and joints. She should be advised to stop her NSAIDs and to take paracetamol as a short-term alternative, and to avoid alcohol. If her blood count and liver function tests are normal 1 week after a 2.5 mg test dose of methotrexate, a weekly dose of 10 mg can be given, with further weekly monitoring of the blood tests initially. The dose can be adjusted every 2–3 weeks until improvement occurs. The skin should show clearance over about 6–12 weeks, but the joints may take longer to respond. Once this has happened, the lowest dose that controls symptoms can be continued as maintenance, with 3-monthly blood tests.

A 24-year-old man presents at the clinic with a 10-year history of plaque psoriasis affecting his elbows, knees and sacral area, with a few small plaques elsewhere. He is otherwise fit and well, but embarrassed by the appearance of his skin when he plays football, as he does regularly. He has tried Betnovate RD ointment (0.025%), which smoothed the plaques a little, and calcipotriol ointment, which removed the scale from the plaques but did not clear them.

Question

What treatment could this patient try next?

Answer

With relatively few plaques to treat, this patient might respond very well to short-contact dithranol creams. These can be started at a concentration of 0.5% in most patients, which can be increased to 1%, 2%, and 3%, every 5–7 days, depending on how well the skin tolerates the treatment. The effect can be enhanced by UVB therapy twice weekly in a dermatology department for up to 8 weeks. The usual staining and burning with dithranol is minimized by short-contact therapy, and any dicolouration fades quickly after the treatment is stopped.

A 45-year-old man has become increasingly disabled with palmoplantar pustular psoriasis; he has frequent crops of inflamed pustules on the palms and soles, which dry up to form crusts and scaling followed by painful fissuring of the skin. This has made his job as a joiner increasingly difficult and he has had prolonged periods of sick-leave; he is afraid that he could be made redundant. He has tried emollients, topical steroid applications and tar and steroid combinations, with only temporary relief.

Question

What are this patient's options for treatment?

Answer

This can be a chronic and very disabling condition for manual workers, and this patient may benefit from systemic therapy.

Oral acitretin works very well in this condition and can be given intermittently or long-term if the patient's fasting lipids and liver function tests remain normal. A rise in lipids may be controlled by diet or medication or reversed by stopping the drug. The major side-effect of retinoids is dry skin, so regular emollient treatment will have to continue.

If there are contraindications to acitretin, an effective alternative is hand and foot PUVA. This involves either applying psoralen paint to palms and soles or taking oral psoralens and then having UVA irradiation, of hands and feet only, twice weekly. The disadvantages are having to wear UVA-screening glasses after oral psoralen on the day of treatment and having to attend hospital regularly, but long-term side-effects on the relatively thick skin of hands and feet seem to be fewer than on thinner skin elsewhere. The major advantage to the patient of both treatments is that he should be able to continue working, using simple emollients only on the skin.

REFERENCES

Boehncke W H, Sterry W, Kaufmann R 1994 Treatment of psoriasis by topical photodynamic therapy with polychromatic light. Lancet 343: 801

British Photodermatology Group 1994 British Photodermatology Group guidelines for PUVA. British Journal of Dermatology 130: 246–255

Camp R D R, Reitamo S, Friedmann P S et al 1993 Cyclosporin A in severe, therapy-resistant atopic dermatitis: report of an international workshop, April 1993. British Journal of Dermatology 129: 217–220

Charman C R 2000 Atopic eczema. Clinical Evidence 3: 797–808

Ellis CN, Fradin M S, Messana J M et al 1991 Cyclosporine for plaque-type psoriasis: results of a multi-dose, double-blind trial. New England Journal of Medicine 324: 277–284

Fung A Y, Look P C et al 1999 A controlled trial of traditional Chinese herbal medicine in Chinese patients with recalcitrant atopic dermatitis. International Journal of Dermatology 38: 387–392.

Kay J, Gawkrodger D J, Mortimer M J et al 1994 The prevalence of childhood eczema in a general population. Journal of the American Academy of Dermatology 30: 35–39

Krutmann J 2000 Phototherapy for atopic dermatitis. British Journal of Dermatology 25: 553–557

Munn S 1999 Use of g-linolenic acid in atopic dermatitis. CME Bulletin of Dermatology 2: 20–22

Roenigk H H Jr, Auerbach R, Maibach H I et al 1988 Methotrexate in psoriasis; revised guidelines. Journal of the American Academy of Dermatology 19: 145–156

Ruzicka T, Bieber T, Schopf E et al 1997 A short-term trial of tacrolimus ointment for atopic dermatitis. European Tacrolimus Multicenter Atopic Dermatitis Study Group. New England Journal of Medicine 337(12): 816–821

Sheehan M P, Atherton D J 1994 One year follow-up of children treated with Chinese medicinal herbs for atopic eczema. British Journal of Dermatology 140: 488–493

Van de Kerkhof P C, Werfel T, Haustein U F et al 1996 Tacalcitol ointment in the treatment of psoriasis vulgaris: a multicentre, placebo-controlled, double-blind study on efficacy and safety. British Journal of Dermatology 135: 758–765

Van Leent E J, Graber M, Thurston M et al 1998 Effectiveness of the ascomycin macrolactam SDZ ASM 981 in the topical treatment of atopic dermatitis. Archives of Dermatology 134(7): 805–809

FURTHER READING

Anon 1994 Immunosuppressive drugs and their complications. Drugs and Therapeutics Bulletin 32: 66–70

Clinical Dermatology Review Series 2000 Atopic dermatitis. Clinical and Experimental Dermatology 25: 522–574

CME Bulletin of Dermatology 1999 2: 4–28

Symposium on Psoriasis 1998 Hospital Medicine 59: 530–542

Williams H C (ed) 2000 Atopic dermatitis. Cambridge University Press, Cambridge

Pressure sores and leg ulcers

56

R. Anderson

Pressure sores

A pressure sore may be defined as any break in skin integrity that results from sustained pressure on the body, with or without the additional stresses of shear and friction. Other patient-specific factors may contribute to skin damage and affect healing ability. The terms 'bed sore' and 'decubitus ulcer' have been used, but these imply that damage can only occur when lying down, whereas the sitting position can equally produce ulceration. The term 'pressure ulcer' is preferable as without pressure the condition cannot develop and, although often sore to the patient with intact sensation, in those with neurological impairment there is no associated soreness.

Epidemiology

Pressure damage occurs in patients whether they are cared for in hospital or the community, and is a distressing and expensive problem to manage. Studies of prevalence have revealed that 5–32% of patients may suffer from pressure ulcers at any one time depending on the patient population studied. Few community-based prevalence studies have been done but a prevalence of 4–7% has been reported. Incidence studies in hospitals show ranges from 2% in 12 months to 66% over 18 months (elderly with hip fractures).

Prevalence in hospice settings from 21% to 37% have been reported, and one community study has shown a 20% incidence over 6 weeks.

Aetiology

Various factors play a role in the development of pressure ulcers.

Pressure

Excess pressure on the skin results in the ischaemia of underlying tissue by mechanical compression of the vascular supply. The critical factor is when pressure on the skin exceeds the average arteriolar pressure (25 mmHg).

Sustained pressure on tissues is most damaging. Low pressure applied for long periods is worse than high pressure for short periods, and some alternating pressure beds work on a high-pressure/short-time cycle principle. Portable equipment is available to measure pressure beneath patients so that the most suitable support equipment (mattress, cushion or chair) can be chosen. However, this approach is not in widespread use.

Shear

All shearing forces will also involve some pressure, but shear caused by patients sliding down beds or chairs will damage the superficial skin layers with resultant stretching of blood vessels, possible thrombosis and damage to the dermis.

Friction

Friction between skin and sheets or seating may cause ulceration by mechanically rubbing off outer layers of skin. Soft and uncreased linen, towels and dressings should be used. Massage and vigorous application of skin preparations should be avoided.

Moisture

In the presence of moisture (due to urine, sweat or faeces), pressure ulcer formation is more likely as skin becomes macerated and traumatized. The excessive use of barrier creams may over-moisten skin and exacerbate the problem.

Combined forces

If shear and friction are applied together, the tissues attached to bony structures move under shear while the epidermal layers may move in the opposite direction due to friction between the skin and supporting surfaces.

The effect of the three combined forces of shear, friction and pressure can result in ulcer formation at lower pressures than would be normally anticipated.

Patient-specific factors and risk assessment

Various concurrent problems may precipitate the development of pressure ulcers; these are summarized in Table 56.1. Pressure ulcers may occur at any age, including childhood, particularly when patient mobility and activity is reduced. It is therefore important that all patients with any of the risk factors shown are assessed for pressure ulcer risk on admission to hospital, and regularly reviewed.

Similarly, chronically ill patients in the community must be monitored.

The Royal College of Nursing (RCN) has produced guidelines on pressure ulcer risk assessment and prevention which have been 'inherited' and published by the National Institute for Clinical Excellence (NICE 2001).

Various risk rating scales are available but these must be used in conjunction with clinical judgement and the scale in use should have been tested for relevance to the population under care. Reliability of scales and respective sensitivities have been investigated to varying degrees. Aspects for consideration within the various scales may include: physical condition; mental condition; activity; mobility; incontinence; nutrition; predisposing diseases; age; and concurrent medication.

Common sites of occurrence

Although any area of the body subjected to unrelieved pressure may ulcerate, certain sites are more susceptible to damage. The five 'classical' locations for pressure ulcers are:

- sacrum
- buttocks (ischial tuberosity)
- hips (greater trochanter)
- heel
- lateral malleolus of foot.

The significance of position in relation to the site of ulceration is shown in Table 56.2.

Pressure ulcers can occur in less common locations that also depend on the position of the patient and include the ear, scalp, elbows and genitalia. In infants and young children pressure injury is more likely on the occipital scalp than the sacrum (Willock et al 2000).

Often the risk to patients who spend most of their time sitting out of bed is not recognized, and regular standing is not encouraged. In contrast, patients nursed in bed are regularly turned to assist in pressure relief.

Table 56.1 Risk factors that may play a role in the development of pressure ulcers

Increasing age
Reduced mobility and activity at any age
Poor nutrition, especially if linked with severe anaemia
Diabetes
Obesity
Cardiac failure
Osteomyelitis
Orthopaedic problems
Drug addiction
Malignancy/cytotoxic therapy
Neurological disorders

Table 56.2. Relationship between position of patient and area at risk of developing a pressure ulcer

Position of patient	Risk areas
Supine	Scapula Sacrum Heels
Prone	Chest Patellae Anterior surface of tibia
Sidelying	Femoral trochanters Malleoli
Sitting	Ischial tuberosities Sacrum Femoral trochanters (posterior surface)

Paraplegics who spend considerable time in wheelchairs should be regularly checked and provided with additional supporting surfaces, such as special cushions, as appropriate. Ring cushions are not appropriate.

Care on transferring patients from bed to chair and on manoeuvring them in bed is vital. Some of the newer pressure-relieving beds reduce the need for such procedures.

Signs of pressure damage

Various warning signs on the skin should immediately indicate the need for additional precautions:

- After sustained pressure, the skin initially turns red due in part to histamine release. This redness is termed blanching erythema, and if gently pressed it will whiten (or blanch). If pressure is relieved at this stage, the skin should return to normal.
- If pressure continues, progression to non-blanching erythema will result. In this situation when the affected area is pressed it will remain red, indicating that a pressure ulcer is developing.
- The next clinical sign is likely to be blistering, which, with sustained pressure, will progress from a soft fluid-filled area to an area of hard, black necrotic tissue, termed an eschar. An eschar may begin to break down and putrify, with formation of a strong odour, usually due to the presence of anaerobic bacteria.

In areas where skin is thin and bony prominences are superficial there may be no warning signs, and progressive damage and full skin thickness necrosis may be the first sign, with underlying bone and muscle exposed to view.

In either case, the necrotic tissue will need to be removed (debrided), and a deep cavity will then exist.

Large volumes of exudate may be produced, particularly if infection is present.

Within deep cavities there may be sinus formation, i.e. narrow tracks may form, which lead into deeper tissue. In such cavities, careful selection of treatment is required to avoid damage to underlying tissue. In patients who have suffered with chronic pressure ulcers, long-standing sinuses may exist, visible on the surface of the skin as only a narrow, often leaking, opening. Normally this is an indication of an unhealed cavity below in which there is risk of abscess formation and chronic infection.

A national grading tool for pressure ulcers is required to achieve standardization in assessment. Pressure ulcers are variously graded from I to IV or V and numerous grading systems have been published in the UK (Harker 2000).

Investigations

If a sinus exists, it is important to establish the extent of the tracking within the body tissue, and this can only be achieved by radiological investigation (a sinogram). The sinogram may indicate the need for surgical intervention to open up the area, drain and treat it as appropriate.

Chronic wounds should be biopsied, especially if the appearance is abnormal, since it is not uncommon for malignancy to develop in non-healing wounds. Such wounds may have a cauliflower-like appearance, suggestive of squamous cell carcinoma, and may bleed very readily. This should not be confused with the phenomenon of over-granulation when excess granulation tissue sometimes develops beneath occlusive dressings.

Treatment

If preventative methods fail, urgent treatment of pressure ulcers is essential. Unfortunately there is little evidence from randomized controlled trials to support current management and treatment.

There is, however, a wealth of evidence to demonstrate the dangers of excessive pressure. Any mechanism which can reduce pressure as well as shear and friction should be considered. Realistic objectives should be established as some pressure ulcers will never heal but may be made more acceptable for patients and their carers.

Deep, infected pressure ulcers carry a high risk of morbidity due to septicaemia. Treatment priorities must be considered, based on the degree of pressure damage and the need for surgical or other intervention with regard to overall prognosis and predisposing factors in the patient. Pressure ulcers on heels can impede rehabilitation by severely restricting mobility. A multidisciplinary approach to treatment will consider all aspects of care and will involve:

- A dietitian, to ensure optimum nutrition for patients with pressure damage, and those at risk.
- A doctor, to assess overall prognosis and patient management.
- A nurse, to regularly reassess patients and their pressure points and to establish a turning/moving routine, regular dressing changes and the provision of moral support to patients and carers. (A variety of risk assessment systems are available but most have been developed with a specific population and cannot be assumed to be applicable to the general population, for example the Norton score for the elderly.)
- A pharmacist, to assist in appropriate product selection and to ensure that staff are familiar with its use and the product is readily available in adequate quantity.
- A physiotherapist, to improve and encourage patient mobility.
- An occupational therapist, to select the most appropriate support, for example bed, chair, mattress or cushion.

Numerous pieces of equipment are promoted for the prevention of pressure ulcers, including fluidized beds and specialized cushions. Unfortunately little evaluative information is available but manufacturers should be able to provide information on minimum and maximum pressures achieved with their own products.

Physiotherapists may treat pressure ulcers with ultraviolet or ultrasound therapy, often in conjuction with topical preparations. This approach should, however, be avoided if the enzyme debriding agent Varidase, containing streptokinase and streptodornase, which are easily inactivated, is being used. The frequency of removal of the topical application will affect the practicality of using combination therapy.

Ultrasound may be performed with dressings in situ, while ultraviolet therapy requires removal of the dressing.

A wound care or tissue viability nurse often coordinates the multidisciplinary team, emphasizes the need for pressure ulcer prevention and coordinates the availability of preventative equipment for hospital and community patients.

Wound management

The holistic approach is essential in pressure ulcer care. Topical applications are only part of treatment, and often surgical intervention will speed healing. No single product is normally suitable for all stages of ulceration. As the ulcer changes, so should the product. However, a fair trial of treatment is essential with accurate documentation to ensure continuity of care.

Clinical infection. Before commencing treatment, any clinical infection should be identified. All wounds will show bacterial growth if swabbed, but this is only significant if present in sufficient numbers to produce clinical infection. When assessing a wound it is necessary to consider whether:

- there is pus formation
- the patient is pyrexial and feeling unwell
- there is surrounding cellulitis (i.e. inflammation of the surrounding skin and tissues with associated heat)
- there is likely to be infection involving bone.

If any of these factors are present, a swab should be taken from the deep part of the wound and appropriate systemic antibiotics commenced. If none of the above factors are present and the wound is progressing well, there is no need for further investigation.

Treatment selection. There are numerous products available for wound care, pressure ulcers and skin trauma. The ideal dressing should:

- create an optimum moist environment for healing
- remove excess exudate from the wound surface
- provide a barrier to microorganisms
- be sterile
- be non-adherent and easily removed
- be free of particulate contamination
- be non-toxic, non-allergenic and non-sensitizing
- be thermally insulating
- allow gaseous exchange
- be easy to use for patients and carers
- be cost-effective
- be available in all necessary sizes for hospital and community use.

Products such as lint, gauze and gamgee do not possess the necessary properties for a dressing because they have limited absorbency and rapidly become saturated with wound exudate which can 'strike through' to the dressing surface and enable bacteria to track down into the wound. As the dressing dries out it will adhere to the wound surface, cause pain and bleeding on removal, and lift newly formed cells from the surface of the wound.

By considering the different groups of wound products available a protocol for pressure ulcer care can be devised, based on the different stages of ulceration and the characteristics of available products. The position of the pressure ulcer will also be relevant to the choice of preparation and the secondary (covering) dressing if needed. Table 56.3 summarizes the possible treatments for pressure ulcers classified as superficial break, partial/full thickness breaks, cavity/sinus, and dependent on the appearance of the ulcer in relation to exudate, slough, odour, etc.

When determining optimum treatment it is necessary to consider the following questions:

- Is the wound clean?
- Is there excessive exudate?

Table 56.3 Management options for different stages of pressure ulcer. Alternative options are shown. Avoid combined use of products as this is expensive and may affect efficacy of individual components

Type of wound	A Epithelializing	B Granulating	C (i) Exuding (light to medium)	C (ii) Exuding (moderate to high)	D Necrotic (dry[a]/moist)	E Sloughy	F Malodorous
Superficial break	Non-adherent dressing	Non-adherent dressing or thin hydrocolloid	Polyurethane foam or hydrocolloid or alginate	Polyurethane foam, alginate or silicone dressing[b]	Hydrocolloid or hydrogel	Hydrocolloid or hydogel	Charcoal dressing or metronidazole gel[c]
Partial/full thickness		Hydrocolloid	Polyurethane foam or hydrocolloid or alginate	Polyurethane foam alginate or silicone, dressing[b]	Hydrocolloid or hydrogel	Hydrocolloid or hydrogel or fibrous hydrocolloid[d]	Charcoal dressing or metronidazole gel[c]
Cavity/sinus (Only loose packing recommended for sinuses, with careful removal) A sinogram will identify any tracking		Hydrogel	Alginate ribbon or hydrogel	Alginate ribbon or silicone dressing[b]	Hydrogel or fibrous hydrocolloid[d]	Hydrogel or fibrous hydrocolloid[d]	Charcoal dressing or metronidazole gel[c]

[a] For dry necrotic areas, a fibrous hydrocolloid is inappropriate.

[b] Mepitel, a silicone dressing, can remain in place for up to 14 days with only an outer absorbent dressing being changed as necessary. Education of users and carers is crucial to cost-effective use of this dressing.

[c] Oral metronidazole should be considered before topical gel for eradication of odour-producing anaerobes, but may be poorly tolerated and the alcohol restriction may be inappropriate. This is less of a problem with the topical gel.

[d] Aquacel, a modified fibrous hydrocolloid, can remain in place for up to 7 days and is suitable for exuding sloughy/necrotic wounds.

N.B. If clinical infection is present, appropriate systemic antibiotics will be required. Do not confuse with wound colonization. Do not swab the wound unless clinical signs of infection are present.

- Is sloughy tissue present?
- Is the wound clinically infected?
- Is the wound malodorous?

Many traditional 'cleansing' agents such as hypochlorite solutions and hydrogen peroxide are now recognized as having harmful effects. Cleaning is needed only if excessive exudate or pus and loose necrotic or sloughy tissue is present. In such cases, warmed sodium chloride solution (0.9%) should be used. Cold solutions can lower the wound surface temperature below body temperature and impair healing by retarding new cell formation.

Methicillin resistant *Staphylococcus aureus* (MRSA). If methicillin-resistant *Staphylococcus aureus* (MRSA) is identified in the wound, special precautions are neeed in the hospital and nursing home situation. Local guidelines should be available, as although this can be grown from wounds which are apparently healing normally, cross-infection to other patients is a risk and some could develop fatal clinical infections. Various options have been tried to both aid healing and reduce cross-infection risks (Young 1996).

Sterile maggots have eradicated MRSA from individual wounds.

Odorous wounds. Although pseudomonal infections can cause odour, the most likely cause is anaerobic bacteria. Charcoal dressings will mask and absorb odour if changed before the charcoal layer is saturated. However, the preferred approach is eradication of the odour-producing anaerobes using metronidazole. This is given orally 200–400 mg three times a day. If poorly tolerated, or if the alcohol restriction is impractical, it can be applied topically as a gel. The alcohol interaction potential will then be reduced.

There are licensing, strength and cost differences between gel products. Those for acne rosacea cost considerably more than those licensed for malodorous wounds, ulcers and tumours. Brand prescribing is therefore recommended for these products. The resolution of the odour is normally dramatic and is reassuring for the patient. Prolonged use may lead to emergence of resistant anaerobes although this is a slower process than with aerobic organisms.

Debridement of the ulcer. Surgical debridement is preferred but is not always practical or available for community patients. Guidance (NICE 2001b) recommends selection of the most cost-effective product. The bio-surgical approach, using sterile maggots of the green bottle fly, is now used in early management by some practitioners. Sharp debridement is a technique practised more widely by nurses in the USA and may increase in the UK if adequate training is made available (Vowden & Vowden 1999). When chemical or bio-surgical approaches are used, including for example the streptokinase-streptodornase product Varidase, and the povidone-iodine containing products Iodoflex and Iodosorb, review dates should be set to assess effectiveness and avoid prolonged use. Re-constitution and application of Varidase requires great care to avoid early inactivation. Excessive use of iodine or povidone-iodine containing products should be avoided, particularly in anyone with a history of thyroid disorder.

Characteristics of interactive wound management products.

Hydrocolloids. Hydrocolloids (e.g. Comfeel and Granuflex) are available as self-adhesive sheets, although if used on the sacrum and buttocks they may need to be taped in place, even if the specially shaped sacral dressings are used. All hydrocolloids contain carboxymethylcellulose and some additionally incorporate pectin and gelatin, the latter being responsible for an unpleasant odour noticeable at dressing changes in the absence of clinical infection.

The dressing liquefies at the wound surface, hydrating soft sloughy tissue and encouraging wound healing. In wounds with low exudate, hydrocolloids may remain in place for 7 days, and, if left in place on a black eschar, marked softening of the necrotic tissue will occur.

Different degrees of gaseous permeability are claimed for the various available products but on initial application most are occlusive and caution should be observed in the presence of anaerobic infection.

Due to this occlusive property, overproduction of granulation tissue may occur beneath hydrocolloids and indicates their use should be discontinued. The excess granulation tissue may be reduced by compression bandaging if appropriate or by use of a particular polyurethane foam dressing, Lyofoam. An alternative is the application of 0.25% silver nitrate solution daily for 5–7 days. Thereafter, epithelialization should be encouraged with an alternative category of dressing appropriate to the wound type.

Modified hydrocolloids (e.g. CombiDERM, Aquacel). These are suitable for medium to heavily exudating wounds and may remain in place for up to 7 days but intially may need more frequent changes. CombiDERM's central wound contact pad contains exudate-retaining polyacrylate granules, while Aquacel is composed of hydrocolloid fibres, sodium carboxymethylcellulose, but no gelatin and hence no odour.

Hydrogels. Hydrogels (e.g. Intrasite, GranuGel) require a secondary covering dressing. Gel formulations are particularly useful for cavity pressure ulcers. These products are composed of a hydrophilic polymer in an aqueous base and serve to hydrate the wound surface and lift slough and necrotic tissue while encouraging moist wound healing. Initially, the gel is normally changed daily, extending to every 3 days in cleaner wounds. Hydrogel-hydrocolloid (e.g. GranuGel) and hydrogel-alginate (e.g. SeaSorb) formulations can stay in place for longer. Hydrogels may be used on black eschars after scoring of the eschar to assist penetration but tend to be rather more rapidly effective on wounds covered with softer necrotic or sloughy tissue. They are inappropriate for heavily exuding wounds. If excessive amounts of gel are applied to an ulcer, maceration will occur at the wound edge with whitening of the surrounding skin.

Alginates. Alginates (e.g. Kaltostat and Sorbsan) are available in a flat or rope form. Most require a secondary dressing but some newer forms incorporate an adhesive border to aid retention on lightly exuding wounds.

The available dressings consist of either calcium alginate alone or a combination of sodium and calcium alginate and the difference in composition is thought to affect the gelling properties of the dressings at the wound surface. In contact with wound exudate the dressing is very absorbent and forms a moist gel over the wound surface. This forms better if the dressing can remain in place for 48 hours.

Alginates are therefore only suitable for exuding wounds, not for dry wounds or eschars where no gelling will occur. In a heavily exuding wound, daily changes may be needed initially but these can be reduced as the exudate lessens, when an alternative dressing may then be considered. The haemostatic properties of some of these dressings may be useful in controlling bleeding on over-granulating pressure ulcers, when daily changes would be needed. Depending on the gelling properties, the dressings are removed from the wound with sterile saline or lifted off with forceps.

Polyurethane foams. Polyurethane foam dressings (e.g. Allevyn and Lyofoam) are not all self-adhesive and some must be held in place with tape. This may be inappropriate on fragile skin, as may be some of the strongly self-adhesive foams. The main characteristic of the foams is high absorbency, making them suitable for exuding wounds. Due to the nature of the dressing, lateral absorption of exudate occurs, avoiding the vertical 'strike through' of traditional dressings. The dressing is initially changed daily. Inspection will reveal if this is inadequate because seepage of exudate will be seen at the edges of the dressing. In wounds producing less exudate, some of the dressings may remain in place for up to 7 days, encouraging healing in a moist environment. The dressings show low adherence but saline may be needed to assist removal.

Cavity dressings. Many of these products are now available, mainly in ribbon form for loose packing into deeper ulcers. Although most are alginates, Allevyn cavity wound dressing consists of small pieces of polyurethane foam dressing encased in a semipermeable membrane produced in various shapes. It is designed for exuding cavities but its usefulness will depend on size and shape of the ulcer and the 'fit' of the dressing.

Film dressings. Film dressings (e.g. OpSite and Cutifilm) are self-adhesive and are inappropriate for use on elderly fragile skin, which can easily be damaged by incorrect application and removal. The films are semipermeable, allowing evaporation of some water vapour, but exudate accumulates beneath and may irritate and macerate the surrounding skin. They are widely used to reduce friction over pressure points in 'at risk' patients when they may be left in place for several days. Careful attention must be paid to the manufacturer's instructions for application and removal of each different film dressing to avoid inflicting skin damage.

Soft silicone wound contact dressings. These products (e.g. Mepitel) can remain in place for up to 7 days and often longer, simply changing the outer dressing which can be of the perforated absorbent type (e.g. Mepore) placed over the silicone gel 'net' of Mepitel. These products are of specific use in blistering skin conditions where non-adhesion is critical but also have a place in exuding pressure sores and in some exuding leg ulcers where compression bandaging may be inappropriate and where infrequent dressing changes are desirable if possible.

Table 56.4 lists some of the common therapeutic problems encountered in the management of pressure

Table 56.4 Common therapeutic problems in pressure ulcers
Inconsistencies between risk assessment schemes used in different settings
Failure to reassess risk as patient's condition changes
Limited availability of preventative equipment and assessments of suitability
Use of the same wound management product for too long with infrequent reviews
Combined use of interactive wound management products
Limited use of portable documentation
Inappropriate use of interactive products, e.g. on non-healing heavily exuding ulcers needing daily changes

ulcers. Figure 56.1 summarizes key steps in the prevention and management of pressure ulcers.

Leg ulcers

A leg ulcer is any break in skin integrity on the lower leg, and normally indicates an underlying circulatory disorder or specific medical condition, even if reported as being initiated by trauma. Many leg ulcers are chronic in nature, with some patients having suffered for 30–40 years. Treatment must be directed at the underlying cause rather than simply the break in the skin.

Epidemiology

It has been estimated that 1% of the population have chronic leg ulcers, with 70% of patients developing the leg ulcer before the age of 65 years, and 25% before the age of 45 years.

Over the age of 50 years, women are more commonly affected. Approximately 75% of healed ulcers may eventually recur. Most leg ulcer patients are managed in the community and the cost has been estimated at between £2700 and £5200 per patient per year. The most recent estimation of annual cost to the UK National Health Service is £300–600 million. With the advent of more specialist leg ulcer treatment clinics and clinical specialists, and with accurate diagnosis and assessment, it may be possible to reduce overall costs and healing times.

Aetiology

There are a number of different types of leg ulcer, which can be classified according to the underlying causation; they include venous, arterial, arteriovenous, diabetic and autoimmune ulcers.

Venous ulcers

Venous ulcers are the most common, accounting for up to 75% of all leg ulcers. They occur as a result of failure of the calf muscle pump, i.e. the calf muscles which squeeze deep venous blood upwards from the legs back to the heart. This pump will not function effectively if there is a back-flow of blood from the deep veins to the superficial veins in the leg. Back-flow may occur due to fatigue or incompetence of the valves in the deep veins and in the perforating veins which connect the superficial and deep veins (as illustrated in Fig. 56.2A).

Restricted mobility may also predispose to venous ulceration. During walking, the action of the foot striking a solid surface facilitates venous return while the

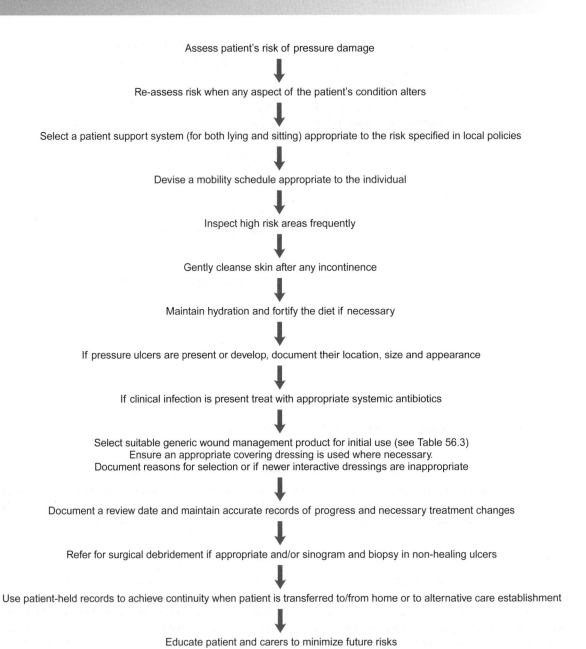

Assess patient's risk of pressure damage

Re-assess risk when any aspect of the patient's condition alters

Select a patient support system (for both lying and sitting) appropriate to the risk specified in local policies

Devise a mobility schedule appropriate to the individual

Inspect high risk areas frequently

Gently cleanse skin after any incontinence

Maintain hydration and fortify the diet if necessary

If pressure ulcers are present or develop, document their location, size and appearance

If clinical infection is present treat with appropriate systemic antibiotics

Select suitable generic wound management product for initial use (see Table 56.3)
Ensure an appropriate covering dressing is used where necessary.
Document reasons for selection or if newer interactive dressings are inappropriate

Document a review date and maintain accurate records of progress and necessary treatment changes

Refer for surgical debridement if appropriate and/or sinogram and biopsy in non-healing ulcers

Use patient-held records to achieve continuity when patient is transferred to/from home or to alternative care establishment

Educate patient and carers to minimize future risks

Figure 56.1 Key steps in pressure ulcer prevention and management.

ankle movement involved in normal walking alternately contracts and relaxes the calf muscle.

As back-flow of blood occurs into the superficial veins and capillaries, leakage of fluid occurs into the interstitial space and oedema results. Haemosiderin from red cell breakdown is deposited in the tissues causing a characteristic brown coloration, particularly in the gaiter or lower area of the leg. Fibrinogen leaks from capillaries and is converted to fibrin, forming a fibrin 'cuff' around the capillaries which may also reduce tissue oxygenation. In the affected area the skin becomes friable as oedema progresses and any slight trauma can precipitate ulceration.

The original cause of perforator valve incompetence may be a deep vein thrombosis which could have occurred many years previously. In elderly women this can often be traced back to a pregnancy.

Patients with valve incompetencies may have a history of varicose veins and approximately 3% of patients with varicosities go on to suffer leg ulcers.

Clinical practice guidelines (RCN 1998) have reviewed available evidence in this area of care and

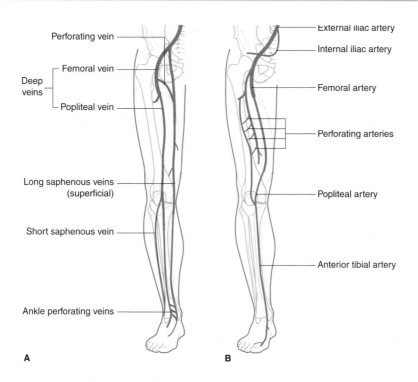

Figure 56.2 **A** Venous circulation – lower limb. **B** Arterial circulation – lower limb.

helped standardize management of patients with venous ulcers and distinguish this from the approaches needed in treating patients with ulcers of differing aetiology.

Arterial ulcers

Figure 56.2B illustrates the arterial circulation. Arterial ulcers arise in a different manner from venous ulcers. Blood fails to reach the superficial tissues as a result of atherosclerosis affecting the medium and large arteries of the lower leg. Oxygen supply to the arterioles is therefore inadequate and breakdown of skin results in a painful ulcer. Arterial ulcers account for approximately 22% of leg ulcers.

An arterial embolism will similarly produce ulceration but in a more rapid and dangerous manner.

Arteriovenous ulcers

Lower leg ulcers may result from a combination of both venous and arterial incompetence and a mixed picture of clinical signs will be seen.

Diabetic leg ulcers

Diabetes is associated with approximately 5% of all leg ulcers. The ulcers of such patients are ischaemic in nature as a result of diabetic vascular disease which affects the small distal arteries, particularly in the weight-bearing areas such as the feet.

Autoimmune leg ulcers

The most common causative factor in this category is rheumatoid arthritis which is present in 8% of patients with leg ulcers. Although associated immobility will limit calf muscle pump activity, the ulceration primarily occurs through arteritis of the small vessels and consequent ischaemia.

Other leg ulcers

Several other conditions may be associated with leg ulcer formation in patients, including burns, infections, haematological disease, lymphoedema and vasculitis. Malignancy can develop in chronic non-healing ulcers or the ulcer may begin as a malignant manifestation. As with chronic pressure ulcers and other non-healing skin problems, biopsy is recommended for long-standing leg ulcers (RCN 1998).

It should be noted that ulcers may be self-inflicted, or an existing ulcer may be further damaged by the patient to maintain contact with health care staff (the 'social ulcer phenomenon').

Clinical signs

In determining the cause of a leg ulcer, observation of clinical signs is important, together with an accurate history from the patient or carer. The characteristic clinical features of venous and arterial ulcers are shown in Table 56.5. Diabetic ulcers often look similar to arterial ulcers. However, in the diabetic ulcer foot pulses may be present if only the microcirculation is damaged while if the deeper arterial system is damaged, as in arterial ulcers, these pulses are absent. The patient with a diabetic ulcer does not always complain of pain, due to loss of sensation resulting from diabetes-induced peripheral neuropathy.

Diagnostic investigation

Before treatment is started, the extent of venous and arterial damage should be determined by use of a portable Doppler machine. This permits calculation of the patient's ankle brachial pressure index (ABPI) by comparing brachial and ankle systolic pressures:

$$ABPI = \frac{\text{systolic blood pressure in the ankle}}{\text{systolic blood pressure in the arm}}$$

The ABPI index should be greater than 1 in people with undamaged arteries.

If compression bandaging is applied to the leg of patients with an ABPI below 0.8, the arterial circulation will be compromised, tissue necrosis may result and amputation could be required (Callam et al 1987). Light compression may be used in patients with an ABPI of between 0.8 and 0.9 and some specialist centres have used this in patients with lower ABPIs (Stevens et al 1997). Erroneous readings can occur in diabetics and compression bandaging should only be used with great caution in such patients.

Ulcer treatment

The treatment regimen must be holistic in approach and must aim to:

- correct the circulation
- provide pain relief
- protect and treat the surrounding skin
- prevent and treat any infection
- heal the ulcer
- prevent any recurrence.

Correction of circulation

If a patient presents with a venous ulcer and severe oedema, total bed rest is required. The affected limb should be elevated above the height of the hip and preferably the heart. If mild oedema is present elevation of the limb at night, achieved by raising the foot of the bed, may resolve the problem.

Venous return to the heart should be encouraged by improving the calf muscle pump. Exercise should be encouraged to the limit of the patient's ability. If severely restricted, regular walking on the spot can help and immobile patients can be taught ankle exercises which may be practised when lying down or sitting. In combination with exercise, graduated compression bandaging applied from the base of the toes to the knee is essential. Various multi-layered compression systems have been used in trials, with the majority consisting of

Table 56.5 Clinical features of venous and arterial ulcers	
Venous	Arterial
Occur in gaiter area (generally above medial malleolus)	Occur around malleolus or on the foot, toes or heels
Often large and shallow with flat edges and copious exudate	Punched-out appearance with steep edges often deep with little exudate. Muscle and tendon exposure occurs
Generalized oedema of leg may be present	Local oedema may occur
Dark staining of lower leg due to red blood cell breakdown	Skin staining rare
Sensitive to touch but not normally very painful unless clinically infected or oedematous. Infection common in chronic venous ulcers	Very painful, especially at night or if leg is elevated Relieved by hanging leg out of bed/sleeping in a chair Pain may be severe on exercise due to muscle tissue ischaemia
Foot pulses are present and foot is warm Surrounding varicose eczema is common	Foot pulses reduced or absent. Foot is cold and shiny with hair loss and degeneration of toe nails Foot may whiten on elevation and colour when dependent

a non-adherent dressing immediately over the ulcer area followed by:

1. orthopaedic padding to protect the bony prominences of the ankle
2. crepe bandage to hold padding in place
3. class 3a compression bandage
4. cohesive outer layer to retain bandages and provide additional compression.

There is no conclusive evidence from randomized controlled trials to confirm that layered systems are more efficient than any other high-compression systems (Cullum 1996, Ruckley 1997, RCN 1998). When interpreting studies it is important to ensure that identical parameters have been compared. Some workers have considered the time to complete healing (i.e. all ulcers healed in all patients), while others have looked at the percentage of individual ulcers healed.

In the absence of strong evidence it has been suggested that cost differences between available methods cannot be overlooked (Torgerson 1999, Vowden et al 2000). The layered components or single layer systems are usually applied weekly but in cases of oedema more frequent changes may be needed as the limb changes shape. Cohesive components cannot be reused but crepe and compression layers can be washed and reapplied. Patient acceptance varies, especially as the layered systems will not fit into a normal shoe.

The correct application of such bandaging is crucial to its success. Incorrect bandaging and its inappropriate use can cause limb necrosis, and is therefore worse than no bandage at all.

In a patient with an arterial ulcer it is essential that the extent of arterial damage is diagnosed and compression bandaging generally avoided. Light bandaging may be used when necessary to hold dressings in place and afford protection. Gentle exercise should be encouraged, limbs should be kept warm, and smoking discouraged. Surgical assessment is important to establish prognosis and the potential for surgical intervention.

There is no clear evidence to support the use of any systemic therapy to improve arterial blood flow and hence treat ulceration, although various vasodilator preparations have been tried (Finnie 2000).

Pain relief

This is an often neglected area of leg ulcer management. Venous ulcers are not generally considered painful but may become extremely painful when first elevated. In addition, applications of compression and the healing process itself can be painful. Regular analgesia may be needed, with an additional dose prior to the dressing change. Anti-inflammatory drugs may help but can interfere with the healing process. Patients with arterial ulcers sometimes require strong analgesia, such as an opioid, particularly at night, when cramping pains may be severe. Opioids may also be needed for some patients with venous ulcers.

Protection and treatment of the surrounding skin

Minimal medication should be applied to a venous ulcer as the surrounding skin is usually extremely sensitive due, in part, to varicose eczema, and also to chronic application of assorted medicaments. So-called barrier creams often contain lanolin and hydroxybenzoate preservatives to which the patient may be allergic and which exacerbate the underlying problem.

Medicated paste bandages (e.g. Icthopaste, Steripaste) or stockings (e.g. Zipzoc) with a zinc oxide base may be used over the chosen ulcer preparation to treat the surrounding chronic eczema and sensitive skin. These can be placed over the primary ulcer dressing prior to application of layered compression. There is a need to be aware of differences in preservative and lanolin content, both of which can cause sensitization, and gelatin content which can cause bandages to harden and impair movement.

In patients with severe eczema on the tissue surrounding the ulcer, a steroid preparation may be needed but care must be taken to avoid contact with the ulcer. Patch testing to identify the causative agent for the eczema may be necessary. Weeping eczema may respond to potassium permanganate soaks. If the surrounding skin of venous ulcers is dry with crusting scales of dead skin (hyperkeratosis), application of olive oil may be helpful.

The skin surrounding an arterial ulcer is often shiny and easily traumatized. The act of rubbing in topical medicaments must be avoided.

Infection

Most ulcers will be colonized with microorganisms and if swabbed, bacterial colonies will be identified. However, only clinical infection is significant. The presence of pus with accompanying odour and the presence of cellulitis in surrounding tissues all indicate the presence of infection. The patient is often unwell and systemic antibiotic therapy is essential. To prevent build-up of exudate and debris in the ulcer, cleansing with water or saline is important. Soaking the leg in warm water is often soothing for the patient.

Healing the ulcer

Without treatment of the underlying condition, topical applications will be ineffective, or effective in the short term only.

If a venous ulcer is present a simple primary dressing can be covered with graduated compression bandaging which aims to correct the circulatory problem as described earlier. In between a paste bandage could be used if the surrounding skin condition is compromised.

For arterial ulcers surgical intervention may be required but the ulcer condition may be improved with a primary dressing selected from Table 56.3 depending on the ulcer assessment, held in place if necessary with light, non-elastic bandaging.

Prevention of recurrence

For all patients with an ulcer, education is essential to prevent recurrence of the problem if and when healing occurs. When a venous ulcer heals, protection is essential together with prescription of accurately fitted, below-knee class II or III compression stockings to avoid future breakdown. These can be obtained in standard sizes but made-to-measure are preferable to achieve an accurate fit and particularly for legs of difficult shape. They should be renewed every 3–6 months and air-dried to maintain elasticity. Class III stockings have been shown to reduce recurrence rates more effectively but Class II are better tolerated (RCN 1998). Patients should be reviewed regularly to encourage compliance with treatment, regular exercise, good nutrition, weight control and appropriate skin care. There is as yet no firm trial evidence to confirm the optimal approach but strategies are based on expert opinion and should be individualized to motivate patients (RCN 1998).

Arterial ulcers must be protected with a light protective dressing to reduce the risk of external trauma when recently healed. Compression should be avoided.

Community leg ulcer clinics. There is some evidence that leg ulcer patients are best managed in specialist community leg ulcer clinics. These clinics are staffed by specially trained community nurses, ideally with access to a vascular surgeon for the referral of patients with arterial ulcers and ulcers of mixed aetiology. Excellent ulcer healing rates have been achieved in these clinics. Recurrence rates also appear to be dramatically reduced as patients receive on-going education about the care of their leg and are often motivated by their peers. An alternative approach is to train district nurses in leg ulcer management techniques.

Some common therapeutic problems in the treatment of leg ulcers are listed in Table 56.6.

Figure 56.3 outlines key steps in leg ulcer management.

The way forward for pressure and leg ulcer management

Compression therapy is likely to remain the mainstay of venous ulcer therapy but research may aid selection of

Table 56.6 Common therapeutic problems in leg ulcers

Reliance on ABPI measurement without adequate clinical assessment when considering bandaging
No access to community leg ulcer clinics
Inadequate support for patients to reduce ulcer recurrence
Use of costly interactive dressings beneath compression therapy is often unnecessary
Limited use of portable documentation

simpler, more universally acceptable regimens which will achieve and maintain adequate pressure.

As growth factors and other tissue engineered products are developed, specific treatments will target different ulcer types, including pressure ulcers. For example, becaplermin, a recombinant human platelet-derived growth factor, is licensed only for use in diabetic neuropathic foot ulcers and only if used in conjunction with good wound care measures, which includes debridement. Dermal replacements have also been developed (e.g. Dermagraft). However, both approaches are costly with limited data on long-term safety. Earlier use of larval therapy for debridement is likely for both pressure ulcers and sloughy, necrotic leg ulcers.

CASE STUDIES

Case 56.1

The 73-year-old patient shown in Figure 56.4 has extensive ulceration of the right foot and malleolar area.

....

Question

What are the worrying aspects of the ulcer's appearance?

....

Answer

The ulcer on the dorsum of the foot shows tendon exposure. Damage to tendons must be avoided during dressing changes otherwise foot mobility will be impaired. Deep ulceration may have led to underlying osteomyelitis which would need to be investigated and treated systemically if present. The apparent over-granulation on the main ulcer area may have been caused by application of an occlusive hydrocolloid as granulation tissue was developing. Dressing choice will need to be reconsidered. The malleolar ulcer appears whitened around the edges suggesting slight maceration which also may be product-related and requires reassessment.

Initial clinical assessment of the patient and their ulcer should suggest whether venous, arterial or mixed aetiology is most likely and should identify underlying conditions and additional risks

Measure ankle and brachial pressure index (ABPI). If less than 0.8, arterial damage is present.
Avoid compression therapy and refer to a vascular surgeon or appropriate specialist.
If less than 0.5 refer urgently, depending on local recommendation. ABPI measurement
can be unreliable in diabetics and those with atherosclerosis. They may have erroneously high readings
and specialist assessment is recommended for them and for the following:
Rapidly worsening ulcers
Ulcers that fail to improve after 12 weeks
Recurrent ulcers
Rheumatoid-related ulcers
Skin sensitivity/contact dermatitis
Ischaemic foot
Infected foot

Document location, number and appearance of the ulceration by photography where possible, incorporating measuring techniques to assist in monitoring progress

Refer for surgical debridement if appropriate

Refer for biopsy in non-healing ulcers particularly if appearance gives concern

If clinical infection is present treat with appropriate systemic antibiotics

If odour present consider appropriateness of systemic or topical metronidazole (see Table 56.3)

Do not neglect pain control which may be needed for either venous or arterial ulcers or those of mixed aetiology. individual assessment of pain is essential

If compression is appropriate, graduated high compression bandaging should be applied to venous ulcers. Patient acceptability and maintenance of compression for 7 days are the main considerations but cost differences between the various layered systems are considerable and in the absence of proven clinical differences between systems, should not be ignored. A non-adherent primary dressing is normally adequate beneath compression bandaging.

When bandages are changed legs can be washed in tap water and dried gently. Olive oil can be used on scaling skin avoiding the ulcerated area

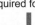

Weekly checks required for signs of deterioration

Significant progress should be expected after 12 weeks of graduated compression bandaging

Patients with healed venous ulcers should be educated in prevention of recurrence. Fitted Class II or III below-knee compression hosiery is recommended. Class II are more likely to be tolerated and recommended for at least 5 years after venous ulcer healing

Figure 56.3 Key steps in leg ulcer management.

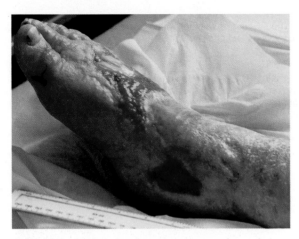

Figure 56.4 Extensive ulceration of the right foot and malleolar area.

The depression higher up on the leg suggests an earlier healed ulcer with considerable dry scaling of the leg which could benefit from olive oil application. The position of the ulcers suggests the need for further investigation of the patient's arterial circulation and the possibility of pressure as an additional factor in ulcer development.

Case 56.2

The middle-aged disabled patient shown in Figure 56.5 has an extensive sacral pressure ulcer which has been debrided and desloughed but is now producing high levels of exudate.

Question

How can the exudate be controlled to improve this patient's quality of life?

Answer

If the exudate is copious, a wound management drainage bag system may be utilized. However, this itself place restrictions on the patient and would depend on the mobility/ability of the patient/carer. Alternatively, or as the exudate lessens, an alginate dressing or a fibrous hydrocolloid product could be utilized and may be able to remain in place for up to 48 hours to minimize disruption for the patient. The choice of product must be in conjunction with a nutritional assessment of the patient and relief of pressure to prevent development of pressure ulcers on the ischial tuberosities and shoulders.

Case 56.3

A 68-year-old woman has extensive leg ulcers (Fig. 56.6) which in the past have been desloughed and cleaned but which deteriorate on discharge from hospital.

Questions

1. What are the likely causes of this patient's ulcers?
2. How could this be confirmed and what professional help should be sought?
3. What services could help in prevention of recurrence?

Answers

1. These appear to be venous ulcers which are chronic in nature and likely to be of many years duration, with sensitive surrounding skin.
2. ABPI (ankle brachial pressure index) will be difficult to assess due to the extent of ulceration and potential pain if the measuring procedure is undertaken. Mixed aetiology is possible and referral to a specialist leg ulcer clinic and/or

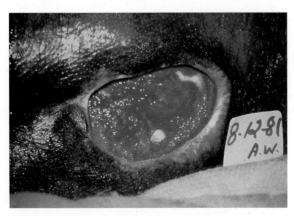

Figure 56.5   Extensive debrided sacral pressure ulcer.

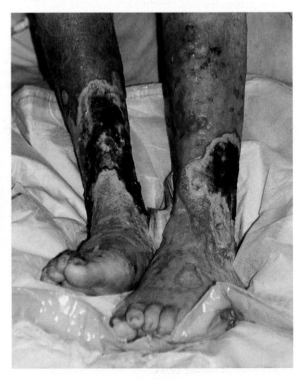

Figure 56.6   Bilateral necrotic leg ulcers, recurrent in nature.

vascular surgeon may be considered. Surgical debridement would help to improve healing potential.

3. Attendance at a community leg ulcer clinic would encourage adherence to management regimens. Involvement of primary care team members could assist with this, including regular input from health visitors, district nurses and encouragement from the local community pharmacist concerning compression hosiery use.

Case 56.4

A 76-year-old man has an ulcer on the malleolar area (Fig. 56.7).

Questions

1. What concerns should there be about the appearance of the ulcer, the edge of the ulcer and the larger area around the ulcer?
2. What assessments should be made:
   - of the patient
   - of the ulcer

and how would these determine future management?

Answers

1. The ulcer itself appears to be infected due to the yellowish exudate. The edge of the ulcer appears to be macerated which may indicate excessive application of hydrogel and/or inadequate absorbency of the covering dressing. The red area surrounding the ulcer suggests presence of cellulitis in the surrounding tissue.
2. The position and 'punched-out' appearance suggest an arterial ulcer but the cellulitis should be dealt with as a priority.
   The patient. Clinical examination of the patient should determine whether the patient feels unwell and is pyrexial and whether the reddened area is warm and extending, all

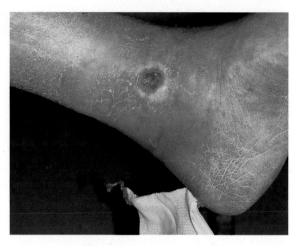

Figure 56.7 Malleolar ulcer with surrounding area of concern.

of which indicate cellulitis. The degree of exudate on previous dressings can be clarified with nursing staff. A would swab would then determine the infecting organisms and results should be awaited prior to commencing systemic antibiotics, depending on the condition of the patient. Pain control should also be considered as arterial ulcers are painful and this will be exacerbated by the accompanying infection.

The ulcer. The ulcer may be of mixed aetiology and may be suitable for light compression bandaging after the cellulitis is treated. Assessment by a vascular surgeon would be necessary to determine arterial blood flow and the risks of compression therapy, and to assess both limbs for other ulcers and/or previous ulceration and the risk areas. If compression is not indicated the patient should be encouraged to exercise appropriately and a foam dressing could be used to absorb exudate. This could remain in place for 4–7 days but more frequent monitoring may be needed initially while the infection settles.

REFERENCES

Callam M J, Harper D R, Dale J J et al 1987 Arterial disease in chronic leg ulceration: an underestimated hazard? Lothian and Forth Valley leg ulcer study. British Medical Journal 294: 929–931

Cullum N 1996 Evaluation of treatments for wounds in clinical trials. Journal of Wound Care 5: 8–9

Finnie A 2000 The SIGN guideline on the care of chronic leg ulcers: an aid to improving practice. Journal of Wound Care 9: 365–367

Harker J 2000 pressure ulcer classification: the Torrance system. Journal of Wound Care 9: 275–277

Ilsley K 2001 Practice devises an effective strategy for venous leg ulceration. Guidelines in Practice 4: 43–50

NICE 2001a Pressure ulcer risk assessment and prevention. NICE, London

NICE 2001b Guidance on the use of debriding agents and specialist wound care clinics for difficult to heal wounds. NICE, London

Royal College of Nursing 1998 Clinical practice guidelines: the

management of patients with venous leg ulcers. Royal College of Nursing, London

Ruckley C V 1997 Evidence-based management of patients with leg ulcers. Journal of Wound Care 6: 442–444

Stevens J, Frank P J, Harrington M 1997 A community hospital leg ulcer service. Journal of Wound Care 6: 62–63

Torgerson D J 1999 The cost-effectiveness of high compression. Journal of Wound Care 8: 215

Vowden K R, Vowden P 1999 Wound debridement. Part 1: sharp techniques; Part 2: sharp techniques. Journal of Wound Care 8: 237–240, 291–294

Vowden K R, Mason A, Wilkinson D et al 2000 Comparison of the healing rates and complications of three four-layer bandage regimens. Journal of Wound Care 9: 269–272

Willock J, Hughes J, Tickle S et al 2000 Pressure sores in children – the acute hospital perspective. Journal of Tissue Viability 10: 59–62

Young T 1996 Methicillin-resistant *Staphylococcus aureus*. Journal of Wound Care 5: 475–477

FURTHER READING

Baeyens T A 2000 Wound care guidelines and formulary for community nurses. Journal of Wound Care 9: 106–108

Baker J 1998 Evidence-based practice in pressure sore reduction. Nursing Times 94: 47–49

NICE 2001 Working together to prevent pressure ulcers: a guide for patients and their carers. NICE, London

Ratcliffy P 1998 Under pressure to update research. Nursing Times 94: 59–63

Simon D A, Freak L, Kinsella A et al 1996 Community leg ulcer clinics: a comparative study in two health authorities. British Medical Journal 312: 1648–1651

Thomas S, Andrews A, Jones M et al 1999 Maggots are useful in treating infected or necrotic wounds. British Medical Journal 318: 807–808

Wilson J 1999 Clinical governance and the potential implications for tissue viability. Journal of Tissue Viability 9: 95–97

APPENDICES

Medical abbreviations

AAA	abdominal aortic aneurysm
	acute anxiety attack
AAAAA	aphasia, agnosia, apraxia, agraphia and alexia
Ab	antibody
abd.	abdomen (abdominal)
	abduction
ABE	acute bacterial endocarditis
ABG	arterial blood gases
ABMT	autologous bone marrow transplant
ABVD	Adriamycin (doxorubicin), bleomycin, vinblastine, dacarbazine
ACAT	acylcholesterol acyltransferase
ACBS	aortocoronary bypass surgery
ACE	angiotensin-converting enzyme
acid phos.	acid phosphatase
AD	Alzheimer's disease
ADC	AIDS dementia complex
ADH	antidiuretic hormone
ADL	activities of daily living
ADP	adenosine diphosphate
ADR	adverse drug reaction
ADU	acute duodenal ulcer
A&E	accident and emergency
AED	antiepileptic drug
AF	atrial fibrillation
AFB	acid-fast bacillus
AFP	α-fetoprotein
AGL	acute granulocytic leukaemia
AGN	acute glomerulonephritis
AHA	autoimmune haemolytic anaemia
AHD	autoimmune haemolytic disease
AIDS	acquired immune deficiency syndrome
AK	above knee
ALD	alcoholic liver disease
ALA	aminolaevulinic acid
ALG	antilymphocyte globulin
ALL	acute lymphocytic leukaemia
ALT	alanine transaminase
AMA	against medical advice
AMI	acute myocardial infarction
AML	acute myeloid leukaemia
AMP	adenosine monophosphate
ANA	antinuclear antibody
ANF	antinuclear factor
ANP	atrial natriuretic peptide
	anti-HbAb anti-hepatitis B antibody
A & O	alert and oriented
A & P	anterior and posterior
	auscultation and percussion
AOB	alcohol on breath
AP	alkaline phosphatase
	angina pectoris
	antepartum
	anterior pituitary
	anterioposterior
	aortic pressure

	apical pulse
	appendectomy
	artificial pneumothorax
APB	atrial premature beat
APC	activated protein C
	atrial premature contraction
APP	amyloid precursor protein
APSAC	anisoylated plasminogen streptokinase activated complex
APTT	activated partial thromboplastin time
AR	aortic regurgitation
	apical/radial (pulse)
ARDS	adult respiratory distress syndrome
ARF	acute renal failure
AS	aortic stenosis
	arteriosclerosis
A–S attack	Adams–Stokes attack
5-ASA	5-aminosalicylic acid
ASB	asymptomatic bacteriuria
ASD	atrial septal defect
ASLO titre	antistreptolysin-O titre
AST	aspartate transaminase
ATG	antithymocyte globulin
ATN	acute tubular necrosis
AUC	area under the curve
AV	aortic valve
	atrioventricular
A-V	arteriovenous
AVR	aortic valve replacement
	augmented V lead, right arm (ECG)
AVS	arteriovenous shunt
A & W	alive and well
AXR	abdominal X ray

BACUP	British Association of Cancer United Patients
BBB	bundle branch block
BBBB	bilateral bundle branch block (ECG)
B Bx.	breast biopsy
BCAA	branched-chain amino acid
BCG	bacille Calmette–Guérin
BDA	British Diabetic Association
BG	blood glucose
BIA	bioelectrical impedence analysis
BJ protein	Bence–Jones protein
BKA	below knee amputation
BM	bowel movement
BMI	body mass index
BMT	bone marrow transplant
BNO	bowels not open
BOR	bowels open regularly
BP	bypass
	blood pressure
BPA	British Paediatric Association
BPD	bronchopulmonary dysplasia
BPH	benign prostatic hyperplasia

BS	blood sugar
	bowel sounds
	breath sounds
BSA	body surface area
BW	body water
	body weight
Bx.	biopsy
C	complement
$C_1, C_2, ...$	cervical vertebrae 1, 2, ...
CA	cancer
	carcinoma
	cardiac arrest
	coronary artery
Ca	carcinoma
CABG	coronary artery bypass graft
CAD	coronary artery disease
CAH	chronic active hepatitis
CAPD	continuous ambulatory peritoneal dialysis
CAT	computerized axial tomography
CAVH	continuous arteriovenous haemofiltration
CBA	cost–benefit analysis
CC	chief complaint
	current complaint
CCF	congestive cardiac failure
CCU	coronary care unit
CEA	cost-effectiveness analysis
CF	cardiac failure
	complement fixation
	cystic fibrosis
CFT	complement fixation test
CGL	chronic granulocytic leukaemia
CGN	chronic glomerulonephritis
CHB	complete heart block
CHD	coronary heart disease
CHF	congestive heart failure
CHO	carbohydrate
CHOP	cyclophosphamide, hydroxydaunorubicin (doxorubicin), Oncovin (vincristine), prednisolone
CI	cardiac index
	cerebral infarction
CIVA	centralized intravenous additive
CK	creatine kinase (same as CPK)
CL	clubbing
CLD	chronic liver disease
	chronic lung disease
CLL	chronic lymphocytic leukaemia
CMA	cost minimization analysis
CML	chronic myelocytic leukaemia
CMV	cytomegalovirus
CNS	central nervous system
CO	cardiac output
c/o	complains of
CoA	coenzyme A
COAD	chronic obstructive airways disease
COD	cause of death
COG	closed angle glaucoma
COLD	chronic obstructive lung disease
COP	capillary osmotic pressure
COPD	chronic obstructive pulmonary disease
COX	cyclo-oxygenase
C & P	cystoscopy and pyelogram
CP	cor pulmonale
	creatine phosphate
CPA	cardiopulmonary arrest
	cerebellar pontine angle
CPAP	continuous positive airway pressure
CPD	continuous peritoneal dialysis
CPK	creatine phosphokinase
CPN	chronic pyelonephritis

CPPV	continuous positive pressure ventilation
CPR	cardiopulmonary resuscitation
CPZ	chlorpromazine
CR	cardiorespiratory
	clot retraction
	colon resection
	conditional reflex
	crown–rump
CRD	chronic renal disease
CRF	chronic renal failure
	corticotrophin-releasing factor
CRP	C-reactive protein
C & S	culture and sensitivity
CSF	cerebrospinal fluid
CSH	chronic subdural haematoma
CSM	carotid sinus massage
	cerebrospinal meningitis
	Committee on Safety of Medicines
CSP	carotid sinus pressure
CSR	Cheyne–Stokes respiration
	correct sedimentation rate
CSS	carotid sinus stimulation
	central sterile supply
CSU	catheter specimen of urine
CT	circulation time
	clotting time
	computerized tomography
	Coombs' test
	coronary thrombosis
CUA	cost–utility analysis
CUG	cystourethrogram
CV	cardiovascular
	central venous
	cerebrovascular
	contingent valuation
CVA	cerebrovascular accident (stroke)
	costovertebral angle
CVD	cardiovascular disease
CVP	central venous pressure
CVVH	continuous venovenous haemofiltration
Cx	cervical, cervix
CXR	chest X ray
d	dead
	deceased
DBP	diastolic blood pressure
D/C	discontinue
D & C	dilatation and curettage
DDx.	differential diagnosis
DH	drug history
DIC	disseminated intravascular coagulation
DIT	diiodotyrosine
DKA	diabetic ketoacidosis
DLE	discoid lupus erythematosus
	disseminated lupus erythematosus
DM	diabetes mellitus
	diastolic murmur
DMARDS	disease-modifying antirheumatic drugs
DNA	did not attend (outpatients)
DOA	dead on arrival
DOB	date of birth
DOD	date of death
DOE	dyspnoea on exertion
D/S	dextrose and saline
DSM	*Diagnostic and Statistical Manual of Mental Disorders*
DTP	diphtheria, tetanus, pertussis (vaccine)
DTs	delirium tremens
DU	diagnosis undetermined
	duodenal ulcer
DUB	dysfunctional uterine bleeding

DUE	drug use evaluation
D5W	dextrose 5%
D & V	diarrhoea and vomiting
DVT	deep vein thrombosis
Dx.	diagnosis
DXT	deep X ray therapy
EBV	Epstein–Barr virus
ECBV	effective circulating blood volume
ECF	extracellular fluid
ECFV	extracellular fluid volume
ECG	electrocardiogram
ECHO	echocardiogram
	echoencephalogram
ECMO	extracorporeal membrane oxygenation
ECT	electroconvulsive therapy
EDD	expected date of delivery
EDV	end-diastolic volume
EEG	electroencephalogram
EENT	eyes, ears, nose and throat
E/I	expiration–inspiration ratio
ELBW	extremely low birth weight
ELISA	enzyme-linked immunosorbent assay
EM	ejection murmur
EMG	electromyogram
EN	erythema nodosum
ENT	ears, nose and throat
EP	ectopic pregnancy
ERCP	endoscopic retrograde cholangiopancreatography
ESM	ejection systolic murmur
ESN	educationally subnormal
ESP	end-systolic pressure
ESR	erythrocyte sedimentation rate
ESRF	end-stage renal failure
ET	endotracheal tube
ETT	exercise tolerance test
FAS	fetal alcohol syndrome
FB	finger breadths
FBS	fasting blood sugar
FCE	finished consultant episode
FEV	forced expiratory volume
FEV_1	forced expiratory volume in 1 second
FFA	free fatty acids
FFP	fresh frozen plasma
FH	family history
FOB	faecal occult blood
FP	frozen plasma
FRC	functional reserve capacity
	functional residual capacity
FSH	follicle-stimulating hormone
FT_4	free thyroxine
FTI	free thyroxine index
FUO	fever of unknown origin
FVC	forced vital capacity
Fx.	fracture
GA	general anaesthesia
	general appearance
GABA	γ-aminobutyric acid
GB	gallbladder
	Guillain–Barré (syndrome)
GBM	glomerular basement membrane
G-CSF	granulocyte colony-stimulating factor
GDM	gastrointestinal diabetes mellitus
GF	glomerular filtration
	gluten-free
GFR	glomerular filtration rate
GGT	γ-glutamyl transpeptidase (transferase)
GIK	glucose, insulin and potassium
GI	gastrointestinal

GLA	γ-linolenic acid
GM seizure	grand mal seizure
GN	glomerulonephritis
GNDC	Gram-negative diplococci
GnRH	gonadotrophin-releasing hormone
grav.	gravid (pregnant)
GS	general surgery
	genital system
g-GT	γ-glutamyl transpeptidase (transferase)
GTN	glyceryl trinitrate
GTT	glucose tolerance test
G6PD	glucose-6-phosphate dehydrogenase
GU	gastric ulcer
	genitourinary
	gonococcal urethritis
GUS	genitourinary system
GVHD	graft-versus-host disease
HAA	hepatitis-associated antigen
HAV	hepatitis A virus
HAS	human albumin solution
HB	heart block
Hb (Hgb)	haemoglobin
HbA_1	glycated haemoglobin
HBAg	hepatitis B antigen
HBsAG	hepatitis B surface antigen
HBD	hydroxybutyrate dehydrogenase
HBDH	hydroxybutyrate dehydrogenase
HBGM	home blood glucose monitoring
Hct. (hct.)	haematocrit
HCV	hepatitis C virus
HDL	high-density lipoproteins
HF	heart failure
HHV	human herpes virus
5-HIAA	5-hydroxyindolacetic acid
Hib	*Haemophilus influenzae* type b
HIE	hypoxic–ischaemic encephalopathy
HIV	human immunodeficiency virus
H & L	heart and lungs
HLA	human lymphocyte antibody
HMD	hyaline membrane disease
HMMA	4-hydroxy-3-methoxymandelic acid
h/o	history of
HO	house officer
HPEN	home parenteral and enteral nutrition
HPI	history of present illness
HPN	home parenteral nutrition
HPV	human papilloma virus
HR	heart rate
HRT	hormone replacement therapy
HS	half strength
	Hartmann's solution
	heart sounds
HSA	human serum albumin
HSV	herpes simplex virus
5-HT	5-hydroxytryptamine (serotonin)
HT, HTN	hypertension
HUS	haemolytic uraemic syndrome
HVA	homovanillic acid
HVD	hypertensive vascular disease
Hx.	history
IADHS	inappropriate antidiuretic hormone syndrome
IBC	iron binding capacity
IBD	inflammatory bowel disease
IBS	irritable bowel syndrome
IC	intercostal
	intracerebral
	intracranial
ICA	islet cell antibody
ICD	*International Classification of Diseases*

ICF	intracellular fluid
ICH	intracerebral haemorrhage
ICM	intracostal margin
ICS	intercostal space
ICU	intensive care unit
ID	intradermal
IDDM	insulin-dependent diabetes mellitus
IDL	intermediate-density lipoprotein
IEP	immunoelectrophoresis
Ig	immunoglobulin
IGT	impaired glucose tolerance
IHD	ischaemic heart disease
IHR	intrinsic heart rate
IMI	inferior myocardial infarction
IMP	impression
Inf. MI	inferior myocardial infarction
INR	international normalized ratio
IOP	intraocular pressure
IPF	idiopathic pulmonary fibrosis
IPP	intermittent positive-pressure inflation with oxygen
IPPB	intermittent positive-pressure breathing
IPPV	intermittent positive-pressure ventilation
IRDS	idiopathic respiratory distress syndrome
ISA	intrinsic sympathomimetic activity
ISDN	isosorbide dinitrate
ISMN	isosorbide mononitrate
IT	intrathecal(ly)
ITT	insulin tolerance test
IUCD	intrauterine contraceptive device
IUD	intrauterine death
	intrauterine device
i.v.	intravenous
IVD	intervertebral disc
IVH	intraventricular haemorrhage
IVP	intravenous push
	intravenous pyelography
IVSD	interventricular septal defect
IVU	intravenous urography
J	jaundice
JVD	jugular venous distension
JVP	jugular venous pressure
KA	ketoacidosis
KCCT	kaolin–cephalin clotting time
KLS	kidney, liver, spleen
KS	Kaposi's sarcoma
KUB	kidneys, ureters, bladder
L	left
	lower
	lumbar
L_1, L_2, …	lumbar vertebrae 1, 2, …
L & A	light and accommodation
LA	left arm
	left atrium
	local anaesthesia
LAD	left anterior descending
LBBB	left bundle branch block
LBM	lean body mass
LBW	low birth weight
LCAT	lecithin–cholesterol acyltransferase
LCT	long-chain triglyceride
LD, LDH	lactate dehydrogenase
LDL	low-density lipoprotein
LFT	liver function test
LH	luteinizing hormone
LHRH	luteinizing hormone-releasing hormone
LIF	left iliac fossa
LK	left kidney

LKS	liver, kidney, spleen
LKKS	liver, kidneys, spleen
LL	left leg
	left lower
	lower lobe
LLL	left lower lobe
	left lower lid
LLQ	left lower quadrant
LMN	lower motor neurone
LMP	last menstrual period
LMWH	low molecular weight heparin
LN	lymph node
LNMP	last normal menstrual period
LOM	limitation of movement
LP	lumbar puncture
Lp(a)	lipoprotein a
LPA	left pulmonary artery
LS	left side
	liver and spleen
	lumbosacral
	lymphosarcoma
LSK	liver, spleen, kidneys
LSM	late systolic murmur
LT	leukotriene
LTC	long-term care
LTOT	long-term oxygen therapy
L & U	lower and upper
LUL	left upper lobe
LUQ	left upper quadrant
LV	left ventricle
LVDP	left ventricular diastolic pressure
LVE	left ventricular enlargement
LVEDP	left ventricular end-diastolic pressure
LVEDV	left ventricular end-diastolic volume
LVET	left ventricular ejection time
LVF	left ventricular failure
LVH	left ventricular hypertrophy
LVP	left ventricular pressure
L & W	living and well
M	male
	married
	metre
	mother
	molar
	murmur
MABP	mean arterial blood pressure
MAC	*Mycobacterium avium* complex
MAI	*Mycobacterium avium-intracellulare*
MAMC	mid-arm muscle circumference
MAO-A	monoamine oxidase A
MAO-B	monoamine oxidase B
MAOI	monoamine oxidase inhibitor
MAP	mean arterial pressure
MBC	minimum bactericidal concentration
MBP	mean blood pressure
MCA	Medicines Control Agency
MCH	mean corpuscular cell haemoglobin
MCHC	mean corpuscular cell haemoglobin concentration
MCP	metacarpal phalangeal (joint)
MCT	medium-chain triglycerides
MCV	mean corpuscular cell volume
MD	mitral disease
	muscular dystrophy
MDI	metered-dose inhaler
MDM	mid-diastolic murmur
MDRTB	multidrug resistant tuberculosis
MEN	multiple endocrine neoplasia
met.	metastatic (metastasis)
MGN	membranous glomerulonephritis

MH	medical history
	menstrual history
MHPG	methoxyhydroxyphenylglycerol
MI	myocardial infarction
	mitral incompetence
MIC	minimum inhibitory concentration
MID	multi-infarct dementia
MIT	monoiodotyrosine
ML	middle lobe
	midline
MOPP	mustine, Oncovin (vincristine), procarbazine, prednisolone
M:P	milk-to-plasma ratio
MPJ	metacarpophalangeal joint
MR	mitral regurgitation
MRDM	malnutrition-related diabetes mellitus
MRI	magnetic resonance imaging
MRRSA	methicillin-resistant *Staphylococcus aureus*
MS	mitral stenosis
	multiple sclerosis
	musculoskeletal
MSL	midsternal line
MSU	midstream urine specimen
MTI	minimum time interval
MTP	metatarsophalangeal
MV	minute volume
	mitral valve
MVP	mitral valve prolapse
MVPP	mustine, vinblastine, procarbazine, prednisolone
MVR	mitral valve replacement
N	normal
NACC	National Association for Colitis and Crohn's Disease
NAD	no appreciable disease
	normal axis deviation
	nothing abnormal detected
NAG	narrow angle glaucoma
NAPQI	*N*-acetyl-*p*-benzoquinoneimine
NARTI	nucleoside analogue reverse transcriptase inhibitor
NBM	nil by mouth
NEC	necrotizing enterocolitis
NG	nasogastric
NHL	non-Hodgkin's lymphoma
NHS	National Health Service
NIDDM	non-insulin-dependent diabetes mellitus
NKHA	non-ketotic hyperosmolar acidosis
NMR	nuclear magnetic resonance
NMS	neuroleptic malignant syndrome
NNRTI	non-nucleoside reverse transcriptase inhibitor
NOF	neck of femur
NS	nephrotic syndrome
	nervous system
	normal saline
	no specimen
NSAID	non-steroidal anti-inflammatory drug
NSFTD	normal spontaneous full-term delivery
NSR	normal sinus rhythm
NSU	nonspecific urethritis
NT	nasotracheal (tube)
N & T	nose and throat
N & V	nausea and vomiting
NVD	nausea, vomiting, diarrhoea
O	oedema
O & A	observation and assessment
O/A	on admission
OA	osteoarthritis
OAD	obstructive airway disease
OAG	open angle glaucoma

OB	occult blood
OD	overdose
O & E	observation and examination
O/E	on examination
OGTT	oral glucose tolerance test
OH	occupational history
OI	opportunistic infection
OKGA	ornithine salt of α-ketoglutaric acid
OPA	outpatient appointment
OPD	outpatient department
OT	occupational therapy
PA	pernicious anaemia
	pulmonary artery
P & A	percussion and auscultation
$P_a\text{CO}_2$	arterial carbon dioxide tension
PACG	primary angle closure glaucoma
PAF	platelet-activating factor
PAH	pulmonary artery hypertension
$P_a\text{O}_2$	arterial oxygen pressure tension
PAPS	primary antiphospholipid syndrome
PAS	*P*-aminosalicylic acid
	pulmonary artery stenosis
PAT	paroxysmal atrial tachycardia
PAWP	pulmonary artery wedge pressure
PB	premature beats
PBC	primary biliary cirrhosis
PBI	protein-bound iodine
PBSCT	peripheral stem cell transplantion
PCA	patient-controlled analgesia
PCAS	patient-controlled analgesia system
$P\text{CO}_2$	partial pressure of carbon dioxide
PCP	*Pneumocystis carinii* pneumonia
PCS	portocaval shunt
PCV	packed cell volume
PD	peritoneal dialysis
PDA	patent ductus arteriosus
PE	physical examination
	pleural effusion
	pulmonary embolism
PEARLA	pupils equal and react to light and accommodation
PEF	peak expiratory flow
PEFR	peak expiratory flow rate
PEG	percutaneous endoscopic gastrostomy
PEJ	percutaneous endoscopic jejunostomy
PEM	prescription event monitoring
PERLA	pupils equal, react to light and accommodation
PERRLA	pupils equal, round, react to light and accommodation
PET	position emission tomography
PF	peak flow
PFR	peak flow rate
PFT	pulmonary function test
PG	prostaglandin
PH	past history
	patient history
	personal history
	prostatic hypertrophy
	pulmonary hypertension
PI	present illness
	protease inhibitor
PICC	peripherally inserted central catheter
PID	pelvic inflammatory disease
PIP	proximal interphalangeal joint
PIVD	protruded intervertebral disc
PJB	premature junctional beat
PJC	premature junctional contraction
PKU	phenylketonuria
PL	product licence

893

PMH	past medical history	RF	renal failure
PMI	past medical illness		rheumatic fever
PMN	polymorphonucleocyte		rheumatoid factor
PMS	premenstrual syndrome	RFT	respiratory function tests
	postmenopausal syndrome	RHF	right heart failure
PMT	premenstrual tension	Rh factor	rhesus factor
PMV	prolapsed mitral valve	rhuEPO	recombinant human erythropoietin
PN	percussion note	rhuGM-CSF	recombinant human granulocyte–macrophage
	peripheral nerve		colony-stimulating factor
	peripheral neuropathy	RHL	right hepatic lobe
PND	paroxysmal nocturnal dyspnoea	RIF	right iliac fossa
	postnasal drip	RIMA	reversible inhibitor of monoamine oxidase type A
Po_2	partial pressure of oxygen	RK	right kidney
POAG	primary open-angle glaucoma	RL	right leg
POMR	problem-oriented medical record		right lung
PPD	purified protein derivative	RLC	residual lung capacity
PPH	postpartum haemorrhage	RLD	related living donor
PPI	proton pump inhibitor	RLL	right lower lobe (lung)
PPNG	penicillinase-producing *Neisseria*	RLQ	right lower quadrant (abdomen)
	gonorrhoeae	RP	radial pulse
PPV	positive-pressure ventilation	RPI	resting pressure index
PROM	premature rupture of membranes	RQ	respiratory quotient
PR	per rectum	RR	respiratory rate
PS	pulmonary stenosis	RR & E	round regular and equal (pupils)
	pyloric stenosis	RS	respiratory system
PSA	prostate-specific antigen	RSF	rheumatoid serum factor
PSG	presystolic gallop	RTA	road traffic accident
PSGN	poststreptococcal glomerulonephritis	rt-PA	recombinant plasminogen activator
PSVT	paroxysmal supraventricular tachycardia	RUL	right upper lobe
PT	parathyroid	RUQ	right upper quadrant
	paroxysmal tachycardia	RV	residual volume
	physical therapy		right ventricle
	physical training	RVH	right ventricular hypertrophy
	posterior tibial (pulse)		
	prothrombin time	SA	sinoatrial (node)
PTC	percutaneous cholangiogram		Stokes–Adams (attacks)
PTH	parathyroid hormone		surface area
PTT	partial thromboplastin time	SB	seen by
PTTK	partial thromboplastin time kaolin		shortness of breath
PTU	propylthiouracil	SBE	subacute bacterial endocarditis
PU	pass urine, per urethra		shortness of breath on exertion
	peptic ulcer	SBO	small bowel obstruction
PUD	peptic ulcer disease	SBP	spontaneous bacterial peritonitis
	pulmonary disease	SCU	*see* SCUF
PUO	pyrexia (fever) of unknown origin	SCUF	slow continuous ultrafiltration
PUVA	psoralen and ultraviolet A radiation	SDD	selective decontamination of the digestive tract
PV	vaginal examination (per vagina)	SEM	systolic ejection murmur
P & V	pyloroplasty and vagotomy	SGOT	serum glutamate–oxaloacetate transaminase
PVB	premature ventricular beat	SGPT	serum glutamate–pyruvate transaminase
PVC	premature ventricular contraction	SH	social history
PVD	peripheral vascular disease	SIADH	syndrome of inappropriate antidiuretic hormone
PVP	pulmonary venous pressure	SIDS	sudden infant death syndrome
PVT	paroxysmal ventricular tachycardia	SLE	systemic lupus erythematosus
Px.	past history	SNRI	serotonin–noradrenaline reuptake inhibitor
	prognosis	SOA	swelling of ankle(s)
		SOAP	subjective, objective, assessment, plan
		SOB	short of breath
QALY	quality-adjusted life year	SOBOE	short of breath on exertion
		SP	systolic pressure
R	respiration	SPA	suprapubic aspiration
RA	renal artery	SPC	Summary of Product Characteristics
	rheumatoid arthritis	SR	sinus rhythm
	right arm		sustained release
	right atrial (atrium)	SSRI	selective serotonin reuptake inhibitor
RAST	radioallergosorbent test	ST	sinus tachycardia
RBBB	right bundle branch block	stat.	immediately (Latin: statim)
RBC	red blood cell	STD	sexually transmitted disease
	red blood (cell) count		sodium tetradecyl sulphate
RBS	random blood sugar	STS	serological tests for syphilis
RDS	respiratory distress syndrome	SV	stroke volume
REMS	rapid eye movement sleep	SVI	stroke volume index

SVT	supraventricular tachycardia	TURP	transurethral resection of the prostate
SWS	slow-wave sleep	TV	tidal volume
Sx	symptoms	Tx.	transfusion
			treatment
		T & X	type and crossmatch
T	temperature		
T$_3$	triiodothyronine	UBIC	unsaturated iron-binding capacity
T$_4$	thyroxine	UC	ulcerative colitis
TB	tuberculosis	U & E	urea and electrolytes
TBA	to be administered	UFH	unfractionated heparin
	to be arranged	URTI	upper respiratory tract infection
TBG	thyroid-binding globulin	US	ultrasound
TBI	total body irradiation	UTI	urinary tract infection
TBW	total body weight	UVA	ultraviolet A
T & C	type and crossmatch	UVB	ultraviolet B
TC	total capacity		
	tricarboxylic acid cycle	VC	vital capacity
TCA	tricyclic antidepressant		vulvovaginal candidiasis
TDM	therapeutic drug monitoring	VD	venereal disease
TEN	toxic epidermal necrolysis (Lyell's syndrome)	VDRL	Venereal Disease Research Laboratory (test for syphilis)
TENS	transcutaneous electrical nerve stimulation		
TGs	triglycerides	VF	ventricular fibrillation
TH	thyroid hormone (thyroxine)	VHD	valvular heart disease
THA	tetrahydroaminoacridine	VLBW	very low birth weight
THC	tetrahydrocannabinol	VLDL	very low-density lipoprotein
TIA	transient ischaemic attack	VMA	vanillyl mandelic acid
TIBC	total iron-binding capacity	VP	venous pressure
TIMP	tissue inhibitor of metalloproteinases	VPC	ventricular premature contraction
TIPSS	transjugular intrahepatic portosystemic shunting	V/Q	ventilation–perfusion ratio
TLC	tender loving care	VS	vital signs
	total lung capacity	VT	ventricular tachycardia
TNF	tumour necrosis factor	VUR	vesicoureteric reflux
t-PA	tissue plasminogen factor		
TPN	total parenteral nutrition	WBC	white blood cell
TP & P	time, place, and person		white blood count
TPR	temperature, pulse, respiration	WCC	white cell count
TRH	thyrotrophin-releasing hormone	WHO	World Health Organization
TSF	triceps skinfold thickness	WPW	Wolff–Parkinson–White (syndrome)
TSH	thyroid-stimulating hormone	WR	Wassermann reaction
TTA	transtracheal aspiration	WTA	willingness to accept
TTO	to take out (to take home)	WTP	willingness to pay
TUIP	transurethral incision of the prostate		
TUR	transurethral resection	ZE	Zollinger–Ellison (syndrome)
TURB	transurethral resection of the bladder	ZIG	zoster immune globulin

Glossary

acanthosis nigricans: diffuse velvety acanthosis with grey, brown or black pigmentation, chiefly in axilla and other body folds, occurring in an adult form, often associated with an internal carcinoma and in a benign, nevoid form, more or less generalized.

addisonian crisis: the symptoms that accompany an acute onset or worsening of Addison's disease, including fatigue, nausea and vomiting, loss of weight, hypotension, fever and collapse.

anoxaemia: reduction of blood oxygen content below physiological levels.

apnoea: cessation of breathing.

arachnoiditis: inflammation of the arachnoidea, a delicate membrane interposed between the dura mater and the pia mater.

atretic: without an opening; characterized by atresia.

azoospermia: absence of spermatozoa in the semen, or failure of formation of spermatozoa.

bacteriuria: the presence of bacteria in the urine.

bronchiectasis: characterized by dilatation of the small bronchi and bronchioles, associated with the presence of chronic pulmonary sepsis. It presents as a chronic cough often with the production of large amounts of purulent, foul-smelling sputum, and may eventually lead to repeated episodes of pneumonia and respiratory failure.

bronchoalveolar lavage: a procedure performed during bronchoscopy in which the bronchial tree is literally washed (lavaged) with a small volume of sterile saline. The saline is then collected and sent for microbiological or cytological examination.

bronchoscopy: the procedure in which a flexible fibre-optic endoscope is inserted into the bronchial tree to allow direct visualization of the bronchi and, if required, the collection of specimens for microbiology or histology.

Budd–Chiari syndrome: symptomatic obstruction or occlusion of the hepatic veins, usually of unknown origin, but probably caused by neoplasms, strictures, liver disease, trauma, systemic infections or haematological disorders.

cachectic: a profound and marked state of general ill health and malnutrition.

cardiogenic emboli: emboli originating from the heart; caused by abnormal function of the heart.

carpal tunnel syndrome: a complex of symptoms resulting from compression of the median nerve in the carpal tunnel, with pain and burning or tingling paraesthesias in the fingers and hand, sometimes extending to the elbow.

cataract: an opacity of the crystalline lens of the eye.

cavitation: formation of cavities. For example in the lungs when the liquefied centre of a tuberculous lesion drains (usually into a bronchus).

Charcot's arthropathy: a destructive arthropathy (disease of any joint) with impaired pain perception or position sense.

cholelithiasis: the presence or formation of gallstones.

chondrocyte: a mature cartilage cell embedded in a lacuna (a small pit or hollow cavity) within the cartilage matrix.

Chvostek's sign: spasm of the facial muscles elicited by tapping the facial nerve in the region of the parotid gland, seen in tetany.

coarctation of the aorta: a localized malformation characterized by deformity of the aortic media, causing narrowing, usually severe, of the lumen of the vessel.

cognitive: pertaining to cognition; that operation of the mind by which we become aware of objects of thought or perception; it includes all aspects of perceiving, thinking and remembering.

cor pulmonale: persistent lung damage eventually leads to increased blood pressure in the pulmonary arteries (pulmonary hypertension), which in turn leads to stress on the right ventricle, right ventricular hypertrophy and heart failure. This process is known as cor pulmonale.

cryptogenic: obscure, doubtful or unascertainable origin.

cytotoxin: a toxin or antibody that has a specific toxic action upon cells of special organs.

denudation: removal of the epithelial covering from any surface.

diarthrodial joint: a joint characterized by mobility in a rotary direction.

dimorphic: occurring in two distinct forms.

disseminated intravascular coagulation (DIC): in this condition vigorous activation of the clotting cascade causes widespread intravascular deposition of fibrin and consumption of clotting factors and platelets. There are numerous potential triggers for this process, including severe sepsis, burns, massive transfusion and placental abruption.

diverticulosis: the presence of circumscribed pouches or sacs of variable size called diverticula that occur normally or are created by herniation of the lining mucous membrane through a defect in the muscular coat of a tubular organ such as the gastrointestinal tract.

Dupuytren's contracture: shortening, thickening and fibrosis of the palmar fascia, producing a flexion deformity of a finger. The term also applies to a flexion deformity of a toe.

dyschezia: difficult or painful evacuation of faeces from the rectum.

dyskinesia: impairment of the power of voluntary movement, resulting in fragmentary or incomplete movements.

dyspareunia: difficult or painful intercourse.

dyspnoea: difficult or laboured breathing.

dystonia: disordered tonicity of muscle.

dysuria: painful or difficult urination.

eclampsia: convulsions and coma occurring in a pregnant or puerperal woman, associated with hypertension, oedema and/or proteinuria.

elliptocytosis: a hereditary disorder in which the majority of erythrocytes are elliptical in shape, and characterized by varying degrees of increased red cell destruction and anaemia.

emphysema: a state in which the alveoli of the lung become dilated, possibly with destruction of the alveolar walls, leading to large empty air spaces which are useless for gas exchange. It is often seen accompanying chronic bronchitis but may be due to inherited disorders such as α_1-antitrypsin deficiency.

encephalopathy: any degenerative disease of the brain.

enterostomy: the formation of a permanent opening into the intestine through the abdominal wall.

enterotoxin: a toxin arising in the intestine.

episcleritis: inflammation of the loose connective tissue forming the external surface of the sclera.

Epstein–Barr virus: a herpes virus originally isolated from Burkitt lymphomas and believed to be the aetiological agent in infectious mononucleosis or closely related to it.

faecal: occult blood in the stools. Called 'occult' because it is partly digested and therefore no longer red in colour. Usually detected by means of a chemical test.

Fanconi's anaemia: a rare hereditary disorder, transmitted in a recessive manner and having a poor prognosis, characterized by pancytopenia, hypoplasia of the bone marrow, and patchy brown discoloration of the skin due to the deposition of melanin, and associated with multiple congenital anomalies of the musculoskeletal and genitourinary systems.

fastidious organism: organism which will only grow with specialist culture media or under certain physiological conditions.

fistula: an abnormal passage or communication, usually between two internal organs or from an internal organ to the surface of the body.

gastroschisis: congenital fissure of the abdominal wall not involving the site of insertion of the umbilical cord, and usually accompanied by protrusion of the small and part of the large intestine.

glossitis: inflammation of the tongue.

granuloma: a tumour-like mass or nodule of granulation tissue, with actively growing fibroblasts and capillary buds; it is due to a chronic inflammatory process associated with infectious disease, or with invasion by a foreign body.

Guillain–Barré syndrome: acute febrile polyneuritis.

haematuria: blood in the urine.

haustral: pertaining to the haustra of the colon denoting sacculations in the wall of the colon produced by adaptation of its length.

Heinz bodies: inclusion bodies in red blood cells resulting from oxidative injury to and precipitation of haemoglobin, seen in the presence of certain abnormal haemoglobins and erythrocytes with enzyme deficiencies.

Henoch–Schönlein purpura: an acute or chronic vasculitis primarily affecting skin, joints and the gastrointestinal and renal systems.

Hirschsprung's disease: congenital megacolon.

Horner's syndrome: sinking in of the eyeball, ptosis of the upper eyelid, slight elevation of the lower lid, constriction of the pupil, narrowing of the palpebral fissure, anhidrosis and flushing of the affected side of the face; caused by paralysis of the cervical sympathetic nerves.

Horton's syndrome: migrainous neuralgia; also called paroxysmal nocturnal cephalalgia.

Huntington's chorea: a rare hereditary disease characterized by chronic progressive chorea and mental deterioration terminating in dementia. The age of onset is variable but usually occurs in the fourth decade of life.

hyaline membrane: a layer of eosinophilic hyaline material lining the alveoli, alveolar ducts and bronchioles, found at autopsy in infants who have died of respiratory distress syndrome of the newborn.

hypersplenism: a condition characterized by exaggeration of the inhibitory or destructive functions of the spleen, resulting in deficiency of the peripheral blood elements, singly or in combination, hypercellularity of the bone marrow, and usually splenomegaly.

ileus: obstruction or lack of smooth muscle tone in the intestines.

immunoblastic: pertaining to or involving the stem cells (immunoblasts) of lymphoid tissue.

index case: the first detected case in a particular series that prompts investigation into other patients.

intussusception: the prolapse of one part of the intestine into the lumen of an immediately adjoining part.

Jod–Basedow syndrome: thyrotoxicosis produced in a patient with goitre, when given a bolus of iodine.

Kayser–Fleischer ring: a grey-green to red-gold pigmented ring at the outer margin of the cornea, seen in progressive lenticular degeneration and pseudosclerosis.

koilonychia: dystrophy of the fingernails, in which they are thin and concave, with edges raised.

Kussmaul's respiration: air hunger.

kwashiorkor: insufficient protein provision.

labyrinthitis: inflammation of the labyrinth; otitis interna.

laminectomy: excision of the posterior arch of a vertebra.

laparoscopy: examination of the interior of the abdomen by means of a laparoscope.

lichenoid: resembling the skin lesions designated as 'lichen' – the name applied to many different kinds of papular skin diseases in which the lesions are typically small, firm papules that are usually set very close together.

Lyme disease: a multisystem tick-borne disorder caused by the spirochaete B*orrelia burgdorferi*. Clinical manifestation includes an erythematous macule followed by systemic disorders such as arthralgias, myalgias and headache followed by neurological manifestations, cardiac involvement and a migratory polyarthritis.

lymphadenopathy: disease of the lymph nodes.

lymphoblastic: pertaining to a lymphoblast.

maculopapular: an eruption consisting of both macules (areas distinguishable by colour from their surroundings, e.g. spots) and papules (small circumscribed, superficial, solid elevations of the skin).

malleolus medialis: the rounded protruberance on the medial surface of the ankle joint.

malrotation: abnormal or pathologic rotation.

marasmus: insufficient energy provision.

melaena: the passage of dark stools stained with blood pigments or with altered blood.

menorrhagia: excessive and prolonged uterine bleeding occurring at the regular intervals of menstruation.

miliary: literally resembling small round millet seeds. Miliary tuberculosis is so called because the chest radiograph usually shows miliary speckling.

morbilliform: resembling the eruption of measles.

mycosis fungoides: a rare, chronic, malignant, lymphoreticular neoplasm of the skin and, in the late stages, the lymph nodes and viscera, marked by the development of firm, reddish, painful tumours that ulcerate.

myositis: inflammation of a voluntary muscle.

necrobiosis lipoidica: a dermatosis usually occurring in diabetics characterized by necrobiosis (swelling and distortion of collagen bundles in the dermis) of the elastic and connective tissue of the skin, with degenerated collagen occurring in irregular patches, especially in the upper dermis.

nystagmus: involuntary rapid movement of the eyeball, which may be horizontal, vertical, rotatory, or mixed.

obligate intracellular pathogen: an organism that cannot be cultured using artificial media since it requires living cells for growth.

orosomucoid: α_1-acid glycoprotein, a glycoprotein occurring in blood plasma.

orthopnoea: difficult breathing except in an upright position.

orthoptic: correcting obliquity of one or more visual axis.

Osler's nodes: small, raised, swollen tender areas, about the size of a pea and often bluish in colour but sometimes pink or red, occurring most commonly in the pads of the fingers or toes, in the palm or the soles of the feet.

osteophyte: a bony or osseous outgrowth.

panmyelopathy: a pathological condition of all the elements of the bone marrow.

paroxysmal nocturnal dyspnoea: difficult or laboured breathing at night that recurs in paroxysms.

pericarditis: inflammation of the fibrous sac (pericardium) that surrounds the heart and the roots of the great vessels.

petechial: characterized by pinpoint, non-raised, round, purplish red spots caused by intradermal or submucous haemorrhage.

phaeochromocytoma: a tumour of chromaffin tissue of the adrenal medulla or sympathetic paraganglia. The cardinal symptom that represents the increased secretion of adrenaline and noradrenaline is hypertension, which may be persistent or intermittent.

pica: a craving for unnatural articles of food.

polymorphic: occurring in several or many forms.

polyp: a protruding growth from a mucous membrane.

pompholyx: a skin eruption on the sides of the fingers, toes, palms or soles, consisting of discrete round intraepidermal vesicles 1 or 2 mm in diameter, accompanied by intense itching and occurring in repeated self-limited attacks lasting 1 or 2 weeks.

porphyria: any of a group of disturbances of porphyrin metabolism, characterized by marked increase in formation and excretion of porphyrins or their precursors.

Prinzmetal's angina: a variant of angina pectoris in which the attacks occur during rest.

pyruvate kinase deficiency: a deficiency in the glycolytic (metabolic) pathway of red blood cells that results in haemolysis.

Raeder's syndrome: a syndrome consisting of the Horner syndrome but without loss of sweating on the affected side of the face.

Reed–Sternberg cells: giant histiocytic cells, typically multinucleate, most often binucleate; the nuclei are enclosed in abundant amphophilic cytoplasm and contain prominent nucleoli.

retinopathy: any non-inflammatory disease of the retina.

retroperitoneal fibrosis: deposition of fibrous tissue in the retroperitoneal space, producing vague abdominal discomfort, and often causing blockage of the ureters with resultant hydronephrosis and impaired renal function.

retrosternal: situated or occurring behind the sternum.

Reye's syndrome: an acute and often fatal childhood syndrome of encephalopathy and fatty degeneration of the liver, marked by rapid development of brain swelling and hepatomegaly and by disturbed consciousness and seizures.

Roth's spots: round or oval white spots sometimes seen in the retina early in the course of subacute bacterial endocarditis.

sarcoidosis: a chronic, progressive, generalized granulomatous reticulosis of unknown aetiology, involving almost any organ or tissue.

sclerotherapy: the injection of sclerosing solutions in the treatment of haemorrhoids or varicose veins.

scotoma: an area of depressed vision within the visual field, surrounded by an area of less depressed or of normal vision.

Sézary syndrome: generalized exfoliative erythroderma produced by cutaneous infiltration of reticular lymphocytes and associated with intense pruritus, alopecia, oedema hyperkeratosis, pigment and nail changes.

Shy–Drager syndrome: orthostatic hypotension, urinary and rectal incontinence, anhidrosis, atrophy of the iris, external ophthalmoplegia, rigidity, tremor, loss of associated movements, impotence, atonic bladder, generalized weakness, fasciculations, and neuropathic muscle wasting.

sickle cell anaemia: a hereditary haemolytic anaemia occurring almost exclusively in Blacks, characterized by arthralgia, acute attacks of abdominal pain, ulcerations of the lower extremities and with sickle-shaped erythrocytes in the blood.

Sjögren's syndrome: a symptom complex of unknown aetiology, usually occurring in middle-aged or older women, in which keratoconjunctivitis is associated with pharyngitis sicca, enlargement of the parotid glands, chronic polyarthritis and xerostomia.

sloughing material: soft, gel-like material often found in ulcer bases. Composed of tissue exudate and cellular debris.

spherocytosis: the presence of spherocytes (thick, almost spherical, red blood cells) characterized by abnormal fragility of erythrocytes, jaundice and splenomegaly.

splinter haemorrhages: linear haemorrhages beneath the nail.

steatosis: fatty degeneration.

stenosis: narrowing or stricture of a duct or canal.

Stevens–Johnson syndrome: a severe form of erythema multiforme in which the lesions may involve the oral and anogenital mucous membranes in association with constitutional symptoms, including malaise, prostration, headache, fever, arthralgia and conjunctivitis.

subchondral: beneath a cartilage.

subluxation: an incomplete or partial dislocation.

supranuclear palsy: pseudobulbar paralysis.

sympathetic ileus: failure of gastrointestinal motility secondary to acute non-gastrointestinal illness, e.g. hyaline membrane disease or septicaemia.

tamponade: surgical use of the tampon; also pathological compression of a part, as compression of the heart by pericardial fluid.

tenesmus: straining, especially ineffectual and painful straining at stool or in urination.

tenosynovitis: inflammation of a tendon sheath.

thalassaemia: a heterogeneous group of hereditary haemolytic anaemias that have in common a decreased rate of synthesis of one or more haemoglobin polypeptide chains and are classified according to the chain involved (α, β, γ). The homozygous form (thalassaemia major) is incompatible with life. The heterozygous form (thalassaemia minor) may be asymptomatic or marked by mild anaemia.

thrombocytopenia: decrease in the number of blood platelets.

thrombocytosis: increased number of platelets in blood.

trephine: biopsy examination of an intact core of tissue (e.g. liver, bone marrow) obtained through a wide-bore needle.

tropical sprue: a malabsorption syndrome occurring in the tropics and subtropics. Protein malnutrition is usually precipitated by the malabsorption, and anaemia due to folic acid deficiency is particularly common.

Trousseau's sign: spasmodic contractions of muscles provoked by pressure upon the nerves which go to them; seen in tetany.

tubular cast: a cast formed from gelled protein precipitated in the renal tubules and moulded to the tubular lumen; pieces of these casts break off and are washed out with the urine.

urethral: pertaining to the urethra, the membranous canal conveying urine from the bladder to the exterior of the body.

variant angina: *see* Prinzmetal's angina.

volvulus: intestinal obstruction due to a knotting and twisting of the bowel.

Wernicke–Korsakoff syndrome: the coexistence of Wernicke's disease (acute onset of mental confusion, nystagmus, ophthalmoplegia, and gait ataxia, due to thiamine deficiency) with Korsakoff's syndrome (a gross disturbance in recent memory, sometimes compensated for by confabulation).

Wilson's disease: characterized by progressive accumulation of copper within body tissues, particularly erythrocytes, kidney, liver and brain, and associated with liver and lenticular degeneration.

xerosis: dry skin.

Changes to the names of certain medical substances

European law has specified requirements for the names of medicinal products and requires the use of the Recommended International Non proprietary Name (rINN). The UK has had its own naming system for many years, utilizing the BP monograph title, British Approved Name (BAN), or Approved Synonym. This naming system has been used in this text book. Whilst the majority of BANs are identical to the corresponding rINN, there are some which differ and for these a change to the use of the rINN will be required over coming years.

A full list of all the affected substances by category is presented below. Whilst most of the names are given in their basic forms many others occur in practice as salts or esters. In such cases their Recommended International Non proprietary Name (rINN) is known formally as a modified rINN (rINNM).

Category A medicines will have dual-labelling (see preface). Both BAN and rINN names must appear on labels, packaging and leaflets until advised by the Medicines Control Agency in the UK. For category B medicines a change to the exclusive use of rINN is required.

Entries shown in italics are for non-marketed, discontinued or abandoned materials but some may still be available on a 'named patient' basis.

List A. Use dual-labelling

UK Name BAN/BANM/BP Title	Recommended INN/INNM
acrosoxacin	rosoxacin
adrenaline	epinephrine
amethocaine	tetracaine
bendrofluazide	bendroflumethiazide
benzhexol	trihexyphenidyl
chlorpheniramine	chlorphenamine
dicyclomine	dicycloverine
dothiepin	dosulepin
eformoterol*	formoterol
flurandrenolone	fludroxycortide
frusemide	furosemide
mitozantrone	mitoxantrone
mustine	*chlormethine*
noradrenaline	norepinephrine

*WHO is intending to change the INN formoterol to eformoterol – the requirement to dual-label is therefore suspended.

oxpentifylline	pentoxifylline
procaine penicillin	procaine benzylpenicillin
salcatonin	calcitonin (salmon)
thymoxamine	moxisylyte
trimeprazine	alimemazine

List B. Change to the INN form

UK Name BAN/BANM/BP Title	Recommended INN/INNM
acepifylline	*acefylline piperazine*
acinitrazole	*aminitrozole*
actinomycin	*cactinomycin*
adenosine phosphate	*adenosine monophosphate*
allyloestrenol	allylestrenol
aloxidone	*allomethadione*
alphadolone	alfadolone
alphaxalone	alfaxalone
amoxycillin	amoxicillin
amphetamine	*amfetamine*
amphomycin	*amfomycin*
amylobarbitone	amobarbital
amylobarbitone sodium	amobarbital sodium
azetepa	*azatepa*
balipramine	*depramine*
barbitone	*barbital*
beclomethasone	beclometasone
benorylate	benorilate
benzathine penicillin	benzathine benzylpenicillin
benzphetamine	*benzfetamine*
benztropine	benzatropine
bethanidine	betanidine
bismuth glycollylarsanilate	*glycobiarsol*
bromocyclen	*bromociclen*
bromodiphenhydramine	*bromazine*
buniodyl	*bunamiodyl*
bupropion	*amfebutamone*
busulphan	busulfan
butamyrate	*butamirate*
butethamate	butetamate
buthalitone sodium	*buthalital sodium*
butobarbitone	butobarbital
butoxamine	*butaxamine*
carbiphene	*carbifene*
carbolonium bromide	hexcarbacholine bromide
carbophenthion	carbofenotion
carphenazine	*carfenazine*
cellacephate	cellacefate
cephalexin	cefalexin
cephaloglycin	*cefaloglycin*
cephalonium	cefalonium
cephaloram	*cefaloram*
cephaloridine	cefaloridine

901

UK Name BAN/BANM/BP Title	Recommended INN/INNM	UK Name BAN/BANM/BP Title	Recommended INN/INNM
cephalothin	cefalotin	ethynodiol	etynodiol
cephamandole nafate	cefamandole nafate	*etifoxin*	*etifoxine*
cephazolin	cefazolin	*fanthridone*	*fantridone*
cephoxazole	cefoxazole	*fenchlorphos*	*fenchlofos*
cephradine	cefradine	*fenethylline*	*fenetylline*
chlophedianol	*clofedanol*	*fetoxylate*	*fetoxilate*
chloral betaine	cloral betaine	flumethasone	flumetasone
chlorbutol	chlorobutanol	*fluopromazine*	*triflupromazine*
chlordantoin	*clodantoin*	flupenthixol	flupentixol
chlorfenvinphos	clofenvinfos	*flurothyl*	*flurotyl*
chlorhexadol	chloralodol	*glycalox*	*glucalox*
chlormethiazole	clomethiazole	glycopyrronium bromide	glycopyrrolate
chlorthalidone	chlortalidone	guaiphenesin	guaifenesin
chlorthenoxazin	*chlorthenoxazine*	*halethazole*	*haletazole*
cholecalciferol	colecalciferol	*halopyramine*	*chloropyramine*
cholestyramine	colestyramine	heptabarbitone	heptabarb
clamoxyquin	*clamoxyquine*	hexachlorophane	hexachlorophene
clomiphene	clomifene	hexamine hippurate	methenamine hippurate
clorgyline	*clorgiline*	*hexobarbitone*	*hexobarbital*
clothiapine	*clotiapine*	*hydroxamethocaine*	*hydroxytetracaine*
co-carboxylase	*cocarboxylase*	*hydroxyamphetamine*	*hydroxyamfetamine*
colistin sulphomethate sodium	colistimethate sodium	hydroxyprogesterone hexanoate	hydroxyprogesterone caproate
corticotrophin	corticotropin	hydroxyurea	hydroxycarbamide
coumaphos	coumafos	indomethacin	indometacin
cromoglycic acid	cromoglicic acid	iodipamide	adipiodone
crotethamide	crotetamide	iophendylate	iofendylate
cumetharol	*coumetarol*	iothalamic acid	iotalamic acid
cyacetazide	*cyacetacide*	*isobuzole*	*glysobuzole*
cyclobarbitone calcium	*cyclobarbital calcium*	isoetharine	isoetarine
cycloprolol	*cicloprolol*	*isometamidium*	*isometamidium chloride*
cysteamine	*mercaptamine*	ketobemidone	cetobemidone
danthron	dantron	*levamphetamine*	*levamfetamine*
deoxycortone	*desoxycortone*	lignocaine	lidocaine
desoxymethasone	desoximatasone	lynoestrenol	lynestrenol
dexamphetamine	dexamfetamine	lysuride	lisuride
diamphenethide	diamfenetide	*malethamer*	*maletamer*
diatrizoic acid	amidotrizoic acid	*meprothixol*	*meprotixol*
diazinon	dimpylate	*methadyl acetate*	*acetylmethadol*
dichlorphenamide	diclofenamide	*methallenoestrol*	*methallenestrol*
dienoestrol	dienestrol	*methallibure*	*metallibure*
dimethicone(s)	dimeticone	*methamphazone*	*metamfazone*
dimethindine	*dimetindine*	*metharbitone*	*metharbital*
dimethisoquin	*quinisocaine*	methenolone	metenolone
dimethothiazine	*dimetotiazine*	*methetoin*	*metetoin*
dimethyl sulphoxide	dimethyl sulfoxide	methimazole	thiamazole
dioxathion	*dioxation*	*methindizate*	*metindizate*
dipenine bromide	*diponium bromide*	*methisazone*	*metisazone*
diphenidol	*difenidol*	*methixene*	*metixene*
disulphamide	*disulfamide*	methohexitone	methohexital
doxybetasol	*doxibetasol*	*methoin*	*mephenytoin*
doxycycline hydrochloride (hemihydrate hemiethanolate)	doxycycline hyclate	methotrimeprazine	levomepromazine
		methsuximide	*mesuximide*
		methyl cysteine	mecysteine
dyclocaine	*dyclonine*	*methylene blue*	*methylthioninium chloride*
epioestriol	*epiestriol*	methylphenobarbitone	methylphenobarbital
epithiazide	*epitizide*	*metriphonate*	*metrifonate*
ethacrynic acid	etacrynic acid	*metyzoline*	*metizoline*
ethamivan	etamivan	monosulfiram	sulfiram
ethamsylate	etamsylate	*naphthalophos*	*naftalofos*
ethebenecid	*etebenecid*	nealbarbitone	nealbarbital
ethenzamide	*etenzamide*	nicoumalone	acenocoumarol
ethinyloestradiol	ethinylestradiol	nitroxynil	nitroxinil
ethoglucid	*etoglucid ethosalamide*	*norbutrine*	*norbudrine*
ethopropazine	profenamine	*norethynodrel*	*noretynodrel*
ethosalamide	*etosalamide*	*noxiptyline*	*noxiptiline*
ethybenztropine	*etybenzatropine*	noxythiolin	noxytiolin
ethyloestrenol	ethylestrenol	*nylestriol*	*nilestriol*

UK Name BAN/BANM/BP Title	Recommended INN/INNM	UK Name BAN/BANM/BP Title	Recommended INN/INNM
octacosactrin	*tosactide*	*sulphamethoxydiazine*	*sulfametoxydiazine*
octaphonium chloride	octafonium chloride	sulphamethoxypyridazine	sulfametoxypyridazine
oestradiol	estradiol	*sulphamoxole*	*sulfamoxole*
oestriol	estriol	*sulphaphenazole*	*sulfaphenazole*
oestriol sodium succinate	estriol sodium succinate	*sulphaproxyline*	*sulfaproxyline*
oestriol succinate	estriol succinate	sulphasalazine	sulfasalazine
oestrone	estrone	*sulphasomidine*	*sulfisomidine*
oxethazaine	oxetacaine	*sulphasomizole*	*sulfasomizole*
oxyphenisatin	oxyphenisatine	sulphathiazole	sulfathiazole
oxypurinol	*oxipurinol*	*sulphathiourea*	*sulfathiourea*
pentaerythritol tetranitrate	pentaerithrityl tetranitrate	*sulphatolamide*	*sulfatolamide*
pentobarbitone	pentobarbital	sulphaurea	sulfacarbamide
pentolinium tartrate	*pentolonium tartrate*	sulphinpyrazone	sulfinpyrazone
phanquone	*phanquinone*	*sulphomyxin sodium*	*sulfomyxin sodium*
phenbenicillin	*fenbenicillin*	*sulthiame*	*sultiame*
phenbutrazate	*fenbutrazate*	tetracosactrin	tetracosactide
phenethicillin	*pheneticillin*	*tetrahydrozoline*	*tetryzoline*
phenobarbitone	phenobarbital	*thiabendazole*	*tiabendazole*
phenoxypropazine	*fenoxypropazine*	*thiacetazone*	*thioacetazone*
phenyl aminosalicylate	*fenamisal*	*thialbarbitone*	*thiabarbital*
phenyramidol	*fenyramidol*	*thiazesim*	*tiazesim*
phthalylsulphathiazole	phthalylsulfathiazole	*thiocarlide*	*tiocarlide*
pipazethate	*pipazetate*	thioguanine	tioguanine
pipothiazine	pipotiazine	*thiomesterone*	*tiomesterone*
polyhexanide	polihexanide	thiopentone	thiopental
potassium clorazepate	dipotassium clorazepate	*thiothixene*	*tiotixene*
potassium menaphthosulphate	*menadiol potassium sulfate*	*thioxolone*	*tioxolone*
pramoxine	pramocaine	thyroxine	levothyroxine
promethoestrol	*methestrol*	*triacetyloleandomycin*	*troleandomycin*
promoxolan	*promoxolane*	*trimustine*	*trichlormethine*
pronethalol	*pronetalol*	*troxidone*	*trimethadione*
proquamezine	aminopromazine	*tyformin*	*tiformin*
prothionamide	*protionamide*	urofollitrophin	urofollitropin
quinalbarbitone	secobarbital	*vinbarbitone*	*vinbarbital*
riboflavine	riboflavin	*vinylbitone*	*vinylbital*
rolicypram	*rolicyprine*	*viprynium embonate*	*pyrvinium pamoate*
salazosulphadimidine	salazosulfadimidine	vitamin A	retinol
secbutobarbitone	*secbutobarbital*	*xanthinol nicotinate*	*xantinol nicotinate*
sissomicin	*sisomicin*	*xanthocillin*	*xantocillin*
sodium calciumedetate	sodium calcium edetate		
sodium cromoglycate	sodium cromoglicate		
sodium diatrizoate	sodium amidotrizoate		
sodium ipodate	sodium iopodate		
sodium ironedetate	sodium feredetate		
sodium picosulphate	sodium picosulfate		
sorbitan mono-oleate	sorbitan oleate		
sorbitan monolaurate	sorbitan laurate		
sorbitan monopalmitate	sorbitan palmitate		
sorbitan monostearate	sorbitan stearate		
stanolone	*androstanolone*		
stilboestrol	diethylstilbestrol		
streptonicozid	*streptoniazid*		
succinylsulphathiazole	*succinylsulfathiazole*		
sulglycotide	*sulglicotide*		
sulphacetamide	sulfacetamide		
sulphachlorpyridazine	sulfachlorpyridazine		
sulphadiazine	sulfadiazine		
sulphadimethoxine	*sulfadimethoxine*		
sulphadimidine	sulfadimidine		
sulphaethidole	*sulfaethidole*		
sulphaguanidine	sulfaguanidine		
sulphaloxic acid	*sulfaloxic acid*		
sulphamethizole	*sulfamethizole*		
sulphamethoxazole	sulfamethoxazole		

List B. (cont'd): The following list concerns names of radicals and groups

UK group name	INN group name
besylate	besilate
camsylate	camsilate
closylate	closilate
edisylate	edisilate
enanthate	enantate
esylate	esilate
ethylsulphate	etilsulfate
isethionate	isetionate
mesylate	mesilate
methylsulphate	metilsulfate
napadisylate	napadisilate
napsylate	napsilate
theoclate	teoclate
tosylate	tosilate

Index

NOTES
Tables and figures are indicated by page numbers in *italics*
Case studies are indicated by references followed by (CS)

To save space, the following abbreviations have been used:

ADR: adverse drug reaction
ALL: acute lymphoblastic leukaemia
AML: acute myeloblastic leukaemia
CHD: coronary heart disease
COX-2: cyclo-oxygenase-2
CHF: congestive heart failure
CLL: chronic lymphocytic leukaemia
CML: chronic myelocytic leukaemia
COPD: chronic obstructive pulmonary disease
LVSD: left ventricular systolic dysfunction
MI: myocardial infarction
NSAIDs: non-steroidal anti-inflammatory drugs
NHLs: non-Hodgkin's lymphomas
PCP: *Pneumocystis carinii* pneumonia
PN: parenteral nutrition
VTE: venous thromboembolism

A

abacavir (ABC) 607
  characteristics *604*
abciximab 349
  acute coronary syndrome therapy 289
abdominal pain
  acarbose ADRs 671
  ulcerative colitis 167
absence attacks 467
absorption (of drugs)
  acute kidney failure 241
  age-related changes 128
  carbamazepine 14
  children 113–115
  definition 6
  digoxin 9
  interactions 23–24
    gastrointestinal effects 23–24
  neonates 101–102
    see also pregnancy
  proton pump inhibitors 154
  type A ADRs 36
  see also individual drugs
ABVD regimen 762, *763*, 764, 771–772 (CS)
acarbose 671
accelerated hypertension 267
acebutolol *286*
aceclofenac 795
ACE inhibitors *see* angiotensin-converting enzyme (ACE) inhibitors
acenocoumarol (nicoumalone) 343
acetazolamide
  ADRs 834–835
  dosage *473*
  epilepsy therapy 473
  glaucoma therapy 834–835
acetylation, type A ADRs 38
acetylcholine, arousal system 424
acetylsalicylic acid *see* aspirin (acetylsalicylic acid)
aciclovir
  drug interactions 30–31 (CS)
  infection prophylaxis *754*
  opportunistic infection therapy *609*
acid–base values 54
α_1-acid glycoprotein 24
acidosis
  acute kidney failure 237
  chronic kidney failure 258
  drug-related 327
  treatment 258
acipimox 369
acitretin
  drug interactions *858*
  psoriasis therapy 865
acneform eruptions 849, *849*, 851–852 (CS)
acquired immunodeficiency syndrome (AIDS) *see* AIDS
action potential, antiarrhythmic drug effect *329*
activated charcoal 201
activated partial thromboplastin time (APTT) 61, 62
active renal tubule excretion, drug interactions 27–28
acuphase *see* zuclopenthixol acetate (acuphase)
acupuncture
  analgesia 498
  antiemetic therapy *513*
  motion sickness therapy 516
acute asthma *see* asthma
acute bronchitis *see* bronchitis, acute
acute coronary syndromes (ACS)
  treatment 288–289
  see also angina; coronary heart disease (CHD)
acute hepatitis *see* hepatitis
acute kidney failure *see* kidney failure, acute
acute lymphoblastic leukaemias (ALLs)
  classification 744–745, *745*
  clinical manifestations 746
  definition 743
  diagnosis *747*
  epidemiology 743
  incidence *743*
  investigations 746
  pathophysiology 744–745
  treatment 747–748, *748*
    maintenance 748
acute myeloblastic leukaemias (AMLs) 757 (CS)
  classification 744, *745*
  clinical manifestations 746
  definition 743
  diagnosis *747*
  epidemiology 743
  incidence *743*
  investigations 746
  pathophysiology 744–745

treatment 748–750
  algorithm *749*
acute renal failure *see* kidney failure, acute
acute schizophrenia *see* schizophrenia
acute sinusitis *see* sinusitis, acute
acyl-CoA cholesterol acyltransferase (ACAT) inhibitors 365
Addison's disease 639–640
adenomas, thyroid 644
adenosine 332
  ADRs *331*
  paroxysmal supraventricular tachyarrhythmia therapy 326
adjuvant chemotherapy 781
adrenaline (epinephrine)
  cardiac arrhythmia therapy 327
  CHF therapy 309
  hypoglycaemia 665
  topical
    ADRs *832*
    glaucoma therapy 832
α adrenoreceptors 130
  receptor antagonists *see* α-adrenergic receptor antagonists
β adrenoreceptors
  receptor agonists *see* β_2 adrenoreceptor agonists
  receptor antagonists *see* β-blockers
adsorption 23
adult onset epilepsy 466
adult polycystic kidney disease 249
adult reference values *47*
adult respiratory distress syndrome (ARDS) (drug-related) 420
  drugs responsible *420*
adverse drug reactions (ADRs) 33–46, 44–45 (CS)
  acute kidney failure *243*
  classification 34–35
  constipation *183*
  definitions 34–35
  delayed 41
  detection/monitoring 41–42
    case–control studies 42
    case reports 41–42
    cohort studies 42
    spontaneous reporting schemes 42
  diarrhoea *186*
  drug interactions 21
  epidemiology 33–34
  geriatric drug therapy 136–137
  identification 42–43
    by patients 43
    by pharmacist 43
  incidence 33
  liver *see* hepatotoxicity
  lungs *see* lung disease (drug-related); *individual diseases/disorders*
  paediatrics 122
  predisposing factors 35–36
  skin *see* skin disorders (drug-related)
  type A *see* adverse drug reactions (ADRs), type A

adverse drug reactions, *continued*
  type B *see* adverse drug reactions (ADRs),
    type B
  withdrawal effects 41
  see also individual drugs
adverse drug reactions (ADRs), type A 34, *35*
  mechanisms 36–38
    pharmaceutical causes 36
    pharmacodynamic causes 38
    pharmacokinetic causes 36–38
  see also individual drugs
adverse drug reactions (ADRs), type B 34, *35*
  mechanisms 38–41
    genetic basis 39, *39*
    immunological causes 41, *41*
    pharmaceutical causes 38
    pharmacodynamic causes 39–41
    pharmacokinetic causes 39
  see also individual drugs
advice *see* education
α-fetoprotein 198
affective disorders 439–454, *451–453* (CS)
  aetiology 440
  age of onset 439–440
  clinical manifestations 441
  drug-related *441*
  epidemiology 439–440
  investigations 441–442
  key points 439
  patient care 450–451
  rating scales 442
  severity 441
  treatment 443–449
    compliance 450–451, 452–453 (CS)
    education 450–451
    problems *451*
  see also depression; mania
Aδ fibres 495
age
  ADRs predisposing factors 35
  COPD risk factor *398*
  hepatotoxicity 193–194
age of onset
  affective disorders 439–440
  rheumatoid arthritis 791
agranulocytosis
  definition *59*
  thionamides ADRs 645
AIDS
  clinical manifestations 600, *601*
  definition 597, 600
  epidemiology 597
  patient care 617–618
    see also opportunistic infections
  terminal care 617
  see also HIV infection; immunocompromised
    patient
AIDS dementia complex 616
AIRE trial
  CHF therapy 305
  MI therapy *290*
airway obstruction (drug-related) 414–417
  see also bronchoconstriction
akathisia 462
alanine transaminase (ALT) 215
  adult reference values *47*
  liver function tests 56–57
  see also liver function tests
alarm symptoms, peptic ulcer disease *147*, 160
  (CS)
albumin
  adult reference values *47*, *121*
  drug interactions 24
  homeostasis 54
  liver function tests 55, 215
  neonatal reference values *121*
  paediatric reference values *121*
  thyroid hormone binding *641*
alcohol abuse 244 (CS)
  dyslipidaemia 358

folate deficiency anaemia 731
  insomnia therapy 430
  methotrexate use 801
  in pregnancy 715 (CS)
  psoriasis 860
aldosterone, CHF 301
alfacalcidol *650*
  hypoparathyroidism therapy 649
  osteoporosis therapy 132
alginates 876
alkaline phosphatase
  adult reference values *47*
  liver function tests 56, 215
    see also liver function tests (LFTs)
alkalosis, diuretic ADRs 311
alkylating agents
  ADRs *769*
  leukaemia development 744
allergies
  airway obstruction 414–415
  contact dermatitis 846, *847*, 854–855,
    866–867 (CS)
  drug-related 844
  emollient bases 857
  lactational drug exposure 713
  type B ADRs 41
Allevyn 876–877
allocative efficiency 98
allogenic stem cell transplantation *see* stem cell
  transplantation
allograft 751
allopurinol
  ADRs 817
  drug interactions 817, *818, 858*
  hyperuricaemia therapy 816–817
  maintenance dose *817*
  pharmacokinetics *819*, 822 (CS)
  toxicity 817
  tumour lysis syndrome therapy 767
all-trans retinoic acid (ATRA) 757 (CS)
  AML therapy 748, 750
alopecia
  cytotoxic drug ADRs 781, 850
  interferon 850
  lymphoma therapy ADRs *768, 769*
  see also hair disorders (drug-related)
α-adrenergic receptor antagonists
  ADRs *270, 833*
  disease interactions *838*
  glaucoma therapy 832–833
  hypertension management 255, 273
  indications/contraindications *272*
α$_1$-antitrypsin
  deficiency 2121
  emphysema 399
alpha-blockers *see* α-adrenergic receptor
  antagonists
alpha-glucosidase inhibitors 671
α$_1$-protease inhibitor, emphysema 399
alteplase *see* tissue plasminogen activator (tPA,
  duteplase, alteplase)
alteplase thrombolysis for acute non-
  interventional therapy in acute stroke
  study (ATLANTIS) 131–132
alternating pressure beds 871
alternative therapies, eczema 859
  see also individual therapies
althesin (ADRs) 414
alveolitis 801
Alzheimer's disease (AD) 130–131
  prevention 702
  therapy 131
amantadine 489
ambulatory chemotherapy 785
ambulatory electroencephalography 468
American College of Rheumatology (ACR) 791
American Psychiatric Organization 441
American Rheumatism Association 792–793
American Society of Anesthesiology (ASA)
  569, *570*

amfebutamone 31 (CS)
amikacin
  ADRs *591*
  tuberculosis therapy *591*
amiloride *219*
amino acids
  conditionally essential 69–70
  essential 69
  PN *see* parenteral nutrition (PN)
aminoglycosides
  ADRs *231*
  aspiration pneumonia therapy 528
  drug interactions *858*
  infective meningitis therapy 559
5-aminolaevulinic acid (ALA) 865
5-aminolevulinate synthase (ALAS) deficiency
  see sideroblastic anaemias
aminophylline 10
  acute asthma therapy 386, *386*, 394–395 (CS)
    dosage *383*
  acute COPD therapy 404
4-aminosalicyclic acid *176*
aminosalicylates 169–171, *171, 176*
amiodarone 331–332
  ADRs *331*
    pulmonary fibrosis 419
    thyroid disease *640*
  drug interactions *335, 346*
  monitoring *203*
  pharmacokinetics *334*
  ventricular tachyarrhythmia therapy 326
  ventricular tachycardia therapy 326–327
amisulpride (ADRs) *459*
amitriptyline
  anxiety therapy *432*
  depression therapy 444
amlodipine
  drug interactions 30–31 (CS)
  properties *288*
ammonia
  hepatic encephalopathy 219
  production 54
amoebiasis *544*
  clinical features 546
  treatment 550
amoxapine 444
amoxicillin
  ADRs 844
  bronchitis therapy 523
  COPD therapy 403
  Helicobacter pylori infection therapy 149
  urinary tract infection therapy *538*
amoxiclav 403
amphotericin B 630–633
  ADRs 564, *628*, 632
    acute tubular necrosis cause *231*
  aspergillosis therapy 754
  candidiasis therapy *609*, 612, 624, 754
  chemical structure 630
  conventional preparation 631–632
    administration 631–632
    dosage *631*, 631–632
    pharmacokinetics 631
  cryptococcal meningitis therapy 563–564,
    609, 612
  drug interactions *627*
  fungal ear infection therapy 626
  general properties 630–631
  lipid formulations 632–633
    colloid *632*
    complex 632
    liposomes 632
  mode of action 630
  spectrum of activity 630–631
ampicillin
  hepatotoxicity 204 (CS)
  infective meningitis therapy *560*
  skin reactions 844
amprenavir (APV) 608
  characteristics *605*

amprenavir, drug interactions *368*
amsacrine 748
anaemias 725–742, 739–741 (CS)
  aetiology *725*, 725–726
  aplastic, leukaemia development 744
  chronic kidney failure association 251–252,
    257–258, *263*, 264 (CS)
  classification 727
  clinical manifestations *726*, 726–727
  epidemiology 725
  haemolytic *see* haemolytic anaemias
  investigations *727*
  iron-deficiency *see* iron-deficiency anaemia
  key points 725
  lymphoma therapy ADRs 768
  megaloblastic *see* megaloblastic anaemias
  normochromic.normocytic, Hodgkin's disease
    759
  sideroblastic *see* sideroblastic anaemias
  therapy 257–258
    problems *739*
  see also erythropoiesis; haemoglobin;
    individual types
anaesthetics *497*
analeptics 405–406
analgesia
  acupuncture 498
  leg ulcers 881
  leg ulcer therapy 881
  osteoarthritis therapy 807
  pharmacological *see* analgesic drugs
  rheumatoid arthritis therapy 795
  stimulation-produced 498
  transcutaneous electrical nerve stimulation
    498
  WHO analgesic ladder 496
analgesic drugs 498–501
  adjuvants 501–503
  epidural 497–498
    local anaesthetics 498
    opioids 498
  MI 289
  peptic ulcer disease 158
  see also individual drugs
analgesic ladder 496
anaphylaxis
  ADRs 414–415
  streptokinase ADRs 345
angina 137 (CS), 295–296 (CS)
  exercise-induced 281
  Prinzmetal's 281
  stable 281
    treatment 285–288
  unstable 281
  variant 281
  see also acute coronary syndromes (ACS)
angiography *293*
angio-oedema 845
angioplasty, primary, MI therapy *291*
angiotensin-converting enzyme (ACE) inhibitors
  ADRs *270*, 305, 313–314
    airway constriction 415–416
    fetal development 709
  CHF therapy 304–305, *306*
  in diabetes mellitus therapy 672
  disease interactions *313*
  drug interactions *312*, 796
  hypertension management 255–256, 271–272
    elderly 134
  indications/contraindications *272*
  LVSD therapy 302
  mechanism of action 304–305
  MI therapy 292
    mortality *292*
    studies *290*
  monitoring *311*
  see also individual drugs
angiotensin II receptor antagonists
  ADRs *270*
  CHF therapy 305–306, *306*

drug interactions *312*
hypertension management 255–256, 271–272
indications/contraindications *272*
LVSD therapy 302
animal models, epilepsy 472
anion exchange resins 368–369, 370–371
  drug interactions *368, 369*
  efficacy *365*
  pruritus therapy 216
anisocytosis *59*
anisoylated plasminogen streptokinase activated
  complex (APSAC) 289
ankle branch pressure index (ABPI) 880
Ann Arbor classification 762
anorexia 781
antacids 157
anthracyclines 747
anti-arrhythmic drugs 328–333
  action potential effects *329*
  ADRs 324–325, *330, 331*
    mortality *325*
  atrial fibrillation therapy *327*
  class I 330
  class II 330–331
  class III 331–332
  class IV 332
  disease interactions *838*
  drug interactions *335*
  electrophysiological effects *329*
  pharmacokinetics *334*
  post-MI 328
  tachyarrhythmia therapy 325–326, *326*
  see also cardiac arrhythmias; *individual drugs*
antibiotics
  administration
    intrathecal 564–565
    intraventricular 564–565
  ADRs 414
  analgesia *497*
  drug interactions 27
  eczema therapy 857
  emollient additives 857
  infection therapy 754
    acute pyelonephritis *538*
    bacteriuria in pregnancy 539
    bronchitis 523
    catheter-associated bacteriuria 539
    COPD 403
    gastrointestinal 547–550
    infective meningitis 558–565, *559, 560*
    inflammatory bowel disease 173, *176*
    neonates 103
    otitis media 521
    pharyngitis 520–521
    unavailable/unsuitable 547–548
    urinary tract 537–538, *538*
  nebulized 529
  prophylaxis
    immunocompromised patients 737
    sickle cell anaemia 737
  in surgery *see* surgical antibiotic prophylaxis
  see also individual drugs
anti-CD33 antibody 750
anticholinergic drugs
  ADRs 322, 415–416, 461
  as antiemetic drugs 516
    characteristics *512*
  asthma therapy, inhaled 381
  COPD therapy 404
  disease interaction *837, 838*
  Parkinson's disease therapy 489–490
  schizophrenia therapy 461
  withdrawal 461
anticipatory emesis 514
anticoagulant drugs 342–345
  acute stroke therapy 132
  ADRs 345
  arterial thromboembolism therapy 348–349
  drug interactions *796, 818*
  MI therapy 292–293

monitoring 61
oral 343–345
see also venous thromboembolism (VTE);
  individual drugs
anticonvulsants *see* anti-epileptic drugs (AEDs)
anticytokine antibodies 752
antidepressant drugs 443–447, 451–453 (CS)
  in analgesia *497*, 501–502
  disease interactions *838*
  drug interactions 27
  metabolization 37
  MI therapy 292
  premenstrual syndrome therapy 684, *685*
  selection 448
  therapeutic problems *451*
  withdrawal 443–444
  see also individual drugs
antidiarrhoeal drugs 173
  see also individual drugs
antidiuretic hormone (ADH) *see* vasopressin
antiemetic drugs 511–516
  administration route 784
  ADRs *512–513*
  characteristics *512–513*
  chemotherapy-induced vomiting therapy
    783–784
  classes 511
  disease interactions *837*
  regimen 511
  see also nausea/vomiting; *individual drugs*
anti-epileptic drugs (AEDs) 468–478
  ADRs *476*
  in analgesia *497*, 501
  chronic epilepsy therapy 471
  cytochrome P450 isoenzyme interaction 25
  different seizure types *469*
    see also seizures
  dosage
    changes 470
    maintenance *473*
  drug interactions *475*
  new *470*, 470–471, 472
  pharmacokinetics *474*
  profiles 472–478
  withdrawal 471
  see also individual drugs
antifungal drugs
  ADRs *628*
  drug interactions 27, *627*
  prophylaxis, in immunocompromised 753
  therapy choice 636, *636*
  see also individual drugs
antihistamines
  in analgesia 502
  as antiemetic drugs *513*, 516
  disease interactions *838*
  drug interactions *627*
  eczema therapy 857
  motion sickness therapy 516
  pruritus therapy 216
  see also H$_2$ receptor antagonists
antihypertensive drugs *270*
  ADRs 358
  placebo-controlled trials *271*
  see also individual drugs
anti-inflammatory agents
  inhaled 379–381
  see also individual drugs
antilymphocyte globulin (ALG), kidney
  transplants 262
antimicrobial drugs
  diarrhoea therapy 188–189, 190 (CS)
  urinary tract infections therapy 536–537
  see also antibiotics; antifungal drugs;
    antivirals; *individual drugs*
antimotility agents 187–188
  see also individual drugs
antimycobacterial drugs 587–592
  ADRs 590–591, *591, 592*
  choice 591–592

antimycobacterial drugs, *continued*
  dosages *588, 591*
  intermittent regimens 589
  toxicity 591–592
  see also individual drugs
antinuclear antibodies (ANA) 794
antioxidants 363
antiplatelet therapy 132
  see also aspirin (acetylsalicylic acid);
    individual drugs
antipsychotic drugs 457–462
  ADRs 458, *459*, 461–462, 463 (CS)
  anxiety therapy 435
  depots 460–461
    comparison *461*
  disease interactions *838*
  dosage 458–460
  drug interactions 461
  mode of action 457
  neuroleptic equivalence 458, 460, *460*
  polypharmacy 458, 463–464 (CS)
  regimen 457
  selection 457–460
  see also neuroleptics
antiretroviral drugs 600–608
  characteristics *603–607*
  clinical trials 602
  entry inhibitors 608
  general principles 601
  guidelines 601–602
  highly active retroviral therapy 600
  integrase inhibitors 608
  toxicity 608
  treatment goals 602
  treatment/monitoring information *602*
  zinc finger inhibitors 608
  see also individual drugs
anti-rheumatic drugs *27*
  see also individual drugs
antiseptics 857
antispasmodic drugs
  in analgesia *497*
  disease interactions *837*
  dysmenorrhoea therapy 686
antithrombin III (ATIII) deficiency 340
antithrombotic therapy
  atrial fibrillation therapy 327
  in cardiac arrhythmias 327
  CHD therapy 284
  see also cardiac arrhythmias
antithymocyte globulin (ATG)
  graft-*versus*-host disease therapy 752
  kidney transplants *261, 262*
antithyroid drugs 645–647
  ADRs 645–646, *646*
  counselling 647, *647*
  see also individual drugs
antivirals
  drug interactions *27, 368*
  retroviral *see* antiretroviral drugs
  see also individual drugs
anxiety 423–438, 436–438 (CS)
  ADRs 425
  aetiology 425
  clinical manifestations 425
  definition 423
  differential diagnosis 426
  investigations 426
  key points 423
  pathophysiology 423–425
  treatment 432–435
    problems *437*
    rational drug choice 435, *436*
    see also anxiolytic drugs
  see also insomnia
anxiolytic drugs 432–435
  ADRs 433–434
  in analgesia 502
  characteristics *432*
  see also anxiety

aplastic anaemia 744
aplastic conditions *59*
apnoea 105
apolipoprotein B-100 358
apomorphine
  ADRs 490
  Parkinson's disease therapy 490
apparent volume of distribution 4
appendicitis 575–576, 580 (CS)
apraclonidine 833
Aquacel 876
aqueous humour
  outflow 825–826
  production 825
  see also glaucoma
arachnoid mater 555
5α-reductase inhibitors 720
are postrema 510
arginine vasopressin *see* vasopressin
arousal systems 423–424, *424*
  emotional 423
  endocrine/autonomic 424
  general 423
  see also insomnia; sleep
arsenic salts 172–173
  inflammatory bowel disease therapy *176*
arsenic trioxide 750
arterial blood gases 401–402
arterial leg ulcers *see* leg ulcers
arterial thromboembolism 347–350, 350 (CS)
  aetiology 347–348
  clinical manifestations 348
  epidemiology 347
  investigations 348
  key points 339
  in lower limb 348, 879
  patient care 349–350
  treatment 348–349
arteriovenous leg ulcers 879
arthritis 133
  acute gouty *814*, 814–815
  rheumatoid *see* rheumatoid arthritis (RA)
arthropathy 862
aseptic techniques 755
asparaginase 747, *748*
aspartate transaminase (AST)
  adult reference values *47*
  CHD diagnosis 282, *283*
  liver function tests 56–57, 215
  see also liver function tests
aspergillosis 636 (CS)
  clinical manifestations *629*
  ear 626
  predisposition *629*
  treatment 754
aspiration pneumonia *see* pneumonia
aspirin (acetylsalicylic acid) 350 (CS)
  ADRs 349
    airway obstruction 415
    asthma 376
    skin reactions 843
  arterial thromboembolism therapy 348–349
  drug interactions *346, 818,* 822 (CS), *858*
  hypertension management 275
  mechanism of action 348–349
  MI therapy *291*
    efficacy *289*
    mortality *292*
  peptic ulcer disease 145–146
  pharmacokinetics *795*
  rheumatoid arthritis therapy 808 (CS)
  stable angina therapy 285
  stroke prevention 132
ASSENT 2 trial 290, *291*
asteatotic eczema 856
asthma 316–317 (CS), 375–396, 393–395 (CS)
  acute 388, 393 (CS), 394–395 (CS)
    immediate management 384, *385,* 386
    prevention 384
    treatment 384–387

aetiology 375–376
  chronic 393–394 (CS)
    treatment 378–384
  clinical manifestations 377–378
  diagnosis 377
  drug-related 376
  epidemiology 375
  extrinsic 376
  intrinsic 376
  investigations 378
  key points 375
  morbidity *397*
  mortality 375
  NSAIDs ADRs 799
  occupational 376
  pathophysiology 376–377
  patient care 387–393
    education 387–388, *388*
    inhalation devices *see* inhalers
    self-management 392, *392*
  patient history 377–378
  prevalence 375
  treatment 378–387
    guidelines *380*
    problems *379*
  trigger factors 375–376, *376*
  see also inflammation
atazanavir *605*
atenolol 331
  drug interactions 31 (CS)
  hypertension management 256
    in pregnancy 710
  MI therapy *291*
  properties *286*
  stable angina therapy 285
atherosclerosis
  leg ulcers 879
  plaques 280–281
atonic seizures 467
atopic eczema 853–854, *854,* 866 (CS)
atorvastatin 365–366
  ADRs 367–368
  characteristics *366*
  drug interactions 30–31 (CS)
atovaqone, opportunistic infection therapy *609*
atracurium 103
atrial arrhythmias 322
  definition *323*
  in pregnancy 325
atrial fibrillation (AF) 336 (CS)
  CHF 300
  epidemiology 322
  treatment 326, 327
    drug types *327*
atrial flutter 322
  treatment 326
atrial natriuretic peptide (ANP) 301
atrioventricular block 325
  degrees 325
atrioventricular node 321
atropine
  ADRs 322
  cardiac arrhythmia therapy 327
auranofin 802
aurothiomalate (ADRs) 417
autograft 751
autoimmunity 879
autologous stem cell transplantation 751
autonomic diabetic neuropathy 661
autonomic dysfunction 484
average costs 92
azapropazone
  ADRs *798*
  drug interactions *346*
  hyperuricaemia therapy 817–818
  pharmacokinetics *795*
azathioprine
  ADRs 850–851
  autoimmune hepatitis therapy 223
  drug interactions *818, 858*

eczema therapy 859
graft-*versus*-host disease therapy 752
inflammatory bowel disease therapy
171–172, *176,* 177 (CS)
kidney transplants 260, *261,* 263–264 (CS)
rheumatoid arthritis therapy 794, *801,* 802,
808–809 (CS)
azimilide
ADRs *331*
pharmacokinetics *334*
azithromycin
ADRs *591*
cryptosporidosis therapy 550, *609*
tuberculosis therapy *591, 609*

B

B19 parvovirus 792
bacampicillin 844
Bacillus cereus infection
clinical features 546
gastroenteritis *544*
bacillus of Calmette and Guérin vaccine *see*
BCG vaccine
back depression inventory 441
baclofen 502
bacterial meningitis *see* meningitis, infective
bacteriuria
asymptomatic 533
of pregnancy 539, 541 (CS)
significant 533
surgical antibiotic prophylaxis 576–577
see also urinary tract infections (UTIs)
balloon tamponade 221
balsalazide *171*
banazol *685*
bandaging 857–858
barbiturates *346*
barium enemas 167
barrier creams 881
basophil count 60
reference values *58*
basophilia *59*
Baxter infusion pump *786*
BCG vaccine 586
tuberculosis prevention 593
BCR-ABL gene 746
beclometasone
ADRs 414
asthma therapy 379, *381,* 393–394 (CS)
COPD therapy 405
inhalers *389*
nebulizers 391
bed sores *see* pressure sores
behavioural disturbances 491
Bence–Jones protein 58
bendrofluazide
ADRs 44 (CS)
CHF therapy *305*
benign clinical enlargement (BCE) 717
benign prostatic hyperplasia (BPH) 717–724,
722 (CS)
aetiology 717
benign clinical enlargement 717
bladder outflow obstruction 717
epidemiology 717
examination 719
digital rectal examination 718
histology 717, *719*
investigations 719
key points 717
lower urinary tract symptoms 717–718
classification 718
irritative 718
obstructive 717–718, *719*
patient care 721
symptoms 717–718

treatment 720–721
minimally invasive techniques 720
non-invasive techniques 720–721
problems *721*
surgery 720
benperidol (ADRs) *459*
benzamides
ADRs *459*
antiemetic characteristics *512*
benzbromarone 818–819
benzodiazepines
action on sleep 426–427, *428*
ADRs 427–429, 438 (CS)
withdrawal reactions 434
in analgesia 502
as antiemetic drugs 516
anxiety therapy 433, 434, 435, *436*
characteristics *432*
drug interactions 428
geriatrics 130
insomnia therapy 426–427, 438 (CS)
mechanism of action 427, *429*
pharmacokinetics 426
during pregnancy 429
profile *427*
see also individual drugs
benzylpenicillin
infective meningitis therapy *560*
Neisseria meningitidis infection therapy 560
pneumococcal pneumonia therapy 525
BEP regimen 787–788 (CS)
β_2 adrenoreceptor agonists
ADRs *382*
asthma therapy 379
acute 386
high-dose 382
long-acting 384
nebulizers 391
COPD therapy 403–404
drug interactions *387*
β-blockers 330–331
adjunctive hyperparathyroidism therapy 652
adjunctive hyperthyroidism therapy 647
ADRs *270,* 285, 314, *331*
airway constriction 416
hyperlipidaemia 358
psoriasis 860
anxiety therapy 435, *436*
CHF therapy *306,* 306–307
disease interactions *313*
drug interactions *312*
hypertension management 256, 271
elderly 133–134
indications/contraindications *272*
LVSD therapy 302
MI therapy 291–292
mortality *292*
monitoring *311*
ocular
ADRs *830, 831*
advantages 830–831
glaucoma therapy 827, *828, 830,* 830–832
pharmacology *831*
oesophageal varices therapy 222
pharmacokinetics *286*
properties *286*
stable angina therapy 285
ventricular tachycardias therapy 326–327
betaxolol
glaucoma therapy 830, *830,* 831
pharmacology *831*
properties *286*
bezafibrate *346*
bicarbonate, serum 54
biguanides 668–669
ADRs 669
pharmacokinetics *667*
bilateral retinoblastoma 776
bile acid sequestrants *365*
biliary tract disease 213

surgical antibiotic prophylaxis 575, 580–581
(CS)
bilirubin
adult reference values *47, 121*
liver function tests 55–56, 215
neonatal reference values *121*
paediatric reference values *121*
bioavailability *(F)* 6
biochemical data *47,* 48–55, 63–64 (CS)
acid–base 54
bicarbonate 54
calcium *see* calcium
cardiac markers *see* cardiac markers
creatinine 54
glucose 54
glycated haemoglobin 55
immunoglobulins 58
potassium *see* potassium
reference ranges *121*
sodium *see* sodium
urea 54
uric acid 55
water *see* water
see also haematology data; laboratory data
biphasic insulin *663*
bipolar disorder 439, 452 (CS), 453 (CS)
clinical manifestations 441
severity 441
therapy 714–715 (CS)
bisacodyl 184
bismuth chelate 156
ADRs 156
bismuth salicylate 188
bismuth salts 172, *176*
bisoprolol
CHF therapy 306, *306*
properties *286*
bisphosphonates
in analgesia *497*
osteoporosis therapy 132–133
bladder outflow obstruction (BOO) 717
bladder training 721
blanching erythema 873
bleomycin
ADRs *769*
pulmonary fibrosis 418
chemotherapy 788 (CS)
in ABVD regimen 762, *763,* 764, 771–772
(CS)
in ChlVPP/PABIOE regimen *763,* 764,
770 (CS)
Kaposi's sarcoma therapy 615
in MACOP-B regimen 765
in m-BACOD regimen 765
in PAdriaCEBO regimen 765, *766*
in PMitCEBO regimen 765, *766*
in ProMACE-CytaBOM regimen 765
blisters 873
'block–replace' regimen 646
blood cultures
gastrointestinal infection diagnosis 547
pneumonia diagnosis 524
blood films 746
blood pressure regulation 266–267
see also hypertension
'blue bloater' 400
body mass index (BMI)
calculation 362
dyslipidaemia therapy 362
screening tool 67
body surface area (BSA)
chemotherapy 780
paediatrics 116–117
bone diseases/disorders
chronic kidney failure *see* renal
osteodystrophy
tuberculosis 589
bone marrow
biopsy, NHL diagnosis 761
transplantation *see* stem cell transplantation

bone metastases, pain management 507
bone pain, in chronic kidney failure 253
Boston Collaborative Drug Surveillance
       Program (BCDSP) 33–34
botulinum toxin, analgesia 502–503
botulism *544*
    clinical features 547
boutonnière deformity 793, *793*
bradyarrhythmias 325
bradycardias *323*
bradykinesia 484
brain tumours 466, 479 (CS)
breast cancer 698
bretylium 331–332
    ADRs *331*
    pharmacokinetics *334*
brimonidine 833
brinzolamide 835
British Association of Cancer United Patients
       (BACUP) 767
British Association of Parenteral and Enteral
       Nutrition (BAPEN) 67
British Hypertension Society (BHS)
    blood pressure guidelines *269*
    management guidelines 267, *272*
British Thoracic Society 375
bromocriptine
    ADRs 420–421
    premenstrual syndrome therapy 684, *685*
broncheoalveolar lavage 524
bronchi 414–417
bronchiestasis 399
bronchiolitis 523
bronchiopneumonia 524
bronchitis, acute 522–523, 531 (CS)
    causative organisms 522
    clinical features 522
    diagnosis 522
    treatment 523
bronchitis, chronic 398, 408–409 (CS), 522
    clinical features 400–401
    definition 397
    pathophysiology 399
    risk factors 398
    see also chronic obstructive pulmonary
       disease (COPD)
bronchoconstriction 415
    see also airway obstruction
bronchodilators
    ADRs 416–417
    asthma treatment 379–387
       comparison *382*
       dosage *383*
       intravenous 386
       oral 381–382
    COPD therapy 403–404
       acute 404
    tolerance development 416–417
    see also individual drugs
bronchopulmonary dysplasia 103–104
    definition 103
    treatment 104
bronchospasm, drug-related *414, 830*
bruxism 425
buccal route 115, 117–118
Budd–Chiari syndrome 212
budesonide
    asthma therapy 379, *381*
    inflammatory bowel disease therapy 176
    inhalers *389*
    nebulizers 391
bulimia 509
bulk forming agents 184
bullous eruptions 846–847, *847*
bumetanide
    ascites therapy *219*
    CHF therapy *305*
buprenorphine 500
Burkholderia cepacia infections 528, 529
Burkitt's lymphoma

chromosomal abnormalities 761
    risk factors 760
burns 505
buserelin 690–691
buspirone
    anxiety therapy 434, *436*
    characteristics *432*
busulfan (ADRs) 418
butyrophenones
    ADRs *459*
    antiemetic characteristics *512*

C

cabergoline 488
caesarean sections 577
caetylcysteine 201
caffeine 105
calcipotriol 863
calcitonin 133
calcitriol *650*
    hypoparathyroidism therapy 649
    osteoporosis therapy 132
calcium 53
    adult reference values *47, 121*
    deficiency *see* hypocalcaemia
    excess *see* hypercalcaemia
    neonatal reference values *121*
    osteoporosis therapy 132
    paediatric reference values *121*
    regulation 53
       see also parathyroid hormone (PTH)
    serum levels 53
    supplements, premenstrual syndrome 682
calcium channel blockers
    acute kidney failure therapy 236
    ADRs *270*
    drug interactions *858*
    hypertension management 255, 272–273
       elderly 134
    indications/contraindications *272*
    properties *288*
    stable angina therapy 288
    see also individual drugs
calcium gluconate 649
calcium homeostasis *253,* 253–254
calf muscle pump 878, 880
campylobacteriosis
    clinical features 546
    diarrhoea 185
    gastroenteritis *544*
    treatment 188, 548
       problems 551
Campylobacter species infections *see*
       campylobacteriosis
cancer
    in children 112
    nausea/vomiting 516
    pain 505–507
    therapy 85
    see also tumours, solid; *specific
       diseases/disorders*
candidiasis 623–625
    clinical presentation 624
    diagnosis 624
    epidemiology 623–624
    neonatal infections 103
    opportunistic 612
       treatment *609–611,* 612
    systemic 637 (CS)
       clinical manifestations *629*
       predisposition *629*
       therapy 635
    therapy 624, 625
    treatment 624–625, 754
       systemic drugs 624–625
       topical drugs 624
cannabinoids

in analgesia 503
    as antiemetic drugs *513*
capacity limited clearance 7–8
capreomycin
    ADRs *591*
    tuberculosis therapy *591*
capsaicin, topical 807
captopril
    ADRs 415–416
    CHF therapy *306*
    MI therapy *291*
carbachol 833–834
carbamazepine
    absorption 14
    ADRs 44–45 (CS), 473, *476*
    distribution 14
    dosage *473*
    drug interactions 30 (CS), *346, 475,* 480
       (CS), 653 (CS), *858*
    elimination 14
    epilepsy therapy 473, 479–480 (CS)
    mania therapy 449
    pharmacokinetics 13–14, *17, 474*
       practical implications 14
    serum concentration–response relationship 14
    withdrawal 469
carbapenems 528
carbimazole
    ADRs 645–646
    CHF therapy 315–316 (CS)
    regimen 646–647
carbomers 173–174
carbonic anhydrase inhibitors
    ADRs *835*
    glaucoma therapy 834–835
    topical 835
carboplatin 781
    chemotherapy 788–789 (CS)
cardiac arrhythmias 321–338, 336 (CS)
    aetiology 322
    atrial 322
    drug induced 324–325, *325*
    epidemiology 322
    key points 321
    patient care 333
       informed consent 333
    signs/symptoms 324, *324*
    treatment 324–328
       after MI 328
       algorithm *329*
       criteria 324
       emergency 327–328, *328*
       hazards 324–325
       problems *335*
       see also anti-arrhythmic drugs;
          antithrombotic therapy
    types 322–323
       description *323*
       see also individual types
cardiac arrhythmia suppression trials (CAST)
       324–325
    class IC anti-arrthymics 330
cardiac block *323*
cardiac disease 85
cardiac fibrillation *323*
cardiac flutter *323*
cardiac glycosides
    CHF therapy 307, *308*
    LVSD therapy 302
    monitoring *311*
    problems 307
    toxicity 307
cardiac markers 57–58
    adult reference values *47*
    see also individual markers
cardiac muscle enzymes 282, *283*
cardiac output
    LVSD 300
    normal 300
cardiomegaly 300

cardiomyopathy (drug-related) *768, 769*
cardiovascular disease, diabetes mellitus 661
cardiovascular drugs
  drug interactions 27
  see also individual drugs
cardioversion
  stroke risk 327
  tachyarrhythmias 326
CARE *367*
carmustine (ADRs) 418
carteolol
  glaucoma therapy 830, *830,* 831–832
  pharmacology *831*
  properties *286*
carvedilol
  CHF therapy *306,* 306–307
  properties *286*
case–control studies 42
case reports 41–42
catatonic behaviour 455
catechol-*O*-methyl transferase inhibitors
    488–489
catheter-associated urinary tract infections 539,
    541 (CS)
causalgia 503
cavity dressings 877
CD4 count 600, *601*
cefalexin *538*
cefotaxime
  infection therapy 754
  infective meningitis therapy *560*
  Neisseria meningiditis infection therapy
    560–561
  spontaneous bacterial peritonitis therapy 219
ceftazidime
  acute pyelonephritis therapy *538*
  infection therapy 754
  noncosomial pneumonia therapy *527*
ceftriaxone
  infective meningitis prophylaxis *562*
  infective meningitis therapy *560*
cefuroxime *538*
celecoxib
  advantages 799
  drug interactions 31 (CS)
  peptic ulcer risk 146
  pharmacokinetics *795*
celiprolol *286*
Centers for Disease Control (CDC) 571, *571*
central nervous system
  ALL infiltration 748
  anatomy *555,* 555–556
  in leukaemias 746
  nausea/vomiting 510
central routes 77
central venous pressure (CVP) 234
centrilobular emphysema 399
cephalosporins
  aspiration pneumonia therapy *528*
  drug interactions *818*
  infective meningitis therapy 559, 560, 561
  nosocomial pneumonia therapy *527*
  pharyngitis therapy 520–521
  streptococcal meningitis therapy 561
cerebral infarction 348
cerebrospinal fluid (CSF) 555
  culture 558
  infective meningitis diagnosis 557–558
  NHL diagnosis 761
  sampling 557
cetrizine *217*
C fibres 495
charcoal dressings 872
Charcot arthropathy 6661
chelation 23
chemical exposure 744
chemoprophylaxis
  infective meningitis 561–563
  tuberculosis prevention 592–593
chemoreceptor trigger zone (CTZ) 510

chemotherapy 780–782, 780–784, 787–789
    (CS)
  adjuvant 781
  ADRs control 783–785
  ambulatory 785
  cellular basis 780–781
  counselling 783
  domiciliary 785
  dose 780
  drugs *see* cytotoxic drugs
  high-dose 781
  in-patient 785
  leukaemia therapy 747–751
  monitoring 782–784, *783,* 785–786
    cumulative dosing 782
    dose modification 782
    drug interactions 782–783
    quality of life 786
    toxicity 785–786, *787*
    treatment response 786
  neo-adjuvant 781
  out-patient 785
  patient education 783
  radiotherapy, with 781
  regimens 780–781
    see also individual regimens
  remission induction 747
  response, classification 786
  scheduling 780
  see also tumours, solid
chemotherapy-induced nausea and vomiting
    (CINV) *see* nausea/vomiting
children
  ADRs predisposition 35
  insomnia 431
  tuberculosis therapy 590
  urinary tract infections 539–540
    epidemiology 533
  see also paediatrics
Chinese herbal medicine 859
Chlamydia pneumoniae infections 524
Chlamydia psittaci infections 524
chloral hydrate 429–430
  characteristics *427*
chlorambucil
  ADRs *769*
  in ChlVPP/EVA regimen *763,* 764
  in ChlVPP/PABIOE regimen *763,* 764, 770
    (CS)
  CLL therapy 750, 757 (CS)
  NHL therapy 770–771 (CS)
chloramphenicol
  ADRs 734
  drug interactions *346*
  infective meningitis therapy 560, *560*
  Neisseria meningiditis infection therapy 560
  streptococcal meningitis therapy 561
chlordiazepoxide
  action on sleep *428*
  characteristics *432*
chloride, reference ranges *121*
chlormethine (mustine)
  MOPP regimen 762, 764
  MVPP regimen 764
chloroquine (ADRs) *860*
chlorphenamine *217*
chlorpromazine
  ADRs *459,* 463 (CS)
  antiemetic characteristics *512*
  anxiety therapy 435
chlorpropamide *667*
ChlVPP/EVA regimen *763,* 764
ChlVPP/PABIOE regimen *763,* 764, 770 (CS)
cholecalciferol *650*
  metabolism 253
cholestasis (drug-related) 195–197
cholestatic hepatitis *see* hepatitis
cholestatic jaundice (drug-related) 40–41
cholestatic lesions 194–195
cholesterol

absorption inhibitors *365*
  reduction 284
  see also HMG-CoA reductase inhibitors
    (statins)
cholesterol ester transfer protein (CETP)
  inhibitors *365*
cholestyramine 173
cholinergic system 130
cholinesterase inhibitors 491
cholinoceptor agonists (ADRs) 415
chondroitin compounds 807
chondroplasia punctata (drug-related) 345
CHOP regimen
  ADRs *768*
  CLL therapy 751
  lymphomas in HIV infection therapy 615
  NHL therapy 765, *766,* 770–771 (CS), 772
    (CS)
chromosomal abnormalities 761
chronic asthma *see* asthma
chronic bronchitis *see* bronchitis, chronic
chronic eczema 853, *854,* 858
chronic epilepsy *see* epilepsy
chronic hepatitis *see* hepatitis
chronic insomnia 431
chronic kidney failure *see* kidney failure,
    chronic
chronic liver disease *see* liver disease
chronic lymphocytic leukaemias (CLLs) 757
    (CS)
  clinical manifestations 746
  definition 743
  diagnosis *747*
  epidemiology 743
  incidence *743*
  investigations 746
  pathophysiology 745
  patient care 752–754
  treatment 750–751
chronic myelocytic leukaemias (CMLs)
    755–757 (CS)
  clinical manifestations 746
  definition 743
  diagnosis *747*
  epidemiology 743
  incidence *743*
  investigations 746
  pathophysiology 745–746
  patient care 752–754
  treatment 750
chronic obstructive airways disease (COAD) *see*
    chronic obstructive pulmonary disease
    (COPD)
chronic obstructive lung disease (COLD) *see*
    chronic obstructive pulmonary disease
    (COPD)
chronic obstructive pulmonary disease (COPD)
    397–412, 408–410 (CS), 522
  acute 405–406
  aetiology 397–399
  classification *400*
  clinical features 400–401
  definition 397
  diagnosis 400, *400*
  epidemiology 397
  investigations 401–402
  key points 397
  morbidity *397*
  pathophysiology 399–400
  patient care 406–407
    domiciliary oxygen therapy 407
    inhaled therapy *404,* 407
    pulmonary rehabilitation 406–407
    smoking cessation 407
  risk factors *398*
  treatment *402,* 402–406
    algorithm *403*
    problems *402*
  see also bronchitis, chronic; cor pulmonale;
    emphysema

chronic plaque psoriasis 861, *861, 868* (CS)
chronic renal failure *see* kidney failure, chronic
chronic tophaceous gout 814
chylomicrons 354
ciclosporin
  ADRs 261
    gout/hyperuricaemia 819
    hyperlipidaemia 359
    skin malignancy 850–851
  distribution 16
  drug interactions 26, 30–31 (CS), *262, 368,*
    627, 858
  eczema therapy 858
  elimination 16
  graft-*versus*-host disease therapy 752
  inflammatory bowel disease therapy 172,
    176
  kidney transplants 260–261, *261,* 263–264
    (CS)
  monitoring 261
  pharmacokinetics 16–17, *17*
  psoriasis therapy 865
  rheumatoid arthritis therapy *801,* 802,
    808–809 (CS)
  serum concentration–response relationship
    16
cidofovir *609,* 615
cilazapril *306*
ciliary ablation, laser 827
cimetidine
  ADRs *151*
  drug interactions 31 (CS), 156, *346, 627, 858*
cinnarizine
  as antiemetic drugs *513*
  motion sickness therapy 516
ciprofloxacin
  ADRs *591*
  drug interactions *346, 858*
  infection prophylaxis *754*
    infective meningitis 561–562, *562*
  infection therapy 754
    acute pyelonephritis *538*
    infective meningitis *560*
    nosocomial pneumonia *527*
    salmonellosis 548
    tuberculosis *591*
    urinary tract *538*
cirrhosis 211–212, 227 (CS)
cisapride *512*
cisplatin 787–788 (CS)
cisplatinum 788 (CS)
citalopram
  anxiety therapy *432*
  depression therapy 447
clarithromycin
  ADRs *591*
  drug interactions *346, 368*
  Helicobacter pylori infection therapy 149
  tuberculosis therapy *591, 609*
clearance *(CL)* 5
  lactation, during 712, *712*
  in pregnancy 709
  proton pump inhibitors 154
clindamycin *527*
  opportunistic infection therapy *609*
  PCP therapy *612*
  toxoplasmosis therapy 613–614
clinical risk management 96–97
Clinimex 78
clinofibrate *346*
Clinomel 78
clobazam
  dosage *473*
  epilepsy therapy 473, 479 (CS)
clofazimine
  ADRs *591*
  tuberculosis therapy *591*
clomethiazole 430
  characteristics *427*
clomipramine

anxiety therapy *432*
  depression therapy 445
clonazepam
  ADRs *476*
  in analgesia 502
  dosage *473*
  epilepsy therapy 473
  pharmacokinetics *474*
clonidine 503
clopidogrel
  acute coronary syndrome therapy 289
  arterial thromboembolism therapy 349
  drug interactions *346*
  stroke prevention 132
Clostridium infections
  clinical features 546
  gastroenteritis *544,* 546
  therapeutic problems 551
  treatment 549
clotting abnormalities, liver disease therapy
  216–218, *217*
clozapine
  ADRs *459*
  schizophrenia therapy 458
cluster headache 505
CMF regimen *780*
coal tar preparations
  eczema therapy 857
  psoriasis therapy 863
co-amoxiclav
  acute pyelonephritis therapy *538*
  urinary tract infection therapy 538, *538*
cocaine abuse 244 (CS)
co-codamol (ADRs) 44 (CS)
codeine 499
  diarrhoea therapy 188
cohort studies 42
colchicine
  ADRs 816
  gout therapy 816, 823 (CS)
  pharmacokinetics 816, *819*
'colds' 519
colestipol 368–369
  drug interactions *346, 369*
colestyramine 368–369
  drug interactions *346,* 369, *369*
  pruritus therapy *217*
colloid amphotericin B 632
colonoscopy 164
colorectal surgery 575–576, 580 (CS)
combivir *604*
ComboDERM 876
Comfeel 876
Committee on Safety of Medicines (CSM)
  ADRs reporting 42
  drug licensing 123
  ocular β-blockers restrictions 830
community-acquired pneumonia *see* pneumonia
comparator choice 92
complete response (CR) 786
Compleven 78
complexing reactions, drug interactions 23
complex partial seizures 467
compliance
  affective disorders 450–451, 452–453 (CS)
  costs 97
  paediatrics 120
  tuberculosis therapy 593
compression systems 880–881
computed tomography (CT)
  angiography 341
  arterial thromboembolism investigation 348
  chronic kidney failure investigation 250
  helical 341
  liver disease diagnosis 215
  spiral 341
conditionally essential amino acids 69–70
congenital abnormality
  in children 112
  definition 707

congestive heart failure (CHF) 299–320,
    315–318 (CS)
  aetiology 300, *304*
  classification 299, *299*
  clinical guidelines 309
  clinical manifestations 301, *301*
  epidemiology 299–300
  investigations 301–302
    physical examination 301
  key points 299
  pathophysiology 300–301
  patient care 309–314
    diet 310
    education 309–310, *311*
    exercise 310
    monitoring 309–310, *311*
  treatment 302–309
    efficacy 310, *312*
    indications *303*
    safety 310–315, *311, 315*
  see also left ventricular systolic dysfunction
    (LVSD)
conjugated bilirubin 56
contraceptives, oral *see* oral contraceptives
CONSENSUS II trial
  CHF therapy 305
  MI therapy *290*
CONSENSUS I trial 305
constipation 179–185, 189 (CS)
  aetiology 180–181, *181*
    drug-related *183,* 500–501
  definition 179
  drug therapy 184–185
    bulk forming agents 184
    emollient laxatives 185
    faecal softeners 185
    osmotic laxatives 184
    stimulant laxatives 184
  in elderly 135, 137–138 (CS)
  incidence 179–180
  investigation
    diagnostic algorithm *182*
    patient history 181–182
  in Parkinson's disease 492
  Rome criteria 179, *180*
    children *180*
  therapy 257
  treatment 181–185
    fibre intake 184
    fluid intake 182, 184
    general management 182
    problems *189*
contact dermatitis 846, *847,* 854
  allergic 846, *847*
contingent valuation (CV) 93
  definition 98
continuous ambulatory peritoneal dialysis
    (CAPD) 259
continuous arteriovenous haemofiltration
    (CAVH) 240
continuous positive airway pressure (CPAP)
    105
continuous venovenous haemofiltration (CVVH)
    240
Coombs' positive haemolytic anaemia 490
Coombs' test 62
copper studies 485–486
coronary artery bypass grafting (CABG) 283
coronary artery disease (CAD) *see* coronary
    heart disease (CHD)
coronary heart disease (CHD) 279–298,
    295–296 (CS)
  aetiology 280–281
  CHF association 300
  clinical manifestations 281
  diagnostic factors 282
  dyslipidaemia 372–373 (CS)
  epidemiology 279–280
  familial hypercholesterolaemia 359
  family history 28

hypothyroidism therapy 643
investigations 282
mortality, location *279*
patient care 293–295
    attack diary 294
    lifestyle changes 294–295
    over-the-counter medicines 294
prevention 701
prognosis 281, *281*
risk factors 280
    modification 283–293, *284*
symptoms 282
treatment 282–283
    algorithm *294*
    pharmacological 283
    problems *295*
    surgery 283
see also acute coronary syndromes (ACS);
        myocardial infarction (MI)
cor pulmonale
chronic bronchitis 399
treatment 406
see also chronic obstructive pulmonary
        disease (COPD)
corpus luteum 679
corticosteroids
acute asthma therapy 386
acute COPD therapy 404
ADRs 856
    hyperlipidaemia 359
    inhaled *382*
    oral *382*
as antiemetic drugs *513*
asthma therapy 379
autoimmune hepatitis therapy 223
COPD therapy 404–405
drug interactions *26, 387*
eczema therapy 856–857
    formulation 857
    potency 856–857
    preparation choice 856–857
    quantities 857
formulations 169
hepatotoxicity therapy 200
inflammatory bowel disease therapy
        168–169, *176*
inhaled 389
oral 384
PCP therapy *612*
respiratory distress syndrome therapy 103
rheumatoid arthritis therapy 803
systemic 865
cost–benefit analysis (CBA) 92–93
cost-effectiveness analysis (CEA) 93–94
cost minimization analysis (CMA) 93
costs
average 92
compliance 97
direct 92
fixed 92
increasing 91
incremental 92
indirect 92
marginal 92
opportunity 92
validation 94
variable 92
cost–utility analysis (CUA) 94
methods 94
quality-adjusted life year (QALY) 94
standard gamble method 94
Coteswold staging 760, *760*
co-trimoxazole
ADRs 613
drug interactions *858*
infection prophylaxis *754*, 757 (CS)
PCP prophylaxis *612–613*
PCP therapy *610, 612*, 618–619 (CS)
in prophylaxis 758
urinary tract infection therapy 537

cough (drug-related) 314
Counhahan model 122
counselling
chemotherapy 783
Hodgkin's disease 767
tuberculosis 593–594
COX-1 inhibitors 796–797
COX-2 inhibitors 796–797, *797*, 799
dysmenorrhoea therapy 686, *687*
peptic ulcer disease 146
Coxiella burnetii infections 524
'cradle cap' 855–856
cranberry juice 539
C-reactive protein (CRP)
rheumatoid arthritis 793–794
values 61
creatine kinase (CK)
adult reference values *47*
as cardiac marker 57
CHD diagnosis 282, *283*
creatinine 54
adult reference values *47, 121*
neonatal reference values *121*
paediatric reference values *121*
serum levels 54
creatinine clearance 8
acute kidney failure 232–233, *233*
Crohn's disease 163–166, 177 (CS)
aetiology 163–164
clinical manifestations 164, *165*
    relation to pathophysiology *164*
epidemiology 163
investigations 164–166
pathophysiology 164
    relation to clinical symptoms *164*
see also inflammatory bowel disease
cromones 379
cryptococcosis 637 (CS)
clinical manifestations *629*, 630
meningitis 637 (CS)
    opportunistic, management *609–610*, 612
    treatment 563–564
    see also meningitis, infective
predisposition 629
cryptogenic epilepsy 466, 479 (CS)
Cryptosporidium infections *see* cryptosporidosis
cryptosporidosis
clinical features 546
gastroenteritis *544*
management 614
opportunistic, management *609*
treatment 549–550
    problems 551
cumulative dose *711*
cumulative dosing 782
CURE trials 289
Cutifilm 877
cyanocobalamin 730
vitamin B$_{12}$ deficiency anaemia therapy 733
cyclic infusions 79
cyclizine *513*
cyclogest 683
cyclo-oxygenase (COX) 796
cyclophosphamide
ADRs *768, 769*
chemotherapy *780*
    ALL 748
    in CHOP *see* CHOP regimen
    CLL 750
    in MACOP-B regimen 765
    in m-BACOD regimen 765
    in PAdriaCEBO regimen 765, *766*
    in PMitCEBO regimen 765, *766*
    in ProMACE-CytaBOM regimen 765
rheumatoid arthritis therapy 802
cycloserine
ADRs *591*
tuberculosis therapy *591*
cyproterone
ADRs 708–709

monitoring *203*
cystic fibrosis 527
cystitis 533
cytarabine
ALL chemotherapy *748*
AML therapy 748
in ProMACE-CytaBOM regimen 765
cytochrome P450 isoenzymes
drug metabolism 24–26
    anti-ulcer drugs 154–155
    prediction 26
induction 24–26, *26*
    drugs *25*
inhibition 26, *27*
    dose-relation 26
    drugs *25, 27*
polymorphisms 24, 154
subfamilies 24
substrates *25*
type A ADRs 37
cytomegalovirus infection 614–615
gastrointestinal tract 615
retinitis 614–615
    therapy *609–612*
therapy *610–612*
cytoscopy, flexible 719
cytotoxic drugs 787–789 (CS)
ADRs 781–782
    control 783–785
analogues 781
drug interactions 782–783, 817
emetogenic levels 514, *515*, 783, *784*
extravasation 785, *785*
formulations 782
leukaemia development 744
monitoring *see* chemotherapy
psoriasis therapy 864–865
resistance 782
see also tumours, solid
cytotoxic lesions 194–195
cytotoxin-associated gene A *(CagA)* proteins
        144

D

dacarbazine
in ABVD regimen 762, *763*, 764, 771–772
        (CS)
ADRs *769*
danaparoid 343
danazol
endometriosis therapy 691, 692 (CS)
menorrhagia therapy *689*
premenstrual syndrome therapy 684
dantrolene
in analgesia 502
monitoring *203*
dantron 184
dapsone *818*
PCP prophylaxis *613*
PCP therapy *610, 612*
daunorubicin
ALL chemotherapy *748*
AML therapy 748, 757 (CS)
Kaposi's sarcoma therapy 615
D-dimers 62
dead space 119
debridement 876
decision analysis techniques 94–96, *95, 96*
decision trees 94–95, *95*, 95–96
decubitus ulcer *see* pressure sores
deep vein thrombosis (DVT) *see* venous
        thromboembolism (VTE)
defibrillators 326–327
dehydration
diarrhoea complications 186
treatment 187, *187*

delavirdine (DLV) 607
    characteristics *603*
delayed emesis 514
δ-waves 424
dementia 130–131
    causes *130*
    see also Alzheimer's disease (AD); multi-
        infarct dementia (MID)
dementia praecox 455
depots, antipsychotic drugs 460–461, *461*
depression 439, 451–452 (CS), 452 (CS), 453
        (CS)
    clinical manifestations 441
    diagnostic criteria *442*
    insomnia 425
    Parkinson's disease 491
    signs/symptoms *442*
    treatment 443–448
        non-pharmacological 447–448
        pharmacology 443–447
            see also individual drugs
        in pregnancy 715 (CS)
dermatitis *see* eczema
dermatophytosis 625–626
    causative organisms 625
    clinical features 625
    diagnosis 625
    epidemiology 625
    therapy 625–626
        systemic 625–626
        topical 625
Dermograft 882
desferrioxamine
    iron poisoning therapy 200
    sideroblastic anaemia therapy 734–735
desitryptamine 37
detrusor instability 135
dexamethasone
    as antiemetic drugs 511, *513*
    bronchopulmonary dysplasia therapy 104
    in m-BACOD regimen 765
    neuropathic pain management 506
    suppression test 442
dexketoprofen *795*
dextromoramide 499
dextropropoxyphene 499
    drug interactions *346*
diabetes mellitus 657–678, 674–677 (CS)
    aetiology 657–658
        classification *658*
    clinical manifestations 659
    complications 660–661
        cardiovascular disease 661
            CHD 280
        chronic kidney failure association 249
        diabetic foot 661, 675–676 (CS)
        dyslipidaemia 357
        eye disease 660
        hypertension *see* hypertension
        infections 661, 675–676 (CS)
        ischaemic ulcers 879
        nerve damage *see* diabetic neuropathy
        urinary tract disease 660
    epidemiology 657
    glycaemic control 673–674
        clinics 673–674
        at home 673
        National Service Framework 674
    insulin-dependent *see* diabetes mellitus type I
    investigations 659–660
    non-insulin-dependent *see* diabetes mellitus
        type II
    pathophysiology 658–659
    patient care 672–674
        education 672, *672*
        management targets 672–673
    PN 85
    therapy 661–672
        carbohydrate intake 661
        diet 661–662, *662*

fat intake 662
    fibre intake 662
    type I *see* diabetes mellitus type I
    type II *see* diabetes mellitus type II
    see also glucose; insulin
diabetes mellitus type I 675–676 (CS)
    aetiology 657–658
    clinical manifestations 659
    complications
        dyslipidaemia 357
        see also diabetes mellitus
    epidemiology 657
    glycaemic control 673
    insulin therapy 662–665
        adverse effects 665
        delivery 664
        dose adjustment 665
        glargine 664
        preparations *see* insulin; *individual types*
        regimens 664–665
        species 662
        storage 665
        types *see* insulin
    investigations *see* diabetes mellitus
    pathophysiology *see* diabetes mellitus
    patient care 673
    patient education *see* diabetes mellitus
    see also diabetes mellitus
diabetes mellitus type II 674–677 (CS)
    aetiology 658
    clinical manifestations 659
    complications
        dyslipidaemia 357, 371–372 (CS)
        see also diabetes mellitus
    epidemiology 657
    glycaemic control 673
    investigations *see* diabetes mellitus
    management 665–671
        algorithm *666*
        insulin therapy 671, 674 (CS)
        treatment choice 665–671
        see also individual drugs
    pathophysiology *see* diabetes mellitus
    patient care 673
    see also diabetes mellitus
Diabetes UK 672
diabetic foot 661, 675–676 (CS)
diabetic ketoacidosis 659
diabetic nephropathy 660
diabetic neuropathy 660–661
    autonomic 661
    distal sensory 661
    proximal motor 661
diabetic proximal motor neuropathy 661
diabetic retinopathy 660
Diagnostic and Statistical Manual of Mental
        Disorders (DSM IV) 441–442
    depression diagnostic criteria *442*
    mania diagnosis *443*
    schizophrenia classification 455
diamorphine 499
diarrhoea 185–189, 189–190 (CS)
    acute-onset 185–186
    aetiology 185
    complications 186
    definition 185
    drug-related 185, *186*
    drug therapy 187–189
        antimicrobials 188–189, 190 (CS)
        antimotility agents 187–188
        bismuth salicylate 188
        codeine 188
        diphenoxylate 188
        loperamide 188
        morphine 188
    incidence 185
    investigations 186
    symptoms/signs 185–186
    treatment 186–189, 189–190 (CS)
        of complications 186–187

hygiene 187
    oral rehydration solution 187, *187*
    problems *189*
    see also gastrointestinal infections
diazepam
    in analgesia 502
    anxiety therapy 434, 435
    characteristics *427, 432*
    drug interactions 154
    epilepsy therapy 473
    neonatal seizure therapy 106
    pharmacokinetics *474*
dibenoxazepine tricyclics (ADRs) *459*
dichloralphenazone 429–430
diclofenac
    gastrointestinal complications risk *798*
    gout therapy 816
    hepatotoxicity 204 (CS)
    pharmacokinetics *795*
    rheumatoid arthritis therapy 808–809 (CS),
        808 (CS), 809–810 (CS)
didanosine (ddt) 607, *627*
    characteristics *604*
dietary fibre
    constipation 184
    diabetes mellitus therapy 662
diets
    CHF therapy 310
    diabetes mellitus therapy 661–662, *662*
    dyslipidaemia therapy 362–363, 370, *370*
    eczema therapy 859
    endometriosis therapy 691
    gout 813–814
    Mediterranean 362
    solid tumours 776
    supplements, premenstrual syndrome therapy
        682–683, *685*
differential white cell count *58*
diflunisal *795*
DIGAMI trial 292
digital rectal examination 718
digitoxin *308*
digoxin 332–333
    absorption 9
    action/uses 9
    ADRs 314, 332, *333*
    CHF therapy 307, *308,* 315–316 (CS), 316
        (CS)
    disease interactions *313*
    distribution 9
    drug interactions *312, 333, 368, 627*
    elimination 9
    geriatrics 130
    LVSD therapy 302
    pharmacokinetics 9, *17,* 18–19 (CS), *334*
        practical implications 9
    problems 307
    serum concentration–response relationship 9
    toxicity 307
dihydrocodeine 499
    rheumatoid arthritis therapy *795*
dihydrotachysterol *650*
dilator muscle theory 826
diltiazem 332
    ADRs *331*
    MI therapy 292
    pharmacokinetics *334*
    properties *288*
diphenoxylate 188
diphenylbutylpiperidines (ADRs) *459*
dipipanone 499
dipivefrine 832
dipyridamole 349
direct costs 92
discoid eczema 856
discounting 94
    definition 98
disease-modifying anti-rheumatic drugs
        (DMARDs) 794, 799–803
    ADRs *801*

combination therapy 802–803
dosage 800, *801*
mechanism of action 800
monitoring *801*
new developments 803–804
patient information 800–801
toxicity 800–801
see also individual drugs
disinhibition
anxiolytic drug ADRs 433
bipolar disorder 441
disopyramide
ADRs 330
drug interactions *335*
pharmacokinetics *334*
Wolff–Parkinson–White syndrome therapy 331
displacement volume 119
disseminated intravascular coagulation (DIC) 746
distal arthritis 862, 868 (CS)
distal interphalangeal joints 806
distal sensory diabetic neuropathy 661
distribution (of drugs)
acute kidney failure 241–242
age-related changes 128
carbamazepine 14
ciclosporin 16
digoxin 9
gentamicin 10
lithium 12
neonates 102
paediatrics 115
protein binding 115
phenobarbitol 15
phenytoin 13
in pregnancy, protein binding 709
theophylline 10
type A ADRs 36
valproate 15
distribution, volume of *4, 4–5*
apparent 4
α phase 5
β phase 5
in pregnancy 709
two-compartment model *5*
dithranol
ingram regimen 863
psoriasis therapy 863, 868 (CS)
short-contact regimen 863
diuretics
ADRs *270*, 310, 311–313
gout/hyperuricaemia 819
hyperlipidaemia 358
induced glucose intolerance 311
ascites therapy 218, *219*
CHF therapy 302–304, *305*
disease interactions *313*
drug interactions *312, 450, 796*
hypertension management 269, 271
indications/contraindications *272*
monitoring *311*
premenstrual syndrome therapy 683, *685*
dizziness 324
DNA testing 485–486
dobutamine
acute kidney failure therapy 236
CHF therapy *308*, 309
docusate sodium 185
dofetilide
ADRs *331*
pharmacokinetics *334*
domiciliary chemotherapy 785
domperidone *512*
donepezil 131
dopamine
acute kidney failure therapy 236
CHF therapy *308*, 308–309
lactational effects 714
premenstrual syndrome 681

dopamine agonists
ADRs 488
Parkinson's disease therapy 488
dopamine D$_2$ post-synaptic receptors 448–449
dopamine theory of schizophrenia 457
dopexamine
acute kidney failure therapy 236
CHF therapy *308*
Doppler ultrasound 348
dorzolamide 835, 839 (CS), 840–841 (CS), 840 (CS)
dose–concentration relationships *8*
lithium 11
dosulepin (dothiepin)
anxiety therapy *432*
depression therapy 445, 453 (CS)
dothiepin *see* dosulepin (dothiepin)
doxapram 405–406
doxazosin 273
doxepin 445
doxorubicin (adriamycin, hydroxydaunorubicin)
in ABVD regimen 762, *763*, 764, 771–772 (CS)
ADRs 768, *769*, 782
in ChlVPP/EVA regimen *763*, 764
in ChlVPP/PABIOE regimen *763*, 764, 770 (CS)
in CHOP *see* CHOP regimen
formulation 782
Kaposi's sarcoma therapy 615
in MACOP-B regimen 765
in m-BACOD regimen 765
in PAdriaCEBO regimen 765, *766*
in ProMACE-CytaBOM regimen 765
doxycyline 403
dressings
cavity 877
film 877
leg ulcers 881
pressure sores 874
soft silicone 877
droperidol
antiemetic characteristics *512*
mania therapy 448–449
drug holidays 458
drug interactions 21–32, 30–31 (CS), 316–318 (CS)
definition 21
epidemiology 22
susceptible patients 22
high-risk drugs 22
mechanisms 22–30
NHL therapy 772 (CS)
pharmacodynamic interactions 28–30
additive/synergistic interactions *28*, 28–29
antagonistic interactions 28
drug transport mechanisms 29
electrolyte balance disturbances 29
fluid homeostasis disturbance 29
indirect 29–30
pharmacokinetic interactions 22–28
absorption *see* absorption
drug displacement interactions 24
drug metabolism 24–26
see also cytochrome P450
elimination *see* elimination
self-therapy 21
see also polypharmacy; *individual drugs*
drug licensing process
marketing authorization 123
paediatrics 123–124
recent legislation 124
product licence (PL) 123
drug metabolism 37
drug reactions *see* adverse drug reactions (ADRs)
drug-related diseases/disorders *see individual diseases/disorders*
drug transport mechanisms 29
drying agents 857

dry-powder inhalers 390–391
dual chamber bags 78
duodenal ulcer *143*
Dupuytren's contracture 6661
dura mater 555
dust mite allergy 375–376
dydrogesterone 683
dysfunctional uterine bleeding 688
dyslipidaemia 353–374, 371–373 (CS)
aetiology 355–359
alcohol abuse 358
chronic renal failure 358
diabetes mellitus 357
drug-related 358–359
see also individual drugs
epidemiology 353–354
population studies 353–354, *354*
hypothyroidism 357
key points 353
nephrotic syndrome 358
obesity 358
patient care 370–371
primary 355–356
pharmacological therapy 363
risk assessment 359
risk assessment 359
screening algorithm *364*
secondary 356–359
associated disorders *357*
drug-related *357*
pharmacological therapy 363–364
risk assessment 359
treatment 359–370
algorithm *364*
body weight 362
diet 362–363, 370, *370*
exercise 363
lifestyle 362
lipid profile 359, 362
pharmacological 363–364, 370–371
see also lipid-lowering therapy
see also individual diseases/disorders
dysmenorrhoea 684–687, 692 (CS)
aetiology 684–685, *685*
epidemiology 684
pain management 505
primary 684–686, 691–692 (CS)
aetiology 684–685
symptoms 684–685
secondary
aetiology 686
symptoms 686
treatment 686–687
treatment 686–687, *687*
dysmorphogenesis
definition 707
drug exposure effects 708
dyspepsia 161 (CS)
peptic ulcer disease 143
dyspnoea
CHF 301
in COPD 405
paroxysmal nocturnal 301
dystonia 462

E

echinocandins 635
echocardiography 301–302
ectopic arrhythmias 336 (CS)
definition 323
eczema 853–859, 866–867 (CS)
acute 853
allergic contact dermatitis 846, *847*, 854–855, 866–867 (CS)
asteatotic 856
atopic 853–854, *854*, 866 (CS)

eczema, *continued*
  chronic 853, *854,* 858
  clinical features 853
  clinical types 853–856
  contact dermatitis 846, *847, 854*
  discoid 856
  flexural *854*
  herpeticum *854*
  key points 853
  leg ulcers 881
  pathophysiology 853
  patient care 859
  primary irritant dermatitis 846, *847,* 855
  seborrhetic 855–856, *856*
  treatment 856–859
    algorithm *860*
    problems *867*
  varicose/stasis 856
  see also skin disorders (drug-related)
eczema herpeticum *854*
education
  affective disorders 450–451
  CHF therapy *311*
  tuberculosis 593
efavirenz (EFV) *603,* 607–608
efficiency 98
eicosanoids *680*
elderly *see* geriatrics
electrocardiography *323*
  cardiac arrhythmias 322–323
  CHD diagnosis 282
  12-lead 282
  PR interval 323
  P wave 323
  QRS complex 323
  QT interval 323
    ADRs *323*
  ultrasound 282
electroconvulsive therapy (ECT) 447
electroencephalograpy
  ambulatory 468
  in epilepsy 466, 467
  video-telemetry 468
electrolyte balance
  chronic kidney failure 252
  drug interactions 29
electrolytes
  adult reference values *47*
  PN 74, *76*
  replacement 547
elimination (of drugs) 5–6
  carbamazepine 14
  ciclosporin 16
  clearance *(CL)* 5
    in pregnancy 709
  digoxin 9
  elimination rate constant (k_e) 5–6
  first order 5, *6*
  gentamicin 11
  half life ($t_{1/2}$) 6
  interactions 26–28
    active renal tubule excretion changes
      27–28
    renal blood flow changes 28
    urinary pH changes 27
  lithium 12
  neonates 102
  phenobarbitol 15
  phenytoin 13
  theophylline 10
  total body elimination 5
  type A ADRs 37
  valproate 15
  zero order 5
elimination rate constant (k_e) 5–6
ELITE trial 306
embryonic stage
  definition 707
  drug exposure effects 708
emesis, acute 511, 514

emetogenic potential 783, *784*
emollient laxatives 185
emollients
  eczema therapy 856
  psoriasis therapy 863
emotional arousal systems 423
emphysema 398–399, 409–410 (CS)
  centrilobular 399
  clinical features 401
  definition 397
  panacinar 399
  pathophysiology 399–400
  see also chronic obstructive pulmonary
    disease (COPD)
enalapril *306,* 316 (CS)
encephalopathy, liver *see* hepatic
  encephalopathy
endocarditis 576
endocrinology 440
endometrial ablation 689–690
endometriosis 690–691, 692 (CS)
  aetiology 690
  epidemiology 690
  infertility link 690
  symptoms 690
  therapy 703 (CS)
  treatment 690–691
endometrium 699
endorphins 495
endoscopy
  oesophageal varices therapy 221
  ulcerative colitis investigations 167
endothelins 685–686
enemas 169, *169*
enoximone *308*
entacapone 488–489
Entamoeba histolytica infections *see* amoebiasis
enteric fever 546–547, 550 (CS)
  therapeutic problems 551
  treatment 548
enteroinvasive *Escherichia coli 544*
enteropathic *Escherichia coli 544*
enterotoxigenic *Escherichia coli 544*
enterotoxins 545
entry inhibitors, antiretroviral drugs 608
eosinophil count 60–61
  reference values *58*
eosinophilia (drug-related) 419–420
eosinophils 377
Epidermophyton species infections *see*
  dermatophytosis
epidural analgesia 497–498
epiglottitis, acute 520
epilepsy 465–482, 479–480 (CS)
  adult onset 466
  aetiology 466
  animal models 472
  chronic 471
    development 465
  clinical manifestations 467
  cryptogenic 466, 479 (CS)
  diagnosis 467–468
  differential diagnosis 467–468
  epidemiology 465–466
  febrile seizures 466
  incidence 465
  key points 465
  mortality 466
  prevalence 465
  prognosis 465
  remission 465
  treatment 468–478
    cessation 471
    general principles 469–471
    long-term 468
    maintenance dosage 469
    monitoring *see* therapeutic drug monitoring
    problems *478*
    regimen changes 469–470
    during seizures 468

    therapy initiation 468, 469, 480 (CS)
  see also seizures
epinephrine *see* adrenaline (epinephrine)
epoetin 258
Epstein–Barr virus
  Hodgkin's disease 759
  NHL involvement 760
  pharyngitis 520
  rheumatoid arthritis association 792
eptifibatide 349
  acute coronary syndrome therapy 289
equity 98
ergocalciferol *650*
erythema
  blanching 873
  multiforme *845,* 845–846
  nodosum 847
  non-blanching 873
erythematous eruptions 844, *844,* 852 (CS)
erythrocyte sedimentation rate (ESR) 61
  reference values *58*
  rheumatoid arthritis 793–794
erythroderma
  atopic eczema 854
  drug-related 844
erythrodermic psoriasis 862
erythromycin
  as antiemetic drug *513*
  campylobacteriosis therapy 548
  COPD therapy 403
  drug interactions *346, 368, 858*
erythropoiesis 726, *726*
  measurement 58
  see also anaemias
erythropoietin 726
  anaemia therapy 257
  sickle cell anaemia therapy 738
eschar 873
Escherichia coli infections
  clinical features 546
  gastroenteritis *544*
  neonates 103
  urinary tract 534
esmolol 331
  properties *286*
esomeprazole (ADRs) *151*
essential amino acids 69
essential fatty acids 681–682
estradiol 681
etanercept 803–804
ethambutol 587, *588*
ethionamide
  ADRs *591*
  tuberculosis therapy *591*
ethosuximide
  ADRs *476*
  dosage *473*
  drug interactions *475*
  epilepsy therapy 473
  pharmacokinetics *474*
  withdrawal 470
etodolac *795*
etoposide
  ADRs *769*
  chemotherapy 788 (CS)
    ALL *748*
    in ChlVPP/EVA regimen *763,* 764
    in ChlVPP/PABIOE regimen *763,* 764,
      770 (CS)
    in PAdriaCEBO regimen 765, *766*
    in PMitCEBO regimen 765, *766*
    in ProMACE-CytaBOM regimen 765
  Kaposi's sarcoma therapy 615
European co-operative acute stroke studies
  (ECASS) 131
evening primrose oil 683
  eczema therapy 859
excipients
  paediatrics 119
  type B ADRs 38

exercise
  CHD therapy 284
  CHF therapy 310
  dyslipidaemia therapy 363
exercise-induced angina 281
exposure estimation, lactation 711–712, 715
  (CS)
exposure timing 708–709
extracellular fluid (ECF)
  osmolarity 48, 49
  paediatrics 115
  sodium homeostasis 48, 49
  water homeostasis 48
extracorporeal membrane oxygenation (ECMO)
  103
extrapyramidal rigidity 484
extravasation
  chemotherapy-induced 785
  cytotoxic drugs 785, 785
extremely low birth weight (ELBW) 101
extrinsic asthma 376
eye disease, diabetes mellitus 660

F

factor V Leiden 340
factor Xa 342
faecal softeners 185
famciclovir 610
familial apolipoprotein C-II deficiency 356
familial combined hypercholesterolaemia 356
familial hypercholesterolaemia 355–356
  genetic basis 355–356
  homozygous form 356
familial lipoprotein lipase deficiency 356
familial type III hyperlipoproteinaemia 356
famotidine (ADRs) 151
fatigue, CHF 301
ω-3 fatty acids 369–370
fatty streaks 280
FDA Modernization Act and Pediatric Rule 124
febrile neutropenia 768
felbamate
  ADRs 478
  characteristics 470
  epilepsy therapy 478
felodipine 288
fenbufen 795
fenoprofen 795
fentanyl 500
  as epidural analgesic 498
ferritin
  iron-deficiency anaemia 728
  reference values 58
ferrous sulphate
  drug interactions 653 (CS)
  iron-deficiency anaemia therapy 729, 739
    (CS)
fetal cell transplantation 491
fetal stage
  definition 707
  drug exposure effects 708–709
fexofenadine (ADRs) 44–45 (CS)
fibrates 367–368
  ADRs 367, 369
  drug interactions 367, 368, 369
  efficacy 365, 368
  mechanism of action 367
fibre see dietary fibre
fibrinolytic drugs 345, 346
  ADRs 345
  see also individual drugs
fibrosis (drug-related) 196, 197
film dressings 877
finasteride
  ADRs 720
  benign prostatic hypertrophy therapy 720

first generation lipid emulsions 72
first metacarpophalangeal joints, osteoarthritis
  806
first order elimination 5, 6
fish oils 369–370
  efficacy 365
  inflammatory bowel disease therapy 173,
    176
fixed costs 92
flecainide
  atrial fibrillation therapy 326
  paroxysmal supraventricular tachyarrhythmias
    326
  pharmacokinetics 334
flexible cytoscopy 719
flexural eczema 854
flexural psoriasis 862
flucloxacillin
  ADRs 195
  aspiration pneumonia therapy 528
  COPD therapy 403
  staphylococcal pneumonia therapy 525
fluconazole 634–635
  ADRs 628, 634
  candidiasis therapy 610, 612, 625
  cryptococcal meningitis therapy 610, 612
  drug interactions 30–31 (CS), 346
  infection prophylaxis 754
  spectrum of activity 634–635
flucytosine 633
  ADRs 628, 633
  cryptococcal meningitis therapy 610, 612
fludarabine 750, 757 (CS)
fluid homeostasis 29
fluid intake 182, 184
fluid overload 118–119
fluid replacement 547
fluid retention
  chronic kidney failure association 251
  in uraemia 256–257
fluorouracil 780
fluoxetine
  anxiety therapy 432
  depression therapy 446–447, 452–453 (CS)
  osteoarthritis therapy 810 (CS)
  in pregnancy 715 (CS)
  withdrawal 443
flupentixol (ADRs) 459
fluphenazine (ADRs) 459
fluroquinolones 548
fluticasone
  asthma therapy 381
  inhalers 389
fluvastatin 365–366
  characteristics 366
fluvoxamine
  anxiety therapy 432
  depression therapy 446
folate, serum 63
folate deficiency anaemia
  aetiology 730, 730
  clinical manifestations 731–732
  drug-related 731
  epidemiology 730
  investigations 732
  pathophysiology 730–731
  patient care 733
  in pregnancy 732–733
  treatment 732
folic acid supplements 732–733
  rheumatoid arthritis therapy 809–810 (CS)
follicular phase 679
fomivirsen 610
fomoterol
  asthma therapy 384
  dosage 383
  inhalers 389
Food and Drug Administration (FDA) 124
forced expiratory volume (FEV)
  in asthma 378

COPD diagnosis 401
forced vital capacity (FVC)
  in asthma 378
  COPD diagnosis 401
formulations
  geriatric drug therapy 136
  pharmacokinetics 3
  theophylline 10
foscarnet
  cytomegalovirus retinitis therapy 610, 615
  Herpes simplex opportunistic infection
    therapy 610
fosinopril 305, 306
4S STUDY 367
fractures 578–579
French–American–British (FAB) classification
  744–745, 745
  ALL 745
  AML 744
friction 872
Friedewald equation 362
fructosamine, serum 673
full blood count
  folate deficiency anaemia investigations 732
  iron-deficiency anaemia 727
fungal infections 623–638, 636–637 (CS)
  deep-seated 628–636
  in immunocompromised 608–613, 628–636,
    637 (CS)
    causative agents 628, 629
    clinical presentation 628, 630
    diagnosis 630
    drug therapy 630–636
      see also individual drugs
    epidemiology 628
    predisposition 628, 629
  key points 623
  superficial 623–626
    ear infections 626
    pityriasis versicolor 626
  therapy see antifungal drugs
  see also individual species; specific infections
fungal meningitis 556
fungi see individual species
fungi, human pathogens 623
  see also fungal infections
furosemide 243–244 (CS)
  acute kidney failure therapy 235–236
  ascites therapy 218, 219
  CHF therapy 305, 315–316 (CS), 316 (CS)

G

gabapentin
  ADRs 476
  characteristics 470
  dosage 473
  epilepsy therapy 473, 479–480 (CS)
  pharmacokinetics 16, 474
galantamine 131
γ-aminobutyric acid (GABA)
  arousal system 424
  in mania 448
  pain transmission 495
gamolenic acid see γ-linolenic acid (GLA,
    gamolenic acid)
ganciclovir 610, 614–615
gastric acidity 545
  receptor stimulation 153
gastric biopsies 147–148
gastric mucosa 510
gastroenteritis 543
  clinical manifestations 545–546, 546
gastrointestinal drugs
  interactions 27
  see also individual drugs

gastrointestinal infections 543–554, 550–552
    (CS)
  aetiology 543–544
  causative organisms *544*
    see also individual organisms
  clinical manifestations 545–547
  cytomegalovirus 615
  epidemiology 543–544
  gastroenteritis *see* gastroenteritis
  in immunocompromised 753
  investigations 547
  key points 543
  pathophysiology 545
  patient care 550
  transmission prevention 550
  treatment 547–550
    problems 551
  see also diarrhoea
gastrointestinal tract
  anatomy 180, *180*
  diseases/disorders *see individual*
    diseases/disorders
  infections *see* gastrointestinal infections
  microflora
    drug interaction effects 23
    infections 545
  motility 23–24
  pH 23
  surgery
    antibiotic prophylaxis 575–576
    post-surgical infections 572–573
  ulceration 135
gastro-oesophageal reflux disease (GORD) 143,
    152–153, 160–161 (CS)
  aetiology 152–153
  complications 152
  symptoms 152
  treatment 152–153
    efficacy *153*
    licensed drugs *155*
  see also peptic ulcer disease
gastrostomy route 118
gemfibrozil, drug interactions *346*
gender
  ADRs predisposing factors 35–36
  COPD risk factor *398*
general arousal systems 423
generalized pustular psoriasis 862
generalized seizures *see* seizures
genetic polymorphism (ADRs) 36
gentamicin
  acute pyelonephritis therapy *538*
  clinical use 10
  distribution 10
  dosage 11
    changing 11
    initial 11
    once daily 11, *12*
  elimination 11
  infective meningitis therapy *560*
  paediatrics *116*
  pharmacokinetics 10–11, *17*, 18 (CS)
    practical considerations 11
  therapeutic range 10
geriatric drug therapy 135–137, 137–138 (CS)
  ADRs 136–137
  avoidance 135
  compliance 137
  concomitant illnesses 136
  dose titration 136
  drug choice 136
  drug history 136
  formulation choice 136
  hypertension management 273, 276 (CS),
    277 (CS)
  monitoring/reviews 136
  packaging/labelling 136
  quality of life effects 135–136
  record keeping 136
  treatment specificities 136

geriatrics 127–139, 137–138 (CS)
  ADRs predisposition 35
  common clinical disorders 130–135
    folate deficiency anaemia 731
    hyperthyroidism 644
    hypothyroidism 642–643
    insomnia 431
    urinary tract infections 533–534
    see also individual diseases/disorders
  drug therapy *see* geriatric drug therapy
  NHS usage 127
  pharmacodynamics 129–130
    α adrenoreceptors 130
    β adrenoreceptors 130
    benzodiazepine response 130
    cholinergic system 130
    cognitive function 129
    digoxin response 130
    orthostatic circulatory responses 129
    postural control 129
    receptor age-related changes 129–130
    reduced homeostatic reserve 129
    thermoregulation 129
    visceral muscle function 129
    warfarin response 130
  pharmacokinetics 127–129
    absorption 128
    distribution 128
    first-pass metabolism 128
    hepatic clearance 128–129
    renal clearance 128
gestrinone
  endometriosis therapy 691
  menorrhagia therapy *689*
Giardia lamblia infections *see* giardiasis
giardiasis
  clinical features 546
  gastroenteritis *544*
  treatment 550
Gilbert's syndrome 213
GISSI-2 study 289–290
GISSI-3 trial *290, 291*, 292
GLA *see* γ-linolenic acid (GLA, gamolenic
    acid)
glargine 664
glaucoma 825–842, 839–841 (CS)
  aetiology 825–826
  clinical manifestations 824
  epidemiology 825
  glucocorticoid 40
    type B ADRs 40
  investigations 824
  key points 825
  low-tension 825
  pathophysiology 826
  patient care 836–837
  primary angle closure (PACG) 825, *826*,
    829, 837, 837, 839–840 (CS)
  primary open-angle (POAG) *828*, 836–837,
    839 (CS), 840–841 (CS)
    in diabetes mellitus 660
  secondary 825
  treatment 827–836
    algorithm *828, 829*
    β-blockers 830–832
    compliance 837–838
    drugs used *828*
    problems *839*
    sympathomimetic agents 832–833
  see also aqueous humour; intraocular pressure
    (IOP)
glibenclamide 676–677 (CS)
  pharmacokinetics *667*
gliclazide, pharmacokinetics *667*
glimepiride, pharmacokinetics *667*
γ-linolenic acid (GLA, gamolenic acid)
  premenstrual syndrome 681–682
  supplements 683, *685*
glipizide, pharmacokinetics *667*
gliquidone, pharmacokinetics *667*

glomerular filtration rate (GFR), acute kidney
    failure 232–233
glomerulonephritis
  acute tubular necrosis cause 230
  chronic kidney failure 249
glucocorticoid glaucoma (drug-related) 40
glucosamine compounds 807
glucose
  adult reference values *47, 54*
  blood 83
  homeostasis 672–674
    monitoring 673–674
    target in diabetes mellitus therapy
      672–673
    see also diabetes mellitus; insulin
  infusion rate 71
  PN 71, *71*, 83
  serum levels 54
glucose-6-phosphate dehydrogenase deficiency
    anaemia 39–40, 740 (CS)
  aetiology 736
  at-risk drugs *40*
  clinical manifestations 737
  drug-related *737*
  epidemiology 39, 735
  investigations 737
  lactational drug use 713, *714*
  pathophysiology 736
  patient care 738
  treatment 738
  types 39–40
glucuronidation (drug-related) 38
glutamate 495
L-glutamine 70
γ-glutamyl transpeptidase
  adult reference values *47*
  drug-related hepatotoxicity 198
  liver function tests 57
glycaemic control *see* diabetes mellitus
glycated haemoglobin
  adult reference values *47*
  glycaemic control monitoring 673
  serum levels 55
glycerol, glaucoma therapy 836, *836*
glyceryl trinitrate (GTN) 287, 336 (CS)
  CHF therapy *306*, 308
  MI therapy *291*
  properties *287*
glycogen storage disease 212
glycoprotein gp 120 598
glycoprotein (GP) IIb/IIIa receptor inhibitors
  acute coronary syndrome therapy 289
  arterial thromboembolism therapy 349
goitre 640
gonadotrophin-releasing hormone (GnRH)
    analogues
  endometriosis therapy 690–691
  menorrhagia therapy 688, *689*
gonioscopy 827
Goodpasture's syndrome 420
goserelin 690–691
gout 813–824, 820–823 (CS)
  acute 814
    arthritis *814*, 814–815
  aetiology 813–814
    uric acid overproduction 813–814
    uric acid underexcretion 814
  chronic tophaceous 814
  clinical manifestations 814–815
  definition 813
  differential diagnosis 815
  drug-related 819
  epidemiology 813
  investigations 815
  nephropathy 814
  patient care 819
  treatment 815–816
    algorithm *820*
    problems *821*
  see also hyperuricaemia

graft-*versus*-host disease (GVHD) 752
'grand mal' seizures 467
granisetron
    antiemetic characteristics *512*
    chemotherapy-induced nausea therapy
        783–784
GranuGel 876
Granulflex 876
granulocyte colony stimulating factor (G-CSF)
    lymphoma therapy 769
    NHL therapy 765
    stem cell transplantation 751–752
granulomatous hepatitis (drug-related) *196*, 197
Graves' disease
    clinical manifestations 644
    epidemiology 643
    eye involvement 648
    see also hyperthyroidism
griseofulvin
    ADRs *628*
    dermatophytosis therapy 625
    drug interactions *346*, 627
growth factors
    in immunocompromised patients 754–755
    lymphoma therapy 768–769
guanethidine 833
GUSTO trial 290, *291*
guttate psoriasis 861, *861*
gynaecology, antibiotic prophylaxis 577
gynaecomastia 214

H

H_2 receptor antagonists 155–157
    ADRs 156
    comparison *156*
    definition 155
    drug interactions 156
    mechanism of action 155–156
    peptic ulcer disease therapy 155–156
    see also antihistamines; *individual drugs*
haem arginate 734
haematocrit *see* packed cell volume (PCV)
haematology data 58–61, 63–64 (CS)
    CHF *302*
    Coombs' test 62
    C-reactive protein values 61
    D-dimers 62
    international normalized ratio (INR) 62
    international sensitivity index (ISI) 62
    iron 62–63
    iron binding 62–63
    monitoring anticoagulant therapy 61
        common pathway 61
        intrinsic pathway 61
    reference ranges *121*
    reference values *58*
    transferrin levels 62–63
    see also biochemical data; laboratory data;
        individual techniques/measurements
haemochromatosis 212
haemodiafiltration 240
haemodialysis *239*, 239–240
    chronic kidney failure 260
    dialysis solution 239–240
    mechanics 239
haemodynamics 302
haemofiltration 240
    clearance rates *241*
haemoglobin
    Bart's 736
    concentration 60
        adult reference values *58*, *121*
        anaemia investigations 727
        neonatal reference values *121*
        paediatric reference values *121*
    electrophoresis 737

H type 736
S type 735–736
see also anaemias
haemolytic anaemias 735–738, 741 (CS)
    aetiology 735–736
    clinical manifestations 736–737
    epidemiology 735
    investigations 737
    pathophysiology 736
    patient care 738
    treatment 737–738
    types *735*
    see also individual types
haemolytic uraemic syndrome 190 (CS)
Haemophilus influenzae infections
    acute epiglottitis 520
    antibiotic resistance 521
    aspiration pneumonia 527–528
    chronic bronchitis 399, 403
    meningitis
        chemoprophylaxis *562*
        treatment 561
    otitis media 521
haemopoiesis *745*
haemorrhage
    streptokinase ADRs 345
    warfarin ADRs 345
    treatment recommendations *347*
haemorrhagic disease of the newborn 105
hair disorders (drug-related) 850, *851*
    see also alopecia; hirsutism
half life ($t_{1/2}$) 6
    phenytoin 13
haloperidol
    ADRs *459*
    antiemetic characteristics *512*
    anxiety therapy 435, 436 (CS), 438 (CS)
    cancer-associated nausea/vomiting therapy
        516
    mania therapy 449, 452 (CS)
halothane (ADRs) 203
Hamilton depression rating scale 442
hand surgery 579
hangover (drug-related) 428
Harvard Medical School 34
Hashimoto's thyroiditis 640
headache, pain management 504, 505
Heaf test 585
heart
    main coronary arteries *283*
    physiology 321–322
        cell potential *321*
        conduction system *321*
        control 321
    surgery, antibiotic prophylaxis 576, 581 (CS)
heart failure 134
Heart Failure Society of America, CHF
        treatment guidelines 309
hebephrenic behaviour 455
Heberden's nodes 815
height 113
Heinz bodies 736
helical computed tomography (CT) 341
Helicobacter pylori infection *144*, 158 (CS),
        161 (CS)
    detection 147–148
        gastric biopsies 147–148
        serology 147
        urea breath tests 147
    epidemiology 144
    eradication 149–151
        clinical studies 149
        compliance 149–150
        licensed drugs *155*
    immunization 157
    iron-deficiency anaemia 729
    pathogenesis 144–145
    see also peptic ulcer disease
heparin-induced thrombocytopenia (HIT) 343
heparinoids 343

heparins 342–343, 350 (CS)
    acute coronary syndrome therapy 289
    ADRs 342–343
    low molecular weight *see* low molecular
        weight heparins (LMWH)
    MI therapy 289–290, *291*
    paediatric PN 86
    treatment guidelines *343*
hepatic encephalopathy 219–221, 227–228
        (CS)
    aetiology 219
    clinical features 220
    grading 220, *220*
    management *220*, 220–221
    precipitating causes *220*
hepatic microsomal enzyme inducers (ADRs)
        359
hepatitis
    acute (drug-related) *196*, 197
    autoimmune 212
        treatment 223
    cholestatic (drug-related) 197
    chronic active (drug-related) *196*, 197
    drug-related 608
    granulomatous (drug-related) *196*, 197
    HIV co-infection 616–617
    viral 210–211
        diagnosis 215
        see also individual diseases/disorders
hepatitis A (HAV) 210–211
    treatment 222
hepatitis B (HBV) 211
    treatment 223
hepatitis C (HCV) 211
    treatment 223
hepatitis D (HDV) 211
hepatitis E (HEV) 211
hepatocellular necrosis (drug-related) 195, 196,
        196
hepatorenal syndrome *231*
hepatotoxicity 193–208, 204–207 (CS),
        212–213
    aetiology 194–196
        cholestasis 195–196
        idiosyncratic (type B) damage 195
        intrinsic (type A) damage 195
        lesion types 194–195
        necrosis 195
        steatosis 195
    clinical manifestations 197–198
    diagnosis 198–199
        algorithm *199*
        drug history 198–199
    differential diagnosis 198
    drugs responsible *194*
        dose related *195*
        herbal remedies 198
    epidemiology 193–194
    investigations 198
    management 200–202
        antidotes 200–202
        coagulation disorders 200
        corticosteroids 200
        pruritus 200
        supportive therapy 200
    paracetamol-induced 2065–207 (CS)
        clearance *201*
        treatment 201–202
    pathophysiology *196*, 196–197
        acute hepatitis *196*, 197
        cholestasis 196–197, (CS)
        chronic active hepatitis *196*, 197
        fibrosis *196*, 197
        granulomatous hepatitis *196*, 197
        necrosis 196, *196*
        steatosis 196, *196*
        tumours 197
        vascular disorders *196*, 197
    patient care 202–203
        counselling 202

hepatotoxicity, *continued*
  risk factors 193–194
    age 193–194
    concurrent disease 194
    enzyme induction 194
    gender 194
    genetics 194
    polypharmacy 194
    pre-existing disease 193
  risk reduction 202–203
  treatment
    algorithm *199*
    drug rechallenge 200
    drug withdrawal 200
    long-term 200–201
  see also liver; paracetamol
herbal remedies (ADRs) *198*
hereditary methanemoglobinaemias (drug-related) 40
heroin abuse 244 (CS)
Herpes simplex infections 857
  opportunistic, management *609–611*
Herpes zoster infections *609–611*
herpetic neuralgia 503
high-density lipoprotein cholesterol (HDL-C) 354
  ideal levels *353*
  lipid transport 354–355
  population studies *354*
high-dose β_2 adrenoreceptor agonists 382
high exposure drugs *713*
highly active retroviral therapy (HAART) 600
  opportunistic infections 614
high resolution computed tomography 417
hips, osteoarthritis 806
hirsutism (drug-related) 850, 851–852 (CS)
  see also hair disorders (drug-related)
hirudins 343
  MI therapy 290–291
histamine release (drug-related) 414–415
HIV encephalopathy 616
HIV infection 597–622, 618–621 (CS)
  clinical manifestations 599–600
    direct manifestations 599
    infections 599
    malignancies 599
  drug therapy 600–617
    combination formulations 607, 619–621 (CS)
    compliance 607, 618
    goals 601
    highly active retroviral therapy 600, 615
    see also antiretroviral drugs; *individual drugs*
  epidemiology 597
  hepatitis co-infection 616–617
  investigations 600
    CD4 count 600, *601*
    infections 600
    viral load 600
  Kaposi's sarcoma *see* Kaposi's sarcoma
  key points 597
  lymphomas 616
  monitoring 600
  neurological manifestations 616
  pathogenesis 598–599
    time course 598–599
    see also opportunistic infections
  patient care 617–618
  transmission 597
  vertical transmission 617
  in women 617
  see also AIDS; immunocompromised patient
HLA-DR4, rheumatoid arthritis 792
HMG-CoA reductase inhibitors (statins) 364–367, 370
  ADRs 367–368
  characteristics *366*
  CHD therapy 293
  drug interactions 366–367, *368, 627*
dyslipidaemia therapy 363–364
  efficacy *365*
  mechanism of action 364
  pleiotropic effects 364–365
  trial outcomes *367*
Hodgkin's disease (HD) 770 (CS), 771–772 (CS)
  aetiology 759
  histopathology 760
  investigations 760
  laboratory findings 759–760
  patient care 767–769
  risk factors 759
  signs/symptoms 759
  staging 760, *760*
  treatment 762–764
    advanced stage 762–764
    algorithm *763*
    early stage 762
    fields *762*
    intermediate stage 762
    patient-specific modifications 767
    relapsed disease 764
homeostatic reserve 129
HOPE study
  CHD therapy 283
  MI therapy 292
hormone replacement therapy (HRT) 696–702, 703–704 (CS)
  applications 700–702
    long-term health 701–702
    menopausal symptom alleviation 700–701
  clinical monitoring 702
  combined 699, *699,* 703 (CS)
  hypertension management 274
  oestrogens 696–699
    administration routes *697,* 697–698
    complications 698–699
    implants *697,* 697–698
    oral administration *697, 697*
    osteoporosis prevention 701–702, 704 (CS)
    topical administration 698
    transdermal administration *697, 697*
    types 696
  osteoporosis therapy 133
  progestogens 699
    complications 699
  raloxifene 700
  tibnolone 699–700
  see also menopause
hormones
  in analgesia *497*
  premenstrual syndrome 681
hospital-acquired pneumonia *see* pneumonia
hospital admissions
  ADRs 34
  drug interactions 22
5-HT *see* 5-hydroxytryptamine (5-HT, serotonin)
human herpes virus 8 (HHV-8) 615–616
human immunodeficiency virus (HIV)
  cellular infection 598
  inactivation 599
  life cycle *599*
  NHL involvement 760
  structure 598, *598*
human T-cell lymphotrophic virus (HTLV) 744
Huntington's disease, Parkinson's disease *vs.* 485–486
hyaline membrane disease (HMD) *see* respiratory distress syndrome (RDS)
hydralazine
  ADRs 308
  CHF therapy *306,* 307–308
  hypertension management 256, 273
  LVSD therapy 302
hydrocolloids 876–877
  alginates 876
  cavity dressings 877
film dressings 877
  hydrogels 876
  modified 876
  polyurethane foams 876–877
  soft silicone dressings 877
hydrocortisone
  acute asthma therapy 386, 394–395 (CS)
  eczema therapy 856, 866 (CS)
  inflammatory bowel disease therapy *176*
hydrogels 876
hydrolysis (drug-related) 38
hydromorphone 499–500
hydroxycarbamide (hydroxyurea)
  ADRs 750
  CML therapy 750
  psoriasis therapy 865
  sickle cell anaemia therapy 737–738
hydroxychlorquine 802
hydroxycobalamin 733
hydroxydaunorubicin *see* doxorubicin (adriamycin, hydroxydaunorubicin)
5-hydroxytryptamine (5-HT, serotonin)
  in affective disorders 440
  pain transmission 495
  premenstrual syndrome 681
5-hydroxytryptamine (5-HT, serotonin) antagonists *512*
hydroxyurea *see* hydroxycarbamide (hydroxyurea)
hydroxyzine *217*
hyoperfusion *231*
hyoscine
  antiemetic characteristics *512*
  motion sickness therapy 516
hyperbilirubinaemia (drug-related) 195–196
hypercalcaemia 53
hypercapnia 378
hypercoagulability
  arterial thromboembolism 348
  risk factors 339–340
  VTE 339–340
hypergammaglobulinaemia 58
hyperglycaemia 659, 660
hyperkalaemia 51–53
  acute kidney failure 237, 244–245 (CS)
  clinical features 51
  drug-related 29, *52*
    ACE inhibitor 313
  gastrointestinal loss 51
  management 237
  renal loss 51
  transcellular movement 51
hyperlipidaemia 348
  see also dyslipidaemia
hypernatraemia 49–50
  chronic kidney failure association *252*
  drug-related 50, *50*
hyperosmotic agents, glaucoma therapy 835–836
  dosages *836*
hyperparathyroidism 649–652
  aetiology 649–650
  clinical manifestations 650, *650*
  epidemiology 649
  investigations 651
  pathophysiology 650
  treatment 259, 651–652
    algorithm *651*
    hormone therapy 651–652
    problems *652*
    surgery 651
hyperphosphataemia 54
  acute kidney failure 238
  chronic kidney failure association 253
  management 258–259
hyperplasia, uterus 699
hypersensitivity pneumonitis 417–418
hypersensitivity reactions (drug-related) 592
hypertension 243–244 (CS), 265–278, 275–277 (CS)

aetiology *266*
assessment 268
CHF association 300
chronic kidney failure association 249, 252–253, *263*
  treatment 255–256
clinical presentation 267
complications *265*
in diabetes mellitus 660, 661
diagnosis 267
drug therapy 268–273
  choice 268–269, *270*
  target blood pressure 268, *269*
  treatment thresholds 268, *269*
  see also individual drugs
in elderly 133–134, 137 (CS), 138 (CS)
epidemiology 266
malignant (accelerated) 267
management 267–275
  benefits 265–266
  in diabetes mellitus 274, 671–672
  elderly 273, 276 (CS), 277 (CS)
  in elderly 133–134
  hormone replacement therapy 274
  kidney disease 274
  lipid-lowering therapy 275
  non-pharmacological 268, 275 (CS)
  oral contraceptives 274, 276 (CS)
  in pregnancy 274, 276 (CS)
  racial groups 273, 275 (CS)
  special patient groups 273–275
  see also blood pressure regulation
hypertensive retinopathy 252
hyperthermia (drug-related) 40
hyperthyroidism 315–315 (CS), 643–648, 652 (CS), 653–654 (CS)
  aetiology 643–644
  clinical manifestations 644, *644*
  in elderly 137–138 (CS)
  epidemiology 643
  investigations 644–645
  localized myxoedema 648
  treatment 645–648
    choice *645*
    counselling 647, *647*
    drugs *see* antithyroid drugs
    problems *652*
    radioactive iodine 647–648
    surgery 647
  see also Graves' disease
hypertrichosis (drug-related) 850
hyperuricaemia
  aetiology 813, 815
  asymptomatic 819
  definition 813
  symptomatic 816–819
  see also gout
hypnotic drugs
  action on sleep *428*
  ADRs 426, 427–429
  drug interactions 428
  insomnia therapy 426–430
hypocalcaemia 53
  acute kidney failure 238
  aetiology *649*
  chronic kidney failure association 253
  hypoparathyroidism 648
  signs/symptoms *649*
hypochromic conditions *59*
hypoglycaemia 676–677 (CS)
  adrenaline (epinephrine) 665
  insulin adverse effects 665
  premenstrual syndrome 682
hypoglycaemic agents *667*
  see also individual drugs
hypokalaemia 51–53
  clinical features 52–53
  drug-related *52*
    amphotericin B 632
    diuretics 29, 311, 313

management 52–53
  emergency 52
  long-term 52–53
  vitamin B$_{12}$ deficiency anaemia therapy 733
hyponatraemia 50
  chronic kidney failure association *252*
  drug-related 50, *50*
    diuretic 313
hypoparathyroidism 648–649
  aetiology 648
  clinical manifestations 648
  epidemiology 648
  investigations 649
  pathophysiology 648
  treatment 649
    problems *652*
hypophosphataemia 53
hypotension (drug-related) 305
hypotensive agents, drug interactions *796*
hypothyroidism 639–643, 652–653 (CS), 654 (CS)
  aetiology 639–640
  classification 639, *639*
  clinical manifestations 641, *641*
  drug-related *642*, 654 (CS)
  dyslipidaemia 357
  epidemiology 639
  investigations 641–642
  mild 642
  pathophysiology 640–641
  patient care 643
  peripheral 639
  post hyperthyroidism therapy 647–648
  prevalence *643*
  prevention 643
  primary 639
  secondary 639
  tertiary 639
  treatment 642–643
    drugs 642–643
    problems *652*
hypoxaemia, chronic bronchitis 399
hypoxic–ischaemic encephalopathy 106
hysterectomy, menorrhagia therapy 689

I

ibuprofen
  ADRs
    gastrointestinal complications risk *798*
    hepatotoxicity 204 (CS)
  pharmacokinetics *795*
ibutilide
  ADRs *331*
  pharmacokinetics *334*
idiosyncrasies *see* adverse drug reactions (ADRs), type B
idiosyncratic drug effects
  in lactation 713
  in pregnancy 708
ifosfamide 787–788 (CS)
imaging techniques
  benign prostatic hyperplasia 719
  liver disease 214–215
  see also individual techniques
imidazoles 633–634
  ADRs 634
  candidiasis therapy 624
  drug interactions *368*, 627
  fungal ear infection therapy 626
  mode of action 633–634
  pharmacokinetics 634
  spectrum of activity 633–634
  topical 858
imipenem *560*
imipramine
  anxiety therapy *432*

depression therapy 444
immunization programmes 113
immunocompromised patient
  infections 753–754, 755–756 (CS)
    prevention 753–754, 757 (CS)
    treatment 754
    see also opportunistic infections
  infective meningitis therapy 563
  tuberculosis 585
    diagnosis 586–587
    investigations 586–587
    treatment 590
  see also AIDS; HIV infection
immunoglobulins, serum 58
immunosuppressive agents 172
  ADRs 172
    acute tubular necrosis cause *231*
  drug-related, lymphoma therapy *768*
  inflammatory bowel disease therapy 171–172, *176*
  kidney transplants 260–261, 263–264 (CS)
  mechanism of action *261*
  primary biliary cirrhosis therapy 223
  psoriasis therapy 865
inbutamol, dosage *383*
incontinence, urinary *see* urinary incontinence
increasing costs 91
incremental costs 92
indapamide (ADRs) 44 (CS)
indinavir (IDV) *605*, 608
  drug interactions *368*
indirect costs 92
indometacin
  ADRs 799, 815–816
    gastrointestinal complications risk *798*
  drug interactions *818, 858*
  gout therapy 815–816
  lactation, during 710
  patent ductus arteriosus therapy 103
  pharmacokinetics *795*
infant dose (D$_{inf}$) 712
infant mortality 111
infant plasma drug concentration (Cp$_{inf}$) 712
infarction, cerebral 348
infections
  acute kidney failure 238
  in children 112
  in diabetes mellitus 661, 675–676 (CS)
  opportunistic *see* opportunistic infections
  post surgery *see* surgical site infections (SSIs)
infective meningitis *see* meningitis, infective
infective mononucleosis 844
infertility 690
inflammation
  airways 376–377
  cellular mechanism 376–377, *377*
  see also asthma
inflammatory bowel disease 163–178, 175 (CS), 177–178 (CS)
  drug therapy 168–175
    aminosalicylates 169–171, *171, 176*
    antibiotics 173, *176*
    antidiarrhoeals 173
    arsenic salts 172–173, *176*
    bismuth salts 172, *176*
    cholestyramine 173
    ciclosporin 172, *176*
    corticosteroids 168–169, *176*
    enemas 169, *169*
    fish oils 173, *176*
    immunosuppressants 171–172, *176*
    lidocaine *176*
    methotrexate *176*
    metronidazole 172, *176*
    monoclonal antibodies 173, *176*
    nicotine 173, *176*
    sodium cromoglicate 172, *176*
    steroids 169
    thalidomide 173
  nutritional therapy 168

inflammatory bowel disease, *continued*
   carbohydrates 168
   food avoidance *168*
   malnourishment 168
  patient care 175
  treatment 168–175
   algorithm *174*
   future work 174–175
   problems *175*
  see also Crohn's disease; ulcerative colitis
inflammatory markers 793–794
inflammatory mediators 556–557
infliximab
  inflammatory bowel disease therapy 173,
   176
  rheumatoid arthritis therapy 803–804
influenza 519
  vaccine 403
informed consent 333
infusion pumps 77–78
infusion rates 119
ingram regimen 863
inhalers 388–392
  children 389–391, *392*
  comparison *407*
  drugs used *389*
  dry-powder 390–391
  metered-dose 388–390
   breath-actuated 390
   with spacer 390
  technique 389–390
  score chart 389–390, *390*
  see also nebulizers
inotropic agents *308*, 308–309
in-patient chemotherapy 785
insomnia 423–438, 436–438 (CS)
  aetiology 425
  chronic 431
  classification 430–431
  clinical manifestations 425
  comorbidities 431
  definition 423
  differential diagnosis 426
  drug-related 423
   benzodiazepines 427–428
  in elderly 431
  epidemiology 423
  investigations 426
  key points 423
  pathophysiology 423–425
  patient care 430–435
  during pregnancy 431
  psychological 426
  short-term 430–431
  transient 430
  treatment 426–430
   drug choice *430*, 431
   drug dosage 431
   drug half life 431
   hypnotic drugs 426–430
    see also individual drugs
   problems *437*
   rational drug treatment 430
  in young 431
  see also anxiety; arousal systems; sleep
insulin
  adverse effects 665
  deficiency 659
  MI therapy 292
  preparations 662–664, *663*
   biphasic *663*
   isophane *663*, 664
   neutral (soluble) 662–664, *663*
   protamine zinc *663*
   zinc suspension (crystalline) *663*
   zinc suspension (mixed) (lente) *663*, 664
  synthesis 658
  see also diabetes mellitus; glucose
insulin-dependent diabetes mellitus *see* diabetes
  mellitus type I

integrase inhibitors 608
interferons
  alopecia 850
  CML therapy 750
  eczema therapy 859
  low-grade NHL therapy 765
  viral hepatitis therapy 223
interleukins 800
intermediate-density lipoprotein cholesterol
  (IDL-C) 354
intermittent claudication 349
intermittent regimens
  antipsychotic drugs 458
  tuberculosis therapy 589
International Association for the Study of Pain
  495
International Classification of Diseases (ICD
  10)
  affective disorders 441
  schizophrenia classification 455
international normalized ratio (INR) 62, 350
  (CS)
  condition-dependent *344*
  warfarin monitoring 343–344
international sensitivity index (ISI) 62
interstitial nephritis
  acute tubular necrosis aetiology 230
  chronic kidney failure association 249, 264
   (CS)
  responsible drugs 230
intestinal motility 545
intracellular fluid (ICF)
  osmolarity 48
  sodium/water homeostasis 48
intracoronary stenting 349
intramuscular route 114
intranasal route 115, 118
intraocular pressure (IOP) 825
  high levels 828, 830
  measurement 824
  safe levels 827
  see also glaucoma
intraosseous route 114
intrarenal acute kidney failure 229–231
Intrasite 876
intrathecal administration 564–565
intravascular volume overload 237
intravenous administration 10
intravenous urography (IVU) 250
intraventricular administration 564–565
intrinsic asthma 376
intrinsic drug toxicity *713*
iodine, radioactive 647–648
Iodoflex 876
Iodosorb 876
ipratropium bromide
  ADRs *382*
  asthma therapy 381, 394–395 (CS)
   acute 386
  COPD therapy 404
  dosage *383*
  inhalers *389*
  nebulizers 391
iron
  absorption 727–728
  binding 62–63
  daily requirements *728*
  dietary 727–728
  reference values *58*
  serum levels 62–63
iron-deficiency anaemia 727–729, 739 (CS),
  741 (CS)
  aetiology 727, *727*
  clinical manifestations 728, *728*
  epidemiology 727
  investigations 728–7
  menorrhagia 687
  pathophysiology 727–728
  patient care 729
  treatment 729

problems *739*
irritant dermatitis, primary 846, *847*, 855
ischaemic heart disease (IHD) 279
ischaemic ulcers , diabetes mellitus 661,
  675–676 (CS), 879
ISIS-1 trial *291*
ISIS-2 trial *291*
ISIS-3 trial 289–290
ISIS-4 trial *290*, *291*, 292
islet cell antibodies (ICA) 657–658
isocarboxazid 446
isoniazid
  monitoring *203*
  tuberculosis therapy 587, *588*, 591–592
isophane insulin *663*, 664
isoprenaline
  ADRs 416
  CHF therapy *308*
  tolerance development 416–417
isosorbide dinitrate (ISDN) 287
  CHF therapy *306*, 308
  properties *287*
isosorbide mononitrate 287
  CHF therapy *306*
  MI therapy *291*
  properties *287*
ispaghula 184
itraconazole 635
  ADRs *628*, *634*
  aspergillosis therapy 635
  candidiasis therapy *611*, 612, 625
  dermatophytosis therapy 625–626
  drug interactions *346*, *368*, *627*, *858*
  infection prophylaxis *754*

J

jaundice 213, *214*, 740 (CS)
  cholestatic 40–41
  drug-related 40–41
  vitamin B_{12} deficiency anaemia 732
joints
  osteoarthritis 806
  psoriasis 862
  replacement surgery 578–579, 581 (CS)
  rheumatoid arthritis 793
  tuberculosis 589
Joint Tuberculosis Committee 587, *589*

K

Kabiven 78
Kaltostat 876
kanamycin
  ADRs *591*
  tuberculosis therapy *591*
kaolin–cephalin clotting time (KCCT) 63
  heparin ADRs 342–343
Kaposi's sarcoma 616
Karnofsky performance index 778, *779*
Kernig's sign 557
ketamine 502
ketoacidosis, diabetic 659
ketoconazole
  ADRs *628*, *634*
  candidiasis therapy *611*, 612
  dermatophytosis therapy 625
  drug interactions *346*, *368*, *627*, *858*
  pharmacokinetics 634
  spectrum of activity 633–634
ketoprofen
  drug interactions *818*
  pharmacokinetics *795*
ketorolac *795*

kidney
  autoregulation 236
  biopsy 250
  blood flow 28
  calculi 249
  clearance 128
  disease
    ACE inhibitor ADRs 305
    hypertension management 274
    PN 84
    tuberculosis therapy 590
  failure 233
    see also kidney failure, acute; kidney
      failure, chronic
  vitamin D metabolism 253
kidney dialysis 239–242, 259–260
  clearance rates 241
  drug dosage 241
  forms 239–240
  haemodiafiltration 240
  haemofiltration 240
  peritoneal dialysis 240, 240
  see also specific methods
kidney failure
  chronic
    dyslipidaemia 358
    hyperparathyroidism 650
    in diabetes mellitus type I 660
    NSAIDs ADRs 799
kidney failure, acute 229–246, 243–245 (CS)
  aetiology 233
    associated factors 232
    course/prognosis 235
  classification 229–231, 231
    intrarenal 229–231
    postrenal 231
    pre-renal 229, 230
  clinical evaluation 232–235, 234
  clinical manifestations 231–232
  definition 229
  diagnosis 232–235
  drug-related 243
  drug use 241–242
    absorption 241
    distribution 241–242
    excretion 242
    metabolism 241
    nephrotoxicity 242
  epidemiology 229
  management 235–236
    dialysis see kidney dialysis
    loop diuretics 235–236
    mannitol 236
    preventative/supportive strategies 235–236
  non-dialysis management 237–239
    acidosis 237
    hyperkalaemia see hyperkalaemia
    hyperphosphataemia 238
    hypocalcaemia 238
    infection 238
    intravascular volume overload 237
    muscle cramps 238
    uraemia 237
    uraemic gastrointestinal erosions 238
  nutrition 238–239
    calorific requirements 238
    parenteral 238–239
  volume depletion 232
  volume overload 232
kidney failure, chronic 247–264, 262–264 (CS)
  aetiology 248, 248–249
    exacerbating factors 254
  calcium homeostasis 253, 253–254
  clinical manifestations 251–254
    acidosis 258
    anaemia 251–252
    bone involvement see renal osteodystrophy
    electrolyte imbalance see individual
      elements
    fluid retention 251

  hypertension see hypertension
  muscle cramps 254
  neurological changes 254, 258
  proteinuria 251
  uraemia 251
  definition 247
  epidemiology 247–248
    race 248
  investigations 249–251
    medical history 249
    physical examination 250
    urine tests 249–250
  phosphate homeostasis 253, 253–254
  prognosis 254
  stages 247
    renal insufficiency 247
    reserve reduction 247
  symptoms 248
  treatment 254–255
    dialysis see kidney dialysis
    problems 263
    symptom relief 255–259
    transplants see kidney transplants
  uraemia 251
kidney transplants
  acute tubular necrosis cause 231
  chronic kidney failure therapy 260–261
  immunosuppressants 260–261, 263–264 (CS)
  methylprednisolone 260
knees, osteoarthritis 806
Koebner phenomenon 860, 860
Kussmaul respiration 659

L

labetalol
  hypertension management 710
  properties 286
laboratory data 47–66, 63–64 (CS)
  liver function tests see liver function tests
  see also biochemical data; haematology data
lactate dehydrogenase (LDH)
  adult reference values 47
  as cardiac marker 57
  CHD diagnosis 282, 283
  Hodgkin's disease 759
lactation
  drug effects on 714
  pharmaceutical drugs 707–714, 715–716
    (CS)
    cumulative dose 711
    exposure estimation 711–712, 715 (CS)
    exposure levels 712, 715 (CS), 716 (CS)
    high exposure drugs 713
    idiosyncratic drug effects 713
    intrinsic drug toxicity 713
    key points 707
    maternal pharmacokinetics 711
    radiopharmaceuticals 713–714
    transfer 710–711
    variation 713
  recreational drugs 714
lactic acidosis (drug-related) 669
lactitol 184
lactulose
  constipation therapy 184
  hepatic encephalopathy therapy 220, 220
lamivudine (3TC) 604, 607
lamotrigine
  ADRs 476, 851 (CS)
  characteristics 470
  dosage 473
  drug interactions 475
  epilepsy therapy 470–471, 473, 475
  pharmacokinetics 16, 474
lansoprazole

  ADRs 151
    drug interactions 154
    peptic ulcer therapy 153
    rheumatoid arthritis therapy 808–809 (CS)
    ulcer therapy 798
laser therapy 720
laser trabeculoplasty 827
latanoprost 827, 835
laxatives
  emollients 185
  osmotics 184
  stimulants 184
leflunomide 800, 801, 803
left ventricular diastolic dysfunction (LVDD)
    300
left ventricular systolic dysfunction (LVSD)
    300
  aetiology 300–301
  cardiac output 300
  treatment 302
    algorithm 304
  see also congestive heart failure (CHF)
leg, circulation 879
Legionella pneumophilia infections see
    Legionnaire's disease
Legionnaire's disease 524
  treatment 525
  see also pneumonia
leg ulcers 877–882, 882 (CS), 884, 884–885
    (CS), 884 (CS), 885
  aetiology 877–879
  arterial 879
    clinical features 880
  arteriovenous 879
  autoimmunity 879
  clinical signs 880
  in elderly 134
  epidemiology 877
  investigation 880
  key points 871
  prevention 882
  treatment 880–882
    algorithm 883
    circulation correction 880–881
    healing 881–882
    infections 881
    pain management 881
    problems 882
    skin therapy 881
  venous 877–879
    clinical features 880
lente insulin 663, 664
lepirudin 343
lesions, cytotoxic 194–195
leucocytosis 59
leucopenia 59
leukaemias 743–758, 755–757 (CS)
  aetiology 743–744
    environmental factors 744
    genetics 744
    haematological disorders 744
  clinical manifestations 746
  epidemiology 743
  incidence 743
  investigations 746, 747
  pathophysiology 744–746
  patient care 752–754
    infections 753–754
      see also immunocompromised patient
    supportive care 752–753
  treatment 747–751
    problems 755
    see also stem cell transplantation
  see also individual types
leukotriene receptor antagonists 384
  ADRs 382
leuprorelin 690–691
levetiracetem
  dosage 473
  epilepsy therapy 476

moisture, pressure sores 872
monoamine-oxidase inhibitors (MAOIs)
  anxiety therapy 432, 434–435, 436
  depression therapy 445–446
  dietary restrictions 445–446
  drug interactions 450
  Parkinson's disease therapy 489
  reversible 446
  traditional 446
  tyramine interaction 29
  withdrawal 443
monoclonal antibodies 173, 176
monocyte count 61
  reference values 58
MOPP regimen 762, 764
moracizine, pharmacokinetics 334
Moraxella catarrhalis infections 399, 403
morning stiffness 793
morphine 499
  cancer pain management 505
  diarrhoea therapy 188
  MI analgesia 289
  neonates 103
motion sickness 516
moxonidine 273
MPTP (1-methyl-4-phenyl-1,2,3,6-
  tetrahydropyridine) 484
mucormycosis
  clinical manifestations 629, 630
  predisposition 629
mucositis
  cytotoxic drug ADRs 781
  lymphoma therapy ADRs 768, 768, 769
mucus production, asthma 377
multi-drug resistant S. typhi (MDRST) 548
multidrug resistant tuberculosis (MDRT) 614
multi-infarct dementia (MID) 130
multiple endocrine neoplasia (MEN) 649–650
muromonab 261, 262
muscle cramps
  acute kidney failure 238
  in chronic kidney failure 254
  insomnia 425
muscle myopathy 367
  Parkinson's disease vs. 486
muscle relaxants 497, 502
musculoskeletal (myofacial) pain treatment 504
mustine see chlormethine (mustine)
MVPP regimen 764
myalgia (ADRs) 419–420
Mycobacterium avium-intracellulare infection
  (MAI) 614
Mycobacterium species 584
  infection see tuberculosis
mycophenolate mofetil 260, 261
Mycoplasma pneumoniae infections 523–524
myelodysplastic syndromes 744
myelosuppression
  cytotoxic drug ADRs 781
  lymphoma therapy ADRs 768, 768, 769
  methotrexate ADRs 802
  therapy 784–785
myocardial infarction (MI) 296 (CS)
  acute 347, 350 (CS)
  cardiac arrhythmia therapy 328
  in diabetes mellitus 661
  dyslipidaemia 371 (CS)
  in elderly 134
  treatment 289–293, 328
    ACE inhibitors 292
    anticoagulants 292–293
    antidepressants 292
    β-blockers 291–292
    insulin 292
    mechanical intervention 293
    nitrates 292–293
    relative benefits 292
    thrombolysis 289–291
    trials 292
  see also coronary heart disease (CHD)

myoclonic seizures 467
myoclonus 425
myxoedema coma 641
  treatment 642

N

nabilone 513
nabutmetone, pharmacokinetics 795
nadolol 286
nafarelin 690–691
nails
  discolouration 850
  psoriasis 861–862, 864
naproxen
  ADRs 798
  drug interactions 818
  gout therapy 816
  rheumatoid arthritis therapy 808 (CS)
nasogastric route 118
National Association for Colitis and Crohn's
  disease (NACC) 175
National Asthma Campaign 389–390
National Eczema Society 859
National Institute for Clinical Excellence
  (NICE)
  drug use in schools 120
  peptic ulcer disease guidelines 146–147, 147
  pharmacoeconomics 91
National Service Framework 674
nausea/vomiting 509–518, 517–518 (CS)
  aetiology 513
  bulimia vs. 509
  carcinomas 516
  chemotherapy-induced 511, 514, 518 (CS),
    781
    acute 511, 514
    anticipatory 514
    control 783–784
    delayed 514
    lymphoma treatment 767, 769
    management 514, 515
    methotrexate 801
  differential diagnosis 509
  drug-related 516
    opioids 500
  epidemiology 509
  key points 509
  labyrinthitis 515–516
  management 511–517
    metoclopramide 257
    problems 517
    see also antiemetic drugs
  migraine 514–515
  motion sickness 516
  pathophysiology 509, 510
    central mechanisms 510
    peripheral mechanisms 510
  postoperative 511, 518 (CS)
    management 514
    risk scores 511
  pregnancy-associated 514, 517 (CS)
  regurgitation vs. 509
  rumination vs. 509
nebivolol 286
nebulizers
  antibiotics 529
  asthma therapy 391–392
    acute 386
  COPD therapy 404
  correct use 391–392, 408
  PCP therapy 612
  see also inhalers
necrosis 849
  hepatocellular, drug-related 195
necrotizing enterocolitis (NEC) 104–105
  aetiology 104–105

  treatment 105
nedocromil sodium
  ADRs 382
  asthma therapy 378, 381, 381
  inhalers 389
nefazodone
  depression therapy 447
  drug interactions 368
nefopam 501
Neisseria meningitidis infection
  aetiology 556
  chemoprophylaxis 562
  treatment 560–561
  see also meningitis, infective
nelfinavir (NFC) 606, 608
neo-adjuvant chemotherapy 781
neomycin 220, 220–221
neonates 101–110, 108 (CS)
  biochemical data 121
  care goals 106–107
    clinical change time-scales 107
    harm avoidance 107
    rapid growth 106
    therapeutic drug monitoring 106–107
  clinical disorders 101–106
    apnoea 105
    haemorrhagic disease of the newborn 105
    hypoxic–ischaemic encephalopathy 106
    seizures 105–106
    see also individual diseases/disorders
  definition 101
  drug absorption see absorption (of drugs)
  drug disposition 101–102
  drug distribution 102
  drug elimination 102
  haematology data 121
  individualized care 107
  infections 104, 104
    treatment 104
  parental involvement 107
  pharmacodynamics 102
  theophylline pharmacokinetics 10
neoral 261
nephropathy, diabetic 660
nephrotic syndrome 358
nephrotoxicity (drug-related) 632
netaglinide 670
  pharmacokinetics 667
neural blockade 497
neurodegenerative diseases, prevention 702
neuroglycaemia 665
neuroleptics
  ADRs 459
  in analgesia 502
  drug interactions 450
  equivalence 458, 460, 460
  mania therapy 448–449
  see also antipsychotic drugs
neuropathy
  diabetic see diabetic neuropathy
  lymphoma therapy ADRs 768, 769
  pain management 505–507, 506
  ulceration 661
  vitamin B_{12} deficiency anaemia 732
neuroprotective agents 132
neurosurgery
  infective meningitis 556
  surgical antibiotic prophylaxis 577–578
neurotoxins 545
neurotransmitters
  pain transmission 495
  Parkinson's disease 484
    see also individual neurotransmitters
neutral insulin 662–664, 663
neutropenia 60
  cytotoxic drug ADRs 781, 784–785
  definition 59
  fungal infections 628, 636 (CS)
  lymphoma therapy ADRs 768
neutrophil count 60

reference values *58*
neutrophilia *59*
nevirapine (NVP) *604*, 607–608
New York Heart Association *299*
nicardipine *288*
nicorandil 287–288
nicotine 173, *176*
nicotinic acid derivatives 369
  ADRs 369
  drug interactions *368*
  efficacy *365*
nicoumalone 343
nifedipine *288*
nisoldipine *288*
nitrates
  CHF therapy *306,* 307–308
  drug interactions *312*
  mechanism of action 285–286
  MI therapy 292–293
  monitoring *311*
  preparations 286–287
  properties *287*
  stable angina therapy 285–287
  sublingual preparations 287
  tolerance 286
nitrazepam 438 (CS)
  characteristics *427*
nitric oxide (NO) 103
  NSAIDs 146
nitrofurantoin
  ADRs 417–418
  urinary tract infection therapy 538, *538*
nitroprusside *306*
nizatidine (ADRs) *151*
no change (NC) 786
nociceptors 495
nodal arrhythmias *323*
non-blanching erythema 873
non-Hodgkin's lymphomas 760–762, 770–771
    (CS), 772 (CS)
  aetiology 760
  Burkitt's lymphoma *see* Burkitt's lymphoma
  classification 761, *761*
  CLL involvement 746
  diagnosis 761
  high grade 772 (CS)
    signs/symptoms 760–761
    treatment 765–766
  histopathology 761
  intermediate grade
    signs/symptoms 760–761
    treatment 765
  laboratory findings 761
  low-grade 770–771 (CS)
    signs/symptoms 760
    therapy 765
  lymphoblastic lymphomas 766
  risk factors 760
  signs/symptoms 760–761
  staging 761–762, 765
  treatment 764–767
    algorithm *764*
    high-dose chemotherapy 766–767
non-insulin-dependent diabetes mellitus
    (NIDDM) *see* diabetes mellitus type II
non-nucleoside reverse transcriptase inhibitors
    (NNRTIs) 607–608
  characteristics *603–605*
  resistance 607–608
  see also individual drugs
non-pulmonary tuberculosis *see* tuberculosis
non-Q wave infarction 288–289
non-steroidal anti-inflammatory drugs
    (NSAIDs)
  ADRs 135, 797–799
    acute tubular necrosis cause *231*
    airway obstruction 415
    fetal development 709
    hypersensitivity pneumonitis 417
    in analgesia 498–499

asthma therapy 316–317 (CS)
  clinical considerations 498
  COX-2 selectivity 498–499, *797,* 799
  drug interactions 31 (CS), *346, 796, 858*
  dysmenorrhoea therapy 686, *687*
  gastrointestinal side-effects 797–799, 807
    mechanism 797
    risk factors 797, *798*
    therapy 797–799
  gout therapy 815–816
  leg ulcer therapy 881
  mechanism of action 796–797, *797*
  menorrhagia therapy 688, *689*
  osteoarthritis therapy 807
  peptic ulcer disease 160 (CS)
    COX-2 inhibitors 146
    epidemiology 145
    nitric oxide NSAIDs 146
    pathogenesis 145–146
    prophylaxis 151–152, *153, 155*
    risk factors *145*
    treatment 151
  pharmacokinetics *795*
  premenstrual syndrome therapy *685*
  rheumatoid arthritis therapy 794, 795–797
  site of action 796
  topical 807
noradrenaline (norepinephrine)
  in affective disorders 440
  CHF therapy 309
  pain transmission 495
norepinephrine *see* noradrenaline
    (norepinephrine)
norfloxacin, drug interactions *346*
normochromic conditions *59*
nortriptyline
  depression therapy 445
  metabolization 37
nosocomial pneumonia *see* pneumonia
novel erythropoiesis stimulating protein (NESP)
    258
nucleoside reverse transcriptase inhibitors
    (NARTs) 607
  characteristics *604–605*
  combination formulations 607
  see also individual drugs
nucleotide reverse transcriptase inhibitors
    (NtRTIs) *607,* 608
nucleus tractus solitarus (NTS) 510
Nutriflex Lipid range 78
nutritional assessment 83
  malnutrition 67, *67*
nutritional requirements 85, *86*
nystatin
  candidiasis therapy 612, 624
  fungal ear infection therapy 626
  infection prophylaxis *754*

O

obesity
  diabetes mellitus type II 658
  dyslipidaemia 358
  metformin role 669
  osteoarthritis 805
obstetrics, antibiotic prophylaxis 577
occupational asthma 376
occupational therapy
  osteoarthritis treatment 806–807
  rheumatoid arthritis 794
octreotide 222, *222*
ocular toxicity 592
odorous wounds 875
oedema 310
oesophageal varices 221–222, 226–227 (CS)
  management 221–222, *222*
    algorithm *221*

oestrogen implants *697,* 697–698
oestrogens
  arterial thromboembolism 348
  hormone replacement therapy *see* hormone
    replacement therapy (HRT)
  VTE 340
'off-label' medicines 123
ofloxacin
  ADRs *591*
  drug interactions *346*
  tuberculosis therapy *591*
olanzapine (ADRs) 45 (CS), *459*
oliguria 232
omeprazole
  ADRs *151*
  drug interactions 154
  peptic ulcer therapy 148, *153*
  ulcer therapy 798
oncovin *see* vincristine (oncovin)
ondansetron
  antiemetic characteristics *512*
  chemotherapy-induced nausea therapy
    783–784
opioid antagonists 216
opioids
  ADRs 500–501
    adult respiratory distress syndrome 420
  in analgesia 499–500
  cancer pain management 505
  clinical considerations 500
  epidural analgesia 498
  gastrointestinal motility effects 24
  potencies *496*
  strong 499–500
  weak 499
  see also individual drugs
opportunistic infections 599–600, 608–617, *753*
  fungi *see* fungal infections
  during HIV infection *601*
  management 600
  treatment 609–612
  see also AIDS; HIV infection;
    immunocompromised patient; *individual*
    diseases/disorders
opportunity costs 92
OpSite 877
oral candidiasis 624
oral contraceptives
  ADRs
    cholestatic jaundice 40–41
    hyperlipidaemia 358–359
    venous thromboembolism 683–684
  drug interactions 26, 31 (CS), 154, *346, 368,*
    627, 858
  dysmenorrhoea therapy 686, *687*
  endometriosis therapy 691
  hypertension management 274, 276 (CS)
  menorrhagia therapy 689
  premenstrual syndrome therapy 683–684,
    685
oral hygiene 753
  candidiasis therapy 612
oral rehydration solution 187, *187*
oral route 113–114, 117–118
oral surgery, antibiotic prophylaxis 579
oral thrush *see* candidiasis
orbit graph *14*
'organizing pneumonia' 419
organogenesis 708
orlistat, drug interactions 30–31 (CS)
Orphan Drug Act (USA) 124
orphenadrine 489–490
orthopaedic surgery, antibiotic prophylaxis
  578–579
orthopnoea 301
orthostatic circulatory responses 129
osalazine *171, 176*
osmolarity
  adult reference values *47*
  extracellular fluid (ECF) 48, 49

osmolarity, *continued*
  intracellular fluid (ICF) 48
  PN 77
osmotic laxatives 184
osteoarthritis (OA) 138 (CS), 804–807, 810
    (CS)
  aetiology 805
  clinical manifestations 806
  epidemiology 804–805
  investigations 806
  key points 791
  pathogenesis 806
  predisposing factors *805*
  treatment 806–807
    algorithm *806*
    drug 806–807
    non-drug 806–807
osteoblasts 648
osteoclasts 648
osteoporosis 132–133
  heparin ADRs 342
  prevention 132
    hormone replacement therapy 701, 704
      (CS)
  treatment 132–133
    alfacalcidol 132
    bisphosphonates 132–133
    calcitonin 133
    calcitriol 132
    hormone replacement therapy 133
    vitamin D and calcium 132
otitis media 521, 529 (CS)
  causative organism 521
  clinical features 521
  diagnosis 521
  treatment 521
out-patient chemotherapy 785
ovarian cancer 788–789 (CS)
ovaries, menopausal changes 695–696
overflow incontinence 135
oversedation (drug-related) 428
over-the-counter medicines
  CHD 294
  monitoring *311*
ovulation 679
oxazepam *432*
oxcarbazepine
  dosage *473*
  epilepsy therapy 470–471, 476
oxitropium
  ADRs *382*
  asthma therapy 381
  COPD therapy 404
  dosage *383*
  inhalers *389*
oxprenolol *286*
oxybutynin
  ADRs 135
  urinary incontinence therapy 135
oxycodone 499–500
oxygen therapy
  acute asthma therapy 386, 393 (CS)
  acute COPD therapy 404
  ADRs 103
  bronchopulmonary dysplasia 104
  COPD therapy 407
  cor pulmonale therapy 406
  respiratory distress syndrome 102–103

P

p53 gene 777
pacemaker 325
packaging 136
packed cell volume (PCV) 59
  adult reference values *58, 121*
  neonatal reference values *121*
  paediatric reference values *121*

paclitaxel 788–789 (CS)
PAdriaCEBO regimen 765, *766*
paediatric drug therapy 116–120, 125–126 (CS)
  absorption *see* absorption (of drugs)
  ADRs 122
  body surface area 116–117
  buccal route 117–118
  compliance 120
  disposition 113–116
  distribution *see* distribution (of drugs)
  dosage 116–117
    selection 124, *124*
  gastrostomy route 118
  intranasal route 118
  licensing *see* drug licensing process
  medication errors 122–123
  metabolism 115–116
  nasogastric route 118
  'off-label' medicines 123
  oral route 117–118
  parenteral route 118–119
    as percentage of adult dose *117*
  pharmacokinetics 113–116
  preparation choice 117–120
  pulmonary route 119–120
  rectal route 118
  renal excretion 116, *116*
  in schools 120–121
    guidelines 120
    policies 120
    responsibilities 120–121
    special-needs schools 121
  theophylline metabolism *116*
  therapeutic index 117
  unlicensed medicines 123
paediatrics 111–126, 125–126 (CS)
  biochemical data *121*
  demographics 111–112
    specific diseases 112, *112*
  drug therapy *see* paediatric drug therapy
  fluid requirements *119*
  haematology data *121*
  immunization programmes 113
  infant mortality 111
  monitoring parameters 121–122
  normal growth/development 112–113, *114*
    indicators 113
  PN *see* parenteral nutrition (PN)
  renal function assessment 122
  vital signs *121*
  see also children; neonates
pain 495–508
  abdominal 167
  acute 496
  aetiology 495
  assessment 495–496
  chronic 496
  gate theory 495
  key points 495
  management 496–498
    adjuvant medication 496, *497*
    analgesic ladder 496
    chemotherapy 784
    neural blockade 497
    patient-controlled analgesia (PCA) 496
    problems *506*
    see also analgesia; analgesic drugs
  neurophysiology 495
  specific syndromes *see individual diseases
    disorders*
palliative care 85
palms, psoriasis 862, *862,* 868 (CS)
palpitations 324
panacinar emphysema 399
pancreatic cancer 507
pancreatitis 84–85
pancuronium 103
pancytopenia *59*
PANDA 618
panic attacks 425

pannus 792
pantoprazole
  ADRs *151*
  drug interactions 154
paracensis 218
paracetamol
  drug interactions *26*
  hepatotoxicity *see* hepatotoxicity
  osteoarthritis therapy 807, 810 (CS)
  overdose 452 (CS)
    see also hepatotoxicity
  rheumatoid arthritis therapy 795, 808–809
    (CS)
paracetamol-induced hepatotoxicity *see*
    hepatotoxicity
paraesthesia (drug-related) 834
paraldehyde 106
paranoid behaviour 455
paraplegics 873
parathyroid gland
  diseases/disorders 648–652
    hyperparathyroidism *see*
      hyperparathyroidism
    hypoparathyroidism *see*
      hypoparathyroidism
  normal functioning 648
parathyroid hormone (PTH) 53
  chronic kidney failure 253–254
  effects 648
  see also calcium
parenteral nutrition (PN) 67–90, 87–89 (CS)
  administration 75, 77–79
    routes 77
    see also individual routes
  amino acids 69–70, *70*
    acute kidney failure 238–239
    adults 70
    conditionally-essential 69–70
    essential 69
    paediatrics 70
  central routes 77
  complications 83–84, *84*
    line blockage 83–84
    refeeding syndrome 84
  components 69–74
  compounded formulations 78
    standardized formulations *vs.* 78
  cyclic infusions 79
  electrolytes 74, *76*
  energy 70–73, *71*
    glucose *71*
  fungal infections 628, 637 (CS)
  indications 68, *68*
  infusion control 77–78
  lipid emulsions 71–73, *72*
  long-term 85
  micronutrients *73,* 73–74, *76*
  monitoring 83
  nutritional assessment 83
  nutrition teams 68–69
  oral equivalents 69
  paediatrics 85–86, 87–88 (CS)
    administration routes 86
    formulation issues 85–86
    heparin 86
    nutritional requirements 85, *86*
    stability issues 85–86
  peripherally inserted central catheters (PICC)
    77
  peripheral routes 75, 77, *77*
    indications/contraindications 77, *77*
  pharmaceutical issues 79–82
    filtration 82
    Maillard reactions 80
    temperature control 82
  shelf-life 82
  specific diseases states 84–85
    acute kidney failure 238–239
    cancer therapy 85
    cardiac disease 85

diabetes mellitus 85
injury 85
kidney disease 84
liver disease 84
palliative care 85
pancreatitis 84–85
respiratory disease 85
sepsis 85
stability
amino acids 80
drugs 82
light protection 82
lipids 79–80, *81*
precipitation 79, *80*
vitamins 80
standardized formulations 78
compounded formulations *vs.* 78
sterility 80
trace elements 73–74
commercial products content *74*
vitamins 74
commercial products content *75*
water volume 69
changes *69*
see also malnutrition
parenteral route, paediatric drug therapy *see*
paediatric drug therapy
parkinsonism 131
antipsychotic drug ADRs 462
drug-related 485, *486*
see also Parkinson's disease
Parkinson's disease 483–494, *492–493* (CS)
aetiology 483–484
clinical features 484
differential diagnosis 484–486, *485, 486,*
492–493 (CS)
drug-related 483, 485, *486*, 492 (CS)
epidemiology 483
investigations 485–486
key points 483
Lewy bodies 484
pathophysiology 484
patient care 491–192
treatment 486–491
general approach 486–487
pharmacology 487–490
see also individual drugs
problems *492*
surgery 490–491
surgical targets *490*
see also parkinsonism
Parkinson's Disease Society 491
PARMA study 766–767
paroxetine
anxiety therapy *432*
depression therapy 447
in pregnancy 715 (CS)
paroxysmal arrhythmias *323*
paroxysmal nocturnal haemoglobinuria 744
paroxysmal supraventricular tachyarrhythmias
326
partial liquid ventilation 103
partial response (PR) 786
partial seizures *see* seizures
partial thromboplastin time kaolin (PTTK) 63
parvoviruses 792
patch testing 846, 855
patent ductus arteriosus (PDA) 103
patient-controlled analgesia (PCA) 496
peak expiratory flow rate (PEFR) 378
peak flow meter 378
penicillamine
rheumatoid arthritis therapy *801*, 802
Wilson's disease therapy 223–224
penicillin
ADRs
airway obstruction 414
hepatotoxicity 195
infection therapy 754
streptococcal meningitis therapy 561

pentamidine isethionate
PCP prophylaxis *612–613*
PCP therapy *611, 612*
pentazocine 500
penthidine 499
peptic ulcer disease 143–162, 158 (CS),
160–161 (CS)
clinical manifestations 146
definition 143
duodenal ulcer *143*
epidemiology 144
investigations 147–148
diagnostic algorithm *148,* 161 (CS)
endoscopy 147
radiology 147
NSAIDs *see* non-steroidal anti-inflammatory
drugs (NSAIDs)
pathogenesis 144–146
patient assessment 146–147
alarm symptoms *147,* 160 (CS)
subgroups *147*
patient care 157–58
stress ulcers 149
surgical antibiotic prophylaxis 575
treatment 148–158
ADRs *151*
algorithm *150*
bleeding ulcers 148
complications 148
costs 157
drugs *see* ulcer-healing drugs
future strategies 157
problems *159*
pyloric stenosis 148
Zollinger–Ellison syndrome 149
see also gastro-oesophageal reflux disease
(GORD); *Helicobacter pylori* infection
percutaneous coronary transluminal angioplasty
(PCTA)
mechanism of action *293*
MI therapy 293
pergolide 488
pericyazine (ADRs) *459*
perimetry 827
perindopril *306*
peripheral infusion tolerance 75, 77
peripherally inserted central catheters (PICC)
77
peripheral lymph nodes 589
peripheral neuropathy 503
peritoneal dialysis 240, *240*
chronic kidney failure therapy 259
clearance rates *241*
complications 259
pernicious anaemia 740 (CS)
epidemiology 730
pathophysiology 731
see also vitamin B_{12} deficiency anaemia
peroxisome proliferator-activated receptor-
gamma (PPARG)
activators *365*
diabetes mellitus type II therapy 670
perphenazine (ADRs) *459*
'petit mal' seizures 467
phantom limb pain 504
pharmacodynamics
drug interactions *see* drug interactions
in elderly patients *see* geriatrics
liver disease 224
neonates 102
type A ADRs 38
type B ADRs 39–41
pharmacoeconomics 91–98
allocative efficiency 98
average costs 92
clinical risk therapy 96–97
comparator choice 92
compliance costs 97
contingent valuation 93, 98
cost minimization analysis 93

decision analysis techniques 94–96, *95, 96*
decision trees 95–96
sensitivity analysis 95
definitions 91–92
direct costs 92
discounting 94, 98
economic evaluations 92–94
cost–benefit analysis *see* cost–benefit
analysis (CBA)
cost-effectiveness analysis *see* cost-
effectiveness analysis (CEA)
cost–utility analysis *see* cost–utility
analysis (CUA)
efficiency 98
equity 98
evaluations 92
guidelines 96
fixed costs 92
glossary 98
increasing costs 91
incremental costs 92
indirect costs 92
marginal analysis 98
marginal costs 92
objectivity/subjectivity 97
opportunity costs 92
validation of costs 94
variable costs 92
willingness-to-accept 93
willingness-to-pay 93
pharmacokinetics 3–20, 17–19 (CS)
absorption 6
bioavailability *(F)* 6
rate constant (k_a) 6
in children *see* paediatrics
clinical applications 8–17
creatinine clearance 8
data interpretation 7–8
capacity limited clearance 7–8
dose–concentration relationships 8
important criteria 7
increasing clearance 8
sampling times 7
therapeutic range 8
definition 3
dosage
alterations 3, 7
initial guidelines 4
loading dose 3, 4
regimens 6–7
drug interactions *see* drug interactions
in elderly *see* geriatrics
elimination *see* elimination
formulation choice 4
general applications 3–4
in lactation 711
liver disease *see* liver disease
maximal response 3
in neonates *see* neonates
orbit graph *14*
paediatrics 113–116
peak and trough levels 7
in pregnancy 709
steady state *3*
therapeutic drug monitoring 4
type A ADRs 36–38
type B ADRs 39
volume of distribution *see* distribution,
volume of
see also individual drugs
pharyngitis 519–521, 530 (CS)
causative organisms 519–520
clinical features 520
diagnosis 520
treatment 520–521
phenelzine
anxiety therapy *432*
depression therapy 446
phenobarbital
ADRs 476, *476*

phenobarbitol, *continued*
distribution 15
dosage *473*
drug interactions *475, 476*
elimination 15
epilepsy therapy 476–477
neonatal seizure therapy 106
pharmacokinetics 14–15, *17*
practical considerations 15
pruritus therapy 216
serum concentration–response relationships 15
withdrawal 469
phenothiazines
ADRs *459*
in analgesia 502
as antiemetic drugs 516
characteristics *512*
phenylbutazone
drug interactions *346*
pharmacokinetics *795*
phenytoin
ADRs *476,* 477
hypernatraemia 50
distribution 13
dosage *473*
drug interactions 154, *346, 368, 475,* 477, *627, 858*
elimination 13
half-life 13
epilepsy therapy 477, 480 (CS)
formulation 477
neonatal seizure therapy 106
pharmacokinetics 13, *17,* 18 (CS), *334, 474*
orbit graph *14*
practical considerations 13
serum concentration–response relationship 13
withdrawal 469, 480 (CS)
Philadelphia chromosome 745–746
phosphate 53–54
adult reference values *47, 121*
homeostasis *253,* 253–254
hyperphosphataemia *see* hyperphosphataemia
hypophosphataemia 53
neonatal reference values *121*
paediatric reference values *121*
phosphodiesterase inhibitors 309
photosensitivity 849, *850*
drug-related 462
phototherapy
eczema therapy 859
psoriasis therapy 863–864
phototoxic reactions 849
physiotherapy
aspiration pneumonia therapy 528
osteoarthritis treatment 806
pressure sores 874
rheumatoid arthritis 794
phytotherapy 721
dyslipidaemia therapy 362–363
pia mater 555
pigmentation 850, *850*
pilocarpine 833–834, 840–841 (CS)
pimozide (ADRs) *459*
pindolol *286*
'pink puffer' 401
pioglitazone *see* thiazolidinediones
piperacillin 754
pipotiazine (ADRs) *459*
piroxicam
ADRs *798*
gout therapy 816
pharmacokinetics *795*
pityriasis versicolor 626
pivampicillin (ADRs) 844
pivmecillinam 537–538
plant sterols 362–363
plaque psoriasis, chronic 861, *861,* 868 (CS)
plasma viscosity (PV), rheumatoid arthritis 793–794

platelet count 60
reference values *58*
pleural reactions, ADRs 420–421
drugs responsible *421*
PMitCEBO regimen 765, *766*
Pneumocystis carinii pneumonia (PCP) 608, 612–613, 618–619 (CS), 620–621 (CS)
diagnosis 608
lymphoma therapy 768
management *609–611,* 612–613
combination therapies 612
prophylaxis 612–613
pneumonia 523–529
aspiration 527–529, 529 (CS)
causative organism 527–528
clinical features 528
in cystic fibrosis 527
treatment *528,* 528–529
atypical 524
community-acquired 523–525
causative organisms 523–524, *524*
clinical features 524
diagnosis 524
treatment 525, *526*
hospital-acquired (nosocomial) 525–527
causative organisms 525, *526*
clinical features 525
diagnosis 525
prevention 526–527
treatment 525–526, *527*
lobar 524
see also Legionnaire's disease
pneumococcal vaccine
COPD therapy 403
sickle cell anaemia therapy 737
poikilocytosis *59*
pollen 376
polyasa *171*
polyclonal antisera, kidney transplants *261*
polycystic kidney disease, adult 249
polycythaemia 399
polyenes 624
polymerase chain reaction (PCR)
infective meningitis diagnosis 558
tuberculosis diagnosis 586
polymyxins 528
polypharmacy 22
ADRs predisposing factors 35
antipsychotic drugs 458, 463–464 (CS)
hepatotoxicity 194
HIV infection therapy 618, 619–620 (CS)
see also drug interactions
polyurethane foams 876–877
polyuria 251
pomphylox 854
population studies
dyslipidaemia 353–354, *354*
high-density lipoprotein cholesterol (HDL-C) *354*
low-density lipoprotein cholesterol (LDL-C) *354*
porphyrias (drug-related) 40
portal hypertension 213–214
portosystemic shunting 224
postamputation pain 504
postherpetic neuralgia (PHN) 503
postmenopausal oestrogen replacement therapy 284–285
postoperative nausea and vomiting (PONV) *see* nausea/vomiting
postoperative pain 504
postremission consolidation chemotherapy 747
postrenal acute kidney failure 231
post-term neonate *101*
postural control 129
postural hypotension
ADRs 314
antipsychotic drug ADRs 462
treatment 492
postural instability 484

potassium 51–53
adult reference ranges *47, 121*
chronic kidney failure 252
excess *see* hyperkalaemia
insufficiency *see* hypokalaemia
neonatal reference ranges *121*
paediatric reference ranges *121*
regulation 51
restriction 256, 257
secretion 51
practolol syndrome 43
pramipexole
ADRs 488
Parkinson's disease therapy 488
pravastatin 365–366
characteristics *366*
prazosin 273
prednisolone
acute asthma therapy 386, 393 (CS)
ADRs 168–169, *768, 769*
autoimmune hepatitis therapy 223
in chemotherapy
ALL 747, *748*
ChlVPP/EVA regimen *763,* 764
ChlVPP/PABIOE regimen *763,* 764, 770 (CS)
CHOP *see* CHOP regimen
CLL 750
MACOP-B regimen 765
MOPP regimen 762, 764
MVPP regimen 764
PAdriaCEBO regimen 765, *766*
PMitCEBO regimen 765, *766*
ProMACE-CytaBOM regimen 765
drug interactions 30–31 (CS)
graft-*versus*-host disease therapy 752
inflammatory bowel disease therapy 168–169, *176,* 177 (CS)
kidney transplants 260
rheumatoid arthritis therapy 803, 808–809 (CS), 808 (CS)
pre-eclampsia treatment 274
pre-embryonic stage
definition 707
drug exposure effects 708
pregnancy
atrial arrhythmias 325
benzodiazepines 429
folate deficiency anaemia 732–733
HIV infection 617
hypertension management 274, 276 (CS)
hyperthyroidism therapy 646
hypothyroidism therapy 642
insomnia 431
iron requirements 728
nausea/vomiting 514, 517 (CS)
pharmaceutical drugs 714–715 (CS), 770–710
clearance 709
effects on fetus 708–709
exposure timing 708–709
idiosyncratic effects 708
key points 707
neonate effects 709
pharmacokinetic changes 709
pharmacological effects 708
placental drug transfer 708
preconception advice 710
protein binding 709
safety/selection 709–710
volume of distribution 709
see also absorption (of drugs)
prenatal development 707
tuberculosis therapy 590
premature contraction arrhythmias *323*
premenstrual dysphoric disorder (PMDD) 680
premenstrual syndrome (PMS) 680–684, 691–692 (CS)
aetiology 681–682
psychological factors *682*

epidemiology 680–681
management 682–684
  dietary supplements 682–683, *685*
  pharmacological 683–684, *685*
  self-help 682
patient care 684
symptoms 682, *682*
pre-renal acute kidney failure 229, *230*
pressure sores 871–877, *884*, 884 (CS)
aetiology 871–872
  patient position 872–873, *873*
  pressure 871–872
  risk factors 871–872, *872*
epidemiology 871
investigations 873
key points 871
signs/symptoms 873
sites 872–873
stages *875*
treatment 873–877
  algorithm *878*
  clinical infections 874
  debridement 876
  odorous wounds 875
  problems *877*
  selection 874–875, *875*
  wound management 874–877
  see also individual products
preterm neonate *101*
primaquine, PCP therapy *611, 612*
primary angle closure glaucoma (PACG) *see* glaucoma
primary biliary cirrhosis (PBC) 212, 227–228 (CS)
treatment 223
primary dyslipidaemia *see* dyslipidaemia
primary dysmenorrhoea *see* dysmenorrhoea
primary hypothyroidism 639
primary irritant dermatitis 846, *847*, 855
primary open-angle glaucoma (POAG) *see* glaucoma
primary sclerosing cholangitis (PSC) 212
treatment 223
primidone
drug interactions *346*
epilepsy therapy 479 (CS)
pharmacokinetics 15, *17, 474*
PR interval 323
Prinzmetal's angina 281
probenecid
drug interactions *818, 858*
pharmacokinetics *819*
procainamide
drug interactions *335*
pharmacokinetics *334*
procarbazine
ADRs *769*
ChlVPP/EVA regimen *763,* 764
ChlVPP/PABlOE regimen *763,* 764, 770 (CS)
MOPP regimen 762, 764
MVPP regimen 764
prochlorperazine 463 (CS)
ADRs *459*
antiemetic characteristics *512*
product licence (PL) 123
progesterone, premenstrual syndrome 681
progestogens
dysmenorrhoea therapy 686, *687*
endometriosis therapy 691
menorrhagia therapy *689*
premenstrual syndrome therapy 683, *685*
progressive disease (PD) 786
progressive nuclear palsy, Parkinson's disease *vs.* 486
prolactin
drug effects 714
premenstrual syndrome 681
ProMACE-CytaBOM regimen 765
promazine (ADRs) *459*

promethazine 430
as antiemetic drugs *513*
characteristics *427*
propafenone (drug interactions) *335*
propanolol
adjunctive hyperthyroidism therapy 647
anxiety therapy *432*, 435
CHF therapy 315–316 (CS)
properties *286*
propylthiouracil (PTU) (ADRs) 645–646
prostaglandin analogues 835
prostaglandins
dysmenorrhoea 685
inhibition 796–797
menorrhagia 688
menstrual cycle 680
premenstrual syndrome 681
prostaglandin synthesis inhibitors 684
prostate gland
enlargement *see* benign prostatic hyperplasia (BPH)
structure 717, *718*
prostate hypertrophy 249
prostate specific antigen (PSA) 57–58, 718
benign prostatic hyperplasia 719
prosthetic implants 569
protamine zinc insulin *663*
prostatectomy, open 720
protease inhibitors *605–606,* 608
  see also individual drugs
protective isolation, immunocompromised 755
protein binding reduction, liver disease 224
protein C deficiency, VTE 340
protein S deficiency, VTE 340
proteinuria
chronic kidney failure 251
in chronic kidney failure 251
prothrombin time (PT) 61–62
liver function tests 215, 217
warfarin monitoring 343–344
proton pump inhibitors 153–155
absorption 154
ADRs 154
clearance 154
clinical use 155, *155*
comparisons *154*
drug interactions 154–155
half-life 154
mechanism of action *153,* 153–154
pharmacokinetics 154
  see also individual drugs
protozoal infections
in immunocompromised 613–614
  see also specific infections
proximal interphalangeal joints
osteoarthritis 806
rheumatoid arthritis 793
pruritus 843–845
hepatotoxicity 200
treatment 216, *217*
in uraemia 257
pseudohypoparathyroidism 649
Pseudomonas aeruginosa infection
aspiration pneumonia 528
treatment 10
urinary tract infections 534
psoralens 864
psoriasiform eruptions 848, *848*
psoriasis 860–865, 868 (CS)
aetiology 860
alcohol abuse 860
arthropathy 862
chronic plaque 861, *861,* 868 (CS)
clinical features 861–862
drug-related 860
erythrodermic 862
flexural 862
generalized pustular 862
guttate 861, *861*
infection 860

Koebner phenomenon 860, *860*
nails 861–862
  therapy 864
palms/soles 862, *862,* 868 (CS)
pathogenesis 861
patient care 865–866
scalp 861, *862*
  therapy 864
smoking 860
stress 860
treatment 862–865
  algorithm *866*
  problems *867*
  systemic 864–865
  topical 863–864
Psoriasis Association 865–866
psychomotor impairment (drug-related) 433
pulmonary arteriography 341
pulmonary embolism (PE)
diagnosis 341
oestrogen replacement therapy 698
in VTE 340–341
  see also venous thromboembolism (VTE)
pulmonary fibrosis (drug-related) 418–419
pulmonary hypertension (drug-related) 419
pulmonary rehabilitation 406–407
pulmonary route 119–120
pulmonary tuberculosis *see* tuberculosis
pulmonary vasculature (drug-related) 419–420
pulmonary vasculitis (drug-related) 420
pulse rate, asthma 378
purpura 847
pustular psoriasis, generalized 862
PUVA (psoralem plus UVA)
adverse effects 864
psoriasis therapy 864
P wave 323
pyelonephritis, acute 533
treatment *533*
pyelonephritis, chronic 533
chronic kidney failure 249
pyloric stenosis 148
pyrazinamide
monitoring *203*
tuberculosis therapy 587, *588*
pyridoxine phosphate 741 (CS)
premenstrual syndrome 681
sideroblastic anaemia therapy 734
supplements 682, *685*
pyrimethamine, toxoplasmosis therapy *611,* 613–614

Q

QRS complex 323
QT interval 323
ADRs *323*
quality-adjusted life year (QALY), cost–utility analysis (CUA) 94
quality of life, chemotherapy 786
quietiapine (ADRs) *459*
quinapril *306*
quinidine
ADRs 330
drug interactions *335*
pharmacokinetics *334*
quinolones
ADRs 188
aspiration pneumonia therapy 528
infective gastroenteritis therapy 188
Q wave 282

R

rabeprazole (ADRs) *151*
radiation 744
radioallergosorbent tests (RAST) 854
radiocontrast media
acute tubular necrosis cause *231*
ADRs 415

radiography
  chest *302*
    COPD diagnosis 402
    tuberculosis 586
  chronic kidney failure investigation 250
  Crohn's disease investigations 165
  ulcerative colitis investigations 167, *167*
radiopharmaceuticals 713–714
radiotherapy
  adverse effects 815
  chemotherapy, with 781
  CLL therapy 751
  Kaposi's sarcoma therapy 615
raloxifene 700
ramipril
  ADRs 44 (CS)
  CHF therapy *306*
  MI therapy 292
ranitidine
  ADRs *151*
  peptic ulcer therapy *153*
  ulcer therapy 798–799
ranitidine bismuth citrate (RBC) 149
rapid eye movement sleep (REMS) 425
rash (drug-related) 608
rate constant (k_a) 6
rebound insomnia 427–428
reboxetine
  ADRs 44 (CS)
  depression therapy 447
reciprocal creatinine plots 250–251, *251*
record keeping 136
recreational drugs 714
rectal route 115, 118
red blood cell count (RBC) 58–59
  reference values *58*
red cell folate, reference values *58*
5 α-reductase inhibitors 135
Reed–Sternberg cells 760
re-entrant arrhythmias *323*
refeeding syndrome 84
reflex sympathetic dystrophy 503
regulatory authorities 43
regurgitation 509
rehabilitation 292
remission 747, 786
remission induction chemotherapy 747
renal failure, acute *see* kidney failure, acute
renal failure, chronic *see* kidney failure, chronic
renal osteodystrophy 253–254
  management 258–259
renin 301
renin–angiotensin–aldosterone antagonists
    271–272
  see also individual drugs
repaglinide 669–670
  ADRs 669
  advantages 669–670
  dosage 669
  drug interactions 669
  mode of action 669
  pharmacokinetics *667*, 669
respiratory depression (drug-related) 500
respiratory disease 85
respiratory distress syndrome (RDS) 102–103
  aetiology 102
  therapy 102–103
respiratory failure, acute 401
respiratory infections 519–532, 529–531 (CS)
  key points 519
  lower tract 522–529
    bronchiolitis 523
  post-surgery 573
  therapeutic problems *530*
  upper tract 519–522
    acute epiglottitis 520
    viral 519
  see also individual diseases/infections
Response Evaluation Criteria in Solid Tumours
    (RECIST) 786

'restless legs syndrome' 425
rest tremor 484
reteplase 345, 347
reticulocytes
  count *58*, 59
  erythropoiesis 726
retinitis, cytomegalovirus *see* cytomegalovirus
  infection
retinopathy, diabetic 660
retinopathy of prematurity 103
revised European–American lymphoma (REAL)
  classification 761, *761*
rhabdomyolysis *231*
rheumatoid arthritis (RA) 791–804, 808–810
    (CS), 810–811 (CS)
  aetiology 792
  age of onset 791
  classification *793*
  clinical manifestations 792–793
  epidemiology 791
  extra-articular features *791*, 793
  investigations 793
  key points 791
  pathophysiology 792
  patient care 804
  prevalence 791
  prognosis *791*
  socioeconomic impact 792
  treatment 794–804
    algorithm *800*
    drug treatment 794–804
    goals 794
    multidisciplinary approach 794
    non-drug 794
    patient education 794
    problems *805*
rheumatoid factors 794
rhodamine–auramine stain 586
ribavirin 223
rifabutin
  ADRs *591*
  drug interactions *346*, 627
  opportunistic infection therapy *611*
  tuberculosis therapy *591*
rifampicin
  ADRs 195–196
  cytochrome P450 isoenzyme interaction 25
  drug interactions *346*, *368*, *627*, *858*
  infective meningitis prophylaxis 562
  infective meningitis therapy 560
  monitoring *203*
  pruritus therapy 216
  tuberculosis therapy 587, *588*, 591–592
risperidone (ADRs) *459*
ritonavir (RTV) *606*, 608
rivastigmine 131
road accidents 112
rofecoxib
  advantages 799
  osteoarthritis therapy 810 (CS)
  peptic ulcer risk 146
  pharmacokinetics 795
Rome criteria 179, *180*
ropinirole
  ADRs 488
  Parkinson's disease therapy 488
rosiglitazone *see* thiazolidinediones
Rosser–Kind matrix 94
rotavirus 185
'rugger-jersey' spine 253, *254*
rumination 509

S

sacroiliitis 862
salbutamol
  asthma therapy 379, 382, 393–395 (CS)
  COPD therapy 403–404

inhalers *389*
salicylic acid
  drug interactions *346*
  psoriasis therapy 863
salmeterol
  asthma therapy 384
  inhalers *389*
Salmonella species infection *see* salmonellosis
salmonellosis
  carriers 548–549
  clinical features 546
  gastroenteritis *544*, 546–547
  treatment 188–189, 548
    problems 551
'salt-sensitive hypertension' 253
sampling times 7
sandimmun 261
saquinavir (SQV) *606*, 608
sarcoma, Kaposi's *see* Kaposi's sarcoma
SAVE trial
  CHF therapy 305
  MI therapy *290*
scalp 861, *862*, 864
Schilling test 732
schizophrenia 438 (CS), 455–464, 462–464
    (CS)
  acute 455–456
    treatment 456
  aetiology 456–457
    developmental model 456
    dopamine theory 457
    ecological model 456
    genetics 456
    transfer abnormality model 456
    vulnerability model 456
  affecting factors 456
  chronic 456
  classification 455
  diagnosis 456
  key points 455
  pharmacological therapy 457–462
    algorithm 458, *460*
    compliance 463 (CS)
    problems *459*
    see also individual drugs
  symptoms 455–456
    common with psychotic illness 455–456
Schlemm's canal 825–826
Schwartz model 122
sclerotherapy 221
scopolamine 516
Scottish Intercollegiate Guidelines Network
    309
seborrhetic eczema 855–856, *856*
secondarily generalized seizures 467
secondary dyslipidaemia *see* dyslipidaemia
secondary dysmenorrhoea *see* dysmenorrhoea
secondary hypothyroidism 639
sedation (drug-related)
  antipsychotic drugs 461
  opioids 500
seizures
  absence attacks 467
  atonic 467
  generalized 467, 468
  'grand mal' 467
  myoclonic 467
  neonates 105–106
  partial 467, 468
    complex 467
    secondarily generalized 467
    simple 467
  'petit mal' 467
  tonic–colonic convulsions 467, 479 (CS)
  treatment *see* anti-epileptic drugs (AEDs);
    epilepsy
  see also epilepsy
selective decontamination of the digestive tract
    (SDD) 526–527
selective serotonin uptake inhibitors (SSRIs)

anxiety therapy *432,* 434–435, *436*
  cost 446
  depression therapy 446–447
    efficacy 446
  drug interactions *450*
  mechanism of action 446
  in pregnancy 715 (CS)
  premenstrual syndrome therapy 684, *685*
  withdrawal 443
selegiline
  depression therapy 445–446
  Parkinson's disease therapy 489, 493 (CS)
self-treatment (drug interactions) 21
senna 184
sensitivity analysis 95
  definition 98
sepsis
  acute tubular necrosis cause *231*
  PN 85
serology
  pharyngitis diagnosis 520
  pneumonia diagnosis 524
serotonin *see* 5-hydroxytryptamine (5-HT,
      serotonin)
serotonin–dopamine antagonists (ADRs) *459*
serotonin–noradrenaline re-uptake inhibitors
      (SNRIs) 447
serotonin syndrome (drug-related) 29–30
sertraline
  anxiety therapy *432*
  depression therapy 447
serum concentration–response relationships
  carbamazepine 14
  ciclosporin 16
  digoxin 9
  phenobarbitol 15
  phenytoin 13
  theophylline 9–10
shear force 872
Sheffield table 359, *360–361*
Shigella infection *see* shigellosis
shigellosis
  gastroenteritis *544*
  treatment 188, 549
    problems 551
short-contact regimen, psoriasis therapy 863
short-term insomnia 430–431
sickle cell anaemia
  aetiology 735–736
  clinical manifestations 736–737
  epidemiology 735
  inheritance *736*
  investigations 737
  pathophysiology 736
  patient care 738
  treatment 737–738
sideroblastic anaemias 733–735, 741 (CS)
  aetiology 734
  clinical manifestations 734
  comorbidities *734*
  drug-related *734*
  epidemiology 733–734
  investigations 734
  pathophysiology 734
  patient care 735
  treatment 734–735
sigmoidoscopy 166, 167
simple partial seizures 467
simvastatin 365–366
  ADRs 367–368
  characteristics *366*
  drug interactions *627*
sinoatrial node 321
sinogram 873
sinus arrhythmias *323*
sinusitis, acute 521–522
  causative organisms 521–522
  clinical features 522
  diagnosis 522
  treatment 522

sinus rhythm 321
sirolimus *261*
skin disorders (drug-related) 843–852, 851–852
      (CS)
  acneform eruptions 849, *849,* 851–852 (CS)
  bullous eruptions 846–847, *847*
  diagnosis 843
  erythema multiforme *845,* 845–846
  erythema nodosum 847
  erythematous eruptions 844, *844,* 852 (CS)
  fixed-drug eruptions 848, *848*
  key points 843
  lichenoid eruptions 847, *848*
  Lyell's syndrome 846, *846*
  malignancies 850–851
  nail discolouration 850
  necrosis 849
  patient care 851
  photosensitivity 849, *850*
  pigmentation 850, *850*
  pruritus 843–845
  psoriasiform eruptions 848, *848*
  purpura 847
  Stevens–Johnson syndrome 846, 851 (CS)
  systemic lupus erythematosus 848–849, *849*
  toxic epidermal necrosis 846, *846*
  treatment 843–851
  urticaria 845, *845*
  vesicular eruptions 846–847, *847*
  see also eczema
sleep
  normal stages *425*
  orthodox 424
  paradoxical 425
  rapid eye movement 425
  slow-wave 424
  systems *424,* 424–425
  see also arousal systems; insomnia
sleep apnoea syndrome 401
small round structured virus (SRSV) 185
SMILE trial *290*
smoking
  cessation 402, 407, 409–410 (CS)
  CHD risk 284
  chronic bronchitis risk factor 398
  in COPD 397–398, *398,* 402
    cessation 407
  in emphysema 399
  psoriasis 860
  solid tumours 775–776
smooth muscle spasm (drug-related) 501
sodium 48–50
  adult reference ranges *47, 121*
  chronic kidney failure 252
  depletion 49
  distribution 49
  excess 49
  extracellular fluid (ECF) 48, 49
  neonatal reference ranges *121*
  paediatric reference ranges *121*
  restriction 256–257
  see also extracellular fluid (ECF);
      hypernatraemia; hyponatraemia;
      intracellular fluid (ICF)
sodium aurothiomalate *801,* 802, 808–809 (CS)
sodium cromoglicate
  ADRs *382*
  asthma therapy 379, 381, *381*
  inflammatory bowel disease therapy 172,
      176
  inhalers *389*
  nebulizers 391
sodium nitroprusside
  CHF therapy 309
  hypertension management 273
sodium valproate
  ADRs 202, *476,* 477
  dosage *473*
  drug interactions *475*
  epilepsy therapy 477, 479–480 (CS), 479 (CS)

mania therapy 448, 453 (CS)
  monitoring *203*
  pharmacokinetics *474*
  withdrawal 469
soft silicone dressings 877
soles, psoriasis 862, *862,* 868 (CS)
solid tumours *see* tumours, solid
soluble fibre 370
soluble insulin 662–664, *663*
SOLVD-P trial 305
SOLVD-T trial 305
somatostatin 222, *222*
Sorbsan 876
sore throat *see* pharyngitis
sotalol 331–332
  ADRs *331*
  properties *286*
  ventricular tachyarrhythmia therapy 326
  Wolff–Parkinson–White syndrome therapy
      332
soybean oil 72
sphincter muscle theory of glaucoma 826
spine, osteoarthritis 806
spiral computed tomography (CT) 341
spirometry 378, *378*
  COPD diagnosis 400
  forced expiratory volume 378
  forced vital capacity 378
  peak expiratory flow rate 378
  see also lung function tests
spironolactone
  ADRs 708–709
  ascites therapy 218, *219*
  CHF therapy *305,* 307
  drug interactions *312*
  LVSD therapy 302
spleen, leukaemia 746
spondylitis 862
spontaneous bacterial peritonitis 219
sputum culture 524
squalene synthetase inhibitors *365*
St. John's wort
  depression therapy 448
  drug interactions 30 (CS), *346, 450*
stable angina 281
  treatment 285–288
stable disease (SD) 786
standard gamble method 94
stanol esters 362–363
stanozolol (drug interactions) *346*
staphylococcal scalded skin syndrome 846
Staphylococcus aureus infections
  acute sinusitis 522
  aspiration pneumonia 527–528, 529 (CS)
  clinical features 546
  in eczema 857
  gastroenteritis *544*
  surgical sites 572–573
stasis eczema 856
statins *see* HMG-CoA reductase inhibitors
      (statins)
stavudine (D4T) *604,* 607
steatosis (drug-related) 195, 196, *196*
stem cell transplantation 751–752
  allogenic 751, 755 (CS)
    AML therapy 750, *752*
    CML therapy 750, *752*
  ALL therapy *752*
  autologous 751, 766
  cell source 751
  complications 752
  NHL therapy 766–767
  Parkinson's disease therapy 491
  peripheral blood 751–752, 766
  principle 751
stenting
  mechanism of action *293*
  MI therapy 293
steroids
  in analgesia *497*

steroids, *continued*
  eczema therapy 858
  gout therapy 816
  Graves' disease therapy 648
  infective meningitis therapy 563
  inflammatory bowel disease therapy 169
  kidney transplants 260, *261*
  osteoarthritis therapy 807
  psoriasis therapy 863
  systemic 858
  topical 863
  tuberculosis therapy 590
steroid-sparing agents 384
Stevens–Johnson syndrome 846, 851 (CS)
STI 571 (GLIVEC™) 750
stimulant laxatives 184
stimulation-produced analgesia 498
stomatitis (drug-related) 801
stool cultures 547
Streptococcus pneumoniae infections
  chronic bronchitis 399, 403
  community-acquired pneumonia 523–524
  meningitis
    aetiology 556
    treatment 561
  otitis media 521
  penicillin resistance 561
Streptococcus pyogenes infection 520
streptokinase 345, 350 (CS)
  ADRs 345
  MI therapy 289–290, *291*
    efficacy *289*
    mortality *292*
streptomycin
  ADRs *591*
  tuberculosis therapy 587, *588, 591*
stress
  anxiety 425
  incontinence 134–135
  psoriasis 860
  ulcers 149
stroke 131–132
  acute treatment 131–132
    anticoagulants 132
    antiplatelet therapy 132
    neuroprotective agents 132
    thrombolytic agents 131–132
  arterial thromboembolism 347
  in atrial fibrillation 327
  primary prevention 132
  secondary prevention 132
sublingual preparations, nitrates 287
substance abuse (drug-related) 433–434
sucralfate 156–157
  ADRs *151, 157*
sudden infant death syndrome (SIDS) 111
sulcinpyrazone, pharmacokinetics *819*
sulfadiazine, toxoplasmosis therapy *611,*
  613–614
sulfasalazine
  ADRs 417
  inflammatory bowel disease therapy
    169–170, *171,* 175 (CS), *176,* 177 (CS)
    formulations 170–171
    mechanism of action 169
    optimal dose 170
    problems *170*
  monitoring *203*
  pharmacokinetics 169–170
  rheumatoid arthritis therapy 794, 801, *801,*
    808–809 (CS)
sulfinpyrazole, drug interactions *346, 818*
sulfonamides, drug interactions *346*
sulindac, pharmacokinetics *795*
sulphonamides, drug interactions *858*
sulphonylureas 666–668
  ADRs 667, *668*
  dosage 667
  drug choice 667
  drug interactions *627, 668*

mode of action 666
  pharmacokinetics 666–667, *667*
sulpiride 463 (CS)
  ADRs *459*
sumatriptin (ADRs) 44 (CS)
supraventricular arrhythmias
  definition *323*
  in pregnancy 325
surfactant, exogenous 103
surgery
  classification *570*
  duration 569, *570*
  endometriosis therapy 690
  glaucoma therapy 827
  hyperthyroidism therapy 647
  infections *see* surgical site infections (SSIs)
  Parkinson's disease therapy 490–491
  pressure sore therapy 873–874
  see also individual procedures
surgical antibiotic prophylaxis 569–582,
  581–582 (CS)
  benefits 570–571
  clinical trials 575
  cost 570
  improvements 579
  in practice 575–579
    minimally invasive 576
    see also individual diseases/disorders
  regimen choice 573–575
    independent policies 574
    local application 574
    short-course 574
    timing 574
  risks 570–571
  therapeutic problems *580*
surgical site infections (SSIs) 580–581 (CS)
  definition 569, 571, *571*
  management 579
    antibiotic prophylaxis *see* surgical
      antibiotic prophylaxis
    problems *580*
  pathogenesis 572–573
    consequences 573
    organisms *572,* 572–573
    sources 572–573
  risk factors 569–570, *570*
    comorbidities 569
    operation 570
    patient 570
suxamethonium apnoea 38
Swan–Ganz balloon catheter 302
swan neck 793
sympathetic nervous system
  cardiac control 321
  nausea/vomiting 510
syndrome of inappropriate secretion of
  antidiuretic hormone (SIADH) 49
synovial fibroblasts, rheumatoid arthritis 792
synovial fluid, gout diagnosis 815
α-synuclein gene 484
systemic lupus erythematosus (SLE) 848–849,
  849
  drug-related 308

T

tacalcitol 863
tachyarrhythmias 325–327
  paroxysmal supraventricular 326
  treatment 325–327
    drugs used *326*
tachycardia 336 (CS)
  definition *323*
  drug-related 322
tacrolimus
  drug interactions *627*
  eczema therapy 859
  kidney transplants *261,* 262

talampicillin (ADRs) 844
tamoxifen, drug interactions *346*
tardive dyskenesia
  ADRs 43
  antipsychotic drug ADRs 462
target blood pressure, hypertension therapy
  268, *269*
technical efficiency 98
teicoplanin 754
temazepam *427*
tenecteplase 345, 347
  MI therapy 290, *291*
tenofovir (TFV) *607*
tenoxicam, pharmacokinetics *795*
teratogens 707, *708*
terazosin
  benign prostatic hypertrophy therapy 720
  hypertension management 273
terbinafine
  ADRs *628*
  dermatophytosis therapy 626
  drug interactions *627*
terbutaline
  asthma therapy 379, 382, 394–395 (CS)
  dosage *383*
  inhalers *389*
terfenadine, drug interactions *627*
terlipressin 222, *222*
tertiary hypothyroidism 639
testicular cancer 788 (CS)
thalassaemias
  aetiology 736
  clinical manifestations 737
  epidemiology 735
  investigations 737
  pathophysiology 736
  patient care 738
  treatment 738
thalidomide
  ADRs 33
  inflammatory bowel disease therapy 173
theophylline
  acute kidney failure therapy 236
  ADRs *382*
  asthma therapy 381–382
  clearance *384,* 404
  COPD therapy 404
  distribution 10
  dosage *383*
  drug interactions 154, *387*
  elimination 10
  intravenous administration 10
  oral administration 10
  paediatrics 116
  pharmacokinetics 9–10, *17,* 17–18 (CS)
  product formulation 10
  serum concentration–response relationship
    9–10
therapeutic drug monitoring (TDM) 4
  epilepsy therapy 471–472
  geriatrics 136
  neonates 106–107
  tuberculosis therapy 590–591
therapeutic index 117
therapeutic range
  gentamicin 10
  pharmacokinetics 8
thermoregulation, age-related changes 129
thermotherapy 720
thiamazole (ADRs) 645–646
thiazide diuretics
  ADRs *819*
  bronchopulmonary dysplasia therapy 104
  CHF therapy 302, *305*
  hypertension management 255
    elderly 133, 273
thiazolidinediones 670–671
  ADRs 670
  advantages 670–671
  dosage 670

drug interactions 670
  mode of action 670
  pharmacokinetics *667*, 670
thienobenzodiazepines (ADRs) *459*
thioguanine *748*
thionamides 645–647
  ADRs 645–646, *646*
  regimen 646–647
thioridazine (ADRs) *459*
thioxanthines (ADRs) *459*
throat swabs 520
thrombocytopenia
  cytotoxic drug ADRs 781
  definition 59
  heparin ADRs 342
thromboembolism
  arterial *see* arterial thromboembolism
  venous *see* venous thromboembolism (VTE)
thrombolytic agents
  acute stroke therapy 131–132
  MI therapy 289–291
    mortality *292*
thrombosis 339–352
  key points 339
thrush *see* candidiasis
thyroid
  adenomas 644
  diseases/disorders 639–648, 652–654 (CS)
    drug-related *640, 642,* 654 (CS)
    hyperthyroidism *see* hyperthyroidism
    hypothyroidism *see* hypothyroidism
    normal functioning *640,* 640–641
    hormone ratios 641
thyroid-binding hormone (TBG) *641*
thyroid-binding prealbumin (TBPA) *641*
thyroid function tests
  hyperthyroidism 644–645
  hypothyroidism 641–642
thyroid storm 647
thyrotoxic storm 645
thyroxine (T$_4$)
  drug interactions *346*
  hypothyroidism therapy 642–643, 652–653
    (CS), 653 (CS)
    overtreatment 643
  metabolization 641
  production 640–641
  protein binding *641*
tiagabine
  characteristics *470*
  epilepsy therapy 477
  pharmacokinetics 16
tibolone
  ADRs 44 (CS)
  hormone replacement therapy 699–700
ticarcillin *528*
ticlopidine
  acute coronary syndrome therapy 289
  ADRs 349
  arterial thromboembolism therapy 349
  drug interactions *346*
time trade-off method 94
TIMI trial *291*
timolol
  glaucoma therapy 830, *830,* 832, 840–841
    (CS)
  pharmacology *831*
  properties *286*
tioguanine 748, 757 (CS)
tirofiban 349
  acute coronary syndrome therapy 289
tissue plasminogen activator (tPA, duteplase,
  alteplase) 345
  arterial thromboembolism therapy 348
  MI therapy 289
    mortality *292*
tocainide, pharmacokinetics *334*
tolbutamide, pharmacokinetics *667*
tolcapone 488
tolerance

anxiolytic drug ADRs 433
  benzodiazepines 427
  nitrates 286
  opioid ADRs 501
tolterodine
  ADRs 135
  urinary incontinence therapy 135
tonic–clonic convulsions 467, 479 (CS)
tonography 824
tophi 815
topical drugs *see* topical therapy; *individual*
  drugs
topical therapy
  adrenaline (epinephrine) *832*
    glaucoma therapy 832
  candidiasis 624
  capsaicin 807
  carbonic anhydrase inhibitors 835
  dermatophytosis 625
  glaucoma 832, 835
  hormone replacement therapy 698
  imidazoles 858
  NSAIDs 807
  oestrogens 698
  paediatrics 114–115
  pruritus therapy 216, *217*
  psoriasis 863–864
  steroids 863
topiramate
  ADRs *476*
  characteristics *470*
  drug interactions *475*
  epilepsy therapy 478, 479 (CS)
  pharmacokinetics 16
torasemide *305*
torsades de pointes 322
  definition *323*
  drug-related 330
total body elimination 5
total cholesterol (TC) 353
  ideal levels *353*
  population studies *354*
total iron binding capacity (TIBC) 62
  iron-deficiency anaemia 728
  reference values *58*
total parenteral nutrition (TPN) 628, 637 (CS)
toxic epidermal necrosis 846, *846*
toxic nodular goitre 644
toxoplasmosis 609, *611,* 613–614
trabeculoplasty 827
trace elements *see* parenteral nutrition (PN)
TRACE trial
  CHF therapy 305
  MI therapy *290*
tramadol
  in analgesia 500
  osteoarthritis therapy 807, 810 (CS)
trandolapril *306*
tranexamic acid 688, *689*
transcutaneous electrical nerve stimulation 498
transdermal oestrogen 697, *697*
transfer abnormality model of schizophrenia
  456
transferrin
  reference values *58*
  serum levels 62–63
transfusions 733
transient insomnia 430
transient ischaemic attacks (TIAs) 348
transjugular intrahepatic portosystemic stent
  shunt (TIPSS)
  ascites therapy 218, *219*
  oesophageal varices therapy 2222
transplants
  kidney *see* kidney transplants
  liver 222, 223
  stem cell *see* stem cell transplantation
transtracheal aspiration 524
transurethral resection of the prostate (TURP)
  720

tranylcypromine 446
Traub and Johnson model 122
traveller's diarrhoea 185, 190 (CS)
trazodone 447
treatment thresholds, hypertension 268, *269*
triazoles 634–635
  ADRs *634*
  candidiasis therapy 624–625
  drug interactions *368, 627*
Trichophyton species infections *see*
  dermatophytosis
triclofos 605
tricyclic antidepressants
  ADRs 322
  in analgesia 501–502
  anxiety therapy 432, *432,* 434–435, *436*
  depression therapy 444–445
  drug interactions *450*
  insomnia therapy 430
  Parkinson's disease therapy 490
  tolerance 445
trifluoperazine (ADRs) *459*
trigeminal neuralgia 503
trigger factors, asthma 375–376, *376*
triglycerides
  PN 72–73
  structure *72*
trihexyphenidyl 489–490
triiodothyronine (T$_3$)
  metabolization 641
  myxoedema coma therapy 643
  production 640–641
  protein binding *641*
trimethoprim
  drug interactions *858*
  PCP therapy *612*
  urinary tract infection therapy *538*
trimetrexate *612*
trimipramine 445
triple chamber bags 78
trizivir 605
tropinin
  adult reference values *47*
  as cardiac marker 58
tropisetron
  antiemetic characteristics *512*
  chemotherapy-induced nausea therapy
    783–784
troponin I 282
troponin T 282
L-tryptophan (ADRs) 419–420
tuberculin reaction 585–586
tuberculosis 583–596, 594–595 (CS)
  aetiology 584–585
  diagnosis 585
  disease control/prevention 592–593
    BCG vaccine 593
    chemoprophylaxis 592–593
  epidemiology 583, *584*
  in immunocompromised 585
    diagnosis 586–587
  investigations 585–587
    chest radiography 586
    Heaf test 585–586
    in immunocompromised 586–587
    Mantoux test 585–586
    microbiology 586
    tuberculin reaction 585–586
    see also individual reactions
  key points 583
  non-pulmonary
    aetiology 584
    bone 589
    disseminated 589
    joints 589
    peripheral lymph nodes 589
  opportunistic, management 609, 614
  patient care 593–594
    counselling 593–594
    education 593

tuberculosis, *continued*
  pulmonary
    aetiology 584–585
    treatment 587–589
  risk groups 585, *585*
  treatment 587–592
    bacterial characteristics 587
    in children 590
    compliance 593
    drug resistance 590
    guidelines 587
    in immunocompromised 590
    intermittent regimens 589
    liver disease 590
    meningitis 589
    monitoring *see* therapeutic drug monitoring (TDM)
    in pregnancy 590
    renal disease 590
    special circumstances 590
    steroids 590
    see also antimycobacterial drugs
tuberculous meningitis *see* meningitis, infective
tubular necrosis, acute (ATN) 230–231
  aetiology 230
  clinical precipitants 230–231, *231*
  see also kidney failure, acute
tubuloglomerular feedback (TGF) 236
tumour lysis syndrome 767, *769*
tumour markers 57–58, 778, *778*
tumour necrosis factor (TNF)
  blockage therapy 800–802
  in rheumatoid arthritis 800
tumour–nodes–metastasis (TNM) system 778
tumours, solid 775–790, 787–789 (CS)
  aetiology 775–777
    environment 775–776
    genetics 776–777
  cellular level 777
  clinical assessment 778
  diagnosis 778
  epidemiology 775
  growth 777
  markers 778, *778*
  metastasis 777
  mortality *776*
  patient management 778–780
  performance status 778, *779*
  presentation 778
  prevention 777
  prognostic factors *779*
  screening 777
  staging 778
  treatment 778–780
    goals 778–779
    guidelines 779
    methods 779–780
    surgery 779–780
    see also chemotherapy; cytotoxic drugs
  see also cancer
two bottle system 78
two-compartment model *5*
tyramine 29

ADRs *151*
drug interactions *152*
H$_2$ receptor antagonists *see* H$_2$ receptor antagonists
see also individual drugs
ulcers
  ischaemic 661, 675–676 (CS), 879
  leg *see* leg ulcers
  NSAIDs *see* non-steroidal anti-inflammatory drugs (NSAIDs)
ultrasound
  benign prostatic hyperplasia 719
  chronic kidney failure investigation 250
  liver disease diagnosis 214
  VTE investigation 341
ultraviolet light 863–864
unconjugated bilirubin 56
undernutrition *see* malnutrition
unfractionated heparins (UFH) 342–343
unipolar disorder 439
United Kingdom Prospective Diabetes Study Group (UKPDS) 671–672
unsaturated iron binding capacity (UIBC) 728, *728*
unstable angina (UA) 281
  treatment 288–289
uraemia
  acute kidney failure 237
  chronic kidney failure 251, 262–263 (CS)
  diuretic ADRs 311
  management 256–257
    diet 256
    fluid retention 256–257
    gastrointestinal symptoms 257
    pruritus 257
uraemic gastrointestinal erosions 238
urea
  adult reference ranges *47, 121*
  breath tests 147
  levels 234
  neonatal reference ranges *121*
  paediatric reference ranges *121*
  serum levels 54
ureidopenicillin
  aspiration pneumonia therapy 528
  nosocomial pneumonia therapy *527*
uric acid
  adult reference values *47*
  overproduction 813–814
  serum levels 55
  underexcretion 814
  see also gout; hyperuricaemia
uricosuric agents
  drug interactions *818*
  hyperuricaemia therapy 818
urinalysis
  benign prostatic hyperplasia 719
  diabetes mellitus diagnosis 660
urinary incontinence 134–135
  detrusor instability 135
  stress 134–135
urinary pH, drug interactions 27
urinary tract
  disease 660
  male *718*
  post-surgical infections 573
  surgery 576–577, 580 (CS)
urinary tract infections (UTIs) 533–542, 540–542 (CS)
  acute pyelonephritis *see* pyelonephritis, acute
  aetiology 534
  clinical manifestations 535
    adults 535
    children 535, 541 (CS)
    elderly 535, 541 (CS)
    infants 535
  cystitis 533
  epidemiology 533–534
  investigations 535–536, 541–542 (CS)
    culture 536

    microscopy 536
    sample collection/preparation 535–536
  key points 533
  pathogenesis 534
    causative organism 534
    host factors 534
    structural abnormalities 534
  prevention 539–540
  prophylaxis 539–540
  treatment 536–539
    adults 537–538
    antimicrobials 536–537
    bacteriuria of pregnancy 539, 541 (CS)
    catheter-associated 539, 541 (CS)
    children 538, 541 (CS)
    non-specific 536
    problems *540*
    relapsing 539
    uncomplicated, treatment 537–538
    see also bacteriuria
urobilinogen 56
urodynamic assessment, benign prostatic hyperplasia 719
ursodeoxycholic acid
  primary biliary cirrhosis therapy 223
  pruritus therapy 216, *217*
urticaria 845, *845*
utility analysis 98

U

UK Parkinson's Disease Brain Bank 485
ulcerative colitis 166–168, 175 (CS), 177 (CS)
  aetiology 166
  classification 166–167
  clinical assessment 167–168
  clinical manifestations 167
  epidemiology 166
  investigations 166, 167, *167*
  pathophysiology 166–167
  see also inflammatory bowel disease
ulcer-healing drugs 153–155, 798–799

V

vaccines 403
  see also individual vaccines
vaginal candidiasis 624
vaginal thrush *see* candidiasis
vagus nerves 510
valaciclovir *610*
valganciclovir *610*
valproate
  distribution 15
  elimination 15
  pharmacokinetics 15–16, *17*
    practical considerations 15–16
valproate semisodium *see* sodium valproate
valve incompetencies 878
vancomycin
  infection therapy 754
    Clostridium difficile 549
    meningitis *560*
    streptococcal meningitis 561
  resistance 549
variable costs 92
variant angina 281
variceal ligation 221
varicose eczema 856
Varidase 876
vascular injury 347–348
vascular surgery 577
vasodilators
  ADRs *270*
  CHF therapy *306*, 309
  hypertension management 256
  indications/contraindications *272*
vasopressin 48, 301
  dysmenorrhoea 685–686
  oesophageal varices therapy 222, *222*
Vaughn–Williams classification 328–332
venlafaxine
  in analgesia 502
  depression therapy 447
venography 341
venous leg ulcers *see* leg ulcers
venous thromboembolism (VTE) 339–347, 350 (CS)
  ADRs 419
  aetiology 339–340
  clinical manifestations 340–341

epidemiology 339
investigations 341
key points 339
leg ulcers 878
oestrogen replacement therapy 698
patient care 347
treatment 341–347
cost analysis 95, 95–96, 96
see also anticoagulant drugs
see also pulmonary embolism (PE)
ventilation–perfusion scanning 341
ventricular arrhythmias 323
ventricular fibrillation (VF) 281
ventricular tachycardias 326–327
verapamil 243–244 (CS), 332, 336 (CS)
ADRs 331
paroxysmal supraventricular tachyarrhythmias 326
pharmacokinetics 334
properties 288
verbal rating scales 496
verotoxin-producing Escherichia coli 544, 546
verotoxins 545
vertical transmission, HIV infection 617
very low birth weight (VLBW) 101
very-low density lipoprotein cholesterol (VDL-C) 354–355
vesicoureteric reflux (VUR) 534
vesicular eruptions 846–847, 847
V-HeFT II trial 305
Vibrio species infections, clinical features 546
vigabatrin
ADRs 476
characteristics 470
dosage 473
epilepsy therapy 478
pharmacokinetics 16, 474
vinblastine
in ABVD regimen 762, 763, 764, 771–772 (CS)
ADRs 769
in ChlVPP/EVA regimen 763, 764
in ChlVPP/PABlOE regimen 763, 764, 770 (CS)
MVPP regimen 764
vincristine (oncovin)
ADRs 768, 769
ALL chemotherapy 747, 748
in ChlVPP/EVA regimen 763, 764
in ChlVPP/PABlOE regimen 763, 764, 770 (CS)
in CHOP see CHOP regimen
Kaposi's sarcoma therapy 615
in MACOP-B regimen 765
in m-BACOD regimen 765
MOPP regimen 762, 764
in PAdriaCEBO regimen 765, 766
in PMitCEBO regimen 765, 766
in ProMACE-CytaBOM regimen 765
viral load 600
viral meningitis see meningitis, infective
viruses 744
visceral muscle function, age-related changes 129
visual analogue scale (VAS)
cost–utility analysis 94
pain assessment 496
vitamin B12
deficiency see vitamin B12 deficiency anaemia

reference values 58
serum measurement 63
vitamin B12 deficiency anaemia 740 (CS), 741 (CS)
aetiology 730
clinical manifestations 732
epidemiology 730
investigations 732
pathophysiology 731
patient care 733
treatment 733
problems 739
see also pernicious anaemia
vitamin D
deficiency 259
metabolism 253, 253
osteoporosis therapy 132
supplements 650
hypoparathyroidism therapy 649
psoriasis therapy 863
vitamin K
haemorrhagic disease of the newborn therapy 105
liver disease therapy 217–218
vitamins
PN see parenteral nutrition (PN)
premenstrual syndrome 681
supplements, uraemia therapy 257
see also individual vitamins
Vitrimex-KV 78
volume of distribution see distribution, volume of
vomiting see nausea/vomiting
vomiting centre 510
voriconazole 635
vulnerability model of schizophrenia 456

West's syndrome 478
white blood cells 60
white cell count (WCC) 60
adult reference ranges 121
neonatal reference ranges 121
paediatric reference ranges 121
reference values 58
willingness-to-accept (WTA) 93
willingness-to-pay (WTP) 93
Wilms' tumour of the kidney 776
Wilson's disease 212
Parkinson's disease vs. 485–486
treatment 223–224
withdrawal
antidepressants 443–444
anti-epileptic drugs (AEDs) 471
carbamazepine 469
monoamine-oxidase inhibitors (MAOIs) 443
phenobarbital 469
phenytoin 469, 480 (CS)
sodium valproate 469
Wolff–Parkinson–White syndrome 331, 332
World Health Organization (WHO)
ADRs definition 34
anaemia diagnosis 725
cytotoxic drug toxicity ratings 787
diabetes mellitus classification 659–660
tumour performance scale 778, 779
WOSCOPS 367

W

warfarin 343–345
ADRs 345
age-related changes 130
atrial fibrillation therapy 327
disease interactions 653–654 (CS)
dosage 344, 350 (CS)
drug interactions 31 (CS), 154, 156, 346, 368, 627, 858
metabolization 344–345
monitoring 61–62, 343–344
structure 343
therapeutic range 344
treatment recommendations 347
'watch and wait' policy 765
water 48–50
balance 48
depletion 48
distribution 48
excess 48–49
extracellular fluid (ECF) 48
minimum daily intake 48
see also extracellular fluid (ECF);
intracellular fluid (ICF)
weight
child development 113
hypertension management 268
PN monitoring 83
Wenckebach block 323

X

X efficiency 98

Y

'yellow card' scheme 42

Z

zalcitabine (ddC) 605, 607
zaleplon 427, 429
zero order elimination 5
zidovudine (AZT) 607
characteristics 605
neurological benefits 616
zidovudine, drug interactions 627, 818
Ziehl–Neelsen stain 586
zinc finger inhibitors 608
zinc protoporphyrin (ZPP) measurement 63
zinc suspension insulin 663, 664
ziprasidone (ADRs) 459
Zollinger–Ellison syndrome 149
zolpidem 427, 429
zonisamide
characteristics 470
epilepsy therapy 478
zopiclone 427, 429, 436 (CS)
zotepine (ADRs) 459
zuclopenthixol acetate (acuphase)
ADRs 459
mania therapy 449